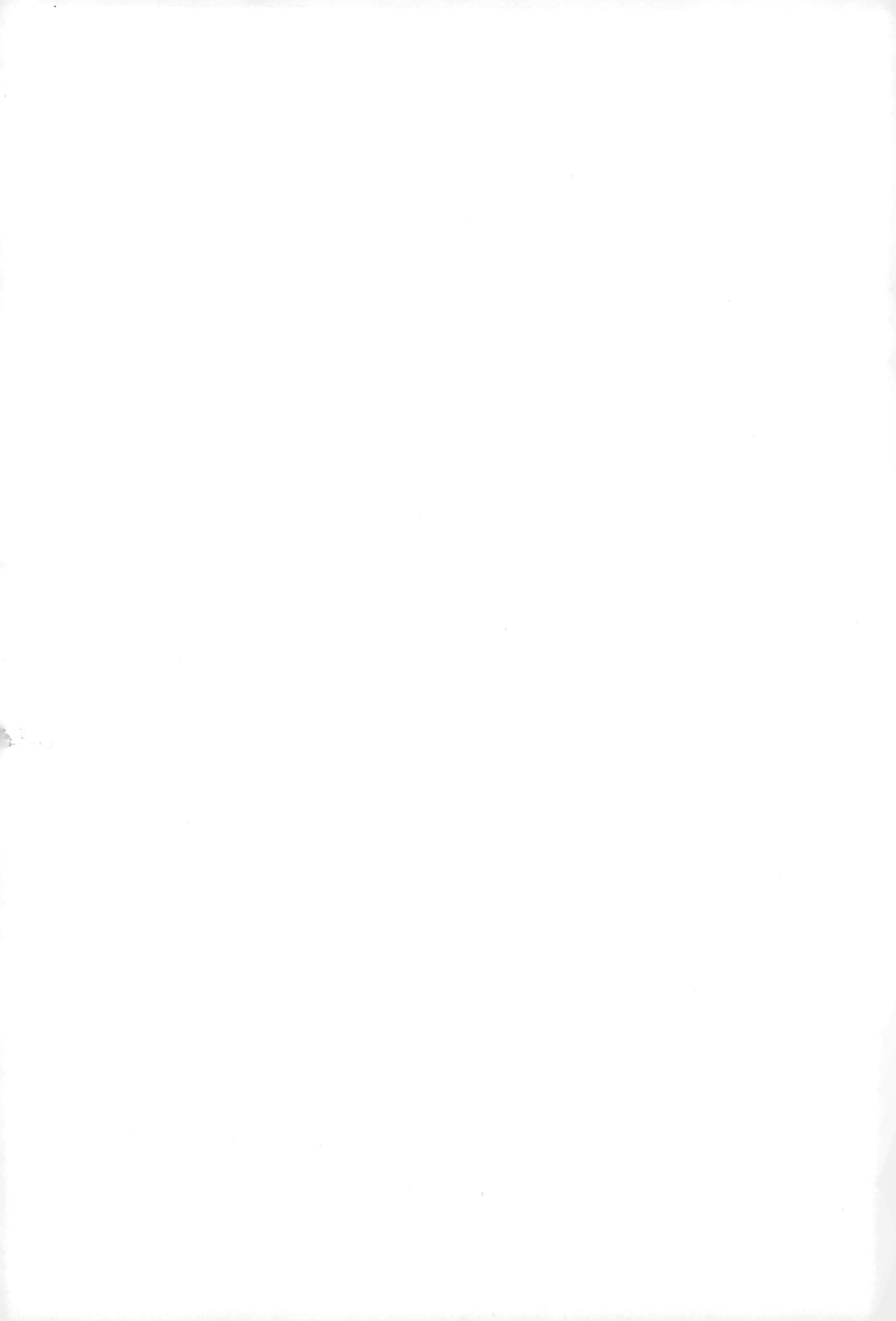

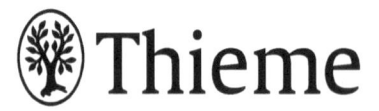

Diagnostic Breast Imaging

Mammography, Sonography, Magnetic Resonance Imaging, and Interventional Procedures

Third edition

Sylvia H. Heywang-Koebrunner, MD
Professor and Head
Reference Center for Mammography Munich
Munich, Germany

Ingrid Schreer, MD
Professor
Radiologic Center Hamburg
Hamburg, Germany

Susan Barter, MB BS, DMRD, FRCR, FRCP
Consultant Radiologist
Cambridge Breast Unit
Addenbrooke's Hospital
Cambridge University Hospitals Foundation Trust
Cambridge, UK

With contributions by

Fleur Kilburn-Toppin, John Kotre, Joerg Naehrig

1,205 illustrations

Thieme
Stuttgart · New York

Library of Congress Cataloging-in-Publication Data are available from the publisher.

Illustrators: Heike Hahn, Berlin, Germany, and Jane Fallows, Cardiff, UK

© 2014 Georg Thieme Verlag KG,
Rüdigerstrasse 14, 70469 Stuttgart, Germany
http://www.thieme.de
Thieme Medical Publishers, Inc., 333 Seventh Avenue,
New York, NY 10001, USA
http://www.thieme.com

Cover design: Thieme Publishing Group
Typesetting by Prepress Projects, Perth, UK
Printed in Germany by CPI, Leck

ISBN 978-3-13-102893-8

Also available as an e-book:
eISBN 978-3-13-150411-1

Important note: Medicine is an ever-changing science undergoing continual development. Research and clinical experience are continually expanding our knowledge, in particular our knowledge of proper treatment and drug therapy. Insofar as this book mentions any dosage or application, readers may rest assured that the authors, editors, and publishers have made every effort to ensure that such references are in accordance with **the state of knowledge at the time of production of the book.**

Nevertheless, this does not involve, imply, or express any guarantee or responsibility on the part of the publishers in respect to any dosage instructions and forms of applications stated in the book. **Every user is requested to examine carefully** the manufacturers' leaflets accompanying each drug and to check, if necessary in consultation with a physician or specialist, whether the dosage schedules mentioned therein or the contraindications stated by the manufacturers differ from the statements made in the present book. Such examination is particularly important with drugs that are either rarely used or have been newly released on the market. Every dosage schedule or every form of application used is entirely at the user's own risk and responsibility. The authors and publishers request every user to report to the publishers any discrepancies or inaccuracies noticed. If errors in this work are found after publication, errata will be posted at www.thieme.com on the product description page.

Some of the product names, patents, and registered designs referred to in this book are in fact registered trademarks or proprietary names even though specific reference to this fact is not always made in the text. Therefore, the appearance of a name without designation as proprietary is not to be construed as a representation by the publisher that it is in the public domain.

This book, including all parts thereof, is legally protected by copyright. Any use, exploitation, or commercialization outside the narrow limits set by copyright legislation, without the publisher's consent, is illegal and liable to prosecution. This applies in particular to photostat reproduction, copying, mimeographing, preparation of microfilms, and electronic data processing and storage.

Contributors

Susan Barter, MB BS, DMRD, FRCR, FRCP
Consultant Radiologist
Cambridge Breast Unit
Addenbrooke's Hospital
Cambridge University Hospitals Foundation Trust
Cambridge, UK

Sylvia H. Heywang-Koebrunner, MD
Professor and Head
Reference Center for Mammography Munich
Munich, Germany

Fleur Kilburn-Toppin, MA, MB, BChir, FRCR
Consultant Radiologist
West Suffolk Hospital
Bury St Edmunds, UK

John Kotre PhD, FIPEM, FInstP
Consultant Clinical Scientist
Head of Imaging Physics and Radiation Safety
Regional Medical Physics Department
Freeman Hospital
Newcastle upon Tyne, UK

Joerg Naehrig, MD
Assistant Professor
Institute of Pathology
Technical University Munich
Munich, Germany

Ingrid Schreer, MD
Professor
Radiologic Center Hamburg
Hamburg, Germany

Preface

Breast cancer remains a life-threatening and frightening disease for millions of women.

Diagnostic breast imaging and intervention has a proven and important role in early detection or exclusion of breast cancer and in the targeted assessment of abnormalities of any size and stage. Modern breast imaging and intervention can thus contribute significantly to both improving women's prognosis by early detection and reducing late breast cancer through screening programs and promoting individualized optimal strategies for successful treatment with the least unavoidable side effects.

This role is associated with a great amount of responsibility. It requires well-founded knowledge, experience, and continuous striving for the best possible solutions. Awareness of the clinical needs and a close integration of imaging in a multidisciplinary team have become increasingly important and today constitute a prerequisite for successful breast diagnosis.

During recent years, increasing data support the value of early detection. Although mammography screening remains the most important tool for early detection, awareness of possible side effects and limitations has increased. The pros and cons of current discussions and controversies are explained in this book. Innovations and advances in mammography, such as digital imaging, tomosynthesis, improved capabilities of ultrasound, and the well-founded contributions of breast magnetic resonance imaging, have been included in this largely rewritten edition.

Increased standardization has been pointed out and will support the reader in the achievement of higher reproducibility, in learning a more systematic way of detection, diagnosis, and assessment.

The chapters are based on extensive literature searching, well-founded results from evidence-based data, and updated guidelines. Based on modern breast imaging and intervention, algorithms are suggested and demonstrated for the workup of typical and atypical findings.

We hope that this updated book will again become a reliable and pragmatic guide for those who try to learn breast diagnostics and intervention in its clinical context and for those who want to update their knowledge or optimize their work based on existing evidence. So, the book was written for radiologists in and beyond their training, clinicians who want to be informed about the capabilities of breast imaging, and technologists and nurses who are becoming increasingly important members in our interdisciplinary teams.

Prof. Dr. Sylvia Heywang-Koebrunner is very proud and happy to present this third edition together with her highly competent team of authors: her dear friend and highly renowned breast diagnostician Prof. Dr. Ingrid Schreer, who has joined her since the very first edition of this book, and Dr. Sue Barter, our new co-author, who complements us ideally by her extensive knowledge, her logical and didactic thinking, her wonderful personality, and her very effective style of working.

We are grateful to our previous co-authors, David Dershaw and Bernd Hoberg, who had set the fundaments of success for this book and who have allowed the use of previous material where needed. Very special thanks go to Prof. Baessler, who—as a highly renowned German pathologist and knowledgeable friend—cooperated in the initial design and contents of this book and advised us like a father.

With evolving new methods and concepts in all fields we have been able to integrate further experts and investigators whose valuable and excellently researched contributions are highly appreciated: the radiologist Dr. Fleur Kilburn-Toppin, the medical physicist John Kotre, and the pathologist Dr. Joerg Naehrig.

All of us would like to thank our diagnostic and multidisciplinary teams including our radiology colleagues, our interdisciplinary partners, and our technologists and non-medical staff. They have continuously supported us in our daily work, the results of which are displayed in this book, and allowed us the time for putting together the knowledge that we share.

Many thanks go to Sabina Wulz-Horber who prepared the case material of an important number of the examples selected.

Sylvia H. Heywang-Koebrunner wants to express her special thanks to her dear friend Despina Schuller and to her family for their constant support, tolerance, and humor.

Ingrid Schreer and Sylvia Heywang-Koebrunner express their deep appreciations to Prof. H.-J. Frischbier, whose work and support constituted an essential basis for this book.

Sue Barter would like to thank Sylvia Heywang-Koebrunner and Ingrid Schreer for the honor of co-authoring this book and for their teamwork and friendship. She would also like to express her gratitude to her family and colleagues at Cambridge Breast Unit for their patience and support.

We would also like to express our appreciation to Cliff Bergman and Stephan Konnry and his team at Thieme who guided us through the various editions of this work.

Sylvia H. Heywang-Koebrunner
Ingrid Schreer
Sue Barter

Abbreviations

ABUS	automated whole breast ultrasound	**ILC**	invasive lobular carcinoma
ACR	American College of Radiology	**LCIS**	lobular carcinoma in situ
ADC	apparent diffusion coefficient	**LN**	lobular intraepithelial atypia
AEC	automatic exposure control	**LP**	line pairs
ADH	atypical ductal hyperplasia	**MIN**	mammary intraepithelial neoplasia
ALH	atypical lobular hyperplasia	**MLO**	mediolateral oblique
ALND	axillary lymph node dissection	**MRI**	magnetic resonance imaging
BCT	breast-conserving therapy	**MTF**	modulation transfer function
BI-RADS	Breast Imaging Reporting and Data System	**NAC**	neoadjuvant chemotherapy
BSE	breast self-examination	**NMR**	nuclear magnetic resonance
CAD	computer-aided diagnosis/detection	**PACS**	picture archiving and communication system
CC	craniocaudal	**PAS**	patient administration system
CCD	charge-coupled device	**PASH**	pseudoangiomatous stromal hyperplasia
CEDM	contrast-enhanced digital mammography	**PET**	positron emission tomography
CNB	core needle biopsy	**PND**	pathologic nipple discharge
CR	computed radiography	**PPV**	positive predictive value
CSL	complex sclerosing lesion	**QC**	quality control
CT	computed tomography	**RI**	radioisotope imaging
DBI	digital breast tomosynthesis	**RIS**	radiologic information system
DCIS	ductal carcinoma(s) in situ	**ROI**	region of interest
DICOM	Digital Imaging and Communication in Medicine	**ROLL**	radioguided occult lesion localization
DWI	diffusion-weighted imaging	**SNB**	sentinel node biopsy
EIC	epithelial invasive cancer	**TDLU**	terminal ductal lobular unit
FEA	flat epithelial atypia	**THI**	tissue harmonic imaging
FNA	fine needle aspiration	**UDH**	usual ductal hyperplasia
GSDF	Grayscale Display Function	**US**	ultrasound
HRT	hormone replacement therapy	**USPIO**	ultrasmall super-paramagnetic iron oxide
IDC	invasive ductal carcinoma	**VABB**	vacuum-assisted breast biopsy

Table of Contents

I Methods — 1

1 Patient History and Communication with the Patient — 3
Scheduling 4
Patient Information 4
Mammography 4
Sonography 4
Magnetic Resonance Imaging with Contrast Medium 5
Interventions 5
Patient History 5
Risk Factors 5
Medical History Data Helpful for Image Interpretation 11
References and Recommended Reading 11

2 Clinical Findings — 15
Purpose 16
Techniques 16
Visual Inspection 16
Palpation 17
Assessment of Clinical Abnormalities 19
References and Recommended Reading 20

3 Mammography — 21
Purpose, Accuracy, Possibilities, and Limitations 22
Indications 22
Accuracy 22
Screening 24
Problem Solving 24
Mammographic Technique 25
Components of the Mammographic Imaging Technique 25
Picture Archiving and Communications Systems (PACSs) 39
Computer-Aided Diagnosis (CAD) 40
Specific Requirements and Solutions 40
Image Sharpness 40
Contrast 41
Noise 49
Radiation Dose 50
Positioning and Compression 52
Compression 52
Positioning for Standard Views 54
Positioning for Additional Views 57
Film Labeling 62
Spot Compression 62
Magnification Technique 64
Positioning of Breasts with Implants 71
Imaging of the Specimen 72
Quality Factors 74
Hardware Factors that Influence Image Quality 74
Influence of the Screen–Film System and Film Processing on Image Quality 75
Additional Factors 76
Quality Assurance in Mammography 76
Reporting and Documentation of Findings .. 78
Clinical Findings 78
Mammographic Report 79
Galactography 85
Duct Sonography and MRI 91
Histopathologic Assessment of Ductal Abnormalities 91
Pneumocystography 92
References and Recommended Reading 93

4 Sonography — 97
Purpose, Accuracy, Possibilities, and Limitations 98
Diagnosing Cysts 98
Differentiating Solid Lesions 98
Diagnosing Carcinoma 98
Imaging Assessment of Younger Women 99
Screening with Sonography 99
Ultrasonography of the Axilla 99
Equipment Requirements 100
Transducer 100
Image Quality 101
Examination Technique 103
Time-Gain Compensation 104
Focusing 105
Examination Technique and Documentation 105
Interpreting and Documenting Sonographic Findings 112
Normal Sonographic Findings 112
Sonographic Lesions 113
References and Recommended Reading 124

Table of Contents

5 Magnetic Resonance Imaging — 127
Purpose, Accuracy, Possibilities, and Limitations 128
MR Technique 129
Dynamic Contrast-Enhanced MRI (DCE-MRI) 129
Unenhanced MRI 131
Diffusion-Weighted Imaging and MR Spectroscopy 132
Scheduling and Performing Breast MRI 132
Performing DCE Breast MRI 132
Performing Plain MRI for Evaluation of Implant Failure 134
Diagnostic Criteria 134
Patient Selection and Indications 151
Contrast-Enhanced MRI 151
References and Recommended Reading 171

6 Emerging Technologies in Breast Imaging — 177
Introduction 178
Mammography 178
Digital Breast Tomosynthesis 178
Dual Energy Mammography (Spectral Mammography) 180
Contrast-Enhanced Digital Mammography 180
Ultrasound 180
Sonoelastography 181
Automated Whole Breast and 3D Ultrasound 181
Magnetic Resonance Imaging 181
Diffusion-Weighted Imaging 181
Magnetic Resonance Elastography 182
Magnetic Resonance Spectroscopy 182
Nuclear Medicine 182
Breast-Specific Gamma Imaging 182
Positron Emission Mammography 182
References and Recommended Reading 183

7 Imaging Assessment and Percutaneous Breast Biopsy — 185
Purpose, Accuracy, Possibilities, and Limitations 186
Purpose 186
Measures Before Histopathologic Assessment 186
Definitions 187
Accuracy 187
Possibilities, Limitations, Choice of Biopsy Method 189
Patient Information, Patient Preparation, and Postbiopsy Care 192
Techniques for Biopsy and Biopsy Guidance 193
Fine Needle Aspiration 193
Core Needle Biopsy 194
Vacuum-Assisted Breast Biopsy 195
Biopsy Under Ultrasound Guidance 197
Stereotactic Biopsy 203
MR-Guided Percutaneous Biopsy 207
Handling the Biopsy Specimen 210
Interpreting the Histopathologic Results 210
References and Recommended Reading 213

8 Preoperative Localization — 215
Purpose, Definition, Indications, and Side Effects 216
Purpose 216
Definition 216
Indication 216
Side Effects 216
Methods and Technique 217
Mammographically Guided Localization Techniques 217
Ultrasound-Guided Localization 221
MR-Guided Localization 222
CT-Guided Localization 222
Galactographically Guided Localization 222
Materials for Lesion Localization 222
Problems and Their Solutions 227
References and Recommended Reading 228

II Appearance — 231

9 The Normal Breast — 233
Anatomy 234
The Adolescent Female Breast 235
Histology 235
Clinical Examination 235

Mammography	235	Macromastia	242
Sonography	235	Accessory Breast Tissue (Polymastia)	244
The Mature Female Breast	235	Inverted Nipple	244
Histology	235	**Pregnancy and Lactation**	246
Clinical Examination	235	Histology	246
Mammography	236	Clinical Examination	246
Sonography	237	Mammography	246
Magnetic Resonance Imaging	237	Sonography	246
Breast Density and Changes with Age	241	Magnetic Resonance Imaging	246
Histology	241	**Breast Response with Hormone Replacement Therapy**	248
Clinical Examination	241	Mammography	248
Mammography	241	Sonography	248
Sonography	241	Magnetic Resonance Imaging	248
Magnetic Resonance Imaging	242	Percutaneous Biopsy	248
Variants of Normal Findings	242	**References and Recommended Reading**	252
Definition	242		
Anisomastia	242		

10 Benign Breast Disorders   255

Definition	256	Diagnostic Strategy and Objectives	260
Pathogenesis	256	Mammography	261
Incidence	256	Sonography	266
Histopathology	256	Magnetic Resonance Imaging	268
Clinical Findings	258	Percutaneous Biopsy	272
Mammographic Density and Risk	258	**References and Recommended Reading**	273

11 Cysts   275

Histology	276	Aspiration of the Cyst	281
Definition	276	Pneumocystography	282
Medical History and Clinical Findings	276	Mammography	282
Breast Examination	276	Magnetic Resonance Imaging	283
Objectives of Diagnostic Studies	276	**Galactoceles and Oil Cysts**	284
Diagnostic Strategy	278	Definitions	284
Sonography	278	**References and Recommended Reading**	286

12 Benign Tumors and Tumorlike Masses   290

Hamartoma or Adenofibrolipoma	290	Angiomas	308
Cowden Syndrome	292	Granular Cell Tumor (Myoblastoma)	309
Fibroepithelial Mixed Tumors	292	Pseudoangiomatous Stromal Hyperplasia	309
Fibroadenoma, Adenofibroma, Juvenile or Giant Fibroadenoma	292	**Benign Fibroses**	310
Papilloma	306	Focal Fibrous Disease or Fibrosis Mammae	310
Lipoma	306	Amyloidosis of the Breast	310
Rare Benign Tumors	306	Steatocystoma Multiplex	310
Leiomyoma, Neurofibroma, Neurilemnoma, Benign Spindle Cell Tumor (Myofibroblastoma), Chondroma, Osteoma	306	Intramammary Lymph Nodes	310
		References and Recommended Reading	312

13 Inflammatory Conditions   316

Mastitis	316	**Abscesses and Fistulas**	321
Etiology	316	Histology	321
Clinical Findings	316	Clinical Findings	321
Diagnostic Strategy and Goals	317	Diagnostic Strategy	321

Granulomatous Conditions 327
Histologic and Microbiological
Confirmation 327
Clinical Findings 327
Diagnostic Strategy 328
References and Recommended Reading 335

14 Lesions of Uncertain Malignant Potential (B3 Lesions)   337

Definition 338
Rationale for Diagnostic Strategy and
Therapeutic Recommendations for
B3 Lesions 338
Diagnostic Strategy and Management 339
Prevalence of Lesions of Uncertain Malignant
Potential, Imaging and Overall Risk 339
Atypical Intraductal Epithelial Proliferations   340
Atypical Ductal Hyperplasia 340
Flat Epithelial Atypia and Columnar
Cell Lesions with Atypia 341
Atypical Lobular Hyperplasia, Lobular
Carcinoma in Situ/
(and Pleomorphic-Type LCIS) 345
Radial Scars 346
Papillary Lesions 348
**Fibroepithelial Lesions of Uncertain
Malignant Potential** 356
Other B3 Lesions 360
References and Recommended Reading 361

15 Carcinoma in Situ   365

Definition, Terminology, and Biological
Context 366
**Lobular Carcinoma in Situ, Pleomorphic
Subtypes (Pleomorphic LCIS)** 366
Incidence 366
Importance 367
Histology 368
Clinical Presentation and History 368
Diagnostic Strategy 368
Ductal Carcinoma in Situ (DCIS) 370
Definition 370
Incidence 370
Histopathology 370
Importance and Natural History 371
Therapeutic Decisions 372
Clinical Findings and History 372
Diagnostic Methods: Value and Goals 372
References and Recommended Reading 386

16 Invasive Carcinoma   391

Epidemiology and Etiology 392
Definition and Problems Posed 392
Spectrum and Detectability 393
Diagnostic Strategy and Goals 394
Histology 400
Breast Cancer and Prognosis 402
Clinical Examination 403
Mammography 405
Radiographic Density of Breast
Carcinomas 405
Direct Signs of Focally Invasive
Breast Carcinoma 407
Indirect Signs (Secondary Criteria of
Malignancy) of Focally Growing Invasive
Carcinomas 417
Signs of Diffusely Growing Carcinomas 420
Value of Follow-up and Prior Studies 420
The Influence of Histology on Mammographic
Presentation 428
Sensitivity and Specificity of
Mammography 431
Differential Diagnostic Considerations 431
Sonography 432
Diagnostic Role 432
Indications 432
Image Presentation of Breast Carcinoma 433
Correlation between Sonographic Image
Presentation and Histology 440
Accuracy and Differential Diagnosis 440
Magnetic Resonance Imaging 441
Diagnostic Role 441
Imaging Presentation of Carcinomas 441
Indications 445
Percutaneous Biopsy Methods 448
Diagnostic Role 448
Indications 450
Disposition after Percutaneous Biopsy 450
References and Recommended Reading 450

17 Lymph Nodes   457

Sentinel Lymph Node Biopsy 458
The Role of Imaging 459
Anatomy 459
Normal Lymph Nodes 459
Pathologic Changes in Lymph Nodes 464
Metastatic Adenopathy 464

Other Causes of Adenopathy 469
Nodal Calcifications 469
Percutaneous Biopsy 471

Further Techniques in Nodal Imaging:
MRI and PET 471
References and Recommended Reading 473

18 Other Semi-Malignant and Malignant Tumors — 475

Phyllodes Tumor (Cystosarcoma Phyllodes) 476
Histology 476
Clinical Findings 476
Diagnostic Strategy and Goals 476
Fibromatosis (= Extra-abdominal Desmoid) 479
Hemangiopericytoma and Hemangioendothelioma 479
Adenomyoepithelioma 480
Sarcomas 480
Histology 480

Clinical Findings 480
Diagnostic Strategy and Goals 480
Malignancies of the Breast of Hematologic Origin 484
Histopathology 484
Clinical Findings 484
Diagnostic Strategy and Goals 485
Metastases 487
Histology 487
Clinical Findings 487
Diagnostic Strategy and Goals 487
References and Recommended Reading 489

19 Post-Traumatic, Post-Surgical, and Post-Therapeutic Changes — 493

Post-Traumatic and Post-Surgical Changes .. 494
Histology 494
Clinical History and Findings 494
Diagnostic Strategy and Goals 494
Reduction Mammoplasty 507
Definition 507
Surgical Procedures 507
Diagnostic Strategy 507
Changes Following Reconstruction 509
Definition 509
Surgical Procedures 509
Diagnostic Strategy 509

Changes Following Breast-Conserving Therapy without Irradiation 512
Definition 512
Clinical and Imaging Findings 512
Differential Diagnosis and Diagnostic Strategy 512
Changes Following Breast-Conserving Therapy with Irradiation 512
Definition 512
Clinical Findings 513
Diagnostic Strategy and Goals 513
References and Recommended Reading 529

20 Radiologic Assessment of Women with Breast Implants — 533

Types of Implants 534
Structure 534
Anatomy 535
Imaging 535
Mammography 535
Ultrasound 539
Magnetic Resonance Imaging 540
Histopathologic Assessment in Women with Implants 540
Complications of Breast Implants 541

Surveillance of Women with an Implant Following Oncoplastic Surgery 544
Screening of Asymptomatic Women who have had Breast Augmentation 547
Imaging Assessment of Women with Implants after Oncoplastic Surgery 547
Imaging Assessment of Women after Augmentation Implant 547
Histopathologic Assessment in Women with Implants 547
References and Recommended Reading 552

21 Skin Changes — 553

Nodular Changes of the Skin and Subcutaneous Tissue 554
Clinical Findings 554
Diagnostic Strategy 554
Skin Thickening 554

Definition 554
Incidence 554
Diagnostic Strategy 555
Clinical Findings 561
References and Recommended Reading 562

22 The Male Breast — 563

- Anatomy — 564
- Clinical Examination — 564
- Mammography — 564
- Ultrasound — 564
- Magnetic Resonance Imaging — 564
- **Gynecomastia** — 565
- Definition — 565
- Histology — 565
- Clinical Findings — 565
- Diagnostic Strategy — 565
- **Breast Cancer** — 567
- Definition — 567
- Histology — 567
- Clinical Findings — 569
- Diagnostic Strategy — 569
- **Miscellaneous** — 571
- **References and Recommended Reading** — 573

III Application of Diagnostic Imaging of the Breast — 575

23 Screening — 577

- Definition — 578
- Quality Assurance — 578
- **The Special Task of Screening** — 578
- **The Data and Discussions** — 579
- Other Age Groups — 581
- Other Tests for Breast Cancer Screening — 582
- Absolute Numbers — 582
- Potential Risks and Limitations — 583
- Expected Advantages — 586
- **References and Recommended Reading** — 589

24 Additional Diagnostic Evaluation of Screening Findings and Solving of Problems in Symptomatic Patients — 593

- **Pathognomonic Findings** — 594
- Imaging Assessment — 595
- Histopathologic Assessment — 596
- **Differential Diagnosis and Assessment** — 597
- Smoothly Outlined Density — 597
- Mass Not Smoothly Outlined, Focal Asymmetry — 604
- Architectural Distortion — 615
- Asymmetry — 626
- The Mammographically Dense Breast — 631
- Other Clinical Abnormalities — 639
- Microcalcifications — 641
- Nipple Discharge — 656
- Inflammatory Changes — 660
- The Young Patient — 662
- **References and Recommended Reading** — 672

I Methods

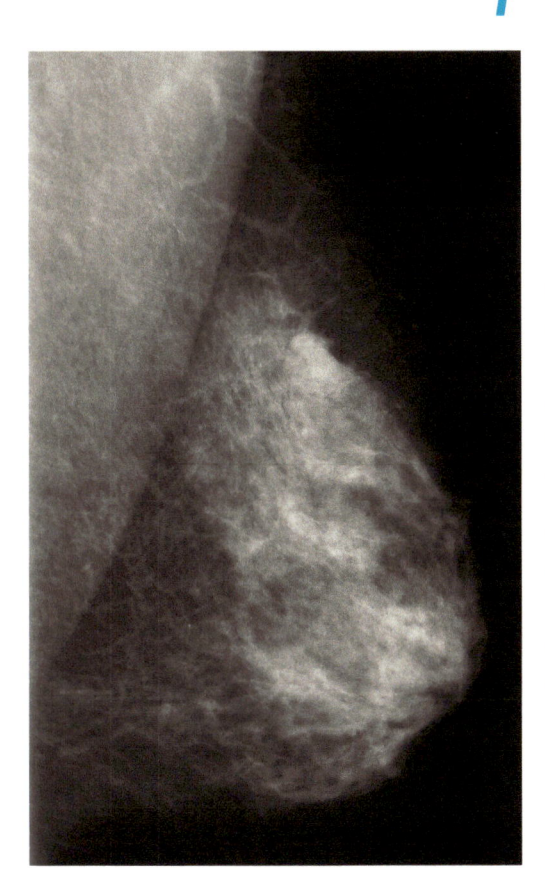

I Patient History and Communication with the Patient

Scheduling → *4*

Patient Information → *4*
Mammography → *4*
Sonography → *4*
Magnetic Resonance Imaging with Contrast Medium → *5*
Interventions → *5*

Patient History → *5*
Risk Factors → *5*
Medical History Data Helpful for Image Interpretation → *11*
References and Recommended Reading → *11*

1 Patient History and Communication with the Patient

S. H. Heywang-Koebrunner, I. Schreer, S. Barter

Providing the patient with some essential information concerning breast imaging may help to gain her understanding and cooperation. Furthermore, obtaining a limited history is very helpful both to separate screening patients from those who need a diagnostic breast study and to support image interpretation in diagnostic breast studies.

Information about both the patient and her history can be obtained orally or by use of an information sheet, a checklist, or a questionnaire.

Scheduling

The issue of whether mammography should be scheduled according to the menstrual cycle is controversial (Hovhannisyan et al. 2009, Morrow et al. 2010). Even though data exist which suggest an impact of the menstrual cycle on breast density and on the accuracy of mammography, (Baines et al. 1997, White et al. 1998, Spratt 1999, Morrow et al. 2010) few international recommendations or guidelines recommend considering this issue in daily practice (Albert et al. 2009). Based on the existing data it may be worth considering the menstrual cycle in younger women, whenever possible. According to our experience the best time span for mammographic imaging is during the second and the beginning of the third week of the menstrual cycle (corresponding approximately to days 7–16 of the menstrual cycle, if the first day of the menstrual bleeding is counted as day 1). We would point out that according to our experience breast changes lag behind the blood parameters of the female hormones. During the above time span the breast is more compressible, and compression is less painful, which is appreciated by the patients. Furthermore, because there is less interstitial fluid during the follicular phase and compression is better, the glandular tissue may even appear less dense on the mammogram, which facilitates diagnosis. Theoretically, it might even be possible to further decrease the radiation risk with such scheduling, since most cells tend to be in the G2 phase (in which they are more sensitive to radiation) during the luteal phase of the menstrual cycle, but not during the follicular (first) phase (Spratt 1999).

With contrast-enhanced (c.e.) magnetic resonance imaging (MRI), nonspecific enhancement in benign tissue may be encountered at the end of the menstrual cycle and during menses, while it is less frequent between day 6 and about day 16 of the cycle. Therefore c.e. MRI should—if possible—be scheduled between days 6 and 16 of the cycle (Kuhl et al. 1997, Müller-Schimpfle et al. 1997, Albert et al. 2009, Sardanelli et al. 2010).

Patient Information

Any specific questions that the patient asks should, of course, be discussed and answered by the technologist or physician. Furthermore, the following essentials concerning the imaging techniques involved may be helpful to gain the patient's understanding and cooperation.

Mammography

- The patient should understand the importance and necessity of compression. Adequate compression helps to visualize small carcinomas, since normal tissue usually can be spread out while carcinomas cannot. Compression also helps to reduce the radiation dose (see Chapter 3, pp. 51–53).
- Any fears that compression might cause cancer should be allayed.
- Possible fear of radiation exposure from mammography should be addressed by putting the risk into proper perspective. For example, the theoretical risk is so small that it can only be extrapolated. The risk of dying of a radiation-induced breast cancer from a screening mammogram after the age of 40 is far lower than the natural annual risk of being affected by breast cancer and dying. Since mammography can save lives, international guidelines have stated that "the radiation risk cannot be accepted as a reason against a quality assured screening mammogram" (Albert et al. 2009; see Chapter 3, p. 50, and Chapter 23, p. 583).

As in any other radiologic examination, pregnancy should be excluded.

Patients who undergo screening mammography should understand that not all cancers can be detected by mammography. Therefore, they should be encouraged to continue to perform breast self-examination. If a change is noted, even if it occurs shortly after screening mammography, the patient should contact her doctor (Berlin 1999).

Sonography

Ultrasound examinations are generally very well accepted by patients. It should, however, be explained that, in general, ultrasonography cannot replace mammography for excluding the presence of cancer. Ultrasound examination alone is not adequate for breast cancer screening (Albert et al. 2009, Lee et al. 2010).

Magnetic Resonance Imaging with Contrast Medium

Contrast-enhanced (c.e.) MRI, like the other methods that do not use ionizing radiation, is well accepted by patients, except for those who suffer from claustrophobia. Contrast-enhanced MRI is used as an additional imaging modality for specific indications. Before performing c.e. MRI, ask for any contraindications and document their absence. These include cardiac pacemakers, intracerebral vascular clips, clips from surgery performed within the last 2 months, implantable drug infusion pumps, and certain types of cardiac valve prostheses (Kanal et al. 2007, Sierra and Machado 2008). Finally, the patient should be informed of the necessity of injecting contrast medium. Contraindications concern rare cases of allergy to paramagnetic contrast medium and severe hepatic or renal insufficiency. Tolerance of this contrast medium is excellent. Allergies occur significantly less frequently than with radiographic contrast media. Another rare side effect concerns NSF (nephrogenic systemic fibrosis). It appears to be avoidable by renal blood testing and strict observation of the recommendations given for individual gadolinium-containing products (ACR Committee on Drugs and Contrast Media 2010).

Interventions

When a needle biopsy is planned the patient should be informed about possible hematoma formation and about the very low risk of infection. The patient should be questioned about any coagulatory disorders, aspirin intake, or other anticoagulation treatment. Provided the direction of puncture is mechanically guided and strictly parallel to the chest wall (usually requiring stereotactic equipment), injury to the chest wall (including pneumothorax) can be excluded, and need not be mentioned. In the other cases, the rare possibility of chest wall injury should be discussed. If a silicone implant is present and might be damaged, the patient must also be informed. In case of axillary punctures, injury to axillary vessels and to the axillary plexus should be discussed. Another very rare complication concerns allergy to local anesthetic. The patient should be questioned concerning any known allergy to local anesthetic and should be informed about such rare side effects.

Other severe diseases should be known. Antibiotic prophylaxis in patients with cardiac failure is only rarely necessary. In patients with infections (hepatitis, HIV [human immunodeficiency virus]) adequate precautions should be considered for the personnel. However, strict observation of hygiene rules is necessary for all patients.

Today, obtaining a standardized informed consent is recommended before carrying out any of these procedures.

Patient History

To save time, many centers have the patient fill out a questionnaire (**Fig. 1.1**). The questions may concentrate on data that are significant for assessing risk and interpreting the images.

Risk Factors

A history of risk factors should be obtained in all patients. Even though improvement in the quality of mammography reporting based on knowledge of the patient's risk has not been proven (Elmore et al. 1997), knowledge of an increased risk may support the decision for the use of additional imaging methods. In addition, the recommendation for screening interval and the starting age may differ from that recommended for women without risk factors. In cases with a strong personal or family history of breast cancer, genetic counseling and intensified surveillance in a dedicated program may be recommended.

With increased risk, additional imaging would in the first place include supplementary ultrasonography. In patients with hereditary breast cancer professional genetic counseling should be considered. If (after counseling) the patient opts against mastectomy and for follow-up by imaging, intensified surveillance should be performed. Internationally, MRI screening is mostly recommended at yearly intervals from ages 25 to 55 and mammography screening is recommended to start at age 30 with yearly intervals (see also Chapter 5, pp. 152–154). (In Germany an additional ultrasound examination is recommended every 6 months.)

The general recommendation internationally for women at intermediate risk is yearly mammography (supplemented by ultrasound examination where indicated) starting at age 40.

For women at low risk most European countries start screening between the ages of 45 and 50. Most European screening programs are biennial; some have shorter intervals (18 months) for those aged 45–55 and longer intervals after age 55. In the United States screening is mostly recommended to start at age 40, thereafter at yearly intervals. However, the optimum recommendations are under discussion.

Even though risk factors are an indicator of increased risk for breast cancer, it is important to realize that an absence of risk factors does not exclude the occurrence of breast cancer. In fact, 70% of breast cancers occur in patients without any risk factors.

The following risk factors for breast cancer have been described (**Table 1.1**) (Lambrechts et al. 2011, Reeves et al. 2011).

- *Personal history:* The personal history of an invasive or in-situ breast carcinoma is significant (with risk factors ranging around 5). The risk increases with decreasing age at diagnosis. Risk factors around 3–5 have been

1 Patient History and Communication with the Patient

Mammography Questionnaire for the Patient

Last name: _____ First name: _____ Date of birth: _____
Address: _____
Phone (home): _____ Phone (work): _____ Insurance provider: _____

Referring physican: _____
(Name, address): _____
Last mammogram (date/facility): _____

Have you had cancer?   No ☐
☐ right breast when? _____ type? _____
☐ left breast when? _____ type? _____
☐ other cancer organ: _____ date: _____

Might you be pregnant?   yes ☐   no ☐

Are you currently nursing?   yes ☐   no ☐

First day of last menstruation? _____

Menopause (since when?) _____ Status after hysterectomy? Yes ☐   No ☐

Are you on hormones (oral contraceptives,
postmenopausal replacement)? _____ If yes, medication/dosage: _____ since when? _____

HISTORY
Age at first menstruation: _____
Have you had severe breast infection? (age/which breast?) _____
Have you had breast surgery? _____
(Which breast/when/result) _____
Have you received radiation therapy? _____
a) to the breast (which breast, when)? _____
b) to the chest (when, why)? _____
c) multiple X-rays, CTs, fluoroscopy of the chest? _____
_____
Was your breast injured (accident?)
   ☐ right   ☐ left   when? _____

FAMILY HISTORY

Family member (age)	Breast cancer (age)	Ovarian cancer (age)
_____	_____	_____
_____	_____	_____
_____	_____	_____
_____	_____	_____
_____	_____	_____

other cancers in family (member/cancer): _____

Have you or your doctor noted an abnormality?   ☐ No
Which abnormality?   Right breast   Left breast   Since when?
Pain   ☐   ☐   _____
Lumpy breast   ☐   ☐   _____
Thickening breast   ☐   ☐   _____
Skin change?   ☐   ☐   _____
Reddening ☐   Retraction ☐   ☐   ☐   _____
Change of nipple   ☐   ☐   _____
discharge: milky ☐   transparent ☐   ☐   ☐
     greenish ☐   red/brown ☐

I have no further questions and consent to the proposed examination

Date: _____   Signature: _____

Fig. 1.1 Mammography questionnaire for patient history.

Technical data

Patient name: _____ Date/examination: _____

Type of unit: _____ Film/screen system _____

Standard views:

	cc:					mlo				
	kV	mAs	kp*	t/f**	AEC	kV	mAs	kp t/f	angle	AEC*
left:										
right:										

* compression   *target/filter   ** automatic exposure control: yes or no

Additional views:

breast/view	retake? (Y/N)	kV mAs kp t/f AEC	spot?	magnification

Reasons for inadequate views? _____

Problems? (pain, compliance?) _____

Technologist: _____   Physician: _____

(Physician's work sheet: see p. 18)

Fig. 1.1 (continued).

1 Patient History and Communication with the Patient

Table 1.1 Risk factors for breast cancer. (Adapted from Kerlikowske et al. 2007, Ortmann et al. 2008, Meindl et al. 2011.)

Risk factor		Approximate relative risk	Remark
Personal history			
	Invasive breast cancer or ductal carcinoma in situ	5	Increases when combined with other risks and/or young age
	Atypias or LIN1–2 (ALH, LCIS)	3–5	Increases when combined with other risks and/or young age
Hereditary monogenic			
	BRCA1, 2, rare syndromes (ataxia telangiectasia, Li–Fraumeni syndrome, Fanconi anemia, Cowden syndrome, Peutz–Jeghers syndrome, or hereditary diffuse gastric cancer syndrome)	> 10	Lifetime risk for breast cancer > 80% Lifetime risk for ovarian and breast cancer and other malignancies often significantly increased
	Genetic alterations under investigation (RAD51C)	Factor being investigated	Lifetime risk being investigated
Polygenic familial			
	90% of all breast cancers	> 3	Risk increases with decreasing age at onset, with number of affected family members, and with presence of further risks
			Combined action of multiple factors suspected
Other important factors			
	Chest radiation before age 20	10	
	Cancer in childhood	> 10	
Breast density			
	Relative risk (related to the risk of women aged 40–69 and ACR1 density), according to Kerlikowske 2007:		
	ACR1	1	Based on data from the Breast Cancer Surveillance Corsortium (Kerlikowske et al. 2007)
	ACR2	2.2	
	ACR3	3.2	
	ACR4	3.5	
Endogenous hormonal factors			
	Menarche before age 11	2–3	
	Menopause > age 54	2	
	First birth > age 40	2–3	
	Hormonal contraceptive	1.2–1.5	
	HRT	1.36	
Body mass index (BMI)	BMI > 30	0.7–2.9	
Nutritional	Fatty acid intake	1.1	
	Unsaturated fatty acids	0.9–1.1	Possibly different influence on pre- vs. postmenopausal women
	Alcohol consumption	2.3	

described for women with previously verified atypias and LIN 2–3. The above risk factors increase in women with multifocal disease, in younger women, and if a positive family history or other risk factors coexist. A personal history of an ovarian, endometrial, or colon cancer also increases the risk for breast cancer (Chuba et al. 2005, Degnim et al. 2007, Zhou et al. 2011, Reeves et al. 2012).

A high risk of breast cancer exists in women with proven monogenic hereditary breast cancer. These include *BRCA1* or *BRAC2* alterations, and other less common genetic disorders such as ataxia telangiectasia, Li–Fraumeni syndrome, Fanconi anemia, Cowden syndrome, Peutz–Jeghers syndrome, or hereditary diffuse gastric cancer syndrome. However, these hereditary breast cancers make up less than 10% of all breast cancers. Further gene alterations (e.g., *RAD51C* or *CHEK2*), however, which have a lower penetrance but may be important in certain constellations, are presently being investigated (Turnbull and Rahman 2008, Meindl et al. 2010, 2011, Walsh et al. 2010).

- *Family history:* A history of breast cancer in first- or second-degree relatives, the number of members affected, their gender (male breast cancer!), and age at detection (early age, premenopausal) are significant. Occurrence of ovarian cancer in first- or second-degree relatives is also important information. Based on the number of family members affected by breast or ovarian cancer and the age at onset, good estimates of the individual lifetime risk and of the risk of being affected by a monogenic hereditary breast cancer are possible for a geneticist. Therefore, in Germany genetic counseling is recommended for constellations which may indicate a risk > 10% of belonging to a high-risk group (BRCA1 or 2). **Table 1.2** gives an overview of the most important constellations (Kutner 1999, Weitzel 1999, Turnbull and Rahman 2008, Meindl et al. 2010, 2011).

Genetic counseling may help the woman to correctly perceive her risk (many affected women indeed overestimate their true risk). In families with a known gene variant (like BRCA1 or 2) a hereditary high risk can even be excluded if the woman does not carry this gene (since she has not inherited it). If she proves to be a carrier of a known pathogenic gene variation or if a known familial syndrome can be identified, she will be counseled concerning the existing choices of prophylaxis and/or surveillance for breast cancer, for ovarian cancer, and for other malignancies associated with the individual constellation. Bilateral prophylactic mastectomy is proven to reduce the risk of breast cancer by 95% and mortality from breast cancer by 90% (Meijers-Heijboer et al. 2001); prophylactic bilateral salpingo-oophorectomy reduces the risk of ovarian carcinoma by 97% and that of breast cancer by 50% (Meindl et al. 2011). Intensified surveillance offers the possibility of early detection, but so far no data are available that confirm whether (or to what degree) intensified surveillance by imaging allows reduction of breast cancer mortality. Counseling may include discussion of prophylactic measures for the patient herself and further family members. Furthermore, psychological support may be given.

- *Radiation or cancer during childhood:* Chest wall radiation during childhood (e.g., mantle field radiation in patients with Hodgkin disease) increases the risk for breast cancer significantly (relative risk factor ranging around 10). These patients are considered to be at high risk. A surveillance following the recommendations of women at high familial risk is recommended today (NICE 2006, Ortmann et al. 2008, Henderson et al. 2010). Also, cancer during childhood indicates a very high risk of being affected by breast cancer (with relative risk factors > 10) (Kaste et al. 1998, Ortmann et al. 2008). The relative risk in a young woman having had cancer in childhood compared with those in the same age group ranges around a factor of 20.

- *Mammographic density:* Data from large studies prove that increased mammographic density is associated with an increased risk of malignancy (McCormack and dos Santos Silva 2006, Boyd et al. 2007). The risk appears to increase continuously from fatty breast tissue (ACR1) through breast tissue with scattered fibro-glandular elements (ACR2) to heterogeneously dense (ACR3) and very dense breast tissue (ACR4) from an odds ratio of 1 to about 4.7. Considering that < 10% of women aged 40–69 have a density of ACR1 and < 10% have a density of ACR4, most women (with normal amounts of breast tissue) have a density of 2 or 3, which corresponds to a 2–3-fold risk compared with predominantly fatty breast tissue (ACR1), which contains very little glandular tissue.

Mammographic density appears to be determined by some genetic predisposition, which may be associated with a variety of genetic polymorphisms, which appear also to contribute to the multifactorial genesis of most breast cancers (Dumas and Diorio 2010, Peng et al. 2011). Even though breast density is an independent risk factor, it may be influenced by other factors such as patient age, menopausal status, and body mass index.

Owing to insufficient standardization, however, breast density does not appear to be sufficiently reliable for predicting an individual's risk (see also Chapter 10).

- *Endogenous and exogenous hormonal factors:* Endogenous factors, such as early menarche, late menopause, and late birth of first child, nulliparity, and the absence of breast-feeding are described as increasing the risk of breast cancer by a factor of 2–3 (Lambrechts et al. 2011).

The increased risk associated with hormone intake appears to be lower than the above endogenous risk

Table 1.2 Probability of being a carrier of a monogenic hereditary gene mutation based on personal and family history (Meindl et al. 2011)

No. of women in family with breast cancers	No. of women in family with ovarian cancer	No. of male breast cancers in family	Probability of being mutation carrier
≥ 3 cases any age	0	0	22%
> 3 cases with 2 cases before age 51	0	0	31%
2 cases with 1 case before age 51	0	0	9%
2 cases both before age 51	0	0	19%
1 bilateral with first event before age 51	0	0	25%
1 case before age 36	0	0	10%
> 1 case any age	> 1 case any age	0	48%
0	> 2 cases any age	0	45%
> 1 breast or ovarian breast cancer		1	42%

factors. However, it can be influenced by the patient herself.

According to the available data, oral contraceptives increase the risk of breast cancer by a factor of 1.2–1.5 on average (Kahlenborn et al. 2006). Hormone replacement therapy (HRT) based on estrogen and progesterone increases the risk of breast cancer on average by a factor of 1.26 (IARC 2007, Kerlikowske et al. 2007, Utian et al. and North American Menopause Society 2008, Farquhar et al. 2009). This corresponds to 8 additional women affected per 10,000 women per year (AWMF 2009). HRT using estrogen only may be associated with a low, statistically non-significant, increase in breast cancer. However, (due to other side effects) this type of HRT can only be recommended to women after hysterectomy.

HRT may also cause increased mammographic density and may be associated with an increased number of benign changes (cyst, fibroadenomas). It thus decreases sensitivity and specificity of mammography and imaging. Knowledge of HRT intake may be important for correctly interpreting observed changes in mammographic density (see Chapter 10).

- *Body mass index, nutrition, other factors:* Obesity (defined as a body mass index above 30) may be associated with an increased risk of breast cancer ranging around a relative factor of 2. Like the above-mentioned endogenous hormonal factors, the increased risk appears to mainly influence the incidence of estrogen or progesterone receptor-positive tumors (Ortmann et al. 2008, Renehan et al. 2008, Yang et al. 2011).

As to nutrition, an increased intake of fat may increase the risk of breast cancer. Unsaturated fatty acids appear to increase the risk in postmenopausal and decrease the risk in premenopausal patients. Existing data, however, are inconsistent (Turner 2011). A reported protective effect of olive oil might be explained by an additional antioxidant effect (Psaltopoulou et al. 2011).

Increased consumption of alcohol (up to five drinks daily) elevates the individual risk by a factor of up to 2.3 (Mørch et al. 2007, Ortmann et al. 2008).

Isoflavones have been suspected to possibly act as protective agents. However, a large meta-analysis could show this effect only in Asian populations (Dong and Qin 2011). Isoflavones may be associated with a slight increase in breast density (Hooper et al. 2010). Vitamin D has been discussed as another potentially protective agent. However, in meta-analyses the effect was reported inconsistently (Chung et al. 2009, Gandini et al. 2011).

To date (possibly due to problems of standardization) and the still inconsistent literature, nutritional factors are not considered when acquiring the patient's history. Hormone intake is considered, however, since it may also have an influence on breast density and on the false positive rate (see below).

Medical History Data Helpful for Image Interpretation

The following data may be helpful in image interpretation:
- Recent pregnancy or breast-feeding. This can be the cause of extensive proliferation of glandular tissue, which may be misinterpreted if the physician is unaware of the patient's history.
- Administration of female hormones. In some postmenopausal patients, HRT may cause extensive proliferation of glandular tissue. Newly occurring or increasing densities can be mistaken for suggestive findings if the physician is unaware of the patient's history. An increase in the size and number of cysts and fibroadenomas has been reported to increase the false positive rate (Banks et al. 2006, Njor et al. 2011).
- Administration of thyroid hormone. Published studies have described that administration of thyroid hormone can promote fibrocystic changes in the breast.
- Surgery or radiation therapy. Changes after surgery or radiation therapy can produce masses, distortions, or microcalcifications that can simulate or obscure a carcinoma (see Chapter 19). Here, careful documentation of scars and their location in the breast is important. Architectural distortion outside the scar area may be a sign of malignancy. Knowledge of the period of time that has elapsed since surgery or irradiation is valuable for correct image interpretation. Comparison with previous films is of utmost importance to identify early changes within scar tissue.
- Furthermore the following symptoms may be a hint to malignancy:
  - Any—even slight—changes of the nipple, such as a recent deviation or inversion of the nipple, are important. Even though deviation or inversion of the nipple can be congenital or can occur following inflammation, new development may be an important and early hint of malignancy.
  - Spontaneous discharge. Significant factors here include color, occurrence over time (association with pregnancy, chronic inflammation, prolactin), number of involved ducts (single vs. multiple), laterality (unilateral vs. bilateral) and the results of cytologic smears where available.
  - It is important to know that only spontaneous nipple discharge is considered pathologic, but not discharge that is provoked by compression. Some women tend to compress their breasts regularly, but this elevates prolactin values and causes discharge.

Significant aspects of any clinical findings (skin dimpling, skin changes, palpable findings) include:
- Time when the condition was first noticed
- Changes since the condition was first noticed (decrease, increase, time span)
- Results of previous examinations (such as surgical biopsy, core biopsy or cytology)

If *previous imaging studies* exist, ask for the name and, if known, the address of the physician who performed them. It may be useful to obtain these films for comparison. Whenever available, *compare findings with earlier imaging studies*, since this might improve diagnostic accuracy.

References and Recommended Reading

ACR Committee on Drugs and Contrast Media. Manual on Contrast Media. American College of Radiology; 2010. Available at: www.acr.org

Albert US, Altland H, Duda V, et al. 2008 update of the guideline: early detection of breast cancer in Germany. J Cancer Res Clin Oncol 2009;135(3):339–354

AWMF (Arbeitsgemeinschaft der Wissenschaftlichen Medizinischen Fachgesellschaften). S3-guideline on HRT during peri- and postmenopause. [In German] German Society of Gynaecology and Obstetrics (DGGG); 2009. Available at: www.awmf.org

Baines CJ, Vidmar M, McKeown-Eyssen G, Tibshirani R. Impact of menstrual phase on false-negative mammograms in the Canadian National Breast Screening Study. Cancer 1997;80(4):720–724

Banks E, Reeves G, Beral V, et al. Hormone replacement therapy and false positive recall in the Million Women Study: patterns of use, hormonal constituents and consistency of effect. Breast Cancer Res 2006;8(1):R8

Boyd NF, Guo H, Martin LJ, et al. Mammographic density and the risk and detection of breast cancer. N Engl J Med 2007;356(3):227–236

Chuba PJ, Hamre MR, Yap J, et al. Bilateral risk for subsequent breast cancer after lobular carcinoma-in-situ: analysis of surveillance, epidemiology, and end results data. J Clin Oncol 2005;23(24):5534–5541

Chung M, Balk EM, Brendel M, et al. Vitamin D and calcium: a systematic review of health outcomes. Evid Rep Technol Assess (Full Rep) 2009;183(183):1–420

Degnim AC, Visscher DW, Berman HK, et al. Stratification of breast cancer risk in women with atypia: a Mayo cohort study. J Clin Oncol 2007;25(19):2671–2677

Dong JY, Qin LQ. Soy isoflavones consumption and risk of breast cancer incidence or recurrence: a meta-analysis of prospective studies. Breast Cancer Res Treat 2011;125(2):315–323

Dumas I, Diorio C. Polymorphisms in genes involved in the estrogen pathway and mammographic density. BMC Cancer 2010;10:636

Elmore JG, Wells CK, Howard DH, Feinstein AR. The impact of clinical history on mammographic interpretations. JAMA 1997;277(1):49–52

Farquhar CM, Marjoribanks J, Lethaby A, Suckling JA, Lamberts Q. Long term hormone therapy for perimenopausal and postmenopausal women. [Review] Cochrane Database Syst Rev 2009; (2):CD004143

Fay MP, Freedman LS. Meta-analyses of dietary fats and mammary neoplasms in rodent experiments. Breast Cancer Res Treat 1997;46(2-3):215–223

Gandini S, Boniol M, Haukka J, et al. Meta-analysis of observational studies of serum 25-hydroxyvitamin D levels and colorectal, breast and prostate cancer and colorectal adenoma. Int J Cancer 2011;128(6):1414–1424

Gandini S, Merzenich H, Robertson C, Boyle P. Meta-analysis of studies on breast cancer risk and diet: the role of fruit and vegetable consumption and the intake of associated micronutrients. Eur J Cancer 2000;36(5):636–646

Giersig C. Progestin and breast cancer. The missing pieces of a puzzle. Bundesgesundheitsblatt Gesundheitsforschung Gesundheitsschutz 2008;51(7):782–786 Review. Erratum in: Bundesgesundheitsblatt Gesundheitsforschung Gesundheitsschutz. 2008;51(8):946

Henderson TO, Amsterdam A, Bhatia S, et al. Systematic review: surveillance for breast cancer in women treated with chest radiation for childhood, adolescent, or young adult cancer. Ann Intern Med 2010;152(7):444–455, W144-54

Hooper L, Madhavan G, Tice JA, Leinster SJ, Cassidy A. Effects of isoflavones on breast density in pre- and post-menopausal women: a systematic review and meta-analysis of randomized controlled trials. Hum Reprod Update 2010;16(6):745–760

Hovhannisyan G, Chow L, Schlosser A, Yaffe MJ, Boyd NF, Martin LJ. Differences in measured mammographic density in the menstrual cycle. Cancer Epidemiol Biomarkers Prev 2009;18(7):1993–1999

IARC Monographs on the evaluation of carcinogenic risks to humans: combined estrogenprogestogen contraceptives and combined estrogen-progestogen menopausal therapy (Volume 91). IARC; 2007. Available at: monographs.iarc.fr

Kahlenborn C, Modugno F, Potter DM, Severs WB. Oral contraceptive use as a risk factor for premenopausal breast cancer: a meta-analysis. Mayo Clin Proc 2006;81(10):1290–1302

Kanal E, Barkovich AJ, Bell C, et al; ACR Blue Ribbon Panel on MR Safety. ACR guidance document for safe MR practices: 2007. AJR Am J Roentgenol 2007;188(6):1447–1474

Kaste SC, Hudson MM, Jones DJ, et al. Breast masses in women treated for childhood cancer: incidence and screening guidelines. Cancer 1998;82(4):784–792

Kerlikowske K, Miglioretti DL, Buist DS, Walker R, Carney PA; National Cancer Institute-Sponsored Breast Cancer Surveillance Consortium. Declines in invasive breast cancer and use of postmenopausal hormone therapy in a screening mammography population. J Natl Cancer Inst 2007;99(17):1335–1339

Kuhl CK, Bieling HB, Gieseke J, et al. Healthy premenopausal breast parenchyma in dynamic contrast-enhanced MR imaging of the breast: normal contrast medium enhancement and cyclical-phase dependency. Radiology 1997;203(1):137–144

Kutner SE. Breast cancer genetics and managed care. The Kaiser Permanente experience. Cancer 1999; 86(11, Suppl)2570–2574

Lambrechts S, Decloedt J, Neven P. Breast cancer prevention: lifestyle changes and chemoprevention. Acta Clin Belg 2011;66(4):283–292

Lee CH, Dershaw DD, Kopans D, et al. Breast cancer screening with imaging: recommendations from the Society of Breast Imaging and the ACR on the use of mammography, breast MRI, breast ultrasound, and other technologies for the detection of clinically occult breast cancer. J Am Coll Radiol 2010;7(1):18–27

McCormack VA, dos Santos Silva I. Breast density and parenchymal patterns as markers of breast cancer risk: a meta-analysis. Cancer Epidemiol Biomarkers Prev 2006;15(6):1159–1169

Meijers-Heijboer H, van Geel B, van Putten WL, et al. Breast cancer after prophylactic bilateral mastectomy in women with a BRCA1 or BRCA2 mutation. N Engl J Med 2001;345(3):159–164

Meindl A, Ditsch N, Kast K, Rhiem K, Schmutzler RK. Hereditary breast and ovarian cancer: new genes, new treatments, new concepts. Dtsch Arztebl Int 2011;108(19):323–330

Meindl A, Hellebrand H, Wiek C, et al. Germline mutations in breast and ovarian cancer pedigrees establish RAD51C as a human cancer susceptibility gene. Nat Genet 2010;42(5):410–414

Mørch LS, Johansen D, Thygesen LC, et al. Alcohol drinking, consumption patterns and breast cancer among Danish nurses: a cohort study. Eur J Public Health 2007;17(6):624–629

Morrow M, Chatterton RT Jr, Rademaker AW, et al. A prospective study of variability in mammographic density during the menstrual cycle. Breast Cancer Res Treat 2010;121(3):565–574

Müller-Schimpfle M, Ohmenhäuser K, Stoll P, Dietz K, Claussen CD. Menstrual cycle and age: influence on parenchymal contrast medium enhancement in MR imaging of the breast. Radiology 1997;203(1):145–149

NICE (National Institute for Health and Clinical Excellence). Familial Breast Cancer: the classification and care of women at risk of familial breast cancer in primary, secondary and tertiary care (Clinical Guideline 41). London: National Institute for Health and Clinical Excellence; 2006. Available at: guidance.nice.org.uk

Njor SH, Hallas J, Schwartz W, Lynge E, Pedersen AT. Type of hormone therapy and risk of misclassification at mammography screening. Menopause 2011;18(2):171–177

Utian WH, Archer DF, Bachmann GA, et al; North American Menopause Society. Estrogen and progestogen use in postmenopausal women: July 2008 position statement of The North American Menopause Society. Menopause 2008;15(4 Pt 1):584–602

Ortmann O, Albert US, Schulz KD. Risikofaktoren. In: Albert US (ed.) Stufe-3-Leitlinie. Brustkrebs-Früherkennung in Deutschland. Munich: W.Zuckschwerst Publ; 2008

Peng S, Lü B, Ruan W, Zhu Y, Sheng H, Lai M. Genetic polymorphisms and breast cancer risk: evidence from meta-analyses, pooled analyses, and genome-wide association studies. Breast Cancer Res Treat 2011;127(2):309–324

Psaltopoulou T, Kosti RI, Haidopoulos D, Dimopoulos M, Panagiotakos DB. Olive oil intake is inversely related to cancer prevalence: a systematic review and a meta-analysis of 13,800 patients and 23,340 controls in 19 observational studies. Lipids Health Dis 2011;10:127

Reeves GK, Pirie K, Green J, Bull D, Beral V; Million Women Study Collaborators. Comparison of the effects of genetic and environmental risk factors on in situ and invasive ductal breast cancer. Int J Cancer 2012;131(4):930–937

Renehan AG, Tyson M, Egger M, Heller RF, Zwahlen M. Body-mass index and incidence of cancer: a systematic review and meta-analysis of prospective observational studies. Lancet 2008;371(9612):569–578

Sardanelli F, Boetes C, Borisch B, et al. Magnetic resonance imaging of the breast: recommendations from the EUSOMA working group. Eur J Cancer 2010;46(8):1296–1316

Sierra M, Machado C. Magnetic resonance imaging in patients with implantable cardiac devices. Rev Cardiovasc Med 2008;9(4):232–238

Spratt JS. Re: Variation in mammographic breast density by time in menstrual cycle among women aged 40-49 years. J Natl Cancer Inst 1999;91(1):90

References and Recommended Reading

Turnbull C, Ahmed S, Morrison J, et al; Breast Cancer Susceptibility Collaboration (UK). Genome-wide association study identifies five new breast cancer susceptibility loci. Nat Genet 2010;42(6):504–507

Turnbull C, Rahman N. Genetic predisposition to breast cancer: past, present, and future. Annu Rev Genomics Hum Genet 2008;9:321–345

Turner LB. A meta-analysis of fat intake, reproduction, and breast cancer risk: an evolutionary perspective. Am J Hum Biol 2011;23(5):601–608

Walsh T, Lee MK, Casadei S, et al. Detection of inherited mutations for breast and ovarian cancer using genomic capture and massively parallel sequencing. Proc Natl Acad Sci U S A 2010;107(28):12629–12633

Weitzel JN. Genetic cancer risk assessment. Putting it all together. Cancer 1999; 86(11, Suppl)2483–2492

White E, Velentgas P, Mandelson MT, et al. Variation in mammographic breast density by time in menstrual cycle among women aged 40-49 years. J Natl Cancer Inst 1998;90(12):906–910

Yang XR, Chang-Claude J, Goode EL, et al. Associations of breast cancer risk factors with tumor subtypes: a pooled analysis from the Breast Cancer Association Consortium studies. J Natl Cancer Inst 2011;103(3):250–263

Zhou WB, Xue DQ, Liu XA, Ding Q, Wang S. The influence of family history and histological stratification on breast cancer risk in women with benign breast disease: a meta-analysis. J Cancer Res Clin Oncol 2011;137(7):1053–1060

2 Clinical Findings

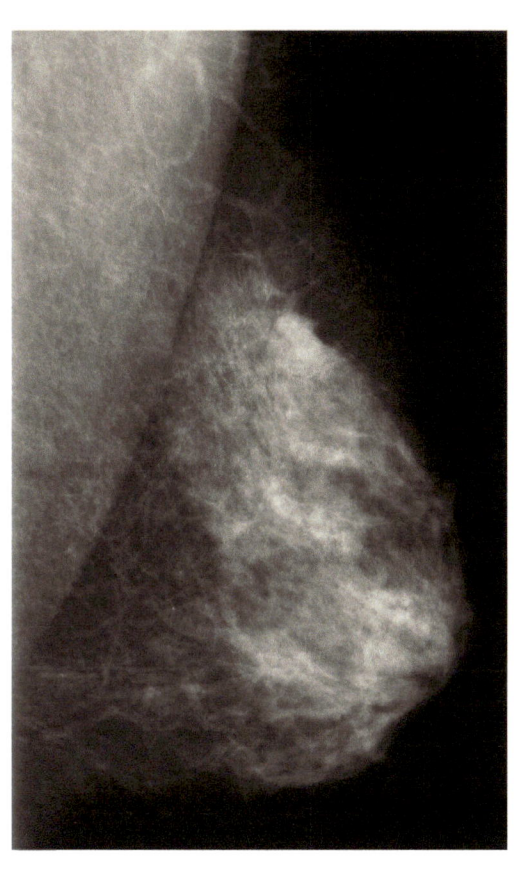

Purpose ⇢ *16*

Techniques ⇢ *16*
Visual Inspection ⇢ *16*
Palpation ⇢ *17*
Assessment of Clinical Abnormalities ⇢ *19*

References and Recommended Reading ⇢ *20*

2 Clinical Findings

S. H. Heywang-Koebrunner, I. Schreer, S. Barter

Purpose

Palpation and inspection yield the first and the easiest information about the breast. It may allow for the detection of breast cancer. This information may be obtained by the woman herself, who should be instructed how to examine her breast (breast self-examination, BSE), or by her physician during a clinical examination.

Based on data from large randomized studies, BSE was not proven to have significant influence on breast cancer mortality (Semiglazov et al. 1993, Thomas et al. 2002). In spite of this finding, most international guidelines recommend that women should be encouraged to examine their breasts regularly for the following reasons:
- Worldwide the majority of breast cancers are still found by the women themselves. Thus BSE should not be discouraged.
- BSE is the main method of detecting interval cancers (which may occur between two screening examinations).
- It is assumed that BSE increases awareness and may in individual cases be of advantage to the woman.

Owing to lack of reliable imaging methods in the younger patient (20–39 years of age) regular BSE (every 3 months) should be encouraged and the woman should be instructed on how to perform BSE.

In several large screening studies, clinical examination (by the physician) detected only about 5% of breast cancers. The reported effect of 5% in the screening setting, however, was not statistically significant (Bobo et al. 2000, Bancej et al. 2003, Weiss 2003, Oestreicher et al. 2005). Also, the mean size of clinically detected breast cancers was reported to range around 21 mm (Mandelson et al. 2000, Kolb et al. 2002).

Thus, clinical examination should not replace mammography screening. But since there is a small effect—as it may enhance breast cancer awareness and interval cancers are usually detected by BSE or clinical examination—clinical examination is considered to be an important component of breast cancer detection (Diratzouian et al. 2005, Ma et al. 2011) and most health systems support it. In the screening setting, clinical breast examination is usually performed not during mammography screening, but by the clinician who generally cares for the patient.

In symptomatic patients, or in patients with an imaging abnormality, clinical breast examination should always be performed as it complements the available information. Correlation of mammographic and clinical findings and vice versa is indispensable; otherwise, in the diagnostic setting, 10–15% of palpable breast cancers might go undetected. It should also be kept in mind that a few unusual cases of cancers exist which may be palpable but not visible by any imaging modality (including MRI).

Competence in physical examination of the breast is therefore a necessary skill for the mammographer.

Techniques

The examination of the breast involves visual inspection and palpation. When the physical examination is abnormal, subsequent diagnostic imaging studies should always be interpreted together with clinical findings. The physician must also ensure that the examination includes the marginal areas of the breast, namely the area close to the sternum, the inframammary fold, the lateral border of the glandular body, and the axilla, which may be poorly imaged at mammography.

Visual Inspection

Observe the breast with the patient's arm raised as well as with her hand placed on her hip. Observe and document any findings with respect to:
- Breast size and symmetry
- Contour
- Skin changes
- Nipples

Findings

The size of the breast can vary considerably among individual patients. Small breasts are easier to examine clinically, while macromastia will limit the amount of information provided by palpation. It is important to determine whether asymmetry in breast size (anisomastia) is an indication of:
- Individual variation
- A postoperative condition, or
- Retraction in the presence of disseminated tumor (reduction in breast size combined with palpable thickening)

The normal *breast contour* is convex. Flattening or dimpling can result from surgery or from retraction due to a subjacent tumor.

Skin changes may be generalized or circumscribed. Examples of such changes include:
- Erythema (mastitis, inflammatory breast carcinoma, or acute radiation reaction)

- Skin thickening
- Peau d'orange (skin thickening with inversion of the pores indicative of lymphedema)
- Prominent veins (supraclavicular, infraclavicular, or mediastinal mass producing venous compression)
- Hyperpigmentation or telangiectasia (sequela of radiation therapy)

Circumscribed skin changes include:
- Verrucae
- Nevi
- Atheromas
- Fibroepitheliomas
- Sebaceous cysts
- Scars
- Long area of retraction associated with thrombophlebitis (Mondor disease)

Inversion of the nipple can be:
- Congenital
- Acquired as a result of surgery
- The result of breast inflammation or a malignant tumor, or
- Associated with retraction

Deviation of the nipple or lack of symmetry when compared with the opposite side can be an indication of the beginning of retraction. Asymmetric depigmentation of the nipple can occur as a result of radiation therapy. Crusty deposits on the nipple can be a sign of pathologic discharge. Eczematous changes in the nipple can be a sign of Paget disease.

Any abnormalities in breast size or contour and any skin or nipple changes should be noted along with the probable causes suggested by the clinical examination or the patient's history. The radiologist should be aware of any benign skin lesions that might simulate a focal lesion at mammography. Cutaneous lesions may calcify, which should be considered in the mammographic differential diagnosis.

Precisely document any scars, since they may explain mammographically detectable structural changes (**Fig. 2.1**).

Palpation

Palpation should be performed gently, allowing for the patient's individual sensitivity to pain.
- Using the fingertips of both hands, separate the glandular tissue from the underlying and surrounding tissue and palpate it. Examine the breasts individually and systematically. Include the whole area from the clavicle to the inframammary fold and from the sternum to the midaxillary line.
- Assess the individual consistency of the gland, looking for circumscribed areas of altered (i.e., firmer) consistency.
- Always palpate both breasts for comparison.
- Normal breast tissue may be nodular or lumpy. However, all nodules should be elastic and the tissue should be easily movable between the fingertips. Search for areas of increased consistency.
- Assess the mobility of the nipple.
- Also assess the mobility of the breast tissue with respect to the skin and chest wall.
- Move your fingers toward each other and grasp the glandular tissue to assess whether a plateau appears as a sign of a desmoplastic reaction in the subjacent tissue (the Jackson sign).

The final procedure is the examination of the lymph drainage routes. These include the axillary tail of the breast, the axilla, the infraclavicular region, and the supraclavicular region. Palpate axillary lymph nodes by examining the patient with her arms hanging down or with her hands placed on her hips. Move your fingertips as far superiorly into the axilla as possible. Applying moderate pressure against the lateral chest wall, move slowly down the lateral chest wall. Lymph nodes will typically slide away under the fingertips. Palpate the axillary tail, the infraclavicular region, and the supraclavicular region using the same technique as for glandular tissue.

Findings

Palpation provides information about:
- The structure of glandular tissue
- Possible asymmetry
- Lumps and their consistency and relation to the surrounding tissue, skin (the Jackson sign), pectoralis muscle, and painful sensation
- The nipple and the subareolar tissue, and
- Lymph drainage routes

The structure of the glandular tissue can be soft or, in the presence of benign breast disorders, firm or granular. Granular texture may be fine, medium, or coarsely nodular. Documenting these palpatory findings is very valuable for interpreting subsequent findings. Asymmetry can be an initial sign of a disseminated or focal carcinoma, but it can also be congenital.

For every circumscribed palpable finding, assess the following parameters:
- Location (laterality, clock position with respect to the nipple, distance from the nipple, depth)
- Size
- Consistency
- Contour
- Mobility, and the relation to surrounding tissue (skin and pectoralis muscle). A malignant tumor can cause a desmoplastic reaction, and/or tumor infiltration may form a plateau accompanied by peau d'orange. This sign can be detected even before a tumor can be reliably palpated

2 Clinical Findings

Physician's Work Sheet

Clinical findings:
Generally **soft** breast: _____ **Firm** glandular tissue: _____
Finely nodular glandular tissue: _____ **Coarsely nodular** glandular tissue: _____

Additional findings:
(please number if more than one)

- Mobile lumps: ○
- Inverted **nipple**: △
- **Retraction** (skin, nipple): □
- Cutaneous **verruca** or similar finding: ●
- Immobile **lumps**: ⌀
- **Thickening**: ▨
- Scar: ┼┼┼┼┼

R L

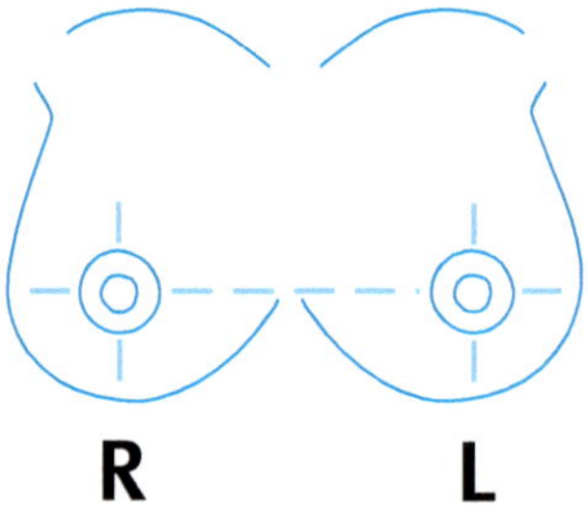

Finding number:	Approximate size:	First noticed when:	Change in size: ↑↓ —
1.	_____	_____	_____
2.	_____	_____	_____
3.	_____	_____	_____
4.	_____	_____	_____

Nipple discharge? N □

	number of ducts	color?	spontaneous?
right □	_____	_____	_____
left □	_____	_____	_____

Pain? N □

	symmetric?	localized*? (where)	type of pain
right □			
left □			

Status of lymph nodes: _____
_____

Physician: _____

Fig. 2.1 Physician's work sheet.

Circumscribed lumps can be soft (lipomas, fibroadenolipomas, partially filled cysts, medullary and mucinous carcinomas, lymphoma) or of firmer consistency (cysts, fibroadenomas, or carcinomas).

Involuted fibroadenomas, oil cysts, chronically inflamed cysts, and circumscribed scarring can have the same hard consistency as a carcinoma.

Fibrocystic masses, distended or chronically inflamed cysts, and hematomas are painful, whereas malignant tumors are less often so. Some women with good body perception will feel localized pain or sense a change at the site of a tumor that may not even be palpable. This may be due to the disturbed parenchymal structure and consistency caused by the tumor. While uni- or bilateral pain is mostly due to hormonal changes, a strictly localized pain, which may be itchy and does not change with the menstrual cycle, should be further investigated. Except for the latter rare sign, pain is usually not indicative of malignancy.

When the nipples are examined, mobility should be assessed. Mobility can be compromised by a tumor in the subjacent tissue or by subacute or chronic mastitis or scarring.

Small (i.e., ≤ 10 mm), smooth, mobile, generally firm lymph nodes can be normal findings in the axilla but are pathologic in the supraclavicular or infraclavicular regions. Enlarged lymph nodes and/or lymph nodes with poor mobility should be regarded as pathologic until proven otherwise.

Ectopic glandular tissue may be present in the axilla, above or below the breast. This will be apparent as relatively soft circumscribed palpable findings. The patient may report changes in size or painfulness related to the menstrual cycle.

Problems

Palpation can reveal small carcinomas in superficial sites or in small breasts. However, tumors exceeding 2 cm in diameter may go undetected in the deeper tissue of large or lumpy breasts. In fact, less than 50% of the tumors smaller than 1.5 cm in size are palpable.

The limitations of early detection by palpation also become obvious when considering that the average size of cancers detected by palpation exceeds 2.1 cm in diameter.

Palpating disseminated carcinomas such as disseminated invasive lobular carcinomas is particularly difficult. More than 90% of intraductal carcinomas are nonpalpable. Extensive nodular breast disorders can greatly limit the diagnostic accuracy of palpation.

Any atypical palpable findings and any findings suggestive of carcinoma should be further assessed by mammography or other diagnostic studies. A clinical examination conducted by a physician familiar with the mammographic findings will permit improved diagnostic interpretation of asymmetries or circumscribed areas of increased density.

Assessment of Clinical Abnormalities

Any clinical abnormality which might indicate malignancy requires further assessment. Further assessment is needed until malignancy is safely excluded. In women up to age 40 years ultrasound should be used as a first step. If malignancy cannot be excluded, mammography should be included. In women above the age of 40, mammography should be performed (unless a recent mammogram is already available). In dense breast tissue (ACR density 2–4) ultrasound examination should be included. Only in women at high risk should MRI be considered in addition. Whenever imaging cannot unequivocally explain the finding as being typically benign, biopsy should be considered. Percutaneous biopsy should, in general, be preferred to open biopsy. In the case of incompatible findings at percutaneous breast biopsy, open biopsy may need to be considered.

Summary

Careful clinical examination is recommended, even with regular mammographic screening. The reasons for this are:

1. Outside the age range for which mammographic screening is recommended, BSE and palpation constitute the first and main methods by which breast cancer may be detected.

2. Mammography has limited sensitivity, especially in radiodense tissue. Approximately 10% of malignancies are discovered only because they are palpable. This means that palpable findings, even with negative mammography, may require further workup or biopsy.

3. Palpation can detect malignant processes along the periphery of the glandular body or in the axillary tail which may escape detection at mammography.

Mammography does not replace careful physical examination. However, whenever questionable or suggestive clinical findings exist, further workup (by mammography, possibly ultrasonography and/or percutaneous biopsy) should follow to avoid missing nonpalpable additional lesions or causing unnecessary biopsy (of lipomas, definite fibroadenomas, hamartomas, oil cysts, or simple cysts).

In the age range for which mammographic screening is recommended, BSE or clinical examination may not replace quality-assured mammographic screening.

References and Recommended Reading

Alexander FE, Anderson TJ, Brown HK, et al. 14 years of follow-up from the Edinburgh randomised trial of breast-cancer screening. Lancet 1999;353(9168):1903–1908

Bancej C, Decker K, Chiarelli A, Harrison M, Turner D, Brisson J. Contribution of clinical breast examination to mammography screening in the early detection of breast cancer. J Med Screen 2003;10(1):16–21

Barton MB, Harris R, Fletcher SW. The rational clinical examination. Does this patient have breast cancer? The screening clinical breast examination: should it be done? How? JAMA 1999;282(13):1270–1280

Bobo JK, Lee NC, Thames SF. Findings from 752,081 clinical breast examinations reported to a national screening program from 1995 through 1998. J Natl Cancer Inst 2000;92(12):971–976

Ciatto S, Rosselli del Turco M, Catarzi S, et al. Causes of breast cancer misdiagnosis at physical examination. Neoplasma 1991;38(5):523–531

Diratzouian H, Freedman GM, Hanion AL, Eisenberg DF, Anderson PR. Importance of physical examination in the absence of a mammographic abnormality for the detection of early-stage breast cancer. Clin Breast Cancer 2005;6(4):330–333

Flegg KM, Rowling YJ. Clinical breast examination. A contentious issue in screening for breast cancer. Aust Fam Physician 2000;29(4):343–346, discussion 348

Kolb T, Lichy J, Newhouse J. Comparison of the performance of screening mammography, physical examination and breast US and evaluation of factors that influence them: an analysis of 27,825 patient evaluations. Radiology 2002;225:165–175

Ma I, Dueck A, Gray R, et al. Clinical and self breast examination remain important in the era of modern screening. Ann Surg Oncol 2012;19(5):1484–1490

McDonald S, Saslow D, Alciati MH. Performance and reporting of clinical breast examination: a review of the literature. CA Cancer J Clin 2004;54(6):345–361

Mandelson MT, Oestreicher N, Porter PL. Breast density as a predictor of mammographic detection: comparison of interval- and screen-detected cancers. J Natl Cancer Inst 2000;92:1081–1087

Miller AB, To T, Baines CJ, Wall C. The Canadian National Breast Screening Study: update on breast cancer mortality. J Natl Cancer Inst Monogr 1997;22(22):37–41

Oestreicher N, Lehman CD, Seger DJ, Buist DS, White E. The incremental contribution of clinical breast examination to invasive cancer detection in a mammography screening program. AJR Am J Roentgenol 2005;184(2):428–432

Reintgen D, Berman C, Cox C, et al. The anatomy of missed breast cancers. Surg Oncol 1993;2(1):65–75

Semiglazov VF, Sagaidak VN, Moiseyenko VM, Mikhailov EA. Study of the role of breast self-examination in the reduction of mortality from breast cancer: The Russian Federation/World Health Organisation Study. Eur J Cancer 1993;29A(14):2039–2046

Shapiro S. Periodic screening for breast cancer: the HIP Randomized Controlled Trial. Health Insurance Plan. J Natl Cancer Inst Monogr 1997; (22):27–30

Smart CR, Byrne C, Smith RA, et al. Twenty-year follow-up of the breast cancers diagnosed during the Breast Cancer Detection Demonstration Project. CA Cancer J Clin 1997;47(3):134–149

Thomas DB, Gao DL, Ray RM, et al. Randomized trial of breast self-examination in Shanghai: final results. J Natl Cancer Inst 2002;94(19):1445–1457

Weiss NS. Breast cancer mortality in relation to clinical breast examination and breast self examination. Breast J 2003;9(Suppl. 2):S86–S89

3 Mammography

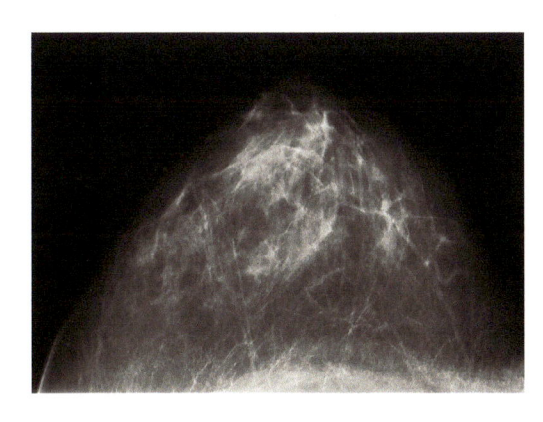

Purpose, Accuracy, Possibilities, and Limitations ⇢ 22
Indications ⇢ 22
Accuracy ⇢ 22
Screening ⇢ 24
Problem Solving ⇢ 24

Mammographic Technique ⇢ 25
Components of the Mammographic Imaging Technique ⇢ 25
Picture Archiving and Communications Systems (PACSs) ⇢ 39
Computer Aided Diagnosis (CAD) ⇢ 40

Specific Requirements and Solutions ⇢ 40
Image Sharpness ⇢ 40
Contrast ⇢ 41
Noise ⇢ 49
Radiation Dose ⇢ 50

Positioning and Compression ⇢ 52
Compression ⇢ 52
Positioning for Standard Views ⇢ 54
Positioning for Additional Views ⇢ 57
Film Labeling ⇢ 62
Spot Compression ⇢ 62
Magnification Technique ⇢ 64
Positioning of Breasts with Implants ⇢ 71

Imaging of the Specimen ⇢ 72

Quality Factors ⇢ 74
Hardware Factors that Influence Image Quality ⇢ 74
Influence of the Screen–Film System and Film Processing on Image Quality ⇢ 75
Additional Factors ⇢ 76
Quality Assurance in Mammography ⇢ 76

Reporting and Documentation of Findings ⇢ 78
Clinical Findings ⇢ 78
Mammographic Report ⇢ 79

Galactography ⇢ 85
Duct Sonography and MRI ⇢ 91
Histopathologic Assessment of Ductal Abnormalities ⇢ 91

Pneumocystography ⇢ 92

References and Recommended Reading ⇢ 93

3 Mammography

S. H. Heywang-Koebrunner, J. Kotre, S. Barter

Purpose, Accuracy, Possibilities, and Limitations

Indications

Mammography is the single most important imaging method in diagnosing breast disease. Its areas of application include:

- **Screening**. Mammography is the only imaging method to date that is suitable for screening of women at low to intermediate risk.
  For women at intermediate risk, screening at yearly intervals and—in the case of dense breast tissue—supplementary ultrasonography is recommended.
  For women at high risk, international guidelines today recommend yearly magnetic resonance imaging (MRI) combined with mammography. Yearly MRI is mostly recommended starting at age 25 up to about age 55 or until mammography exhibits low breast density (ACR1 or 2) (see also Chapter 5). Yearly screening mammography of women at high risk is recommended to start at age 30 or 5 years before the youngest age of involvement in the family. Owing to the low sensitivity of mammography in young carriers of the *BRCA1* mutation and an increased sensitivity of breast tissue to radiation below age 40, the added use of screening mammography before age 40 may require further data and continuous re-evaluation.
- **Problem solving**. Aside from a few exceptions (such as unequivocal sonographic diagnosis of a cyst, unequivocal clinical diagnosis of an abscess, and very young patients) mammography is indicated as a diagnostic method in the majority of symptomatic patients over the age of 40.
  In symptomatic women above age 40, bilateral mammography should usually be performed, or a recent mammogram should be available to exclude the presence of malignancy in the area of concern or in other quadrants of the same or the contralateral breast. This recommendation takes into account the increasing incidence of breast cancer after age 40, and the increasing sensitivity of mammography with increasing patient age. This approach will avoid missing a mammographically visible breast cancer (even in other quadrants) in women who undergo assessment for one specific problem, since any false reassurance could lead to delayed diagnosis.
  Before the age of 40, assessment should usually start with sonography. If the problem is solved by using ultrasound (e.g., by demonstration of a simple cyst or of homogeneous echogenic tissue in a young woman without increased risk), mammography may not be necessary.

A basic knowledge of the accuracy of mammography is a prerequisite to properly judge its value in screening and clinical use.

Accuracy

General Aspects

The sensitivity and specificity of the method cannot be precisely quantified. While high image quality and experienced examiners are essential, accuracy also depends on the following factors:

- **Patient selection**. Screening versus diagnostic problem solving, type of screening (number of views, use of clinical data, and screening interval), prevalence of findings in the study group, and the extent to which other methods of preoperative diagnosis are used.
- **Threshold of the individual examiner**. Experience being equal, a low threshold will lead to a high sensitivity at the expense of specificity, whereas a high threshold increases specificity and the positive predictive value at the expense of sensitivity.
  An individual's threshold represents a compromise arrived at by assessing the tradeoff between the false negative rate and the false positive rate. It is also influenced by other factors such as the limited funds of the screening program and restrictions concerning the accepted rate of imaging or histopathologic assessment.

Sensitivity

Realistically, mammography has a sensitivity of about 85%; that is, around 15% of carcinomas which are otherwise symptomatic at the time of the mammographic examination are not detected initially by mammography.

When mammographic screening is performed, in good-quality assured programs with 2-year intervals, about 20–30% of carcinomas become apparent between two screening examinations (i.e., up to 24 months after the examination!), usually by manifesting clinical symptoms. They are called *interval carcinomas*. Their number depends on the length of the screening interval and on other factors of the particular screening program or the screened population.

Interval carcinomas consist of cancers that grow and thus become detectable during the interval between scheduled screening mammograms (Boyer et al. 2004, Porter et al. 2006, Hofvind et al. 2008, Caumo et al. 2010). They include cancers which (even in retrospect) are not visible on the initial screening mammogram (*type 1: occult carcinomas*), cancers which are visible on the initial screening mammogram in retrospect, frequently as a nonspecific change that could not be expected to have been diagnosed prospectively (*type 2: minimal sign*), and cancers which are visible on the initial screening mammogram and could/should have been diagnosed prospectively (*type 3: false negative calls*).

Type 1 carcinomas include new tumors which have grown during the interval and carcinomas which are not visible by mammography (limitation of mammography). Some of the latter are not visible even on the diagnostic mammogram at the time of clinical presentation.

Distinguishing between type 2 and 3 carcinomas may be quite difficult and requires significant experience with both evaluation of interval cancers and screening of asymptomatic women. The fact that some uncharacteristic change is visible in retrospect on a screening mammogram is not equivalent to a miss.

At first sight this may be difficult to understand. However, retrospective interpretation of a mammogram knowing the result or even the location of a clinical finding is not at all comparable to prospective detection of a clinically occult abnormality. The reason is that countless normal variations and benign changes exist. Finding a significant abnormality among the many benign changes prospectively and without knowledge of a clinical change (which by definition is the task of screening) is a difficult task and may be comparable to that of not being able to "see the wood for the trees."

Thus the sensitivity of mammography screening is different from that of diagnostic mammography, where targeted evaluation is performed based on overlapping information from clinical examination and mammography with targeted and multimodality interpretation.

The threshold of detection of screening mammography depends on tumor size, tumor type and surrounding tissue, and patient age. Since both the surrounding tissue and histology of the cancer determine its mammographic visibility, it must be understood that depending on the type of breast cancer and the surrounding tissue there may be varying size thresholds for detectability of breast cancers. In some unfortunate cases even large tumors (often diffusely growing tumors or tumors located within dense tissue) may not be detectable by mammography. This issue may be difficult to understand for people who are not familiar with breast imaging.

Even though a significant number of symptomatic breast cancers which are mammographically occult are known to be visible by other methods, it is uncertain how many asymptomatic carcinomas which are occult at screening mammography might prospectively be detectable by other methods in the screening situation (i.e., prospectively without any clinical suspicion).

So far, mammography is the only method for which reproducible and reliable detection of a prognostically relevant number of nonpalpable carcinomas has been proven at an acceptable rate of false positive calls and at acceptable expense. No other method is presently considered capable of reproducing these results (Heywang-Köbrunner et al. 2008). Whether or for which subgroups of women the *added* use of further methods (such as ultrasound or MRI) might allow a reproducible increase in sensitivity at acceptable specificity and costs for society remains a topic for future research.

Prognosis of interval cancers depends on tumor size, grading, lymph node involvement, and ER/PR (estrogen/progesterone receptor) status at detection. It is usually worse than that of screen-detected breast cancers, but comparable to the prognosis of clinically detected breast cancers in women who do not undergo screening mammography (Caumo et al. 2010).

Overall sensitivity of mammography in fatty tissue is excellent, ranging around 98% in the completely fatty breast (ACR1) and around 50–60% in the very dense breast (ACR4). It decreases as radiodensity increases. This means that mammography has a lower sensitivity in radiodense tissue and, therefore, a negative mammogram does not eliminate the need for further workup of otherwise indeterminate or suggestive clinical findings in dense tissue (Rosenberg et al. 1998, van Gils et al. 1998).

Mammography is highly sensitive in detecting carcinomas containing microcalcifications, and this sensitivity is largely uninfluenced by the radiodensity of the surrounding tissue. These carcinomas account for about 50% of all cancers, including some 30%–40% of all invasive carcinomas and about 90% of carcinomas in situ currently detected. Since these are generally not palpable but have excellent cure rates, mammography plays a decisive role in early detection.

Specificity

In the screening situation mammography is the only method for which (with sufficient training) a good sensitivity is combined with the required high specificity. For subsequent screening rounds in European screening programs it ranges around 95–98% (calculated by counting a recall for a finding that eventually proved benign as a false positive call). In the United States higher recall rates are reported. If histopathologic assessment is considered a false positive call, the specificity can be as high as 99%. These high specificities are needed for any screening, since false positive calls accumulate during the 20 years for which screening is offered to the woman. Low specificities leading to high numbers of biopsies within the screened population might not be acceptable to the woman and might lead to unacceptable costs.

Specificity of mammography in symptomatic cases is limited:
- Absence of malignancy can be diagnosed reliably in fatty breasts (provided the area in question is included on the mammogram).
- A definitive diagnosis of a benign lesion is possible for a typical oil cyst, a hamartoma, a lipoma, a typically calcified fibroadenoma, or lymph nodes with typical mammographic features.
- A relatively reliable diagnosis of a benign tumor or cyst (> 98% correct) is possible in the case of a typical well-circumscribed mass.

However, in the majority of clinically or mammographically detected changes, mammography is nonspecific and permits only statements of likelihood.
- The specificity of the diagnosis of a carcinoma is quite high for spiculated masses, as well as for pleomorphic and casting microcalcifications with ductal distribution. However, a spiculated mass can also be caused by an area of fat necrosis or a radial scar. Rarely, even suspicious microcalcifications are associated with papillomatosis, papilloma, fibroadenoma, plasma cell mastitis, or fat necrosis.

In addition to the factors already mentioned (patient selection and examiner threshold), the physical size of the findings decisively influences the expected specificity of the mammographic study. In fact, most nonpalpable carcinomas, in particular small carcinomas, appear as nonspecific changes (Liberman et al. 1998). Unless the examiner is only looking for large, obvious findings, one has to be aware that only 1 of every 5 to 10 mammographically suspicious changes will correspond to malignancy (Perry et al. 2006, Elmore et al. 2009).

Further diagnostic studies, including additional views, sonography, and percutaneous biopsy, can improve this rate so that more than half of the excisional biopsies of nonpalpable abnormalities will be performed for a malignancy (Perry et al. 2006).

Screening

Owing to the high sensitivity of mammography in fatty tissue and its ability to reveal microcalcifications, mammography can detect small carcinomas at an early and prognostically favorable stage.

Mammographic screening has resulted in a significant reduction in mortality (see Chapter 23). To date, neither physical examination nor any other diagnostic test or method has been able to achieve comparable results. It is estimated that half of the achieved mortality reduction today is due to early detection (mostly by mammography screening) while half of the effect is probably due to improvement of therapy (Berry et al. 2005). Early detection furthermore allows improved treatment (more breast conservation, fewer axillary dissections, less use of chemotherapy).

Mammography is the only imaging modality suitable for screening. In addition to good sensitivity and acceptable specificity, it offers the following important advantages:
- It is the most cost-effective noninvasive examination method.
- Mammographic studies are reproducible and easily documented.
- It requires relatively little physician time (in contrast to breast sonography).
- It is the only technique that reliably visualizes microcalcifications which are associated with approximately 30% of the invasive breast cancers and almost all presently detected intraductal cancers.

Yet despite the many advantages, limitations and potential side effects need to be considered. To maximise the effect and limit side effects, systematic quality assurance and regular training are necessary.

Problem Solving

Problem solving begins when clinical data, the patient's medical history, or imaging studies (usually mammography) reveal an abnormality. The most important objective is to verify or exclude the presence of a carcinoma with the highest possible degree of certainty.

For this purpose multi-modality imaging assessment (including state-of-the-art two-view mammography, additional mammographic views when needed and ultrasound examination) should be performed before deciding on further steps. MRI is not part of the standard imaging assessment, but may be helpful in selected cases (see Chapter 5, p. 158–170).

If malignancy cannot be excluded by standard imaging assessment, histopathologic assessment represents the next step, which should be performed, whenever possible, using percutaneous breast biopsy.

Overall, a high degree of certainty is necessary to exclude a suspected malignancy.

The following should be remembered for problem solving:
1. The sensitivity of mammography is excellent (approaching 100%) in fatty breasts or in all fatty areas of the breast. This means that in the absence of mammographic findings, malignancy can be excluded with a high degree of certainty, even in the presence of palpable abnormality in this area. This applies only if the palpable findings in question:
   - Have been included mammographically (note that the axillary tail and areas close to the chest wall can be a problem), and
   - Lie entirely within fatty tissue

For this reason it may be useful to place a radiopaque marker over palpable lesions to localize them on the mammogram.
2. It is particularly important to remember that the sensitivity of mammography is significantly reduced in areas containing a high proportion of glandular or connective tissue. Carcinomas without microcalcifications can be overlooked in such areas. Thus, in tissue that is not mammographically equivalent to fat, any suggestive palpable findings require further workup.
3. Only a few entities have such a distinct mammographic appearance that no further diagnostic studies are necessary. These include:
   - Lipomas
   - Typical hamartomas
   - Characteristically calcified fibroadenomas
   - Oil cysts and some galactoceles
   - Intramammary lymph nodes
4. Whenever a mammographically, clinically, or otherwise detected abnormality does not exhibit a pathognomonic appearance, further workup is necessary.

Another important task of mammography concerns detection of secondary lesions. For this reason, even in women with palpable lesions undergoing surgical biopsy (except very young women), mammography is always indicated preoperatively to be certain that a second nonpalpable lesion that requires biopsy is not present.

Mammographic Technique

Compared with radiographic studies of other parts of the body, mammography places particularly stringent demands on equipment and image quality. The stringent demands of technique and positioning make mammography one of the most difficult examinations in conventional radiology.

The specific requirements can be *summarized as follows*:

- Extremely fine microcalcifications and fibrotic strands (tiny structures with a size of approximately 100 µm with only slight differences in density compared with the surrounding tissue) must be imaged sharply, with high contrast and with a low level of image noise.
- Despite the highest possible contrast, mammography must permit adequate assessment of areas of greatly varying density. These include fatty areas behind the nipple or close to the skin in small breasts, areas of radiodense fibrocystic tissue in large breasts, and the tissue overlying the pectoralis muscle. This requires an imaging system with a wide object range.
- In view of the sensitivity of mammary tissue to radiation (especially in younger women), the examination should involve the minimum dose of radiation sufficient to produce an image of acceptable quality.
- Imaging the complete body of the gland is imperative for an accurate assessment in both screening examinations and diagnostic problem solving. This is possible only with a consistent effort to achieve optimum standard positioning. Knowledge and application of additional views, whenever indicated, are necessary.

These stringent requirements apply to the choice of equipment and film as well as to the level of training and experience of physicians and technical staff. Radiologists and radiologic technologists must ensure a standard of image quality that permits detection of early malignancy.

It is therefore *essential that radiologists and radiologic technologists* be thoroughly familiar with mammographic technique and constantly monitor quality. Studies have shown that only optimal imaging technique ensures early detection of breast cancer (Boyd et al. 1993). Where this is not the case, early stage carcinomas with excellent cure rates will not be detected with sufficient certainty. This has serious negative repercussions because the mammographic examination will give the patient and her referring physician a false sense of security, and both may underestimate the significance of early clinical signs of malignancy.

Components of the Mammographic Imaging Technique

(See **Fig. 3.1**.)

The X-ray Tube

Mammography requires special tubes that produce particularly *low-energy radiation* in comparison with other diagnostic X-ray tubes. This is achieved by the use of special targets and filters. Mammography requires low-energy radiation to achieve the required high tissue contrast.

Since the radiation needed originates in a small focal spot and the exposure time should be as short as possible (to avoid motion blurring), the tubes used for mammography must incorporate a high heat capacity target.

Sharpness: Focal Spot Size and Geometry (Source to Image-Receptor Distance = SID)

To achieve the required sharpness (spatial resolution), mammography tubes must have an extremely small focal spot. A *nominal focal spot size smaller than 0.4* is required today.

3 Mammography

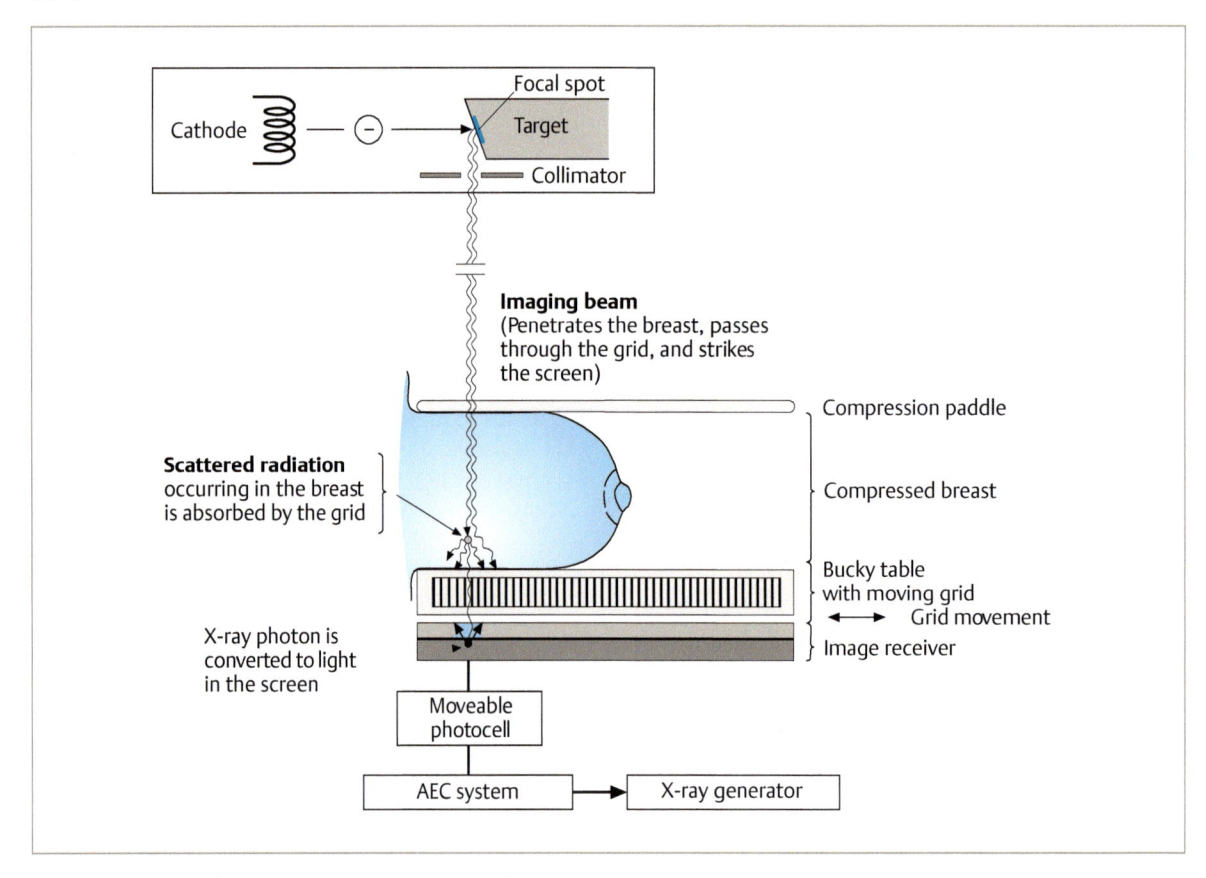

Fig. 3.1 Mammographic imaging technique. Overview of components.

Note: A nominal focal spot size of 0.4 means that the diameter in each direction will be between 0.4 mm and 0.6 mm. The local projection of the width of the focal spot will vary according to:
- Its distance from the chest wall
- The angulation of the tube

In addition to minimal focal spot size, the proper geometric configuration of the focal spot, object, and image receptor is important in achieving the necessary sharpness. Use of a *small focal spot, the shortest possible distance between the object and the film, and the longest possible distance between the focus and the film* will minimize the penumbra (geometric blurring) (**Fig. 3.2**).

Radiation Spectrum: Penetration and Contrast

The radiation produced in X-ray tubes is not monoenergetic but consists of a spectrum of radiation energies. This spectrum comprises X-ray bremsstrahlung and the characteristic radiation determined by the target material.

Since the spectrum of imaging radiation greatly influences contrast and radiation dose, the following physical aspects should be considered:

- With *low-energy radiation,* slight differences in the radiodensity of soft tissue of the breast that would otherwise remain undetected can be visualized with *high contrast.*
- *Increasing energy* of the radiation *decreases soft-tissue contrast.*
- But the radiation spectrum must have *sufficiently high energy for adequate penetration* of thick breasts and breasts with abundant fibrotic or glandular tissue.
- Radiation with insufficient energy will not penetrate the breast even with long exposure time. Such radiation is not suitable for imaging at all. It will unnecessarily increase the radiation dose and, since dense tissue cannot be penetrated, will produce an inadequate image.

Thus, *higher-energy* radiation is required in *dense breasts* (in the presence of abundant fibrotic or glandular tissue) and in *thick breasts.*

With the optimum radiation energy selected, the *absorption is higher in radiodense tissue (fibrotic tissue, glandular tissue, and malignant tissue) than in radiolucent tissue (fat or loose connective tissue)*. These *differences in absorption* produce the image pattern.

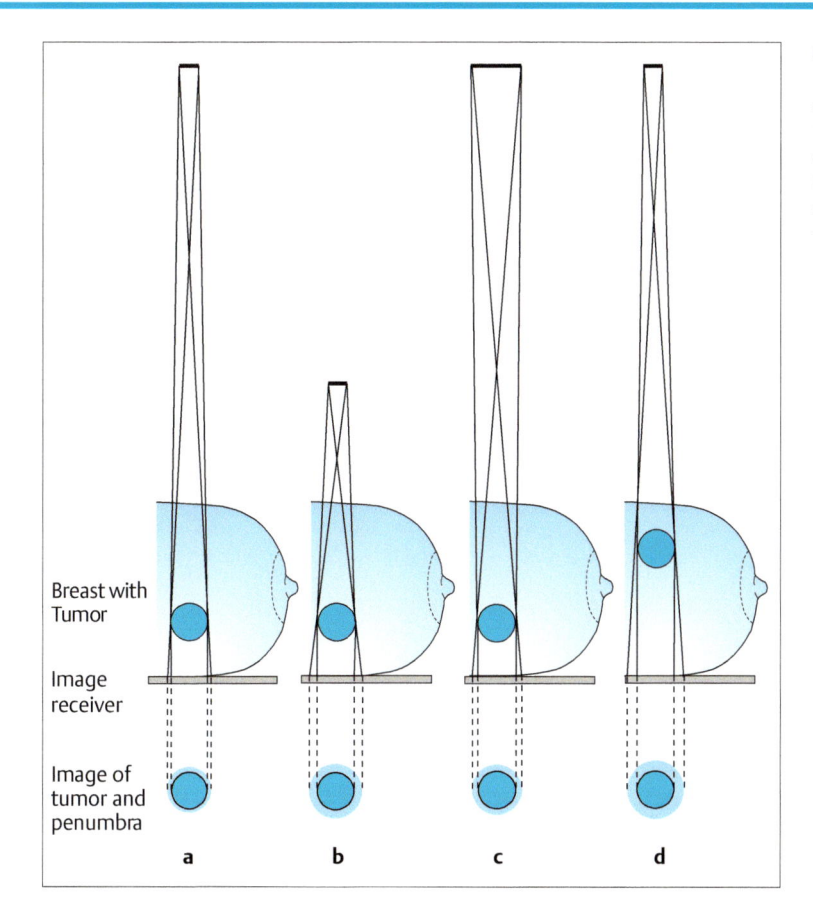

Fig. 3.2a–d A long SID (source to image-receptor distance), small focal spot, and short distance between the object and the image receiver minimize penumbra and optimize image definition (**a**). The penumbra increases with a short SID (**b**), large focal spot (**c**), and a long distance between object and film (**d**).

Since too large a component of high energy reduces the contrast and too high a component of low energy results in excessive radiation exposure, it is advisable to adapt the radiation spectrum as closely as possible to the thickness and density of the breast.

The radiation spectrum is determined by the following factors:
1. The *target/filter combination* of the X-ray tube
2. The *peak kilovoltage (kVp)* setting on the X-ray unit

Target/Filter Combination

The radiation spectrum created at the target depends on the kVp setting and on the *target material*.

The radiation spectrum of molybdenum targets contains a higher proportion of low-energy radiation (including characteristic peaks at 17.5 and 19.6 keV) than do the spectra of tungsten or rhodium tubes.

Selective filtering is used to adapt the radiation spectrum of a given target as closely as possible to the specific requirements.

Selective filtering:
- Suppresses the low-energy components of the spectrum that would represent unnecessary radiation exposure because they are absorbed in the breast (e.g., the standard aluminum filter).
- Reduces the energy components above the K absorption edge characteristic of the selected filter material, essentially permitting a narrow spectral range directly below the K absorption edge to pass. Any filter is particularly efficient at absorbing that part of the radiation whose energy exceeds a limit, referred to as the K absorption edge, specific to the filter material.

The effective spectral range can thus be defined by selecting the target and filter material and the thickness of the filter (**Fig. 3.3**).

Commercially available *target/filter combinations* include molybdenum/molybdenum, molybdenum/rhodium, rhodium/rhodium or tungsten/molybdenum, and tungsten/rhodium.
- The radiation quality from a molybdenum/molybdenum or tungsten/molybdenum target/filter combination is suitable for most breasts.
- The combinations tungsten/molybdenum, molybdenum/rhodium, tungsten/rhodium, and rhodium/rhodium provide, in this order, increasingly high-energy radiation spectra. They permit better penetration of large and dense breasts with abundant glandular, fibrotic, and connective tissue, resulting in higher image quality and a reduction in unnecessary radiation exposure.

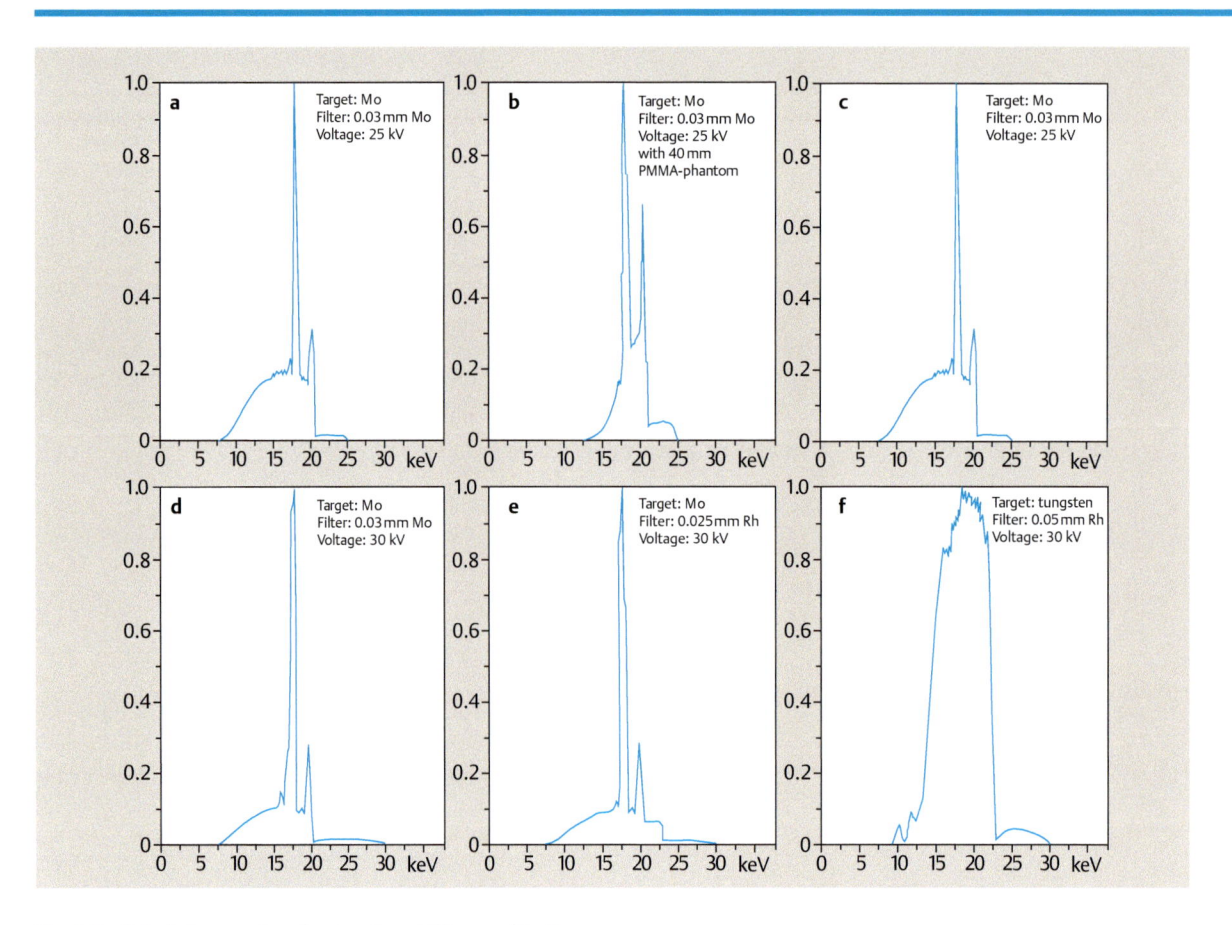

Fig. 3.3a–f Radiation spectra of various target/filter combinations.

a,b The illustration shows the photon spectrum of a molybdenum/0.030-mm molybdenum filter combination at 25 kV peak kilovoltage as it is emitted from the X-ray tube (**a**), and as it is measured at the image receptor after penetrating a 4-cm breast phantom (**b**). The correspondings spectra of radiation in the right and left pictures are normalized according to the maximum energy (= 100%) present in the spectrum.
Comparing left and right illustrations reveals that the low energies are absorbed in the breast. Thus, they cannot contribute to visualization but only increase the dose. The more breast thickness increases, the more low-energy components of the spectrum are absorbed in the glandular tissue.

Increasing the average energy of the spectrum in proportion to breast thickness and density is recommended to achieve sufficient penetration and avoid an excessive dose due to absorption of the low-energy radiation.

c–f One way of increasing the high-energy components in the spectrum is to increase the kVp setting. Changing the filter material and/or filter thickness or choosing another target material makes it possible to adapt the radiation spectrum even more closely to the thickness and density of the breast. (This increases the high-energy components in the spectrum and better filters out the low-energy components, which increase the dose, particularly in dense breasts.) This may be illustrated in the spectra of various target/filter combinations.

Peak Kilovoltage (kVp)

A higher kVp setting increases the relative proportion of high-energy radiation in the spectrum, whereas a lower kVp setting increases the relative proportion of low-energy radiation.

Selecting the proper kVp setting, target material, and filter material according to breast thickness and density: Since the optimum kVp for a target/filter combination is not applicable to others, automatic exposure control systems are provided to make it easier to match kVp to breast thickness and density. Depending on the manufacturer, the system can select or suggest the proper settings (see pp. 30 and 47).

Penetration: Heel Effect

The heel effect of the X-ray tube is also exploited to compensate for varying penetration in the chest wall and nipple.

The heel effect (**Fig. 3.4**) means that the intensity of rays emitted by the target is not uniform throughout the beam.

More of the rays that leave the target at obtuse angles will be absorbed by the target than those leaving the target at acute angles, owing to the longer path they have to travel in the target.

Since the thickness of the breast is greater close to the chest wall than near the nipple, it is best when the area

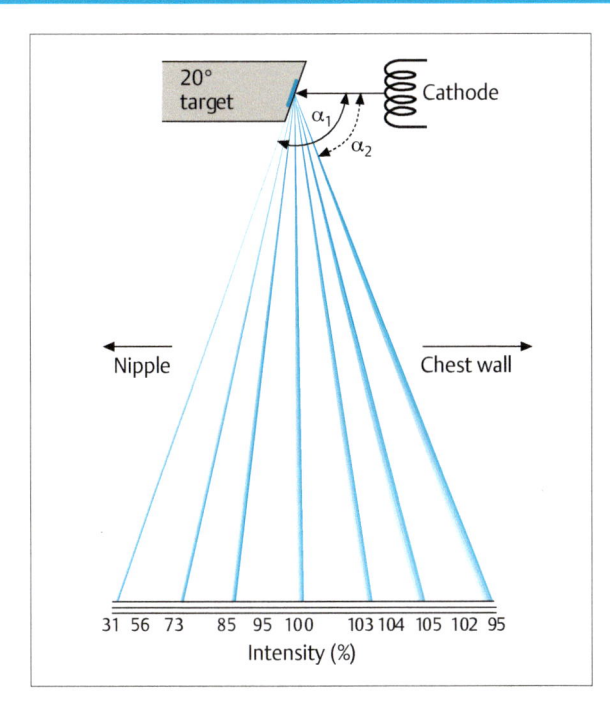

Fig. 3.4 Heel effect. The beam created at the target focus is weaker on the target side than on the cathode aside. The illustration shows the radiation intensity referred to the central ray (100%). The intensity varies depending on the angle of egress of the radiation from the target. This effect is used in mammography by locating the cathode closer to the chest wall than the anode. Thus the radiation intensity will be greater close to the chest wall and less near the nipple, where the breast is thinner.

of maximum radiation intensity lies near the chest wall. This is achieved by positioning the target opposite the cathode, which is closer to the chest wall. The intensity distribution of the radiation can be influenced by slightly angling (i.e., tipping) the X-ray tube. However, this alters the projection of the focal spot.

Scattered Radiation

In every radiograph of the breast, *scattered radiation* is produced in the tissue. More scattered radiation occurs in denser and thicker glandular tissue than in the thinner, fatty, transparent tissue. Increasing amounts of scattered radiation result in progressive loss of contrast.

Scatter Reduction: Grids

The grid is placed between the breast and the image receptor (screen–film system) to reduce undesired scattered radiation that impairs image quality.

Grids (see **Fig. 3.1**) consist of strips of lead that absorb obliquely oriented radiation, whereas radiation parallel to the lead strips passes through. The lead strips are focused on the focal spot.

During the exposure, the grid rapidly moves perpendicular to the path of the beam and to the orientation of the strips to prevent the strips from appearing on the mammogram as thin lines that mar the image. A variation on this design is the 'cellular' grid, which is composed of hexagonal cells. A more complex grid motion (with a minimum exposure time) is required to blur the grid structure with this design.

The efficiency of the grid depends on the height of the strips and the strip spacing. The ratio of strip height to strip spacing is known as the grid ratio. The larger the grid ratio, the greater the efficiency of the grid, but also the greater the required radiation dose. For this reason, only grid ratios of 4:27 or 5:30 are recommended for mammography (Kimme-Smith et al. 1992).

Since the grid absorbs both scattered radiation and a small proportion of useful radiation, a longer exposure time and, therefore, an increased radiation dose is required if the optical density on the film is to be maintained. Exposures with a grid require a *grid exposure factor* of approximately 2.5. The use of more sensitive screen–film systems has compensated for this increased dose, compared with earlier gridless mammographic techniques. Digital receptors are more flexible in what receptor dose they can operate with, but an increased patient dose is still required when using a grid. This is dictated by the signal-to-noise ratio needed in the image rather than the sensitivity of the receptor.

The significant *increase in image quality fully* justifies the increased radiation dose required by the grid, and *grid mammography* has superseded gridless mammography.

Gridless mammography can be performed without significant loss of quality only in very small, compressed, and fatty breasts in the interest of reducing radiation exposure, or in magnification mammography where the "air gap" between the breast and image receptor acts to reduce the amount of scattered radiation detected.

Scatter Reduction: Compression

The second important method of *reducing scattered radiation* consists of sufficient *compression of the breast*. By reducing breast thickness, compression reduces the proportion of scattered radiation, thus reducing the dose and improving the image contrast (Barnes and Brezovich 1979, Kimme-Smith et al. 1992).

Other options for reducing scattered radiation include the air-gap technique. The air gap, which is effective only in conjunction with good collimation, is used for scatter reduction in magnification mammography. Slot mammography represents another effective method of scatter reduction (see p. 47).

Image Receptor System

After passing through the breast and the grid, the imaging radiation reaches the *image receptor system*. In modern screen–film mammography, this system consists of either a *single intensifying screen* with luminescent coating and

3 Mammography

a *special single-emulsion film* (**Fig. 3.5a**) or, increasingly, one of several designs of digital receptor. Both of these types of receptor will be described in detail.

Screen–Film Systems

The film emulsion and the coated side of the screen face each other. To obtain a sharp focus, the two must be in direct contact. Insufficient screen–film contact will cause significant local blurring.

Screen–film systems with dual-emulsion mammographic films should not be used because the light photons, which are emitted from the film emulsion facing away from the screen, cause additional blurring (crossover effect). Since the low-energy X-ray photons used in mammography would furthermore be significantly attenuated in a front screen, a single screen that lies behind the film (back screen) is used. This geometry also maximizes image definition (**Fig. 3.5b,c**). Because the film emulsion lies in front of the screen, and the mean X-ray photon energy is low, a significant contribution to film blackening (~15%) is made by direct absorption of X-rays in the film emulsion.

Every quantum of radiation absorbed in the luminescent layer of the screen excites the phosphorus, causing it to emit several quanta of light. The resulting intensifying effect of the screen depends on the intensifying substance, the density of the luminescent layer, the distribution of the coating, and the screen dye. All the currently available intensifying screens contain gadolinium oxysulfide as an intensifying substance.

While greater screen thickness and coarse crystal structures increase the intensifying effect of the screen, they also decrease the resolution. In addition to this, high intensification is accompanied by a significant increase in image noise (owing to the lower number of X-ray photons that are needed). Thus to achieve the resolution required in mammography, only very high-definition intensifying screens (speed class 12) should be used.

While the *sharpness* of a screen–film system is determined primarily *by the screen,* the *contrast* of the system is determined *by the film* and by the processing. Since the differences between the currently available high-resolution screens of the same class are slight, the sensitivity of a screen–film system and thus the required dose are then influenced by the choice of film.

The contrast behavior of a mammographic film is shown in its *characteristic curve.* The characteristic curve shows the relationship between film density and the dose of radiation incident on the film. Optical density (blackening) is plotted against the logarithm of the radiation dose (**Fig. 3.6**).

The steeper the curve, the higher is the contrast. The contrast is decisive not only in the medium-density range. In dense breasts or dense areas of the breast, the contrast (and thus visualization) in the lower-density range (0.5–1.5) is even more important.

For diagnostic purposes, uniformly high contrast in every density range would be desirable. Since the film curves flatten out significantly below an optical density of 0.6 and the human eye cannot distinguish differences at densities exceeding 2.2 (2.8–3.0 maximum in bright light), *the useful range of every film is limited to optical densities between 0.6 and 2.2–2.8.*

The exposure range (x-axis of **Fig. 3.6**) in which density differences can be visualized with good contrast, i.e., the useful optical density range (y-axis in **Fig. 3.6**), is known as the *imageable object range or latitude.*

If the film contrast is too high, the latitude will be too narrow. This means that the imageable object range will not include areas of very high or of very low density in the breast, and these areas can no longer be visualized in the useful density range. Density differences in these relatively *overexposed or underexposed areas* will no longer be adequately visualized (despite or because of the particularly high contrast in areas of medium density). Such overexposed or underexposed areas can appear particularly in large or dense breasts since their differences in absorption are especially high. To minimize these problems, the resulting contrast must be carefully optimized but should not be too high.

The contrast of screen–film mammography is essentially determined by the choice of film, the quality of radiation (exposure voltage, target and filter), and the film processing.

Exposure

After selecting the proper screen–film system and after adapting the radiation quality to the thickness and density of the breast, the film must be exposed in such a manner that all details relevant to the diagnosis are visualized in the optimum optical density range. This means that the mean optical density should lie approximately in the middle of the useful optical density range. (A systematic evaluation has shown a higher mean density preferable to the mean density of 1.2–1.6 mentioned in previous medical guidelines [Young et al. 1997].) The practice in European screening programs is now to set a target mean optical density in the range 1.5–1.9.

Film density ranges below 0.6 and above 2.2 (or 2.8 in bright light) permit only limited visualization at best.

The *exposure* is the *product of tube current (mA) and exposure time (second),* expressed as the milliampere-second product, or mAs product. One method of adjusting the exposure is by selecting the settings manually, that is, all exposure parameters can be freely selected. However, this requires a fair amount of experience because the exposure varies with both breast thickness and breast density.

Even experienced radiologists and radiologic technologists will use *automatic exposure control systems* to minimize the chance of incorrect exposure. The purpose of an automatic exposure control system (a required feature

Mammographic Technique

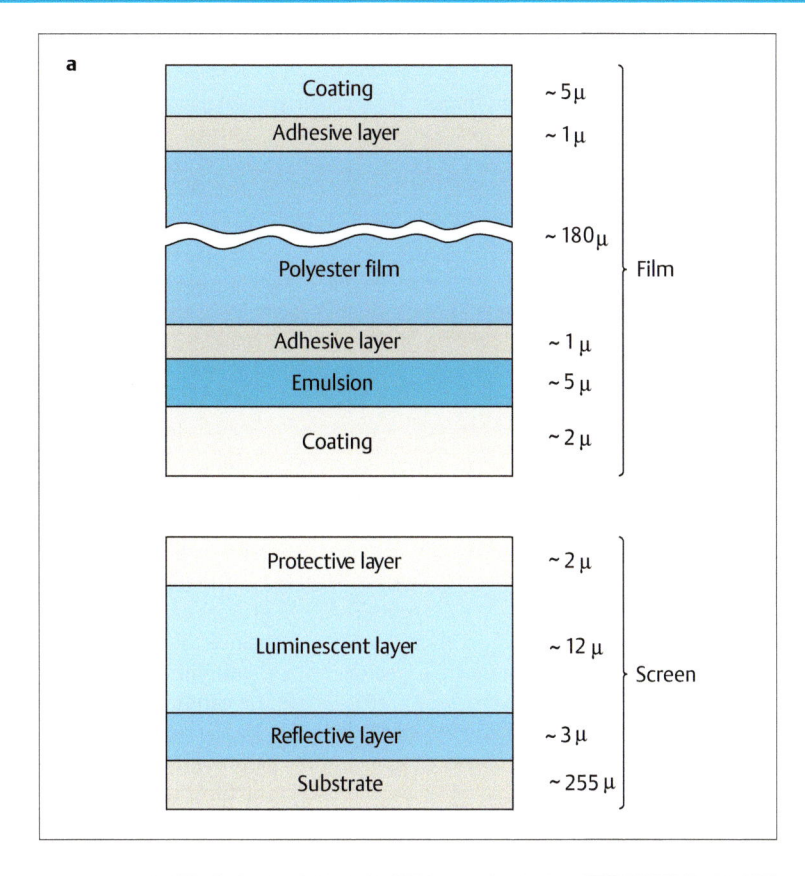

Fig. 3.5a–c Influence of the arrangement of film and intensifying screen on image sharpness.

a Mammography film and screen.
b The photons released from the luminescence centers of the intensifying screen are nondirectional in contrast to X-ray beams. For this reason, the diameter of the dense spot will increase with the distance between the film emulsion and the screen. This is illustrated by the diagram of a dual-emulsion film with a screen behind the film. Because of this phenomenon, only single-emulsion films are used in mammography.
c Owing to absorption of the X-ray beam within the intensifying screen, the majority of luminescence centers contributing to the image will be on that side of the screen, where the X-ray beam enters the screen. If a front screen were used, the majority of luminescence centers would be farther away from the film than if a back screen (behind the film) were used. Therefore, a front screen produces more blurring than a back screen. For this reason, only single-emulsion films with a back screen are used in mammography.

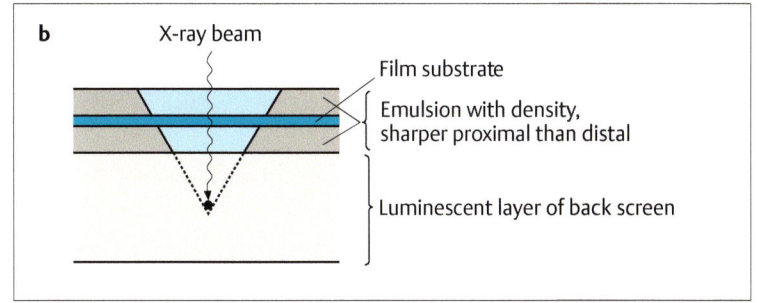

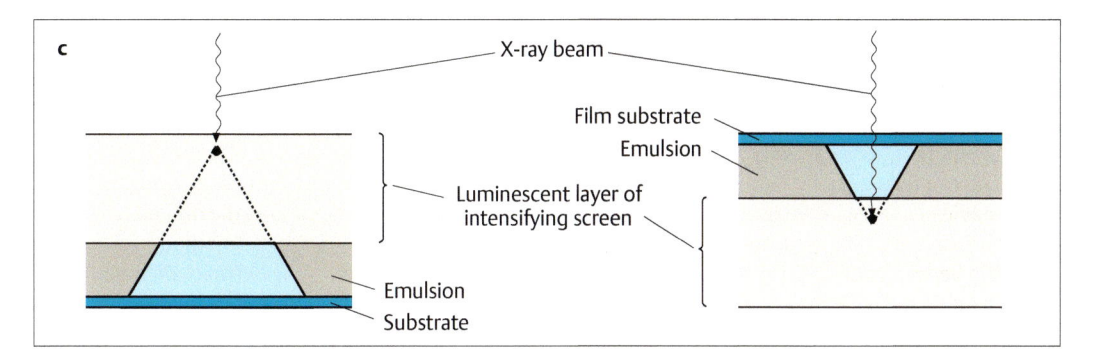

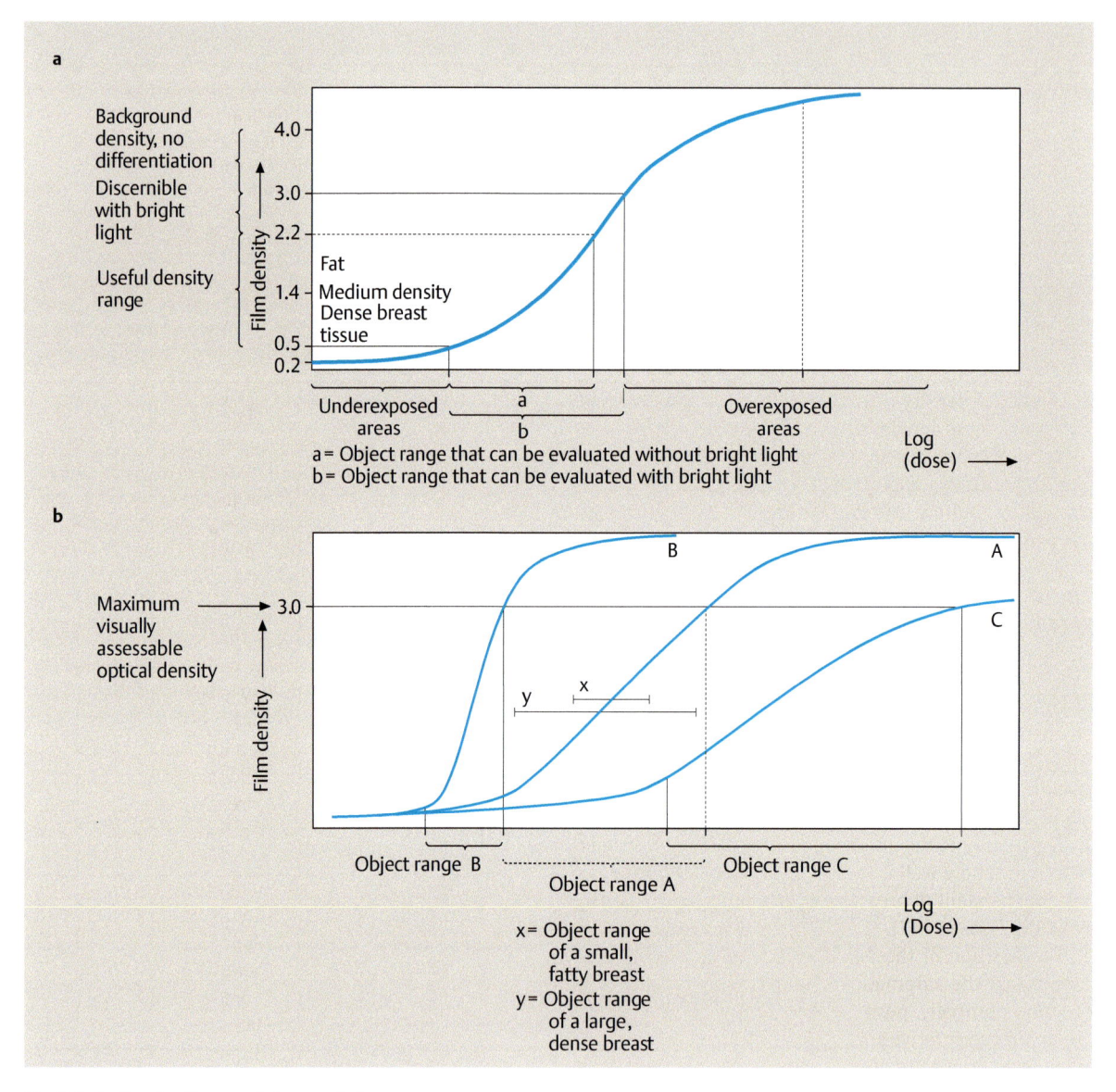

Fig. 3.6a,b The significance of characteristic curves.
a Principal curve.
b Exaggerated gradation curves of different films:
Film A shows a wide object range within which details are visualized with good contrast and can be easily discerned.
Film B is more sensitive (left shifted) and images the details in the center section of the curve with greater contrast. However, its object range is narrower so that details beyond this range are visualized with poor contrast (underexposed or overexposed).
Film C requires a high dose yet images a narrower density range. In spite of this, it visualizes a wide object range with uniform albeit relatively low contrast.
Imaging a small breast requires a narrower object range than imaging a large, dense breast.
The mean exposure (center of the object range of the breast to be imaged) is adapted to the sensitivity of the screen–film system by selecting a higher or lower mAs product (right or left shift in the object range of the breast to be imaged). Changing the mAs product will not influence the width of the object range. This means that a small breast can be imaged with all three films. At optimum exposure settings, film B will produce the highest-contrast image. This image will be perceived as the sharpest, although there is no objective difference in the definition of films A, B, or C.

Film B cannot adequately image a dense breast. The object range of this film is narrower than that required for imaging dense breasts, and overexposed and underexposed areas will result. For this reason, film B should not be used although it produces better images of small breasts. Film A is the optimal film since it can image both large, dense breasts and small breasts with good contrast. Here, precise exposure settings are essential to avoid overexposed or underexposed areas since its object range is only slightly larger than a large, dense breast requires. Film C can image both small breasts and large, dense breasts in an acceptable range, albeit with slightly less contrast. This film should be considered if achieving precise exposure is a problem (as can occur with older automatic exposure control systems with insufficient density compensation). Experience has shown that both microcalcifications and structures relevant to the diagnosis can be discerned, although they are less obvious.

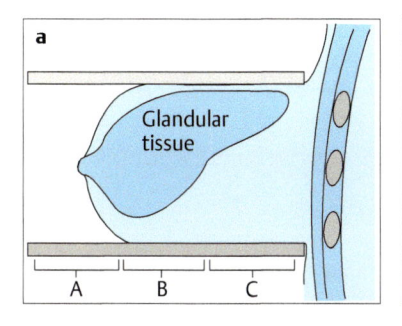

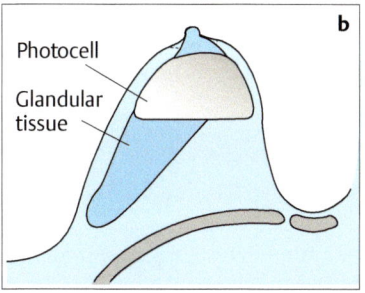

Fig. 3.7a,b Positioning the photocell.
a Lateral view of the compressed breast.
Position A is poor (beam must pass through too much air).
Position B is optimal.
Position C is poor (beam must pass through too much fat).
b View of breast from above showing optimal photocell position.

on every mammography unit) is to ensure a reproducible mean optical density of 1.2–1.6 on the film regardless of breast thickness and density.

The automatic exposure control system (see **Figs. 3.1 and 3.7**) utilizes a *photocell* placed beneath the cassette containing the film and screen. The chamber measures the dose behind the image receptor in a representative area. When the *cutoff dose* for the selected mean optical film density is reached (this depends on the screen–film system used), the system *switches off the exposure.*

Since the sensitivity of the photocell varies with different radiation energies (which result from beam hardening behind breasts of different thickness or density and behind the image receptor), the automatic exposure control system must compensate for the variable breast thickness and density when determining the optimum cutoff dose.

The quality of the automatic exposure control system determines how well it can achieve a constant film density independent of breast thickness and density (Young et al. 1997) (see p. 47).

The position of the photocell has to be adjusted. To ensure that the automatic exposure control system will function optimally, position the *photocell* so that it lies *under a representative part of the glandular tissue (which is in the anterior third of the breast)*. The correct position of the photocell will depend on the size of the breast. Incorrect positioning of the photocell will result in incorrect exposure. Problems may occur with very small breasts that cannot cover the photocell or with silicon implants (see p. 47).

Film Processing

Since deviations in chemical composition or developing time and temperature can cause problems with image contrast, noise, sensitivity, and fog, *it is essential to process the film strictly according to the manufacturer's recommendations and regularly monitor processing* (see pp. 49 and 52). Carefully controlled film processing becomes all the more important when it is understood that most acute changes in image quality are caused by deviations in film processing (Yaffe 1990).

Viewing the Image

Proper evaluation of the complete density range of a well-exposed mammogram requires a viewbox that *provides* homogeneous illumination at the required intensity. Viewboxes must provide adjustable luminance in the range of 2,000–3,000 cd/m^2 at a color temperature of 4,500–6,500 K. An additional bright spotlight must be available for illuminating areas of high exposure. This light should provide luminance up to 20,000 cd/m^2. Focused illumination of images that cover a wide density range with bright light will make details in highly dense areas appear more readily visible. However, this is only possible up to an optical density of 2.8. Focused illumination provides important additional information, although this is always limited and is usually not able to compensate for incorrect exposure, an excessively high-contrast film, or excessively high contrast due to errors in processing the film.

All viewing areas for mammography, including the work area for technologists, should be furnished with identical illumination. All light bulbs should be changed routinely throughout these viewing areas and the viewboxes cleaned weekly. The films are to be read in a darkened room with masking of the viewbox to the size of the film, when possible. These techniques minimize ambient light, and resulting structured and unstructured reflections (Robson 2008), and thereby increase contrast when viewing the films. A *magnifying lens* with magnification by at least a factor of 2 should be available for evaluating the mammogram.

Digital Mammographic Receptors

Digital mammography has until recently lagged behind the widespread move to digital imaging which has transformed the rest of radiology, owing to the demanding specification of an imaging modality that must deliver high spatial resolution for imaging microcalcifications and fine soft tissue strands (requiring a pixel size of around 0.05–0.1 mm), low image noise for imaging subtle differences between glandular and adipose tissues, and all of this at the low radiation dose required especially in breast cancer screening. Digital technology was first introduced into mammography as "small-field digital mammography" for needle and core biopsy guidance using detectors between about 5 × 5 cm and 5 × 9 cm in size. Full-field digital mammography, with detector sizes up to the equivalent of the 24 × 30 cm film cassette size, developed later, but proof was needed that the performance was adequate to replace the fully mature technology of screen–film.

Early trials in Colorado indicated no significant difference in cancer detection between digital and screen–film mammography (Lewin et al. 2001, 2002), and similar results were obtained in two Swedish trials based in Oslo (Skaane et al. 2003, Skaane and Skjennald 2004). The large Digital Mammographic Imaging Screening (DMIST trial), performed on 49,500 women across the United States and Canada, showed that the diagnostic performance of full-field digital mammography in terms of screening accuracy is very similar to that of the screen–film mammography that it is intended to replace, and that digital mammography has a significantly better diagnostic accuracy in women aged under 50 years and in those with relatively glandular breasts. These trial findings taken together have encouraged national breast-screening programs to move toward digital mammography (Pisano et al. 2005, Skaane 2009, Vinnicombe et al. 2009).

The imaging advantages of digital mammography include a wide dynamic range and the separation of the image capture and image display functions (a film combines both), so that the image display can be varied to optimally show the full range of recorded X-ray intensities. This provides good visualization of the skin line and nipple, and has advantages when imaging dense breasts and younger women. In the United Kingdom, for example, breast screening using digital mammography was targeted at younger women first. At the time of writing, the move from screen–film to digital mammography is rapid and worldwide. The market for mammographic film is shrinking quickly and this seems likely to further drive the move to digital mammography.

General Features of Digital Mammographic Images

A digital image is not a continuous distribution of bright and dark, but is composed of a finite number of points (or "pixels"), where each pixel has a value of brightness dictated by a stored numerical value. Digital images have the advantages that they can be enhanced and manipulated by computer to extract the maximum amount of diagnostic information, and that they can be stored, transferred, copied without detriment, and retrieved in a very efficient manner using computer mass data storage techniques. They have the disadvantage of a limit to spatial resolution caused by the pixel size. Unlike the sigmoid characteristic curve that defines the contrast and latitude of screen–film mammography (**Fig. 3.6**), digital mammography receptors usually have a linear response between pixel value and the radiation dose incident on the pixel over a very wide dynamic range, typically a factor of some 10,000 : 1. The choice of what patient dose is required for digital mammography is therefore driven by the signal-to-noise ratio required for a diagnostic image rather than being dictated by the limited exposure latitude of the screen–film receptor.

Image Capture Technologies

A range of competing image-capture technologies for digital mammography is available, and the choice of technology depends to some extent on the imaging task, be it screening or symptomatic, and the size and format of the hospital or clinic environment in which it will be operated. The range of technologies described below fits the state of the market at the time of writing, but this is an area where progress is still rapid.

All of the imaging considerations regarding the use of anti-scatter grids, breast compression, and positioning apply equally to digital as to screen–film mammography. The design and performance of the associated X-ray tubes is also generally similar, but higher-energy target/filter combinations such as rhodium–rhodium and tungsten–rhodium are more commonly employed, as well as higher tube voltages in the range 30–35 kVp.

The Direct Digital Detector—Amorphous Selenium

In direct conversion detectors the X-ray interaction is converted directly to an electrical signal using an amorphous selenium (a-Se) layer, behind which lies an amorphous silicon micro-circuit layer, which in turn is supported by a rigid substrate (**Fig. 3.8a**). Selenium is a photoconductor, so is an electrical insulator in the dark, and a conductor when exposed to light or X-rays. The amorphous selenium is employed as a mammographic image receptor in the form of a thin layer (0.5 mm) with a voltage applied between a large-area electrode across the front surface, and an array of charge collection electrodes, one per pixel, on the back surface. These are linked to capacitors to accumulate the charge released during the exposure. These are linked in turn to thin-film transistor switches to provide a line-by-line read-out arrangement in which the charge stored for an individual pixel is passed pixel by pixel along the line until it can be measured by electronics external to the imaging sensor. Incoming X-ray photons interact photoelectrically in the a-Se layer, producing electrons and "holes" (the vacancy where an electron should be). Because of the high-voltage gradient across the thin a-Se layer, the electrons move toward the positive surface electrode and the holes toward the negative charge collection electrodes. The electrons and holes do not move sideways as they have to follow the direction of the electric field gradient, so image blurring from this source is minimal and the spatial resolution of the detector is good. At the end of the exposure, the charge signals (proportional to the radiation detected) from each pixel are read out via the thin-film transistor switches and data lines. The charge signals are converted to digital values via charge amplifiers and a digital-to-analog converter, and sent to the computer for assembly into an image.

The a-Se layer has good photon capture characteristics in the mammographic energy range, and the lack of sideways spread of the electrons and holes carrying the image information allows the a-Se layer to be made relatively thick, resulting in an efficient detector. As the receptor is mounted rigidly in the breast support table of the mammography unit, it is always in the same position with respect to the X-ray beam, allowing the use of "flat-fielding." This is an important image calibration in which the receptor is exposed to the unattenuated X-ray beam under test conditions, so that variation in the X-ray intensity across the field and variations in pixel-to-pixel sensitivity can be removed from subsequent images. The removal of these fixed noise sources further improves the efficiency of the receptor.

The Indirect Digital Detector—Scintillator and Amorphous Silicon

This type of receptor is similar to that commonly employed in digital radiography, and consists of a thin crystalline scintillator layer closely coupled to an amorphous silicon micro-circuit layer which is supported by a rigid substrate (**Fig. 3.8b**). Indirect conversion detectors work by first converting the incident X-ray distribution into a light image, then converting the light distribution into electrical signals addressable to a pixel location on the detector. The most successful scintillator is thallium-activated cesium iodide. This has excellent X-ray absorption characteristics and can be grown in a channeled crystal structure that acts like a fiberoptic guide to prevent light spreading sideways, and this gives the detector improved spatial resolution. It is similar to the input phosphor material of X-ray image intensifiers (**Fig. 3.8c**). The scintillator layer is deposited onto an amorphous silicon micro-circuit array of light-sensitive photodiodes and associated electronics to measure the signal from each photodiode. After the X-ray exposure is completed,

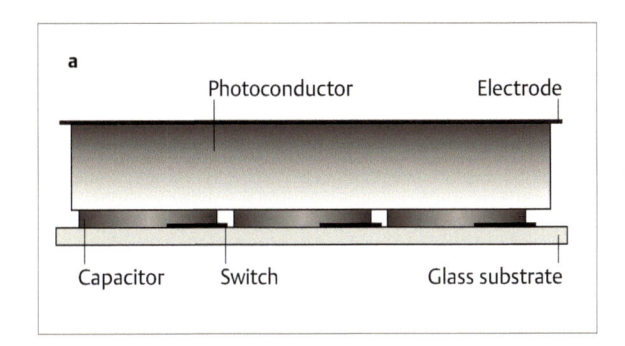

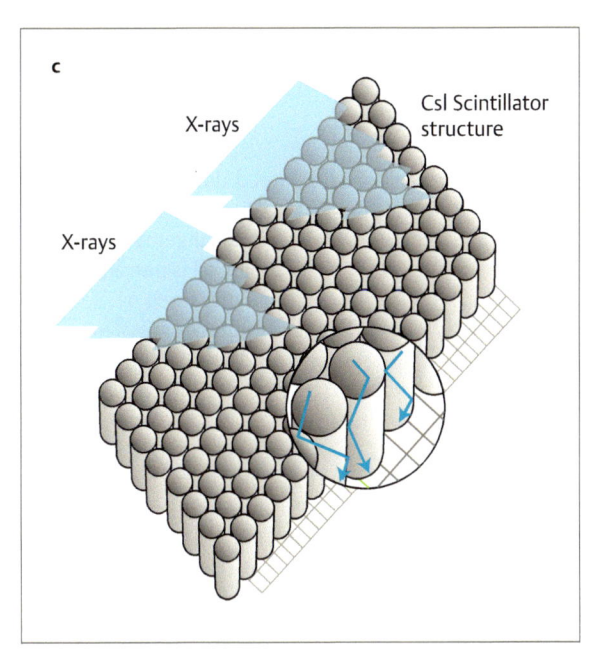

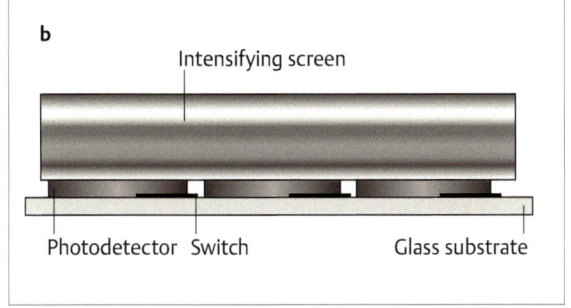

Fig. 3.8a–f

a Cross-section through a direct digital mammography image receptor. The photoconductor is a layer of amorphous selenium that allows electrons to flow across it when exposed to X-ray photons. The capacitor builds up a charge, proportional to the X-ray exposure for that pixel. The charge is transferred out of the device via the switch at the end of the exposure and converted to a numerical pixel value.
b Cross-section through an indirect digital mammography receptor. The intensifying screen (scintillator) produces light when exposed to X-ray photons. The photodetector measures the amount of light for that pixel and stores the signal as a charge. The charge is transferred out of the device via the switch at the end of the exposure and converted to a numerical pixel value.
c Much magnified view of a cesium iodide scintillator layer. The CsI crystals grow in columns which prevent light spreading sideways even though the scintillator layer is relatively thick.

Fig. 3.8 d–f ▷

d X-ray exposure / Erasure

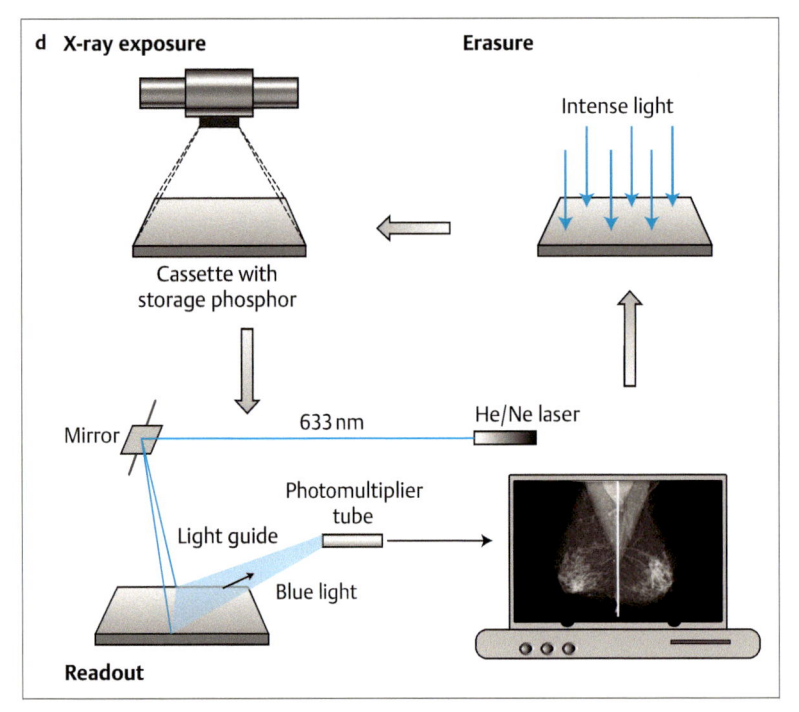

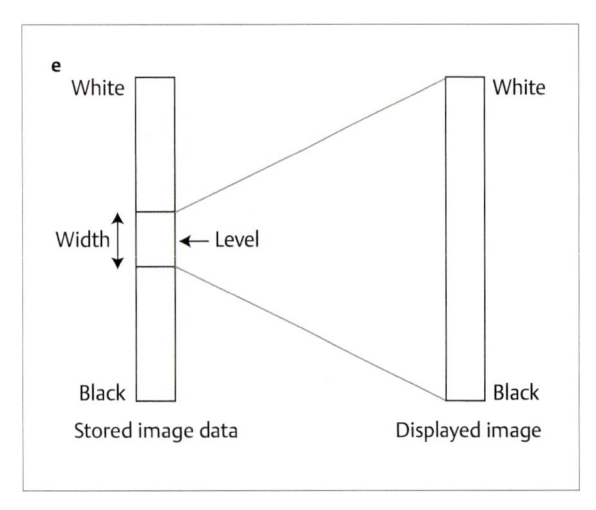

(Figure 3.8d: Diagram showing cassette with storage phosphor, He/Ne laser at 633 nm, mirror, light guide, photomultiplier tube detecting blue light, and erasure by intense light)

e Image display windowing diagram: Stored image data (White to Black) mapped via Width and Level to Displayed image (White to Black).

◁ continued

d The cycle of mammographic image production using computed radiography. The image plate is initially erased, exposed in a conventional mammography unit, then read out by a scanning laser beam that stimulates the plate to produce light proportional to the X-ray exposure at that point. The small light signal is amplified by the photomultiplier and converted to a pixel value. The plate is re-used.

e Image display windowing. The stored image data may consist of 4,000 or more shades of gray, but the image display black to white range is only 256 shades of gray (which is still more than the observer can perceive). To make all of the contrast recorded observable, a subset of the stored brightness range can be displayed, and varied to the observer's requirements by altering the window level and width.

f Example of image display windowing. Image **f2** is the same as image **f1**, but windowed to show contrast within the implant that could not be assessed on **f1**.

a switching array of thin-film transistors and associated data lines allow the signals from the photodiodes to be fed out of the receptor array in sequence. These signals are then digitized and transferred to the computer to be assembled into an image.

This type of receptor is also mounted rigidly in the breast support table of the mammography unit, so the important flat-fielding correction described above can also be used, with the same removal of fixed pattern noise and resulting efficiency improvement.

Computed Radiography

Computed radiography (CR) is based on the phenomenon of photo-stimulable luminescence (**Fig. 3.8d**). When X-rays are incident on a material such as europium-doped barium fluorohalide, they produce high-energy photoelectrons, which in turn produce ionization that results in a large number of lower-energy electron–hole pairs. In conventional screen–film mammography this happens in a screen in close contact with the film where the electron–hole pairs recombine to emit light that then exposes the film. In photo-stimulable luminescence, however, less than 50% of the electron–hole pairs recombine; the others are trapped apart owing to the presence of the doped sites in the phosphor. These electron traps are crystal lattice defects where halogen ion vacancies occur in the otherwise regular ionic lattice. These so-called "F" or "Color" centers are created during manufacture by prolonged irradiation of the imaging plate with high-intensity X-rays and ultraviolet light. Following exposure, electrons can remain trapped at these defects for many hours or days, although the stored image gradually fades with time. The concentration of trapped electrons is proportional to the locally incident X-ray exposure. The electrons are trapped in this state until they are stimulated by light of a suitable wavelength in a CR plate reader, whereupon they are free to travel to the holes, recombine, and emit light. The emitted light, which is linearly proportional to the locally incident X-ray intensity over four decades (i.e., 10,000 : 1), is then detected by a photomultiplier and digitized to form an image.

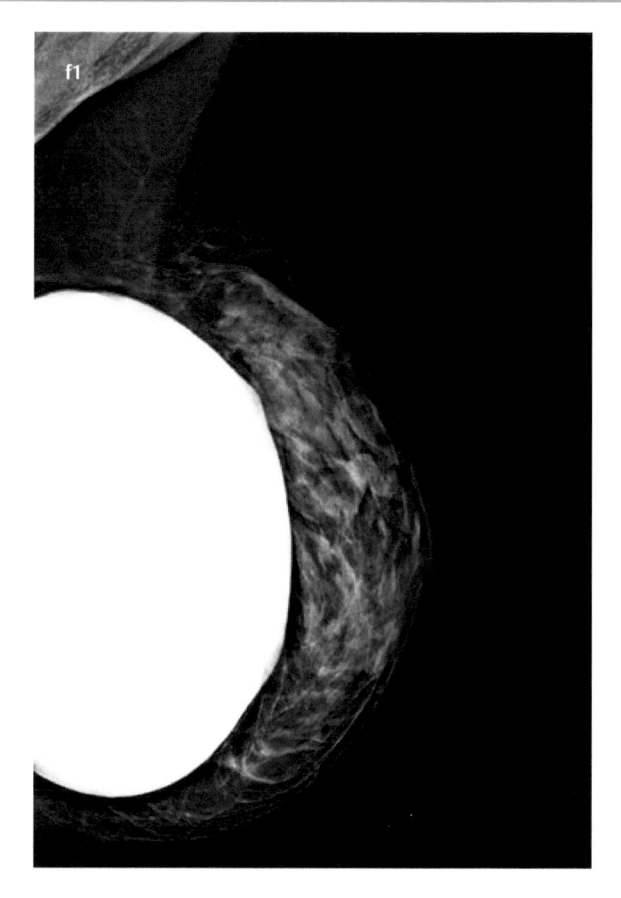

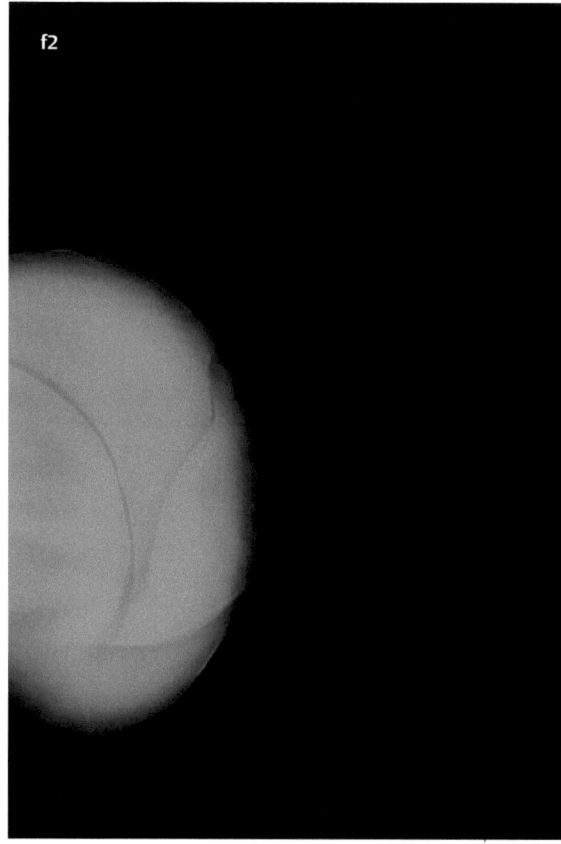

The CR cassette housing the image plate looks much like a screen–film cassette and can be used in substantially the same way. The read-out is performed in a plate reader, which works by scanning an intense laser beam across the image plate on a line-by-line basis while the plate is slowly drawn through. A red laser is used to add enough energy to get the trapped electrons out of their traps and into the conduction band of the material. They can then move and recombine with a positive ion, dropping back to the ground energy state and in doing so emit their excess energy as a photon of blue light. This weak light signal is picked up by a light guide and sent via a blue filter (to keep out the red light of the stimulating laser) to a photomultiplier tube that measures the amount of light. This signal is then digitized to produce the raw "pixel value" associated with that particular location on the image plate.

The scanning laser is focused to a diameter of approximately 0.1 mm to define the pixel of the image (although note that the imaging plate is continuous and not divided into physical pixels). Following read-out, the image plate is exposed to high-intensity light to completely erase any traces of the previous image, then reloaded into the cassette and ejected from the reader ready for reuse.

Because the CR cassette is not mounted rigidly in position, and several cassettes will normally be used in rotation, it is not possible to apply flat-fielding corrections in CR mammography, and the efficiency of the detector is reduced by the fixed pattern noise in the image arising from non-uniformity of the crystalline photo-stimulable phosphor. There is also an element of light spread in the phosphor from the read-out laser that leads to some blurring. New developments in 'needle plate' (cesium bromide) phosphors which have a channeled crystalline structure similar to that of cesium iodide (above) promise to improve the efficiency of CR mammography provided these delicate phosphors can be made robust enough for routine use.

Scanned Slit Linear Detectors

A quite different type of digital mammography unit that is increasing its share of the market is that employing a scanning fan beam of X-rays coupled to a moving one-dimensional detector. This geometry is attractive in terms of its ability to reject scattered photons using a slit collimator at the detector, so no anti-scatter grid is required. Also the one-dimensional detector can be made relatively complex and its signal transfer to the external electronics more direct than with a thin-film two-dimensional array. One commercial design employs a photon-counting detector based on those used in high-energy experimental physics. Using this approach, individual photons are counted in each pixel of the image and the pixel brightness is dictated by the total photons counted during the time the X-ray beam was swept over the pixel position. This has the advantage that low-level fluctuations caused by thermal excitation in the amplifiers and electronics can be rejected, leaving only the higher-energy photon counts, so a source of image noise can be negated. The motorized movements of the scanning beam are complex, the X-ray tube loading tends to be high, and the scan time is generally longer than the exposure time for a two-dimensional receptor, but the overall performance of this technology is directly competitive with the more common amorphous selenium detectors.

Charge-Coupled Devices

Charge-coupled devices (CCDs) are rarely used in full-field digital mammography owing to the size limitations on the image receptor array, which is fabricated on a conventional silicon wafer. These are, however, common in devices designed for "small field mammography" where the application is primarily to provide image guidance for biopsy procedures. A layer of scintillator, such as cesium iodide, is directly coupled to the light-sensing CCD array in the small field device. Designs giving larger field sizes by coupling a larger area scintillator layer to the CCD using fiberoptic bundles or systems of mirrors and lenses have been produced, but the efficiency is generally reduced by light losses in these coupling systems.

Image Presentation and Processing

Display Monitors

With a pixel size of 0.05–0.1 mm, and a typical field size for full-field digital mammography of 24 × 30 cm, a digital mammography image may well be composed of over 10 million pixels. Specialist medical-grade display monitors are required to provide an adequate display for primary reporting, and standards in the United States (ACR-AAPM-SIIM practice guideline 2007) and Europe (Perry et al. 2006) provide a basis for specification. Lower-specification displays may be used as "review" monitors in the mammography room for the technologist to confirm the quality of image acquisition, but these should not be used for primary reporting. Most digital mammography monitors are now LCD flat-panel displays, although some legacy equipment based on cathode ray tubes is also in use.

Although there can be some flexibility in the format of simultaneous image display, in general two high-resolution monitors in portrait orientation will be required for a reporting workstation, as usually two images need to be compared, but other monitors may be added to allow simultaneous comparison of prior screening mammograms. An additional low-resolution monitor may be required to display patient information, work lists, and other textual diagnostic reports.

It is not generally expected that the display monitor will be capable of displaying the full resolution of the recorded image as a complete frame, but that magnification, pan, and zoom within the image will be used to display all of the pixels when this is needed. Presently 5 megapixel monitors are recommended (2000 × 2500 pixels) (Perry et al. 2006, ACR-AAPM-SIIM practice guideline 2007), so that 50% or greater area of the breast image can be displayed at full resolution.

An important distinguishing feature of medical-grade displays is their maximum luminance. Ideally this should be 450 cd/m^2 or higher (much brighter than standard computer displays) so that a large ratio between maximum and minimum can be maintained, and susceptibility to the effects of ambient lighting is reduced. Careful consideration to the design of the viewing room is still required, however, as the brightness of the monitor itself will light up the room (as well as more obvious light sources such as open doors and windows) and structured reflections of room surroundings and indeed the observer superimposed on the viewed image will reduce its contrast and may introduce distracting features. With the monitor switched off, the ambient light in the room at the position of the observer should not be greater than 10 lux (Perry et al. 2006).

Display workstations would be expected to provide a user interface providing an efficient throughput of images and a range of display tools typically including:

- Magnification, zoom, and pan (roam)
- Contrast and brightness adjustment (windowing)
- Image flip and rotation
- Black/white inversion
- Spatial measurement
- Edge enhancement and noise reduction (spatial frequency filtering)

Some of these features are further explained below.

The DICOM Grayscale Display Function

DICOM (Digital Imaging and Communications in Medicine) is a medical image interchange standard that allows vendors to transmit images between their imaging systems and PACS (the picture archiving and communication system). One element to DICOM that is particularly important from the radiologic reporting standpoint is the Grayscale Standard Display Function (GSDF) (Samei and Badano 2005). This is based on a psychophysical model of the human visual system and is designed to maximize the number of "just noticeable differences" that a given display can reproduce, and to give a perceptually linear grayscale, with the same small change in contrast visible in a dark part of the image as in a light part. Usually the GSDF boosts the signal in the white, but it will be different for cathode ray tube flat screen displays and (if this is used) hardcopy film. If the GSDF is correctly implemented for a given monitor, it should give the best display which that monitor is capable of in the viewing conditions where it is used. The GSDF attempts to make the best of the display's capabilities but cannot make a cheap display in poor viewing conditions as good as an expensive megapixel grayscale monitor in good viewing conditions.

Windowing

Postprocessing of digital images by windowing is a very powerful feature of digital imaging that also applies to computed tomography (CT), MRI and radioisotope imaging (RI). Because in a digital image the brightness of a pixel is dictated by an integer number (the "pixel number"), there is a finite number of values that the brightness level can take. Digital mammography systems might typically digitize to 12 bits (4,096 gray levels), whereas the display monitor will probably only have a capability of displaying 256 levels of luminance (8 bits). In addition, the human visual system is only capable of distinguishing about 100 gray levels in an image, even under ideal viewing conditions, so it follows that if all the information present in a digital image were displayed on the monitor at once, small differences in contrast, although recorded successfully, would not be distinguishable. The solution to this problem is to display only a selected range of pixel values, thus increasing the displayed contrast for that subset of levels. This "window" of pixel number values is defined by a window "width" and window "level" (**Fig. 3.8e**). By altering the display window width and level settings, the observer can optimize the display of the range of gray levels for the diagnostic task being undertaken, and any contrast recorded in the image can be displayed (**Fig. 3.8f**), but the time taken to make many such adjustments could become a factor in reporting high volumes of images. The user interface for window width and level adjustment is usually quite intuitive, using computer mouse or trackball, and preset window preferences can also save time.

Spatial Frequency Filtering

Images can be thought of and analyzed as sets of spatial frequencies. In general, low spatial frequencies are associated with uniform grayness or slowly changing gradients, while high spatial frequencies are associated with sudden changes in brightness, such as at sharp edges or patterns of dots or lines. By applying a spatial frequency filter, ranges of spatial frequencies can be enhanced or attenuated. Enhancing high spatial frequencies enhances the contrast of sharp edges—for example, due to microcalcifications and linear structures—and generally "sharpens" the image. Unfortunately, high-frequency enhancement comes at the price of also boosting the noise that lies in this frequency band, so subtle enhancement is the most effective. Attenuating high frequencies effectively blurs the image, and this can be used to reduce the appearance of quantum noise in some situations. Various layers of image processing, including spatial frequency filtering, are routinely used in digital mammography. While this processing can make improvements to clinical images, it can also cause problems with quality assurance of phantom images, for which the image processing often has to be deselected.

Picture Archiving and Communications Systems (PACSs)

One driver for the development of digital mammography has been the goal of the filmless radiology department. Although the capital costs are high, the advantages are seen as lower running cost, flexible transmission, recovery and multiple viewing of images, multimodality reporting, and long-term image storage without degradation. Although this has been a target since the early 1980s, the cost and availability of the technology has made it feasible only relatively recently. Now the move toward filmless departments is rapid and seen as inevitable.

A PACS requires a hospital-wide network of high-speed optical fiber cables, many viewing monitors, at least one server computer but probably more than one, mass storage devices of various types (e.g., hard drives, RAID arrays, optical disk jukebox), and communications links to all modalities and to the outside world (other hospitals and regional "hubs" of mass storage, so-called data warehouses). System architectures vary, but there is often a split between the PACS database of images and the RIS (Radiologic Information System) of patient demographic information and reports. There may also be a PAS (Patient Administration System) running in parallel with these and there is the potential for problems with these databases becoming out of agreement on the records of individual patients. There are moves toward an Electronic Patient Record incorporating all patient data, but presently the separate systems from different vendors tend to coexist on any given site. The large image sizes associated with digital mammography and requirements of screening centers may make a PACS dedicated to mammography the preferred solution at some centers.

The transfer file format for communicating between different medical imaging devices and the PACS network is DICOM. This defines a set of recognized codes in the "header" of the image file that describes the images contained (e.g., picture height and width in pixels, modality: MRI, CT, US, CR, DR [digital radiography], MAMMO, image processing applied, last used window settings, etc.). There are hundreds of possible fields of information defined for the header and not all are used at present, but some (e.g., radiation dose) have potential for the future. For digital mammography, the initial image display will be on the display device of the mammography unit itself, after which images approved as being diagnostic by the operator will be annotated and "pushed" to PACS for reporting. Once there, they can be accessed from many locations and viewed using a PACS "browser" which will incorporate some search tools as well as image manipulation such as windowing, zoom, invert, etc. The image should be viewed via a DICOM GSDF display so that it looks the same wherever it is viewed.

Computer-Aided Diagnosis (CAD)

Computer-aided diagnosis (CAD) is well suited to digital mammography. The digital image can automatically be fed to an image-processing computer system programmed to identify areas possibly representing carcinoma for special attention by the interpreting radiologist. This technology functionally operates as a second reading of the mammogram.

To date, double reading with arbitration or consensus reading is the standard of care in most organized screening programs. Double reading of mammograms by radiologists has been shown to increase the detection rate for breast cancer by 3–14% with a mostly stable or slightly decreased recall rate compared with single reading (Dinnes et al. 2001, Taylor and Potts 2008, Houssami et al. 2009).

CAD is capable of detecting malignancy that was missed by a single reader (Gromet 2008, Karssemeijer et al. 2009, Noble et al. 2009). To date—even though considerable variation appears to exist between the studies—on average this gain of sensitivity appears to be smaller than that of double reading and it is achieved at the cost of a significantly increased recall rate (Taylor and Potts 2008, Houssami et al. 2009). Thus for screening programs with established double reading, further improvements appear necessary before double reading by CAD systems could become cost-effective. The major drawback of CAD remains the 1–1.5 hits per screening mammogram and their very low positive predictive value (Guerriero et al. 2011). Overall, however, computer-assisted detection remains a promising field.

Whereas most efforts have concentrated on mammography and will certainly be further improved with the rapidly increasing digital databases of benign and malignant changes, breast imaging/CAD using a multimodality approach and computer-aided diagnoses emerge as further fields of research.

Specific Requirements and Solutions

The ability to recognize structures on the mammogram is determined by:
- Resolution
- Image noise
- Contrast

These variables must be optimized using the lowest possible radiation dose.

The following sections will explain factors that influence these variables.

Image Sharpness

Image sharpness is determined by motion blur, geometric blurring, and the blurring of the image receptor system (**Table 3.1**).

Motion blurring is caused by patient motion and, less pronounced, by arterial pulsation. It can be minimized by:
- **Adequate compression**. This eliminates motion of the breast if the patient moves. Adequate compression will also suppress arterial pulsation.
- **Short exposure time**. This in turn depends on the X-ray tube rating, the size of the focal spot, the focus–film distance, the sensitivity of the image receptor, and density and thickness of the object (breast compression!)

As a general rule, exposure times should not exceed 1 second (some guidelines still specify 2 seconds).

Geometric blurring can be reduced by:
- Using a small focal spot
- Maintaining the largest possible focus–film distance
- Optimizing breast compression (see **Fig. 3.2**)

Breast compression not only reduces motion blur (see above), it also reduces geometric blurring of structures that are farther away from the image plane by reducing the distance to the image receptor. The minimum focal spot size and maximum focus–film distance are limited by the capacity of the X-ray tube, the resulting extended exposure times, and the motion blurring that can occur.

When using a standard technique, according to the ACR standard, 30 the focus–film distance *should not be less than 55 cm* for a focal spot size of 0.4. For magnifica-

Table 3.1 Minimizing blurring

Goal	Recommendation	Limiting factors
Motion blurring	Short exposure time	Power
	Intense compression	Patient's pain tolerance
Geometric blurring	Long SID[a,c]	Focus load rating, power
	Small focus	
	Intense compression (to reduce distance to objects farther from the film)	Patient's pain tolerance
Screen–film blurring	High-resolution screen,[b] sufficient dose (quantum noise), single-emulsion film	High radiation dose
	Good contact between film and screen	Exposure time

[a] SID, source–image receptor distance.
[b] Rarely relevant.
[c] Film granularity is not relevant because the screen blurring is always more important.

tion imaging, the distance should be ≥ 60 cm. In magnification mammography, smaller focal spot sizes (0.1–0.15, depending on the power of magnification) are required to minimize the penumbra.

The resolution of the screen–film system is primarily determined by the resolution of the intensifying screen, since film resolution is always higher than that of the screen. With very low-dose screen–film systems, the increased image noise that occurs can reduce the clarity of details (**Fig. 3.9**).

Differences between screens are almost always due to differing densities of the luminescent layer and the dye used for selective filtering of components of the green spectrum. Thinner, more finely structured screens almost always produce *higher resolution* but are less sensitive, that is, they require a *higher dose*.

Since the loss of definition resulting from the cross-over effect is not acceptable for standard mammographic technique, only single-emulsion films with a back screen are used.

To minimize loss of definition due *to insufficient screen–film contact* as the imaging radiation passes from the screen to the film, always wait at least 2 minutes after loading the cassette before performing mammography. Always ensure that a sufficient number of cassettes is available.

Most screen–film systems achieve a high-contrast resolution of 14–18 *line pairs per millimeter* (LP/mm), which can be verified using a lead line grid. This value matches the high-contrast resolution that mammography units achieve by adjusting focal spot size, focus–film distance, and object–film distance.

However, the clarity of detail of microcalcifications is determined only in part by the spatial resolution. When present in areas of dense breast tissue, microcalcifications may show only very slight differences in density. Therefore, whether they can be detected is highly dependent on contrast and image noise. The clarity of details as a function of their size is expressed by the modulation transfer function (MTF) (see **Fig. 3.10**). This means that for a given image receptor system, large objects will appear with high contrast, whereas fine objects will be imaged with low contrast and will thus have poor resolution. Thus, despite its capability for a high-contrast resolution of 14–18 line pairs, an optimum technical system will be limited to detecting microcalcifications measuring *0.1–0.2 mm* or larger (corresponding to 10 or 5 LP/mm).

The high-contrast resolution of digital mammographic receptors is primarily limited by the pixel size and pitch (the distance between pixel centers), so that there is a limit (the Nyquist limit) beyond which rapid spatial variations cannot be reproduced. In terms of high-contrast line-pairs patterns, this can be thought of as the limit where one pixel is black (corresponding to a lead bar the same width as the pixel) and the adjacent one is white (corresponding to the space between the bars). A line-pairs pattern of N LP/mm will therefore require $2N$ pixels/mm to display it, and higher line frequencies than this not only will not be reproduced, but will degrade the image by introducing lower-frequency artifacts by "aliasing." Digital receptors generally give a lower high-contrast resolution in terms of LP/mm than do screen–film systems, but the MTF in the 5 cycles/mm range is comparable, and this is thought to be the more relevant performance measure when the imaging task is that of detecting microcalcifications or fine soft-tissue strands.

Contrast

Contrast can be defined as the relative difference in optical density or digital pixel value between an object and its surroundings referred to the surrounding density:

$$\text{Contrast} = \frac{\text{Density}_{obj.} - \text{Density}_{surroundings}}{\text{Density}_{surroundings}} \times 100$$

3 Mammography

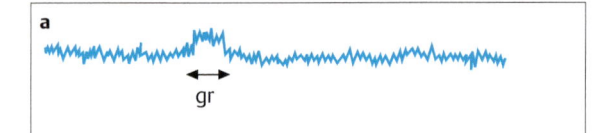

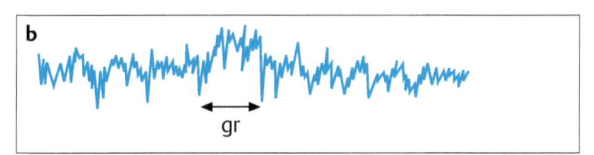

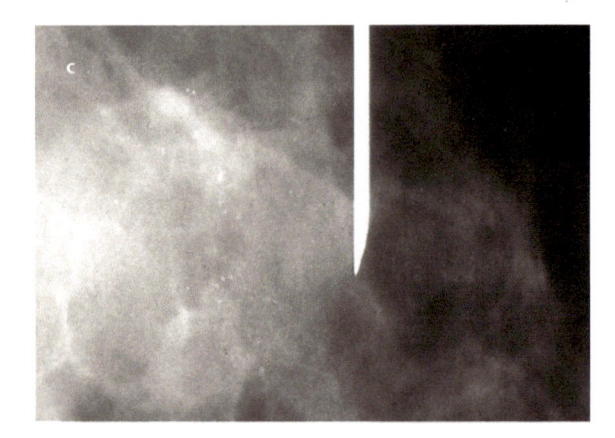

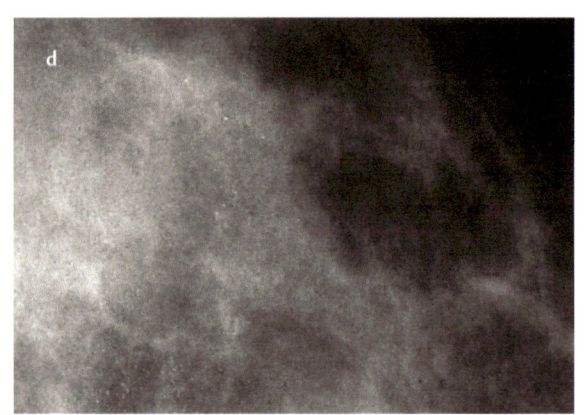

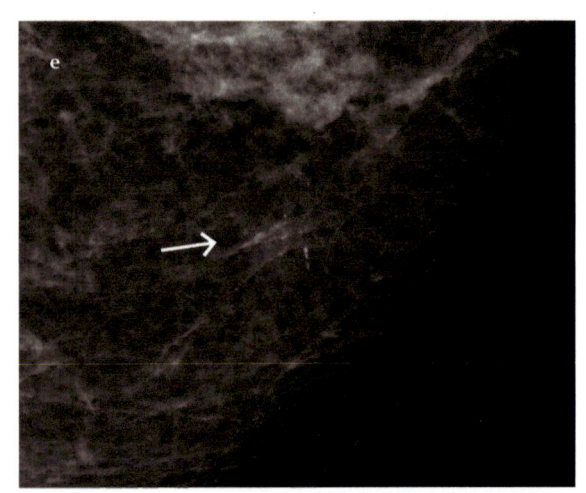

Fig. 3.9a–f Noise can interfere with the clarity of detail in particularly low-dose screen–film systems.

- **a** Theoretical principle of an image detail within a line.
- **b** The same detail as in (**a**) is much more difficult to discern in the presence of intense noise. If it were smaller, it might even go unnoticed.
- **c,d** Extremely fine microcalcifications, a sign of a ductal carcinoma, are readily apparent with a high-contrast and high-resolution screen–film system (**c**), but are hardly discernible with the low-dose screen–film system (**d**).
- **e** Influence of noise on image quality: Suspicious microcalcifications shown on a screening mammogram obtained with a full-field digital unit.
- **f** The same patient underwent an additional mediolateral mammogram before vacuum-assisted breast biopsy. In spite of a more than 2-fold dosage this computed radiography image is noisier and the group of microcalcifications is less obvious. (Note also the change of contrast in the subcutaneous breast tissue, which is due to an algorithm that enhances the skin.) *Histology* yielded flat epithelial atypia.

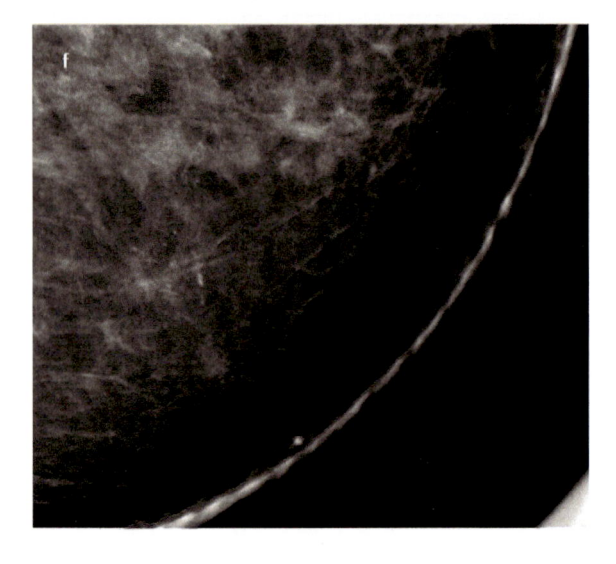

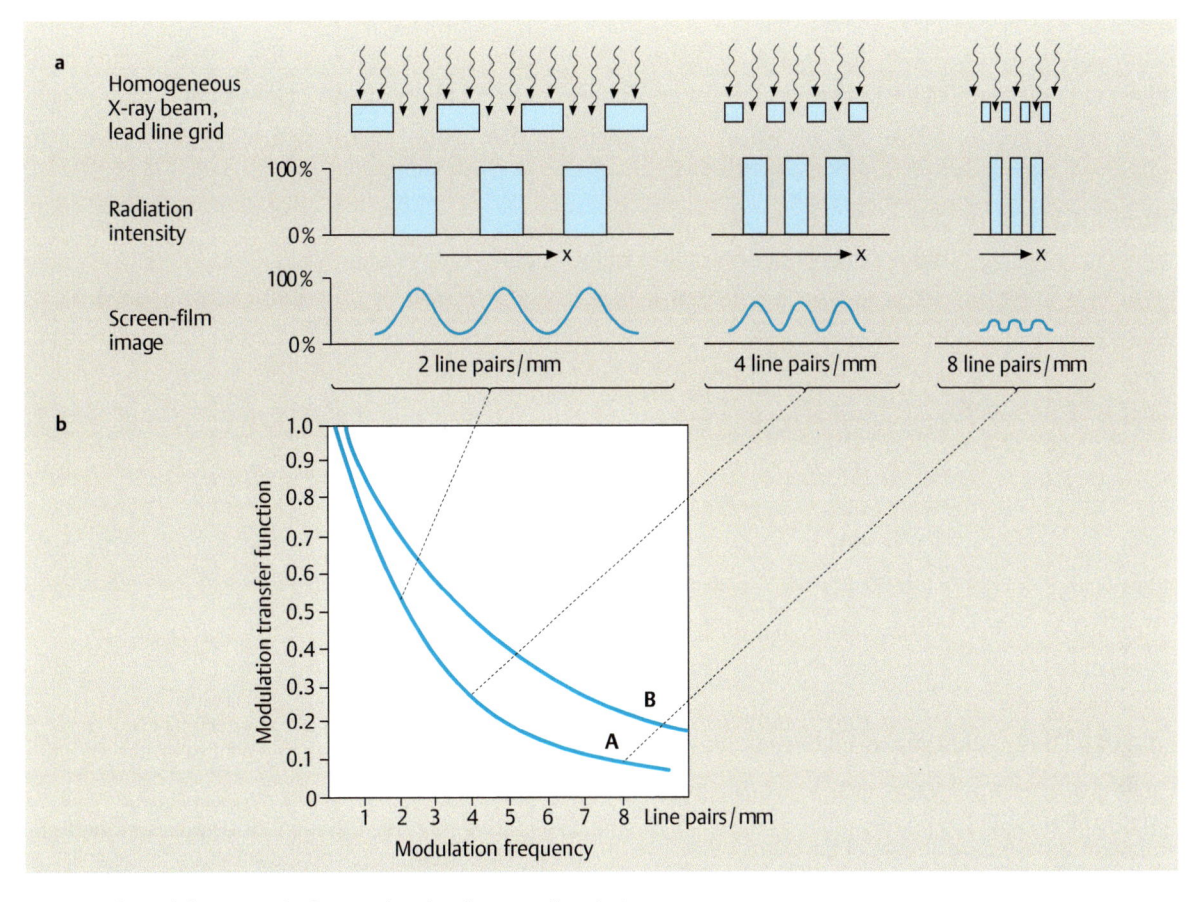

Fig. 3.10 a, b Modulation transfer function (MTF) and structural resolution.

a A lead line grid imaged with a homogeneous beam. The radiation density in the image of the line grid is alternately 0 and 100%. Light scattering in the screen–film system in particular causes the sharp edges of the grid to appear fuzzy. The finer the grid, the more the differences in intensity will be equalized in the image.

b The resulting relationship that renders structures less detectable as they become finer (local modulation frequency of intensity) is described by the modulation transfer function (MTF) of a component (in this case, the screen–film system). As the fineness of the lines increases, the MTF decreases from an initial value of 1 (no loss of information), thus limiting the resolving power of the components.
Curve B shows a better MTF than curve A.

Fundamental Considerations

High contrast is always required to differentiate very fine structures with slight differences in optical density or pixel value, such as microcalcifications. However, as was discussed on page 26, this contrast should *not be excessive* either. For screen–film systems (as described on pp. 30–32), the flat part of the curve at the foot of the characteristic film curve (foot gradient) limits contrast in the low-density range (dense breast tissue). In the high-density range, the eye can no longer perceive differences over a density of 2.4. Even in bright light, recognition of differences is limited to densities below 2.8. Beyond the optimum exposure range (optical density of 0.6 to ~2.4), image quality is significantly limited in that underexposed and overexposed areas begin to appear (see **Fig. 3.6**). When high-contrast films are used, these limits are reached sooner, and details in the high and low density ranges can be lost due to underexposure or overexposure, respectively (Young et al. 1997).

With digital receptors, the characteristic curve is essentially a straight line, and the image acquisition and display functions are separated, so that any recorded contrast can be demonstrated by suitable choice of display window width and level. It is still possible, however, for inappropriate image processing to reduce the displayed contrast.

Whereas low-contrast images appear to the eye to be "poor" or "flat," high-contrast images appear particularly "sharp." Here the physician must critically examine the images to verify that in the majority of breast studies, *no overexposed or underexposed areas appear*.

3 Mammography

Table 3.2 Optimizing contrast

Goal	Recommendation	Limiting factors
High-contrast image	1. Select a radiation spectrum with the lowest possible energy by using appropriate target material, filter material, and kVp setting	Unit design, breast penetration (dense breast), radiation exposure
	2. Compensate for breast thickness with compression (to reduce the density range that has to be imaged)	Compliance
	3. Reduce scattered radiation with compression, grid technique, low-energy radiation	Patient compliance, penetration, radiation dose
	4. Air gap (magnification mammography, see p. 64) Collimation (spot compression and magnification)	Dose, small section
	5. Use digital mammography instead of screen–film	
	6. High-contrast film	Film latitude limited (overexposure, underexposure), limited exposure range, increased noise, fogging
	7. High-contrast development (time, temperature, activity of the chemicals)	
	8. Avoiding: • Increased fog (film storage and processing) • Exposure to external light	Applicable only to screen–film mammography

Factors that Determine Contrast

Contrast is determined by various factors. These factors include (Table 3.2):
- Breast thickness and density of the breast tissue
- Radiation quality (target/filter combination, kVp)
- Breast compression, scatter-reducing techniques (such as grids)
- Choice of a suitable screen–film system, and film processing
- Choice of suitable digital image processing and display optimization

Proper exposure is a prerequisite.

Radiation Quality

The *energy spectrum* of the X-ray radiation greatly influences radiation contrast. *Low-energy radiation increases the contrast.* However, if the radiation *energy is too low, penetration* of the breast will be significantly *poorer.* This means that if the energy radiation used is too low in thick, dense breasts, even a long exposure time will fail to sufficiently expose the film, resulting in underexposure. Instead, this radiation is absorbed in the breast, and radiation exposure is increased unnecessarily.

Target/Filter Combination

The energy spectrum of the radiation depends on the *target and filter material,* the thickness of the filter, and the *kVp applied.*

Whereas normal-sized and small breasts of moderate density usually can be optimally imaged with a *molybdenum target* and a *0.03 mm molybdenum filter* at 25–30 kVp, the combinations molybdenum/rhodium, tungsten/molybdenum, rhodium/rhodium, and tungsten/rhodium may improve the image in large and dense breasts (Fig. 3.11). Recently developed units with bifocal tubes permit the selection of different target/filter combinations for thick and dense breasts or normal-sized and less dense ones. This means that the quality of the radiation is optimized not only by preselecting the maximum voltage, but also by selecting the most suitable target/filter combination.

Peak Kilovoltage (kVp)

Increasing the kVp setting increases the mean energy of the radiation and thus its penetrating power, whereas decreasing the kVp setting decreases the mean energy and penetrating power. However, contrast is increased at a low kVp.

Choosing the Optimum Target/Filter Combination and kVp Setting

A sophisticated automatic exposure control system is usually provided to aid the radiologic technologist in selecting a target/filter combination and the corresponding kVp setting appropriate to the breast density and compressed thickness. Some systems automatically select the target and filter material, kVp, and mAs product (according to low-dose, standard, or high-contrast exposure settings) after a short test exposure; other systems provide push-

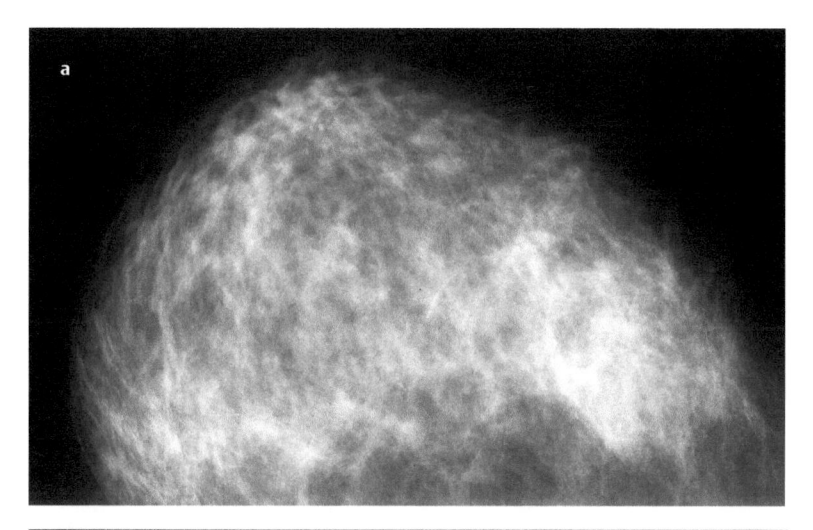

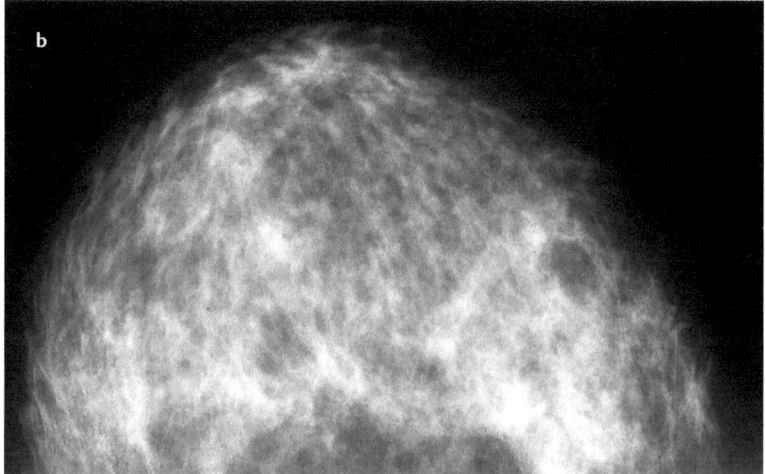

Fig. 3.11a,b The breast image obtained using a molybdenum target and rhodium filter at automatic exposure control settings of 29 kV and 51 mAs shows a slight improvement in penetrating dense areas over the image obtained using a molybdenum target and molybdenum filter at automatic settings of 29 kV and 78 mAs. In this case, the rhodium filter system achieved a slightly higher-quality image with a dose reduction of approximately 40%. Published studies report dose reductions in dense breasts of up to 50% over molybdenum/molybdenum images at the same kVp setting, depending on the composition of the glandular tissue (Küchler and Friedrich 1993).

a Craniocaudal mammogram, molybdenum/molybdenum.
b Craniocaudal mammogram, molybdenum/rhodium.

button program selection (for fatty, normal, or dense tissue). Once the selection is made, the unit suggests the suitable target/filter combination and corresponding kVp, taking into account the compressed breast thickness. As usual, the beam is switched off as soon as the mAs product required for the correct mean film density or desired digital receptor dose has been reached. Some automatic systems adjust the kVp during the exposure. In general, digital mammography systems are optimized to use higher kVp (around 32 kVp) and target/filter combinations that give more penetrating beams (e.g., tungsten/rhodium) than screen–film technology.

In the semiautomatic mode, the radiologic technologist selects the target and filter material and the kVp, and the automatic exposure control system then selects the mAs product as usual. Finally, all mammography units must permit manual exposure control, whereby the radiologic technologist can freely select every parameter. This feature is useful in special cases, such as very small breasts that do not cover the photocell or with augmentation implants, but considerable experience is required.

Reducing Scattered Radiation

Scattered radiation is an undesirable effect in breast imaging, since it causes opacification without diagnostic information and thus limits the information available on the film. Most of the scattered radiation is produced as the beam penetrates the breast tissue.

The most important means of effectively reducing scatter radiation are adequate breast compression and use of grid technique or collimation (spot compression and air-gap magnification mammography).

Breast Compression

The best possible breast compression contributes decisively to increasing contrast:
- It reduces the thickness through which the beam passes, significantly reducing scattered radiation, thus improving contrast. According to model calculations by Barnes, the ratio of scattered radiation to primary radiation in a breast compressed in thickness from 6 cm to 3 cm decreases from 1.0 to 0.4, resulting in an

improvement in contrast by a factor of 1.43 (Barnes 1994).
- In addition, healthy tissue usually spreads, whereas true masses will persist. This improves visualization of true masses and diminishes the likelihood of falsely identifying a lesion.
- It decreases motion of the breast during the X-ray exposure.
- Finally, breast compression also permits a significant reduction in radiation dosage (see p. 51).

Grid Technique

The grid technique significantly reduces scattered radiation (**Fig. 3.12**). This makes the technique indispensable with glandular normal-sized and large breasts; it is indicated as the standard technique despite the fact that the required radiation dose is increased by a factor of around 2.5 (see **Fig. 3.12**).

Gridless mammography could be considered only in small, low-density breasts in light of the lesser quantities of scattered radiation encountered in these patients.

However, today the grid is removed only during magnification mammography.

Grids are not used in magnification mammography because a significant reduction in scattered radiation can be achieved with the air gap in conjunction with good collimation.

In standard mammographic technique, however, the increased dose required by the grid is acceptable in light of the significant improvement in image quality, and it is more than offset by the reduced dose requirements of current image receptors.

Other Techniques for Scatter Reduction

When spot films using a contact technique (coned-down views without collimation) are taken, the scattered radiation from the surrounding tissue is reduced by the collimation to a small area of interest.

In *magnification mammography,* good collimation in combination with the air gap effectively reduces scattered radiation, which is why this technique does not require a grid. The grid would only increase the dose unnecessarily

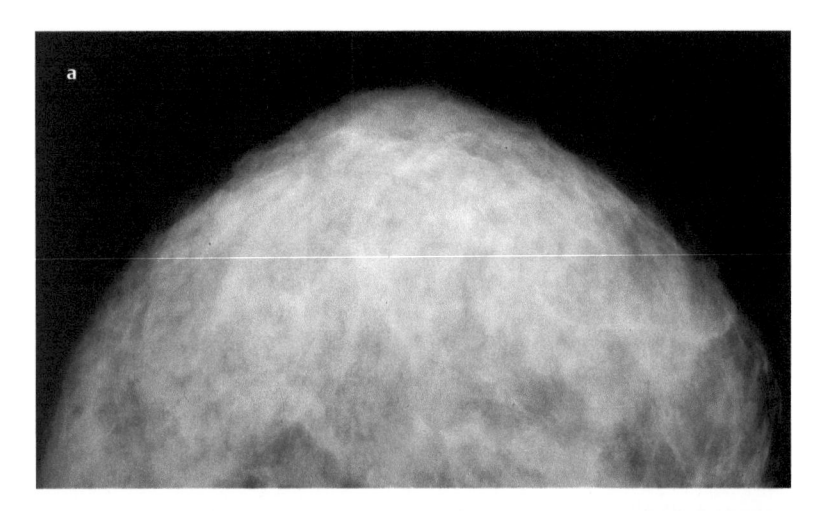

Fig. 3.12a,b The comparison shows that the significantly reduced scattered radiation in grid mammography permits significantly better visualization of the structures in the glandular tissue and of microcalcifications, which are located in the glandular tissue.
a Mammogram without grid.
b Mammogram taken 1 year later with grid.

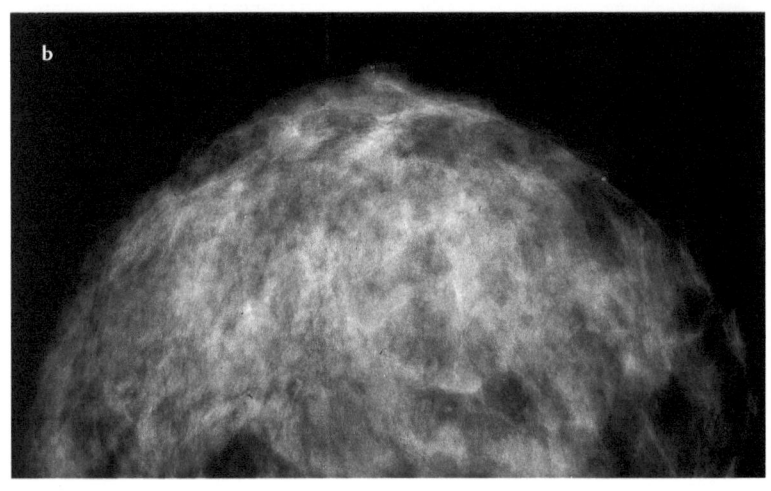

and require significantly longer exposure times, leading to motion blurring.

Slot mammography produces an image by exposing the breast line by line through a slit. Each exposed line is read behind the breast by an image receptor, which is collimated to the slit. By moving the slit over the breast, the complete breast is scanned. The technique effectively reduces scatter, thus improving image contrast. The additional dose which is needed by a grid due to absorption within the grid can be reduced. This technique is used in some designs of full-field digital mammography systems.

A very recent new DR technology removes the signal of scattered radiation from the image by a filtering algorithm. This allows the grid to be removed and saves about 30% of the radiation dose.

Automatic Exposure Control System

The *automatic exposure control system* uses a *photocell placed underneath the cassette*, to determine the radiation dose. The photocell switches the beam off once the dosage required for the desired mean optical film density or digital pixel value has been reached.

With respect to automatic exposure control, there are definite *differences in system quality* that influence image quality. Not every automatic exposure control system is equally effective in achieving the desired optimum mean optical density on the film or digital pixel value irrespective of the energy spectrum of the incident radiation. There are two reasons for this:

1. The required radiation energies vary with each patient owing to differences in the thickness and density of the breasts imaged. In particular, the degree to which the lower-energy components of this spectrum are weakened depends on breast thickness and density. This means that the extent to which the radiation is hardened in the breast varies. To varying degrees, the radiation also undergoes further hardening in the grid table and cassette before it enters the photocell. Since the sensitivity of the photocell is dependent on the energy spectrum of the incident radiation, failure to compensate for thickness in dense and thick breasts can cause the unit to switch off too soon, producing an underexposed image.
2. With longer exposure times, the optical density of the film no longer increases in proportion to the exposure time (reciprocity law failure; see p. 48). This means that insufficient optical density is achieved with long exposure times, that is, the image is underexposed. This is not a problem with digital receptors as these do not exhibit reciprocity law failure.

The designs of modern automatic exposure control systems attempt to compensate for both effects as successfully as possible. Some use a pair of photocells either side of a thin metal filter and employ the ratio between the signals from the two sensors to estimate the hardness of the beam exiting the breast. Some digital mammography units use the signal from areas of the image receptor itself to control the exposure. Digital units may be configured not to produce a constant pixel value, but instead to maintain constant a more relevant image quality metric such as contrast-to-noise ratio. Phantom images, usually of varying thicknesses of Plexiglas (polymethyl methacrylate) can be used to verify the quality of compensation achieved and thus assess the performance of the automatic exposure control system.

Positioning the Photocell

It is important to position the photocell under a representative part of the glandular tissue. Never position the photocell so that the breast does not completely cover it. Otherwise the photocell will receive unattenuated radiation and will switch off too soon, producing an underexposed image. The central part of the anterior third of the breast has proven to be the optimum region for placing the photocell, since it usually contains relatively uniform glandular tissue. In contrast, variations in the distribution of glandular and fatty tissue are greater in the areas close to the chest wall, increasing the risk that the photocell would lie under an area not representative of the rest of the breast (see also **Fig. 3.7**). Improper positioning of the photocell (unfortunately sometimes due to the design of the unit) is the most frequent source of error that causes incorrect exposure.

Manual Exposure

Since very *small breasts* and breasts with *silicone implants* do not generally permit positioning the photocell under a representative area, manual exposure is required. When adjusting the exposure manually, the radiologic technologist sets the mAs product according to breast thickness and the estimated radiodensity. In the absence of previous mammograms, the radiologic technologist essentially estimates radiodensity according to tissue consistency. This requires experience. Recorded exposure values from previous examinations are helpful. This is one reason why it is worthwhile recording the thickness and degree of compression, the mAs product, kVp setting, and the target/filter combination at every mammographic examination. If breasts with implants are radiographed, the exposure setting that provides optimum exposure of the glandular tissue adjacent to the implant should be selected. The soft radiation cannot penetrate a silicone-filled implant. Adequate penetration of a silicone-filled implant would cause overpenetration of the glandular breast tissue. The same principle applies to saline-filled implants.

Film Selection

When selecting the film, high contrast is important for visualizing details, but excessive contrast will limit the visibility of details in the areas of high and low density. Especially in large and dense breasts, excessive contrast will manifest itself in the simultaneous presence of underexposed and overexposed areas (overexposed tissue in thin areas near the skin and underexposed in dense areas of the breast tissue) (**Fig. 3.13**). Moreover, a very high-contrast screen–film system will be more sensitive to slight fluctuations in the development process, to an automatic exposure control system with less than optimum thickness and density equalization, and to suboptimal photocell positioning. This means that even slight deviations will lead to incorrect exposures that can affect the diagnosis (i.e., exposure tolerance is reduced) (Friedrich 1993). For these reasons, high-contrast films require an optimally adjusted automatic exposure control system, a precisely positioned photocell, and constantly optimized film processing.

It is also important to understand that the increased image noise associated with particularly *low-dose screen–film systems* (screen noise and quantum noise) diminishes the clarity of detail (see **Fig. 3.9**). Sometimes the very short exposures (necessary for small breast) are not possible on some equipment, leading to overexposure. Finally, with extremely short exposure times, the grid strips themselves will often be imaged when the grid does not move fast enough for the short exposure time (**Fig. 3.14**). If problems of this sort occur, a slightly lower voltage or a less sensitive screen–film system must be used. If this does not solve the problem, then the mammography unit should be upgraded.

Screen–film systems with extremely low sensitivity can result in disproportionately *long exposure times* when used with high breast densities and low voltage (reciprocity failure law; see p. 47). Since low-sensitivity films are no longer used today, these problems will occur only when the radiation energy selected is too low for the breast thickness and density. In magnification mammography, long exposure times may occur as a result of the reduced power of the small tube focal spot. Particularly with low kVp settings when the automatic exposure control system does not compensate sufficiently, this can lead to incorrect exposure (as explained above) or it can result in motion blurring. Problems of this nature can be compensated for by selecting a higher voltage or by using a more sensitive screen–film system.

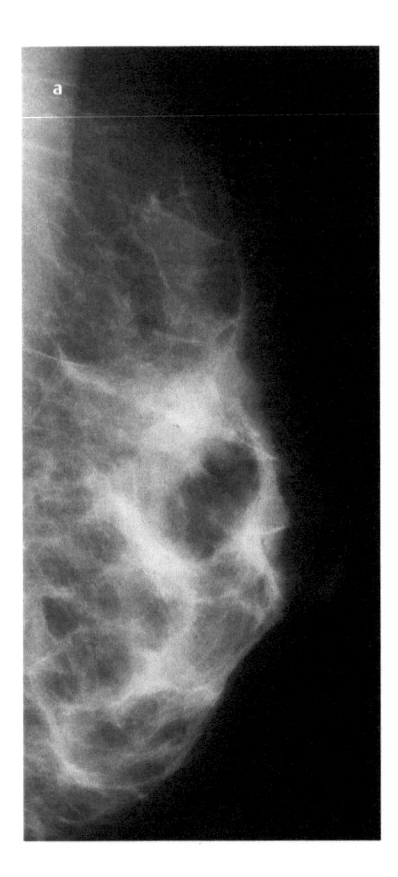

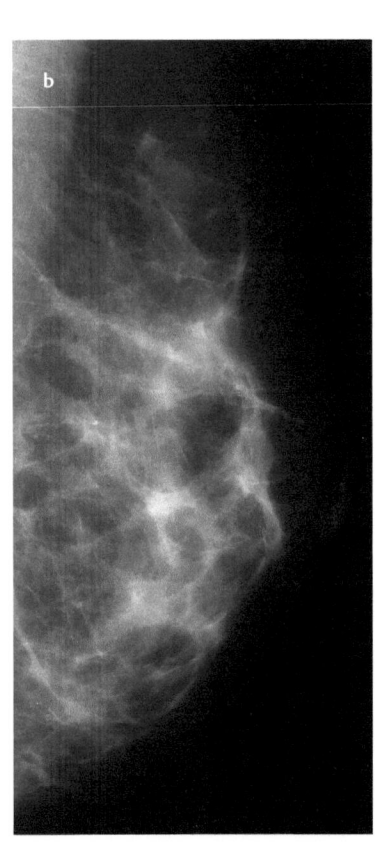

Fig. 3.13a,b Breast images using a high-contrast film (**a**) and a lower-contrast film (**b**).

a The high-contrast film shows parts of the glandular tissue in the relatively flat section of the characteristic curve. Contrast within the glandular tissue is therefore low, making these areas difficult to diagnose, although the breast as a whole is correctly exposed. (The subcutaneous tissue is just barely discernible with the bright light.)

b The glandular tissue can be much better evaluated with the slightly lower-contrast film. (Note that positioning is significantly better than in **a**.)

Specific Requirements and Solutions

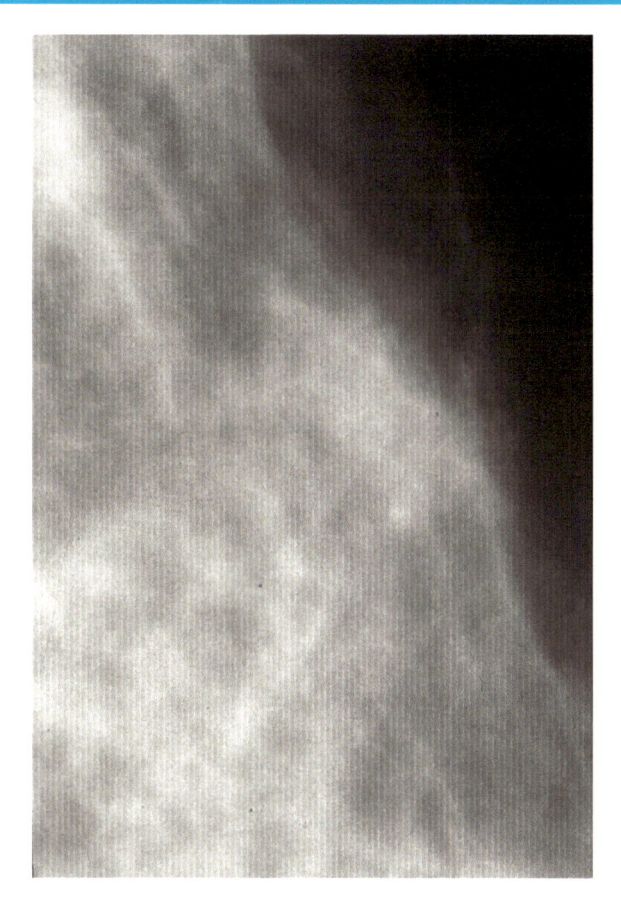

Fig. 3.14 Particularly when imaging thin and fatty breast, using extremely sensitive films may result in the grid strips themselves being imaged as parallel lines because of the short exposure times required (partial view).

Film Processing

Film processing influences contrast, fog, sensitivity, and noise.

The rule is that increasing developing time or temperature will increase fog, noise, and film sensitivity, whereas contrast reaches its maximum at a certain development temperature and time. It follows from this that the *optimized processing parameters recommended by the manufacturer* must be strictly observed. *Quality control testing should verify consistent processing daily.* It should be noted that a sufficient degree of consistency can be achieved only with a minimum throughput of over 20 films per day.

With some films, *extending the developing time can further increase contrast and sensitivity.* Since the maximum contrast varies with the type of film, consultation with the manufacturers regarding such decisions may be advisable. Aside from this, a film's maximum contrast does not necessarily represent the optimum that a specific mammography system requires. No generalized recommendations can be made.

Improper or defective darkroom lighting may be an additional factor that influences contrast. For this reason, darkroom light should be checked once every year.

Noise

Noise is a general term borrowed from engineering and refers to the random fluctuation of a variable about some mean value. If that variable contains a non-random signal which is to be detected, then the minimum detectable signal will be governed by the amount of noise present. In mammography, the signal to be detected is the variation in X-ray attenuation between tissues, and the minimum contrast that can be visualized will be limited by the random variation in displayed image brightness due to noise.

The noise visualized in the image consists of the combined effect of several sources of variation, arising from quantum noise (fundamental to imaging with X-rays) and noise sources within the image receptor and display. *Quantum noise* occurs as a result of statistical fluctuations that exist in the X-ray beam which become visible when only a few X-ray quanta hit the receptor. With extremely sensitive (i.e., low-dose) receptors, the effects of quantum noise become more clearly visible. This is more pronounced in areas of dense breast tissue, where even fewer X-ray quanta reach the image receptor.

The *structural noise* of the screen generally increases with more sensitive screen–film systems. The same applies to the granularity of the film.

Digital receptors also exhibit *structural noise*, which depends on the design of system. Direct and indirect digital detectors can have most of their structural noise calibrated out by the process of flat-fielding, but this cannot be done with computed radiography. Digital systems may also exhibit electronic noise from the amplifiers and electronics associated with their operation, although this should always be at much lower amplitude than the quantum noise. Photon-counting digital systems largely eliminate electronic noise at the receptor by ignoring any signal fluctuations below a threshold minimum photon energy.

Noise becomes particularly apparent and can interfere with the diagnostic study, especially in high-definition images and with high contrast. Although the trained eye can learn to distinguish relevant differences in density, this is possible to only a limited extent (see **Fig. 3.9**).

For this reason, it is important that noise does not exceed a certain level, which may vary individually. This means that when considering extremely low-dose receptor systems, the radiologist should carefully weigh the disadvantages of increased noise against the advantages of the reduced radiation dose. Automatic exposure control systems for digital mammography may be optimized to maintain a target signal-to-noise ratio.

3 Mammography

Radiation Dose

Studies of patients whose breasts were exposed to high doses of radiation either for therapeutic reasons or following the atomic bomb explosions in Hiroshima and Nagasaki (National Academy of Sciences BEIR VII report 2006; SSK report 2010) have demonstrated that the glandular tissue of the breast is sensitive to radiation. As in other radiographic studies, it is important to keep the dose used in mammography as low as possible without compromising the quality required for diagnosis.

Regrettably, initial reports *greatly overestimated* the *presumed cancer risk*. This in turn has unfortunately caused a great deal of uncertainty about mammography on the part of some patients and physicians. For this reason, we shall explicitly address the risk of cancer from mammography.

Radiation Dose from Mammography

A certain dose of radiation is necessary to obtain a high-quality mammogram.

The absorbed glandular dose depends on various individual factors, such as the thickness and density of the breast, and can be measured via the entrance exposure. It can also be estimated on the basis of phantom images when the thickness of the breast is known.

Applicable statutes and regulations require that mammography units, screen–film systems, imaging technique, and development be selected and monitored so that the radiation dose at the image receptor does not exceed 300 μGy for a normal breast image. This dose is very small. It is less than the dose previously required for screenless film mammography by at least a factor of 10. Today, the total dose for mammography of both breasts of normal size in two planes is calculated to range around 4 mGy. Today the lowest dosage is achieved using DR mammography, followed by screen–film mammography and CR mammography.

Assessing the Risk

At such low radiation doses, a possible cancer risk could only be demonstrated by comparing several million patients with and without mammography, all other factors being kept equal. Obviously, this is not feasible.

Not surprisingly, previous comparative assessments involving several hundred thousand patients who underwent mammography have not demonstrated any increase in the incidence of cancer.

For this reason, we can only extrapolate from the data on high-dose exposure to low doses. However, this ignores the body's repair mechanisms that are possible at low-dose exposures. Thus the results of such estimates that assume a linear dose–response curve represent the worst case. In this worst case, mammography in two planes (4 mGy) performed at age 50 years theoretically could produce cancer in 1 of 100,000 patients (Hendrick 2010, National Academy of Sciences BEIR VII report 2006).

Assuming varying scenarios with annual to biennial **screening** performed on patients between age 40 and 80 years and a mortality reduction of 15–30%, it has been calculated that 50–80 times more deaths can be prevented than could be caused by annual mammography (Hendrick 2010, O'Connor et al. 2010, Yaffe and Mainprize 2011). For women above age 50, the risk of dying of breast cancer induced by mammography is so slight that it is considered to be essentially too small to calculate. It is approximately equivalent to the risk of dying of lung cancer from smoking about three cigarettes.

Owing to the lower breast cancer incidence at age 40 and the higher sensitivity of breast tissue to radiation at younger age, the risk–benefit ratio is much better for screening after age 50 than between ages 40 and 49. Based on the existing evidence it is, however, assumed that the benefit safely exceeds the risk after the age of 40, even if a higher sensitivity to radiation is assumed for low-energy radiation (Law et al. 2007, Albert et al. 2009, Heyes et al. 2009, O'Connor et al. 2010).

In patients *below* the age of 40 years, routine mammographic screening examinations are not usually recommended for the following reasons:

- The overall incidence of cancer is significantly less.
- The tissue is more sensitive to radiation (Law et al. 2007).
- Mammography may be less effective in young, dense tissue.

If mammography is indicated before age 40, as may be the case for patients with high genetic risk, it is recommended that it is performed in centers with strict quality control and a high level of expertise (Law 1997). Also, research is still needed to address benefit–risk ratios for the individual subgroups of women at high risk, since both detection rates of mammography and sensitivity of the breast tissue to radiation may differ between these subgroups.

In case of **symptoms** the use of mammography is justified for most age groups except very young patients. Overall the risk of malignancy is much higher in symptomatic patients than in the screening population. Therefore mammography should not be dispensed with where clinical or diagnostic findings require clarification and a malignant process cannot be excluded.

However, besides the positive predictive value of a clinical or sonographic finding, age-dependent probability of malignancy, detection rate of mammography, and sensitivity of the breast tissue to radiation need to be considered.

A general recommendation may be to use mammography first in symptomatic women above age 40 and use sonography first below age 40 (Albert et al. 2009). Each method has to be complemented by the other method or further tests unless malignancy can definitely be ruled out.

Summarizing, for women above age 40–50 the expected benefit of screening mammography appears to safely exceed the risk. Therefore radiation dose should not be an argument against mammography screening above age 40. In symptomatic women mammography should not be dispensed with where clinical or diagnostic findings require exclusion of malignancy. Before age 40, however, sonography should be considered first.

Owing to the low but existing oncogenic risk, use of mammography always requires adequate quality assurance. Strict quality assurance is mandatory for any screening indication and very strict quality assurance and particular expertise is needed for young women at high risk.

Dose-related Optimization of the Exposure Technique

Exposure technique and strategy (e.g., the number of images) should be optimized with respect to the dose for the reasons mentioned in the previous sections. At the same time, *quality should not be sacrificed to reduce the dose, and restricting the maximum number of images should never compromise the required information.*

The following section discusses *factors influencing the radiation dose* which, when optimized, permit further dose reduction (**Table 3.3**).

Radiation Quality

Selecting *optimum radiation quality* permits optimizing both image quality and dose. In particular, *too high a proportion of low-energy radiation* must be avoided since it tends to be absorbed in dense glandular tissue and in thick breasts and contributes only slightly, if at all, to information on the mammogram.

The quality of radiation depends on the *target/filter material* and on the selected *maximum tube voltage.* Optimum adjustment of radiation quality is most easily achieved using *newer mammography units* that automatically select both voltage and *target/filter material* matched to the type of breast. Here, it is important that the *mammography unit has sufficient capacity.* If the *output is too low* (as with some inexpensive units), the only way to achieve the dose necessary is by extending the exposure time. To avoid this, the capacity of a mammography unit should never be below 1 kW at 30 kV. This is only a minimal requirement. Units of higher capacity are important for achieving adequate image quality in dense breasts and for reducing the radiation dose.

Breast Thickness

The *dose* required to penetrate the breast is highly dependent on the *thickness and density of the breast.* The density increases with a high proportion of glandular tissue containing large quantities of cells, fluid, and/or connective tissue. Good compression can markedly reduce the thickness, *significantly reducing the required radiation dose.* Thus, penetrating a breast compressed to 4 cm requires only 80% of the dose required to penetrate a breast compressed to 4.5 cm.

Film Density

Mammography using screen–film should always try to achieve the recommended optimum *mean film density* of 1.5–1.9 (Young et al. 1997, Perry et al. 2006). An optical density that is too low significantly limits *the content of diagnostic information.* An excessively high optical density can also limit the diagnostic information but in any case is associated with *an unnecessary increase in the required dose.*

Table 3.3 Minimizing dose

Goal	Recommendation	Limiting Factors
Minimizing dose	Sufficient radiation energy (appropriate selection of kVp and target/filter combination) for: • Good penetration • Avoiding reciprocity law failure	Depends on mammography unit Occurs only with screen–film mammography
	Breast compression • Reduce the thickness to be penetrated	Compliance
	Use sufficient power to avoid reciprocity law failure	Depends on mammography unit
	Correct exposure • Avoiding overexposure • Avoiding repeats	Depends on mammography unit (automatic exposure control system) and technologist's experience
	Use full-field digital radiography instead of computed radiography or screen–film mammography	

Grid

Since the proportion of scattered radiation in thick and dense breasts is significant, a *grid* is required. Although the grid *increases in dose by a factor of approximately 2.5,* it is indispensable for achieving adequate image quality in these breasts. Theoretically, reducing the dose in patients with very small and fatty breasts by not using the grid technique could be discussed. However, practical considerations have prevented frequent switching between gridless and grid techniques from becoming common practice.

Screen–Film System

The selection of a screen–film system also has a decisive influence on the dose. Among the new screen–film systems, we differentiate between systems with *low* and *extremely low dose* (speed class: 12 or 25, respectively) requirements. The latter are often marketed as "screen–film systems for mammographic screening." The required doses differ by a factor of about 2. The extremely low-dose screen–film systems are subject to significantly higher noise levels, generally at very high contrast. This can impair visualization, particularly in the lower-density range of dense breast tissue. Here, image noise can interfere with detection of microcalcifications. Optimum exposure and film processing are more critical here than with other screen–film systems. Depending on the mammography unit, extremely short exposure time settings may fall below the unit's minimum switching intervals (resulting in incorrect exposure) or cause the visualization of grid lines. This may make adequate imaging with these films difficult.

Film Processing

Extending the processing time or increasing the processing temperature can increase the sensitivity of some films, permitting a further *reduction in dose* by as much as one-third. However, since this is frequently associated with a *further increase in contrast,* such modifications are not always desirable and should be considered in relation to other factors determining contrast. Moreover, an increase in processing temperature is frequently accompanied by a decline in quality.

Optimization of Digital Mammography

The linear response and wide dynamic range of digital mammographic receptors means that images can be successfully acquired over a large range of doses. This provides several possibilities for optimization and dose reduction, but equally also allows suboptimal systems to acquire images at higher patient doses than are necessary.

Since digital image receptors can adapt the image density to the received dosage at the receptor, with digital mammography there is a direct relationship between signal to noise (which leads to better image quality) and radiation dose. For reasons of radiation protection, however, dose must be limited and should not compensate for insufficiencies of the digital mammography system.

The phenomenon of "exposure creep" has been identified in general digital radiography, where average patient doses can rise due to the natural human inclination to make the images look better, and the fact that images are not rejected for being "too good." In digital mammography a universal approach to dose optimization is still a distant goal (although much research is in progress), but initial findings in well-controlled programs with properly calibrated automatic exposure devices are that average patient doses with new digital units are lower than those for the screen–film systems they replaced. Modern automatic exposure control software may offer alternative combinations of automatic exposure factors that optimize either for contrast (at the expense of dose) or for dose (at the expense of poorer contrast-to-noise ratio).

Number of Images

In the interest of *reducing the radiation dose,* an effort should be made to *avoid* repeating images by ensuring optimal technical conditions, continuous quality assurance, and well-trained personnel. When adjusting exposure manually, the technologist should initially take only one mammogram, with the remaining images taken only after correct exposure has been verified.

Sites that intend to perform screening will invariably require a grid table for large breasts in addition to the standard grid table. If mammograms of large breasts are routinely obtained by combining small views, significantly increased doses can result (for mammography in two planes, up to four times as much). This should be considered unacceptable.

Positioning and Compression

Mammographic positioning involves obtaining *the best possible compression* and correct *positioning* to ensure that the entire glandular body is imaged.

Compression

As explained in the previous sections, adequate *breast compression* is one of the main prerequisites for obtaining high-quality mammograms with the best possible visualization of pathologic changes (Barnes 1994).

The contributions of compression to quality mammography are summarized here:
- Good compression improves the *resolution* by reducing the distance between the image receptor and objects, which are farther from the image receptor. This reduces geometric blurring.
- It reduces motion blurring.

- It improves *contrast* since the reduced thickness of the breast significantly *reduces scattered radiation.*
- It improves *contrast* since low-energy radiation, which provides higher image contrast, can be utilized in penetrating tissue of reduced thickness.
- It permits higher *contrast* in the area of interest since, by *equalizing the thickness of the tissue,* it reduces the necessary object range.
- It permits *visualization of small areas of pathology buried in the glandular tissue* since normal tissue can be spread, whereas malignant foci will persist due to their firmer consistency.
- It permits a significant *reduction in the dose* by reducing the thickness of tissue to be penetrated.

These mentioned advantages illustrate the importance of achieving the best possible *compression*. As a prerequisite for high image quality, *early cancer detection* may depend on it (**Fig. 3.15**).

Naturally, the best possible breast compression can only be achieved with the patient's cooperation and must never be obtained against her will. Despite every effort to achieve optimum image quality, the technical staff must appreciate that the sensitivity of the glandular body to pressure varies. Patients differ in their willingness to endure pain or discomfort for good diagnostic results.

It is thus essential to *briefly discuss the need for compression* with the patient and to obtain her understanding, cooperation, and *motivation.* For this reason, the patient should be informed that some of the *smallest and earliest cancers can only be visualized with compression* and that compression significantly *reduces the dose of radiation.* She should be told that *there is no way in which compression can cause a carcinoma*, which is a common concern.

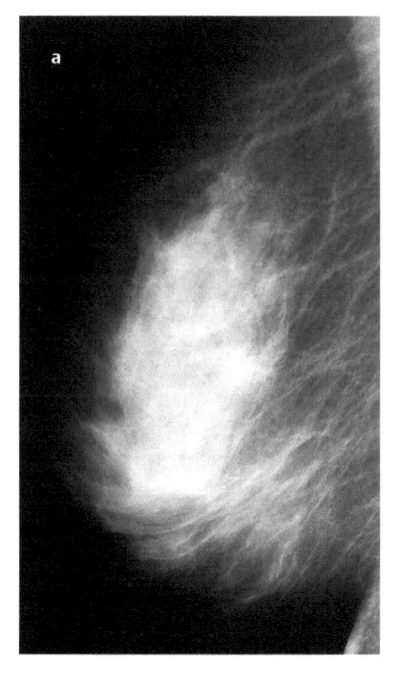

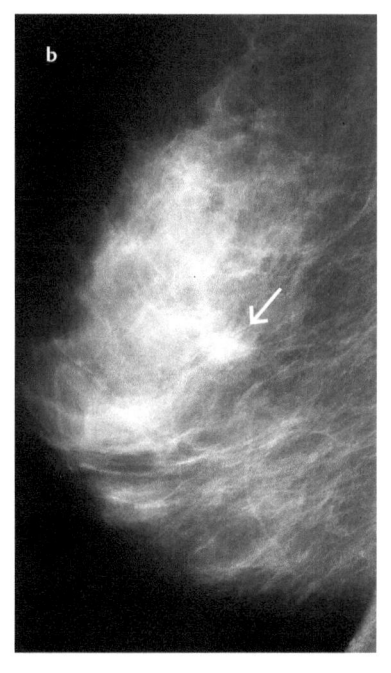

Fig. 3.15a–d Importance of compression.
a Mediolateral mammogram with poor compression where the glandular tissue has not been sufficiently spread out. The carcinoma in the glandular tissue is difficult to discern.
b With better compression and better spreading of the tissue, the carcinoma (arrow) and its spiculations are considerably easier to discern.
c Section of a mediolateral oblique view with poor compression. The glandular tissue structures are dense and blurred because of insufficient compression. Several calcifications are faintly visible in the poorly compressed tissue.
d A repeat mediolateral oblique view with good compression reveals significantly sharper visualization of the glandular tissue structures. Several more highly suggestive calcifications are now discernible.

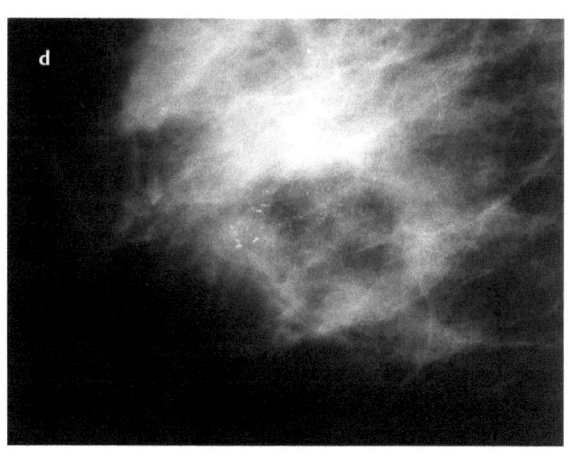

Since compression of tissue with low interstitial water content is less painful, and the density of the breast decreases and image quality improves as the water content decreases, *the mammographic examination may be more comfortable for women during the first half of the menstrual cycle.* When compressing the breast, it is important that all of the *glandular tissue is spread as evenly as possible and that no skin folds are present.* Compression of unevenly distributed glandular tissue is more painful, and the folds may cause densities that interfere with the diagnosis.

Positioning for Standard Views

In mammography, we differentiate between standard views and *additional views*.

Number of Views in Standard Mammography

Except in unusual instances, all mammographic examinations should be obtained in two planes.

So-called single-view mammography, which essentially consists of only the mediolateral oblique view, has been used for screening, because of the lower costs involved. Because of its reduced sensitivity and specificity, most mammography experts do not regard single-view mammography as sufficient for diagnostic purposes or cost-effective. Many patients require repeated examinations. For this reason, mammography in only one plane should be reserved for exceptional cases (such as a limited examination in the presence of known findings, in young patients, or during pregnancy).

Whereas standard views permit reliable identification or exclusion of malignant processes in most patients, additional views should be used liberally whenever mammograms in the standard imaging planes are inconclusive or do not visualize the findings completely. Any additional view is preferable to an unnecessary biopsy or a carcinoma that goes undetected.

Standard Views

The *mediolateral oblique view* and the *craniocaudal view* used in combination have become the international standard views (Young et al. 1997, Perry et al. 2006).

Mediolateral Oblique View

Purpose

The mediolateral oblique view is regarded as the most important view since it best visualizes the tissue adjacent to the chest wall and the axillary tail. It is the view that is most likely to include all the breast tissue. It is designed to maximize visualization of the lower axilla and the upper outer quadrant. If tissue is not included on this view, it is most likely in the inferomedial breast. Most carcinomas can be visualized in the mediolateral oblique view.

Conducting the Examination (Fig. 3.16a,b)

Rotate the X-ray tube and the film holder to permit positioning the film cassette between the patient's pectoralis muscle and latissimus dorsi. This can be achieved with 30°–70° inclination, depending on the patient's habitus. For short, stocky women, positioning will be more horizontal, and for tall, slim women, more vertical. The beam will travel from medial and superior to lateral and inferior, hitting the film cassette perpendicularly. Positioning the cassette and compression paddle parallel to the pectoralis in this manner allows optimum mobilization of the glandular tissue away from the chest wall.

Place the cassette posterior to the anterior axillary line. Place it so that it mobilizes the lateral breast medially and upward. This makes it possible to pull the breast away from the chest wall to achieve optimum positioning. Placing the film cassette inferior to the breast or too far laterally increases the tension on the medial tissue, which is painful and prevents adequate pulling of the breast onto the film cassette.

Do not push the cassette too high into the axilla. Note that the imaging table should be set about 2 cm lower for the mediolateral oblique view than for the craniocaudal view. A table position that is too high tenses the pectoralis, making it difficult to pull the breast forward. If part of the humerus appears on the image or if major parts of the image are occupied by axillary tissue or the pectoral muscle, adequate compression is not possible and the breast may not be held in position. It may drop, leading to a "camel nose" shape of the breast.

The patient's arm should rest lightly on the cassette, since this also permits better mobilization of the glandular tissue. Turn the patient so that she faces the mammography unit. Thus the medial parts of the breast tissue will be included, and the inframammary fold will become visible on the image. Now pull the breast forward firmly so that as much tissue as possible lies on the cassette. Unlike compression, pulling the breast forward is not painful but visualizes another centimeter of glandular tissue anterior to the chest wall. Pull the breast anteriorly and superiorly to separate the glandular tissue as much as possible. Otherwise, small carcinomas will be easily concealed. Once the breast is spread out, it is easily compressible and compression is less painful.

When lowering the compression paddle, the breast should be pulled until the compression paddle holds the breast in position. Make sure that the compression does not produce any folds in the skin that might interfere with the diagnosis. Be certain that the inframammary fold is open and the abdomen is not superimposed. Inadequate visualization of the inframammary fold is an important cause of missed cancers.

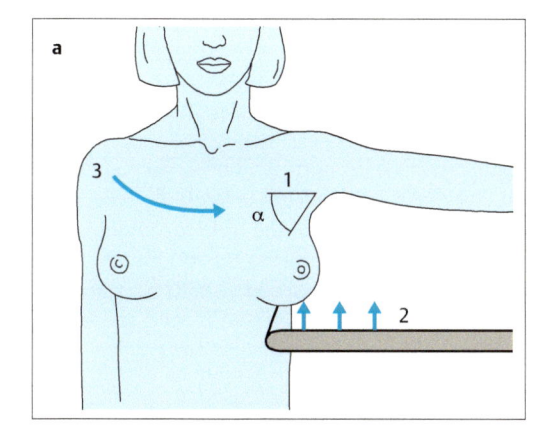

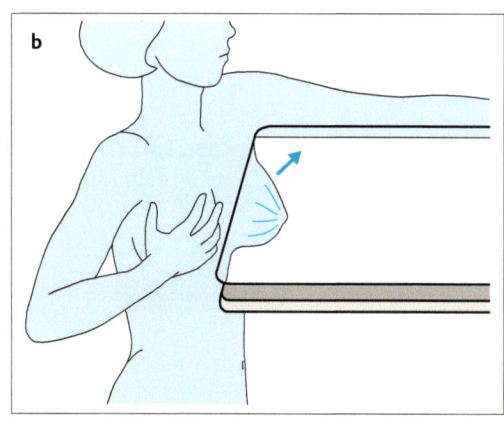

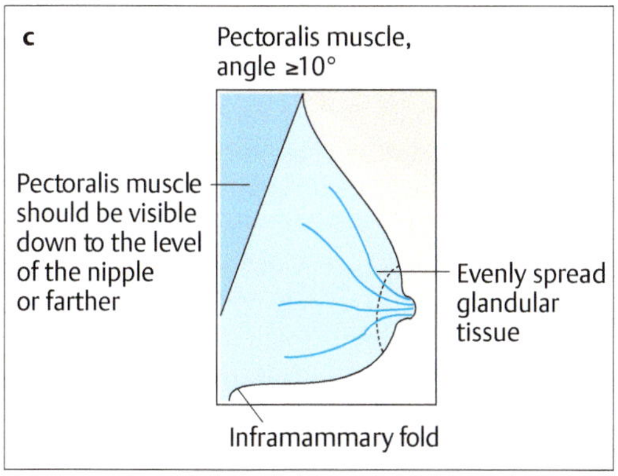

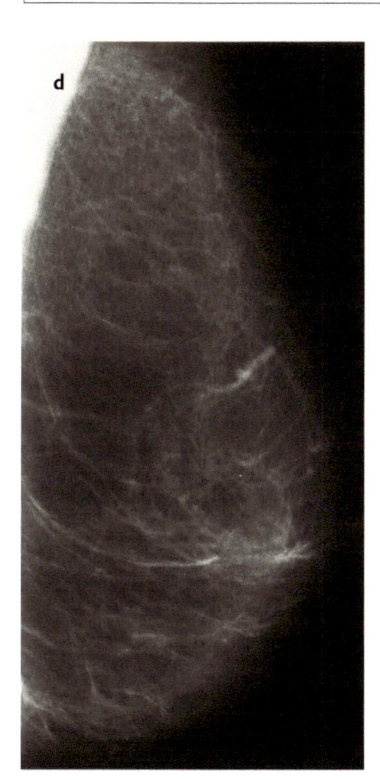

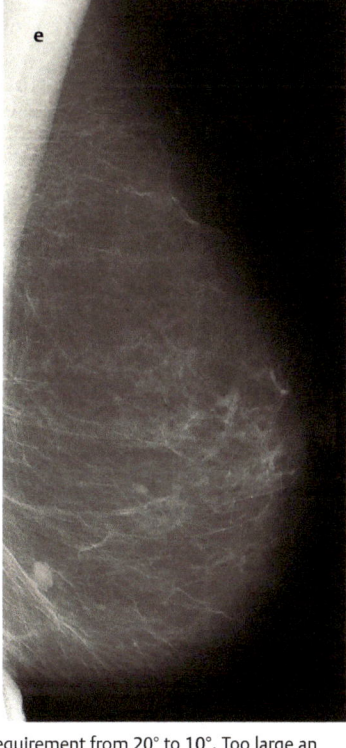

Positioning and Compression

Fig. 3.16 a–e Mediolateral oblique view.

a Check that the image table is not moved too high in the axilla. (Usually the table needs to be ~2 cm lower than for the craniocaudal view; the humerus should not be included in the image.) Correct positioning is achieved by rotating the tube arm to an angle corresponding to the course of the pectoralis (1). Then the bucky is placed under the breast so as to mobilize the breast medially and superiorly as much as possible (2). Finally (3), the patient is turned toward the unit and the technologist pulls the breast onto the film holder. That way as much medial breast tissue as possible is included, when the compression paddle (not shown) is lowered.

b With the breast correctly positioned, the technologist pulls the breast tissue anteriorly and superiorly (arrow), moving it forward and spreading it as much as possible. The patient's ipsilateral arm (shown here) should rest on the film holder while she holds the contralateral breast back with her other hand.

c A good mediolateral oblique view fulfills the following quality criteria: The pectoralis muscle should course diagonally along the superior and lateral border of the image (at an angle of at least 10°)*. The pectoralis should be visible in the image at least as far as the level of the nipple. The glandular tissue should appear well spread out, and the image should include the inframammary fold. The latter should be visualized without superimposition, which is best achieved when the breast is pushed anteriorly and superiorly until the compression paddle grasps the breast.

d A small, not entirely smoothly contoured density close to the chest wall was only barely visualized in this poorly positioned mediolateral oblique view and thus was overlooked (the inframammary fold was not visualized).

e The medial lesion is readily discernible in the mediolateral oblique view with better (but still not optimal) positioning (the patient was turned toward the mammography unit).
Histology: Fibroadenoma.

*Some screening programs have changed this requirement from 20° to 10°. Too large an angle leads to the inclusion of too much of the pectoral muscle. Thus, the breast tissue cannot be adequately compressed, and in some patients the breast may even drop, leading to the so-called "camel's nose" appearance of the breast and an inadequate display of the inframammary fold.

Quality Criteria for Optimum Positioning in the Mediolateral Oblique View (Fig. 3.16a–e)

- The pectoralis muscle should be visible in the image at least to the level of the nipple.
- It should course superiorly along the lateral border of the image at an angle of about 20°. (Since visualization of too much pectoral muscle may interfere with good compression, some screening programs are presently changing to recommend an angle of 10–20°.)
- The inframammary fold should be included inferiorly. This is achieved by having the patient turn far enough toward the mammography unit.
- The glandular tissue should appear well spread out in the image.

Optimization

The view can be optimized by rotating the tube to an angle corresponding to the course of the pectoralis. The position of the image receiver should not be too high in the axilla. The following steps include lifting the breast, pulling it forward firmly, turning the patient toward the mammography unit, spreading out the glandular tissue, and achieving the best possible compression.

Craniocaudal View

Purpose

The mediolateral oblique view is routinely supplemented by the craniocaudal view in which the beam travels from superior to inferior (**Fig. 3.17**).

Conducting the Examination

To pull the breast as far away from the chest wall as possible, lift the breast from below to shift the inframammary fold as far superiorly as possible. It is possible to lift the inframammary fold by several centimeters. Then adjust the table to the height of the upwardly mobilized inframammary fold and lay the breast on the table. Pulling the breast forward and compressing it at the original height of the inframammary fold would increase tension on the skin and subcutaneous tissue superior to the nipple, limiting forward mobility. This also is painful. After achieving correct cassette and breast positioning, firmly pull the breast away from the chest wall until it is held in place by the compression paddle.

In the craniocaudal view, the nipple should be centered or pointing slightly medially. It is important to visualize the medial glandular tissue (which sometimes cannot be completely visualized in the mediolateral oblique view) as completely as possible. If this is problematic, it may be helpful to include the most medial aspect of the other breast to assure inclusion on the film of the breast being examined (see also cleavage view; p. 60). The craniocaudal view also serves as the second plane for imaging the axillary tail. This structure is rich in glandular tissue and should be carefully analyzed since it is a frequent site of cancer. To maximize visualization of the axillary tail, some authors recommend firmly pulling it forward before completely lowering the compression paddle. For this view, it is helpful to let the arm on the side being imaged hang down. This way, the outer quadrant of the relaxed pectoralis muscle will lie on the bucky, and it will be easier to pull it forward and visualize it. Here, too, make sure that the glandular tissue is well spread out before compression and that skin folds are avoided.

Quality Criteria

Ideally, the craniocaudal view should include the entire body of the gland with the medial and lateral retromammary fat. In particularly high-quality images, the pectoralis will just barely be visible along the edge of the mammogram. If the medial edge of the image includes the medial fold (which is not always possible) one can be sure that the body of the gland has been optimally visualized. Visualization of the medial breast is sometimes optimized by including the medial aspect of the opposite breast. If the pectoralis muscle is not included on the craniocaudal view, adequacy of inclusion of posterior tissues is determined by comparison with the mediolateral oblique view. On the mediolateral oblique view, a measuring line is drawn at a 90° angle to the pectoralis muscle and through the nipple. This line, which starts at the nipple and ends at the pectoralis muscle, is called the pectoralis–nipple line, and on the craniocaudal view the distance from the nipple to the posterior edge of the image should not be less than the length of the pectoralis–nipple line minus 1.5 cm.

Positioning the Photocell

Once the correct settings have been selected, choosing the proper position for the photocell is crucial to ensure proper functioning of the automatic exposure control system. The photocell is optimally positioned under the anterior third of the breast (behind the nipple) since this area contains relatively uniform, representative glandular tissue. Make sure that the photocell is completely covered by glandular tissue, which should extend beyond the photocell by about 1 cm (see **Fig. 3.7**).

Importance of Optimum Breast Positioning

Optimum positioning for standard views is important because:

- Compression is *less painful* with good positioning.
- Good positioning will visualize considerably more tissue adjacent to the chest wall. In particular, since it is poorly accessible to palpation, this tissue is *especially*

Positioning and Compression

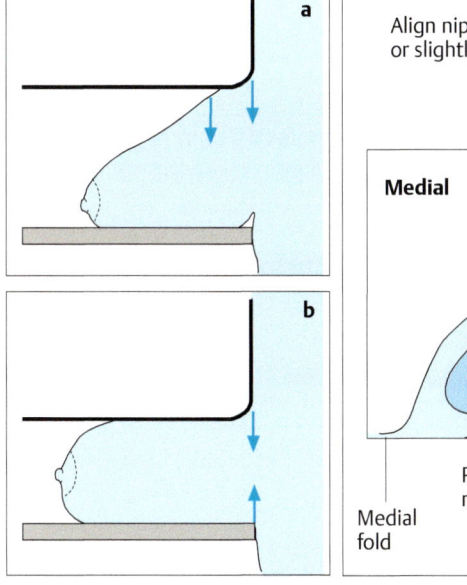

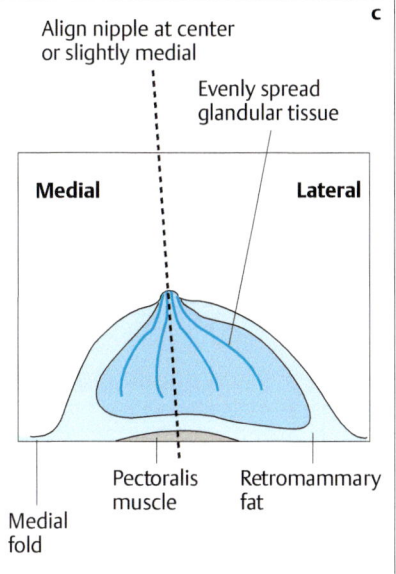

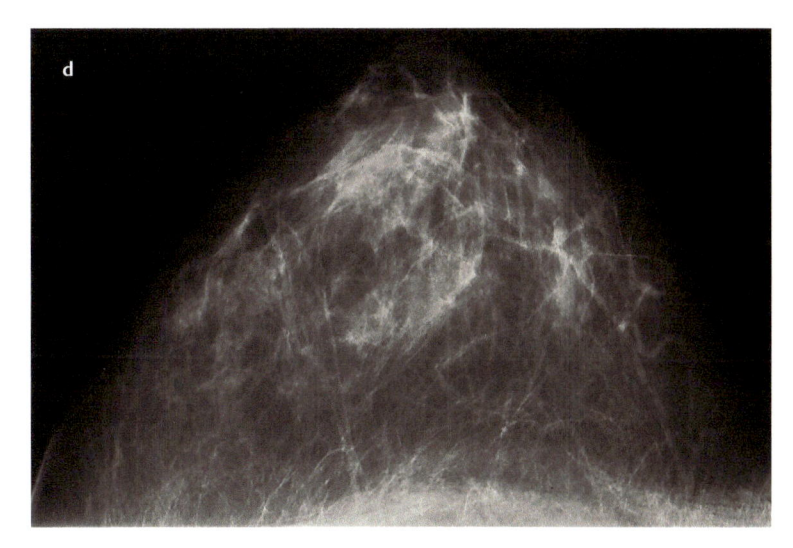

Fig. 3.17a–d Craniocaudal view.
a If the breast is not lifted, compression will cause painful tension (arrows) on the superior breast tissue, which also hinders pulling the breast forward from the chest wall.
b Correct positioning requires mobilizing the breast as far superiorly as possible. Raise the film holder accordingly. This makes it possible to pull the breast forward to achieve optimum positioning while making compression far less painful.
c A good craniocaudal view fulfills the following quality criteria: The image should include the entire body of the gland with the retromammary fat. This is best achieved with the nipple centered or positioned slightly medially. In particularly high-quality images, the pectoralis will just barely be visible along the edge of the mammogram and/or the medial border of the image will include the medial fold. Inclusion of the pectoral muscle is, however, only possible in some patients. It is therefore not considered a general requirement.
d Craniocaudal view with proper positioning.

important for early diagnosis (**Fig. 3.16**). The strip of fat usually present in this tissue makes it particularly suitable for detection of cancer by mammography.

Experienced staff can achieve very good positioning in as many as 90% of all cases. However, extensive scarring that does not permit sufficient mobilization of the glandular tissue can cause problems. Similar problems can occur in the presence of chest deformities such as pectus excavatum or rotatory scoliosis. In patients with severe scoliosis a caudocranial view may achieve better positioning than the standard craniocaudal view.

Further Procedure

No additional mammograms will be required if the standard views clearly reveal or exclude malignant findings and all breast tissue has been completely imaged. An additional view in the mediolateral projection is helpful even in the case of clear findings when a lesion is nonpalpable and preoperative needle marking is indicated.

However, if there is any uncertainty, obtaining additional views is the first step in arriving at a diagnosis (Logan and Janus 1987, Sickles 1988, Eklund and Cardenosa 1992).

Positioning for Additional Views

The most important *additional views* include:
- Spot compression and magnification views
- The 90° true lateral view
- The exaggerated lateral craniocaudal and the exaggerated medial craniocaudal views
- So-called rolled views

3 Mammography

- The tangential view and oblique views with (customized) settings for visualizing findings in atypical locations

Rare applications include:
- The axillary view
- The so-called "cleavage" view

The special views required with implants are discussed on pp. 71–72 and in Chapter 20.

90° Lateral View

Significance

The 90° lateral view (**Fig. 3.18**) is used in the following situations:
- As a third imaging plane when a *questionable superimposed structure* cannot be clearly distinguished from a genuine lesion.
- For *initial assessment of indeterminate microcalcifications*. The typical layering of milk of calcium in microcysts *(the so-called teacup phenomenon)* is visible only in a 90° lateral view. This pattern of layering is an important criterion for benign microcalcifications (see Chapter 10). For this reason, this projection (often with magnification) is frequently used in the assessment of microcalcifications.
- As an aid to localizing the true position of nonpalpable lesions in the breast prior to marking or percutaneous biopsy.

Conducting the Examination

When imaging the breast in the 90° projection, *the questionable structure* should be positioned as *close to the film* as possible to improve definition and minimize magnification. This means that a medial finding requires a *lateromedial view*, and a lateral finding requires a *mediolateral view*.

Exaggerated Lateral Craniocaudal View

(See **Fig. 3.19a,b**.)

Conducting the Examination

The mammography unit is positioned as for the craniocaudal view parallel to the floor. However, the patient is turned so that the lateral breast is pulled onto the film cassette, compressed, and imaged. The medial position of breast is therefore sacrificed on the image.

Purpose

This view is used to visualize changes in the axillary tail of the breast in the craniocaudal plane. It is indicated in the presence of suspicious clinical findings in this area or to localize or further clarify uncertain or suspected findings which may be visible on the mediolateral oblique view but are not seen on the routine craniocaudal view.

Even in the absence of clinical findings, it can be used to supplement the standard views if these views do not adequately visualize the axillary tail.

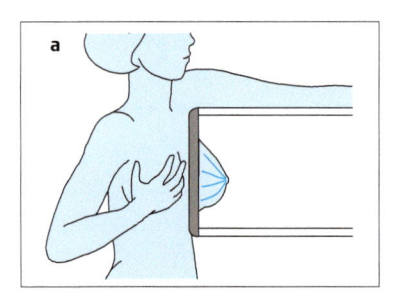

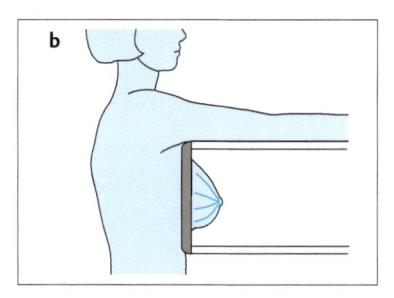

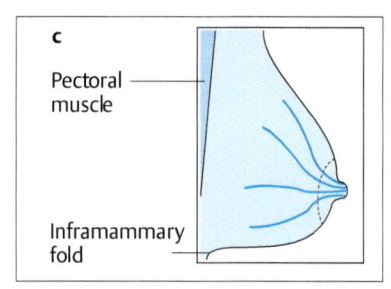

Fig. 3.18a–c 90° lateral (true lateral) view. The 90° lateral mammogram is prepared using a mediolateral or lateromedial beam with the mammography unit positioned at a 90° angle. Make sure that the structures of interest are positioned as close to the film as possible.

a   In the mediolateral view the patient stands directly in front of the unit facing it. The upper outer corner of the bucky lies in the patient's axilla; her arm rests lightly on the film holder. Support the patient's back so that she will not withdraw when compression is applied. Lift the breast superiorly, pulling it away from the chest wall and spreading it to achieve good tissue separation until the breast is held in place by the compression paddle.

b   In the lateromedial view the medial aspect of the patient's breast is positioned along the film holder. The arm of the side being imaged lies parallel to the upper edge of the compression cone. As in the mediolateral view, the technologist lifts the breast, pulls it forward, and holds it until it is held in place by the compression cone.

c   A good mediolateral view fulfills the following quality criteria: the image should include the entire body of the gland with the retromammary fat. The pectoralis should also be visible as a narrow band at least in the upper half of the image. The body of the gland should be well spread out, and the inframammary fold should be discernible.

Positioning and Compression

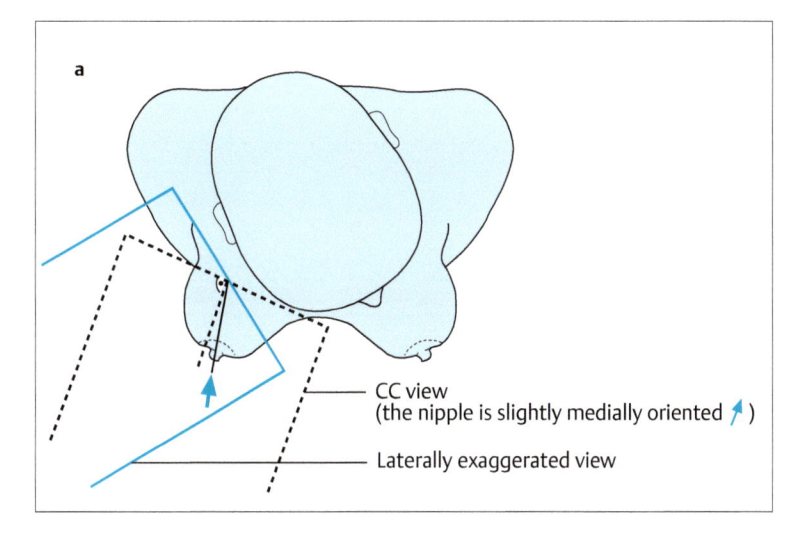

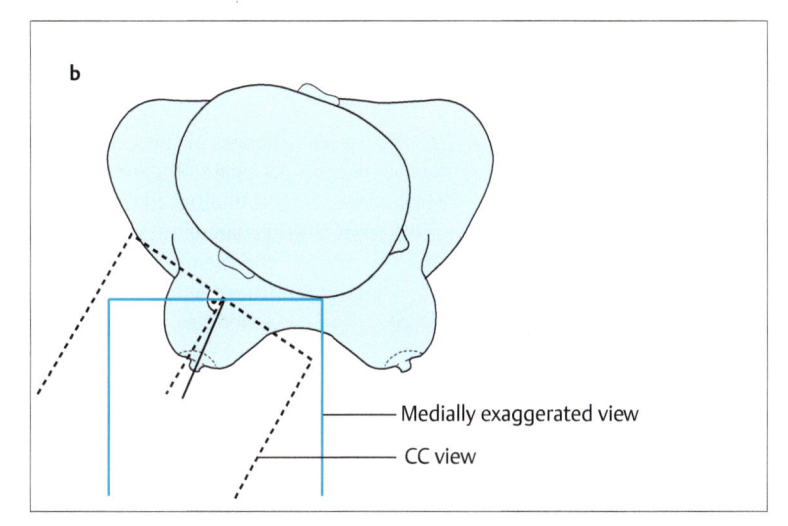

Fig. 3.19a–c

a The laterally exaggerated craniocaudal view is performed like the routine craniocaudal (CC) view, but the patient is rotated and faces the film holder obliquely so that the lateral breast tissue is included in the field of view. In contrast to the routine craniocaudal view, the medial breast tissue is excluded.

b The medially exaggerated view is performed with the patient rotated in the opposite direction to bring the medial breast tissue into the field of view.

c This externally exaggerated CC view reveals a small breast carcinoma that was projected over the pectoral muscle in the mediolateral oblique view. Only the externally exaggerated view could exactly localize the small breast carcinoma by visualizing it in a second projection.

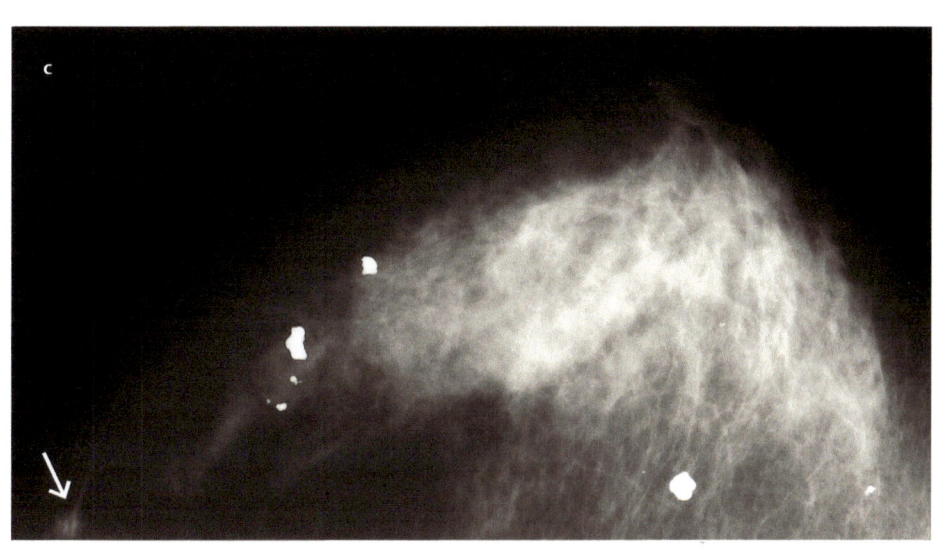

Exaggerated Medial Craniocaudal View

Purpose

The exaggerated medial craniocaudal view can be used to image medial findings very close to the chest wall that are difficult to include on the correctly positioned craniocaudal view.

Conducting the Examination

The image is obtained with the mammography unit in the same position as for the craniocaudal view. However, the patient is turned so that the medial breast is pulled onto the film holder, sacrificing the lateral aspect on the image.

Tangential View

Significance

Tangential views are valuable for detecting subcutaneous calcifications (**Fig. 3.20**). If the calcifications are in the skin or in the subcutaneous tissue, benign calcifications can be assumed. For this reason, definite intracutaneous or subcutaneous localization provides important information for the differential diagnosis of calcifications. The tangential view is also useful for displacing masses away from an overlying implant.

Conducting the Examination

When skin lesions are being assessed, phototiming may overexpose the skin. Therefore manually adjusting exposure settings may be appropriate in this situation.

Various options are available to localize calcifications clearly in subcutaneous or cutaneous tissue. One can attempt to find the true tangential view by taking several exposures. This method is not recommended because it is imprecise and exposes the patient to unnecessary radiation. Alternatively, a localizing plate with an alphanumeric grid can be used to compress the breast instead of the standard compression paddle. The selected breast projection (craniocaudal, caudocranial, mediolateral, or lateromedial) should have the area of calcifications nearest the fenestrated plate (**Fig. 3.20**). With the breast still compressed, this image is used as a guide and the area in which the calcifications are projected is marked. The gantry is then rotated and/or the breast rolled until this marker, with the localizing lights on, casts a shadow on the plate on which the breast is resting in this position. Then the beam is incident precisely tangential to the marked skin. If the calcifications in question are in the skin, they will be visualized in this location.

If only a small part of the body of the gland is fixed for a tangential view, *the breast may slip out of the compression device. A strip of double-sided adhesive tape, which is applied to the compression paddle and/or grid holder, may be helpful to avoid this.*

Cutaneous localization can also be achieved by stereotaxy. Using standard stereotactic images, the z-axis of the target point is calculated as lying at the surface of the skin.

Oblique View with Customized Settings

Although positioning for the standard views should include all the glandular tissue in screening examinations, palpable changes occasionally occur in locations that render visualization next to impossible (especially in locations close to the chest wall). Here, the radiologist may use almost any *customized angle of the mammography unit and patient position* that can hold the breast in a fixed position and visualizes the findings in question for interpretation.

Axillary View

This view is used to evaluate findings in the lower portion of the axilla not visualized in the oblique view (this is rare). It is usually done as a 30° oblique, using a small, rectangular compression paddle. The chest wall is not included. The exposure can be phototimed.

Cleavage View

The cleavage view (**Fig. 3.21**) is a rarely used one that visualizes the medial breast close to the chest wall particularly well. In this view, both breasts and the medial fold (cleavage) between them are compressed and imaged using a craniocaudal beam and a small compression cone. Since the photocell is not covered by the breast in this view, the exposure must be set manually.

Rolled Views

The rolled views can be used to determine the depth of a lesion detectable only in one plane.

If, for example, we roll the upper breast medially from a craniocaudal position, lesions in the superior quadrants will move medially, that is in the direction of the roll, whereas lesions located in the inferior quadrants will move laterally in the opposite direction.

Today, the imaging modalities for determining the depth of a lesion detectable in only one plane include mammographic stereotaxy, sonography, and contrast-enhanced MRI.

Rolled views can still be extremely helpful in determining whether dense areas detected primarily in one plane are real or represent superimposed structures (**Fig. 3.22**).

Positioning and Compression

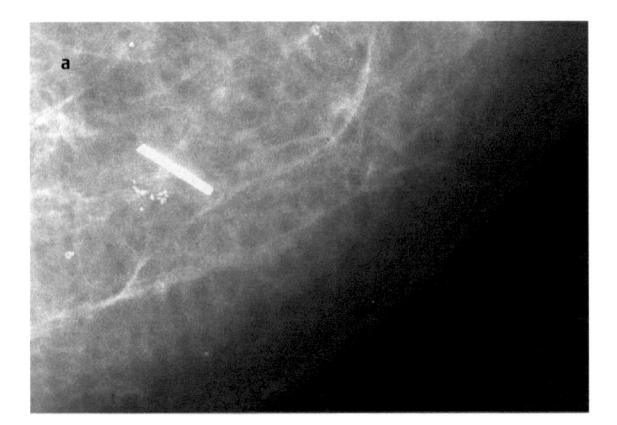

Fig. 3.20 a–d Mammogram demonstrating subcutaneous calcifications.

a The mediolateral oblique view shows a small cluster of presumably benign microcalcifications very close to the chest wall (arrow), which in the craniocaudal view appeared to be in the medial glandular tissue.

b To verify the subcutaneous location of the microcalcifications assumed on the basis of its morphology, the breast was compressed for a mediolateral oblique view. Using a fenestrated compression cone, a small marker was fixed against the skin above the cluster of microcalcifications.

c Then another mammogram was performed with the patient positioned in a craniocaudal view with the tube at a 15° angle. The direction of the beam and compression was selected so that the skin marker was imaged tangentially to the beam next to the breast.

d This craniocaudal view (magnifying a section of the skin) verifies that the microcalcifications are subcutaneous.

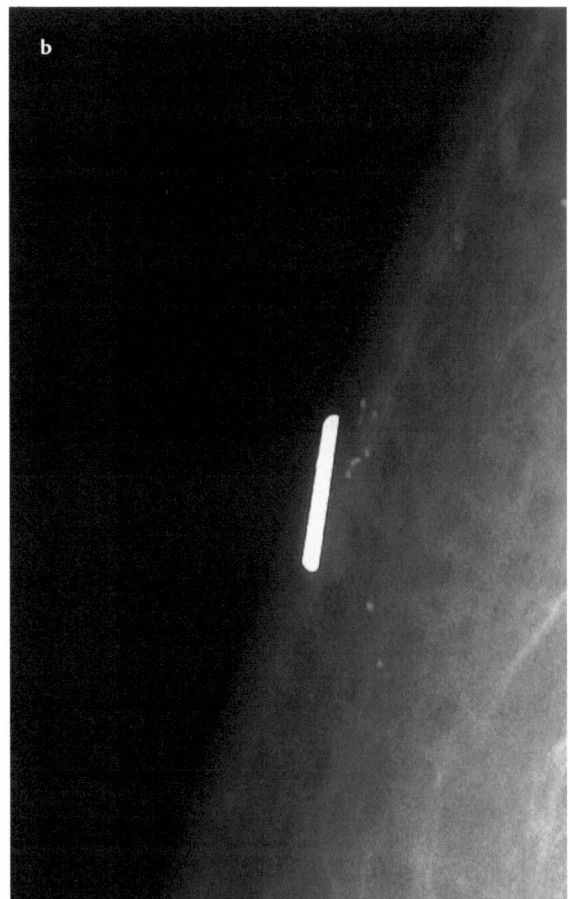

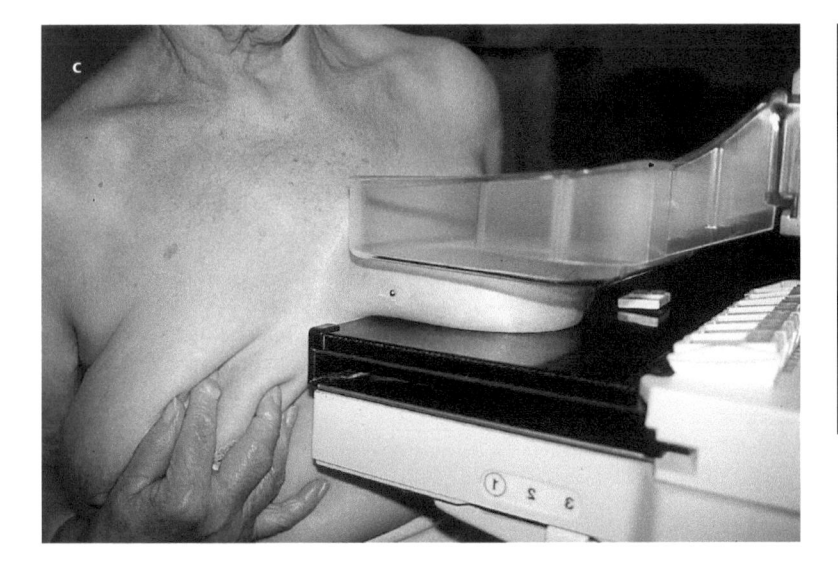

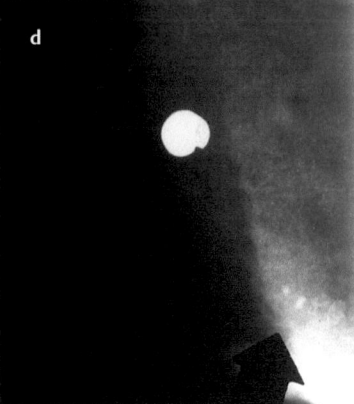

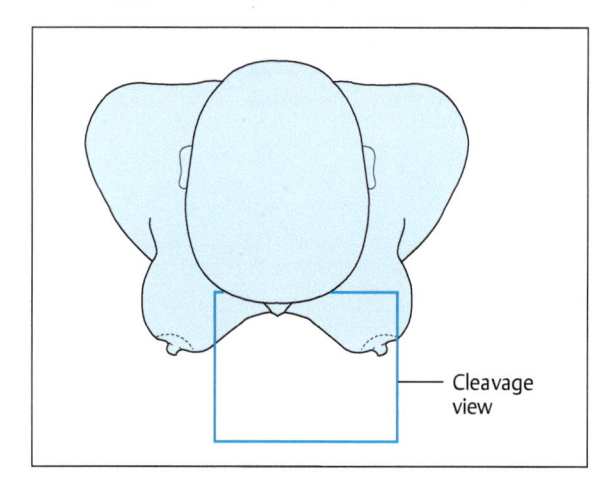

Fig. 3.21 In the cleavage view, both breasts and the medial fold between them are compressed and imaged. This view visualizes medial lesions very close to the chest wall.

Film Labeling

Mammograms have to be labeled with a permanent identification label containing the name and address of the institution, the patient's name and a unique patient identification number (e.g., medical record number, social security number, date of birth), and the date of the examination. Each film should be labeled left or right and the view should be specified with radiopaque markers placed on the film near the axilla.

The labeling abbreviations for positioning recommended by the American College of Radiology are as follows.

Right	R
Left	L
Mediolateral oblique	MLO
Craniocaudal	CC
90° lateral:	
• Mediolateral	ML
• Lateromedial	LM
Magnification	M (used as a prefix before the projection)
Exaggerated craniocaudal	XCC or Ext CC
Cleavage	CV
Axillary tail	AT
Tangential	TAN

Rolled views should be marked as such (e.g., rolled CC). We also recommend that the direction of rolling is indicated (e.g., by an arrow).

The film should also be labeled with the unique initials of the technologist who performed the mammogram. Each screen should be labeled with a unique identifying number or letter, so that dusty or defective screens can be identified readily.

Films should be labeled by flashing information on the film or using a sticker. It is recommended that the dose, or technical factors from which the dose can be calculated (kVp, mAs, target/filter combination, and compressed breast thickness), and parameters which allow the positioning to be reproduced (compression force, angle of obliquity on the mediolateral oblique view) should be included. If a facility has more than one unit, it is desirable to identify which unit was used. A paper sticker with the date of the examination is recommended so that different studies are easily identifiable.

Spot Compression

Definition

In spot compression (**Fig. 3.23a**), a small compression paddle is used to compress only the area of the breast of interest, with the beam collimated on this area of interest. We recommend not using too small a paddle and collimating in a way that allows visualization of sufficient surrounding tissue to countercheck whether the field of view was correctly chosen. Otherwise a significant risk of misinterpretation may exist. Spot compression can be performed in any imaging plane.

Advantages

(See **Figs. 3.23 and 3.24**.)
- *Dense areas resulting from summation of superimposed images can be spread out*; malignant foci and architectural distortion will mostly remain.
- Spreading of the surrounding parenchyma means that the outline of masses (possibly also of microcalcifications) is less obscured by superimposed tissue and may be better visualized. *Note*: Magnification may add information about the contours of masses.
- Better localized compression (reduction in the thickness to be penetrated) and, to a lesser extent, the collimation reduce scattered radiation and improve contrast.
- The increased compression makes its possible to decrease the distance between some structures and the image receptor and thus to decrease geometric blurring.
- Occasionally, findings close to the chest wall are more accessible with a small, round cone.

Positioning and Compression

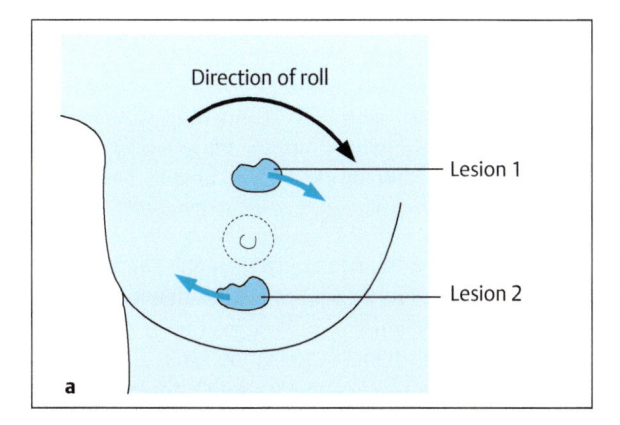

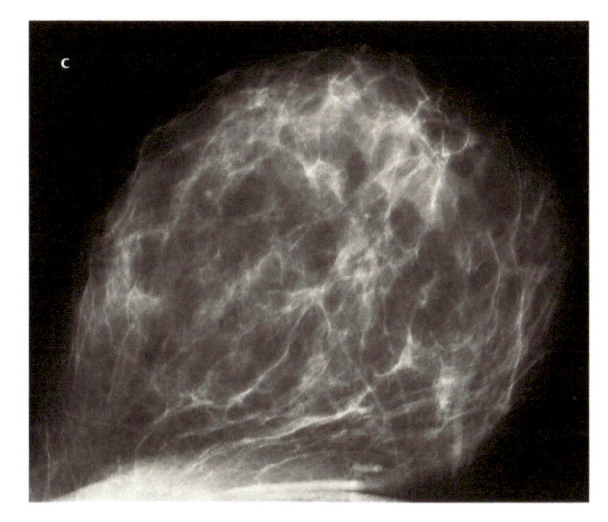

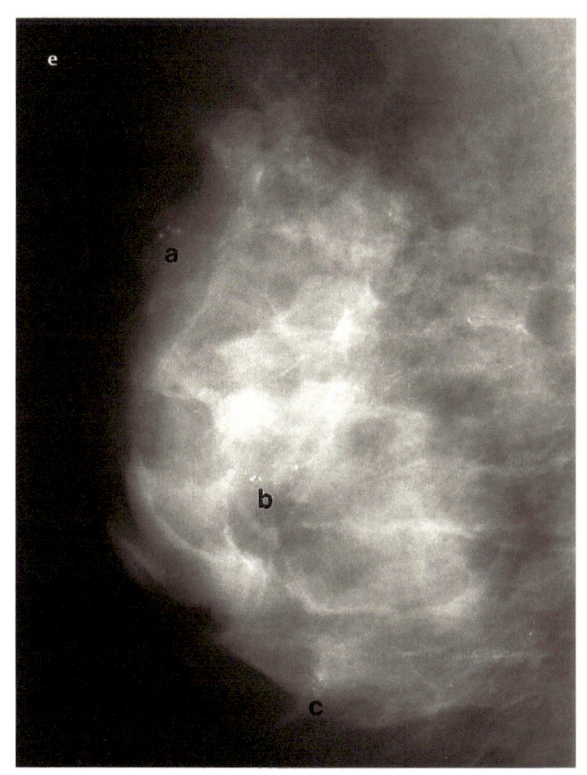

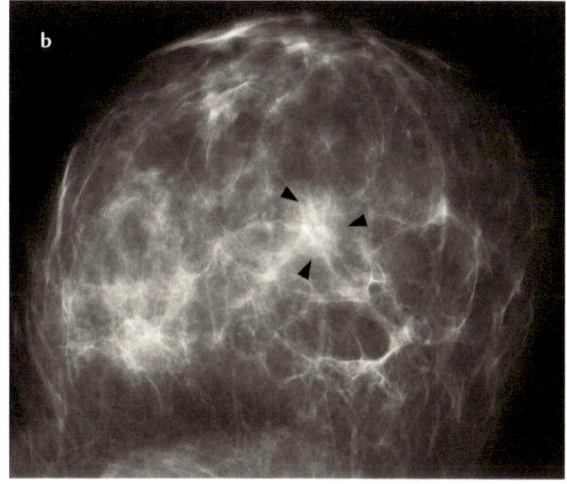

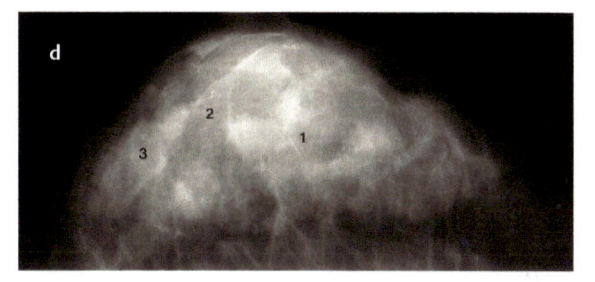

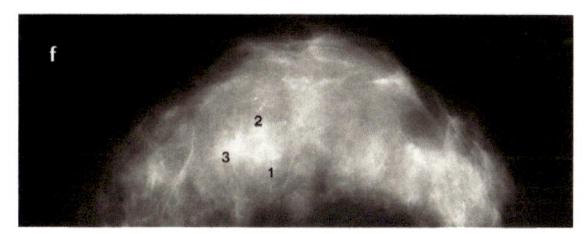

Fig. 3.22a–f

- **a** Principle of the rolled view shown with a craniocaudal view. If the upper breast is rolled medially, superior lesions (lesion 1) will move in the direction of the roll, whereas inferior lesions (lesion 2) will move in the opposite direction.
- **b** Patient with an uncertain density that appears in only one plane.
- **c** The rolled view reveals that the density was caused by superimposition.
- **d,e** This patient presented with three groups of indeterminate microcalcifications. **d** Craniocaudal view shows three groups of microcalcifications: 1, 2, and 3. **e** Oblique view also shows three groups of microcalcifications: a, b, and c. However based on the views and the morphology of the microcalcifications it was not clear which groups on the craniocaudal and oblique views corresponded. Thus, an exact localization was not possible. To choose the most appropriate approach for percutaneous biopsy, however, exact localization was needed.
- **f** Therefore, another craniocaudal view was obtained, for which the upper breast was rolled medially (the double arrows indicate direction of rolling). Group 1 rolls medially and therefore corresponds to group a (in the upper breast); group 2 stays and therefore corresponds to group b (mid-breast); group 3 rolls laterally and therefore is located in the lower breast (corresponding to group c). Such problems may be elegantly and reliably solved by tomosynthesis, where available.

63

Limits

(See **Fig. 3.25** and **Fig. 24.6d–f**.)

Unfortunately, some early cancers, including some lobular cancers, may also spread out using strong compression and may thus be missed. Furthermore, in large breasts it may be difficult to correctly position small compression paddles. To be sure that the correct area is identified we recommend that collimation is not too narrow.

Because of the above limits we also recommend combining compression views with other views such as mediolateral or rolled views.

Indications

- Differentiating dense areas resulting from summation of superimposed structures from real masses (**Figs. 3.23 and 3.24**)
- Imaging findings close to the chest wall

Magnification Technique

Definition

Magnification mammography involves the following:
- The breast is placed on a platform located at a defined distance from the grid holder (**Fig. 3.26**).
- The area of interest is compressed and the image field is collimated as described with spot compression.
- A small focal spot is selected and the grid removed.

Fundamental Considerations

The total resolution (definition) in an unmagnified image is limited by geometric blurring, resolution of the screen–film system and, in applicable cases, motion blurring.

Total resolution is also influenced by the contrast of the detail being imaged and by image noise.

Magnification mammography has the following effects (Berkowitz et al. 1989):

1. Magnifying details by the factor f and projecting them on the screen–film system improves that proportion of the resolution (definition) determined by the screen–film system by precisely this factor f.
2. Increasing the magnification while keeping the size of the focus constant would significantly increase the geometric blurring owing to the larger penumbra (geometric blurring). The geometric threshold resolution has definitely been reached when the size of the penumbra equals or exceeds that of an imaged detail. For this reason, magnification mammography requires a *microfocus with a nominal maximum value of 0.1–0.15* (depending on the magnification factor). The size of the focus in turn limits the maximum feasible *magnification factor to 1.4–2.0 on standard units*.
3. The minimal size of the focal spot is currently limited by the load rating of the microfocus.
4. Bearing in mind the limited power of the microfocus, we recommend the following measures to minimize exposure time (in the interest of reducing motion blurring and dose, and avoiding reciprocity law failure of the film):
   - Use a faster low-dose screen–film system (e.g., sensitivity class 25. At the given magnification factor, the screen–film system no longer influences maximum resolution).
   - Increase the peak kilovoltage by about 2 kVp compared with the corresponding nonmagnified exposure. This allows a decrease in the exposure time (mAs) while the density remains comparable to the nonmagnified view. Otherwise, the small focal spot would require a long exposure, and patient motion may be a problem.
5. To maintain an adequate signal-to-noise ratio, the dose required to produce the image increases as the square of magnification factor. If all other parameters are kept constant, magnifying the image by a factor of 1.4 will double the dose, and magnifying the image by a factor of 2 will quadruple the dose. Minimizing the dose is necessary in the interest of minimizing the patient's exposure to radiation and to avoid exceeding the load rating of the microfocus. This is achieved by increasing the voltage by about 2 kV and eliminating the grid.

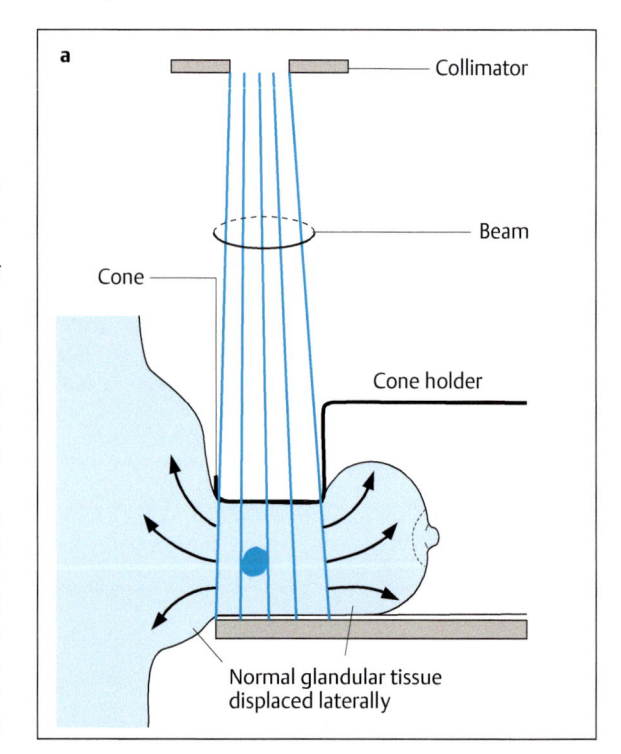

Fig. 3.23a–e

a Spot compression in the craniocaudal (CC) view.

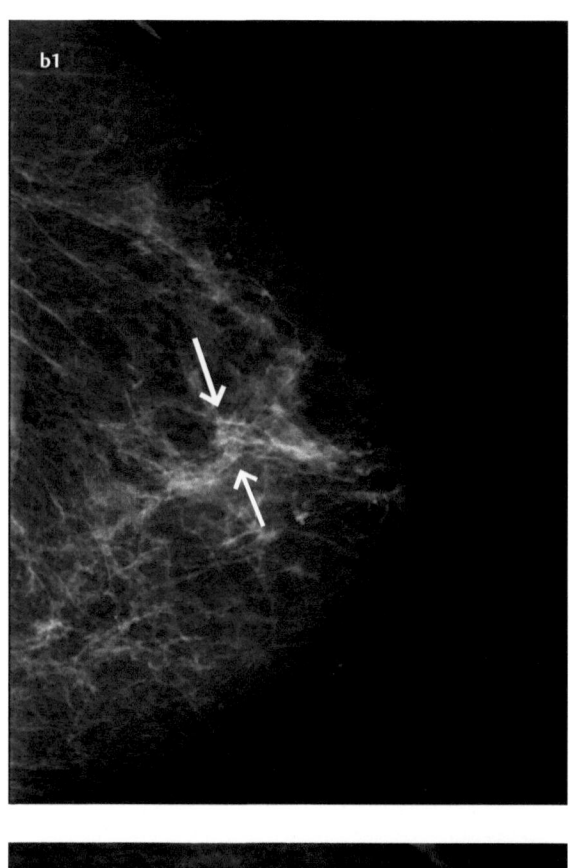

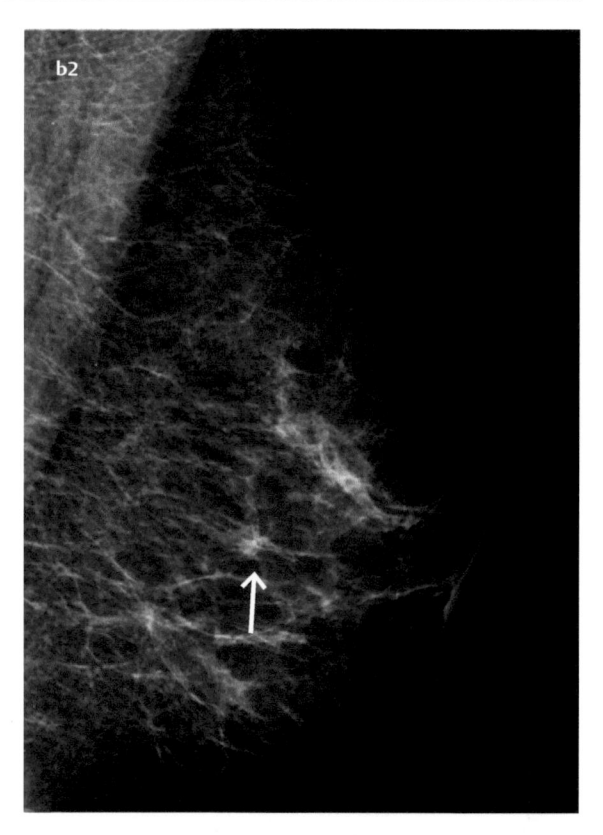

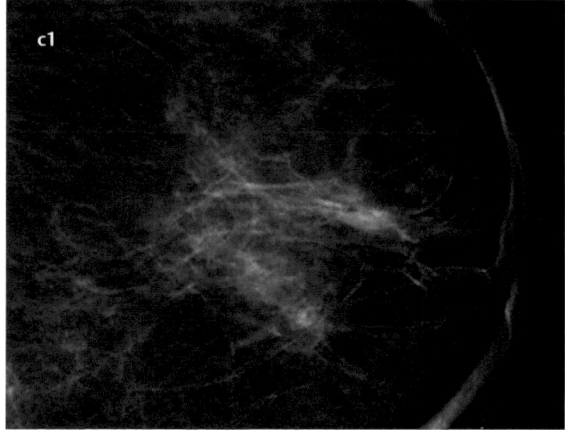

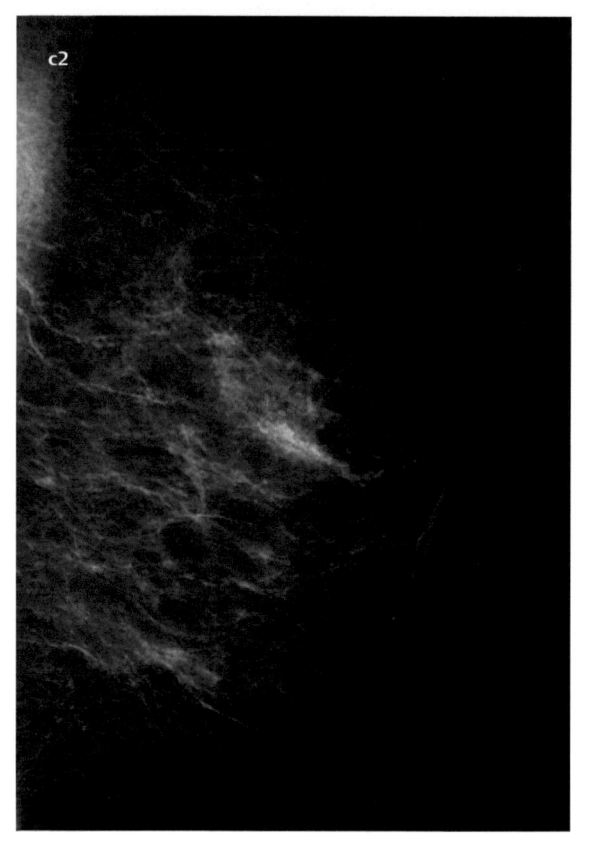

Positioning and Compression

b1 Questionable architectural distortion: CC view.
b2 Mediolateral oblique view (arrows point to the questionable abnormality).
c1 On the CC spot view the questionable architectural distortion resolves completely.
c2 It also resolves completely on the left mediolateral view and can thus be explained as superimposition (proven by follow-up).

Fig. 3.23 d–e ▷

◁ continued

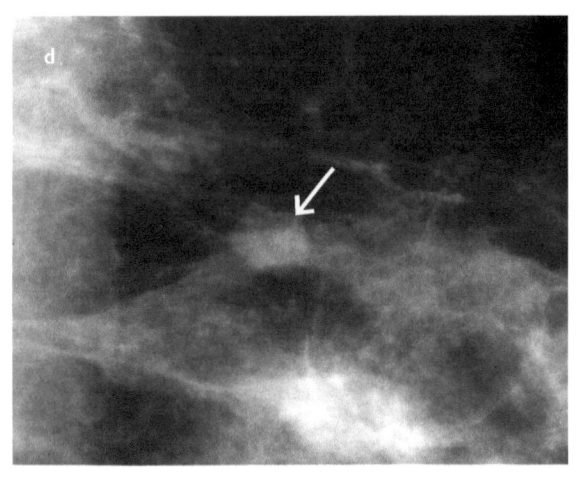

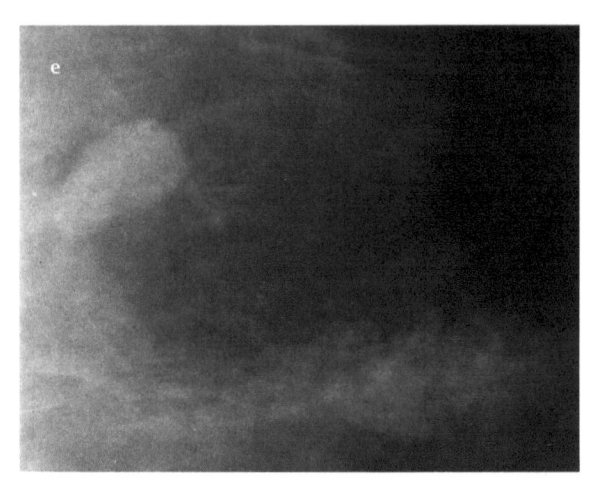

d,e The mediolateral oblique view shows an indeterminate mass measuring 7 mm located at the superior margin of the parenchyma (**d**). Spot compression reveals this to be a smooth-contoured lesion, compatible with a lymph node (**e**).

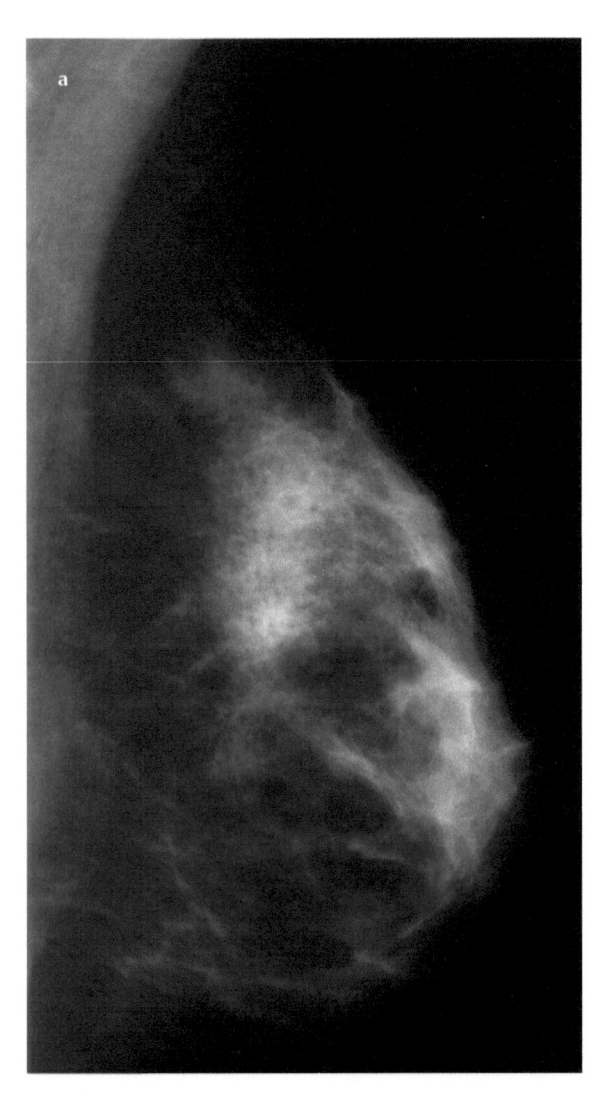

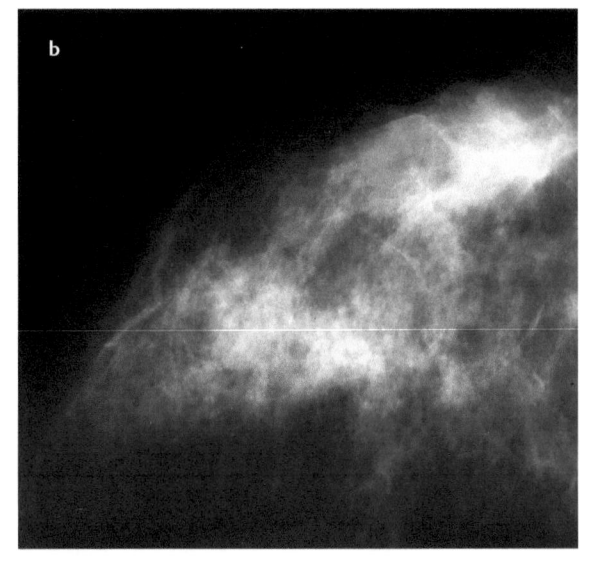

Fig. 3.24a–d

a On the mediolateral oblique view of this screening mammogram a discrete architectural distortion was noted about 4 cm behind the nipple.
b On the craniocaudal view the architectural distortion cannot be clearly identified. Therefore, craniocaudal spot compression views were performed beginning laterally.
c This craniocaudal compression view of the patient's left lateral breast allows identification of a starlike architectural distortion. The area was excised after preoperative wire localization.
d The specimen radiograph demonstrates the architectural distortion even more clearly.
Histology: Radial scar with intermediate-grade ductal carcinoma in situ.

Fig. 3.24 c–d ▷

Positioning and Compression

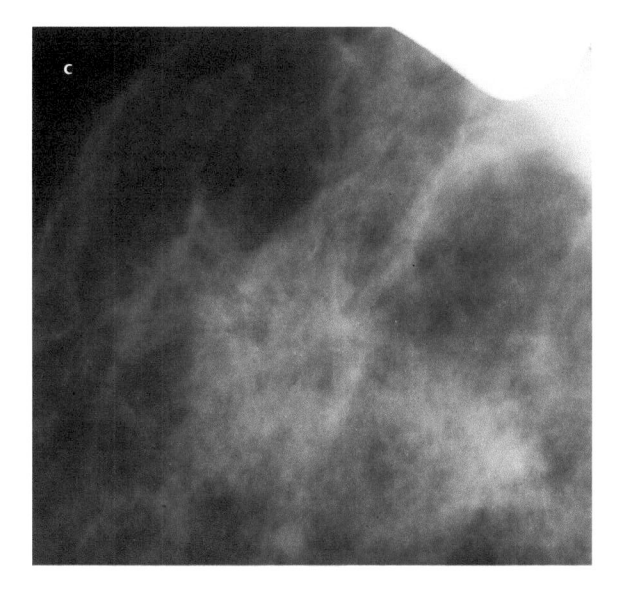

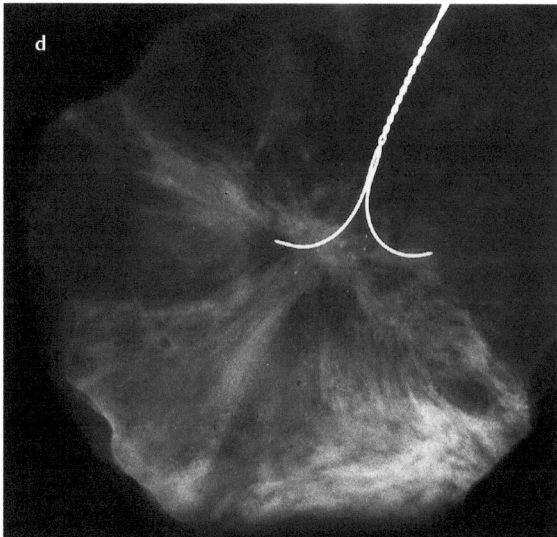

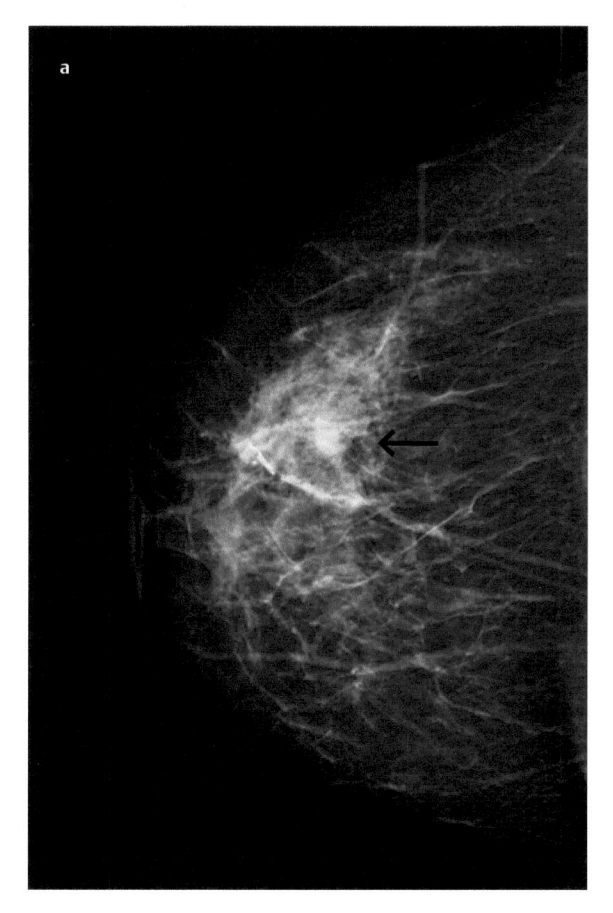

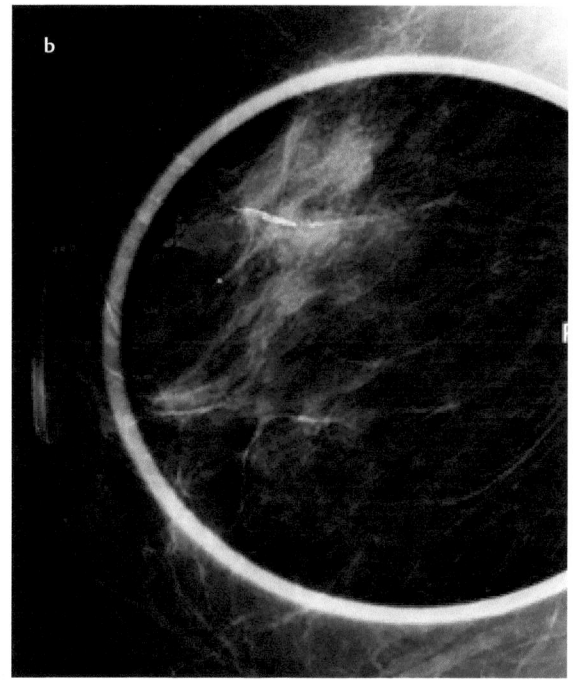

Fig. 3.25a–f Misleading result of spot view.

a On the craniocaudal view a nodular density is noted laterally.
b On the spot view the nodular density spreads out well and appears to resolve. The spot view suggests that there is just nodular benign tissue, no prominent lesion. Ultrasound imaging, however, showed a hypoechoic density which by core needle biopsy proved to be a papillary ductal carcinoma in situ (see also **Fig. 15.6**).

Fig. 3.25 c–f ▷

◁ continued

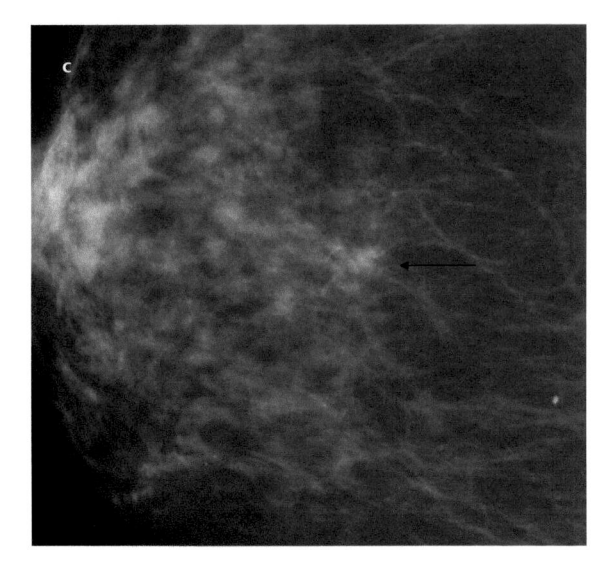

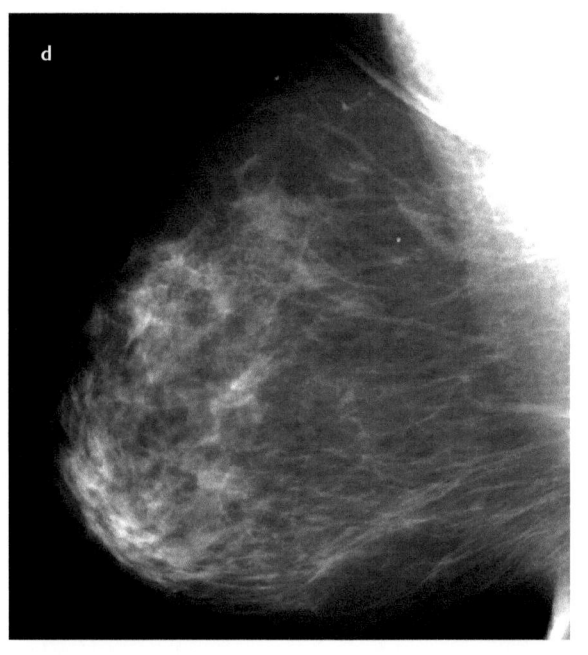

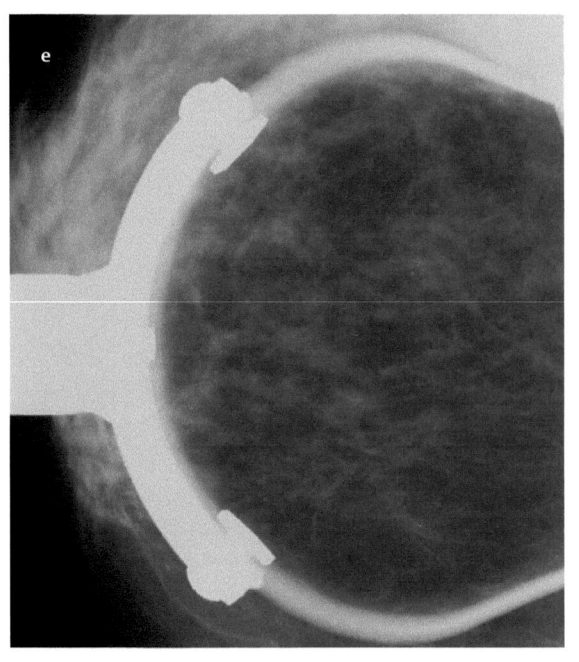

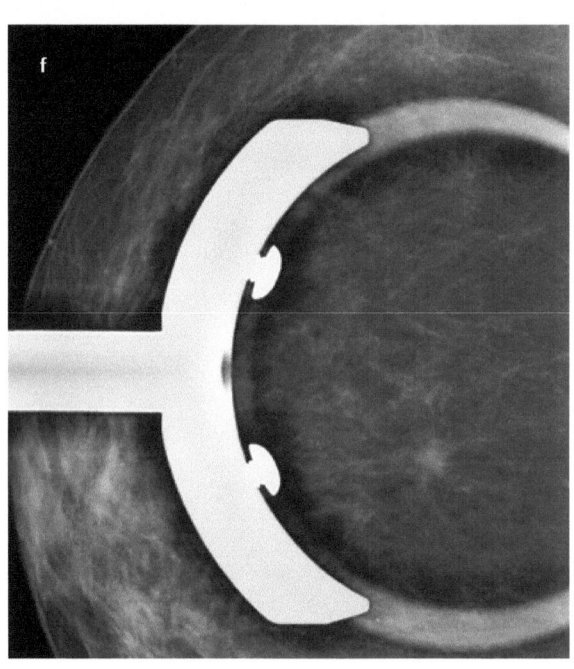

c On the craniocaudal view of the screening mammogram a faint density or architectural distortion was suspected on this view only.

d No abnormality was noted on this mediolateral oblique view.

e On the spot compression the faint density and suspected architectural distortion disappeared completely. The ultrasound examination was negative, too. Therefore no further views (mediolateral) were obtained (possibly a wrong decision). However short-term follow-up at 6 months was recommended.

f Six months later a density persisted on the craniocaudal spot view. The lesion could then be detected on ultrasound as well and proved to be a 5-mm lobular carcinoma.
Note: Small lobular carcinomas may disappear with strong compression, so spot views in particular may be misleading in very early lesions.

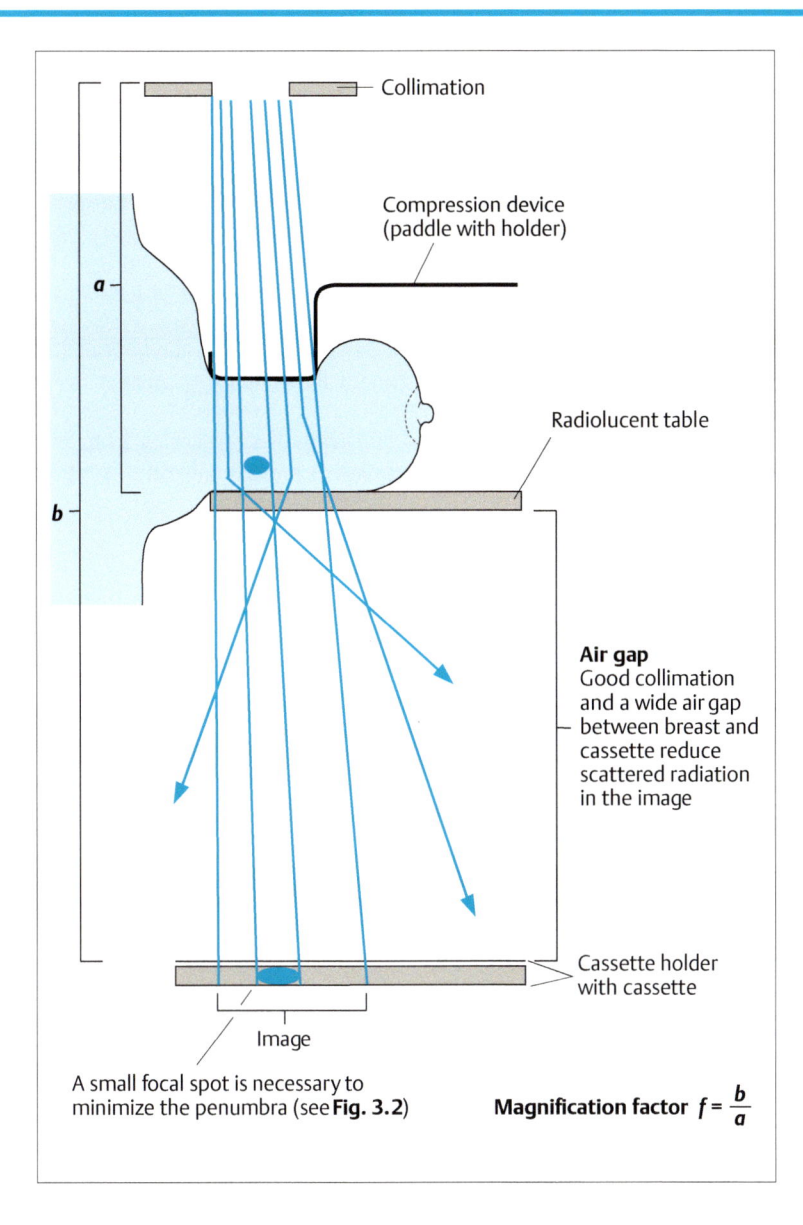

Fig. 3.26 Magnification mammography.

Labels in figure:
- Collimation
- Compression device (paddle with holder)
- Radiolucent table
- Air gap: Good collimation and a wide air gap between breast and cassette reduce scattered radiation in the image
- Cassette holder with cassette
- Image
- A small focal spot is necessary to minimize the penumbra (see **Fig. 3.2**)
- **Magnification factor** $f = \dfrac{b}{a}$

6. For magnification mammography, the grid is removed. This is necessary to limit the radiation dose to the breast and to reduce the exposure time, which otherwise might become very long (because of the increased dose required for magnification and because of the limited load rating of the small focus). To avoid motion blurring and reciprocity law failure, the exposure time should not be too long. Removing the grid results in decreased radiation and shorter exposure time with less patient motion.
7. Scatter reduction, which improves contrast in magnification mammography, is achieved by the "air gap" combined with good collimation. The air gap itself allows reduction of scatter since part of the scattered radiation will pass beyond the film. Even though magnification without collimation is possible, good collimation significantly enhances the effect of the air gap. Only with good collimation (≤ 5 cm) can the lack of the grid be compensated by the air gap.

Advantages

- Improved resolution of fine details by overcoming blurring due to the screen–film system.
- Magnified details are easier to observe, that is, there is more information on the image receiver of the area imaged.
- When spot compression is used along with magnification, structures are less obscured by displacing the superimposed tissue.

- Dense areas representing summation of superimposed tissue can be differentiated from real findings (see also Spot Compression).

Disadvantages

- Magnification mammography increases the dose required, but this is largely compensated for by using a low-dose screen–film system, increasing the kVp, and eliminating the grid.
- Contrast could be decreased owing to the lack of a grid and the higher kVp setting. This can largely be compensated for with good compression of the area of interest (pushing superimposed tissue aside) and good collimation (air gap reduces scattered radiation).

Indications

- Determining whether microcalcifications are present.
- Analyzing the geometry and distribution of microcalcifications (**Fig. 3.27**).
- Detecting additional fine calcifications for improving the differential diagnosis of microcalcifications.
- Excluding or verifying the presence of multiple foci and assessing the extent of carcinomas with microcalcifications (**Fig. 3.28**).
- For analysis of the contours of masses and for their differentiation as smooth, lobulated, or spiculated

For summation of superimposed structures from real masses, spot compression is preferred, because it offers higher image contrast (see **Fig. 3.23d,e**).

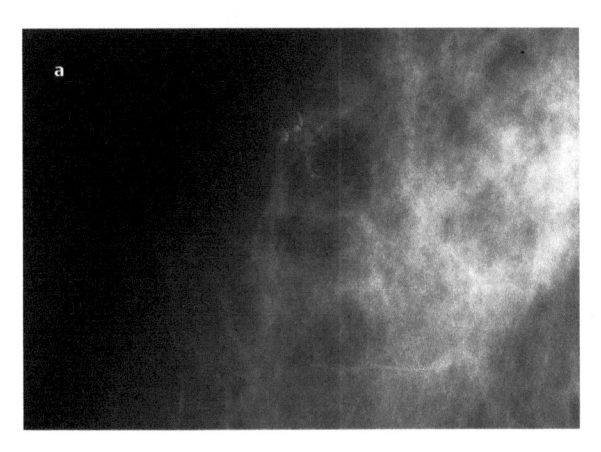

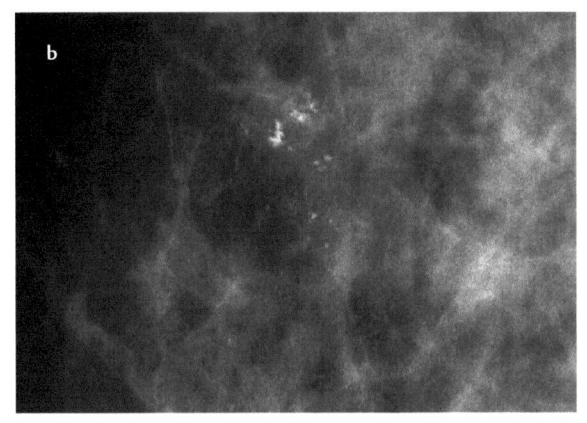

Fig. 3.27a,b The craniocaudal view shows a group of pleomorphic microcalcifications at the margin of the parenchyma (**a**). An additional magnification view (**b**) clearly reveals them to be suggestive of malignancy.

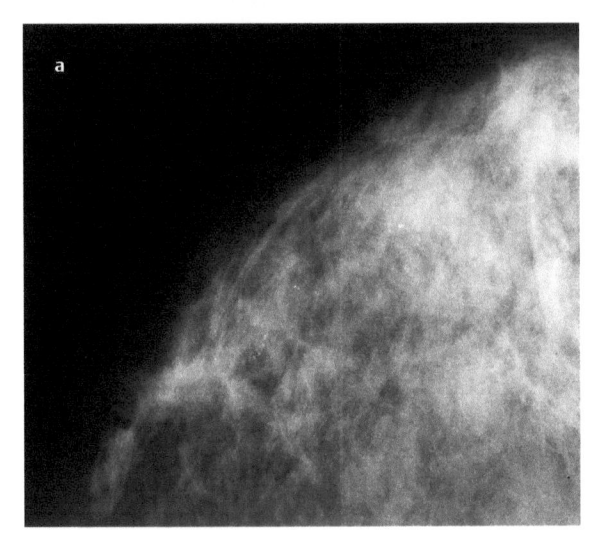

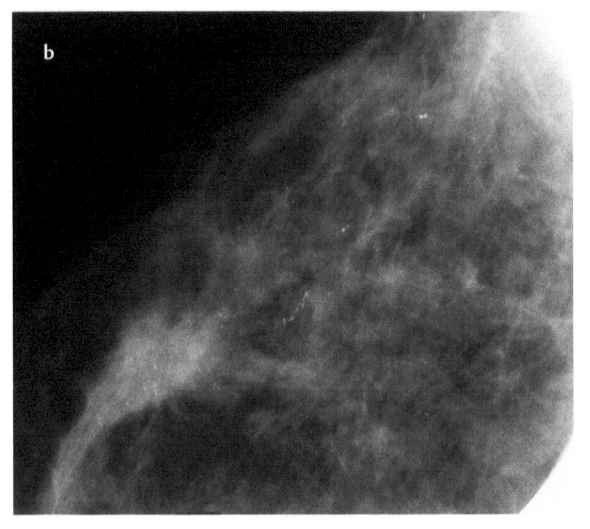

Fig. 3.28a,b The craniocaudal view reveals a focal density with ill-defined contour with central and marginal microcalcification (**a**). The magnification mammogram (**b**) with spot compression clearly demonstrates highly suspicious spiculations. In addition to the above-mentioned suspicious microcalcifications, more pleomorphic microcalcifications are shown on this magnification view extending toward the nipple.

Positioning of Breasts with Implants

Surgical technique and type and location of the implant determine the available mammographic imaging options. Following subcutaneous mastectomy and implant placement, usually only a small amount of tissue will remain around the implant. If the breast tissue has been completely removed, mammography is usually not necessary. The distribution and architecture of the breast parenchyma can vary considerably. After augmentation mammoplasty, all of the breast tissue that was originally present will usually be superficial to the implant. Achieving good results in mammography depends upon the type of previous surgery and the type and position of implant material.

Standard mammography of these women usually requires manual exposure settings for those views that include the implants, since the implant usually overlies the phototimer, attenuating the X-ray beam and causing the image to be overexposed.

The augmented breast should not be imaged as a two-view screening study but should be adapted to the individual anatomy. Full imaging of the augmented breast may require up to four views, not just the routine two views. Depending on the anatomy and the mobility of the breast tissue surrounding the implant, a combination of standard mediolateral oblique and craniocaudal views of the breasts, including and/or excluding the implant, may be considered. Whatever combination is chosen, the goal should be to image as much breast tissue as possible without superimposed implant.

Compression used should be adequate to stabilize the breast so that there is no motion on the image. Compression beyond this should not be used for fear of rupturing the implant. The risk of implant rupture increases with increasing age of the implant and with increased capsular contracture.

Technologists performing mammograms on patients with implant should be aware of possible complications. Also, patients should be informed likewise.

The above-mentioned views excluding the implant should be performed according to the procedure described by Eklund and Cardenosa (1992): pull the glandular tissue anteriorly away from the implant, push the implant posteriorly, and gradually slide the compression paddle over the breast tissue anterior to the implant. This pushes the implant posteriorly, allowing better compression of the glandular tissue itself (**Fig. 3.29**). Imaging should be done in the craniocaudal and mediolateral oblique or 90° lateral projections. It should be possible to obtain these displacement views in around 80% of women with implants. In those women who have hard, noncompressable implants (capsular contracture) or for whom the displacement maneuver is painful, it will not

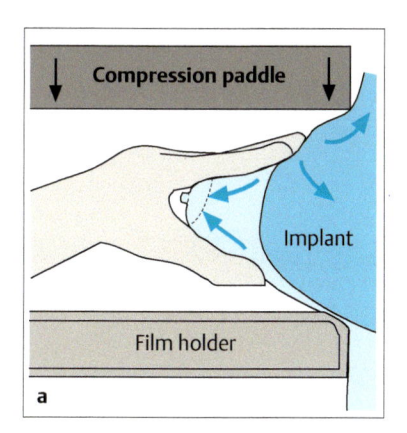

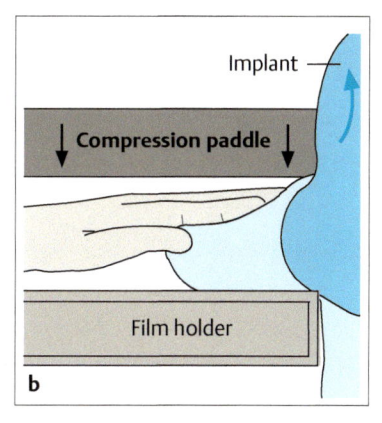

Fig. 3.29a–d Displacement method of imaging a breast with an implant following augmentation mammoplasty.

a,b The glandular tissue is pulled forward away from the implant, which is displaced posteriorly, as the technologist lowers the compression paddle over the breast tissue and compresses it.
c This displaces the implant posteriorly so that it no longer covers the glandular tissue.
d The nondisplaced view including the implant is shown.

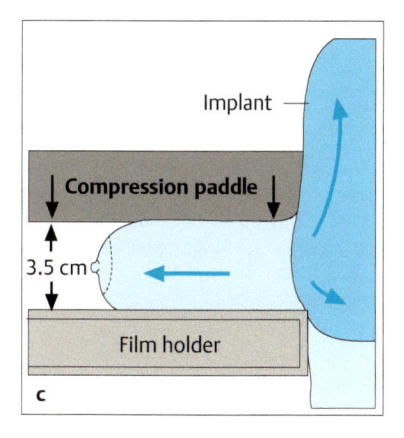

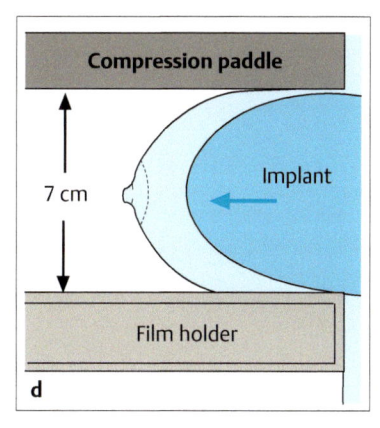

3 Mammography

be possible to obtain these additional two views. Since these views are done with the implant out of the way, phototiming can be used.

Mammography as described by Eklund is generally no longer possible after subcutaneous mastectomy and breast reconstruction. Mammography can still be performed to clarify clinical findings, but the radiologist should be aware that only the tissue layers tangential to the beam which are not obscured by the implant can be assessed. For this reason, mammography is usually performed in several planes, though it will not be possible to image all of the tissue surrounding the implant in these patients. If mammographic imaging of all or part of the breast is not possible, supplementary sonography may be considered. If malignancy or recurrence is suspected, MRI may also be very helpful (Heinig et al. 1997).

Imaging of the Specimen

(See **Fig. 3.30**.)

Nonpalpable, mammographically confirmed lesions requiring excision must be localized preoperatively (see Chapter 8). After excision, specimen radiographs—that is, radiographs of the surgical specimen—are obtained to verify whether the mammographic findings leading to

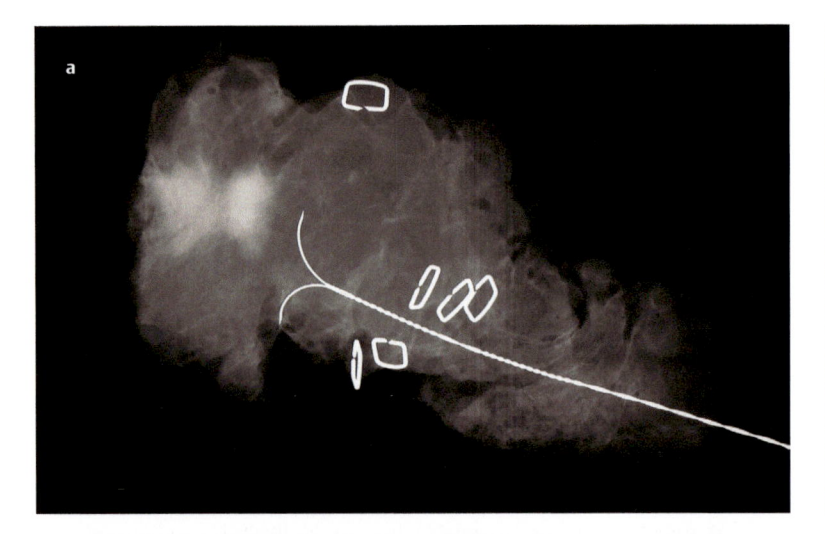

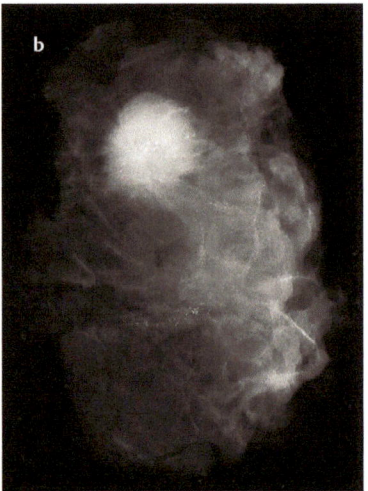

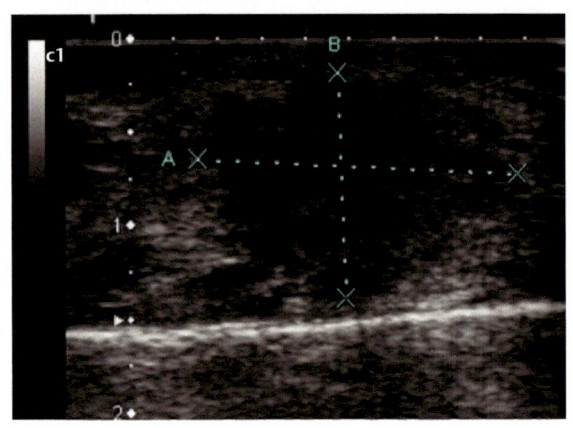

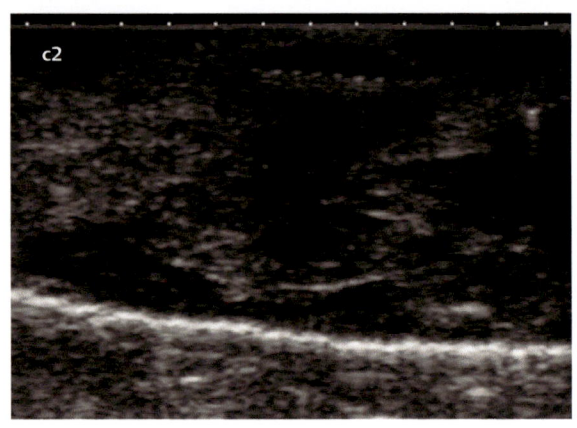

Fig. 3.30a–e Specimen imaging.

a The specimen radiograph should be oriented as agreed with the cooperating surgeon. Some surgeons indicate the different margins (e.g., anterior margin, lateral margin, margin adjacent to the nipple) by clips; others use threads of different colors. In this case the tumor is located eccentrically in the specimen and touches its margin. Knowledge of the exact orientation is important to give a correct recommendation for further excision.

b This specimen radiograph shows a 17-mm mass and two remote foci of microcalcifications. Histologically the mass corresponded to an invasive ductal carcinoma. It was surrounded by an extensive intraductal component. Furthermore another focal ductal carcinoma in situ was verified 15 mm from the invasive tumor.

c Specimen ultrasound imaging: view showing a central slice (**c1**) of an excised tumor. (The bright echo shows the support, on which the specimen was placed for the ultrasound examination.) In a more peripheral slice of the tumor, part of the wire with multiple windings is seen.

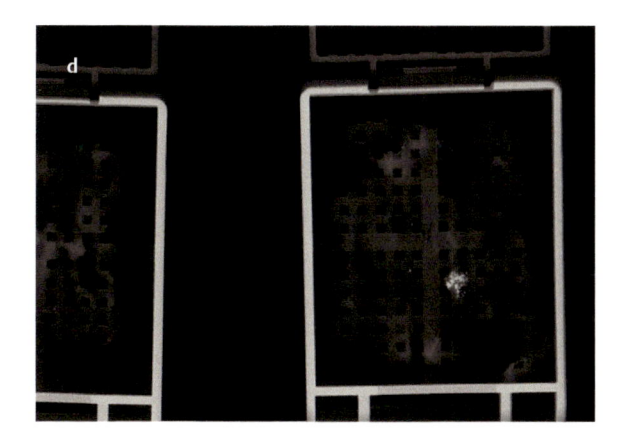

d After vacuum-assisted breast biopsy, specimen radiography of the acquired cores should always be performed, if the lesion in question consisted of or contained microcalcifications. Some small lesions may be completely visualized within one or a few cores, as in this case of a small fibroadenoma with dystrophic microcalcifications.

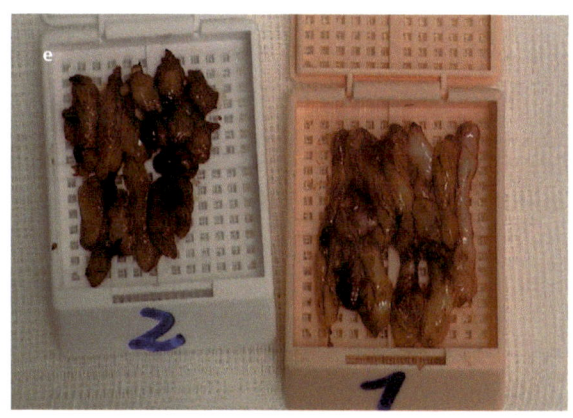

e We arrange the specimens in small plastic boxes which are provided by the pathology department and which (after being closed) can be automatically processed. Parallel orientation of the cores may be helpful to the pathologist for interpreting ductal pathology and extension. When imaged unclosed, the pattern of the box does not interfere with the radiologic interpretation. If several boxes are filled with specimens (as this is mostly the case) the boxes are numbered.

the excision are confirmed and to identify the location of the lesion in the specimen for histologic analysis. If the biopsied lesion is malignant and it extends to the margin of the specimen, specimen radiography can also be used to suggest the need for further surgical excision (Samuels et al. 1990, Rose et al. 1991, Graham et al. 1994).

Specimen radiography is also indicated for specimens obtained from percutaneous biopsies of microcalcifications. The specimen radiograph or a high-quality copy of it should accompany the biopsy specimen to the pathology department. That way the pathologist can verify the type, number, and arrangement of microcalcifications to be correlated within the specimens obtained. If, with the standard preparation, he or she cannot correlate the findings, the specimen should be further analyzed. If necessary the complete material may have to be worked up. The arrangement and preparation of the specimens should always be agreed with the cooperating pathologist.

Specimen radiography can be performed using a mammography unit or a Faxitron—a tabletop X-ray unit designed for specimen radiography. If a mammography unit is used, manual settings instead of automatic exposure settings should be employed.

Compression of the specimen improves the image, especially when the biopsy has been performed for an uncalcified mass. Compression equalizes differences in thickness, reduces scattered radiation, and spreads out the overlying tissue.

A radiograph in a second plane might help to localize small foci of disease or to determine whether the lesion has been transected during surgery. Owing to the geometry of the specimen, a specimen radiograph in the second plane is, however, often not possible and is not standard. Areas in the specimen that require histologic analysis should be indicated for the pathologist so they will not be overlooked.

For specimen radiography the specimen should be oriented as agreed with the interdisciplinary team. For optimum orientation, the surgeon may attach threads of different color or length to the specimen and indicate the cranial and lateral margins as well as the margin pointing toward the nipple. Alternatively, differing numbers of suture clips may be used to indicate the margins.

Specimen radiography after surgery of microcalcifications should be performed using magnification. This provides additional information about further extremely small microcalcifications and their relationship to the margins. In breast-conserving treatment of carcinoma, this is important for determining the extent of tumor and its proximity to the margin of the excised specimen. However, assessment of a mass surrounded by dense breast tissue may be difficult. Furthermore, areas removed because of asymmetry may not be identified with certainly on the specimen radiograph.

In cases where a mass is visible only on ultrasound examination, specimen sonography may be considered to countercheck for correct excision.

Finally, it must be remembered that in some cases the full extent of tumor may be visible only histologically. Therefore, correct and complete excision can only be assessed by combined evaluation of the preoperative mammogram, the specimen radiograph, and the histopathologic result.

Radiologic examination of the paraffin blocks is indicated whenever histopathologic examination of a biopsy performed for mammographically detected microcalcifications fails to reveal these calcifications since the standard procedure involves microscopic examination of only representative sections of the biopsy. Radiologic examination of the paraffin block will reveal whether microcalcifications are present in the part of the biopsy that was not examined under the microscope. Histopathologic workup has to continue until correlation of the histopathologic and the imaging finding is assured or until the complete specimen has been worked up.

If any doubts exist concerning correct or complete excision, a repeat mammogram is recommended.

Mammography may be performed in the early postoperative period without causing any undue pain. However, only compression sufficient to stabilize the breast should be used. Rarely, microcalcifications may be washed out with the blood (e.g., during vacuum-assisted breast biopsy) or microcalcifications may be lost during cutting of the specimen in the pathology department. If the specimen is completely worked up and if the microcalcifications are removed from the breast (as shown on the postoperative or postinterventional films), no further measures are needed, since after complete workup of the histopathologic specimen, malignant changes causing the microcalcifications would reliably have been detected.

If, owing to postoperative changes, removal of the mass or density in question is uncertain, MRI shortly after surgery (optimally within the first 10 days) may be helpful.

Quality Factors

Hardware Factors that Influence Image Quality

The American College of Radiology (ACR) as well as European Guidelines have recommended specifications for new mammography equipment. These requirements and other important hardware factors that influence image quality are summarized and discussed in the following section. More detailed information is available in the applicable literature (Perry et al. 2006, ACR-AAPM-SIIM practice guideline 2007).

Generator and Tube Power

Adequate generator or tube output is required to achieve sufficiently short exposure times, particularly for thick and dense breasts and for magnification mammography. Most quality mammography units achieve 4–5 kW.

The required power also depends on the target and filter material used. When tungsten and rhodium targets are used, the change in radiation quality is enough to penetrate even thick and dense breasts using less power than with conventional molybdenum tubes and filters.

Insufficient power requires excessively long exposures times (> 2 seconds), which result in motion blurring. Moreover, insufficient power disproportionately increases the exposure time and radiation dose required for adequate optical density (reciprocity law failure) when using screen–film. If the automatic exposure control system is unable to compensate for this effect, then an underexposed image will result.

Before installing a mammography unit, it is advisable to check the electrical system on the premises for voltage fluctuations. Mammography units cannot compensate for voltage drops; fluctuations in radiation quality will result, even when settings remain constant.

Because of the need to keep the voltage constant over time and, furthermore, because of the short exposure times required for low-dose screen–film systems, newer units are equipped with high-frequency generators.

Resolution

The ACR requires measurement of a bar pattern 45 mm above the breast support surface of the unit, within 1 cm of the chest wall and centered laterally. At this point resolution should be 11 lp/mm when the pattern is oriented with the bars perpendicular to the cathode–anode axis of the X-ray tube, and 13 lp/mm when parallel to this axis.

For digital mammography the use of bar patterns is less reliable since the frequency of bars resolved will depend on the orientation of the pattern to the pixel matrix. Consequently, more routine use is being made of the modulation transfer function as a quantitative measure of resolution.

Magnification Technique

Magnification mammography has become increasingly important. Studies have demonstrated that magnification mammography permits better analysis of microcalcifications, better visualization of the extent of carcinomas, and more reliable exclusion of malignancy. Most importantly, magnification mammography can reduce the number of unnecessary diagnostic biopsies. For this reason, breast imaging facilities, which are used for problem solving, must be able to perform magnification mammography. This requires an additional focus with a rated size less than or equal to 0.1–0.15 depending on the magnification factor, an insert for positioning the breast at a distance from the cassette, and a collimator. Magnification should be between 1.5× and 2.0×. Greater magnification may result in blurring due to long exposure times and increased geometric blurring. The dose also may become excessive.

Radiation Quality

The requirement that voltage must be regulated emphasizes the importance of radiation quality adapted to match the thickness and density of the breast.

The voltage settings required to achieve a certain desired radiation quality will vary depending on the mammography unit, target, filter, and generator, and thus are not necessarily comparable.

The ACR recommends that the X-ray source assembly include a molybdenum target, a beryllium window of 1.5 mm thickness or less, and a molybdenum filter. Alternate combinations can be used if they can achieve comparable diagnostic quality with equal or reduced radiation dose.

Most modern mammography units offer a choice of various target/filter combinations to achieve the ideal radiation energy for the breast thickness and density to be penetrated. An autoselect mode is provided to aid in selecting the optimum parameter combination.

Radiation Protection and Field Limitation

Use of a moving grid is specified in the regulations to achieve the reduction in scattered radiation necessary to ensure sufficient contrast.

Grid lines should not be evident and should not degrade images obtained of the ACR phantom. Grids should be available in both 18 × 24 cm and 24 × 30 cm sizes.

The required collimation of the useful beam is intended to protect the chest wall from excessive radiation exposure. This value is verified during the acceptance inspection and in routine quality control testing.

The image receptor must be completely exposed on the side close to the chest. The X-ray field may not extend more than 3 mm beyond the edge of the image receptor on the chest wall side (to protect the chest wall from excessive radiation).

X-ray attenuation in the compression paddle, grid table, and film or CR cassette vary between manufacturers. Exact specifications should be obtained, since high attenuation in the grid table and cassette unnecessarily increases the radiation exposure of the breast. The ACR recommends that all materials between the X-ray filter and the breast should not absorb the X-ray beam by more than 20%.

Exposure

The option of an automatic exposure control system is mandatory for mammography equipment, because it minimizes the number of incorrect exposures for routine mammography. The manual adjustment option is required as well. It is needed for achieving good exposure with small breasts that do not completely cover the photocell, and breasts with implants.

The quality of the automatic exposure control system greatly affects image quality. Only a good automatic exposure control system can achieve a reproducible, constant mean optical density regardless of the thickness and density of the breast. Failure to sufficiently equalize differences in thickness and density will mean that voluminous breasts and breasts with dense glandular tissue will be underexposed. Where the automatic exposure control system does not compensate sufficiently, an experienced radiologic technologist must make manual adjustment with the correction key. This makes it more difficult to achieve reproducible optimum exposure settings.

A medical physicist can verify the quality of an automatic exposure control system by using it to image Plexiglas plates of varying thickness. Differences in the mean optical density may not exceed agreed action limits and should produce reproducible exposures.

Even an optimally functioning automatic exposure control system will produce correctly exposed mammograms only when the photocell lies under a representative area of the breast (generally in the anterior third of the breast). Unfortunately, sometimes the design of the unit itself restricts the options for positioning of the photocell. In routine use, these design restrictions can have a detrimental effect similar to that of an automatic exposure control system that cannot properly compensate for differences in breast thickness and density.

In modern digital units the automatic exposure control can be set up to provide a constant contrast-to-noise ratio with increasingly compressed breast thickness, or a compromise "low-dose" configuration in which the contrast-to-noise ratio is allowed to decrease slowly with increasingly compressed breast thickness in return for a dose saving for the largest breasts. These functions are achieved using a complex set of relationships between kVp, target/filter combination, and phototiming, which use inputs from the compression paddle position as well as energy-sensitive measurements of radiation transmission through the breast. Some designs use the output from the image receptor itself to provide a signal to the automatic exposure control, and this can be configured in several ways using software to provide a range of sensor patterns or automatically locate the densest area of the breast to provide a reference signal.

Influence of the Screen–Film System and Film Processing on Image Quality

In addition to hardware factors, the choice of screen–film system and proper film processing greatly influences image quality.

Screen–Film System

Visualization of fine details requires high contrast. Yet contrast must not be too high to avoid relative underexposure of those areas with low optical density. Low-contrast films must be used when less sophisticated automatic exposure control systems, or problems in achieving consistent film processing, cause the mean optical density to fluctuate. High-contrast film does not tolerate such fluctuations in mean optical density, and overexposed and underexposed areas will result.

Extremely sensitive screen–film systems, which usually are of very high contrast, are marketed by manufacturers as so-called screening systems. They exhibit increased noise that is further intensified by the greater contrast. Excessive noise can make it difficult to discern details.

With their extremely short exposure time settings, highly sensitive screen–film systems can result in the grid itself being imaged, particularly when used in older mammography units. When their exposure time settings fall below the unit's minimum exposure times, small breasts can be overexposed.

There are differences in film quality. Sensitivity fluctuations between film batches should not exceed 10%, but the acceptable range for each manufacturer may vary. This range can be obtained from the film manufacturer. Inexpensive films may exhibit greater fluctuations in fog and sensitivity between film batches. They produce different optical densities at the same exposure settings that may interfere with the interpretation. Sensitometric testing is indicated whenever such fluctuations are suspected.

Film Processing

As has been mentioned, films should always be processed according to the manufacturer's recommendations. Since aberrations of the film processing are the most frequent cause of acute fluctuations in quality, consistent processing should be verified daily. If the processor is used for both mammography films and other films, then consistency must always be established with mammography films as well as with the type of other films most often used. Processor consistency should be checked before mammography begins each day.

Separate film processing for mammography has certain advantages because processing can be optimized for this specific film.

Processors for mammography films should be equipped with soft rubber rollers to minimize tears (pickoffs) in sensitive mammography films. Separate film processing for mammography is recommended only if at least 20 mammography films are developed per day because otherwise the chemicals cannot be maintained at a constant level of activity. To keep the darkroom free of dust it should be cleaned daily. Weekly cleaning of screens is also necessary, but they should be cleaned more often, whenever dust appears on films.

Additional Factors

The minimum exposure times of the automatic exposure control system and the speed of the moving grid of a mammography unit are also important.

If particularly low-dose receptor systems requiring extremely short exposure time are used, the system will image a slow-moving grid. This interferes with image interpretation and should always be avoided.

Exceeding the machine-specific minimum exposure time can lead to overexposure of small or fatty breasts.

Quality Assurance in Mammography

In the United States quality assurance in mammography is controlled under the federal legislation entitled the Mammography Quality Assurance Act (MQSA), which is administered by the Food and Drug Administration (FDA). All mammography facilities in the United States must meet the criteria established under MQSA. In Europe, national screening programs have broadly similar quality assurance criteria, and for digital mammography the European Commission guideline document provides a centrally agreed basis for quality assurance.

Quality assurance entails procedures that guarantee the quality of all facets of mammography practice. This includes equipment, radiation exposure, and image interpretation. A subset of this is quality control (QC), which involves the technical procedures that guarantee a quality mammogram. The steps involved in QC include acceptance testing, establishment of baseline performance of equipment, assessing the reasons for change in the performance of equipment before they impact on the quality of the image, and documentation that appropriate corrections have been made whenever necessary.

The quality assurance program of a facility has procedures that are the responsibility of the radiologist, the radiologic technologist, and the medical physicist. The ultimate responsibility for quality assurance lies with the radiologist. The radiologist's responsibilities include assuring that appropriate education and training have been met by all those involved in mammography, delegating appropriate responsibilities to technologists and medical physicists, being certain that QC measures have been performed, assuring that established criteria are met by the facility, and keeping appropriate records.

The medical physicist's responsibilities include acceptance testing of equipment. In addition, a regular examination of facility equipment includes assessment of the mammographic unit assembly, assessment of collimation, assessment of focal spot performance, testing of kVp accuracy and reproducibility, measuring the beam quality (half-value layer measurement), testing automatic exposure control, testing radiation dose, and an overall evaluation of image quality and of artifacts.

Radiologic technologists are responsible for a variety of tests. These include:
- Daily: Evaluating darkroom cleanliness and processor quality control, simple block test for automatic exposure control operation.
- Weekly: Cleaning screens and viewboxes and evaluating viewing conditions, assessment of image quality using a suitable test phantom.
- Quarterly: Critical analysis and analysis of fixture retention in film.
- Semiannually: Assessing darkroom fog, screen–film contact, and compression.

Documentation that quality control measures have been met is required by federal legislation or by the quality standards of breast screening programs and symptomatic services in Europe. Facilities in the United States are subject to annual inspection to ensure that they meet the requirements established by law.

In addition to the quality control measures mandated in an ongoing fashion, the radiologist interpreting the films should monitor the quality of those images and institute corrective action as needed on the basis of image quality. The radiologist should also appreciate that the QC measures required by the radiologic technologist entail a significant amount of time and training. A technologist should be designated as the quality control technologist. This technologist should be given adequate time in his or her schedule to perform the required procedures.

Medical Physicist's Responsibilities

The medical physicist's responsibilities include the following:
1. **Mammographic unit assembly evaluation**. This is to determine that all locks, angulation indicators and the mechanical support of the system operates properly. This includes visual inspection of the entire assembly, verification that moving parts operate appropriately, testing of locks to be certain they prevent mechanical motion, and determination that the image receptor holder assembly is secure and slides smoothly into appropriate position. Verification that the compressed breast thickness scale, if one is provided, is accurate and to be certain that in normal operation neither patient nor operator is exposed to hazards from sharp or rough edges or dangerous electrical wiring.
2. **Collimation assessment**. This testing is done to ensure that the collimator or cone does not allow significant radiation beyond the edges of the imager receptor.
3. **Evaluation of focal spot performance**. This is done by measuring the dimensions of the focal spot perpendicular and parallel to the anode–cathode axis. Slit camera measurement of the focal spot size is performed as well as high-contrast resolution pattern measurement.
4. **kVp accuracy and reproducibility**. This testing is done to assure that kVp is accurate within 5% of the indicated kVp and is reproducible with a coefficient of variability ≤0.02. European standards stipulate kVp accuracy to within 1 kV (Perry et al. 2006).
5. **Beam quality assessment (half-value layer measurement)**. This is done to determine that half-value layer of the X-ray beam is adequate so that radiation exposure of the patient is minimized without loss of necessary contrast.
6. **Automatic exposure control (AEC) system performance assessment**. This is done to ensure that the AEC system performs appropriately. The range of operation and reproducibility of the AEC is tested using uniform slabs of Plexiglas (polymethyl methacrylate) in various thicknesses so that the automatic selection of mAs, target/filter, and kVp can be assessed. For screen–film systems the uniformity of resulting film optical density is measured, and for digital systems the average pixel value, noise, and relative contrast of a small area of aluminum are used to test the signal.
7. **Patient dose**. The radiation dose (average glandular dose [AGD] in the United States, mean glandular dose [MGD] in Europe) is assessed for a "standard breast" phantom exposed under AEC to give a comparative measure of typical radiation dose for the unit. Also, the doses to a sample of patients can be assessed to give more realistic information on the range of patient doses being used. Some mammography units record the exposure factors for patients, or the data can be retrieved from the header information in digital mammograms. The dose to the radiosensitive tissue of the breast (a risk-related quantity) is estimated using standard methods for AGD and MGD (Hendrick et al. 1999, Dance et al. 2000).
8. **Image quality evaluation**. This is done to assess the quality of the mammographic image and to detect any changes over time in the quality of image. A range of phantoms is available, but most combine high-resolution tests (e.g., line-pairs patterns) with low-contrast test features of different sizes that have to be assessed for their visibility in the image noise. Some phantoms for digital mammography can be read automatically by image-processing software to decrease the variability on serial measurements.
9. **Artifact evaluation**. Images should be assessed for the presence of artifacts and, if artifacts are identified, their source determined.

The Radiology Technologist's Responsibilities

In a department using screen–film mammography, the radiology technologist's responsibilities include:
1. **Darkroom cleanliness**. This minimizes film artifacts due to dirt and dust. Daily cleaning of the darkroom is required.
2. **Processor quality control**. This assures that the film processor chemical system is working optimally. Testing is done daily before the initiation of clinical imaging by inserting a sensitometric strip to check film density and base-plus-fog level. In addition, processor quality control operating levels need to be established when the quality control program is initiated or when there has been an important change made in film, chemicals, or processing conditions. To ascertain that the system is stable, testing of the processor should be conducted on five consecutive days after such changes are made.
3. **Screen cleanliness**. To minimize dust and dirt particles in the screen, it should be cleaned at least weekly.
4. **Phantom images**. Weekly/monthly testing with phantom images should be performed once baseline levels of performance are established within a department. Requirements state that sensitometric control strips need to be run daily for the processor.
5. **Darkroom fog**. This testing is done to be certain that light inside and outside the darkroom does not fog mammographic films. A visual inspection of the darkroom should be done semiannually. Clinical films are also exposed to tests for film fogging.
6. **Screen–film contact**. This testing is to determine that optimal contact is maintained between the film, the screen, and the cassette. A film is exposed with a copper mesh placed on top of the screen. No grid is used. Image quality is evaluated.
7. **Compression**. Semiannual test of compression is made using a bathroom scale to measure pounds of compression. Compression force should range between 20 lb and 40 lb (200 N maximum in Europe) (Perry et al. 2006).
8. **Repeat analysis**. The number of and reason for repeated mammograms is determined.
9. **Viewbox viewing conditions**. This is checked to be certain that viewbox and viewing conditions are optimal throughout the department. Viewboxes should be kept clean and illumination levels uniform.
10. **Analysis of fixture retention in film**. As an indicator of maintained quality, the quantity of residual fixture in process film is determined. Test solution is placed on film and compared with a standard to make this determination.
11. **Visual checklist**. This is done to determine that the mammography unit indicator light, displays, and locks are working appropriately. Visual inspection of the equipment is made.

In a department using digital mammography, the radiology technologist's responsibilities include:
1. Daily/weekly checking of system imaging operation and automatic exposure control using a simple block phantom. Adherence to manufacturer's recommendations on periodic flat-fielding procedure.
2. Periodic checking of the condition of the review and reporting display monitors. Various self-checking and remote calibration tools are available, and some systems may employ a visual challenge at log-in as a crude check of ambient lighting conditions.
3. Compression testing as above.
4. Repeat analysis as above. Digital systems with PACS may provide tools to aid repeat analysis.
5. Visual checklist as above.

Reporting and Documentation of Findings

(See also American College of Radiology: Practice Guidelines and Technical Standards 2006)

Clinical Findings

A complete breast examination is necessary for all symptomatic patients and in all women requiring further assessment of a screen-detected or imaging abnormality.

It involves a physical examination of the breast in addition to mammography.

The physical examination begins with the *visual inspection*. The examining physician inspects the breasts for asymmetry in size (anisomastia), changes in shape or contour, generalized skin changes (such as erythema, skin thickening, peau d'orange, dimpling, hyperpigmentation, or vascular anomalies), focal skin lesions (such as lipomas, atheromas, nevi, or warts), or scarring (localization and cause).

Palpation provides information on the structure of the glandular tissue (soft, thickened, nodular). It also provides information on possible differences between the breasts, namely location and consistency of lumps and the relationship of these lumps to the surrounding breast tissue, the skin (the Jackson sign), and to the pectoralis muscle. Palpation can also assess pain and mobility of the nipple and the region posterior to it, and it reveals palpable changes in the lymph drainage routes.

These findings should be recorded. Information from the findings on physical examination is useful in interpreting or tailoring the mammogram.

Documentation of any abnormalities will help to check whether:
- An area of clinical abnormality (if present) was included on the mammogram, and
- An imaging method is positive or negative in this area and whether this is reliable

Mammographic Report

The mammographic report should be based on the present study and, if available, on previous studies.

Importance of previous studies and follow-up. Whenever possible, the radiologist should compare the findings with prior mammograms (Harvey et al. 1993, Varela et al. 2005, Roelofs et al. 2007). Comparison with mammograms that are 2 or more years old may be even more informative than the comparison with more recent mammograms. Discrete changes may go undetected with too short a follow-up period, whereas they become more obvious when older mammograms are compared, provided mammographic technique is comparable. Comparison with previous studies is useful for correct interpretation of asymmetries and for earliest possible detection of newly developing or increasing discrete densities or microcalcifications.

Malignancy should always be considered when a new finding develops or when a finding increases, particularly in a postmenopausal patient. However, even an increasing or newly developing lesion cannot be considered as proof of a malignant process. New fibroadenomas can occur, particularly with hormone replacement therapy. Furthermore, hormone replacement can induce a changed parenchymal structure and increased density.

Absence of a perceivable increase in size is not necessarily sufficient for excluding a malignant process, although it is true that absence of change with increasing time of follow-up makes a benign process more and more probable. It must, however, be remembered that some cancers are slow growing and may show little or no change for several years. Also some malignant processes lead to retraction and even decrease in size.

Finally, a decrease in pre-existing microcalcifications may indicate the presence of an invasive carcinoma. This phenomenon is caused by the decreased pH in invasive tumorous tissue.

The report of a diagnostic mammogram should first include information concerning the indication and any specific question that was asked.

It should include major risk factors (from family history or individual history) and clinical findings that may be important for image interpretation (e.g., scarring due to surgery; if benign/malignant finding, in which breast/location).

Finally, abnormal clinical findings need to be documented.

The report should include information as to whether previous mammograms were available for interpretation.

Overall breast density and parenchymal pattern should be classified according to the categories suggested by the ACR.

Parenchymal Pattern

The overall composition of the breasts (e.g., fatty, heterogeneously dense, extremely dense) should be described, as this will influence the sensitivity of the mammography.

The ACR suggests the following categories and recommends that—for consistency—breast composition should be mentioned in every report:
- ACR1: The breast is almost entirely fatty (< 25% glandular).
- ACR2: There are scattered fibro-glandular densities (~25–50%).
- ACR3: The breast tissue is heterogeneously dense, which could obscure detection of small masses (~51–75% glandular).
- ACR4: The breast tissue is extremely dense. This may lower the sensitivity of mammography (> 75% glandular).

Description of Abnormalities

The radiologist's role is to describe the radiologic morphology without using histologic terms. However, there are certain entities that have characteristic mammographic and sonographic findings allowing histologic diagnoses. These include lipoma, fibroadenolipoma, oil cysts, calcified fibroadenoma, and lymph nodes.

Overall it is recommended that the nomenclature suggested by the ACR be used. However, the ACR states that for quality assurance and auditing the use of the nomenclature is not mandatory (whereas the use of BI-RADS [Breast Imaging Reporting and Data System] categories for classification of the final result and outcome *is* considered mandatory.)

Whenever a lesion is present, the type of lesion should be indicated, such as:
- Mass (with or without microcalcifications)
- Density (with or without microcalcifications). The term density used to describe a masslike lesion that is visible on only one view (see below). The category "density" has meanwhile been eliminated. According to the BI-RADS lexicon, such changes should be included in the term "asymmetry."
- Asymmetry (with or without microcalcifications)
- Architectural distortion (with or without microcalcifications)
- Microcalcifications

3 Mammography

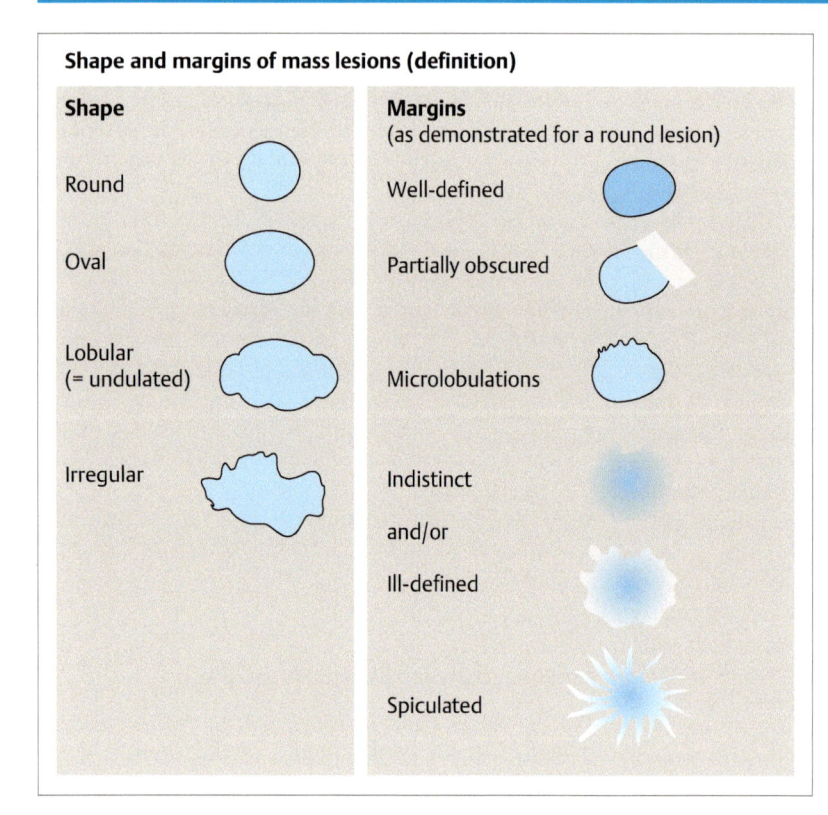

Shape and margins of mass lesions (definition)

Shape	Margins (as demonstrated for a round lesion)
Round	Well-defined
Oval	Partially obscured
Lobular (= undulated)	Microlobulations
Irregular	Indistinct and/or Ill-defined
	Spiculated

Fig. 3.31 Interpreting and documenting masses and masslike lesions.

Definition: A *mass* is a space-occupying lesion that is visible in two views. A change seen *on one view only* is usually called a focal asymmetry. It may represent:
- Superimposition
- A normal finding
- A potential true mass

Further assessment: A *focal asymmetry* may be dismissed after careful consideration. if:
- It is stable for > 2–3 years.
- It is included on both views and spreads out on the second view.
- It exhibits fatty inclusions.

(Exceptions to the above criteria exist.)
In case of any doubts further assessment is indicated.

A *mass* should be analyzed based on its shape, margins, density, and stability over time:
- Stability over > 2–3 years supports benignity
- High *density* of a mass is associated with a higher probability of malignancy than low density.

However, many cancers are isodense with surrounding breast tissue. Few (mostly early) malignancies exhibit quite low density.

Only well-circumscribed margins which are not obscured in > 75% of the circumference are associated with low probability of malignancy.

Oval and round shape are more probably associated with benign disease. This criterion alone, however, is unreliable.

Mass

By definition a mass is a three-dimensional structure with convex borders that is evident on two orthogonal views (e.g., craniocaudal and mediolateral oblique)

A description of a mass should include (**Fig. 3.31**):
- Size, contour, (roentgen-)density, presence or absence of associated changes

Descriptions for shape in the BI-RADS lexicon include:
- Oval or round
- Lobular
- Irregular

Margins can be further described as:
- Circumscribed
- Microlobulated
- Obscured (partially hidden by adjacent structures)
- Indistinct or ill defined
- Spiculated

The (roentgen-)density of a mass is described by comparing it with the density of normal breast tissue:
- High density
- Isodense or equal density
- Low density
- Fat-containing

Special cases which can be specifically described:
- Solitary dilated duct
- Intramammary lymph node

Density (as Lesion Type)

This term was used in the first three editions of the BI-RADS lexicon. In the fourth edition (D'Orsi et al. 2003) it has been included in the term "asymmetry." Nevertheless, the authors feel that—even though a clear distinction from asymmetry may not always be possible—it may be valuable to use this term as formerly intended: a density described as a masslike finding that is visible on one view

Reporting and Documentation of Findings

a Certain types of calcifications should be known:

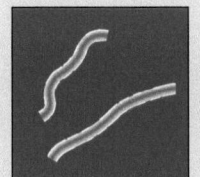

Vascular calcifications*

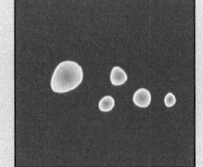

Liponecrosis* (smooth calcifications often with central lucency)

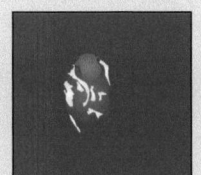

Eggshell

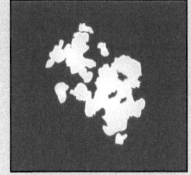

Popcorn-like large calcifications* (typically benign in fibroadenomas)

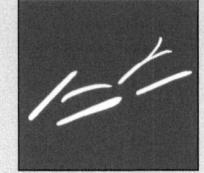

Rod-like calcifications (ductal smooth elongated non-fragmented rods) typical of benign secretory disease

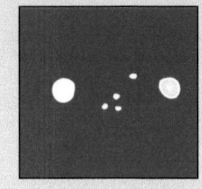

Coarse or smooth round* (sometimes with a lucent center)

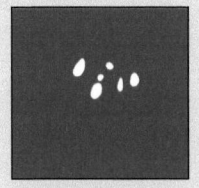

Milk of calcium Typical of microcystic benign changes as seen on the CC view

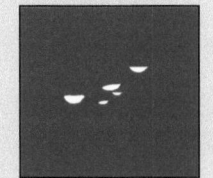

Milk of calcium Typical of microcystic benign changes as seen on the lateral view

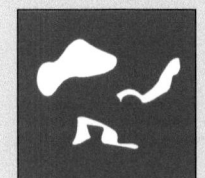

Coarse large (dystrophic) macrocalcifications

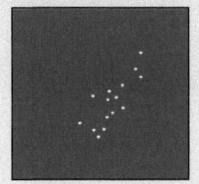

Punctate

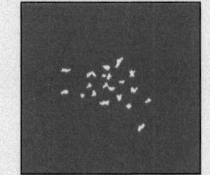

Fine granular

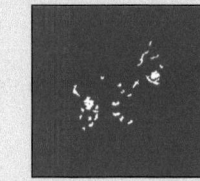

Coarse granular

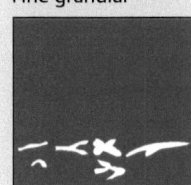

Casting (suspicious)

Fig. 3.32a,b Interpreting and documenting microcalcifications.

a Calcifications are described and interpreted based on their individual shape, their size and their distribution in the breast.

Fig. 3.32b ▷

b Typical distribution pattern of microcalcifications

Skin calcifications

Grouped

Regional

Scattered

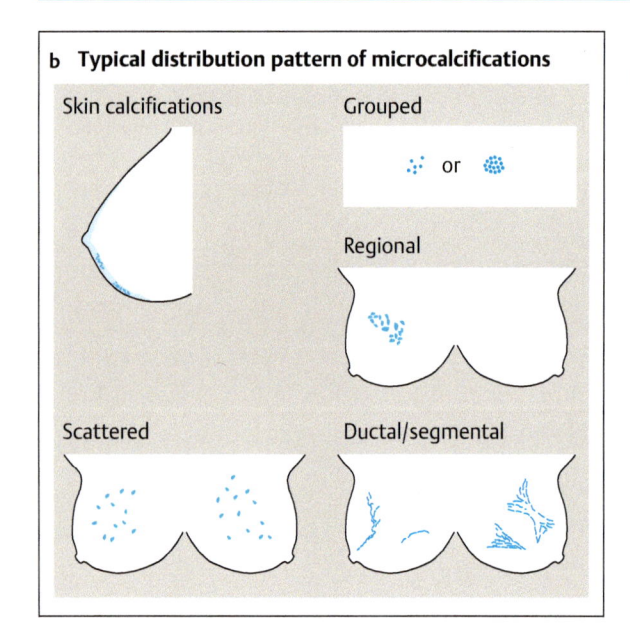

Ductal/segmental

◁ continued

b Microcalcifications should be assessed using a true lateral view and magnification views.
Grouping must be proven three-dimensionally. If visible on only one plane (unless the area is not included in further projections) superimposition may mimic grouping of microcalcifications.

only. Thus it may indicate the presence of a true mass (that might be obscured on the other view). Or it may be caused by superimposition of normal structures mimicking a mass. Overall it is associated with a lower probability of malignancy than a mass.

Asymmetry

Asymmetry (with or without microcalcifications) may include larger areas or smaller focal asymmetries and may be characterized as:
- Asymmetric breast tissue, or
- Asymmetric focal density

For focal changes, size measurements should be given; for diffuse changes, the approximate extent should be mentioned.

Architectural Distortion

Architectural distortions (with or without microcalcifications) have a dense or lucent center. The former is associated with a higher probability of malignancy than the latter.
If possible the approximate size may be given.

Calcifications

Localization, number, distribution pattern, and morphology of calcifications are described. Clusters of calcifications must be visualized in two planes to be regarded as a true cluster. If a "cluster" is visible in one plane only, it may not be a real cluster but caused by superimposition of single calcifications in different locations.
With respect to *localization*, a differentiation has to be made between calcifications outside the breast paren-

chyma (i.e., skin or subcutaneous tissue) and calcifications within the parenchyma.
If calcifications can be specifically characterized as benign, they should be described as such. These calcifications include (**Fig. 3.32**; see also Chapter 22):
- Skin calcifications
- Vascular calcifications
- Coarse, "popcorn" calcifications
- Large, rodlike calcifications
- Round calcifications, which can be described as punctate if they are smaller than 0.5 mm
- Centrally lucent calcifications
- Rim or (eggshell) calcifications, as seen in the walls of cysts
- Milk of calcium
- Suture calcifications
- Dystrophic calcifications

Calcifications classified as indeterminate include those that are amorphous or indistinct or fine granular. Calcifications suspicious for malignancy include pleomorphic or heterogeneous microcalcifications, as well as irregular linear, branching, or casting calcifications.
The distribution of calcifications should be described as:
- *Grouped or clustered*, occupying less than 2cm^3 of breast volume
- *Segmental*, occupying more than 2cm^3 but less than regional
- *Regional*, occupying a large volume of the breast, not in a ductal or segmental distribution, and not the entire breast
- *Diffuse or scattered*, distributed throughout the breast in a random fashion
- *Linear*, corresponding to a ductal pattern

Furthermore, a lobular distribution describes the presence of multiple punctate, generally round, calcifications within a small area (2–3 mm). Such calcifications are usually located within the lobule and are arranged like a small morula or flower (rosette).

Associated Changes

These can be added to descriptions of masses or calcifications or can be used independently. They include:
- Skin retraction
- Skin thickening
- Trabecular thickening
- Nipple retraction
- Axillary adenopathy
- Architectural distortion
- Increased vascularity

In addition, the mammogram can show a diffuse increase in breast density.

If previous studies are available, whether or not a finding represents an interval change, a new or increasing finding should be reported.

For both any change and stability the time interval of observation (e.g., stability since …) should be mentioned.

Lesion Location

The radiologist must indicate the location of any significant mammographic finding based on the information from both mammographic views. This can be done by specifying the quadrant or (as mostly done) noting the corresponding hour on the face of a clock. Findings located in the retroareolar region or on the axis behind the nipple are special cases. If only the craniocaudal and mediolateral oblique views are available or if a lesion is seen on only one view, the location should be described as laterally or medially in the breast or as superiorly or inferiorly in the breast.

Lesion location should also include whether the lesion is in the anterior, middle, or posterior third of the breast. More commonly the distance from the nipple is measured and indicated.

Whenever a location is determined based only on the craniocaudal and mediolateral oblique views it should be borne in mind that errors concerning the true location may occur, since the latter view is not perpendicular to the former view.

The location can usually be determined by using a scheme as shown in **Fig. 3.33**.

To avoid errors targeting a lesion, a lateral view (mediolateral or lateromedial) should be obtained before stereotactic procedures (performed for percutaneous breast biopsy or needle localization).

Final Diagnosis and Recommendation

The report has to conclude with a final diagnosis, which should be categorized according to definite categories.

The most widely used system is the BI-RADS system (see below). Each category is associated with a recommendation on how to proceed.

In the conclusion the initial questions need to be addressed. For each clinical or mammographic abnormality a BI-RADS category should be assigned and a recommendation on how to proceed given.

The BI-RADS recommendation for the breast in question or for the patient results from the highest BI-RADS category of the breast in question or of the patient.

The recommendation should be categorized as follows:
- BI-RADS 1: Normal findings (negative examination), back to screening (usual age- and risk-adapted interval).
- BI-RADS 2: Benign finding (no increased risk compared with BI-RADS 1), back to screening (usual age- and risk-adapted interval).
- BI-RADS 3: Probably benign finding. Short-term follow-up (usually at 6 months) recommended. This recommendation should be given only after completed standard assessment with additional views and ultrasound examination.
- BI-RADS 4: Suspicious finding. Histopathologic assessment recommended for an abnormality of low (BI-RADS 4a), intermediate (BI-RADS 4b), or high suspicion (BI-RADS 4c).

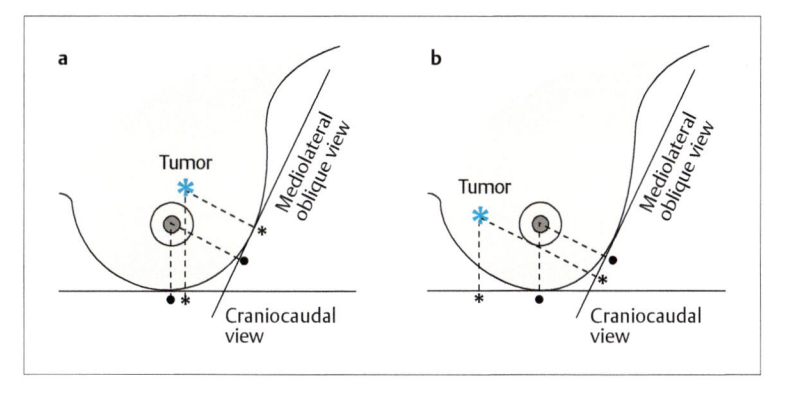

Fig. 3.33a,b Localizing a tumor by means of the craniocaudal view and mediolateral oblique view. Aside from some uncertainty caused by the mobility of the breast parenchyma, the tumor can be localized by its different vertical projections in both views (**a**). It should be noted that a tumor located above and medial to the nipple can appear "below" the level of the nipple in the mediolateral oblique view (**b**).

3 Mammography

Table 3.4 Most important parameters and thresholds for assessing the quality of the screening process according to the European guidelines for quality assurance in mammography screening, 4th ed. (Perry 2006)

Parameter	Calculation (as defined)	Acceptable (round 1)	Desirable (round 1)	Acceptable (subsequent rounds)	Desirable (subsequent rounds)
Participation rate	Proportion of women invited that attend for screening			> 70%	> 75%
% eligible women re-invited within the desired screening interval (or within the screening interval plus < 6 months)	% of timely re-invitation (as defined)			> 95% (> 98%)	100%
Technical repeat	Percentage per women screened	< 3%	< 1%	< 3%	< 1%
Recall rate	Women recalled per women screened	< 7%	< 5%	< 5%	< 3%
Short-term follow-up (may only be recommended after completed imaging assessment)	Number of screenees with recommendation for short-term follow-up per women screened	< 1%	0	< 1%	0
Detection rate	Rate of DCIS and invasive breast cancers per number of screened women	3 × IR[a]	> 3 × IR[a]	1.5 × IR[a]	> 1.5 × IR[a]
Interval cancer rate first year (for biennial screening)	Number of interval cancers observed during the first year after a screening mammogram per number of incident invasive cancers per year	0.3 × IR	< 0.3 × IR	0.3 × IR	< 0.3 × IR
Interval cancer rate second year (for biennial screening)	Number of interval cancers observed during the second year after a screening mammogram per number of incident invasive cancers per year	0.5 × IR	< 0.5 × IR	0.5 × IR	< 0.5 × IR
Proportion of screen-detected cancers that are stage II+	Screen-detected stage II+ cancers per number of screen-detected DCIS plus invasive breast cancers	NA	< 30%	25%	< 25%
Proportion of screen-detected invasive cancers that are node negative	Screen-detected node-negative cancers per number of screen-detected invasive cancers	NA	> 70%	75%	> 75%
Proportion of screen-detected cancers that are DCIS per total cancers	Screen-detected DCIS per screen-detected DCIS and invasive cancers	10%	10–20%	10%	10–20%
Screen-detected cancers < 10 mm	Invasive screen-detected cancers < 10 mm in size per number of screen-detected invasive cancers	NA	≥ 25%	≥ 25%	≥ 30%
Screen-detected cancers < 15 mm	Screen-detected invasive cancers < 15 mm	50%	> 50%	50%	> 50%
Proportion of screen-detected cancers with a preoperative diagnosis of malignancy	Cancers with preoperative diagnosis of malignancy per number of screen-detected DCIS and invasive breast cancers	> 70%	> 90%	> 70%	> 90%

Parameter	Calculation (as defined)	Acceptable (round 1)	Desirable (round 1)	Acceptable (subsequent rounds)	Desirable (subsequent rounds)
Waiting time between screening exam and result < 15 wd (desirable: < 10 wd)	Percentage of screened women in whom the condition is fulfilled	95%	> 95%	95%	> 95%
Waiting time between screening result and offered assessment < 5 wd (desirable: 3 wd)	Percentage of screened women in whom the condition is fulfilled	90%	> 90%	90%	> 90%

DCIS, ductal carcinoma in situ; wd, waiting days.
NA, not applicable.
[a] The incidence rate (IR) is calculated using the incidence of invasive breast cancers before the start of a screening program.
Note: Parameters may vary with differing regional conditions (prevalance of opportunistic screening).

- BI-RADS 5: Abnormality highly suggestive of malignancy. Histopathologic assessment and probably appropriate treatment for malignancy required.
- BI-RADS 0: Further imaging assessment and/or prior studies needed before a final category can be assigned.
- BI-RADS 6: Histopathologically verified malignancy. Appropriate action has to be taken.

BI-RADS 3 should be avoided whenever possible, since short-term follow-up is usually associated with uncertainty and psychological stress to the patient for at least 6 months and since absence of a change during 6 months cannot exclude that malignancy is present.

Based on existing experience (Sickles 1999, Baum et al. 2011) follow-up should not stop before 2 years has elapsed. A good protocol appears to be follow-up at 6, 12, and 24 months.

In the United States communication of results to the patient is required. It is advisable to document this communication in the written report. Finally, it may be helpful to give advice concerning the mode of histopathologic workup (type of needle biopsy, open biopsy, preoperative wire localization).

To reduce costs and save time, screening findings can be documented in a brief form to facilitate computer processing. However, screening involves more than documenting findings; it also requires documentation and evaluation of histologic results of both screen-detected and interval cancers. For this purpose the European guidelines propose parameters which allow monitoring and thresholds. **Table 3.4** gives an overview of the parameters and the recommended thresholds.

Galactography

Definition

Galactography refers to the examination of lactiferous ducts using a contrast medium (Tabár et al. 1983, Kindermann 1985, Ciatto et al. 1988, Dinkel et al. 2000, Hou et al. 2001).

Injecting a water-soluble contrast medium permits mammographic imaging of the lactiferous duct system belonging to the excretory duct into which the needle is introduced. After the duct is filled with contrast medium, the breast is imaged in the craniocaudal and mediolateral planes. Oblique views or magnification mammograms may also be required.

Indications

Today the indications for galactography are decreasing. First, duct sonography is able to visualize a dilated duct and target it and thus may be able to guide biopsy to the area of concern.

Second, although galactography may show the ductal system of concern, it rarely eliminates the need for further investigation. If additional information is needed, MRI appears to be a promising tool as it is presently the most sensitive imaging method and allows visualization of lesion extent beyond occluded ducts.

Overall, galactography should only be used if:
- Pathologic nipple discharge is present
- Mammography and sonography cannot define an abnormality that would require histopathologic assessment

The role of MRI is presently still under investigation (Sardanelli et al. 2010).

If galactography shows an abnormality, immediate galactography-guided vacuum-assisted breast biopsy (in case of a clearly defined focal area) and/or clip marking (in case of suspected diffuse changes) might be considered.

Galactography should be performed only in the presence of pathologic secretion, which itself makes it possible to detect the opening of the excretory duct. Absence of secretion precludes any ductal probing.

Pathologic discharge includes:
- Spontaneous, nonmilky discharge (clear serous, cloudy, or brownish from a single or several ducts, usually unilateral)—this does not include discharge that is expressed under firm pressure, since such a discharge can be provoked in many women
- Bloody discharge
- Any discharge with suggestive cytologic findings (Groups IV or V) (Montroni et al. 2010)

Galactography is not indicated in the presence of:
- Galactorrhea, that is, milky discharge that is not due to pregnancy or breast-feeding. Galactorrhea is always a sequela of primary and/or secondary hyperprolactinemia and may occur bilaterally or unilaterally.
- Bilateral, bloodless discharge from multiple ducts (serous or green) without cytologic abnormality. This too can be the result of hormonal imbalance or duct ectasia with chronic inflammation.

Contraindications

Galactography is contraindicated in the presence of inflammation, which can be exacerbated by the procedure.

Hypersensitivity to contrast medium is a relative contraindication. To date duct sonography and MRI should be considered in these patients first. The physician may also consider intraoperative probing of the duct or, after injecting methylene blue, excision of the lactiferous duct without galactography.

Side Effects

Since a pathologic discharge is usually associated with duct ectasia, galactography can lead to *galactophoritis* or mastitis. This has been observed in only rare cases since the introduction of water-soluble contrast media.

Allergic reactions to contrast media are rare with galactography. For patients with known allergies other methods need to be considered first and the indication for galactography should be counterchecked. Prophylactic antihistamine and steroid medication must be considered in patients with known allergies if galactography cannot be avoided. Furthermore, the indication should be checked and appropriate precautionary measures taken (see previous section).

If a mild, acute reaction occurs, it can be treated with antihistamines. Severe reactions should be treated with intravenous cortisone and, in applicable cases, intravenous epinephrine, as with other contrast reactions.

If the injection pressure is too high or if too much contrast medium has been instilled, extravasation of contrast medium can occur, with contrast medium seen outside the duct system in breast parenchyma. In this setting lymphatic vessels may be imaged. The patient will usually perceive this as *pain*, although this has no serious effects other than insufficient or obscured visualization. The galactogram needs to be terminated, if this occurs. Contrast medium will be reabsorbed and the procedure can be repeated after a few days.

Procedure

Comfortable patient positioning and good lighting are important for this procedure. A magnifying lens or an eyepiece mounted on an eyeglass frame can be helpful in locating the excretory duct.
- Cytologic smears of the discharge may be taken before galactography.
- In the presence of profuse discharge, the breast should be expressed prior to galactography to remove coagulated blood or thickened secretion that might interfere with contrast medium injection or appear as filling defects that can lead to misdiagnosis.
- After disinfecting the nipple and the surrounding skin, the physician carefully inserts the probe into the nipple, first pressing out a small drop of secretion to better locate the opening of the secreting lactiferous sinus. Once the orifice is located, the physician will be able to insert the cannula without any difficulty. Use a thin (25–30 gauge), blunt, short cannula (such as the lymphography cannula or galactography catheter, or a 30-gauge sialography needle). Using a thin cannula minimizes the necessity for painful dilation of the orifice. The tubing connecting the cannula to the syringe containing the contrast medium should be filled with contrast medium and free of air bubbles before positioning in the duct.
- Local anesthesia may be applied to the nipple in particularly anxious patients. After applying a topical anesthetic, the physician inserts a thin needle next to the areola and injects a local anesthetic behind the areola. After about 10 minutes, the nipple is completely insensitive, and the physician can begin the cannulation.
- Using a nonionic contrast medium is recommended because of its very low incidence of allergic reactions and particularly good patient tolerance. Nonionic contrast media have the added advantage of causing the least amount of unpleasant sensations during the examination.

- After the canula has been positioned in the duct, it can be secured in place with adhesive tape.
- Next, 0.1–0.5 mL of contrast medium without air bubbles is injected slowly into the duct. Injection has to be stopped as soon as slight resistance is noted. Otherwise extravasation may occur, which may impair evaluation of the images.
- After the ducts have been filled, it is recommended the excretory duct is compressed with a swab during mammography until the moment of exposure. If the ductal system is only mildly dilated, it can be closed with vaseline or 4% collodion.
- Next, mammograms are obtained in two planes with additional magnification mammograms if necessary.
- It is important to use only moderate compression in galactography. Excessive compression can displace secretion from the ducts in the central breast (where compression is best) and simulate filling defects.
- If the ductal system is not sufficiently filled with contrast medium, the filming is repeated using a slightly greater quantity of contrast medium.
- Insufficient filling with contrast medium can be due to debris or coagulated blood within the ductal system. If this is the case, the ductal system should be expressed and again injected with contrast medium.
- Care should be taken not to introduce any air when injecting the contrast medium. If air has been inadvertently injected, the bubbles can be identified by their beadlike arrangement along the superior margin of the lactiferous duct in the lateral plane. For this reason, we prefer to use the 90° lateral view as the second imaging plane as opposed to the mediolateral oblique view. If any doubt remains, air bubbles can be identified by their mobility after a second injection.

Difficulties and Possible Solutions

Unsuccessful *cannulation* may be due to *an intraductal mass located near the nipple.* This will cause rapid reflux of the injected contrast medium. Sometimes the excretory ducts are extremely narrow or go into spasm when cannulation is attempted. In this case, we recommend applying a warm moist towel to relax the muscles.

Lifting the nipple helps extend a *kinked lactiferous duct* behind the nipple and facilitates cannulation.

Galactography is usually difficult in *retracted nipples.* Here, an attempt should be made to pull the nipple outward or spread out the areola with two fingers so that the orifice becomes visible.

Findings

Pathologic secretion can be caused by chronic inflammation, papilloma, papillomatosis, or, rarely, an intraductal or invasive carcinoma.

In Kindermann's material (1,694 galactographies), no intraductal mass but only duct ectasia was present in 65% of the cases. Biopsies were done in 35% of all cases, and malignant tumors were found in only 4.3%. The majority of pathologic findings were caused by papillomas or papillomatosis. With bloody secretion, the incidence of malignancy increased to as high as 37% (Kindermann 1985). Overall the reported rate of malignancy among patients undergoing galactography ranges around 5–30%, probably depending on the preselection and the intensity of preceding imaging assessment (Dinkel et al. 2000, Hou et al. 2001, Montroni et al. 2010).

The principal findings are:
- Normal ductal system (**Fig. 3.34**).
- Duct ectasia (**Fig. 3.35a,b**). This condition involves more or less pronounced distension of the ducts up to cystic distension. It occurs primarily in the presence of fibrocystic changes and subacute or chronic plasma cell mastitis (a preliminary stage of the familiar calcifying plasma cell mastitis) or secretory disease.
- Filling defects or cutoff of the duct. Once filling defects due to debris are excluded, inflammatory changes or proliferative changes should be considered, including papillomatosis, papilloma, and carcinoma.

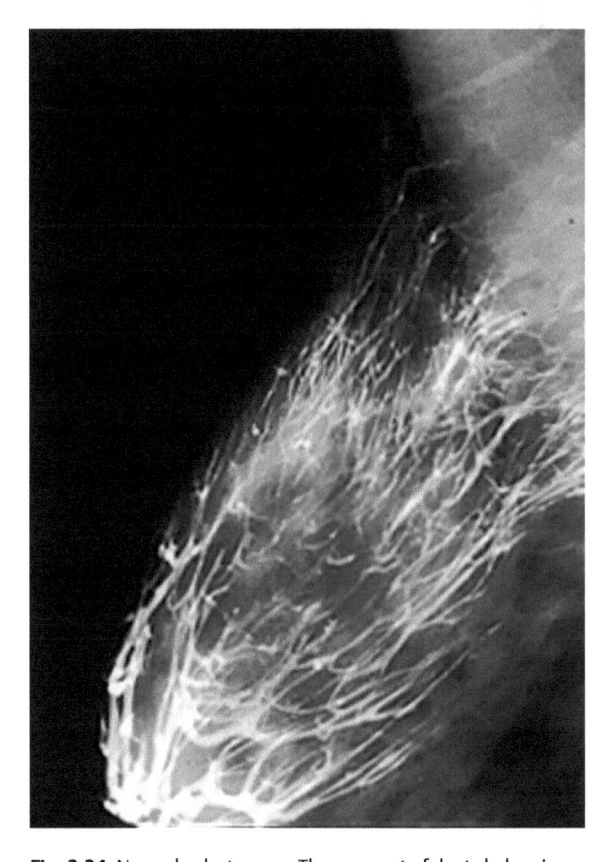

Fig. 3.34 Normal galactogram. The segment of ducts belonging to the injected lactiferous duct will appear as a tree-shaped structure that extends from the excretory duct and divides into increasingly narrower branches toward the periphery.

3 Mammography

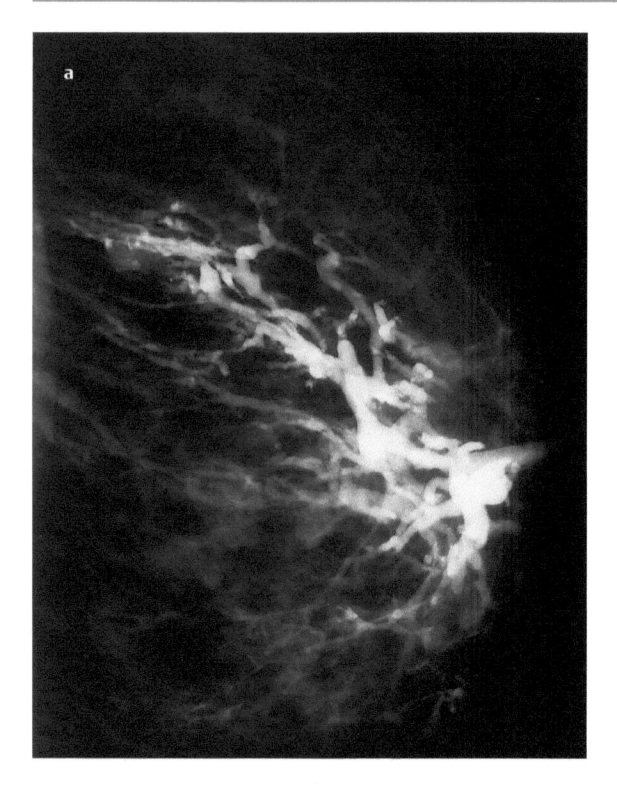

Fig. 3.35a,b
a Duct ectasia. No evidence of an intraductal mass.

b Besides normal ducts a conglomeration of small cysts as well as several further small cysts are filled with contrast agent.

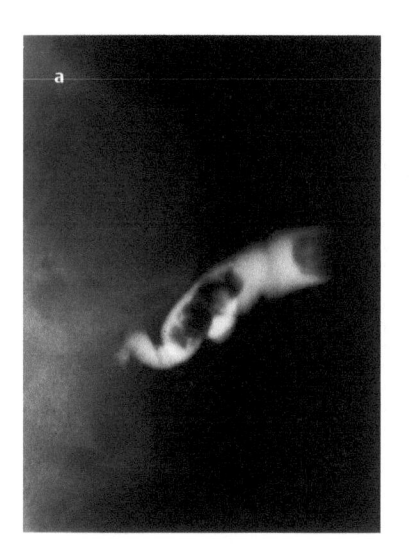

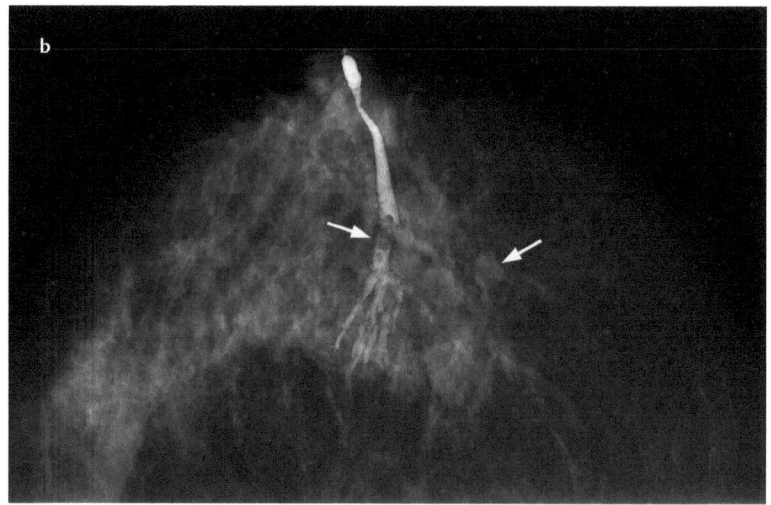

Fig. 3.36a,b
a Intraductal masses lead to isolated or multiple filling defects, that is, the contrast medium flows around the intraductal mass in an arc-shaped pattern.

b Multiple round filling defects in a distended lactiferous duct, histologically confirmed as papillomatosis. The small, smooth-contoured, focal lesion in the parenchyma also corresponds to a papilloma.

Galactography

Galactography is not suitable for diagnosing the nature of the filling defect. These changes require excision and histo-pathologic examination. However, galactography can be useful in localizing the site of the lesion causing the nipple discharge (**Figs. 3.36, 3.37, 3.38, 3.39**).

Figures 3.40 and 3.41 demonstrate common artifacts caused by extravasation or air bubbles. The former may impair assessment in the area of extravasation; the latter may be recognized by the very low density, by their sharp margin, and by their arrangement at the top of the duct, as visualized on the 90° lateral view.

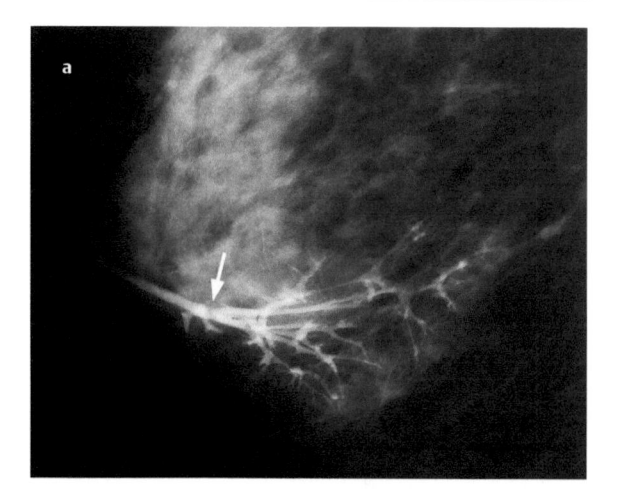

Fig. 3.38a–c Various intraductal processes are shown. ▷
- **a** Marginal filling defects that interrupt the contour of the wall: ductal carcinoma in situ.
- **b** Tiny round filling defects arranged like a string of beads in a main excretory duct. *Histology*: DCIS.
- **c** Multiple irregular filling defects with loss of the contour of the wall: papillomatosis in transition to an invasive carcinoma.

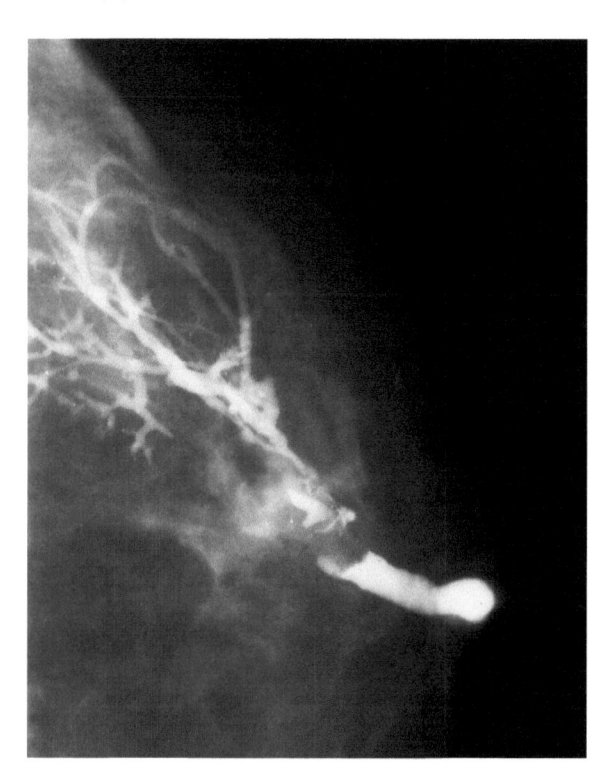

Fig. 3.37 Where an intraductal mass completely blocks the lactiferous duct, the galactogram will show a filling defect with partial truncation of the duct.

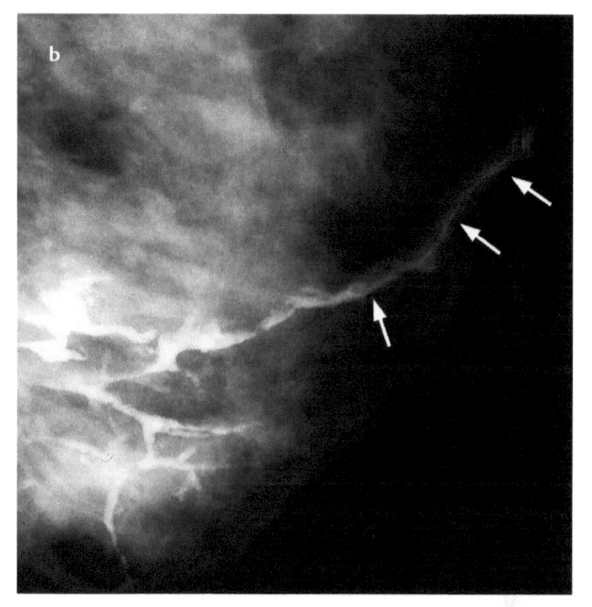

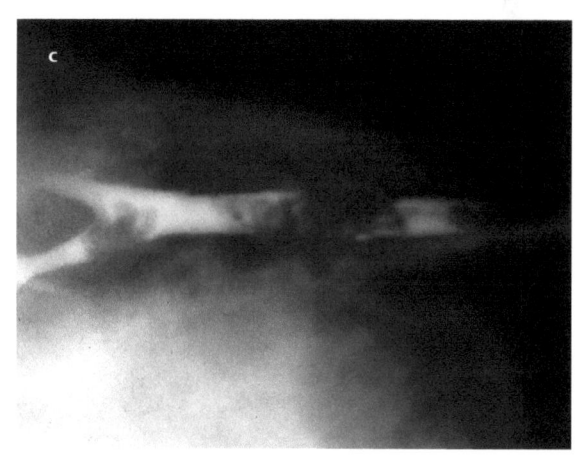

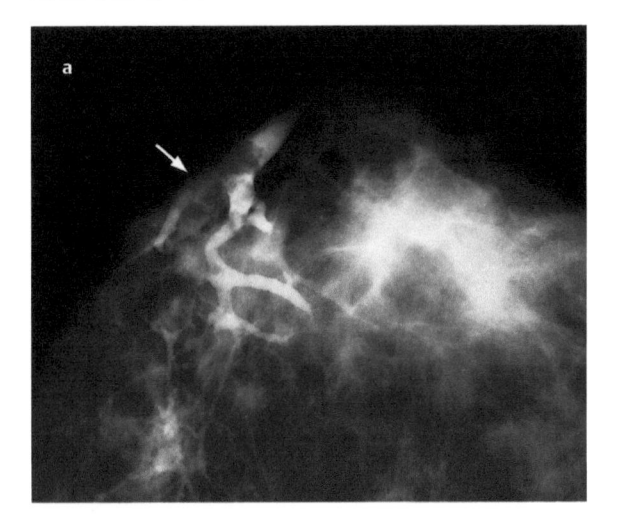

Fig. 3.39a,b
a Lobulated filling defect in an ectatic lactiferous duct: papillomatosis.

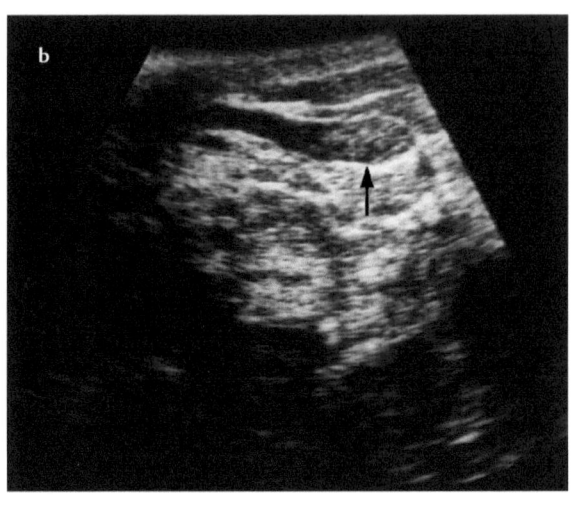

b Good sonographic image (13.5-MHz technique) of a distended duct containing a tiny hyperechoic mass.

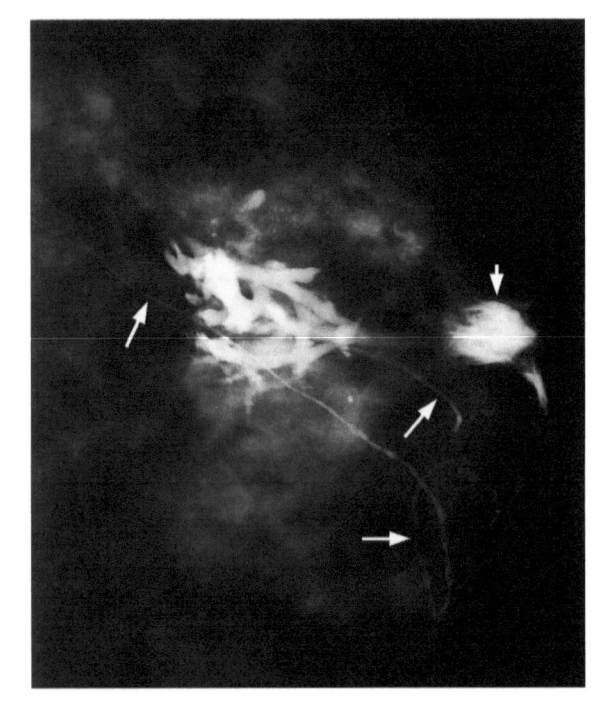

Fig. 3.40 Extravasation of contrast medium (short arrow) and several fine winding lymph vessels (long arrow).

Galactography

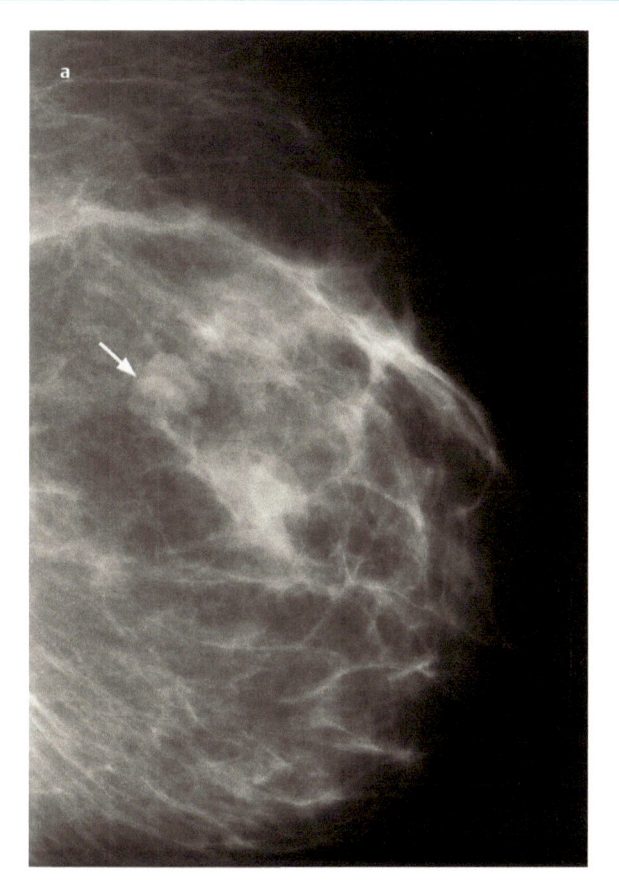

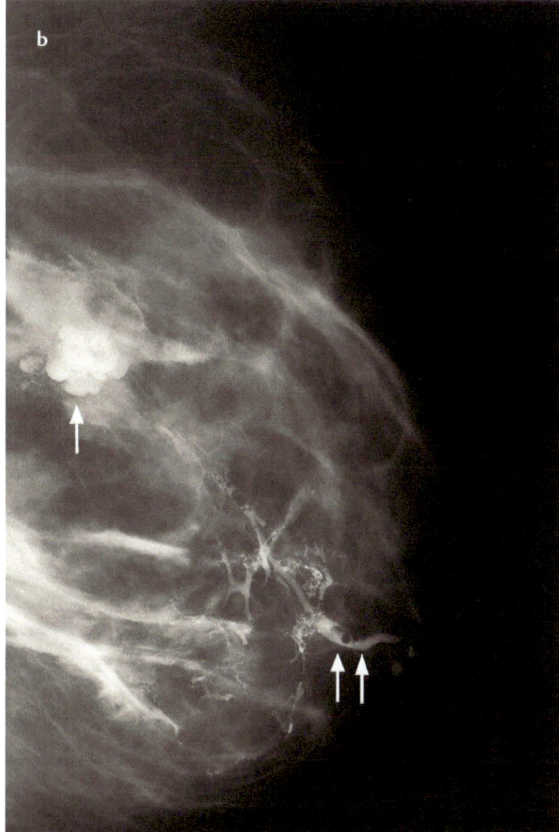

Fig. 3.41a,b

a Lobulated focal density is shown laterally on this mediolateral mammographic view.

b Galactography revealed this to be a small convoluted cyst (single arrow). Air bubbles in the lactiferous duct system can be identified by their uniform round shape and their varying localization on several views. On the mediolateral view, they can be identified by their localization along the superior wall of the ducts (double arrows). Leakage of contrast is seen in the inferior aspect of the breast.

Duct Sonography and MRI

With the increasing resolution of high-frequency ultrasound transducers, duct sonography is increasingly being used to evaluate the ductal system (Ballesio et al. 2007, Rissanen et al. 2007). Duct sonography is performed by imaging the breast and retroareolar area using radial planes. That way the course of ducts may be followed and intraductal abnormalities may be recognized as such (**Fig. 3.39**). Using high-resolution ultrasound (US) the proximal 3–5 cm of the ducts can thus be visualized. Sometimes (but not regularly) even peripheral dilated ducts may be recognized. If duct sonography shows an intraductal abnormality, US-guided percutaneous breast biopsy or needle localization becomes possible. Since intraductal changes may be quite small and subtle, US-guided vacuum-assisted breast biopsy (VABB) is preferable to core needle biopsy for the assessment of focal lesions (Torres-Tabanera et al. 2008). For diffuse, regional or segmental ductal changes surgery after US-guided marking is the method of choice.

If duct sonography is negative, galactography or MRI remains necessary.

Based on the limited data available, MRI might become an alternative to galactography (Sardanelli et al. 2010). Currently MRI is indicated whenever duct sonography is negative and galactography is not possible.

Histopathologic Assessment of Ductal Abnormalities

Further assessment of ductal abnormalities depends on the extent of the changes and on the mode of detection.

Focal abnormalities may be well suited for percutaneous breast biopsy. Since most ductal abnormalities are small or concern papillary lesions (for which core needle biopsy may not be representative) VABB should be considered the method of choice. VABB may be used under sonographic, galactographic, or (if a lesion is visible only by MRI) MR guidance.

For segmental lesions excision of the involved segment will mostly be preferable, since (in the case of larger lesions) excision will usually yield a representative result and will eliminate the symptom. Excision should be performed after preoperative marking of the area in question.

There are essentially several ways of marking nonpalpable intraductal findings that are not visualized by ultrasound:

1. The physician can perform repeat galactography of the suspicious duct immediately preoperatively. The duct is filled with a mixture of 50% contrast medium and 50% methylene blue. Since methylene blue diffuses rapidly, the blue-dyed ductal system must be excised shortly after injection.
2. After repeat galactography with contrast and methylene blue has been performed, the galactographically suspicious area is marked under mammographic guidance (see Mammographic Localization Procedure, Chapter 8). If a wire is used for marking, timing of surgery directly after the marking (with a well-positioned and fixed wire) is not as critical as it is if methylene blue were used.
3. Clip marking is possible directly after detection and may thus even help avoid repeated galactography. Timing of surgery is independent of the time of clip marking.
4. Changes that are visible by MRI only require MR-guided preoperative marking (using MR-compatible wires or clips).
5. For planning surgery and preoperative marking it should be remembered that intraductal disease may extend into the periphery beyond a galactographic or galactoscopic stop.

Summary

Galactography is still considered the method of choice for imaging assessment of pathologic nipple discharge or those changes that are not visible by mammography or ultrasound including duct sonography.

Galactography allows localization of intraductal masses. It may help to better assess the extent of these lesions. Only when nipple discharge is due to duct ectasia can a definitive diagnosis be made. Biopsy is indicated for any intraductal mass detected by galactography because this imaging modality cannot reliably distinguish between benign and malignant filling defects.

Pneumocystography

Definition

Pneumocystography refers to mammographic imaging of an aspirated cyst that has been filled with air. It has been used to diagnose and to treat cysts, that is, bring about their involution.

Indications

With increasing capabilities of ultrasonography, the application of pneumocystography for workup of *sonographic findings that are suspicious but inconclusive for cysts* is decreasing and is now only very rarely utilized (e.g., if there is uncertain differentiation between hyperechoic debris in the cyst, intracystic mass, and a hypoechoic solid mass). In current practice aspiration of a suspected cyst is attempted. If this is not possible and the lesion proves to be (completely or partly) solid, core needle biopsy is usually indicated instead.

The use of pneumocystography for treatment of symptomatic cysts is controversial. Since large cysts can cause a sensation of pressure and pain, decompressing the cyst will relieve these symptoms. However, frequently after decompression of one cyst others will appear.

Indications no longer applicable. Cysts with sonographically detected *irregularities in their walls* or intracystic masses. For these cases, pneumocystography has been replaced by biopsy.

Aspirating a cyst containing a small intracystic mass can even be detrimental. The lesion might disappear—at least for a limited time—and thus cannot be targeted for percutaneous biopsy or for surgery. However, this sort of complicated cyst will generally fill again if a papilloma or carcinoma is actually present, and the cyst will then again become visible, enabling percutaneous breast biopsy (core needle biopsy or VABB) or surgery to be performed.

Whenever unequivocal sonographic diagnosis of a simple cyst is possible, no further histo-pathologic assessment is indicated.

Contraindications

- Acute inflammation
- Coagulopathies or anticoagulant therapy (relative contraindication)

Side Effects

Puncturing a hardened, chronically inflamed cyst wall may be painful, but may be alleviated by use of local anesthetic. Inflammatory reaction after aspiration is extremely rare. Hematomas due to injury of a vascular structure are rare but possible. The indication must be carefully checked in patients with coagulatory disorders or on anticoagulant therapy or aspirin. Pneumothorax has been observed in very rare cases. For this reason, the needle should always be introduced parallel to the chest wall and—whenever close to the chest wall—under sonographic guidance.

Procedure

- Palpable superficial lumps can be aspirated without guidance.
- Aspiration under sonographic guidance is recommended for nonpalpable or confluent cysts. Aspirate after disinfecting the skin. Select a needle that is not too thin (a 20-gauge needle will usually be sufficient) since the contents of the cyst may vary in viscosity.
- Empty the cyst completely. With the needle still in place, attach a new syringe and insufflate the cyst with a slightly smaller volume of air than the volume of fluid that was removed (note that the air will expand at body temperature). Non-milky fluid should be examined cytologically. However, negative cytology does not eliminate the need for futher investigation of residual or suspicious lesions (by percutaneous or open biopsy).

Any suspicious intracystic mass is an indication for biopsy. Negative cytologic examination of the aspirated fluid should not prevent biopsy because false negative results are possible in the presence of necrotic material.

> **Summary**
>
> Diagnostic pneumocystography has become a very rare procedure for assessment of sonographically inconclusive findings. It should usually be replaced by cyst aspiration, percutaneous biopsy, or, rarely, surgery. It may sometimes be used to decompress a painful cyst.
>
> The introduction of air is believed by some to prevent refilling of the cyst by facilitating shrinkage of the cyst walls. If pneumocystography shows no pathologic findings, standard sonographic follow-up examinations will be sufficient.
>
> When bloody fluid is aspirated from the cyst, yet cytologic results are negative, a short interval (e.g., 3 months) follow-up sonographic examination may be desirable.

References and Recommended Reading

ACR-AAPM-SIIM practice guideline for determinants of image quality in digital mammography. American College of Radiology; 2007. Available at: www.acr.org

Albert US, Altland H, Duda V, et al. 2008 update of the guideline: early detection of breast cancer in Germany. J Cancer Res Clin Oncol 2009;135(3):339–354

American College of Radiology BI-RADS Atlas and MQSA. Frequently Asked Questions (updated 4/11/08). American College of Radiology; 2008. Available at www.acr.org

American College of Radiology. Practice Guidelines and Technical Standards. Breast Imaging and Intervention. American College of Radiology; 2006. Available at: http://www.acr.org

Ballesio L, Maggi C, Savelli S, et al. Adjunctive diagnostic value of ultrasonography evaluation in patients with suspected ductal breast disease. Radiol Med (Torino) 2007;112(3):354–365

Barnes GT. Mammography equipment: compression, scatter control and automatic exposure control. In: Haus AG, Yaffe MJ, eds. Syllabus: A categorical course in physics: Technical aspects of breast imaging, 3rd ed. Oak Brook: RSNA Publications; 1994:75

Barnes GT, Brezovich IA. Contrast: effect of scattered radiation. In: Logan WW, Muntz EP, eds. Reduced dose mammography. New York: Masson; 1979

Baum JK, Hanna LG, Acharyya S, et al. Use of BI-RADS 3-probably benign category in the American College of Radiology Imaging Network Digital Mammographic Imaging Screening Trial. Radiology 2011;260(1):61–67

Berkowitz JE, Gatewood OM, Gayler BW. Equivocal mammographic findings: evaluation with spot compression. Radiology 1989;171(2):369–371

Berry DA, Cronin KA, Plevritis SK, et al; Cancer Intervention and Surveillance Modeling Network (CISNET) Collaborators. Effect of screening and adjuvant therapy on mortality from breast cancer. N Engl J Med 2005;353(17):1784–1792

Boyd NF, Jong RA, Yaffe MJ, Tritchler D, Lockwood G, Zylak CJ. A critical appraisal of the Canadian National Breast Cancer Screening Study. Radiology 1993;189(3):661–663

Boyer B, Hauret L, Bellaiche R, Gräf C, Bourcier B, Fichet G. Retrospectively detectable carcinomas: review of the literature. [Article in French] J Radiol 2004;85(12 Pt 2):2071–2078

Caumo F, Vecchiato F, Strabbioli M, Zorzi M, Baracco S, Ciatto S. Interval cancers in breast cancer screening: comparison of stage and biological characteristics with screen-detected cancers or incident cancers in the absence of screening. Tumori 2010;96(2):198–201

D'Orsi CJ, Bassett LW, Berg WA, et al. Breast Imaging Reporting and Data System: ACR BI-RADS-Mammography (ed. 4). Reston, VA: American College of Radiology; 2003

Dance DR, Skinner CL, Young KC, Beckett JR, Kotre CJ. Additional factors for the estimation of mean glandular breast dose using the UK mammography dosimetry protocol. Phys Med Biol 2000;45(11):3225–3240

Dinkel HP, Trusen A, Gassel AM, et al. Predictive value of galactographic patterns for benign and malignant neoplasms of the breast in patients with nipple discharge. Br J Radiol 2000;73(871):706–714

Dinnes J, Moss S, Melia J, Blanks R, Song F, Kleijnen J. Effectiveness and cost-effectiveness of double reading of mammograms in breast cancer screening: findings of a systematic review. Breast 2001;10(6):455–463

Eklund GW, Cardenosa G. The art of mammographic positioning. Radiol Clin North Am 1992;30(1):21–53

Elmore JG, Armstrong K, Lehman CD, Fletcher SW. Screening for breast cancer. JAMA 2005;293(10):1245–1256

Elmore JG, Jackson SL, Abraham L, et al. Variability in interpretive performance at screening mammography and radiologists' characteristics associated with accuracy. Radiology 2009;253(3):641–651

Friedrich M. The technique and results of mammography. [Article in German] Radiologe 1993;33(5):243–259

Graham RA, Homer MJ, Sigler CJ, et al. The efficacy of specimen radiography in evaluating the surgical margins of impalpable breast carcinoma. AJR Am J Roentgenol 1994;162(1):33–36

Gromet M. Comparison of computer-aided detection to double reading of screening mammograms: review of 231,221 mammograms. AJR Am J Roentgenol 2008;190(4):854–859

Guerriero C, Gillan MG, Cairns J, Wallis MG, Gilbert FJ. Is computer aided detection (CAD) cost effective in screening mammography? A model based on the CADET II study. BMC Health Serv Res 2011;11:11

Harvey JA, Fajardo LL, Innis CA. Previous mammograms in patients with impalpable breast carcinoma: retrospective vs blinded interpretation. 1993 ARRS President's Award. AJR Am J Roentgenol 1993;161(6):1167–1172

Heinig A, Heywang-Köbrunner SH, Viehweg P, Lampe D, Buchmann J, Spielmann RP. Value of contrast medium magnetic resonance tomography of the breast in breast reconstruction with implant. [Article in German] Radiologe 1997;37(9):710–717

Hendrick RE. Radiation doses and cancer risks from breast imaging studies. Radiology 2010;257(1):246–253

Hendrick RE, Bassett L, Botsco RT, et al. Mammography quality control manual. American College of Radiology; 1999

Heyes GJ, Mill AJ, Charles MW. Mammography–oncogenicity at low doses. J Radiol Prot 2009;29(2A):A123–A132

Heywang-Köbrunner SH, Schreer I, Heindel W, Katalinic A. Imaging studies for the early detection of breast cancer. Dtsch Arztebl Int 2008;105(31-32):541–547

Hofvind S, Geller B, Skaane P. Mammographic features and histopathological findings of interval breast cancers. Acta Radiol 2008;49(9):975–981

Hou MF, Huang TJ, Liu GC. The diagnostic value of galactography in patients with nipple discharge. Clin Imaging 2001;25(2):75–81

Houssami N, Given-Wilson R, Ciatto S. Early detection of breast cancer: overview of the evidence on computer-aided detection in mammography screening. J Med Imaging Radiat Oncol 2009;53(2):171–176

James JJ, Gilbert FJ, Wallis MG, et al. Mammographic features of breast cancers at single reading with computer-aided detection and at double reading in a large multicenter prospective trial of computer-aided detection: CADET II. Radiology 2010;256(2):379–386

Karssemeijer N, Bluekens AM, Beijerinck D, et al. Breast cancer screening results 5 years after introduction of digital mammography in a population-based screening program. Radiology 2009;253(2):353–358

Kimme-Smith C, Bassett LW, Gold RH. Workbook for quality mammography. Baltimore: Williams & Wilkins; 1992

Kindermann G. Diagnostic value of galactography in the detection of breast cancer. In: Zander J, Baltzer J, eds. Early breast cancer. Berlin: Springer; 1985:136–139

Küchler A, Friedrich M. Progress in mammography technics. Bimetal anode tubes and selective filtration technic. [Article in German] Fortschr Rontgenstr 1993;159(1):91–96

Law J. Cancers detected and induced in mammographic screening: new screening schedules and younger women with family history. Br J Radiol 1997;70:62–69

Law J, Faulkner K, Young KC. Risk factors for induction of breast cancer by X-rays and their implications for breast screening. Br J Radiol 2007;80(952):261–266

Lewin JM, Hendrick RE, D'Orsi CJ, et al. Comparison of full-field digital mammography with screen-film mammography for cancer detection: results of 4,945 paired examinations. Radiology 2001;218(3):873–880

Lewin JM, D'Orsi CJ, Hendrick RE, et al. Clinical comparison of full-field digital mammography and screen-film mammography for detection of breast cancer. AJR Am J Roentgenol 2002;179(3):671–677

Liberman L, Abramson AF, Squires FB, Glassman JR, Morris EA, Dershaw DD. The breast imaging reporting and data system: positive predictive value of mammographic features and final assessment categories. AJR Am J Roentgenol 1998;171(1):35–40

Logan WW, Janus J. Use of special mammographic views to maximize radiographic information. Radiol Clin North Am 1987;25(5):953–959

Montroni I, Santini D, Zucchini G, et al. Nipple discharge: is its significance as a risk factor for breast cancer fully understood? Observational study including 915 consecutive patients who underwent selective duct excision. Breast Cancer Res Treat 2010;123(3):895–900

National Academy of Sciences. Health risks from exposure to low levels of ionizing radiation: BEIR VII–phase 2. Washington DC: National Academies Press; 2006

Noble M, Bruening W, Uhl S, Schoelles K. Computer-aided detection mammography for breast cancer screening: systematic review and meta-analysis. Arch Gynecol Obstet 2009;279(6):881–890

O'Connor MK, Li H, Rhodes DJ, Hruska CB, Clancy CB, Vetter RJ. Comparison of radiation exposure and associated radiation-induced cancer risks from mammography and molecular imaging of the breast. Med Phys 2010;37(12):6187–6198

Perry N, Broeders M, De Wolf C, et al, eds. European Guidelines for quality assurance in mammography screening, 4th ed. Luxembourg: Office for Official Publications of the European Communities; 2006

Pisano ED, Gatsonis CA, Hendrick E, et al; Digital Mammographic Imaging Screening Trial (DMIST) Investigators Group. Diagnostic performance of digital versus film mammography for breast-cancer screening. N Engl J Med 2005;353(17):1773–1783

Porter GJR, Evans AJ, Burrell HC, Lee AH, Ellis IO, Chakrabarti J. Interval breast cancers: prognostic features and survival by subtype and time since screening. J Med Screen 2006;13(3):115–122

Rissanen T, Reinikainen H, Apaja-Sarkkinen M. Breast sonography in localizing the cause of nipple discharge: comparison with galactography in 52 patients. J Ultrasound Med 2007;26(8):1031–1039

Robson KJ. An investigation into the effects of suboptimal viewing conditions in screen-film mammography. Br J Radiol 2008;81(963):219–231

Roelofs AA, Karssemeijer N, Wedekind N, et al. Importance of comparison of current and prior mammograms in breast cancer screening. Radiology 2007;242(1):70–77

Rose A, Osborne J, Wright G, Billson V. Is what you see what you get? Breast specimen handling re-visited. Australas Radiol 1991;35(2):145–147

Rosenberg RD, Hunt WC, Williamson MR, et al. Effects of age, breast density, ethnicity, and estrogen replacement therapy on screening mammographic sensitivity and cancer stage at diagnosis: review of 183,134 screening mammograms in Albuquerque, New Mexico. Radiology 1998;209(2):511–518

Samei E, Badano A. Chakraborty et al. Assessment of display performance for medical imaging systems. Report of the American Association of Physicists in Medicine (AAPM) Task Group 18 (AAPM On-Line Report No. 03). Madison, WI: Medical Physics Publishing; 2005

Samuels T, Kerenyi N, Taylor G, Savilo E, Ehrlich L. Practical aspects of mammographic-pathological correlation: experience with needle localization. Can Assoc Radiol J 1990;41(3):127–129

Sardanelli F, Boetes C, Borisch B, et al. Magnetic resonance imaging of the breast: recommendations from the EUSOMA working group. Eur J Cancer 2010;46(8):1296–1316

Sickles EA. Practical solutions to common mammographic problems: tailoring the examination. AJR Am J Roentgenol 1988;151(1):31–39

Sickles EA. Probably benign breast lesions: when should follow-up be recommended and what is the optimal follow-up protocol? Radiology 1999;213(1):11–14

Sickles EA, Ominsky SH, Sollitto RA, Galvin HB, Monticciolo DL. Medical audit of a rapid-throughput mammography screening practice: methodology and results of 27,114 examinations. Radiology 1990;175(2):323–327

Skaane P. Studies comparing screen–film mammography and full-field digital mammography in breast cancer screening: updated review. Acta Radiol 2009;50(1):3–14

Skaane P, Skjennald A. Screen–film mammography versus full-field digital mammography with soft-copy reading: randomized trial in a population-based screening program—the Oslo II Study. Radiology 2004;232(1):197–204

Skaane P, Young K, Skjennald A. Population-based mammography screening: comparison of screen–film and full-field digital mammography with soft-copy reading—Oslo I study. Radiology 2003;229(3):877–884

Strahlenschutzkommission SSK. Evaluierung von Nutzen und Risiken im qualitätsgesicherten Mammographie-Screening in Deutschland. Empfehlung der Strahlenschutzkommission; 2010. Available at http://www.ssk.de

Tabár L, Dean PB, Péntek Z. Galactography: the diagnostic procedure of choice for nipple discharge. Radiology 1983;149(1):31–38

Taylor P, Potts HW. Computer aids and human second reading as interventions in screening mammography: two systematic reviews to compare effects on cancer detection and recall rate. Eur J Cancer 2008;44(6):798–807

Torres-Tabanera M, Alonso-Bartolomé P, Vega-Bolivar A, et al. Percutaneous microductectomy with a directional vacuum-assisted system guided by ultrasonography for the treatment of breast discharge: experience in 63 cases. Acta Radiol 2008;49(3):271–276

van Gils CH, Otten JD, Verbeek AL, Hendriks JH, Holland R. Effect of mammographic breast density on breast cancer screening performance: a study in Nijmegen, The Netherlands. J Epidemiol Community Health 1998;52(4):267–271

Varela C, Karssemeijer N, Hendriks JH, Holland R. Use of prior mammograms in the classification of benign and malignant masses. Eur J Radiol 2005;56(2):248–255

Vinnicombe S, Pinto Pereira SM, McCormack VA, Shiel S, Perry N, Dos Santos Silva IM. Full-field digital versus screen-film mammography: comparison within the UK breast screening program and systematic review of published data. Radiology 2009;251(2):347–358

Yaffe MJ, Mainprize JG. Risk of radiation-induced breast cancer from mammographic screening. Radiology 2011;258(1):98–105

Yaffe MJ. AAPM tutorial. Physics of mammography: image recording process. Radiographics 1990;10(2):341–363

Young KC, Wallis MG, Blanks RG, Moss SM. Influence of number of views and mammographic film density on the detection of invasive cancers: results from the NHS Breast Screening Programme. Br J Radiol 1997;70(833):482–488

4 Sonography

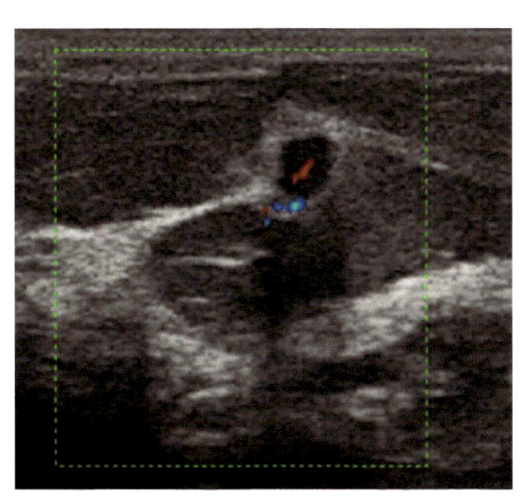

Purpose, Accuracy, Possibilities, and Limitations ⇢ *98*
Diagnosing Cysts ⇢ *98*
Differentiating Solid Lesions ⇢ *98*
Diagnosing Carcinoma ⇢ *98*
Imaging Assessment of Younger Women ⇢ *99*
Screening with Sonography ⇢ *99*
Ultrasonography of the Axilla ⇢ *99*

Equipment Requirements ⇢ *100*
Transducer ⇢ *100*
Image Quality ⇢ *101*

Examination Technique ⇢ *103*
Time-Gain Compensation ⇢ *104*
Focusing ⇢ *105*
Examination Technique and Documentation ⇢ *105*

Interpreting and Documenting Sonographic Findings ⇢ *112*
Normal Sonographic Findings ⇢ *112*
Sonographic Lesions ⇢ *113*

References and Recommended Reading ⇢ *124*

4 Sonography

I. Schreer, S. H. Heywang-Koebrunner, S. Barter

Purpose, Accuracy, Possibilities, and Limitations

After mammography, sonography is the most important breast imaging modality. Its most important roles include:
- Diagnosing cysts
- Characterizing masses that are incompletely assessed by mammography (BI-RADS [Breast Imaging Reporting and Data System] 3, 4 and 5)
- Characterizing palpable masses that are obscured by dense tissue on mammography
- Complementary assessment in women with dense tissue and high risk
- First imaging choice in symptomatic women under the age of 40 years
- First imaging modality for visualization of the axilla
- Imaging guidance for percutaneous biopsy and localization

Diagnosing Cysts

Diagnosing cysts is one of the most important contributions of sonography to breast imaging. The diagnosis of a simple cyst makes it possible to assure that a mass is benign and requires no additional workup for definitive diagnosis. Sonography is the most accurate method in this regard, and can correctly diagnose the vast majority of simple cysts. Therefore, sonography is very useful in the workup of any palpable or nonpalpable lesion that could be due to a simple cyst. It is important to be quite diligent with this diagnosis. There are a few malignant lesions that may appear almost anechoic and can thus be confused with a simple cyst. Lesions that are not anechoic, do not exhibit adequate through-transmission, or show irregular margins may require further evaluation. Tissue harmonic imaging, Doppler imaging, or elastography may help with the distinction. In case of doubt the lesion should be punctured.

Differentiating Solid Lesions

Sonography is helpful as a modality in addition to mammography in assessing the internal texture and shape of the margins of masses that are partially or completely obscured by dense tissue on mammography. Palpable lesions that are located in dense tissue and cannot be clearly or completely visualized mammographically can often be further characterized by sonography. In interpreting sonographic results, the following considerations should be kept in mind:
- If a lesion is not a simple cyst and a mammogram has not been performed, this should be done to further characterize the mass, for example to demonstrate possible diagnostic patterns of calcifications.
- Benign sonographic findings in the presence of suspicious mammographic findings do not exclude malignancy.
- A mass that cannot be seen sonographically should be considered not to be a cyst and therefore solid. This implies that these lesions may also be caused by a carcinoma.
- If there are any doubts about the benignity of a lesion after complete imaging assessment, further diagnostic procedures (short-term follow-up or biopsy) are indicated.

Diagnosing Carcinoma

Although many carcinomas are seen sonographically as hypoechoic masses, the echogenicity of carcinoma is variable. Some carcinomas are hyperechoic with fat and some are isoechoic with breast tissue.

The sonographic visibility of carcinomas also depends on the surrounding tissue. Since fat is hypoechoic compared with glandular tissue (as are most carcinomas), carcinomas may be missed sonographically within fatty tissue. Hypoechoic fat lobules may, furthermore, mimic malignancy.

Because of these factors, some cancers will not be seen with sonography, although they may be easily found mammographically. This pitfall may occur in any type of breast tissue, but is more frequent within fatty breast tissue than in mixed breast tissue or dense hyperechoic glandular tissue.

Hypoechoic carcinomas are readily identified when they are located within more echogenic breast parenchyma. In these situations, where cancers may be obscured by surrounding breast tissue mammographically, sonography can be very useful, especially in assessing a palpable lesion.

Some anatomical structures in the breast can be confused with worrisome lesions. These include shadowing Cooper ligaments and hypoechoic fatty lobules. Considerable time and effort is necessary in the sonographic examination of some breasts to reliably distinguish normal structures from malignancy. Diligent evaluation of sometimes numerous hypoechoic areas and shadowing is needed; this includes verification of the finding in two planes and compressibility checks.

Imaging Assessment of Younger Women

In the imaging assessment of younger women (below age 40), sonography should usually be the first imaging study in the workup of a palpable mass. If diagnosis of a simple cyst is possible, no further workup is needed. If a simple cyst cannot be diagnosed, mammography should be performed to attempt to gain additional information before deciding upon the need for biopsy. In women below age 30 it may be decided to proceed directly from sonography to ultrasound (US)-guided biopsy if the underlying lesion is likely to be a fibroadenoma and no other indications for mammography exist (high risk). If the expected specific benign and compatible diagnosis is not obtained by US-guided biopsy, mammography should be re-considered.

Screening with Sonography

The only imaging study that has been demonstrated to be effective for screening is mammography. Based on the limited sensitivity of ultrasound concerning the detection of small and in-situ carcinomas—even if high-frequency transducers are used—ultrasonography cannot replace mammography. Only limited evidence suggests that sonographic screening added to mammography may allow reliable detection of additional carcinomas with acceptable side effects.

In selected groups of women with dense breast tissue and negative clinical and mammographic examination, an incremental cancer detection rate ranging from 2.8 to 4.6 cancers per 1,000 women has been reported. Owing to differing selection of the examined women (concerning age distribution, indication, and risk factors) these results cannot be transferred to the usual screening population (age 50–69, low to moderate risk). The existing results suggest that the false positive rate (concerning recommendation for biopsy or for short-term follow-up) may be unacceptably high with sonography (Buchberger et al. 1999, Kaplan 2001, Gordon 2002, Kolb et al. 2002, Crystal et al. 2003, Berg et al. 2008, Nothacker et al. 2009, Lee et al. 2010, Corsetti et al. 2011). The examination is also very operator dependent and time consuming (Berg et al. 2006, Lazarus et al. 2006, Abdullah et al. 2009).

The feasibility of quality assurance (technique and interpretation), which would be indispensable for any type of additional ultrasound screening, is not established. Thus, based on the existing evidence, *there are no recommendations for the use of sonography for screening for breast cancer*. The Standards of the American College of Radiology specifically state that sonography is not a screening study for the breast (American College of Radiology Practice Guideline 2011).

Even though reduction in the rate of interval cancers and improved detection of malignancy (without microcalcifications) in mammographically dense tissue may be very desirable, establishment of a nationwide quality assurance system and specific testing concerning the added value and side effects in the screening situation would be needed before the role of ultrasonography in breast cancer screening should be discussed.

Ultrasonography of the Axilla

Ultrasound examination of the axilla is indicated:
- As the first imaging method, whenever a clinical finding of the axilla is noted or reported (palpable abnormality, pain) or for the assessment of impaired vascular or lymphatic drainage.
- For complementary evaluation of axillary changes detected by mammography, magnetic resonance imaging (MRI), positron emission tomography (PET) or other tests.
- To screen the axilla in patients with a known breast cancer (surveillance after breast cancer).
- To countercheck for suspicious lymph nodes in patients with an imaging abnormality of the breast that requires histopathologic assessment. The reason for axillary evaluation before histopathologic assessment (or verification of a malignancy) is that specificity of ultrasonography after biopsy might be decreased due to postinterventional reactive changes of the lymph node(s).

Apart from lymph nodes, ectopic breast tissue including benign and malignant breast disease and rarely other changes or disease (like vascular abnormalities, inflammation, haematoma, benign and malignant tumors of the soft tissues, nerves, skin, etc.) may be detected (Kim et al. 2009). Further assessment is possible by mammography, computed tomography, MRI, image-guided biopsy, or surgery.

The accuracy of ultrasonography of axillary breast disease is expected to be similar to that of breast imaging. To date, axillary ultrasonography (usually combined with US-guided biopsy) is increasingly used for locoregional staging. The rationale is that, if malignancy is proven by ultrasonography and US-guided biopsy, sentinel node biopsy (which—if positive—would currently be followed by axillary dissection) can be averted. This may save unnecessary stress to the patient and unnecessary costs by avoiding two axillary surgical procedures. For this special indication the limited sensitivity of imaging for the detection of early lymph node involvement is acceptable. The reported specificity of combined ultrasonography and US-guided biopsy is > 97% (Sidibé et al. 2007). According to the published literature the sensitivity and specificity of for evaluation of all lymph nodes (palpable or nonpalpable) range around 60–80% and 85–85%, respectively. Sometimes even large lymph nodes may not be adequately visualized (Neal et al. 2010) and the sensitivity for detection of malignancy in nonpalpable lymph nodes ranges only around 40% (Alvarez et al. 2006, Sidibé et al. 2007, Mainiero et al. 2010, Mills et al. 2010). However, the diagnostic accuracy of MRI or PET is no better. The specificity of ultrasonography is increased by combining it with percutaneous breast biopsy, mainly US-guided fine needle biopsy. For the above goal, ultrasonography with US-guided fine needle biopsy has to date proved to be the best combination.

If, however, the need for axillary staging or surgical treatment (as presently discussed by some epidemiologists) might be questioned, the role of axillary imaging will also have to be re-assessed.

Guiding Biopsy

Whenever a lesion requires histopathologic assessment and the lesion is visible by ultrasound imaging, ultrasonography should be the preferred method of guidance. The reason is that this technique allows real-time monitoring. It allows access from almost any direction. Furthermore it is the simplest and fastest method. US-guided biopsies are thus usually excellently tolerated and are most cost-effective. US guidance should also be used for palpable lesions, since a better accuracy has thus been achieved.

> **Summary**
>
> Ultrasonography is the most important breast imaging modality after mammography. It is excellent in diagnosing simple cysts, eliminating the need for biopsy of unequivocal cysts.
>
> Definitive sonographic diagnosis of solid masses is less certain, although certain characteristics can increase the likelihood that a mass is malignant or benign. There are criteria based on which biopsy can be avoided and follow-up is justified. In many cases biopsy will be required for a definitive diagnosis.
>
> When a mass is palpable and no focal sonographic findings are present, the lesion should be considered to be solid, increasing the possibility of it being malignant. When a cyst is seen to correspond to a palpable mass, care should be taken to make certain that the palpable lesion and the cyst are the same mass.
>
> When younger women (below age 40) present with a breast mass, the initial step in the evaluation of the mass is usually sonography. If the lesion is a cyst, no further imaging is needed. Sonography is not a proven tool for breast cancer screening. Its use in this setting is not encouraged. Ultrasonography combined with US-guided biopsy may be useful to avoid unnecessary sentinel node biopsy (followed by axillary surgery) in cases with a high probability of axillary involvement (T2–T4 stages).

Equipment Requirements

In spite of the expected advantages of automated breast sonography (contiguous imaging of the breast tissue, analysis of symmetry in bilateral examinations, potential of improved standardization, time-savings for the radiologist) it so far has not been able to replace hand-held ultrasonography, which in Europe is usually performed by the trained physician.

Considering the direct and obviously indispensable interaction of the examiner, so far hand-held ultrasonography has proved to be superior to the automated technique. This interaction concerns adaptation of transducer angulation to avoid shadowing, examination in varying planes, combined evaluation of palpable and sonographic findings, testing of elasticity, and mobility.

Therefore, to date hand-held ultrasonography remains the state-of-the-art method of performing breast ultrasound imaging.

Transducer

Breast sonography requires the use of hand-held, high-frequency, linear-array transducers. These should be able to be focused in the near field, and have a capacity for variable focus, so that the ultrasound beam can be focused at the level of interest in the breast. Transducer frequency should be at least 7.5 MHz. Transducers with a higher frequency may improve resolution. However, with increasing frequency the ability of the soundbeam to penetrate tissue decreases. Therefore, very high-frequency transducers may not be able to fully penetrate large breasts. The minimum acceptable penetration must allow visualization of all the breast tissue from the skin to the chest wall in all slices of the examined breast. Exceptions should be made only for targeted ultrasound examination of superficial lesions in very large breasts.

Furthermore very high-frequency transducers may also have a smaller field of view. With a very small field of view a significant risk exists that a small lesion may escape a systematic check and may thus be missed. Also, a too small field of view may lead to overestimation of very small changes and might impair assessment of diffuse changes. Optimum possibilities exist with larger transducers (> 5 cm), which provide an adapted range of frequencies to image both superficial and deep structures. Transducers with a field of view < 5 cm are usually needed for evaluation of the axilla, since with larger transducers coupling may be impaired owing to the curved surface of the axilla.

Image Quality

Factors determining the image quality of a breast sonography unit are spatial resolution, contrast resolution and contrast, image quality in the near field, reduction of noise and artifacts, slice thickness (focusing), and temporal resolution (multifocus realtime imaging, etc.).

Spatial Resolution, Contrast Resolution

Resolution is determined by axial resolution, lateral resolution (**Fig. 4.1**), and contrast resolution.

1. *Axial resolution* (resolution along the direction of sound travel) is determined by the length of the ultrasound pulse, which is generally about two wavelengths. The minimum axial resolution is half of this value. Generally, for a 7.5-MHz transducer, resolution is around 0.4 mm.

2. *Lateral resolution* (the width of the ultrasound pulse) is determined by the size of the transducer element or its aperture, the frequency, and the focus. Transducer designs have different abilities to focus the soundbeam. Fixed-focus transducers have a concave arrangement of transducer elements or use an acoustic lens. To change the focus of the soundbeam when using transducers of this configuration, the transducer must be changed. This design is largely archaic and is not part of modern ultrasound technology.

Modern transducers are designed to have a variable focus that is electronically controlled (**Fig. 4.1**). Depending upon the timing of excitation of various elements in the transducer, the focus can be altered to a variety of distances from the transducer surface. Electronic focusing makes it possible to focus the soundbeam during transmission (multiple transmit focusing) and during reception (dynamic focusing).

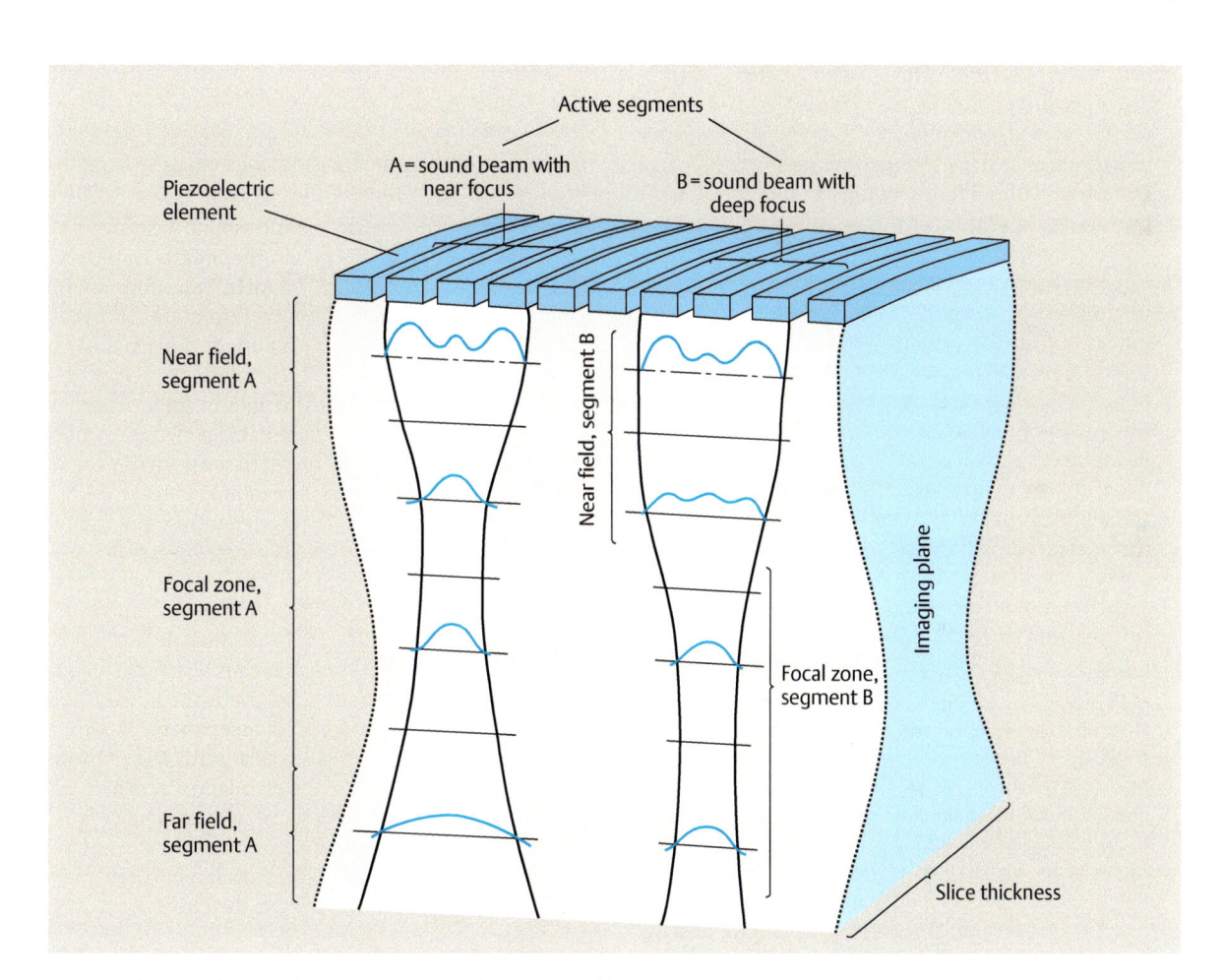

Fig. 4.1 Schematic diagram showing the ultrasound beam emitted by a transducer.
The depth of focus (shown here for segments A and B) is set by delaying the excitation of the central transducer element accordingly. The ultrasound signal (depicted in the diagram as individual echoes in the ultrasound beam) shows artifacts in the near field due to interference. A fixed focus can be achieved by a concave arrangement of the piezoelectric elements.

This makes is possible to improve lateral resolution over a wide range of distances from the transducer surface.

Further improvement in focusing is possible by electronically adjusting the aperture (the area of the active piezoelectric element array).

While dynamic focus capability improves resolution simultaneously at various depths, multiple transmit focusing decreases the possible frame rate (images per second). Depending on the individual equipment, dynamic lesion evaluation (compressibility test, monitoring of interventions) may be impaired to a varying degree. If such a multifocus capability is not desirable and therefore not chosen, the examiner must adjust the depth of the focus to the depth of the tissue area in question. Dynamic focusing is always active during reception and no control element is necessary.

3. Contrast resolution is a major factor in determining the quality of the image. Among other factors, it is a measure of the sharpness of the lateral definition of the pulse and of how well a weak echo can be discerned next to a slightly stronger echo. Contrast resolution depends upon the transducer and signal processing within the sonographic unit.

Compared with earlier sonographic units, newer units provide significantly finer grayscale definition (> 8 bits, corresponding to 256 shades of gray). These units can produce high-contrast images of the varying echo intensities occurring in tissue. They may also elicit echoes within the proteinaceous or serosanguinous contents of many cysts. Over-sensitive demonstration of echoes in cysts, however, may interfere with the capability of correctly identifying cysts with ultrasound.

Apart from varying algorithms of image processing, compound imaging is being used to optimize soft tissue contrast and reduce artifacts. With compound scanning a slice is electronically interrogated from slightly different angles and a compound image is calculated from this information. This allows increasing image contrast by decreasing noise and artifacts and reducing disturbing shadowing from oblique or perpendicular structures like Cooper ligaments or side walls of cysts or solid lesions. Too much compounding, however, may also reduce the diagnostic information that is gained from shadowing that, for example, may occur behind a malignancy.

Another approach to gain further information from the obtained ultrasound beam is tissue harmonic imaging (THI). With THI, harmonic echo frequencies rather than the original (fundamental) transmit frequency are used to generate the image. The second and higher harmonic frequencies are contained in the reflected ultrasound echo signals due to the nonlinear tissue response to the incident ultrasound beam. A prerequisite for THI is the efficient suppression of other components in the echo signals. This is achieved by inverting the phase between two consecutive transmit pulses (phase inversion technique). When the echoes from these two pulses are added, the fundamental echo components cancel each other and the harmonic echo signals are enhanced. This technique, of course, can be achieved with high precision only by all-digital beam-forming electronics, as provided by state-of-the-art high-end equipment. The information may be used to further improve spatial resolution and gain novel contrast information.

So far THI has proven helpful by better visualization of the needle during breast interventions. Also simple cysts may be better recognized. However, so far this information has not yet significantly influenced the differential diagnosis of solid breast masses.

Image Quality in the Near Field

Aside from optimal overall resolution, the image quality in the near field is important for breast sonography. Because the thickness of most breasts is only a few centimeters during sonography, many lesions will be located close to the transducer. High image quality in the near field is necessary to accurately assess these lesions. Unfortunately, transducer design and other factors can make it difficult to image these areas. While most modern units allow good image quality in the near field, resolution should be counterchecked with older units.

Some (older) transducers have difficulty focusing the soundbeam within a few millimeters of the transducer. For these transducers it remains necessary to use a standoff pad between the transducer and the breast to achieve good images of the subcutaneous tissues and the superficial breast tissue. These pads physically move the near field of the transducer away from the breast surface, placing the breast within a distance from the transducer at which the soundbeam can be reliably focused.

For all pads, sufficient coupling agent (gel or oil) must be used to eliminate air between the transducer and the pad and between the pad the breast surface. Reverberation echoes can be caused by the repeated reflection of sound between the pad and the transducer (**Fig. 4.2**). These produce lines of echoes that run parallel to the transducer and repeat one, two, three, or more times at a given distance from the transducer. They add artifact to the image, and compromise the ability to make an accurate diagnosis.

Reverberation echoes may occur at the skin (as in the above case). They may also occur at the anterior wall of a cyst. Since they originate from multiple reflexions (between the surface of the transducer and the cyst wall), these reverberation echoes are projected into the anterior part of the cysts as multiple repetitions (of the original echoes from the cyst wall). They resemble waves which repeat at the same distance from each other and which decrease from anterior to posterior.

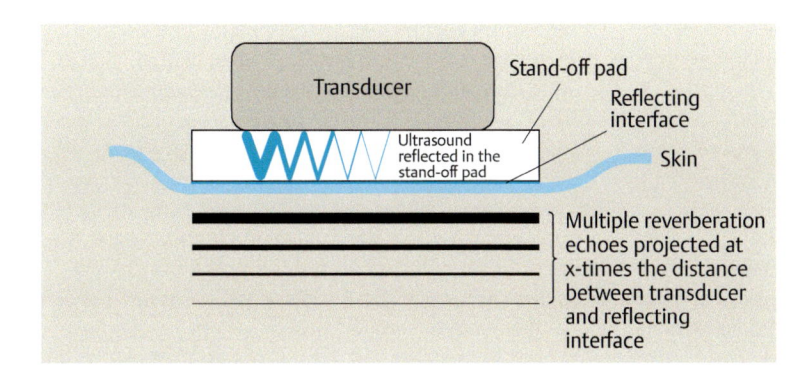

Fig. 4.2 Reverberation echoes resulting from insufficient contract between stand-off pad and skin.

Slice Thickness

Slice thickness is a function of quality and design of the transducer and should be considered when purchasing equipment; furthermore, the appropriate transducer has to be chosen. If slice thickness is too thick, cysts that should appear echo free will not be reliably imaged due to the inclusion of adjacent solid tissue within the tissue slice. Accurate diagnosis may not be possible in these cases, particularly when cysts are small.

Equipment Quality Control

Each facility should have in place a quality control program to maximize the quality of its breast sonography. Ongoing monitoring and evaluation of equipment should be a part of this program. A routine preventive maintenance program is desirable. Records should be kept to document this program. Efforts undertaken to improve quality of care should also be documented. Equipment performance monitoring may be done following the ACR Guidelines and Standards Committee of the Commission on Ultrasound.

Special phantoms are available for assessing relevant image quality parameters for breast sonography.

> **Summary**
>
> Linear transducers with a nominal frequency of at least 7.5 MHz should be used for breast sonography. Imaging detail is determined by axial, lateral, and contrast resolution. Lateral resolution is significantly influenced by focusing. Special attention must be paid to adequate resolution in the near field. The transducer and the magnification factor should be chosen to assure adequate visualization of the complete tissue between skin and chest wall.
>
> Care must be taken to always image the area in question using the appropriate focus. This is possible by diligent manual adaptation of the focus depth by use of multiple transmit focus or dynamic focusing.
>
> Slice thickness will also have an impact on the quality of the study, particularly when imaging small cysts. A quality control program is desirable to maximize patient care and safety.

Examination Technique

Sonography of the breast is usually best performed with the patient supine. When the outer quadrants are being scanned, the patient should extend the ipsilateral arm over the head and elevate the ipsilateral shoulder (contralateral posterior oblique position). It is helpful to place a cushion or pillow under the ipsilateral shoulder to help the patient maintain this position. This positioning flattens the breast against the chest wall, decreasing the amount of tissue that must be penetrated by the soundbeam and reducing breast mobility. When the inner quadrants are being examined, a straight supine position accomplishes the same results for the inner quadrants.

When scanning a palpable mass, it can be helpful to bracket the lesion with two fingers of one hand and slip the transducer between these two fingers. This ensures that the volume of the breast being imaged corresponds to the site of the palpable mass.

A sufficient amount of gel should be used between the transducer and the skin (and the stand-off pad, if one is being used) to eliminate air between these structures, thereby minimizing reverberation artifact. The use of slight compression on the transducer is also helpful.

Slight compression and flat positioning of the breast also help to position tissue interfaces as parallel as possible to the transducer. Diagonal tissue interfaces such as Cooper ligaments can cause part of the soundbeam to be reflected away from the transducer, resulting in acoustic shadowing. These shadows can be diagnostically confusing and can obscure lesions distal to the shadowing structures (**Fig. 4.3a,b**). Slight compression of the breast tissue and variation of the angulation of the transducer usually allows these shadows to be identified as unimportant "non-persisting" shadowing.

Whenever a finding that requires histopathologic assessment is detected, and in all patients with known breast cancer, ultrasound examination of the axilla should be performed. Even though other draining lymph nodes are also known (internal mammary lymph nodes, supraclavicular lymph nodes, and lymph nodes of the neck), standard examination of these lymph nodes is not considered necessary. The reason is that detection of any asymptomatic finding in these areas is not associated with a change of treatment (since either these nodes are not accessible or the disease is too progressed to be accessible to therapeutic surgery).

It is recommended that scanning of the axilla is performed before a planned interventional procedure, since reactive changes after biopsy might mimic lymph node involvement.

Systematic assessment of the axilla should cover the complete axilla with its boundaries, as indicated:
- Lateral border: humerus
- Posterior border: posterior axillary line (lateral margin of the latissimus dorsi muscle)
- Anterior border: pectoralis major and minor muscles
- Superior border: clavicle
- Inferior border: inframammary fold
- Medial border: anterior serratus muscle with the lateral thoracic vessels (the medial border of the axilla blends into the area covered by breast ultrasonography)

We usually scan the axilla in tracks with the transducer orthogonal to the anterior and posterior axillary folds. We usually start in the posterior axilla in a cranial–caudal direction and progress anteriorly and medially. We then cover the area below the clavicle by moving the vertically oriented transducer from laterally to medially.

The most important area to be examined in asymptomatic women with breast cancer concerns the lower axilla, which reaches down to the level of the axillary fold. It usually harbours the sentinel lymph node, which is usually one of the lowest lymph nodes of the axilla.

Anatomically the axilla is divided into three parts (**Fig. 4.3c**):
- Level 1 comprises the lymph nodes inferior and lateral to the pectoralis minor muscle.
- Level 2 comprises the lymph nodes posterior to the pectoralis minor muscle.
- Level 3 comprises the lymph nodes anterior, cranial and medial to the pectoralis minor muscle.

Time-Gain Compensation

Time-gain compensation adjusts the visual presentation of the reflected soundbeam to an image of equalized brightness and intensity, despite decreased energy of the beam as it travels farther from the transducer. For a 7.5-MHz beam, the soundbeam loses about 50% of its energy through every centimeter of tissue it traverses. Time-gain

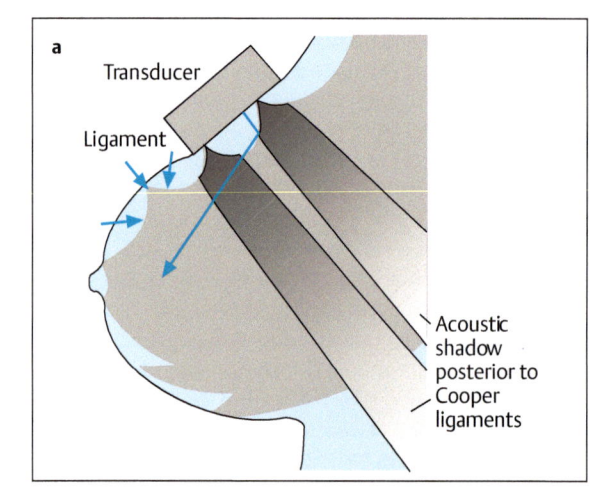

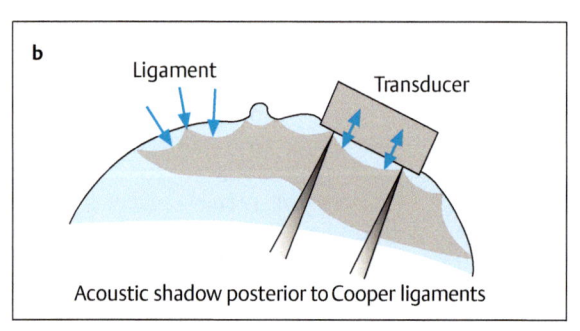

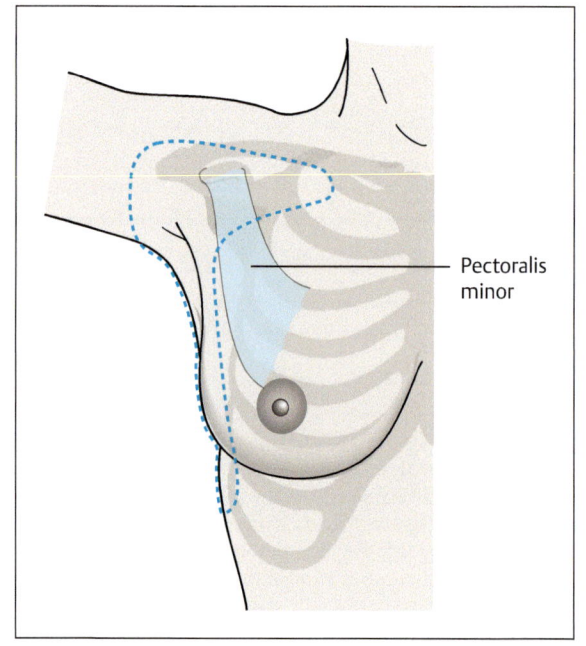

Fig. 4.3a–c

a,b Positioning the patient supine and applying slight compression helps to orient the interfaces parallel to the transducer (**b**). Less ultrasound energy is reflected away from the transducer than in a hanging breast (**a**).

c The axillary area to be scanned (surrounded by broken line). Levels I, II and III of the lymph nodes are defined according to the position of the lymph nodes with respect to the pectoralis minor muscle.

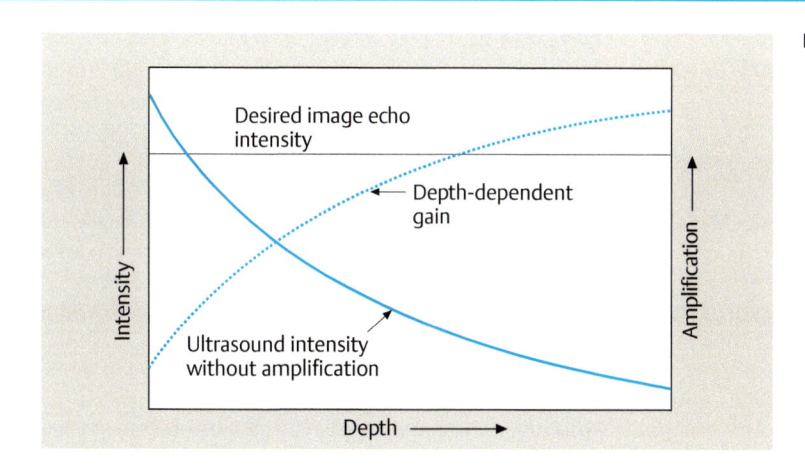

Fig. 4.4 Time-gain compensation.

compensation allows the beam to appear to be at equal intensity at all distances from the transducer (**Fig. 4.4**). However, equalization of the intensity of echoes throughout the image requires matching image compensation to ultrasound absorption throughout the image. Although modern equipment is produced with programs to automatically compensate for decreasing intensity of the beam at greater distances from the transducer, variability in absorption patterns in different patients—due to the variable amounts of fatty, glandular, and fibrotic tissue in the individual breast—often necessitates optimization of the image manually.

The echoes that make up the sonographic image are produced in two different ways:
- *Specular echoes.* Specular echoes are strong echoes caused by reflection at interfaces between two tissues with sufficient difference in impedance. These interfaces must be sufficiently large (larger than the wavelength) and have a smooth surface. The angle of incidence equals the angle of reflection. Echoes striking diagonal interfaces can be reflected away from the transducer. Such echoes are not visualized on the ultrasound image.
- *Scatter echoes.* Scatter echoes occur at small interfaces with irregular surfaces. The size of these interfaces is of the same magnitude as the wavelength of the soundbeam. The sound wave is scattered in variable directions, and the intensity of the echo returned to the transducer is weak. Most echoes in glandular and fatty tissue are scatter echoes, produced by microscopic tissue interfaces.

Focusing

Optimal imaging of the lesion requires focusing the soundbeam at the depth from the transducer at which the lesion is located. This requires adjusting the focal zone to this site. As noted, this can be done by using a variable focus transducer and electronically adjusting the focal zone. In some cases, a stand-off pad will be required. Focusing is important, since only in the focal zone is imaging within a thin slice achieved. Outside the focal zone thin slice thickness increases and partial volume with surrounding tissue may decrease lesion contrast of small lesions and may falsely display echoes within small cysts. If during a biopsy procedure the lesion is out of the focal zone, a needle that passes behind or in front of a small lesion may falsely be displayed as if it has crossed the lesion.

Examination Technique and Documentation

Sonographic examination makes it possible to study the breast in an infinite number of planes. Standardization of the examination and appropriate labeling of images makes these studies interpretable by those who have not performed them, and also makes them reproducible.

Examination of the breast should be performed systematically so that the complete tissue is analyzed. In principle different techniques may serve this purpose.

Some investigators examine the breast tissue in a "lawnmower pattern." This means that, for example, the longitudinally oriented transducer is moved from left to right in a cranial track. It is then moved back from right to left in a track that slightly overlaps but is caudal to the first track, and so on.

Commonly the breast is imaged in anti-radial and radial planes. The anti-radial plane allows "shoveling" or compression of the breast tissue toward the nipple. It matches well with the anatomy and helps to avoid missing areas of the tissue. The radial plane follows the course of the ducts and may thus help to distinguish the varying ductal anatomy from small lesions. It is also the preferred plane to detect and analyze intraductal changes. The radial and anti-radial planes correspond to spokes of a wheel extending from the nipple and right angle to these axes.

4 Sonography

Whatever technique is chosen, all the breast tissue should be analyzed. To avoid missing a lesion, the tracks should overlap.

If no abnormality is seen scanning the breast, usually one representative slice of each breast is documented to demonstrate the type of breast tissue.

When a lesion is detected, its position should be labeled at o'clock axes (clock position and distance from the nipple).

All suspected lesions need to be analyzed and documented in at least two orthogonal planes, optimally the radial and anti-radial planes. This usually makes it possible to differentiate real lesions from breast anatomy. For example, fat lobules typically appear as elongated structures in the second plane. Often, a connection to the subcutaneous or retromammary fat layers can be demonstrated (**Fig. 4.5a,b**).

Palpable findings should be correlated under sonographic monitoring. This is possible by, for example, performing ultrasound examination while the lesion is fixed between two fingers of one hand. Direct correlation is very important to countercheck whether a palpable finding corresponds to a potentially suspicious hypoechoic area or whether the hypoechoic area directly adjacent to homogeneous hyperechoic tissue just corresponds to an adjacent soft fat lobule. The latter situation might help rule out a suspicion.

Real-time testing of mobility and compressibility may yield further significant information and should therefore regularly be applied in areas that are difficult to assess and in case of any suspicion.

Mobility of the breast tissue and any suspected lesion should be counterchecked directly, as shown in **Fig. 4.5c,d**. Fibroadenomas are, for example, readily mobile. If mobility cannot be confirmed, malignancy should be considered even if the mass is well circumscribed with homogeneous internal echoes. Even though excellent mobility is one of the features of benign fibroadenomas, mobility alone cannot guarantee benign origin of an ill-circumscribed lesion or even of a well-circumscribed mass, if it is hard or increases in size.

Compressibility is also counterchecked directly by compressing a suspected lesion or area of tissue by the palpating finger or by moving the transducer to exert

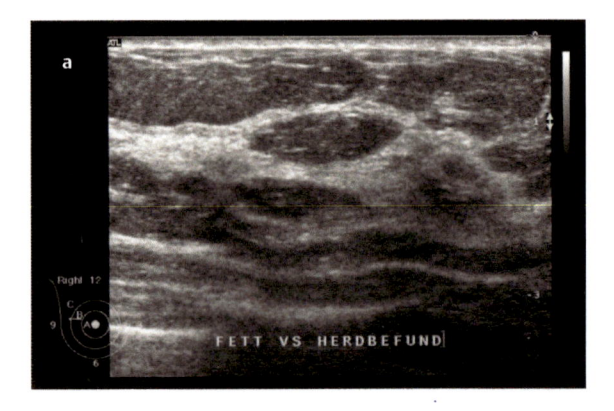

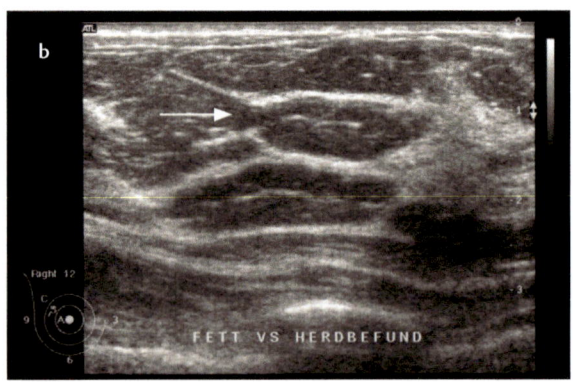

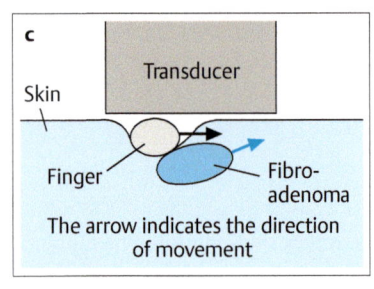

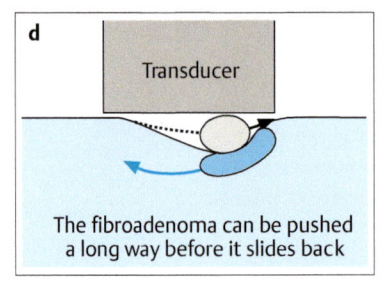

Fig. 4.5a–d

a,b Imaging in two planes: Interspersed fat lobules can simulate a hypoechoic tumor (**a**). As the transducer is turned, the same fat lobule appears as an elongated structure (arrow). The image in this plane also reveals that the fat lobule is connected to subcutaneous fat (**b**).

c,d Assessing mobility (diagram). To assess mobility, insert a finger underneath the transducer. Fibroadenomas usually are far more mobile than carcinomas.

pressure on the underlying tissue. Excellent compressibility is usually observed with interposed fat lobules, hamartomas, lipomas, and with many cysts and fibroadenomas. Malignancy should be considered if compressibility is decreased. In spite of known overlap the above information may represent an important piece of information that should not be ignored.

Overall, mobility and compressibility give additional information that always needs be considered both in the clinical context and in correlation with other imaging findings.

Elastography

Considering the known diagnostic importance of tissue elasticity (only few cancers are known to be elastic, while most cancers exhibit decreased elasticity compared with normal tissue or benign changes) some manufacturers have developed a new mode of ultrasound imaging, which allows display of tissue elasticity. This mode is called elastography.

There are two different principles to measure and image tissue elasticity:

- With the initially developed mode (*strain elastography*) strain is applied to the tissue by use of slight (repeated or even vibrating) compression. The compression may be exerted manually by slightly pressing the transducer on the breast (a motion that may be operator dependent and requires some training). Some manufacturers also use the patient's respiratory or cardiac motion to calculate tissue elasticity. Tissue elasticity or stiffness is calculated from the slight shift of the echoes on the B-mode image. Tissue elasticity is then displayed in a separate image or superimposed as color coding on the usual B-mode image.
- One company has developed a different way of elastographic imaging—*shear wave elastography*—whereby tissue is excited by a focused ultrasound pulse wave. This wave induces a slow shear wave in the tissue. The speed of the shear wave is proportional to the elasticity of the tissue from which it originates. It is read out by ultrafast imaging and the elasticity information is superimposed on the usual B-mode images by color coding. In contrast to strain elastography, shear wave elastography is not operator independent. Furthermore it yields quantitative information on tissue elasticity. Since shear waves propagate only in elastic media, no signal is received from simple or complex cysts. Such a phenomenon may also occur in very stiff carcinomas. These should, however, be easily recognized on the B-mode image by their posterior shadowing.

Unfortunately, there is no agreement on the color coding, and different vendors color-code elasticity information differently.

For visual evaluation of elasticity images a five-step scoring has been suggested for strain elastography (Itoh et al. 2006):

- Score 1: Homogeneously soft
- Score 2: Mosaic of soft and stiff areas
- Score 3: Soft periphery and decreased elasticity in a central part that is smaller than the lesion
- Score 4: Low elasticity throughout the lesion
- Score 5: Area of low elasticity larger than the lesion visible on the corresponding B-mode image

Scores 1 and 2 are considered benign, score 3 probably benign. Scores 4 and 5 are considered suspicious or highly suspicious. The cutoff level that so far has achieved the best accuracy is a score between 3 and 4.

For evaluation of shear wave elastography quantitative values may be used.

Initial results show that elastography may help improve the sensitivity and specificity of breast ultrasonography. It may add valuable information. However, owing to false negative and false positive calls, which occur with either method, elasticity alone cannot be considered sufficiently reliable to avoid biopsy (Wojcinski et al. 2010) (**Fig. 4.6**).

Power Doppler Imaging

Because breast carcinoma is often hypervascular and various benign lesions are hypovascular, it was hoped that the determination of blood-flow patterns within a lesion would be helpful in differentiating malignant from benign processes.

It has been suggested that breast cancers tend to show higher vascularity. An irregular vascular pattern has been described to occur in malignancy. Furthermore vessels penetrating into the tumor have been described in malignancy, whereas vessels stretching around the tumor are considered characteristic of benign fibroadenomas. Peak velocity and resistance indices have been measured. However, so far differentiation of solid masses by power Doppler has not proven superior to differentiation based on B-mode imaging.

In spite of these disappointing results power Doppler imaging may be helpful in selected cases (Stavros 2003):

- It may demonstrate vascular signal in very hypo- to anechoic lesions that could otherwise be misinterpreted as cysts. Some medullary or anaplastic carcinomas and some lymph node metastases may be so hypoechoic that they could be mistaken for cysts. Thus power Doppler may be useful to *countercheck presumed cysts with discrete abnormalities* (e.g., cysts with a slightly irregular margin, a suspected halo, or suspected internal echoes). In these rare cases power Doppler may help avoid misinterpretation.
- It may be useful to *distinguish debris in cysts or ducts from papillomas and papillary carcinomas*. Both papillomas and papillary carcinoma usually have a highly

4 Sonography

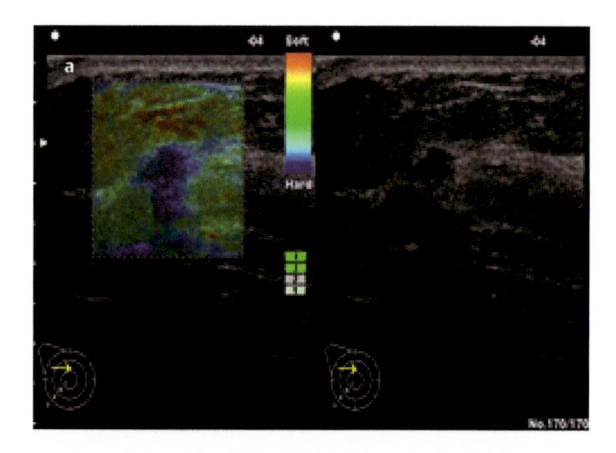

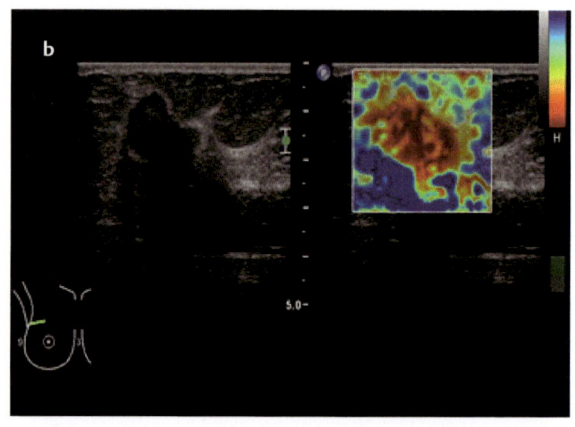

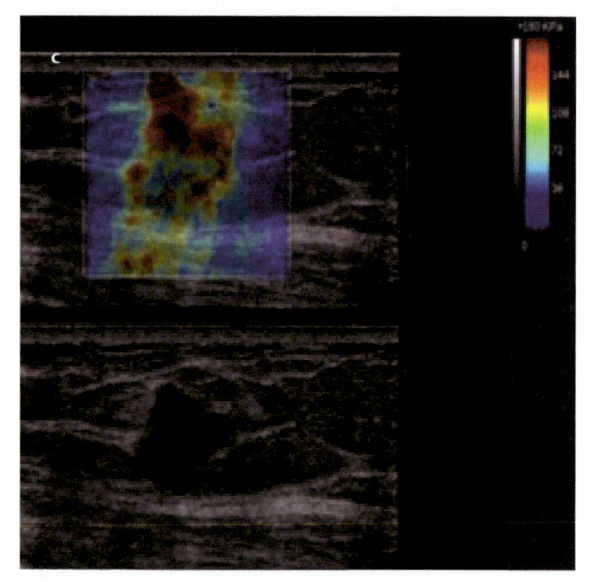

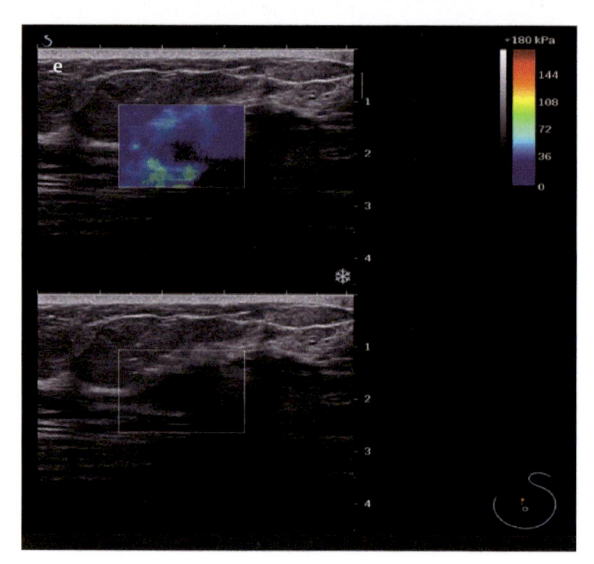

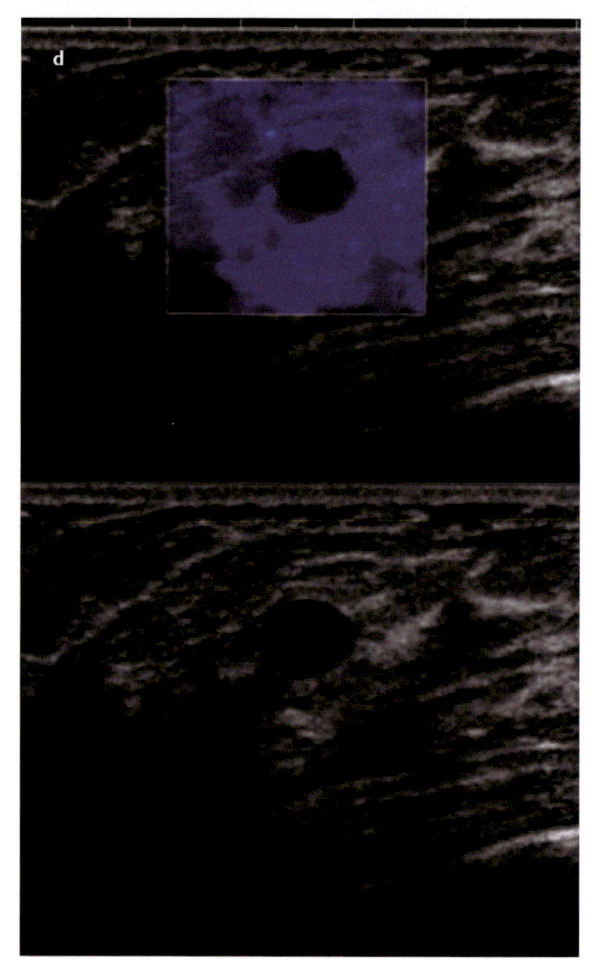

Fig. 4.6a–f Strain images may be acquired by different methods of elastography imaging. **a–c** show different cases with invasive ductal carcinomas imaged using three different types of equipment.

a Manual freehand compression.
b Soft compression using spontaneous (respiratory or cardiac) displacement.
c Use of a focused ultrasound pulse wave or shear wave elastography.
d In simple and complex cysts the shear waves do not propagate, and the lesion remains black.
e Shear wave image of a benign (fibroadenoma) lesion.

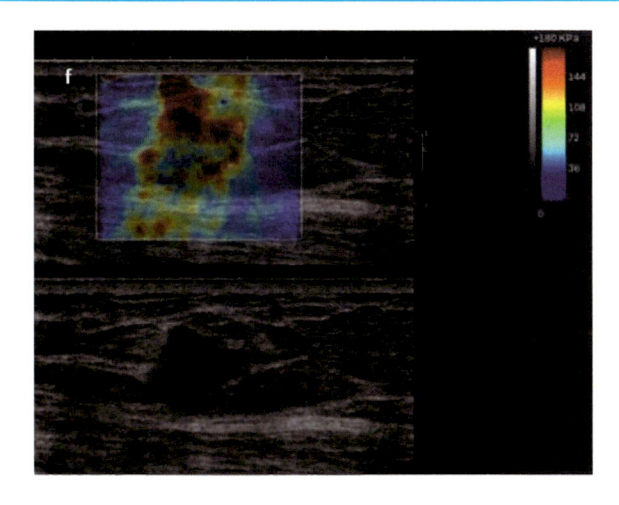

f Typical malignant lesion on strain imaging: the color spectrum is heterogeneous; the lesion contour is irregular, not corresponding to the B-mode image, and the size is larger in elasticity mode than in B-mode.

vascularized stalk and can thus be recognized as lesions that require histopathologic assessment. (In contrast, absence of Doppler signal in suspected cysts may increase confidence that the change is benign but is not completely reliable, since some early and low-grade malignancies exhibit little or nondetectable perfusion.)
- It may allow demonstration of vascular signal in hypervascularized lymph node metastases. Malignancies that are highly vascularized are usually associated with highly vascularized lymph node metastases. Demonstration of a strongly vascularized hypoechoic area in a lymph node can *confirm (but not exclude) a malignant involvement in lymph nodes with indeterminate findings on B-mode imaging.* Another sign which strongly supports malignant involvement (as opposed to inflammatory change) of a lymph node is visualization of transcapsular vessels. Other than the usual central feeding vessels of a lymph node that enter through the hilum, transcapsular vessels penetrate from outside into the lymph node.
- The use of power Doppler imaging to follow response to chemotherapy has also been suggested. In highly vascularized tumors, a decrease in the vascularity may precede tumor shrinkage.

Overall, power Doppler plays a limited role in breast imaging (**Fig. 4.7**). It may be helpful to increase confidence and even exclude some pitfalls in selected constellations. It is important to understand that demonstration of increased or abnormal vascular signal represents quite valuable diagnostic information. Its absence, however, is not reliable for exclusion of malignancy.

When Doppler imaging is performed, care must be taken not to exert too much pressure on the transducer, since pressure may suppress blood flow and can thus reduce the Doppler signal.

For this reason, the use of Doppler or power Doppler interrogation of breast masses has not been found to be useful by most experts in determining which lesions require biopsy and which are benign.

The use of microbubble contrast agents has also been described in several studies in an attempt to better define vascular patterns within lesions. Use of these agents remains experimental.

Image Labeling

Owing to the variability of examination technique that is possible during sonographic study, precise labeling of images is necessary so that sonographic examinations are reproducible and lesions can be found on repeat study. Labeling of sonographic studies of the breast should include:
- Patient identification: Name and unique identifying number such as medical record number, birth date, and social security number
- Examination date
- Breast laterality (right or left)
- Breast quadrant
- Axis, indicated by o'clock designation
- Distance of the lesion from the nipple (some guidelines also recommend documentation of distance from the skin surface)
- An indication as to whether the lesion is palpable

It is also desirable to include the initials of, or otherwise identify, the technologist or physician performing the study.

If a breast icon is present on the equipment, it should be used to record the position of the transducer on the image.

4 Sonography

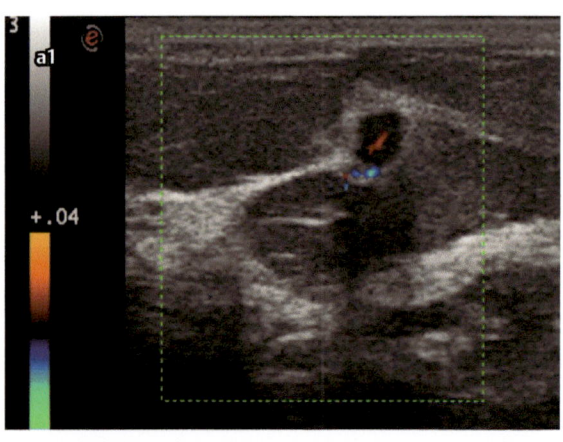

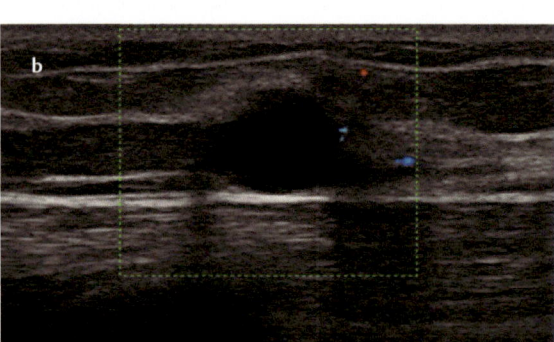

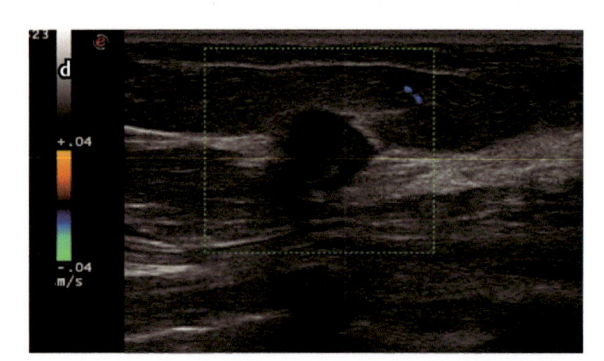

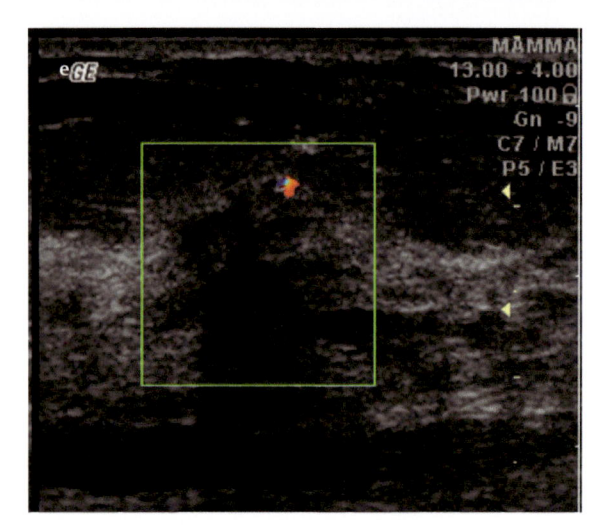

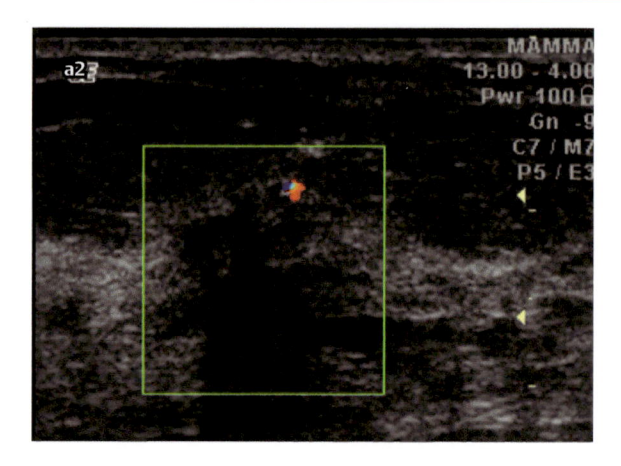

Fig. 4.7a–g Power Doppler of different breast lesions.

a   Two quite different carcinomas are shown. On the left (**a1**) the carcinoma appears as a round mass with a central feeding vessel. On the right (**a2**) the carcinoma exhibits only a vessel in its periphery. It is visible as a highly suspicious architectural distortion. Both lesions proved to be invasive ductal carcinomas.
b   An ill-defined strongly hypoechoic lesion with posterior enhancement without vascularization is demonstrated. *Histology*: Medullary cancer.

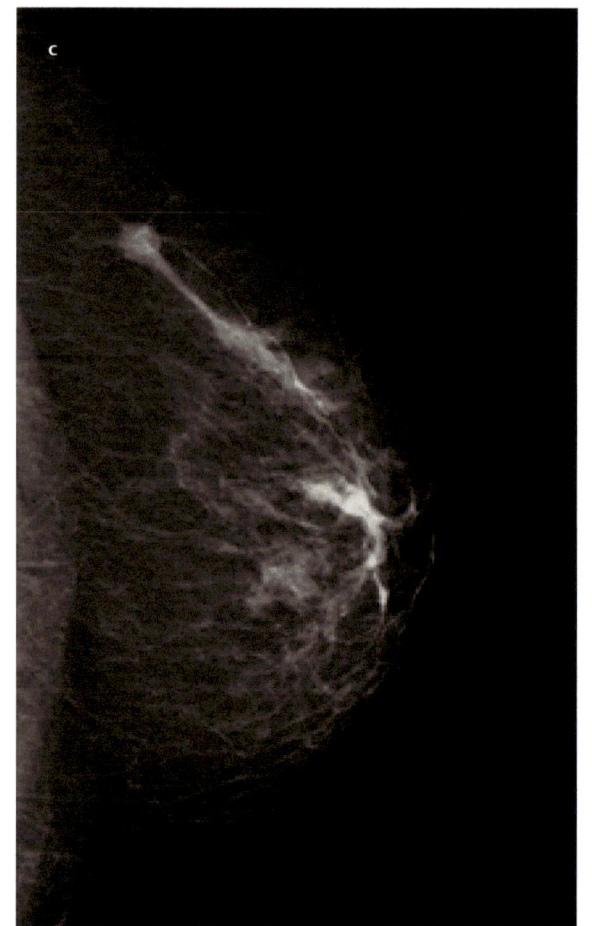

Examination Technique

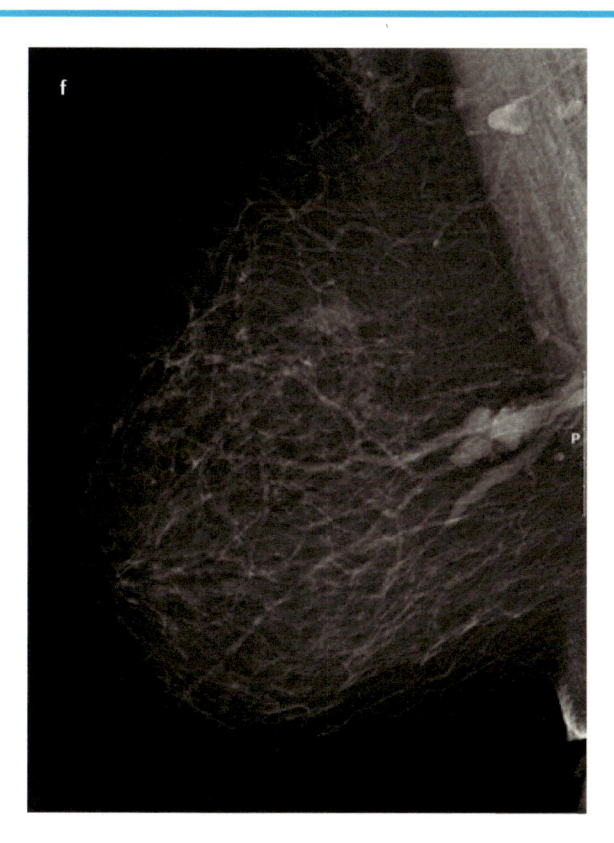

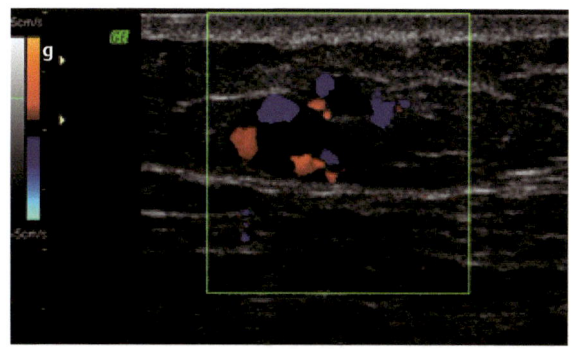

f,g Mammography (MLO view) with a multinodular mass anterior to the pectoral muscle (**f**), corresponding to a bundle of vessels (**g**).

◁ **c,d** Mammographic craniocaudal view showing a suspicious lesion located laterally (**c**). Using power Doppler (**d**) it presents without vascularization, corresponding histologically to another ductal invasive cancer.
e This invasive ductal carcinoma showed only a few vessels at the periphery of the tumor.

Interpreting and Documenting Sonographic Findings

Normal Sonographic Findings

As in the mammographic pattern of the normal breast, there is broad variation in the normal sonographic pattern of the breast. Subcutaneous fatty tissue appears hypoechoic with echogenic bands of Cooper ligaments coursing through the fat. Glandular tissue has an echogenic pattern, interrupted by hypoechoic fatty lobules.

Worrisome sonographic patterns can be caused by shadowing fibrous bands and by hypoechoic fat lobules mimicking a mass. Scanning in multiple projections will usually identify these findings as part of the normal anatomy of the breast (**Fig. 4.5a,b**). Furthermore normal and benign changes mostly exhibit good compressibility and mobility.

According to the BI-RADS lexicon it is recommended that the echotexture of the underlying breast tissue is described, since it may influence sensitivity and specificity of the examination.

Whereas homogeneous hyperchoic breast tissue allows excellent detection of those malignancies present-

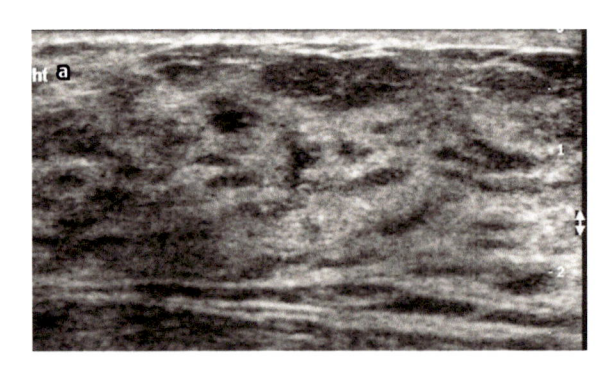

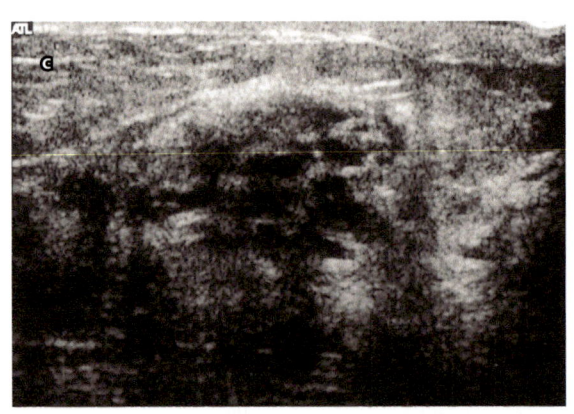

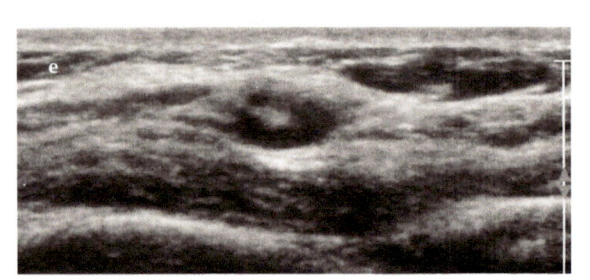

Fig. 4.8a–e Examples of normal breast tissue.
- **a** Homogeneous, dense and regular breast tissue.
- **b** Homogeneous hypoechoic breast tissue due to involution.
- **c** Heterogeneous tissue, dilated ducts, interspersed with echo-rich fibrous structures and shadowing.
- **d** Typical intramammary lymph node with symmetric and hypoechoic cortex and echo-rich hilum.
- **e** Example of a regular axillary lymph node: the cortex does not exceed 3 mm in width; the hilum looks homogeneously dense.

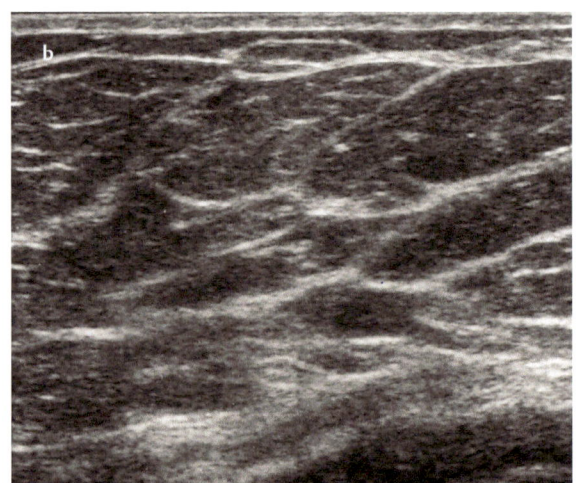

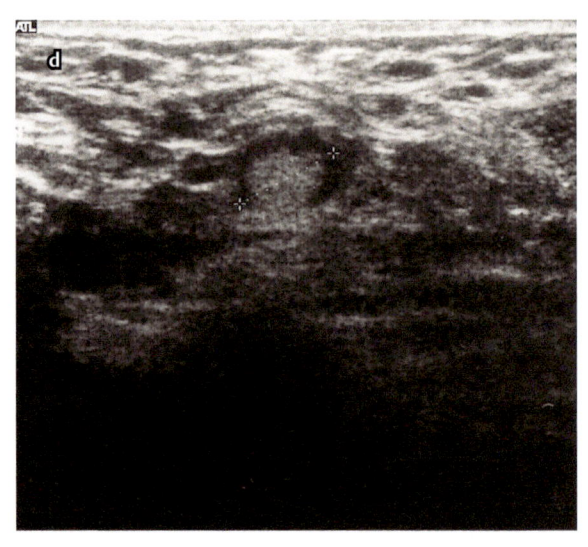

ing as hypoechoic masses, heterogeneity owing to interposed fat lobules, dilated ducts, hypoechoic periductal structures, or adenosis may interfere with the detection of malignancy.

Shadowing may also impair diagnostic assessment and may strongly interfere with the detection of those malignancies that present as architectural distortion or shadowing. The heterogeneity can be focal or diffuse. There is no measure of the degree to which assessment may be impaired. The only measure to improve diagnostic accuracy is scanning with different compression, in multiple planes and with differing angulations of the transducer, and testing mobility. These measures will aid in identifying shadowing from normal versus suspicious structures and distinguishing true masses from interposed fat or dilated ducts.

We usually characterize the underlying tissue as hyperechoic (like breast tissue) or hypoechoic (like fat), homogeneous or heterogeneous, and indicate whether there is disturbing shadowing (**Fig. 4.8**). According to the BI-RADS lexicon, tissue composition should be characterized as:
- Homogeneous, or
- Heterogeneous

To date there is no evidence for or against one or other of the proposed nomenclatures.

In the clinical setting patients often present with uncharacteristic palpable findings or "lumps." Mammography and ultrasonography are applied to detect malignancy and direct biopsy in the case that a suspicious finding is confirmed. It is recommended that a suspicious clinical finding should undergo histopathologic assessment even if mammography and ultrasonography are negative.

For the innumerable findings of low suspicion, however, biopsy may represent overtreatment.

Based on current data short-term follow-up is considered justified for findings of low clinical suspicion, if mammography and ultrasonography are negative. Findings that are most consistent with a benign entity include:
- Absence of any signs of malignancy on ultrasonongraphy and mammography
- Intense homogeneous hyperechogenicity (if the echotexture is not uniform or if it contains hypoechoic areas other than fat lobules that are larger than normal ducts or terminal ductal-lobular units [> 4 mm], this criterion is not fulfilled)

According to the existing literature the above constellation is associated with a high negative predictive value of 97–100% (Stavros et al. 1995, Dennis et al. 2001, Soo et al. 2001, Raza et al. 2010).

Thus, negative sonographic and mammographic findings cannot exclude malignancy, but the likelihood of malignancy is so low that in experienced hands this constellation can support the diagnostic decision for short-term follow-up and can thus help avert unnecessary biopsy.

Normal axillary findings include visualization of vessels and normal lymph nodes. As a normal variant ectopic (hyperechoic) breast tissue may be visualized with or without interposed fat in the axilla.

Many normal lymph nodes are not visible by ultrasonography, since they are isoechoic to fat and/or very small. Other normal lymph nodes may be visualized as bean-shaped or kidney-shaped masses with a hyper- or isoechoic hilum and a cortex or rim that may be hypoechoic, but sometimes even hyperechoic (due to post-inflammatory changes). The cortex or rim should be < 3 mm and should not be thickened. (Lymph nodes with a thin regular cortex may be considered normal even if they are quite large, i.e., > 1 or 2 cm.) (**Fig. 4.8d,e**).

Sonographic Lesions

Significant abnormalities (simple cysts that explain a mammographically or clinically suspicious finding or an abnormality that might require follow-up or histopathologic assessment) have to be documented in two orthogonal imaging planes.

Its location (o'clock position, distance to the nipple, distance from the skin surface*) should be indicated on the image and/or in the written report. Its extent should be indicated in three dimensions.* Its degree of suspicion should be indicated using the BI-RADS categories. It should be correlated with clinical findings and mammography and a final recommendation should be given, as suggested in the BI-RADS lexicon (Madjar et al. 2006, American College of Radiology Practice Guideline 2011).

Most lesions present sonographically as focal mass lesions. However, benign and malignant changes may also present as architectural distortion without a mass or as a diffuse change.

An *architectural distortion* may present as interruption of ligaments or normal structures. Normal structures such as the fascia, the retromammary fat layer, the subcutaneous fat layer and the glandular tissue usually course horizontally when the patient lies prone. Interruption of these structures is defined as architectural distortion. Architectural distortion mostly occurs with malignancy, but may also be caused by scarring or fat necrosis. It is often associated with shadowing and may or may not be associated with a mass. If a mass can be identified, it is usually located proximal to the shadowing (with respect to the transducer). Both the mass and the architectural distortion may sometimes be quite discrete. Some architectural distortions are best seen on coronal reconstructions (**Fig. 4.9**).

---

* Recommendation by DEGUM (German Association of Ultrasound in Medicine; Madjar 2006).

4 Sonography

Fig. 4.9a–f ▷
- **a** Architectural distortion.
- **b** With Doppler mode one vessel is visible in the center of the lesion.
- **c** Using 3D mode and coronal reconstruction the typical stellate character of the lesion is demonstrated. *Histology*: Invasive ductal carcinoma.
- **d** A tiny architectural distortion with shadowing.
- **e** In the second plane (a radial scan) this architectural distortion presented as a small angular lesion with some posterior shadowing, highly suspicious of malignancy, which was confirmed histologically.
- **f** This woman presented with a palpable tumor measuring 4 cm. Sonographically, it corresponded to an area of diffuse architectuaral distortion within very dense parenchyma; no definite mass could be visualized. Histologically, a lobular carcinoma was diagnosed.

Diffuse changes may be associated with benign disease, with inflammation or with diffusely growing malignancy. Diffuse changes affect larger areas of tissue. The distribution of diffuse changes may be segmental, regional or throughout the breast. Diffuse changes may include diffuse ductal dilatation, diffuse shadowing or edema of the breast with or without involvement of the subcutaneous tissue and the skin (**Fig. 4.10**).

Focal sonographic lesions comprise simple or complex cystic lesions or solid masses.

Cysts

Simple cysts can be diagnosed as benign lesions by sonography (**Fig. 4.11a,b** and **Fig. 4.12a**). Their characteristics include:
- Round or oval shape.
- Smooth, thin echogenic wall. It is important that the thin, smooth wall is preserved in all slices. Irregularities of the contour are not compatible with the diagnosis of a simple cyst.
- Absence of changes within the surrounding tissue. (An echogenic halo in all or part of the cyst is not compatible with the diagnosis of a simple cyst, but could indicate either a directly adjacent carcinoma or that the lesion itself represents a very hypoechoic or largely necrotic malignancy.)
- Absence of internal echoes (except for artifactual echoes such as reverberation echoes). With the increasing resolution of the latest transducer technology, echoes (caused by proteinaceous or serosanguinous contents in the cysts) may become visible in many cysts which formerly had been considered and eventually proven to be simple cysts. Owing to this change in technology a low level of monomorphous echoes may be acceptable in cysts. The exact level will depend on the equipment used and requires sufficient experience on the part of the examiner. Under real-time study, echoes within cysts will often be seen to be moving, representing debris within the cystic fluid. Sedimented debris in the dependent portion of the cyst will often move with a change in patient positioning (**Fig. 4.12b1, b2**). In case of doubts, additional methods such as power Doppler imaging, elastography, or even needle biopsy may need to be applied.

To avoid misinterpretation care must be taken to always view the image with sufficient gain and brightness to be able to recognize low-level echoes.

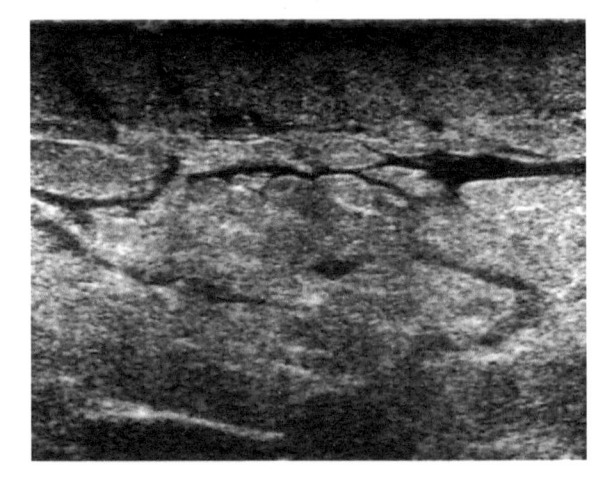

Fig. 4.10 Diffuse changes. Homogeneously dense structures without delineation of the subcutaneous fat layer, widening of the lymph channels, and skin thickening due to edema of the breast early after irradiation (no malignancy).

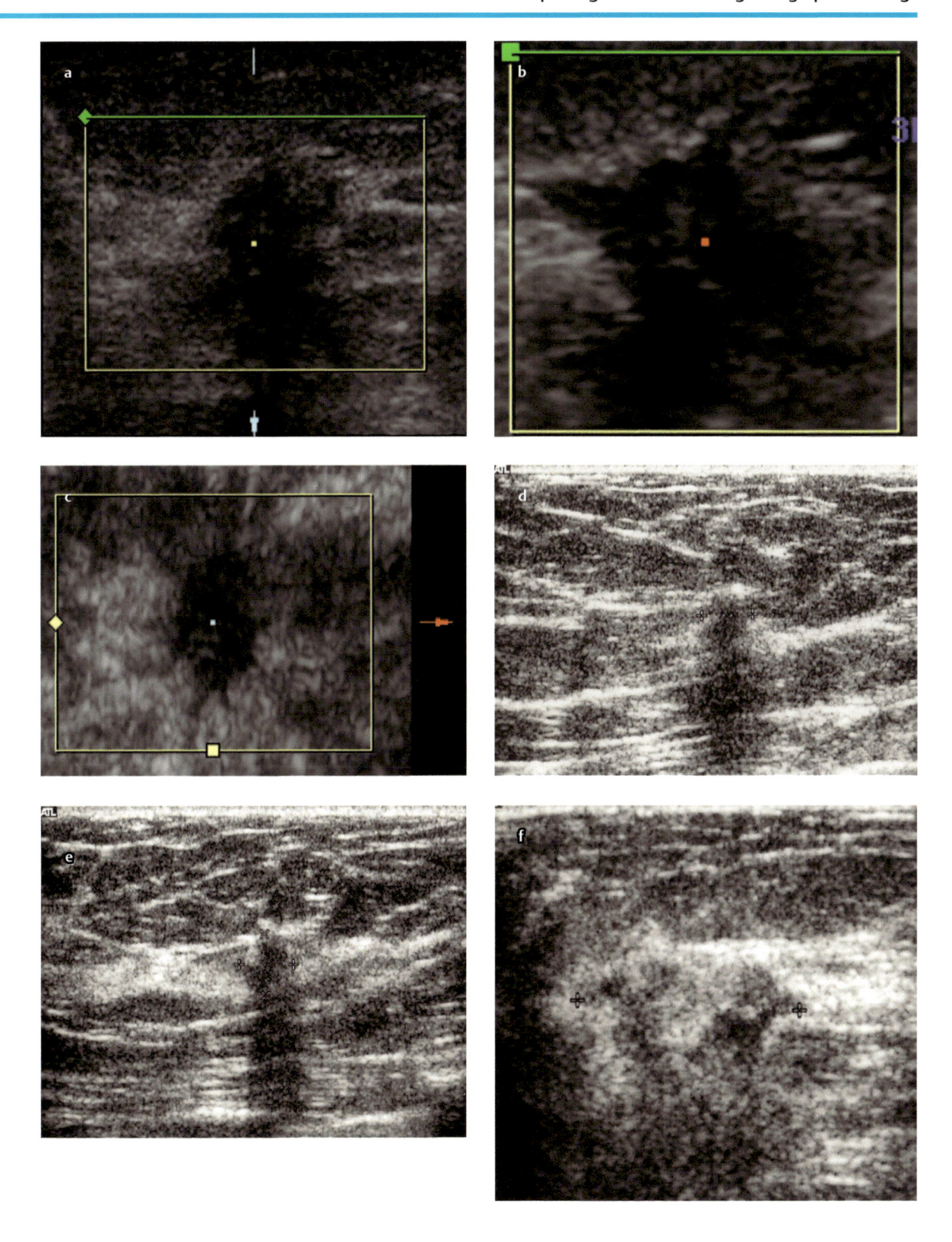

Interpreting and Documenting Sonographic Findings

115

4 Sonography

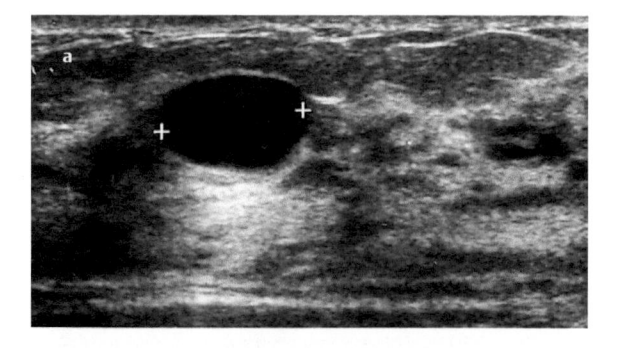

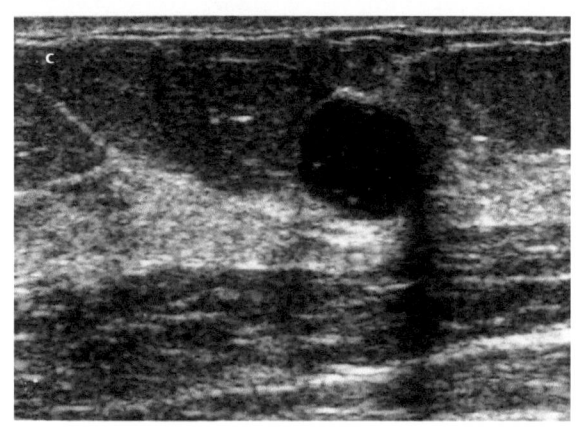

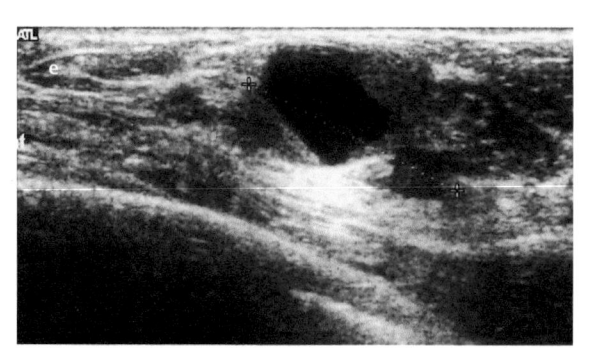

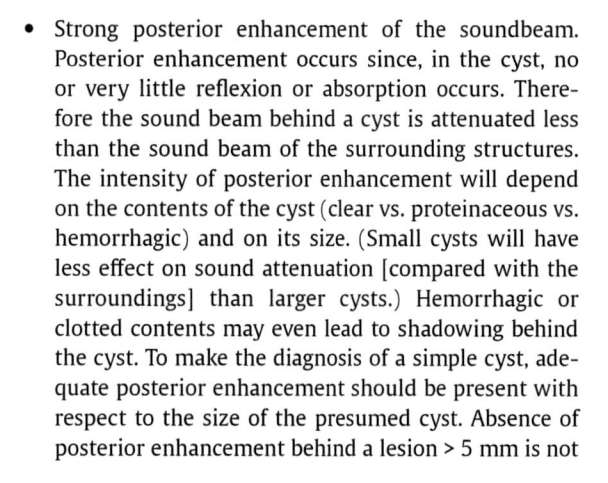

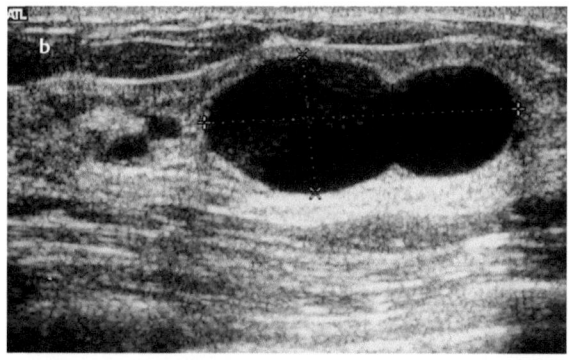

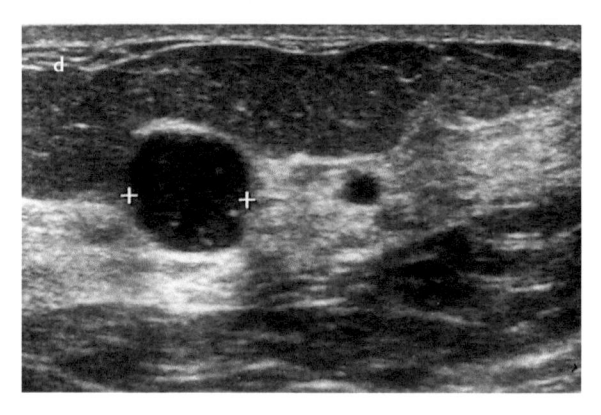

Fig. 4.11a–e

a This simple cyst can be definitively diagnosed sonographically by its oval shape, thin wall, absence of internal echoes, and far wall enhancement of the soundbeam.
b Bulging simple cyst.
c,d Complex cyst: This oval mass is partially smooth-walled and shows posterior enhancement of the soundbeam and asymmetric lateral shadowing. However, multiple internal echoes make this a complex cyst. (**d**) Using spatial compounding the contour is distinct, the lateral shadows disappear. This mass was a cyst with hemorrhage.
e An oval, lobulated lesion with hyperechoic parts. *Histology*: Papillary intracystic carcinoma.

- Strong posterior enhancement of the soundbeam. Posterior enhancement occurs since, in the cyst, no or very little reflexion or absorption occurs. Therefore the sound beam behind a cyst is attenuated less than the sound beam of the surrounding structures. The intensity of posterior enhancement will depend on the contents of the cyst (clear vs. proteinaceous vs. hemorrhagic) and on its size. (Small cysts will have less effect on sound attenuation [compared with the surroundings] than larger cysts.) Hemorrhagic or clotted contents may even lead to shadowing behind the cyst. To make the diagnosis of a simple cyst, adequate posterior enhancement should be present with respect to the size of the presumed cyst. Absence of posterior enhancement behind a lesion > 5 mm is not compatible with the diagnosis of a simple cyst, if the ultrasound imaging parameters were correctly chosen (sufficient gain, sufficient contrast, imaging in the focal zone).
- *Thin edge shadows:* These were initially described as a sign of benign lesions or cysts. Thin edge shadows may occur at any smooth wall that is parallel to the soundbeam, since—as a result of the angle of incidence—the echo from that structure is reflected away from the transducer. With modern compound technique thin edge shadows are seen less frequently. Since they might also arise from the lateral wall of a well-circumscribed malignancy, they are redundant to other signs and are no longer considered a diagnostically important feature.

Interpreting and Documenting Sonographic Findings

Fig. 4.12a–c

a This simple cyst can be definitively diagnosed sonographically because of its oval shape, thin wall, absence of internal echoes, and far wall enhancement of the soundbeam.

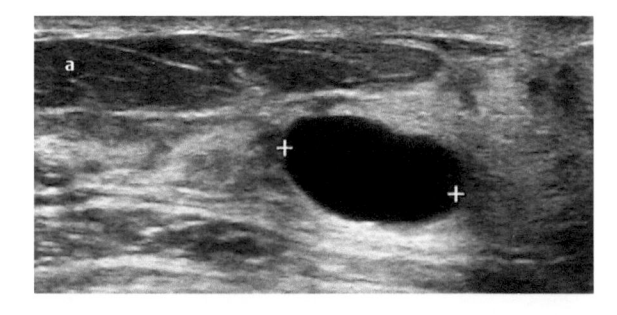

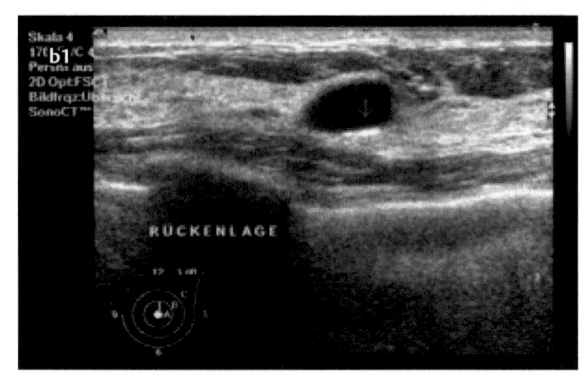

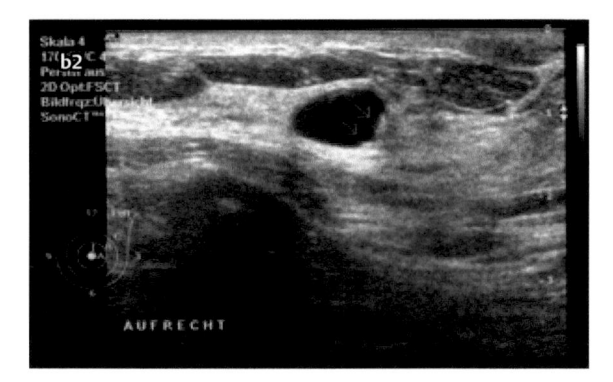

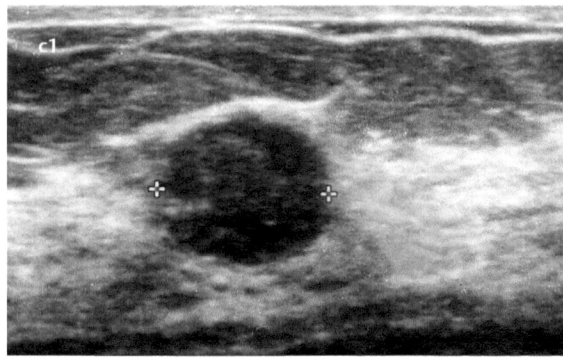

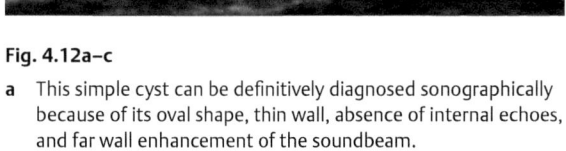

b1 This cyst exhibits some internal echoes owing to some proteinaceous contents and some debris.

b2 This image (of the same cyst) was acquired with the patient sitting upright to demonstrate the sedimentation. The dependent portion is shown on the right. Arrows mark the level of the sedimentation.

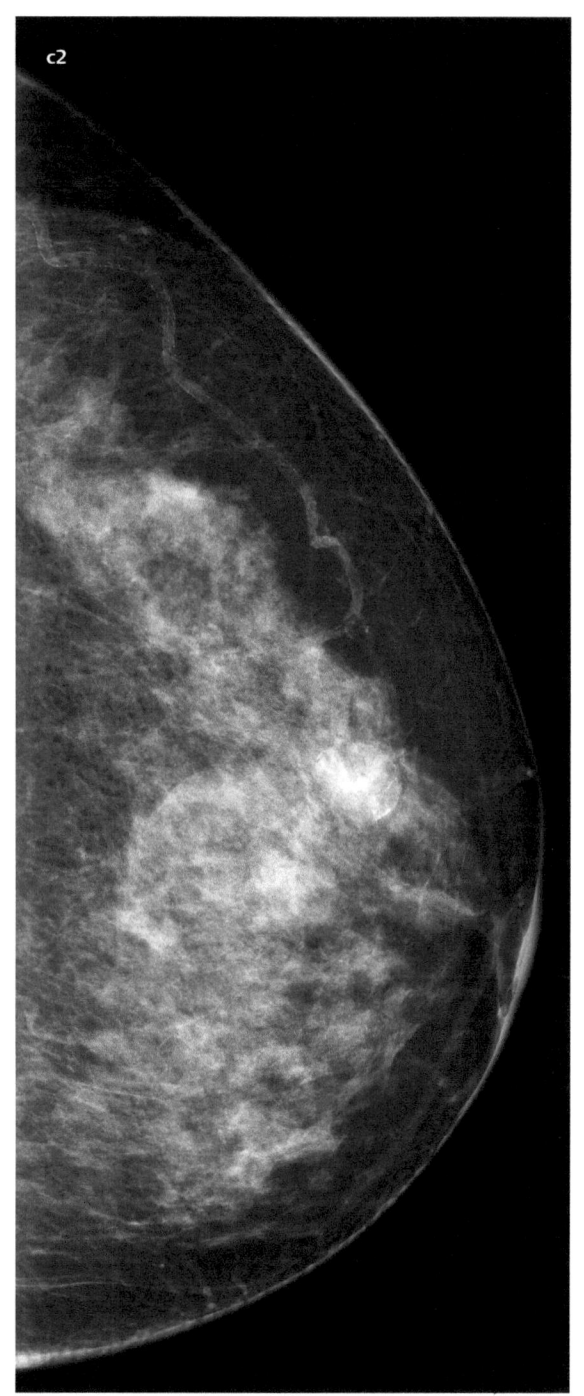

c1 Ultrasound demonstrates a well-circumscribed round hypoechoic lesion. The ultrasound image would require further assessment. However, correlation with mammography (**c2**) demonstrates that the lesion corresponds to a partly calcified cyst with thickened contents (no further assessment required).

If the above findings are present throughout the lesion, a simple cyst can be diagnosed (see **Fig. 4.11a,b**). A simple cyst corresponds to a BI-RADS 2 lesion and does not require further assessment or short-term follow-up.

In the breast, cysts commonly are clustered or may have thin septations. Thin septations are a normal finding and do not indicate malignancy.

Cysts are common in the breast. If there is a worrisome lesion on mammography that might be explained as a cyst, it is important that the cyst seen on ultrasound imaging corresponds to the worrisome lesion on mammography. When the mass is seen on mammography and does not correlate with the sonographic finding for certain, a marker can be placed over the mass seen on sonography and the mammogram can be repeated. If there is still uncertainty, the cyst can be aspirated, and, if necessary, the mammogram may be repeated. This should show that the mass has resolved. As noted above, when a palpable mass is scanned it can be bracketed with two fingers and the transducer slipped between the bracketing fingers to ensure that the sonographically identified cyst corresponds to the palpable mass.

Masses that do not contain all the characteristics of simple cysts require additional workup: cyst aspiration (in case of a suspected cyst) or (if the lesion proves to be solid) percutaneous biopsy.

If a lesion is suspected to be a cyst but contains echoes, does not exhibit adequate posterior enhancement, or shows some irregularities of the wall or a thickened wall, or if a lesion contains liquid parts but contains solid elements as well, the lesion may be named a *complex cystic lesion* (**Fig. 4.11c–e**).

Complex cystic lesions may correspond to benign cysts with debris or clotted contents; they may correspond to an infected cyst or an oil cyst, to a cyst with benign or malignant (mostly papillary) proliferation, or to malignancy with liquefied necrotic parts. Some malignancies which consist of very homogeneously arranged cells (e.g., some medullary or anaplastic carcinomas) may present as very hypoechoic or, rarely, anechoic lesions. This large differential diagnosis explains why further workup is necessary for all complex cystic lesions (**Fig. 4.13**). Usually, this workup should include an additional mammogram (to exclude signs of malignancy or prove the typical appearance of an oil cast, for example). Unless a benign change is unequivocally proven based on the mammographic–sonographic appearance, cyst aspiration or histopathologic assessment (usually by core needle biopsy) is needed.

Solid Masses

Definitive diagnosis of the histology of a solid mass is not usually possible based on its sonographic pattern. However, certain characteristics are helpful in determining whether a solid mass might be malignant or whether it very probably represents a benign lesion (**Figs. 4.13, 4.14, 4.15**).

In the latter case follow-up can be justified instead of percutaneous breast biopsy, which formerly had been recommended for verification of any solid lesion.

The characteristics observed by ultrasonography and their diagnostic significance (as reported in the literature) are summarized in **Table 4.1** (Stavros et al. 1995, Kolb et al. 1998, Skaane and Engedal 1998, Graf et al. 2004, Hong et al. 2005, Mainiero et al. 2005, Madjar et al. 2006, Raza et al. 2010).

When solid lesions are assessed, the above features should be systematically checked.

Features of low specificity and significance according to our own experience include echotexture and vascularity.

Echotexture of solid lesions (homogeneous vs. heterogeneous) seems to be unspecific with significant overlap between malignant and benign changes.

Since absent or low vascularity cannot exclude malignancy, we usually do not include Doppler imaging in our differential diagnostic considerations.

Even though presence of calcifications within a mass is more common among malignant than benign masses, the discriminating capability of this feature is limited according to our experience.

The features with the highest positive predictive value of malignancy include echogenic halo, architectural distortion, spiculated and angulated margins, microlobulated contour, and anti-parallel orientation (Stavros et al. 1995, Skaane and Engedal 1998). The echogenic halo in fact represents an increased number of interfaces caused by spiculations that extend into surrounding tissue. Angulated margin describes a margin that is acute, obtuse, or 90°.

Many malignancies appear to have some (sometimes slight) posterior attenuation. However, absence of this sign does not exclude malignancy.

Whenever any sign with low-to-intermediate, intermediate, or high risk of malignancy (as mentioned in **Table 4.1**) is present and cannot be unequivocally proven to be a benign condition (as proven by a mammographically pathognomonic appearance or by unchanged presentation on mammographic–sonographic follow-up), further assessment is required. That is, the lesion should be classified as BI-RADS 4 and should then undergo histopathologic assessment (usually by core needle biopsy).

For lesions with a high or very high probability of benignity short-term follow-up may be considered instead of histopathologic assessment. Before such a diagnosis is possible, the following checks are recommended:

- *First*, any sign indicating malignancy on ultrasonography must be absent.
- *Second*, mammography should be performed for complementary assessment whenever follow-up of a solid lesion is considered instead of biopsy. Rare exceptions,

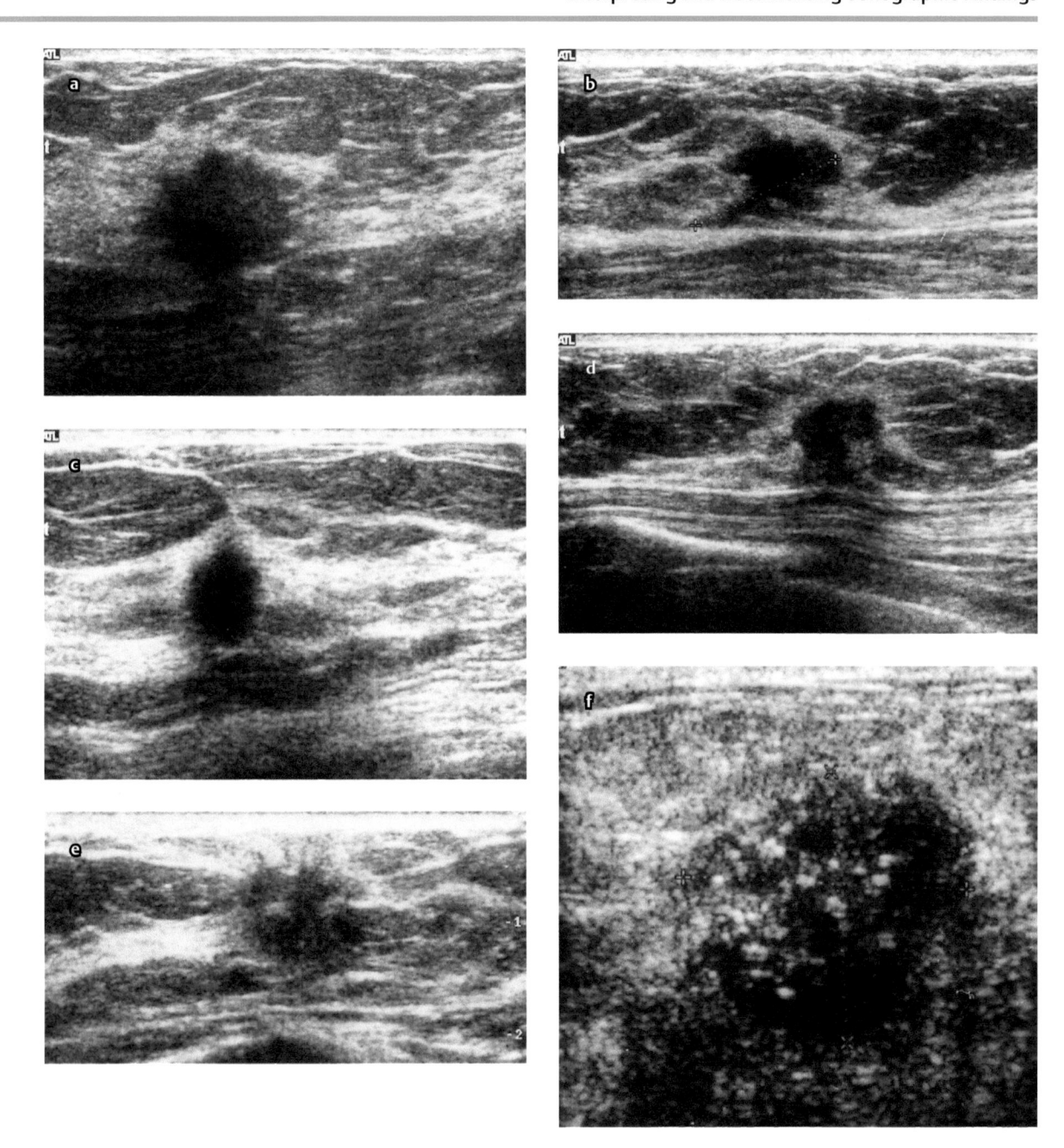

Fig. 4.13a–f Sonographic patterns that are highly suspicious for malignant lesions.

a The shape of this lesion is roundish, the margins are irregular and spiculated, the echo pattern hypoechoic, some discrete posterior shadowing. *Histology*: Infiltrating ductal carcinoma.
b The shape of this malignant lesion is irregular, the echo pattern hypoechoic, the margins are indistinct and angular with destruction of the normal parenchymal surrounding structure.
c This small invasive ductal carcinoma is extremely hypoechoic, the shape is taller than wide, the margins are microlobulated and show an abrupt interface.
d Typically malignant lesion with a broad hyperechoic rim and disruption of the Cooper ligaments.
e Invasive ductal carcinoma with irregular shape, spiculated margins, complex echo pattern, and abrupt interface.
f Invasive ductal carcinoma with ductal microcalcifications.

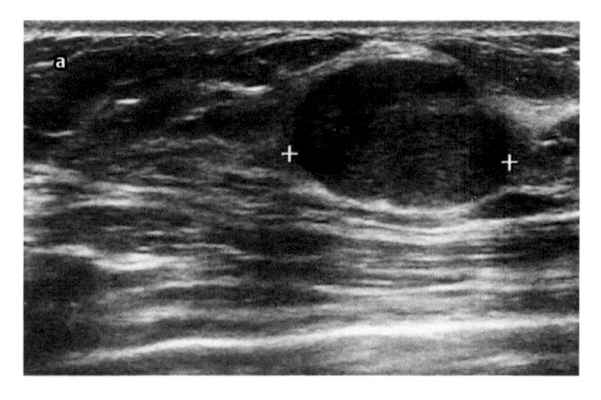

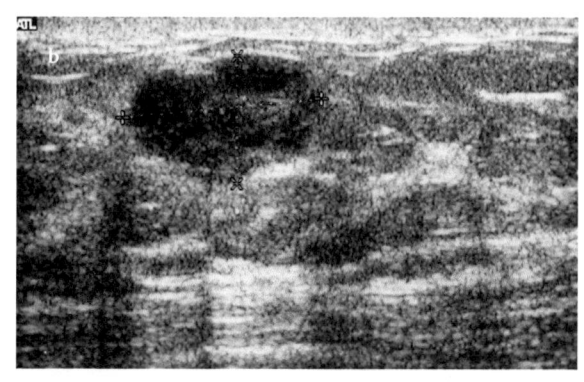

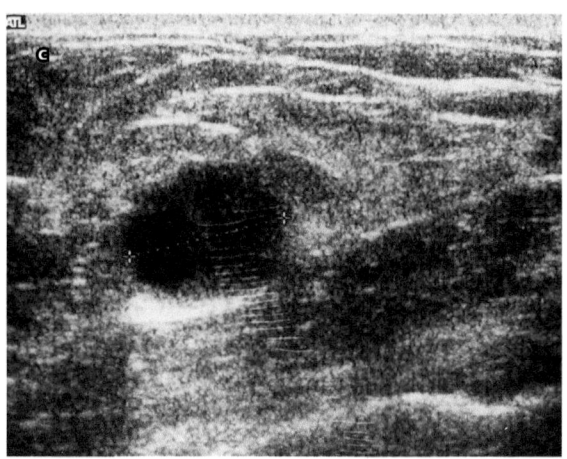

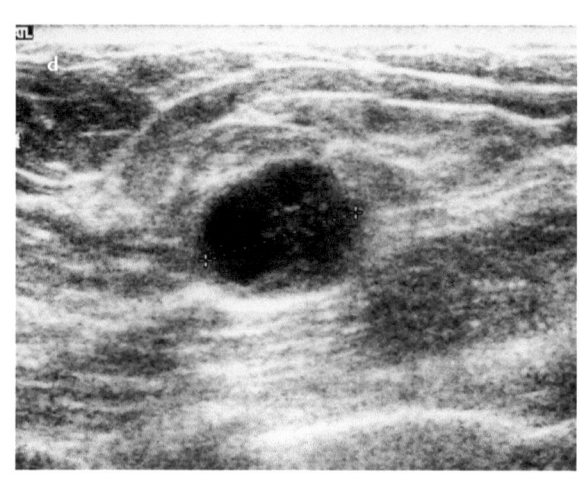

Fig. 4.14a–d

a A well-defined mass is shown. With a single gentle lobulation, its homogeneous echotexture, its thin echogenic pseudocapsule, and excellent mobility (as checked during real-time imaging), it is a typical example of benign fibroadenoma. Its oval shape and width greater than its height (ratio > 1.5) further support this diagnosis.

b This oval mass is not completely well defined at its posterior contour. The internal echo pattern is heterogeneous and posterior acoustic enhancement is present together with some shadowing. The sonographic findings are nonspecific, but might suggest a benign lesion. The lesion underwent biopsy and was found to be a high-grade invasive ductal carcinoma.

c,d This oval complex mass showed indistinct margins, but a strong posterior enhancement (**c**). With compound imaging (**d**) the margins falsely appeared to be better defined. However, the echogenic structure inside the cystic lesion is better demonstrated. Excisional biopsy proved the mass to be an intracystic papillary carcinoma (ductal carcinima in situ). Images **b** and **c** were acquired without use of the compound mode.

where mammography may not be necessary, may concern very young women without increased risk and lesions that fulfil all the below criteria of a probably benign lesion.

- *Third*, a combination of signs should be present that strongly supports the presence of a benign change.

Whereas single feature descriptors allow an increase in the level of suspicion, only systematic assessment of the combination of important signs, including clinical information, patient age, and information from mammography, should be used to downgrade a solid lesion (recommending short-term follow-up) and avert biopsy.

The single most reliable indicator of a benign mass appears to be presence of a fine pseudocapsule (Stavros et al. 1995, Skaane and Engedal 1998, Stavros 2003). A smooth margin without a fine pseudocapsule, however, may also be present in malignancy and should therefore be considered only an uncertain indication of benignity.

According to Skaane, a sufficiently *high level of certainty* can be reached when presence of a pseudocapsule is combined with good through-transmission (posterior enhancement), absence of an echogenic halo, or architectural distortion (Skaane and Engedal 1998).

Other authors consider the following combination of signs as a sufficiently reliable indicator of a benign mass: oval shape, smooth wall (optimally a pseudocapsule, no irregularity of the margin), transverse axis (long to short axis > 1.5), absence of changes in the surrounding tissues and homogeneous good through-transmission.

Interpreting and Documenting Sonographic Findings

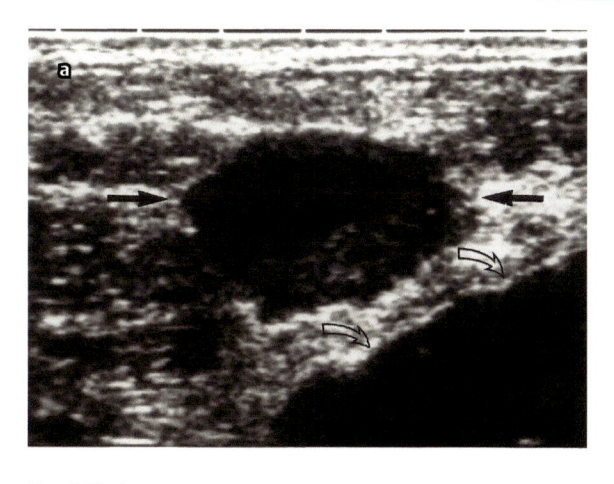

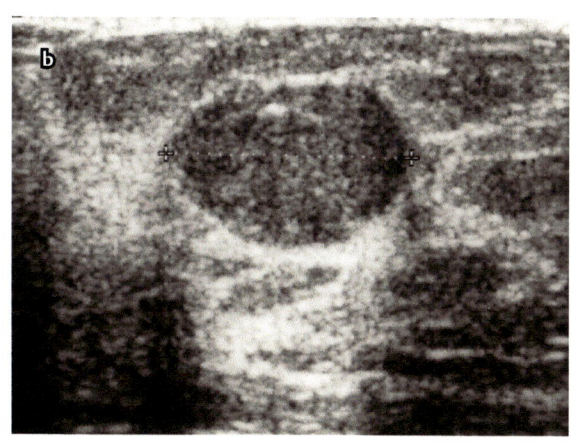

Fig. 4.15a,b

a There can be a considerable overlap in the sonographic characteristics of benign and malignant lesions. In this patient the superficial mass (solid arrows) has an oval shape and is partially well defined. However, there is a heterogeneous internal echo pattern, some irregularity of its margins, and microlobulation in the far wall. The deeper lobulated mass underneath it (curved, open arrows) corresponds to a silicone-filled augmentation prosthesis. The lesion proved to be an invasive ductal carcinoma.

b This oval heterogeneous lesion seemed to be rather well defined; nevertheless, the strong heterogeneity of the echo structure and a small hyperechoic rim suggested malignancy. Histologically, an invasive ductal carcinoma was diagnosed.

Table 4.1 Lesion characteristics on ultrasonography and diagnostic implication[a]

Lesion characteristics	Feature	Suspicion of malignancy	Remark
Shape	Oval	Low	
	Round	Low (to intermediate)	
	Irregular	High	
Orientation	Parallel (to the transducer)	Low	Ratio of horizontal to AP axes > 1.5
	Anti-parallel (taller than wide)	High	
	Indeterminate	Intermediate to high	
Margins	Fine pseudocapsule	Very low	Most important single sign of benign etiology
	Circumscribed	Low to intermediate	
	Smooth lobulation	Low to intermediate	
	Indistinct	Intermediate to high	
	Microlobulation	High	
	Angulated margin	High	
	Spiculated	Very high	
Surrounding tissue: echogenic halo	Present	Very high	Important indicator of malignancy
	Absent	Indeterminate	
Surrounding tissue architectural distortion	Present	High to very high	Important indicator of malignancy
	Absent	Indeterminate	

continued ▷

Table 4.1 (continued)

Lesion characteristics	Feature	Suspicion of malignancy	Remark
Echogenicity	**Anechoic** combined with good posterior enhancement	Benign	**(Simple cyst)**
	Hypoechoic	Indeterminate	Echogenicity as compared with fat
	Isoechoic	Low	Echogenicity as compared with fat
	Hyperechoic	Low	Echogenicity as compared with fat
Internal echo pattern	Homogeneous	Low to intermediate	Low diagnostic value
	Heterogeneous	Intermediate to high	Low diagnostic value
Sound absorption	Shadowing	Intermediate to high	
	Posterior enhancement	Low	
	Indifferent	Indeterminate	
Surrounding tissue	Architectural distortion	High (except for scarring)	Structures interrupted; optimally seen on coronal reconstructions
	Displaced surrounding structures	Low (to intermediate)	
Calcifications	Within the lesion	Intermediate to high	
Compressibility (elasticity)	High (= soft)	Low	
	Low (= hard)	High	
	Not examined	–	
Mobility	High	Low	
	Low	High	
	Not examined	–	
Vascularity	Increased		Increased vascularity of a lesion is considered associated with increased risk of malignancy
	Tangential	Low	Moderately reliable
	Radial	High	
	Irregular	High	
	Not examined	–	
Special cases	Conglomeration of microcysts	Indeterminate	According to the DEGUM consensus (Madjar et al. 2006) BI-RADS 3 category is suggested
	Dilated ducts with irregularities or occlusion	Intermediate to high	Possible sign of DCIS
	Presence of suspicious regional lymph nodes	(High)	
Further signs	Cooper ligaments interrupted, thickened or straightened		
	Coopers ligaments pushed		
	Edema of skin		
	Edema of breast tissue		
	Infiltration of chest wall		

AP, anteroposterior; DCIS, ductal carcinoma in situ.
[a]The most important features are highlighted in bold italic letters.

Mobility and elasticity have also been used in addition by most experienced investigators. Hard lesions (even if mobile) or immobile lesions should lead to further assessment and are not compatible with BI-RADS 3 lesions. Soft and mobile lesions support the above-mentioned combined signs that rule in a benign lesion.

The latest literature on elastography supports the importance of elasticity. Based on the fact that soft carcinomas are uncommon (< 10%), elasticity measurement may provide another important feature that may support benignity in combination with other features. However, further data confirming the role of this technology in combination with other features will be needed.

With a combination of several signs biopsy can be avoided for some solid masses. *These masses may be classified as BI-RADS 3 lesions*. Usually short-term follow-up after 6 months should be considered for solid masses with benign features.

A BI-RADS 2 category is appropriate for solid masses for which no change is proven by follow-up of 2–3 years, or for which pathognomonic benign features exist on mammography.

However, patient age, high family risk, or increasing size should require special consideration. With increasing age the risk of malignancy increases even for well-circumscribed lesions. A significant number of cancers in *BRCA1* mutation carriers present as well-circumscribed lesions.

Therefore, in mutation carriers or women at high risk, solid lesions should usually undergo percutaneous breast biopsy even if they fulfill the criteria of BI-RADS 3.

For elderly women with solid lesions histopathologic assessment is preferred to short-term follow-up.

Increase in size should usually lead to histopathologic assessment and thus to classification as BI-RADS 4 (or 5).

BI-RADS Lexicon

The BI-RADS lexicon uses the following categories to classify abnormalities:
- Masses
- Calcifications
- Special cases
- Vascularity

Masses are described by their shape, margins, echo pattern, posterior acoustic features, and effect on surrounding tissue (echogenic halo, architectural distortion).

Calcifications are classified as macro- or microcalcifications and calcifications within or outside a mass.

Special cases describe clustered microcysts, complicated cysts, masses in or on the skin, foreign bodies, lymph nodes (intramammary or in the axilla).

Vascularity may be present or not, immediately adjacent to a lesion or diffusely increased in the surrounding tissue. Absent vascularity is not a specific finding.

The BI-RADS lexicon recommends briefly reporting the imaging findings of each modality. However, the final recommendation should be based on the integrated information, including clinical information, history, scope of the examination (targeted or survey), comparison with previous studies, correlation with the physical and mammographic (or if available also MRI) findings.

The final categories, which it is recommended are used, are:
- BI-RADS 0: Further imaging required
- BI-RADS 1: Normal, no suspicion of malignancy; usual screening recommended (as appropriate for the patient's age and risk)
- BI-RADS 2: Benign lesion (e.g., cyst, internal mammary lymph node or fibroadenoma, as proven by follow-up); usual screening recommended
- BI-RADS 3: Probably benign; short-term follow-up (usually at 6 months) recommended (solid lesion with typically benign features,* conglomeration of microcysts)
- BI-RADS 4: Suspicious finding (all solid lesions without typically benign features); histopathologic assessment recommended
- BI-RADS 5: Highly suspicious of malignancy; histopathologic verification recommended
- BI-RADS 6: Proven malignancy

For lesions that are only seen on ultrasound imaging and exhibit no mammographic features of malignancy the following recommendation may be given:
- BI-RADS 2 may be assigned to lesions fulfilling all criteria of a simple cyst and to lesions for which benignity is proven by long-term follow-up or previous histopathologic assessment.
- BI-RADS 3 category may be considered:
  - For unspecific, probably benign, palpable findings if ultrasonography exhibits no sign of malignancy in homogeneously echogenic tissue (with or without mobile and compressible interposed fat lobules or regular ductal structures)
  - For solid masses without sonographic signs of malignancy that fulfil one of the accepted combinations of benign features.* In addition, such lesions should be mobile and soft.
- BI-RADS 4 category should be assigned to:
  - All solid lesions with benign features that increase in size
  - Any lesion that does not belong to category 2 or 3
  - Any lesion that is considered indeterminate or does not fulfill the criteria for 2 or 3 category.
- BI-RADS 5 category should be considered for solid lesions with features of high or very high probability of malignancy. The most frequent signs implying

---

* In women at high risk, biopsy should be considered, even of completely well-circumscribed masses.

a high probability of malignancy include echogenic halo, lesion taller than wide, irregular or angulated margin, posterior shadowing (combined with further signs), immobile lesion.

Suspicious Findings of the Axilla

The presence of a solid or complex cystic mass in the axilla has to be considered suspicious and requires further assessment.

Lymph nodes that are suspected of being involved with malignancy or require further assessment include lymph nodes with diffuse or focal thickening of the cortex > 3 mm, with replacement or effacement of the hyperechoic fatty hilum.

References and Recommended Reading

Abdullah N, Mesurolle B, El-Khoury M, Kao E. Breast imaging reporting and data system lexicon for US: interobserver agreement for assessment of breast masses. Radiology 2009;252(3):665–672

Alvarez S, Añorbe E, Alcorta P, López F, Alonso I, Cortés J. Role of sonography in the diagnosis of axillary lymph node metastases in breast cancer: a systematic review. AJR Am J Roentgenol 2006;186(5):1342–1348

American College of Radiology Practice Guideline for the Performance of a Breast Ultrasound Examination 2011. Available at: www.ACR.org

Berg WA, Blume JD, Cormack JB, Mendelson EB. Operator-dependence of physician-performed whole breast US: lesion detection and characterization. Radiology 2006;241(2):335–365

Berg WA, Blume JD, Cormack JB, et al; ACRIN 6666 Investigators. Combined screening with ultrasound and mammography vs. mammography alone in women at elevated risk of breast cancer. JAMA 2008;299(18):2151–2163

Buchberger W, DeKoekkoek-Doll P, Springer P, Obrist P, Dünser M. Incidental findings on sonography of the breast: clinical significance and diagnostic workup. AJR Am J Roentgenol 1999;173(4):921–927

Corsetti V, Houssami N, Ghirardi M et al. Evidence of the effect of adjunct ultrasound screening in women with mammography-negative dense breasts: interval breast cancers at 1 year follow-up. Eur J Cancer 2011;47(7):1021–1026

Crystal P, Strano SD, Shcharynski S, Koretz MJ. Using sonography to screen women with mammographically dense breasts. AJR Am J Roentgenol 2003;181(1):177–182

Dennis MA, Parker SH, Klaus AJ, Stavros AT, Kaske TI, Clark SB. Breast biopsy avoidance: the value of normal mammograms and normal sonograms in the setting of a palpable lump. Radiology 2001;219(1):186–191

Gordon PB. Ultrasound for breast cancer screening and staging. Radiol Clin North Am 2002;40(3):431–441

Graf O, Helbich TH, Fuchsjaeger MH, et al. Follow-up of palpable circumscribed noncalcified solid breast masses at mammography and US: can biopsy be averted? Radiology 2004;233(3):850–856

Hong AS, Rosen EL, Soo MS, Baker JA. BI-RADS for sonography: positive and negative predictive values of sonographic features. AJR Am J Roentgenol 2005;184(4):1260–1265

Itoh A, Ueno E, Tohno E, et al. Breast disease: clinical application of US elastography for diagnosis. Radiology 2006;239(2):341–350

Kaplan SS. Clinical utility of bilateral whole-breast US in the evaluation of women with dense breast tissue. Radiology 2001;221(3):641–649

Kim EY, Ko EY, Han BK, et al. Sonography of axillary masses: what should be considered other than the lymph nodes? J Ultrasound Med 2009;28(7):923–939

Kolb TM, Lichy J, Newhouse JH. Occult cancer in women with dense breasts: detection with screening US—diagnostic yield and tumor characteristics. Radiology 1998;207(1):191–199

Kolb TM, Lichy J, Newhouse JH. Comparison of the performance of screening mammography, physical examination, and breast US and evaluation of factors that influence them: an analysis of 27,825 patient evaluations. Radiology 2002;225(1):165–175

Lazarus E, Mainiero MB, Schepps B, Koelliker SL, Livingston LS. BI-RADS lexicon for US and mammography: interobserver variability and positive predictive value. Radiology 2006;239(2):385–391

Lee CH, Dershaw DD, Kopans D, et al. Breast cancer screening with imaging: recommendations from the Society of Breast Imaging and the ACR on the use of mammography, breast MRI, breast ultrasound, and other technologies for the detection of clinically occult breast cancer. J Am Coll Radiol 2010;7(1):18–27

Madjar H, Ohlinger R, Mundinger A, et al. BI-RADS-analogue DEGUM criteria for findings in breast ultrasound—consensus of the DEGUM Committee on Breast Ultrasound. [Article in German] Ultraschall Med 2006;27(4):374–379

Mainiero MB, Goldkamp A, Lazarus E, et al. Characterization of breast masses with sonography: can biopsy of some solid masses be deferred? J Ultrasound Med 2005;24(2):161–167

Mainiero MB, Cinelli CM, Koelliker SL, Graves TA, Chung MA. Axillary ultrasound and fine-needle aspiration in the preoperative evaluation of the breast cancer patient: an algorithm based on tumor size and lymph node appearance. AJR Am J Roentgenol 2010;195(5):1261–1267

Mendelson EB. Problem-solving ultrasound. Radiol Clin North Am 2004;42(5):909–918, vii

Meissnitzer M, Dershaw DD, Lee CH, Morris EA. Targeted ultrasound of the breast in women with abnormal MRI findings for whom biopsy has been recommended. AJR Am J Roentgenol 2009;193(4):1025–1029

Mills P, Sever A, Weeks J, Fish D, Jones S, Jones P. Axillary ultrasound assessment in primary breast cancer: an audit of 653 cases. Breast J 2010;16(5):460–463

Neal CH, Daly CP, Nees AV, Helvie MA. Can preoperative axillary US help exclude N2 and N3 metastatic breast cancer? Radiology 2010;257(2):335–341

Nothacker M, Duda V, Hahn M, et al. Early detection of breast cancer: benefits and risks of supplemental breast ultrasound in asymptomatic women with mammographically dense breast tissue. A systematic review. BMC Cancer 2009;9:335–344

Raza S, Goldkamp AL, Chikarmane SA, Birdwell RL. US of breast masses categorized as BI-RADS 3, 4, and 5: pictorial review of factors influencing clinical management. Radiographics 2010;30(5):1199–1213

Sidibé S, Coulibaly A, Traoré S, Touré M, Traoré I. Role of ultrasonography in the diagnosis of axillary lymph node metastases in breast cancer: a systematic review. [Article in French] Mali Med 2007;22(4):9–13

Skaane P, Engedal K. Analysis of sonographic features in the differentiation of fibroadenoma and invasive ductal carcinoma. AJR Am J Roentgenol 1998;170(1):109–114

Soo MS, Rosen EL, Baker JA, Vo TT, Boyd BA. Negative predictive value of sonography with mammography in patients with palpable breast lesions. AJR Am J Roentgenol 2001;177(5):1167–1170

Stavros AT, Thickman D, Rapp CL, Dennis MA, Parker SH, Sisney GA. Solid breast nodules: use of sonography to distinguish between benign and malignant lesions. Radiology 1995;196(1):123–134

Stavros AT. Breast ultrasound. Philadelphia: Lippincott Williams and Wilkins; 2003

Tohno E, Cosgrove DO, Sloane UP. Ultrasound diagnosis of breast diseases. Edinburgh: Churchill Livingstone; 1994

Wojcinski S, Farrokh A, Weber S, et al. Multicenter study of ultrasound real-time tissue elastography in 779 cases for the assessment of breast lesions: improved diagnostic performance by combining the BI-RADS®-US classification system with sonoelastography. Ultraschall Med 2010;31(5):484–491

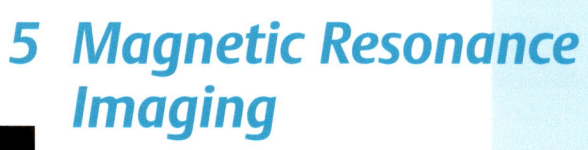

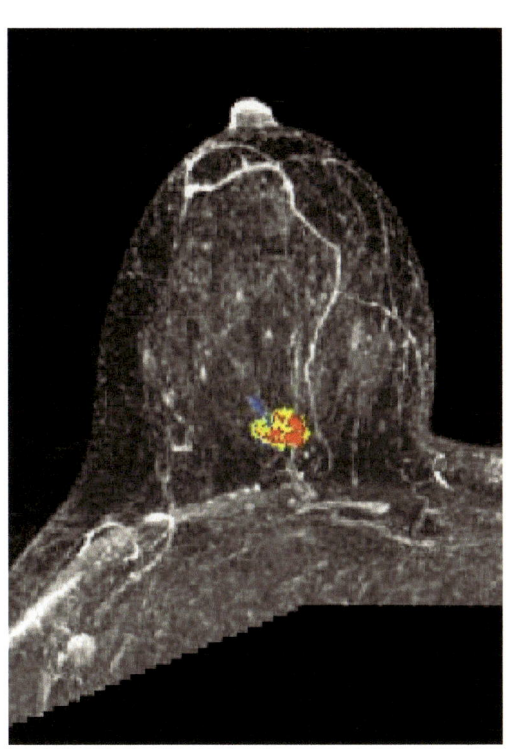

5 Magnetic Resonance Imaging

Purpose, Accuracy, Possibilities, and Limitations ⇢ *128*

MR Technique ⇢ *129*
Dynamic Contrast-Enhanced MRI (DCE-MRI) ⇢ *129*
Unenhanced MRI ⇢ *131*
Diffusion-Weighted Imaging and
MR Spectroscopy ⇢ *132*

Scheduling and Performing Breast MRI ⇢ *132*
Performing DCE Breast MRI ⇢ *132*
Performing Plain MRI for Evaluation of Implant Failure ⇢ *134*

Diagnostic Criteria ⇢ *134*

Patient Selection and Indications ⇢ *151*
Contrast-Enhanced MRI ⇢ *151*

References and Recommended Reading ⇢ *171*

5 Magnetic Resonance Imaging

S. H. Heywang-Koebrunner, S. Barter

Early studies using magnetic resonance imaging (MRI) for breast imaging were performed without contrast agents (unenhanced MRI). However, unenhanced MRI with various combinations of pulse sequences has not proved helpful for detection or diagnosis of breast cancer.

The use of contrast agents, as initiated by Heywang in 1986 and 1988, is now considered mandatory for detection and diagnosis of breast cancer by MRI. Contrast-enhanced breast MRI today implies that both breasts are imaged with high spatial resolution before and at least two or three times after intravenous administration of a standard MR contrast agent (so-called "dynamic contrast-enhanced breast MRI"). Both morphology of a lesion (before and after contrast administration) and its enhancement dynamics contribute to the diagnostic information that may be provided only by MRI.

Unenhanced MRI using specific sequences has proven useful for detection or exclusion of implant failure. Novel MR techniques such as proton spectroscopy or diffusion-weighted MRI are being evaluated currently as additional tools. Preliminary results will be summarized at the end of this chapter.

Unless explicitly stated otherwise, this chapter will discuss the use of dynamic contrast-enhanced breast MRI for detection, diagnosis, or exclusion of breast cancer.

Purpose, Accuracy, Possibilities, and Limitations

Dynamic contrast-enhanced MRI (DCE-MRI) is probably the most sensitive breast imaging method available today. The added information gained from the morphology and dynamics of contrast enhancement makes it a very valuable additional tool for appropriate indications. Its specificity varies depending on the indication.

Owing to the large number of false positive studies, short-term follow-up recommendations, and its high costs, MRI does not appear to be appropriate for any type of low-risk screening. Using contrast-enhanced MRI as the sole imaging modality or interpreting contrast-enhanced MRI without conventional breast imaging (usually mammography supplemented by ultrasound as indicated) does not represent sound diagnostic practice. Also, owing to limitations of its sensitivity, MRI is in general not appropriate to replace histopathologic assessment of suspicious lesions. The best results have been achieved by combining MRI with mammography and ultrasound, and by limiting its use to selected appropriate indications.

In most published studies the sensitivity of MRI ranges around 90–95% for the detection of invasive breast cancer; for the detection of ductal carcinoma in situ (DCIS) published sensitivity values vary from 50% to 90%. Specificities vary markedly between the studies, but most report a range of around 60–95%. For MR screening some authors have reported specificities as high as 95%. These reported numbers, however, refer only to biopsy indications as false positive results. Short-term follow-up examinations are not included and are often not mentioned. They range around 10% and the resulting patient concern needs to be considered as an important side effect of MR screening.

Caution is necessary when interpreting results from different studies, as different factors may affect the accuracy of results. The varying factors which may influence both the achievable and the reported sensitivities and specificities include:
- MR technique
- Interpretation criteria
- Patient selection
- Other important factors related to study design and statistics

The following paragraphs will elucidate the above-mentioned factors.

MR Technique

Today, state-of-the-art DCE-MRI allows the combination of high spatial resolution (in-plane optimally < 1 mm^2, slice thickness < 3 mm or even isotropic) and sufficient temporal resolution (3D imaging every 1–2 min covering up to 5–6 min post injection of contrast medium). These techniques with some variations have been used by several research groups for up to 10 years. Technical progress and—most importantly—increasing standardization contribute to secure reproducibility of the results and further optimization of accuracy. The main advantages and limitations of MRI, however, may be defined by the biology of contrast media uptake within the breast tissue.

Image Interpretation Criteria Employed

The information provided by DCE-MRI of the breast is based on lesion morphology, the presence of enhancement, and its dynamics.

Lesion morphology on MRI is assessed in a similar way to that of mammography. Absence of *enhancement* or very little enhancement is associated with very low probability of invasive malignancy. However, absence of enhancement can exclude neither the presence of DCIS nor 100% of invasive malignancies. Evaluation of *enhancement dynamics* may support diagnosis of a benign or a malignant change, although overlap exists for this feature as well as for interpretation of lesion morphology.

Various interpretation rules, which synthesize the three types of information outlined above, have been suggested. None of the rules allows optimum sensitivity and specificity. As for all diagnostic tests, depending on the chosen interpretation rules and thresholds, high specificity may be obtained with some loss of sensitivity and vice versa.

Patient Selection and Choice of Indications

As with any other complex imaging method, careful selection of the appropriate indications is an absolute prerequisite for obtaining good results. Appropriate and inappropriate indications will be treated in detail later in this chapter. In scientific studies patient preselection may have a strong influence on the obtained results. Without clearly defined selection that excludes significant bias, results may not be reliable. Do not rely on reproducing results that were obtained with different patient selection or otherwise different conditions.

Factors to Be Considered

The following factors may have an important influence on reported results: Patient selection (preselection bias), study design (prospective vs. retrospective, evaluation of MRI alone vs. MRI combined with other information and imaging results, multicenter vs. single institution), the exact definition of a positive and a negative finding, sensitivity and specificity calculation used and verification of the results (verification bias).

Overall, the influence of the above-mentioned factors tends to be underestimated. Reliable information may be expected only from studies with a well-defined design and a clear and homogeneous patient selection. Depending on differences in design, comparison between studies is usually difficult and often impossible. Extrapolation from studies with a design that differs from the intended method of application should be avoided.

Conclusion

Overall, MRI has proved to be the most sensitive method for the detection of invasive breast cancer, with reported sensitivities for invasive breast cancer ranging around 85–97%. The sensitivity for DCIS is lower, and in this context MRI is complementary to mammography. The specificity of MRI is lower than that of mammography.

It is essential that MR-guided interventions must be available to further assess lesions that are detected and visible only by MRI. Without diligent patient selection with appropriate indications there may be an underestimated problem of availability and resources. Even though the accuracy of MRI is not sufficient to replace biopsy, in experienced hands the addition of MRI may in some instances allow improvement of sensitivity and/or specificity and better select patients who require biopsy.

MR Technique

Dynamic Contrast-Enhanced MRI (DCE-MRI)

Optimum technique is an important requirement to achieve high accuracy. Optimum technique should allow imaging of both breasts with high temporal and spatial resolution with maximum reduction of artifacts.

> During the first 15 years of use, MR protocols usually represented a compromise between high temporal and high spatial resolution. Thus some research groups preferred protocols with higher spatial resolution (which usually yielded higher sensitivity at the cost of specificity), while others preferred protocols with higher temporal resolution (which mostly yielded higher specificity at the cost of sensitivity). During the past 5 years both high temporal resolution and high spatial resolution have become widely available, thus improving the available information.

Today, excellent image quality is possible with state-of-the-art 1.0 and 1.5 tesla MR equipment. Few data exist on DCE-MRI performed at 0.5 or 3 tesla.

The use of dedicated breast coils is mandatory. Double breast imaging carries the advantage of detecting additional unsuspected malignancy in the contralateral breast of women with breast cancer or other risk factors. It also permits comparison of symmetry of the enhancement pattern and may thus provide additional diagnostically useful information.

Interventional breast coils should allow sufficient immobilization of the breast to prevent any movement when introducing a needle or biopsy probe. Furthermore adequate resolution and good access to the breast in question (optimally access from medially and laterally) is required. Therefore most interventional coils image just one breast. Interventional coils need to be delivered with adequate software that allows for planning and monitoring of the intervention.

For DCE-MRI the slice thickness should be ≤ 3 mm. Isotropic imaging allows reformatting of the images in other planes retrospectively. For small enhancing ducts and small lesions partial volume effects are reduced with thinner slices. However, patient motion will limit the advantages of high resolution.

Even though good results have been published for 2D or 3D imaging, today 3D imaging (with or without fat saturation) may offer more possibilities for further optimization. (Previously reported problems with artifacts caused by the acquisition mode have been mostly eliminated.) Overall 3D sequences permit imaging of thin slices with excellent signal-to-noise ratio and without gaps between the slices.

In-plane resolution should be as good as possible. With the latest technology, with double breast coils, in-plane resolution can be ≤ 1 mm (optimally around 0.7 mm).

Temporal resolution (i.e., imaging at different time points after administration of contrast agent) is useful for the following reasons. Soon after contrast administration (1–3 min post injection) the best contrast exists between malignancy and surrounding tissue. Later after contrast injection (> 3 min), unspecific enhancement within benign tissue and decreasing enhancement of most malignant masses may cause false negative and false positive results. Early peripheral enhancement, an important morphologic sign of malignancy, may be detected only within the first few minutes after injection. In general three or more sequences should be acquired and 6–7 minutes postinjection should be covered by the dynamic series. Even though it may be possible to acquire 3D datasets every minute or even more frequently, no data exist to prove any significant diagnostic advantage of such protocols.

Remaining imaging time should be invested in spatial rather than temporal resolution (preferring in-plane resolution over slice thickness below 2–3 mm). Good spatial resolution is important to correctly assess lesion borders and internal architecture, which is as important diagnostically as information on enhancement dynamics.

Every effort should be made to avoid motion, since movement degrades spatial resolution and may significantly impair evaluation of enhancement dynamics (see below). For this reason:
- Ensure that the patient is fully informed. Insert an intravenous cannula before the precontrast sequences and do not change positioning during imaging.
- Immobilize the breast as much as possible. Immobilization is best achieved by using a breast coil with an integrated or add-on compression mechanism. If this is not available, cotton may be packed between the breast coil and the breast, but this is less effective. Do not over-compress the breast. Too much compression may impair contrast enhancement in malignancy as a result of increased interstitial pressure.

Care should be taken to exclude artifacts from cardiac motion in the diagnostic field of view, by switching the direction of frequency and phase encoding. Artifacts from cardiac motion can also be avoided by imaging in the coronal plane, since in this plane cardiac artifacts run parallel to the spine and thus cross neither the breast nor the axilla. If the breast is imaged in the axial (transverse plane), which may be the acquisition plane of choice, artifacts should not cross the left breast. This is achieved by choosing a phase-encoding direction from left to right, which minimizes motion artifacts across the breasts, but the axillary tails may still be affected. A very elegant new development is 3D isotropic image acquisition in the coronal plane combined with image calculation in the axial plane.

The most widely used pulse sequences are fast 3D gradient-echo pulse sequences with or without fat saturation. The majority of published cases have been examined using these or similar gradient-echo pulse sequences. Other sequences have also been described, but are not commonly used.

Suppression of the signal from fat is considered essential for improved detection of enhancement, since both enhancing lesions and fat display high signal intensity on postcontrast MR images. Detection of enhancement therefore depends either on exact comparison of corresponding precontrast and postcontrast slices or on effective suppression of the fat signal. Elimination of fat signal is achieved either by use of spectrally selective fat saturation or water excitation, or fat nulling, or by image subtraction. Pulse sequences used for image subtraction are usually faster and thus may allow higher in-plane and temporal resolution.

Unless spectrally selective pulse sequences are used, breast MRI must be performed using an in-phase condition. The in-phase condition is fulfilled when echo times of 3.6 to 6.0 milliseconds (= 4.8 ms ± 25%) at 1.5 tesla or of about 5.4 to 8.0 milliseconds (= 7.2 ms ± 25%) at 1 tesla are used.

In-phase condition means that fat and water vectors need to point in the same direction. If this condition is not fulfilled (in an opposed image), the fat and water vectors are opposite each other. If partial volume of fat and water occurs within the pixel (which is frequent with small carcinomas growing along ducts) due to changing cancellation effects in the precontrast and postcontrast images, uptake of contrast medium (Gd-DTPA) may become invisible on (so-called) opposed images. In fact, in small carcinomas and DCIS surrounded by fat, uptake of Gd-DTPA may lead either (as expected) to an increase of signal or to unchanged signal, or even to a decrease of signal after contrast medium administration (Heywang-Köbrunner et al. 1996). (Opposed images—which may be observed in non–fat-saturated images that were acquired with inappropriate echo times—can in general be easily identified, since "frames" of low signal intensity are seen between the borders of fatty and nonfatty tissue.)

The recommended dosage of Gd-DTPA ranges from 0.1 to 0.2 mmol/kg body weight. The same dosage of Gd-DTPA should always be used and should be indicated in the report or on the images.

Both phantom and patient images have shown that with 3D imaging no saturation effect following contrast occurs with flip angles of 20–35°. (With 2D imaging, however, saturation may occur. That is, with intermediate or high dosages the signal will not increase further with increasing concentration of the contrast medium!) The main advantage of higher dosages (as these can be used with 3D imaging) is that even in the presence of motion or motion artifacts (which may be unavoidable depending on the individual patient) small lesions are more obvious and may thus be better detected and differentiated.

We strongly recommend a standardized window setting and a standardized imaging order for evaluating the large number of images. Standard PACS (picture archiving and communication system) allows simultaneous viewing of corresponding anatomic slices before and at different time points after intravenous injection of contrast medium. This capability is crucial for reading DCE-MRI studies, to enable correct interpretation in the event of motion occurring between the acquired image sets. Since CD viewers and software do not allow such simultaneous viewing of different sequences, these viewers are usually not appropriate for reading dynamic breast MRI studies.

Quantitative evaluations may be helpful in the differential diagnosis of lesions. They are usually obtained from selected regions of interest (ROIs). For representative results such ROIs should be chosen as large as possible (usually larger than 3–4 pixels), but small enough to include only the area with the most suspicious enhancement (which usually has to be selected visually). The result of such a quantitative evaluation, which is possible with standard MR software, is an enhancement curve. Since the signal intensity strongly depends on the location of a voxel within the coil, measurements curves used for diagnostic purposes in DCE breast MRI should always display relative enhancement changes (i.e., percentage increase compared with the precontrast image), not absolute values, because of differing reception of signal within surface coils.

Relative enhancement is defined as:

$$\frac{(\text{Signal after contrast} - \text{Signal before contrast})}{(\text{Signal before contrast})} \times 100\%$$

It should be understood that any quantitative evaluation may be strongly influenced by the relation of lesion size to slice thickness (partial volume effect) and by patient motion (changing partial volume effect). Significant errors may occur for any lesion whose diameter is smaller than two slice thicknesses, since significant partial volume may occur depending on the location of the lesion within or between slices. Owing to changing partial volume, motion may disturb any curve measurement, and this increases with decreasing lesion size. Relying on ROI measurements or curves that cannot warrant measurement of the same anatomic area at different time points may lead to marked diagnostic errors.

Automated programs are being developed to correct for patient motion. However, their use cannot replace critical visual evaluation and careful consideration of partial volume effect and patient motion. Further research in this field should, however, be supported.

Overall, high image quality and critical assessment of the obtained images is of great importance for DCE breast MRI.

Unenhanced MRI

Unenhanced MRI using a combination of appropriate pulse sequences is presently considered the method of choice for detection and diagnosis of small implant leaks.

For this indication, too, careful examination technique is essential. The use of a dedicated breast coil is mandatory, as it is for DCE-MRI.

Slice thickness should always be 5 mm or less, desirably ≤ 3 mm. The protocol should contain at least one pulse sequence with slice thicknesses of 2 mm or less.

Images should be obtained in at least two imaging planes; alternatively, isotropic imaging and reconstruction in different planes can be considered.

First a combination of pulse sequences is recommended to obtain the best possible contrast between implant, surrounding scar or breast tissue, and fluid (such as cysts, silicone deposits, or reactive serous or serosanguinous fluid surrounding the implant). This is usually possible by a combination of a T1-weighted (or proton density-weighted) and a T2-weighted pulse sequence with or without fat saturation. Any combination of sequences can be used that allows the capsule to be imaged as a thin, low-signal-intensity line in contrast to silicone.

Whenever abnormal fluid is identified outside or adjacent to the implant, differentiation of a cystic lesion with or without protein or serosanguinous contents or of reactive fluid collections from silicone is necessary.

For this purpose the additional use of so-called "silicone only" and "silicone-suppressed" sequences with selective excitation (or suppression) of silicone is necessary. These sequences are also particularly helpful for recognition of extracapsular silicone.

Further possible pulse sequences or combinations can be found in the relevant published studies.

Cardiac artifacts should be eliminated as described above.

Diffusion-Weighted Imaging and MR Spectroscopy

Diffusion-weighted imaging (DWI) is a newly described functional MR technique which provides information about the extent and direction of random water motion in tissues. Restricted diffusion of water molecules corresponds to less signal loss, giving rise to hyperintense areas, whereas high diffusion gives rise to greater signal loss, which is seen as hypointense areas. Several studies have shown that DWI could potentially provide information on tumor biology and physiology.

The apparent diffusion coefficient (ADC) is a quantifiable measurement of the molecular movement of water. Diffusion of water molecules predominantly occurs in the extracellular space, and is therefore influenced by cellular density, extracellular matrix, and fibrosis. Therefore it is postulated that increasing cellularity with decreased extracellular space, as found in malignant masses, restricts water motion, leading to low ADC values.

Studies have shown high ADC values in benign lesions and normal fibro-glandular breast tissue, and low values in malignant lesions, although there is considerable overlap of ADC values between benign and malignant lesions. ADC values have also been reported to be lower in invasive tumors than in DCIS.

DWI sequences should be obtained after standard pre-contrast sequences and before contrast is administered.

MR imaging using proton (and less commonly phosphorus) spectroscopy have been recently described. Formerly only large voxels could be measured, but novel techniques, which have mainly been used at 3 tesla, allow measurement of small voxels and multivoxel imaging. The differing groups of molecules are identified by spectral evaluation of the signal within each voxel. Within this signal a spectrum of slightly differing precession frequencies can be identified depending on the chemical binding of the protons within the voxel. The most interesting molecular components which have been identified within MRI spectra are phosphocholines, which appear to be elevated in malignant tumors, glycine components and lactate. Whereas the value of this information for lesion differentiation has not yet been fully assessed, its most interesting application may concern monitoring of the response to neoadjuvant chemotherapy (see p. 166).

Scheduling and Performing Breast MRI

Performing DCE Breast MRI

DCE-MRI should, whenever possible, be scheduled considering potential hormonal influences:

- According to our experience, hormonal influences often lead to diffuse, sometimes patchy, enhancement. They may even cause asymmetric regional enhancement, focal areas of enhancement, or masslike enhancement. Even though most of this enhancement will be delayed (progressive) or plateau-type while invasive cancers mostly enhance fast, the distinction is uncertain. Some invasive cancers and many in-situ cancers exhibit progressive enhancement; therefore, hormonal influences may unnecessarily either obscure or mimic malignancy.
- *Whenever possible, MRI should be scheduled approximately on day 7–16 of the menstrual cycle* in premenopausal patients. (Day 1 is the first day of the menstruation bleeding.) Shorter time frames (e.g., day 7–14) should be considered in women with short menstrual cycles. In perimenopausal patients and in patients after hysterectomy a hormonal blood test may be necessary to avoid imaging during the luteal phase. According to our experience scheduling MRI about 5–8 days after measuring a low blood level of progesterone works very well. This also takes into account that MR enhancement lags behind hormonal blood levels by 5–8 days.
- Most contraceptive pills pose no problem when MRI is performed during the correct part of the menstrual cycle.
- Postmenopausal patients taking *progesterone-containing hormone replacement therapy should be advised to stop taking it for at least 4 weeks prior to the MRI*, according to current experience. In our own experience tibolone or pure estrogens appear to have little or no disturbing influence on DCE-MRI.
- **Fig. 5.1** demonstrates the influence of hormones on normal breast tissue.

We strongly recommend taking a *history*, which should include information on

- Recent surgery, percutaneous biopsy, or radiation therapy
- The diagnostic question (as far as this is known to the patient), and
- Individual risk factors

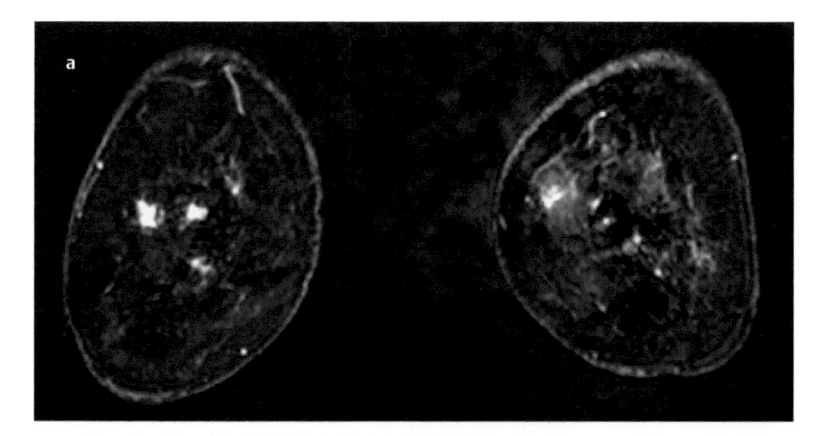

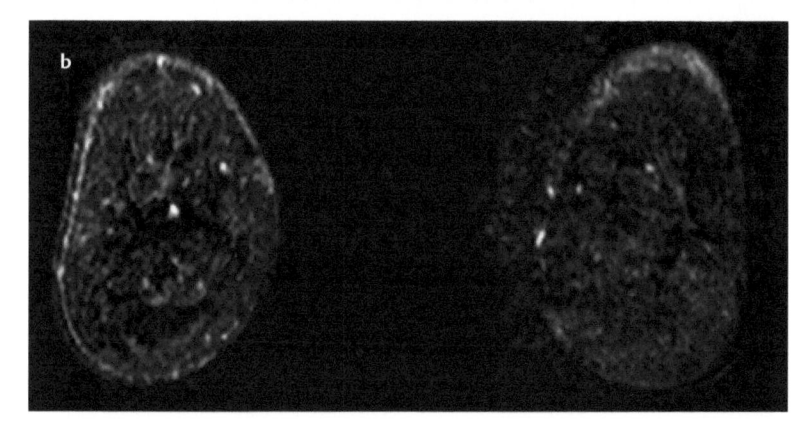

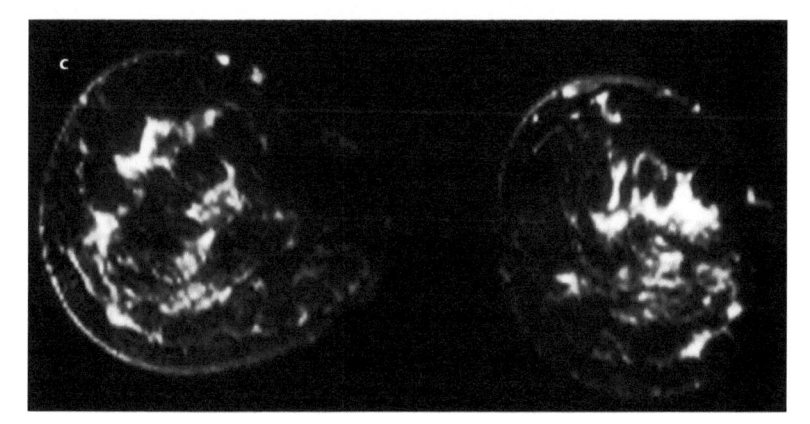

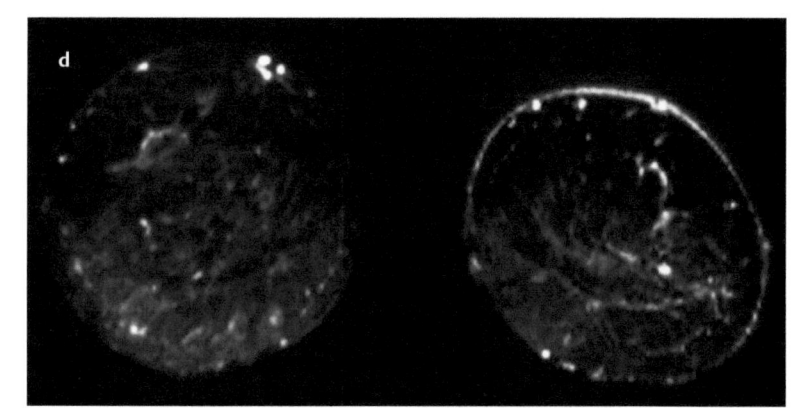

Fig. 5.1a–d Influence of hormones on MRI of the breast.

a,b Images from a 40-year-old patient are shown, who underwent breast MRI because of her family history of breast cancer. Normal findings were proven by more than 5 years of follow-up. (From Heywang-Köbrunner SH, Hacker A, Sedlacek S. Kontrastmittel MRT der Brust bei Staging und Früherkennung: wo benötigen wir sie? [Contrast-enhanced MRI for early detection and staging of breast cancer: Do we need it?] Geburtsh Frauenheilk 2010;70(3):184–193). **a** Subtraction image (representative slice), obtained on day 27 of the menstrual cycle, shows several foci with strong plateau-type enhancement. Malignancy cannot be excluded. **b** Subtraction image (representative slice), obtained on day 9 of the menstrual cycle, shows regression of the different foci.

c,d This 58-year-old patient underwent MRI because of a questionable architectural distortion. The problem was solved and absence of malignancy was proven by more than 4 years of follow-up. **c** Subtraction image (representative slice), obtained at the time of presentation. The patient was on combined estrogen–progesterone hormone replacement therapy (HRT). **d** Subtraction image (representative slice) obtained 6 weeks after stopping HRT medication.

History concerning recent surgery, percutaneous biopsy, or radiation therapy should include information on the type of the diagnostic or therapeutic action, the time elapsed since then, and its location in the breast and laterality. This information is important, since fresh granulation tissue may lead to focal enhancement and thus may cause a false positive result. Early after surgery or after radiation therapy, the scar or treated tissue, respectively, may enhance diffusely, sometimes inhomogeneously, leading to a false positive result.

Therefore, unless there is a strong clinical indication, we generally recommend performing MRI more than 4–6 months after surgery or more than 12 months after radiation therapy.

Finally, we demand that *conventional imaging* has already been performed (at least within the preceding 6 months). We routinely request the results *and* the images of the preceding conventional studies *or schedule the patient for the indicated studies.* We also ask for all available images from previous studies. We do not usually perform DCE-MRI without state-of-the-art assessment by conventional imaging. If a patient undergoes MRI without conventional images being provided, we inform the patient in advance that she can expect her final report only after the necessary baseline information is obtained.

Performing Plain MRI for Evaluation of Implant Failure

For evaluation of implant failure it is not so imperative to consider hormonal influences. However, it is useful to acquire the following history data, if possible:
- Type of implant if known (double lumen vs. single lumen). Some patients may have a "passport" for their implant or they can name the surgeon and year when the implant was inserted.
- Have there been previous implants?
- Have there been previous implant complications?
- Do previous studies exist? (If yes, these should be made available for comparison.)

The information may be helpful, since in rare cases it may be difficult to distinguish a ruptured single lumen implant from a double lumen implant. Also, silicon deposits from previous implants should not lead to surgery of an intact present implant.

Diagnostic Criteria

As for every diagnostic method, standardization and the use of systematic diagnostic criteria are prerequisites for assurance of high diagnostic quality and for achieving reproducibility of the results. However, as for mammography, breast ultrasound, or other diagnostic tests no unique, simple scheme exists. The final diagnosis must consider individual information and requires sufficient experience and training.

To standardize the description of MR findings the American College of Radiology (ACR) has recommended the use of a standardized MRI lexicon. **Table 5.1** gives an overview of the most important features as defined in the ACR lexicon and as described in the current literature. A comment on their predictive value based on our own experience and data from the literature has been added in the right column.

Overall the ACR lexicon may be understood as a very complete and detailed nomenclature. Systematic analy-

Table 5.1 MRI features and positive predictive value (PPV)

Classification	PPV	Comment	Author/Reference?
(a) Lesion size			
< 5 mm	Low	3–15%	Gutierrez 2009, Liberman 2006
< 10 mm	Low to intermediate	~20%	Gutierrez 2009, Liberman 2006
> 10 mm	Intermediate	~30%	Gutierrez 2009, Liberman 2006
(b) Degree of enhancement			
None to low	Very low	–	Schnall, Liberman
Moderate	Intermediate	–	Schnall, Liberman
Strong	High to very high	–	Schnall, Liberman
(c) Enhancement dynamics			
No or very low enhancement	Very low	–	Kinkel, Heywang-K
Continuous (delayed)	Low	–	Kinkel, Heywang-K, Liberman
Plateau	Intermediate	–	Kinkel, Heywang-K, Liberman
Washout	Very high	–	Kinkel, Heywang-K

Diagnostic Criteria

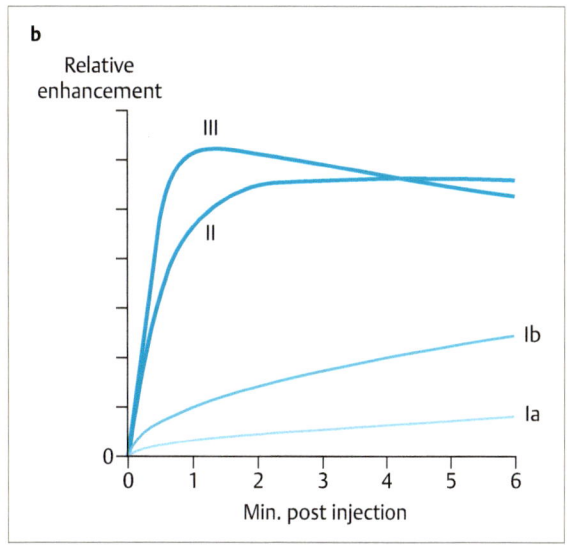

Fig. 5.2a–c Schematic diagrams showing the different enhancement curves, which may be observed with invasive malignancy (**a**), with ductal carcinoma in situ (**b**), and with benign tumorous or nontumorous changes (**c**). The thickness of the curve gives some hint concerning the probability frequency of the curve among the indicated pathologic changes.

a About 85% of invasive breast cancers exhibit enhancement curves of type II or III. Another 10% exhibit progressive enhancement (type Ib), whereas absent enhancement is an unusual finding occurring in a few percent of the cases.

b Ductal carcinoma in situ (DCIS) may exhibit enhancement of type II–III in ~60% of the cases, depending on the selection and size of the lesions. The remaining cases of DCIS will show progressive or absent enhancement. Even though curves II–III are more frequent among high-grade DCIS, even extended high-grade DCIS may not enhance and DCIS grade 1 and 2 may sometimes enhance strongly and fast. Furthermore, absent or progressive enhancement may occur more often among small lesions. Thus, a tendency for increasing enhancement with increasing grade exists. This is, however, not reliable, and histopathologic assessment of lesions suspicious of malignancy remains necessary.

c Most benign changes exhibit enhancement curves of type I or II. Type III curves are infrequent (approximately 5%). If present, they are mostly associated with proliferative changes (or benign tumors), with hyperplastic changes such as adenosis, or with acute or subacute inflammation.

sis of MR features and knowledge of their approximate positive or negative predictive values will support diagnostic considerations. However, no direct translation from features or combinations of features to a final diagnosis is given in the ACR lexicon or is presently available worldwide.

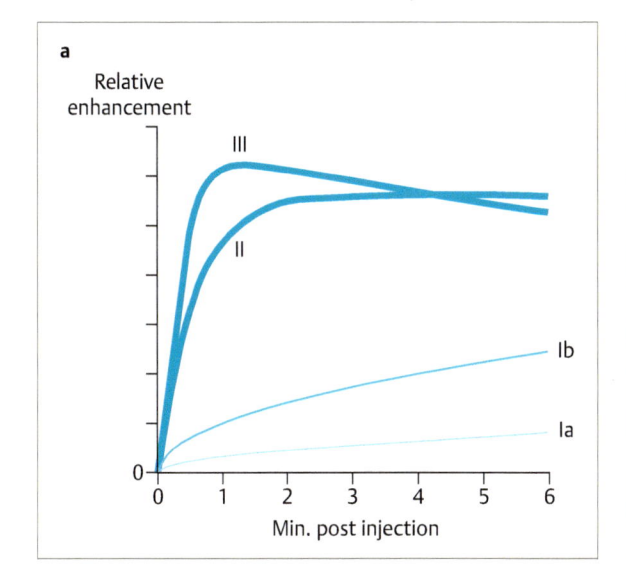

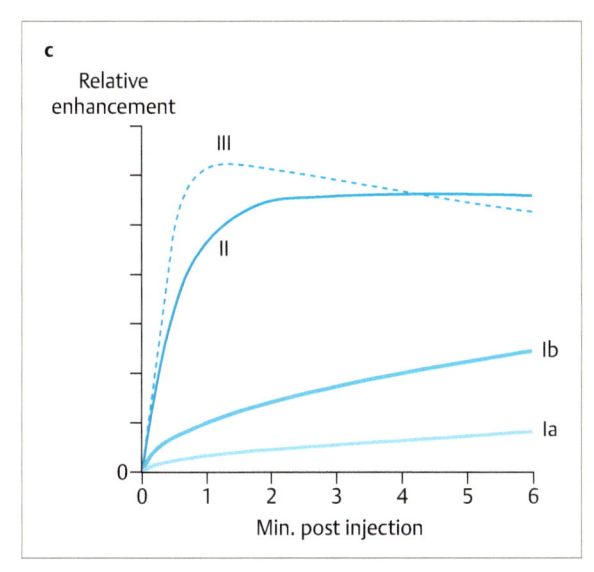

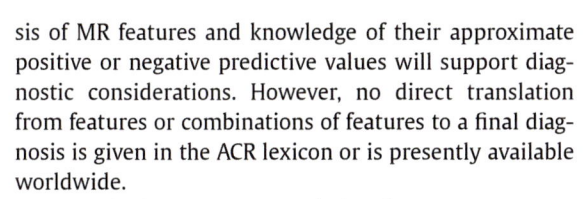

Fig. 5.2 demonstrates typical enhancement curves seen with DCE-MRI.

Figs. 5.3 and 5.4 give an overview of the most frequent morphological presentations of invasive breast cancer and of DCIS, respectively, as compared with benign masslike (Fig. 5.5) or non-masslike (Fig. 5.6) lesions. The development of a generally applicable algorithm for the distinction of benign from malignant lesions is not possible, owing to the overlap of benign- and malignant-type features; false negative and false positive diagnoses cannot be avoided.

Initial attempts to distinguish benign from malignant disease based on either quantitative parameters or lesion morphology alone have not been reproducible; however, during the last 5–10 years, most groups have used or developed algorithms, which consider all information available from DCE-MRI:
- *Presence (amount) of enhancement*
- *Morphology of enhancement*
- *Enhancement dynamics*

5 Magnetic Resonance Imaging

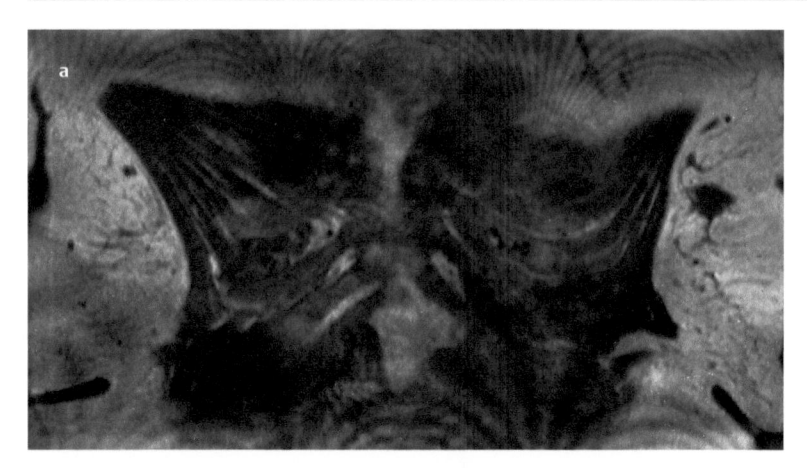

Fig. 5.3a–o This series gives an overview of presentations of invasive breast cancer.

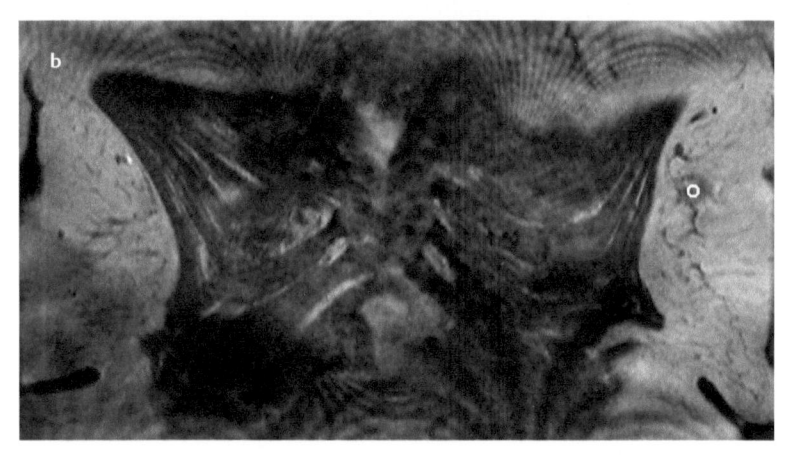

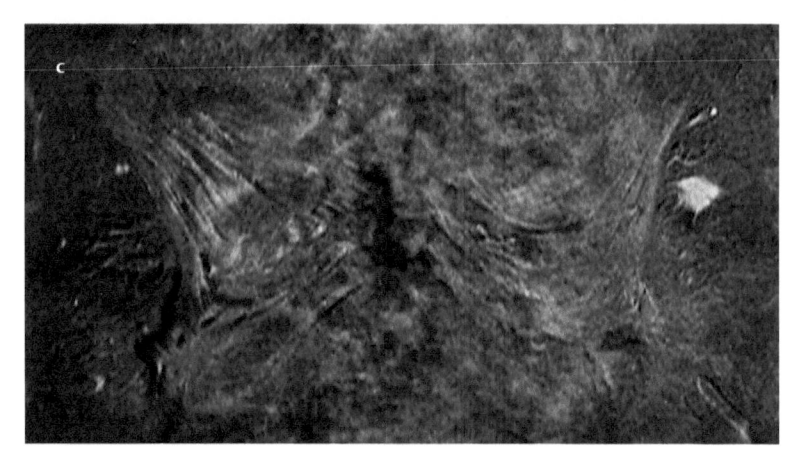

a–c Precontrast, postcontrast, and subtraction images of the central slice through this invasive ductal carcinoma (pT1, G2). The lesion is identified by its spiculated margins. The major part of the lesion exhibited a delayed enhancement curve. Most ductal cancers, however, exhibit washout or plateau-type enhancement.

Diagnostic Criteria

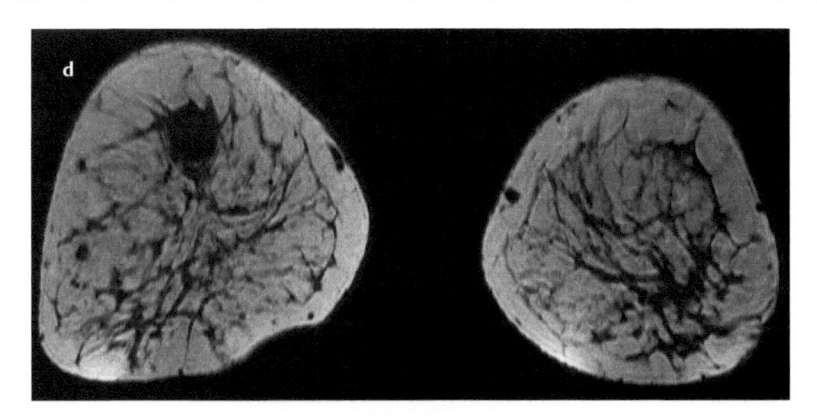

d–f Precontrast, postcontrast, and subtraction images of another invasive ductal carcinoma. This lesion presented as an ill-circumscribed mass with inhomogeneous enhancement and a washout curve. The small focus laterally (arrow) proved to be a small focus of DCIS of intermediate grade.
g–i This oval mass appeared fairly well

Fig. 5.3 g–o ▷

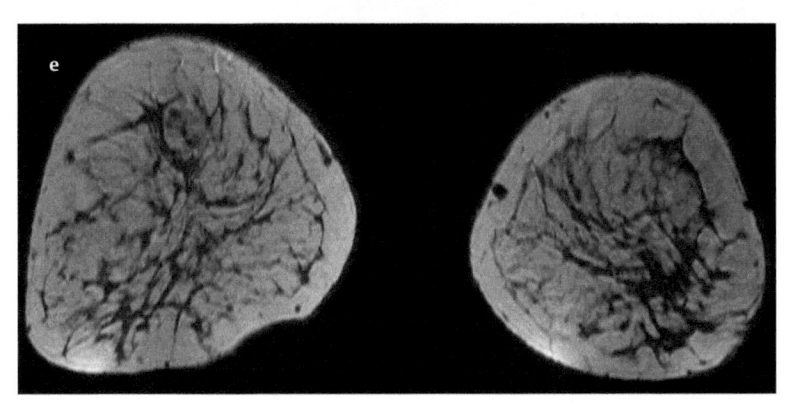

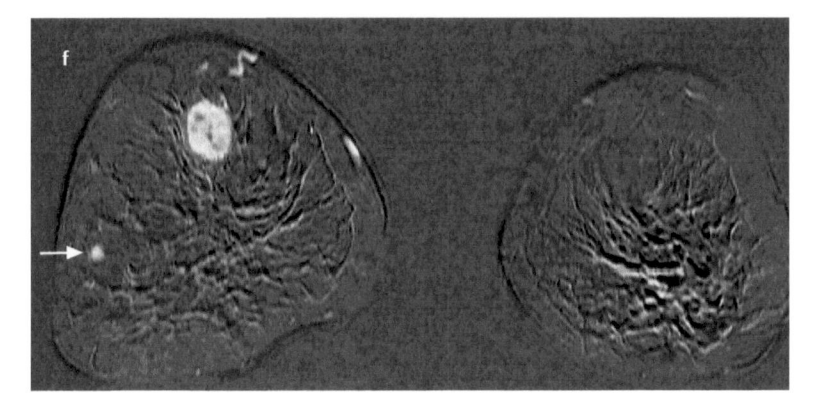

137

◁ continued

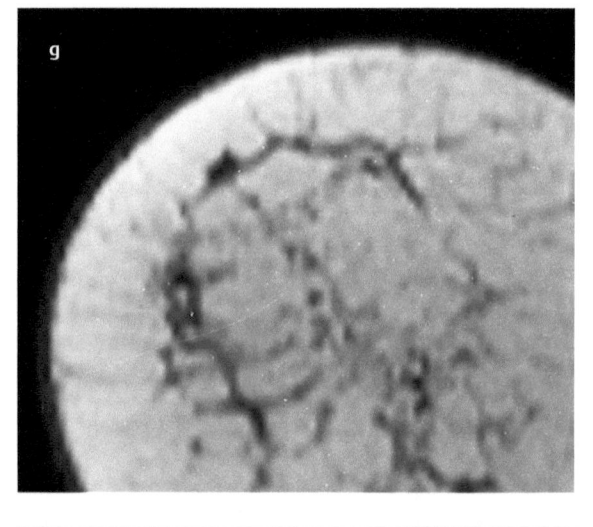

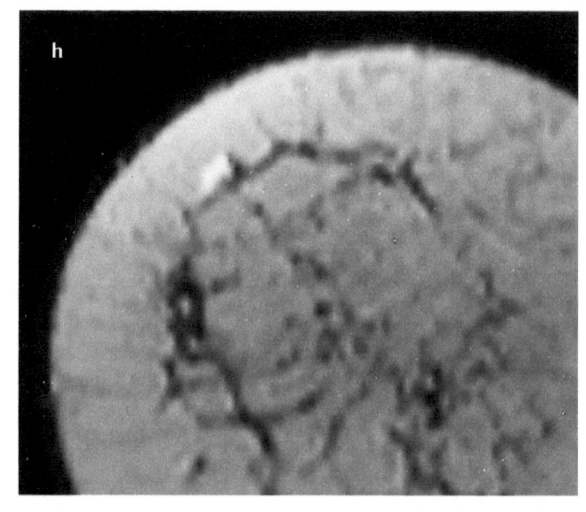

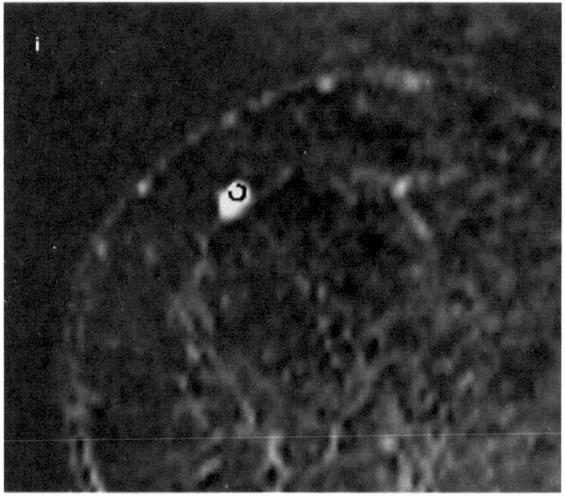

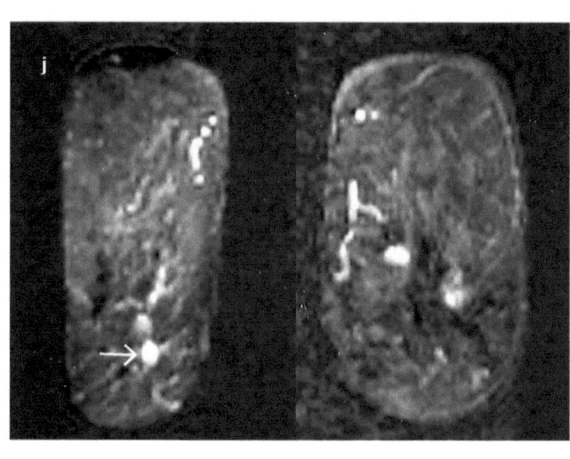

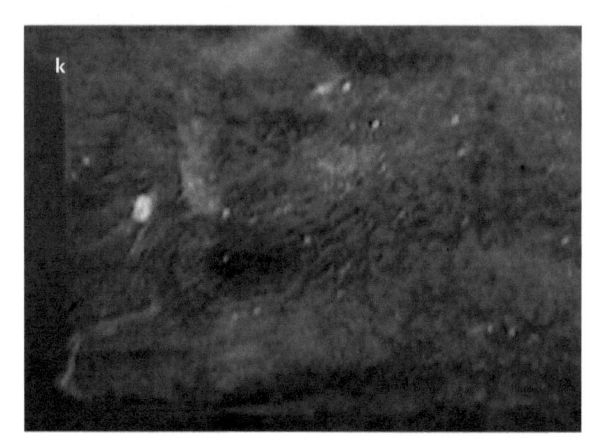

circumscribed. A slight irregularity may be suspected on the postcontrast image. The lesion, which exhibited progressive enhancement, proved to be a 5 mm invasive ductal carcinoma.

j   Four oval masses are shown (some only partly contained in the slice) in a young patient carrying the BCRA1 mutation. All masses exhibited plateau-type enhancement, no washout, no rim enhancement. The arrow points to the mass that proved to be a medullary carcinoma (G3). The other masses proved to be fibroadenomas. Well-circumscribed malignancies usually occur in less than 5% of the cases. In patients carrying BRCA1, however, oval and fairly well-circumscribed cancers are a quite common finding.

k   Well-circumscribed malignancy. Even though this ductal invasive carcinoma is located in the axillary tail, it should not be confused with an axillary lymph node. Based on its morphology, it should not be confused with a fibroadenoma. (The hypointense structure centrally corresponds to central fribrosis, not a septum.) It was recognized as it exhibited early enhancement and washout.

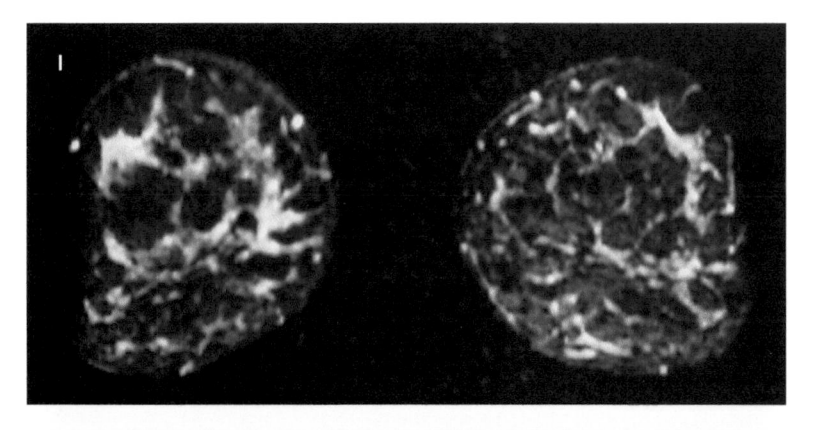

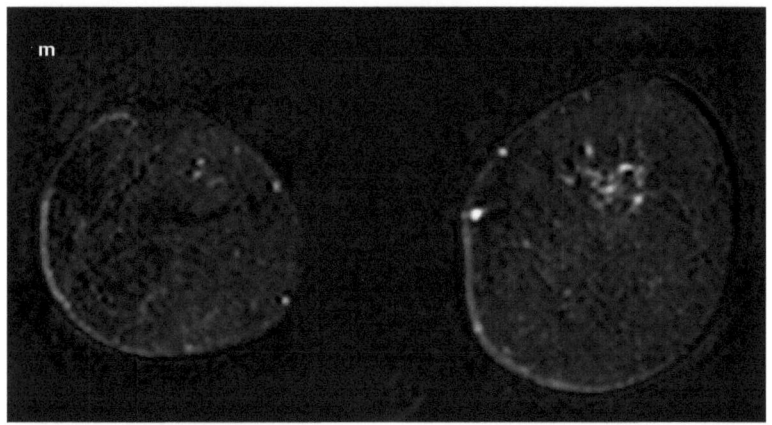

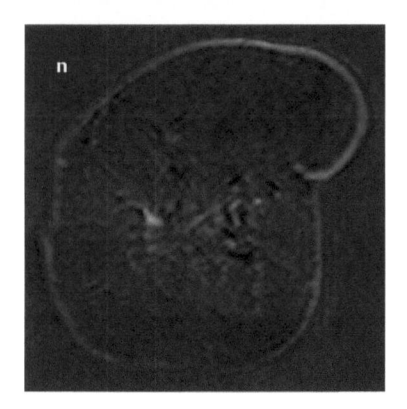

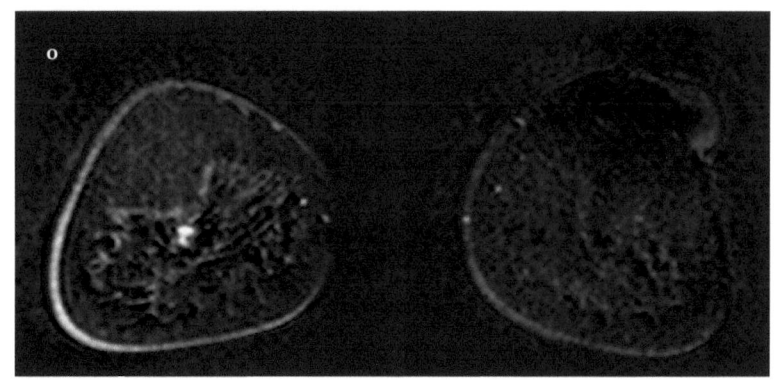

l Diffusely growing cancers may be difficult to detect and to delineate. Furthermore, diffuse enhancement of surrounding tissues may obscure malignancy. This patient, who was on hormone replacement therapy, presented with a 4-cm palpable thickening in her right breast medially. The enhancement curves of various areas in the right and left breast exhibited progressive to plateau-type enhancement curves.
Histology (from bilateral mastectomy, as explicitly desired by the patient) proved a T2 infiltrating lobular breast cancer in the right breast medially, but no malignancy laterally or in the left breast.

m This breast cancer presented with an area of ductal-type enhancement with a dendritic distribution in an asymmetric area of ~2 mm in diameter. This pattern might be confused with a vascular enhancement. Histologically the enhancing ductal structures corresponded to DCIS grade 3, which contained a small focus of invasive carcinoma grade 3.

n In this patient a small ductal type enhancement was the only hint of this small carcinoma. Even though morphology of this lesion might rule in a ductal carcinoma or DCIS, this lesion proved to correspond to a small invasive lobular carcinoma (pT1b).

o Small nodular, possibly ductal enhancement in a patient who was at intermediate risk of breast cancer (family history). MR-guided vacuum-assisted breast biopsy (VABB) was performed, since the patient presented with a swollen lymph node, which eventually proved to be benign. Histology of MR-VABB and subsequent surgery yielded an invasive lobular breast cancer (ILC) with a final unsuspected extent of 5 cm. Major parts of this lobular carcinoma consisted of fibrosis, which contained small numbers of cells typical of ILC. This histopathologic appearance explains the low degree of enhancement within the large area.

5 Magnetic Resonance Imaging

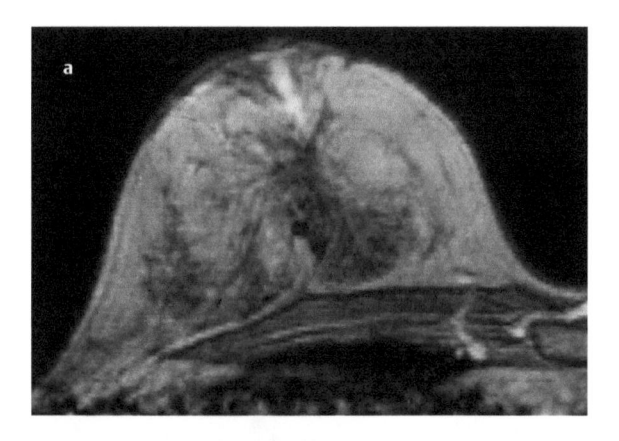

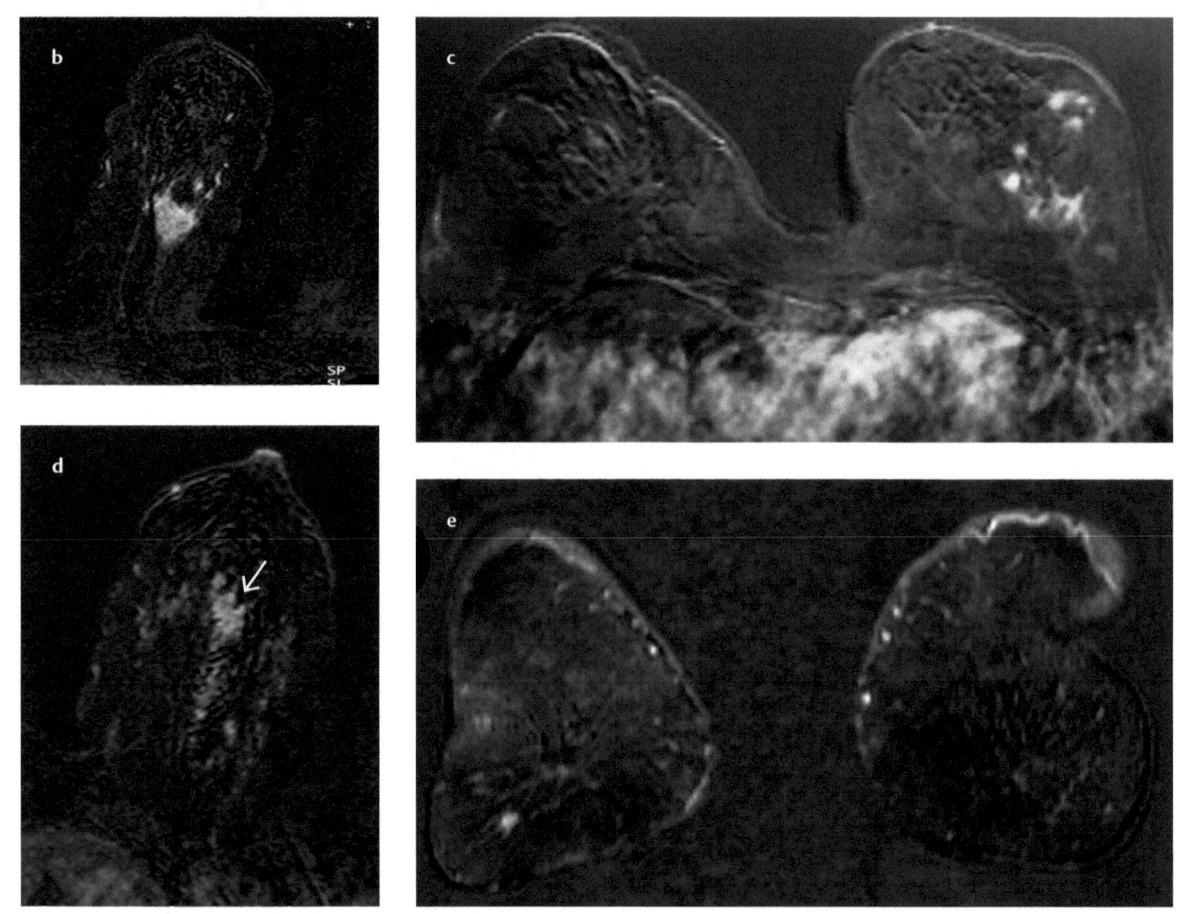

Fig. 5.4a–i This series gives an overview of presentations of ductal carcinoma in situ (DCIS).

a Ductal enhancement is shown on the postcontrast image of this high-grade DCIS, which was detected in the ducts between the nipple and the centrally located scar several years after breast-conserving therapy. The DCIS was not associated with microcalcifications and was mammographically occult. Reproduced with kind permission of Springer Science+Business Media from Heywang-Köbrunner SH, Beck R. Contrast-Enhanced MRI of the Breast. 2nd ed. Berlin: Springer; 1995: 154.)

b Segmental inhomogeneous enhancement in a patient with a solid DCIS of intermediate grade.

c Segmental dendritic enhancement in another patient with mammographically occult high-grade DCIS.

d In this patient a regional area of fast enhancement (arrow) surrounded by some diffuse stippled enhancement was detected. Histologically the regional enhancement corresponded to a low-grade DCIS, which was surrounded by diffuse benign changes.

e This focal, ill-circumscribed enhancement correlated with another low-grade DCIS, which was incidentally detected by MRI.

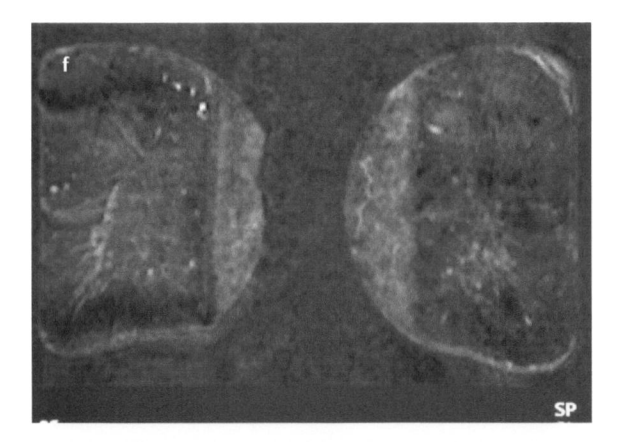

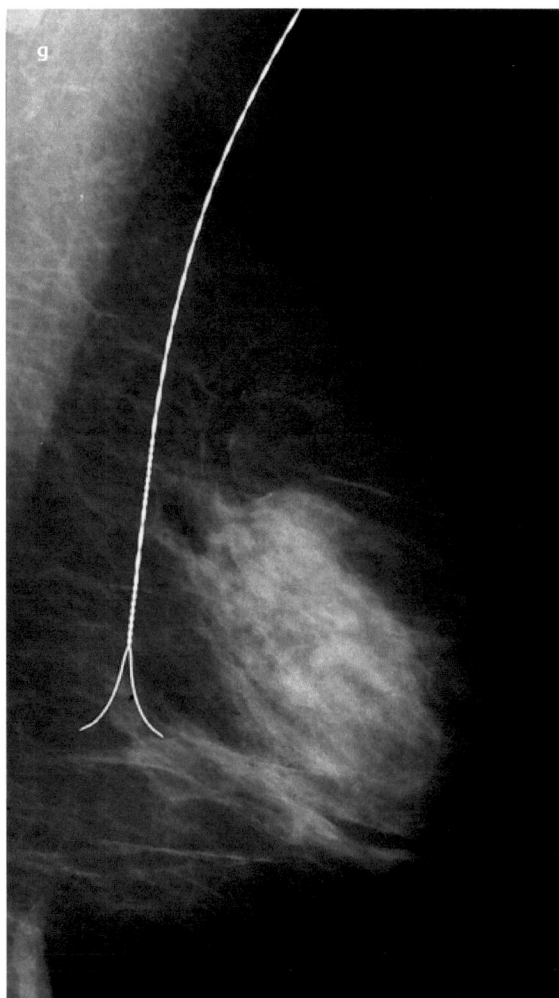

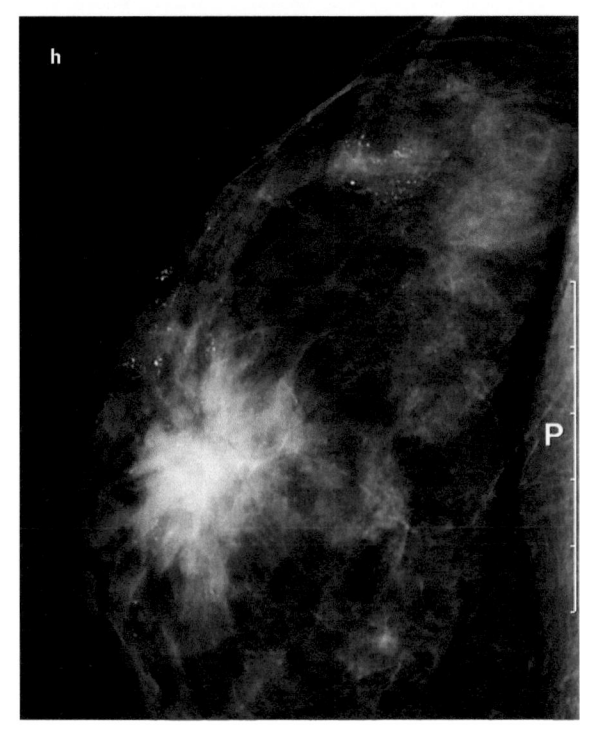

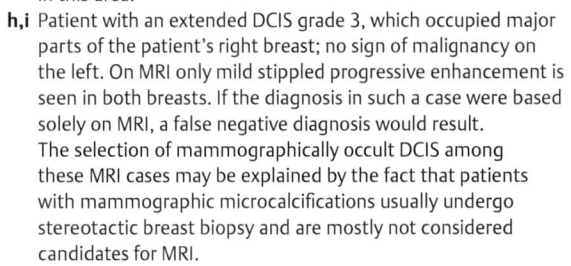

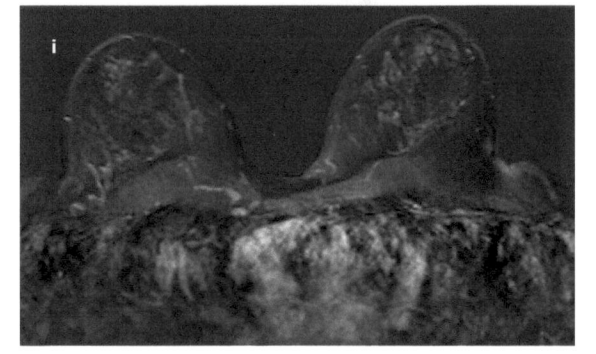

f,g Mammographically this intermediate-grade DCIS became apparent as a neodensity. On MRI no enhancement was seen in this area.

h,i Patient with an extended DCIS grade 3, which occupied major parts of the patient's right breast; no sign of malignancy on the left. On MRI only mild stippled progressive enhancement is seen in both breasts. If the diagnosis in such a case were based solely on MRI, a false negative diagnosis would result.
The selection of mammographically occult DCIS among these MRI cases may be explained by the fact that patients with mammographic microcalcifications usually undergo stereotactic breast biopsy and are mostly not considered candidates for MRI.

5 Magnetic Resonance Imaging

Fig. 5.5a–j This series gives an overview of tumorous and tumorlike benign changes.

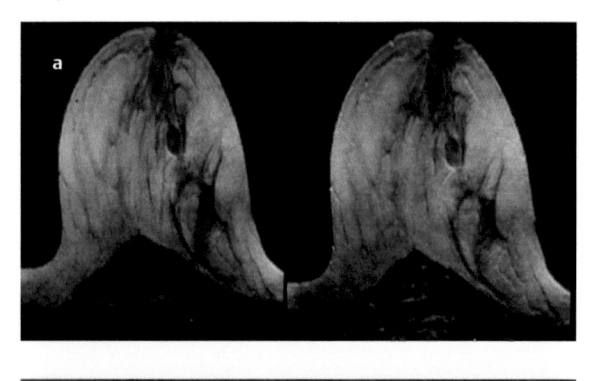

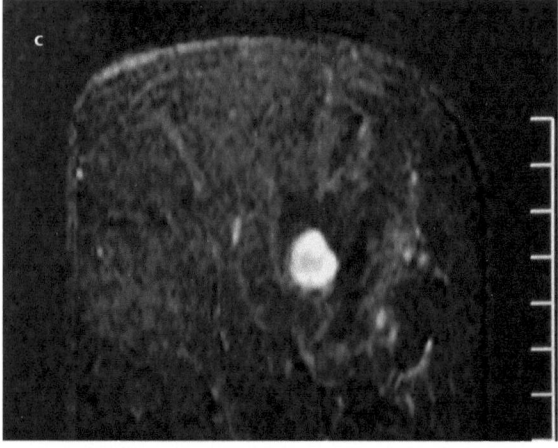

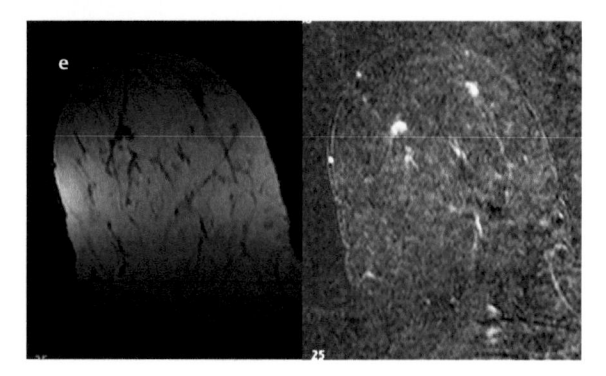

a Nonenhancing fibrosed fibroadenoma: an oval well-circumscribed mass is shown on the precontrast and second postcontrast images.

b Varying presentations of enhancing fibroadenomas (postcontrast images are shown) include an oval well-circumscribed mass (left upper), a well-circumscribed mass with macrolobulation (right upper), a rounded mass with dark, fine central septation (left lower), and a mass with irregular margin (right lower). In the last case further assessment is absolutely necessary. Further assessment should also be considered if central septation might be confused with central necrosis or for lesions that increase in size. Benign fibroadenomas mostly exhibit plateau-type or progressive enhancement. Some fibroadenomas enhance quite strongly. Washout occurs rarely.

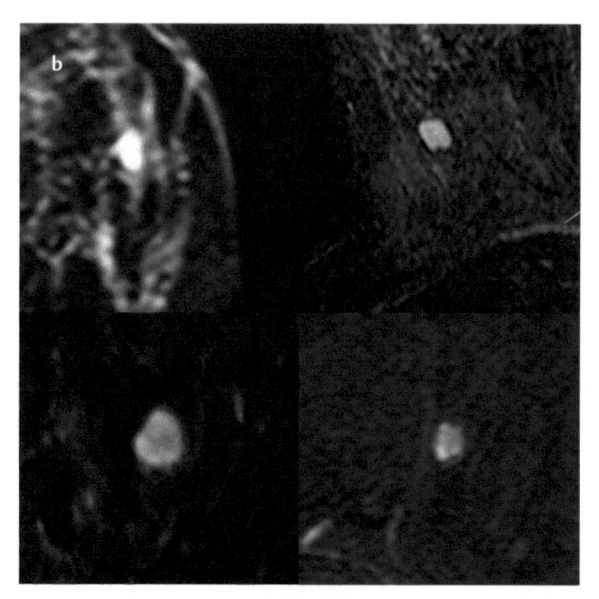

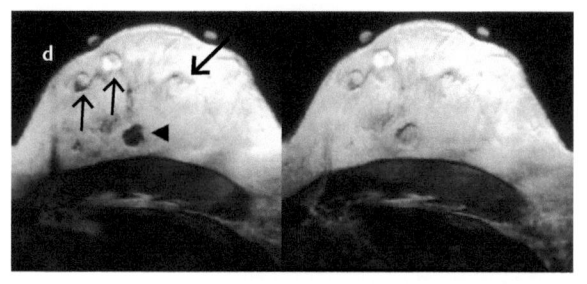

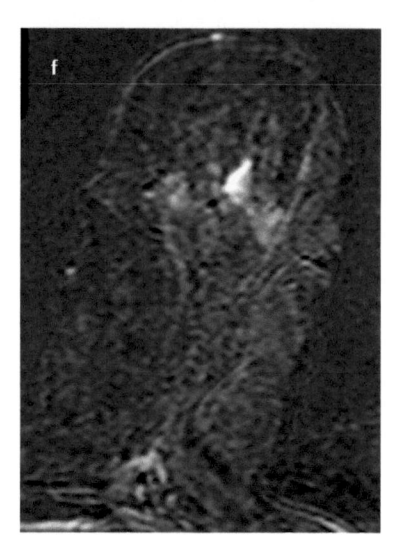

c This fibroadenoma with fine septations and progressive enhancement may be appropriate to follow (subtraction image 2 min post injection).
d Papillomas may present as masses with or without associated cyst. In this breast several papillomas are visualized (as precontrast and postcontrast images). Only the papilloma posteriorly (arrowhead) is not associated with a cyst. Owing to sero-sanguinous contents, the associated cysts (arrows) of the other papillomas present with high signal before and after contrast. On the right (long arrow) only the sero-sanguinous cyst is seen (the papilloma is imaged on another slice). The visualized papillomas exhibit low signal on the precontrast image and mild progressive or no enhancement after contrast medium, compatible with fibrosed papillomas.
e Most papillomas exhibit moderate to strong early enhancement; some may even show a washout. Papillomas may present as well-circumscribed or (like the papillomas shown here) as irregular masses (precontrast and subtraction images).
f This early enhancing ductal lesion histologically corresponded to a small intraductal papilloma (subtraction image).
g Two granulomas are shown: one nonenhancing granuloma (arrowhead) presents as signal void—probably due to some metallic residual after electrocautery; the other granuloma presents as a strongly and early enhancing 5-mm lesion (histologically proven).
h Typically benign lymph nodes present with progressive to plateau-type enhancement. The fatty hilum typically does not enhance, while the rim of the lymph node usually enhances moderately, sometimes strongly, giving the typical beanlike shape. The rim of a normal lymph node usually does not exceed 3 mm in diameter.
i This axillary lymph node in a patient with breast cancer was considered suspicious because of its strong enhancement, the increased thickness of the margin, and its disappearing hilum. *Histology*: Benign lymph node.
j This 1-cm lymph node exhibited washout and proved to be involved with breast cancer. Washout rules in malignancy, but may sometimes be seen with inflammatory changes, too. Progressive or plateau-type enhancement rules in benign changes but cannot exclude malignancy.

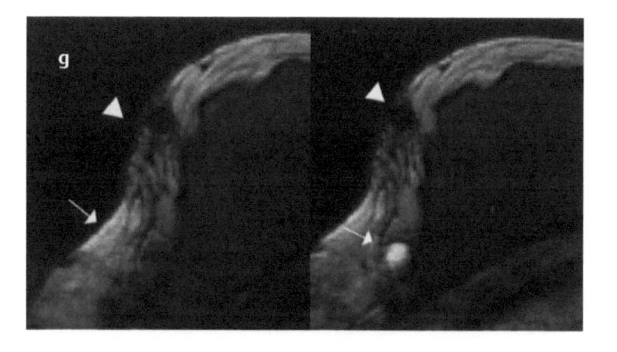

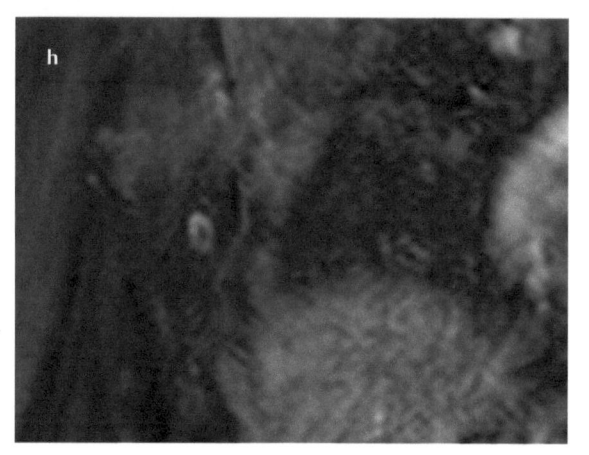

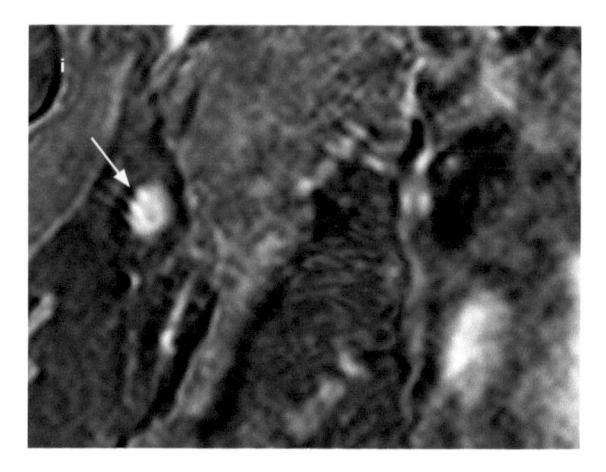

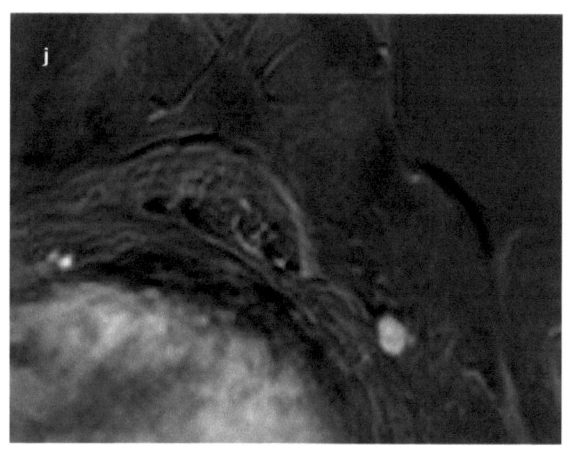

> For obtaining optimum results we strongly recommend that:
> - The reports and images of the indicated conventional studies be available for interpretation of MRI.
> - DCE-MRI is interpreted only by radiologists with significant experience with conventional breast imaging and intervention.
> - Percutaneous MR-guided intervention must be available within an acceptable time-frame, whenever a lesion is detected by MRI.

Such recommendations have been integrated in official guidelines, recommendations and consensus statements.

Following the desire for a simplified algorithm, Baum et al. (2002) proposed a simplified scheme that supports establishment of a diagnosis by attributing 0–2 points of suspicion for several features that should be checked for in an enhancing lesion. Depending on the overall sum of points, each lesion in question is then categorized as BI-RADS (Breast Imaging Reporting and Data System) 2, 3, 4 or 5 (**Tables 5.2** and **5.3**). Even though assignment of points to arbitrary cutoff values (e.g., 100%) cannot realistically be expected to directly reflect biology, the algorithm has been successfully used by several groups and may be useful as a simplified scheme initially. However a major disadvantage of this algorithm is the resultant classification of a fairly high number of BI-RADS 3 lesions, which have been reported to include a varying number of malignancies (up to several percent).

Today, no perfect simplified algorithm can be suggested to make an MR diagnosis. Considering the fact that an important number of cases referred to MRI are considered "diagnostically difficult," over-simplification may be unable to meet the goal of achieving the best possible diagnosis for each individual case.

Whatever rules are used, these must be applicable for *all* expected histologies. It is not sensible to refer to different rules for the detection of invasive versus in-situ cancer (as has been suggested). If we could predict the histology of the imaged lesion, we would not need further imaging.

The following paragraphs describe the rules which we follow when elaborating a final diagnosis.

1. *All MR diagnoses should be based on knowledge of the diagnostic question* (from clinical information and conventional imaging) *and of the individual risk factors.*
   This information helps to narrow down the differential diagnosis and to choose a sensible and balanced "threshold" for the final diagnostic decision (for or against further assessment or follow-up) with an acceptable risk of unavoidable false negative or false positive calls.
   Considering, for example, the superior sensitivity and specificity of percutaneous biopsy, *we generally do not use MRI to replace histopathologic assessment of lesions considered to be BI-RADS 4 or 5 by conventional imaging*, if these can be targeted. Rare exceptions may be lesions which following MRI all information concordantly explains the findings as signs of a benign entity. *For lesions detected by MRI only*, a decision always needs to be made as to whether the lesion is benign or might require short-term follow-up or even histopathologic assessment. This decision should be based on *all available MR information and on an algorithm or threshold that promises the best possible decision for the individual diagnostic setting and risk.*

2. Before analyzing the MR study, we recommend first *checking for the presence of enhancement in the vessels and in the cardiac region*. In the case of a complete or partial paravenous injection, vessel enhancement and enhancement of the cardiac artifact may be weak, absent, or delayed. Any such suspicion should lead to a repeat examination.

3. *Absence of enhancement excludes malignancy with high probability, if no other suspicion exists.* Since about 5% of invasive malignancies and > 20% of DCIS (including parts of high-grade DCIS, as confirmed by numerous publications) may not enhance, absence of enhancement should not be used to rule out malignancy in the presence of a suspicious mammographic, sonographic, or clinical finding that could be targeted and thus could be histologically assessed. However, absence of enhancement may strongly support a benign diagnosis in well-selected cases, where assessment by conventional imaging is impaired (e.g., diagnostic problems within scarring) and where the need for percutaneous biopsy is unclear.
   In addition, a well-circumscribed non-enhancing mass with low signal intensity on T1- and T2-weighted images is likely to correspond to a fibrosed fibroadenoma. This knowledge may be helpful in the presence of multiple nodules or in rare cases with contraindications to biopsy. In case of doubt, however, percutaneous biopsy remains necessary.

4. *Whenever enhancement is detected:*
   - *True enhancement needs to be distinguished from pseudo-enhancement* which does not reflect contrast uptake in breast tissue but can be explained as an artifact (**Fig. 5.7**).
     On subtraction images *incorrect subtraction due to patient motion* may easily mimic or obscure true enhancement. Therefore, if patient motion occurs, diligent comparison of corresponding and neighboring pre- and postcontrast slices is needed. Confusion of true versus pseudo-enhancement is according to our experience the most frequent source of unnecessary false positive calls (except for those due to hormonal enhancement).
   - *Overlying enhancing cardiac artifacts* may, for example, mimic confluent patchy enhancement, which might also obscure malignancy. In the cor-

Diagnostic Criteria

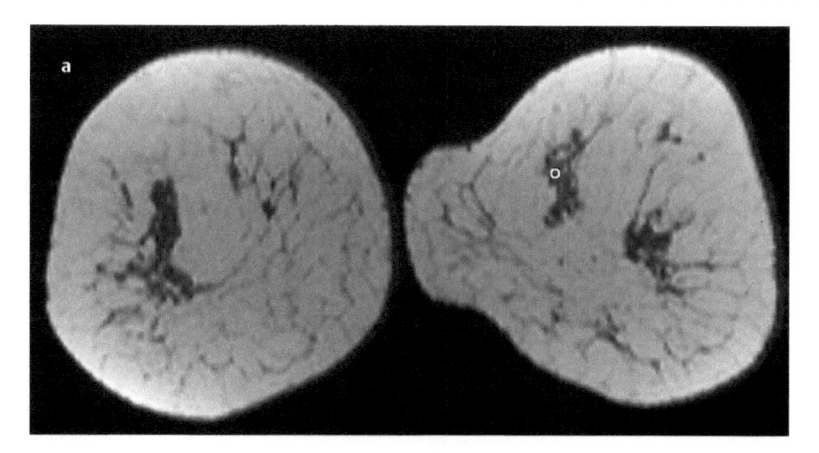

Fig. 5.6a–g This series gives an overview of nontumorous benign changes.

a–c Patient with a somewhat striking asymmetry on mammography. Precontrast, postcontrast (2–3 min postinjection), and subtraction images are shown. No enhancement is seen, ruling in benign asymmetry.

Fig. 5.6 d–g ▷

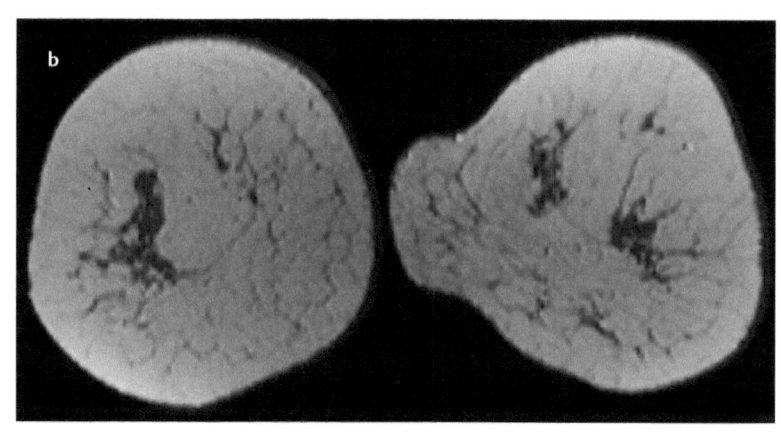

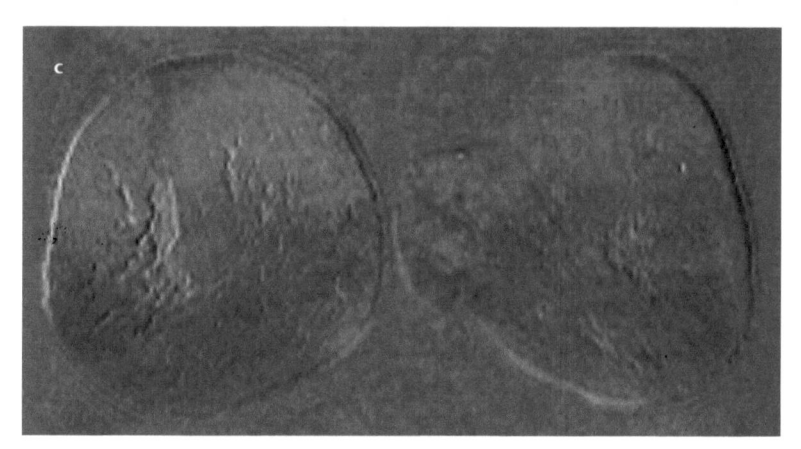

responding anatomic areas this requires diligent analysis (**Fig. 5.8**).
- *Hormonal influence* may be another possible cause of uncharacteristic enhancement. If doubts exist, a repeat MR study in the correct phase of the menstrual cycle or after stopping hormonal replacement with progesterone should be considered (see **Fig. 5.1**).
- In patients after surgery or biopsy it should be checked whether the enhancement may correspond *to granulation tissue or fresh fat necrosis*.

5. Next, true enhancement may be classified according to its *morphology* as:
   - *Focus*
   - *Mass*
   - *Nonmass: ductal or linear*
   - *Nonmass: segmental*
   - *Regional, multiple regions or focal area*
   - *Diffuse*

Assessment of any focus, mass, ductal, or linear enhancement should always include a comparison of original

◁ continued

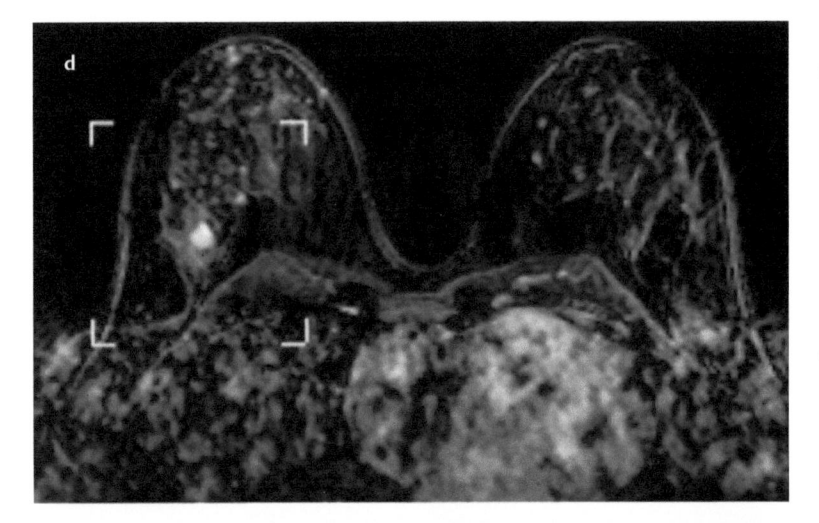

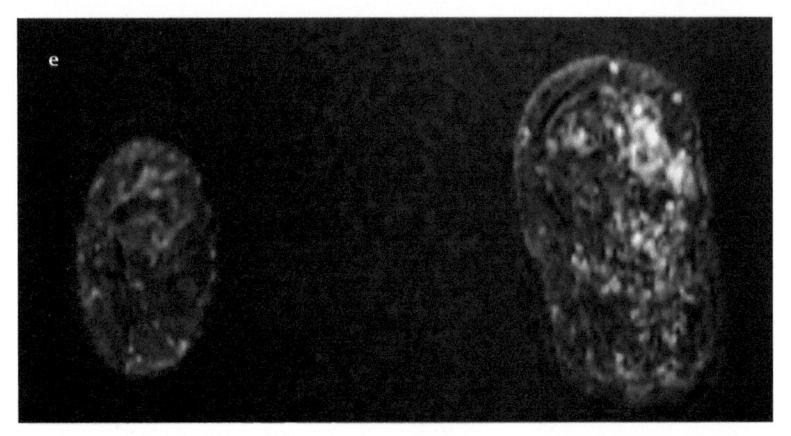

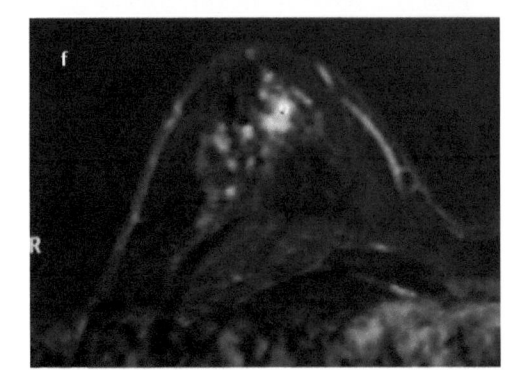

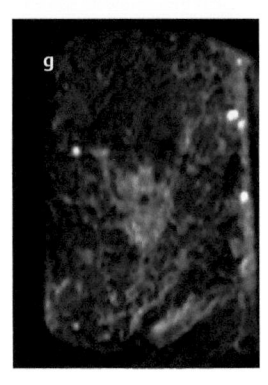

d The subtraction image demonstrates stippled diffuse enhancement (which enhanced progressively) in both breasts and a round MR-detected lesion with strong progressive enhancement. Since the patient was at high risk, MR-guided vacuum-assisted breast biopsy was performed, proving a benign fibroadenoma and benign hyperplastic and proliferative changes without atypias.

e Unilateral patchy enhancement with progressive enhancement dynamics on the left. Absence of a focal or segmental distribution rules in benign changes, as proven by more than 4 years of follow-up. *Note*: No significant enhancement is seen in the right breast > 1 year after irradiation (status after breast conservation).
Note also: Even stronger and more confluent enhancement is shown in **Fig. 5.3l**. The strong enhancement in the left breast corresponds to proven benign changes. The diffusely growing cancer on the right (medially) cannot be distinguished from enhancing benign tissue in the lateral quadrants.

f Focal enhancement with plateau-type dynamic curve caused by benign sclerosing adenosis and papillomatosis (subtraction image).

g Focal ill-defined progressive enhancement in an area of a palpable thickening. Considering that lobular carcinoma may present with a similar appearance, the finding requires further assessment. *Histology* (open surgery) showed benign chronic inflammatory changes.

Table 5.2 Points attributed to various features

Feature	0 points	1 point	2 points
Shape	Round or oval	Dendritic or irregular	–
Margin	Well-defined	Ill-defined	–
Internal pattern	Homogeneous	Inhomogeneous	Rim
Initial enhancement[a]	< 50%	50–100%	> 100%
Postinitial enhancement	Continuous increase	Plateau	Washout

[a] Using a dosage of 0.1 mmol Gd-DTPA/kg.

Table 5.3 BI-RADS category depending on number of points

BI-RADS	1	2	3	4	5
Points	0–1	2	3	4–5	> 6

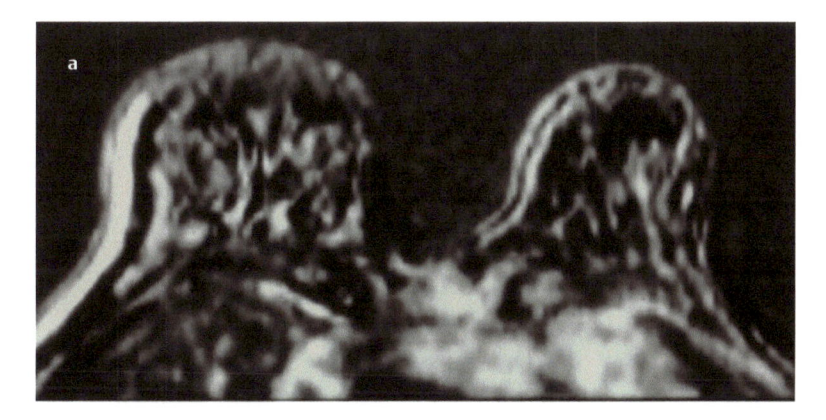

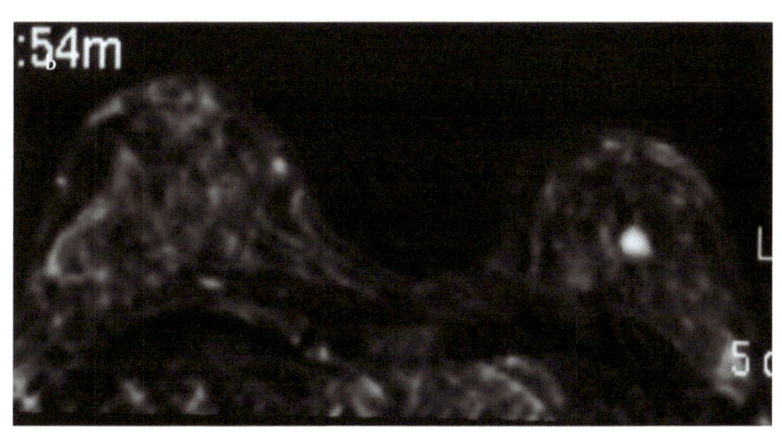

Fig. 5.7a,b Effect of patient motion on subtraction images.

a Subtraction image (same area as in **b**). Owing to strong motion anatomically different structures are subtracted. This leads to the white and black lines parallel to the interfaces between glandular and fatty structures. (Bright lines occur when nonenhancing glandular tissue is subtracted from fatty tissue. Dark lines occur when fatty tissue is subtracted from nonenhancing glandular structures.) The width of these lines indicates the millimeters of shift and gives a hint to the range of possible error. Subtraction of noncorresponding structures may thus mimic or obscure enhancement. Owing to the strong motion artifacts this examination was repeated on the following day.

b Subtraction image (same patient as in **a**) shows a breast cancer surrounded by normal breast tissue, a finding which was completely obscured by artifacts on the initial examination.

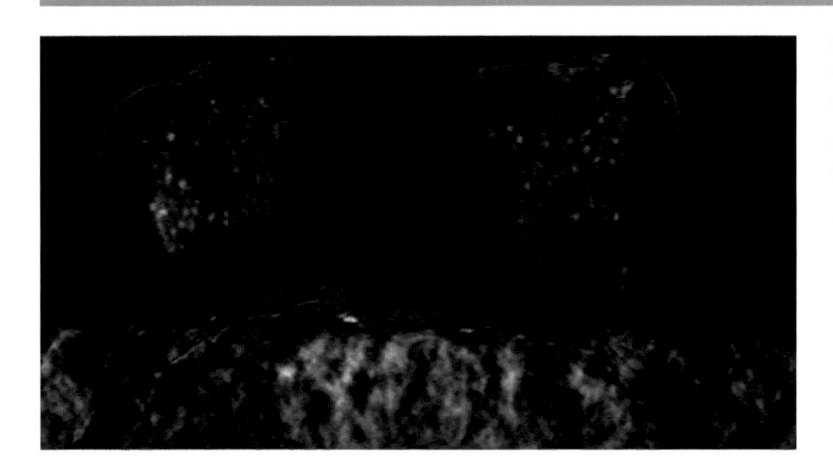

Fig. 5.8 Cardiac artifacts are crossing both axillary tails, making assessment of these areas impossible. Further motion artifacts lead to ghost images between and lateral to both breasts. Stippled enhancement within benign breast tissue (no change in right breast on follow-up; benign changes in left breast verified by histology).

pre- and postcontrast images, since on subtracted images margins may be blurred due to patient motion. The distinction between a pseudo-lesion and a true lesion is best perceived on the original scans.

6. *Focus.* The ACR lexicon defines a focus as a spot of enhancement < 5 mm in size that cannot be otherwise characterized. An approximate size of < 5 mm appears to be a sensible cutoff value, since the probability of malignancy decreases with smaller sizes. Also, for such small foci an attempted analysis of enhancement dynamics (and enhancement curve measurements in particular) may be unreliable or even spurious owing to varying partial volume effect, caused by patient motion between pre- and postcontrast measurements. For *very small lesions* we recommend proceeding as follows:
   - Check for *signs of high suspicion* such as spiculated or irregular margins or a new developing indeterminate lesion (e.g., in a scar or in otherwise nonenhancing tissue). If present, histopathologic assessment should be recommended (**Fig. 5.9**).
   - For lesions with *indeterminate morphology* we recommend *retrospective sonographic correlation*. If visible with ultrasound, US-guided biopsy should be considered. For the *remaining lesions* either short-term follow-up or usual follow-up should be considered depending on the morphology of the lesion and the individual risk. In general, the probability of malignancy of a benign-appearing or uncharacteristic MR-detected focus is quite low in patients at low to moderate risk. In addition, presence of multiple lesions favors benign changes.

7. *Mass.* MRI should in general not be used to avoid biopsy of an otherwise suspicious mass that can be approached by percutaneous biopsy.
   - Check for signs of high suspicion, such as irregular (spiculated or micro-lobulated) margin, rim enhancement of a noncystic lesion, wash-out, newly developing lesions, or lesion with increasing size. Such changes should usually prompt histopathologic assessment (irrespective of the other features of the lesion).
   - If the above signs of high suspicion are absent, check for signs indicating a low probability of malignancy, such as a well-circumscribed margin (oval or with large lobulations), fine nonenhancing septations,* a well-circumscribed fat-containing lesion (e.g., lymph node or hamartoma). For the latter lesions usual follow-up is recommended; for the former, short-term follow-up should be considered.
   - For any other (uncharacteristic) MR-detected mass, retrospective ultrasound is recommended. If visible with ultrasound, US-guided biopsy is recommended. If not visible with ultrasound, short-term follow-up or biopsy under MR guidance may be considered depending on the patient's overall risk and the exact size and shape of the lesion.

8. *Nonmass linear enhancement.* True linear enhancement is rare. Linear enhancement is distinguished from ductal enhancement, since it does not follow the course of ducts.
   Linear enhancement may be due to pseudo-enhancement caused by an artifact, or to enhancement within a vessel or vascular abnormality. This pattern of enhancement is usually not suspicious. Linear enhancement may also occur within a scar. If ductal enhancement remains a differential diagnosis, short-term follow-up may be considered.
   (Owing to expected partial volume effect and expected washout of vessels, dynamic curves are often not helpful.)

9. *Nonmass ductal enhancement.* Ductal enhancement may be caused by benign intraductal changes (e.g., papillary lesions) or by malignancy such as DCIS or

---

* This sign is indicative of a fibroadenoma. High-resolution images may, however, be necessary to distinguish between septations and other inhomogeneities of low signal intensity (e.g., central fibrosis, which is indicative of malignancy!).

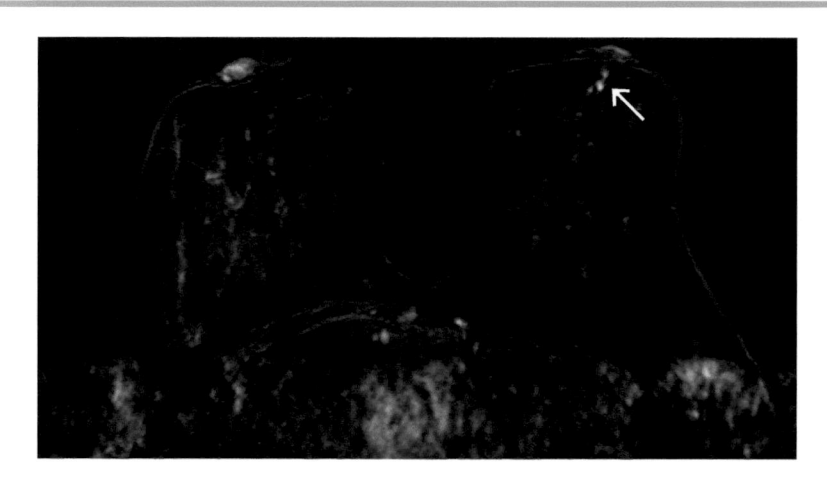

Fig. 5.9 In this patient with a proven, small, breast cancer, excision of this retroareolar duct (arrow) was recommended, since this nodular enhancement clearly followed a duct, and appeared earlier than the enhancement within surrounding benign changes. *Histology*: 3-mm invasive ductal carcinoma. (Considering the stippled enhancement within the surrounding tissue, however, this may have been a somewhat fortuitous decision.)

invasive malignancy. Since DCIS and early malignancy (Viehweg et al. 2000, Heywang-Köbrunner et al. 2001, Schnall et al. 2006) may exhibit quite variable amounts and dynamics of enhancement—including low and progressive enhancement—ductal enhancement *should usually prompt histopathologic assessment.*

10. *Nonmass segmental enhancement.* Segmental enhancement may be considered to be a more extended variant of ductal enhancement, since it describes enhancement of part of the ductal tree. Usually segmental enhancement is a type of triangular enhancement, where the tip of the triangle points toward the nipple. (The triangle may be small; it may include one or several quadrants or segments.)

    The differential diagnosis is similar to that of ductal enhancement. Based on the differential diagnosis, here, too, low enhancement and progressive enhancement dynamics cannot exclude malignancy. The reason is that DCIS often grows in a segmental or ductal pattern, but may in part just exhibit low to moderate progressive enhancement. Overall the probability of malignancy is higher for segmental enhancement than it is for regional or for ductal enhancement.

    Therefore, histopathologic assessment is usually indicated in cases that exhibit ductal or segmental enhancement (see **Fig. 5.4**).

11. *Nonmass regional enhancement and nonmass focal area enhancement.* Both these descriptions concern enhancement that corresponds neither to a mass (a 3D space-occupying lesion) nor to a segmental enhancement.

    - *Regional enhancement* is described as enhancement within a larger area of the breast that does not follow a segmental pattern.
    - *Focal area enhancement* describes enhancement within a smaller (nonsegmental) area that does not correspond to a mass, as it may also contain nonenhancing normal or fatty tissue and does not appear as a 3D "ball-like" lesion.

Their differential diagnosis is difficult, since both are often seen in proliferative changes or adenosis. They may, however, also be seen in areas of diffusely growing invasive carcinoma or may be associated with areas of DCIS.

All mentioned entities may display variable amounts and dynamics of enhancement ranging from low to strong enhancement with a progressive or fast rise. While the positive predictive value (PPV) of reticular, dendritic, heterogeneous, or clumped enhancement is quite high, it is lower for homogeneous or stippled enhancement.

If washout is seen or worrisome patterns of enhancement (reticular, dendritic, heterogeneous, or clumped) are present, usually biopsy should be considered.

Close correlation with clinical findings and conventional imaging should always be ensured.

Any clinically, mammographically, or sonographically suspicious area should be histologically assessed. For the remaining cases with uncharacteristic homogeneous or heterogeneous regional or focal area enhancement, an individual assessment considering all methods, overall risks, symmetry, and change with time need to be made. Whatever decision is made based on MRI, errors may occur.

12. *Nonmass diffuse enhancement.* Diffuse enhancement by definition occupies major parts of both breasts. Overall, the differential diagnosis includes the same entities as regional enhancement. However, owing to the symmetry and the similar appearance of all breast tissue, benign changes are far more likely than malignant changes provided no other suspicion exists (clinically or by conventional imaging).

    If washout enhancement or clumped or reticular enhancement is seen within all or major parts of the enhancing tissue or if other possible signs of malignancy exist (skin thickening, retraction of the skin or breast tissue, nipple retraction), histopathologic assessment needs to be considered.

In all cases with moderate to strong diffuse enhancement, assessment by MRI is impaired, since a significant percentage of malignancies (mainly those with low to moderate or delayed enhancement) might go undetected. Unfortunately, background diffuse enhancement is a frequent finding. In most cases it represents just one possible presentation of benign changes.

Overall, low to moderate enhancement, monomorphic and symmetric appearance, and progressive dynamics support a benign diagnosis.

13. *Changes on plain MRI.* Depending on the composition of benign and malignant changes we have noted significant overlap of appearances on unenhanced MRI. On T2-weighted images, for example, low signal intensity may occur in fibrosed carcinomas, old scarring, or in benign fibrotic changes, whereas high signal intensity may occur in myxoid fibroadenomas, in mucinous carcinomas, in many ductal carcinomas, in inflammatory changes, or in areas of benign adenosis. Other authors have reported that high signal intensity on T2-weighted images significantly increases the probability of malignancy among enhancing lesions.

Based on the large multicenter study conducted by Schnall et al. (2006) using multivariate analyses, however, this appears to be redundant to the more specific information gained following contrast enhancement. Decreased signal intensity on T1-weighted images appears to increase the probability of malignancy. Absence of this sign, however, cannot exclude malignancy.

Summarizing the existing data, there is still no reliable evidence that unenhanced MRI contributes significant information. *The use of contrast medium thus remains indispensible for the diagnosis of malignancy by MRI.*

14. *The following other findings should be described if present:*
    - Abnormal signal void (e.g., in scarring). Signal void in scarring may be due to artifacts after electrocautery or to powder residue from surgical gloves (**Fig. 5.5g**).
    - Cysts, hematoma or blood, precontrast high ductal signal. The last may indicate a duct filled with proteinaceous or serosanguinous contents and therefore only rarely indicates a nonenhancing malignancy (intraductal DCIS or mucinous carcinoma) (**Fig. 5.10**).
    - Nipple retraction, skin retraction, skin thickening (focal or diffuse), edema, lymphadenopathy.
        – The differential diagnosis of these signs mainly includes post-therapeutic changes, inflammation, or diffuse malignancy (**Fig. 5.11**).
    - If a lesion is demonstrated, the presence of nipple invasion, skin invasion, muscle invasion should be described.

15. *Information on surrounding tissue.* As for mammography or breast ultrasound, where a description of the tissue surrounding a lesion in question is given, it is important to describe the pattern and dynamics

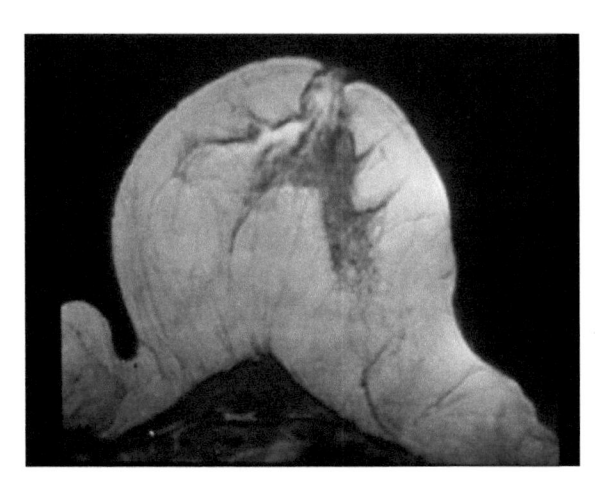

Fig. 5.10 In this patient bright signal intensity was seen in some retroareolar ducts on the T1-weighted pre- and postcontrast images. The bright signal may occur in ducts with increased protein content or with serosanguinous contents, which leads to T1-shortening and thus increased signal. Owing to pre-existing T1-shortening, enhancement with MR contrast agent may be obscured. Therefore in such cases subtraction images may (falsely) not enhance. In most cases the bright signal within retroareolar ducts is caused by secretory disease. Rarely mucinous carcinoma or papillary DCIS might also cause such findings.

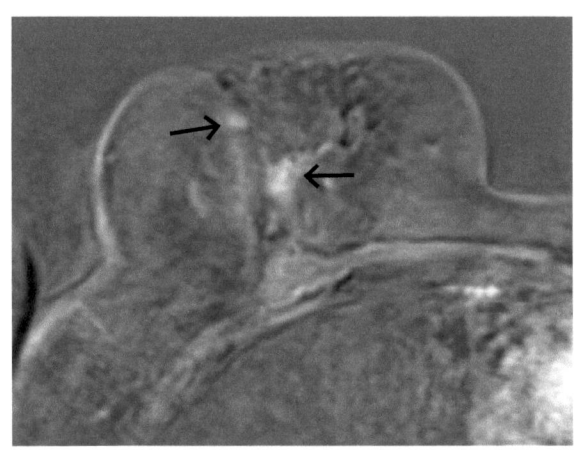

Fig. 5.11 In this patient skin thickening and nipple retraction are explained by status after breast-conserving therapy of malignancy. Representative MR-guided vacuum-assisted breast biopsy of the focal enhancement centrally yielded papillomatosis and post-therapeutic inflammatory changes.

of enhancement seen in surrounding tissue. The reason is that enhancement of surrounding tissue may obscure or mimic lesions and thus may have significant impact on the reliability and accuracy of MRI in each individual case.

Usually assessment is excellent if no surrounding enhancement is present. Assessment (and thus the capability of MRI to detect or exclude malignancy) decreases with increasing, rapid and inhomogeneous enhancement in surrounding tissue.

It is important to understand that the quantity and dynamics of enhancement of benign surrounding tissue on MRI do not correlate with mammographic density or echogenicity of the tissue on ultrasound. It appears to correlate with the extent of hyperplastic or proliferative changes or with chronic inflammatory changes within the benign tissue. The quantity and dynamics of enhancement, however, do not correlate with presence or absence of atypia.

Minimal background enhancement may be expected in postmenopausal patients who are not on hormone replacement therapy, in breasts more than 1 year after radiation therapy, in areas of dense fibrosis, and in many premenopausal women—if the latter are examined during the correct phase of the menstrual cycle (optimally day 7–15).

16. *BI-RADS categories.* The American College of Radiology (ACR) has recommended use of the BI-RADS categories for MRI, as they are currently used for mammography and sonography.

    The suggested categories are as follows:
    - BI-RADS 0 = additional imaging (or clinical) evaluation needed. This may include repeat MRI due to a technically insufficient scan, additional pulse sequences, additional conventional imaging (such as retrospective ultrasound correlation), clinical correlation, or comparison with previous imaging.
      – No definitive diagnosis yet possible.
    - BI-RADS 1 = normal, no finding.
      – Usual follow-up as recommended for the specific age and risk groups.
    - BI-RADS 2 = definitely benign finding (cyst, scar, fibrosed fibroadenoma, etc.)
      – Usual follow-up as recommended for the specific age and risk groups.
    - BI-RADS 3 = probably benign finding. Malignancy highly unlikely, but stability should preferably be established.
      – Short-term follow-up recommended.
    - BI-RADS 4 = lesion with a low to moderate probability of being malignant.
      – Histopathologic assessment recommended.
    - BI-RADS 5 = lesion highly suggestive of being malignant.
      – Adequate further diagnostic and therapeutic steps recommended (usually percutaneous biopsy followed by adequate surgical and/or oncological treatment).
    - BI-RADS 6 = known biopsy-proven malignancy.
      – Appropriate action should be taken.

> We strongly recommend that a final diagnosis is always established, which is based on a conclusion from all available information (clinical information, mammography, sonography, MRI) and which leads to a final recommendation for the patient.

Patient Selection and Indications

Contrast-Enhanced MRI

In all fields of medicine selection of patients and selection of indications may heavily influence the results. The additional information provided by MRI may be extremely valuable in selected difficult cases.

Unfortunately, MRI is associated with a significant rate of false positive calls leading to biopsy or at least short-term follow-up. Even though the addition of MRI may help to detect more malignancies than conventional imaging, possible advantages (earlier detection) must be weighed against side effects (increased false positive rate, increased rate of difficult MR-guided interventions and surgery, increased rate of short-term follow-up, unknown rate of over-diagnosis). When MRI is used, histopathologic assessment of lesions visible by MRI alone must be available. Unfortunately, to date there is a significant lack of specialized equipment and personnel to enable all centers to have this capability.

> Considering strengths and weaknesses of MRI as an additional imaging tool, selection of the appropriate indications appears of utmost importance for obtaining the best possible and clinically most valuable results for our patients and for a responsible use of available resources. The choice of appropriate indications should be based on the critical appraisal of the existing evidence. Such evidence can only be expected from literature which is based on clearly defined patient preselection, on multimodality comparison using state-of-the-art methods, and on adequately verified data.

At present, MRI is not recommended for the following indications:

- *Screening of women at low to moderate risk* (e.g., women with dense breast tissue or lifetime risk < 15%). Here the prevalence of cancer is generally so low (< 0.5% per year) that the additional workup or short-term MR-follow-up of false positive MR findings that occurs in 15–20% of the examined patients (> 150–200/1,000 patients per year) cannot be justified.
- *Workup of lesions that could instead be appropriately assessed by percutaneous biopsy.* MRI is not cost-effec-

tive because of its much higher rate of false positive results compared with percutaneous biopsy and also to the high rate of MR-detected incidental findings, which in the low-risk population mostly prove to be benign. Furthermore, based on the fact that a significant percentage of invasive cancers and parts of DCIS do not enhance, the negative predictive value (NPV) of MRI is inferior to that achieved by state-of-the-art percutaneous (or open) biopsy.

Indications for which MRI has been recommended or discussed include:
- Search for tumor when the primary is unknown and breast cancer is suspected.
- "MRI screening" of women at high risk for breast cancer
- Staging of the local tumor extent and exclusion of multicentricity in the same or contralateral breast
- Problem-solving after breast-conserving therapy or after silicon implant
- Monitoring of neoadjuvant chemotherapy
- Selected cases in which state-of-the-art workup performed by experienced breast imagers cannot answer the diagnostic question

> The following paragraphs summarize the present knowledge concerning the above-mentioned recommended or discussed MR indications.

Search for Primary Tumor

Cancer of unknown primary accounts for a small percentage of breast cancers. These cancers become apparent by finding enlarged nodes, mostly axillary nodes, sometimes by enlarged lymph nodes outside the axilla, and sometimes by distant metastases. Particularly when only axillary nodes are involved, detection of the primary tumor is desirable, since some of these patients are still in a curable stage and since knowledge of the primary may influence treatment strategies. If the primary is not detectable by any method and breast cancer is still suspected, the chance of cure appears to be equal for patients undergoing radiation therapy and patients who undergo mastectomy.

The initial diagnosis of malignancy in these cases is thus usually made based on the histology of an enlarged lymph node. The breast may be suspected to be the original site of the primary based on the location of the lymph nodes in the axilla, based on the histologic type of the tumor cells, based on suspicious mammographic microcalcifications contained in the lymph node, or based on immunohistochemistry that is hormone receptor or Her-2neu positive. The probability of breast cancer may best be estimated based on the discussion of such individual cases by the interdisciplinary team.

The search for a primary breast cancer should first include clinical examination, mammography, and ultrasound. If all are negative, MRI has been reported to detect a primary cancer of the breast in 24–80% of the cases (mostly in about two-thirds of cases). In the remaining cases the primary may be outside the breast. According to the data in the literature and our own experience, in most of the remaining cases the primary has remained occult or was located in another organ. In a few cases the primary of the breast may become apparent later. We are aware of just one publication reporting a primary that was occult to MRI but was detected by positron emission tomography (PET).

Whenever an enhancing lesion is detected by MRI, the usual workup is recommended (retrospective sonographic correlation to check if percutaneous US-guided biopsy is possible. If not, MR-guided percutaneous biopsy should be preferred over MR-guided surgery.) Preoperative histology is desirable since, according to the literature benign enhancing lesions may give false positive results in 20–30% of these patients.

Based on the existing data search for primary tumor is generally considered an accepted indication for DCE-MRI in most health systems (**Fig. 5.12**).

MRI Screening in Women at High Risk

Definition: Screening asymptomatic women systematically and periodically using gadolinium-enhanced MRI to detect clinically occult breast cancer.

So far the expression *MR screening* has been used in a wider sense than the strict definition of mammographic screening, as given in the European guidelines. MRI screening mostly implies that women participate in a program (or study) with *intensified surveillance*, which includes contrast-enhanced MRI, mammography, and clinical examination at yearly intervals. Only some programs have also included ultrasound. To our knowledge only the German program includes ultrasound and clinical examination at 6-month intervals.

The current existing *national programs for intensified surveillance of high-risk groups* restrict participation to exactly defined high-risk groups and age ranges (based on the age-dependent difference in remaining risk) with some variations between the programs. Based on existing evidence in the literature, both risk–benefit and cost–benefit considerations, European programs have so far strictly limited the use of MRI screening to true high-risk groups (usually lifetime risk > 30%), whereas US recommendations apparently also include patient groups at moderately high risk (usually lifetime risk > 20%).

Fig. 5.12a–e In this patient with histologically proven malignant axillary involvement, MRI was performed, since clinical examination and conventional imaging did not allow locatation of the suspected primary tumor.

- **a** Mammogram (mediolateral oblique view).
- **b** Mammogram (craniocaudal view).
- **c** Representative ultrasound image showing hyperechoic breast tissue. No sign of malignancy.
- **d,e** Two small enhancing masses of 7 mm and 4 mm (plateau enhancement) were seen as the only abnormalities and underwent MR-guided vacuum-assisted breast biopsy (subtraction image, early series, post intravenous contrast media). *Histology*: Two foci of invasive ductal breast carcinoma.

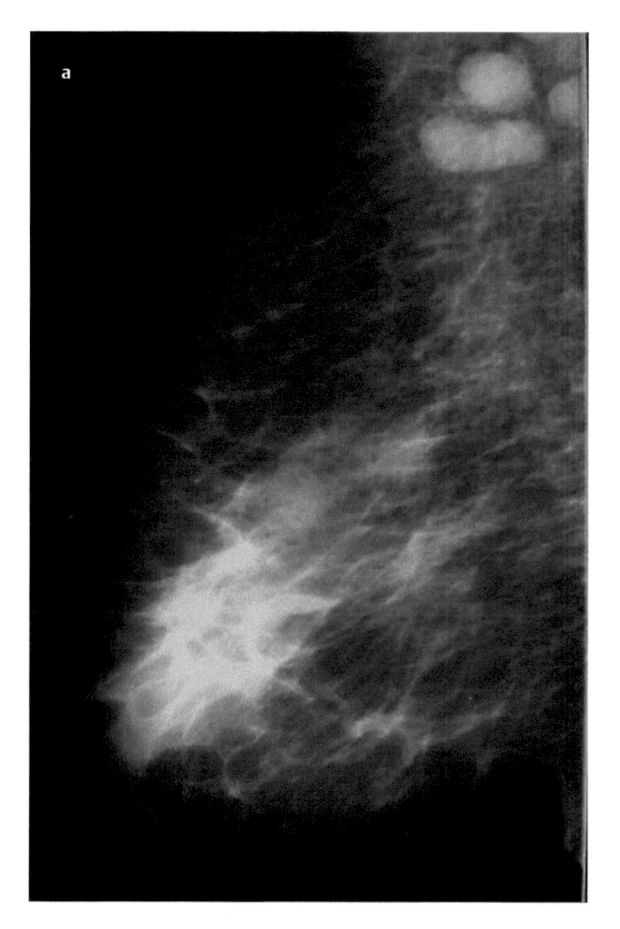

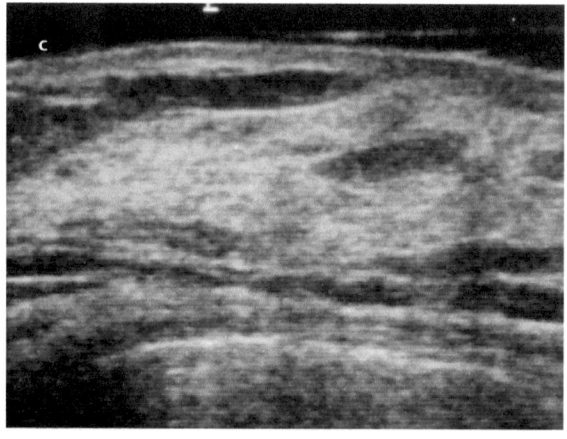

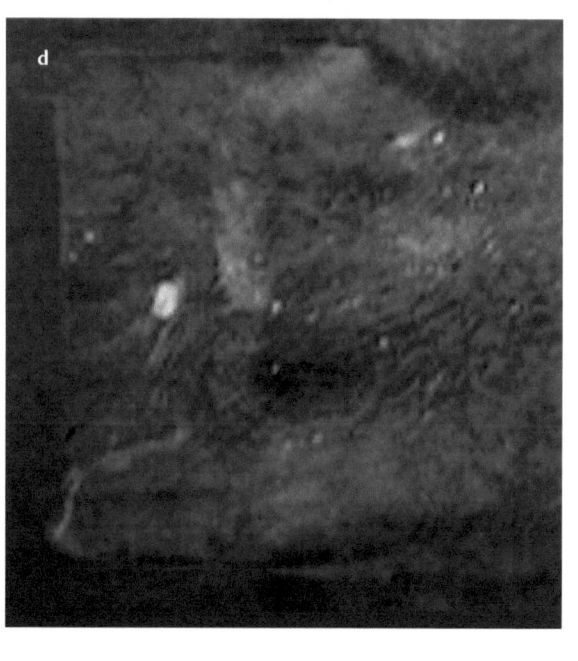

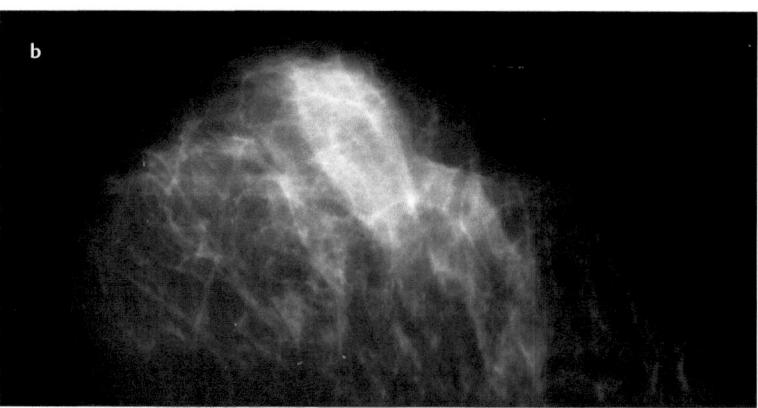

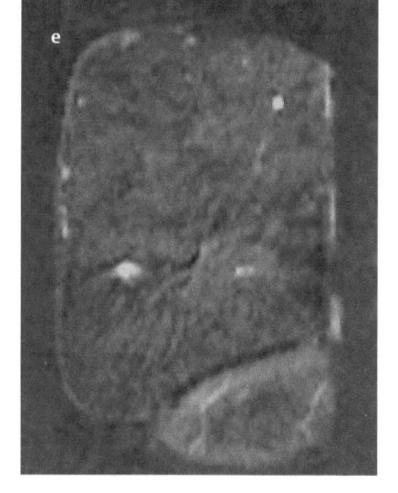

For the following *risk groups* official recommendations (with mentioned national differences) exist:
- Carriers of *BRCA1 or BRCA2* gene mutations
- *Carriers of other mutations* at very high risk for breast cancer such as women with changes in the *TP53* or the *PTEN* genes (Li–Fraumeni, Cowden, or Bannayan–Riley–Ruvacaba syndromes)
- Women who are BRCA mutation negative but with a high risk based on *strong family history* (of breast and/or ovarian cancer), as calculated from well-known algorithms by geneticists
- Women who have received *previous mediastinal radiotherapy* for Hodgkin disease or other childhood tumors ≤ age 30 years.

Recommended Age Range, Intervals, Methods

- Yearly intervals are recommended for MRI and mammographic screening. Some programs include ultrasound and clinical examinations. (Only the German program includes sonography and clinical examination at 6-month intervals.)
- Start of surveillance is generally recommended at age 30 years.
- Some guidelines recommend starting MRI screening at age 25, or 5 years before the age at which the youngest relative presented with breast cancer.
- Programs usually include women up to 50–55 years of age.

Evidence for High-Risk Screening

The initial evidence for the efficacy of MR screening has been gained from six prospective multicenter studies. These studies are summarized in **Table 5.4**. Furthermore, systematic reviews have been published on this topic (Lord et al. 2007, Warner et al. 2008, Sardanelli et al. 2011). In spite of some differences in patient selection, study design, and results, all studies showed that the additional use of MRI increased sensitivity significantly and that cancers could be detected at a better stage of prognosis. Overall sensitivity levels ranged from 77% to 100%.

A comparison of the reported sensitivities of the single methods shows that in these selected patients about 33% of malignancies are detected by MRI alone, about 11% are detected by mammography alone, while only 3% are detected by ultrasound alone.

While some studies included only gene carriers or high-risk patients, others also included patients at somewhat lower risk. The majority of included patients and overall evidence, however, concerns women at high risk. Owing to the small numbers of women with uncommon genetic disorders (such as TP53 carriers and women with Li–Fraumeni syndrome) evidence concerning these entities cannot be expected yet. Evidence is also limited for women who received previous mediastinal radiotherapy for Hodgkin disease or other childhood tumors in their second or third decade. Knowing about the increased risk, which for TP53 carriers starts at an even younger age (> age 20), these groups have been included in national recommendations based on expert consensus. The risk after mediastinal radiation seems to mainly concern a time period lasting from 10 to 30 years after irradiation.

It is still unclear whether early detection by MR imaging will translate into improved disease-free and overall survival, but data should emerge from the United Kingdom in the near future as data on this group of patients are collected and audited nationally.

Table 5.4 Published results for MRI screening in women with high familial breast cancer risk (see References and Recommended Reading, Indications—MRI Screening)

Study and year	Study name or known as	No. of centers	No. of women	Cancers detected	MR		Mammography	
					Sensitivity (%)	Specificity (%)	Sensitivity (%)	Specificity (%)
Kriege 2004	Netherlands	6	1909	50	80	90	33	95
Warner 2004	Canadian	1	236	22	77	95	36	99
Leach 2005	MARIBS	22	649	35	77	81	40	93
Kuhl et al. 2005, 2010	EVA	1 (3)	529 (687)	43 (27)	91 (93)	97	33 (34)	97
Lehman 2005	International Breast MRI Consortium	13	390	4	100	25	95	98
Sardanelli 2011	HIBCRIT	9	278	18	100	99	59	Not stated

Insufficient Evidence For or Against MRI Screening

Currently there is not sufficient evidence to advise whether or not to screen with MRI women in the following groups:
- Those with a lifetime risk above 15% and below 20–30% due to family history
- Those with increased risk due to personal history of lobular carcinoma in situ (LCIS) or atypical lobular hyperplasia (ALH), or atypical ductal hyperplasia (ADH)
- Heterogeneously or extremely dense breast on mammography

The very limited existing evidence on MR screening in this risk category indicates that the ratio of MR-detected additional cancers versus MR-initiated additional assessment may be less convincing than has been proven for women at high risk. The large studies which included women at intermediate risk have not evaluated this subgroup separately.

MRI Screening Not Recommended

Women with a lifetime risk of less than 15% should not be enrolled in MR screening programs, based on expert consensus opinion and on all existing guidelines.

Risks and Benefits

As with any screening program there are benefits and risks to be considered. Even in the high-risk population the *yearly* rate of cancers is low, ranging around 2%.

There are substantial concerns about limited availability of *high-quality MRI breast screening services* for women with familial and other risk factors for breast cancer. Besides recommended standards on quality assurance of breast MRI, Quality Assurance Guidelines have been published in the United Kingdom and those also recommend that all screening breast MRI should be double-read by experienced readers who are also involved in mammographic screening. In the United States an ACR accreditation process has been announced which will stipulate a minimum number of examinations that must

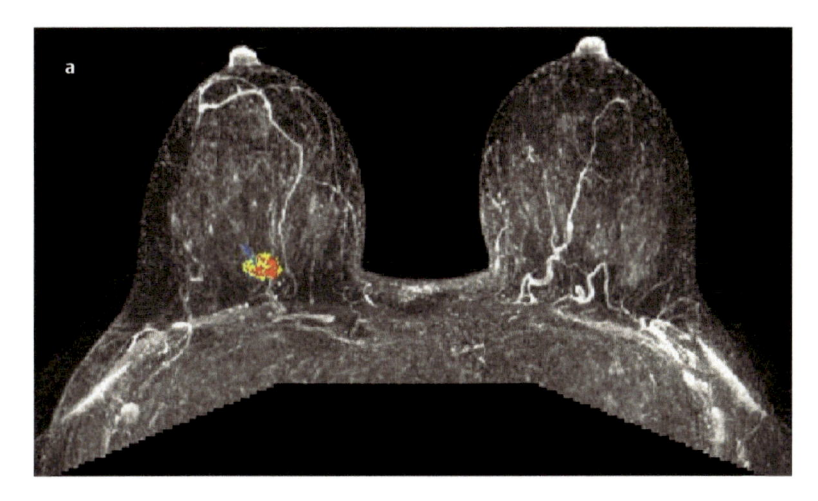

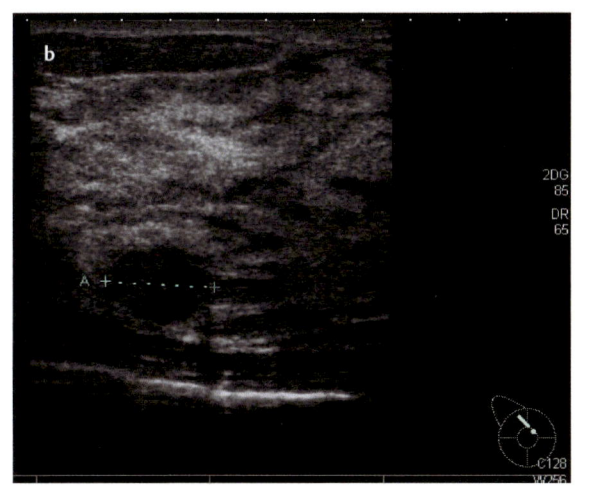

Fig. 5.13a,b A 32-year-old patient carrying the *BRCA1* gene underwent her first MRI screen.

a Centrally and posteriorly in the right breast is a well-defined mass which measures 13 mm by 13 mm by 11 mm. It is of low signal intensity on T1- and T2-weighted imaging. It demonstrates avid enhancement with a type III curve. The morphology of the lesion was suggestive of a fibroadenoma. (CAD-generated color map: red is rapid strong enhancement, and washout; blue is moderate enhancement, and plateau; yellow indicates slow rising enhancement.)
Mammograms show dense breast tissue only.

b By ultrasonography, the lesion appeared as a fairly well defined hypoechoic mass. US-guided core biopsy revealed a grade 3 invasive ductal carcinoma.

be read for training purposes and a minimum number interpreted for ongoing accreditation.

It is only by providing a high-quality MRI screening service that results at least equivalent to published data will be achieved.

Although the sensitivity for breast cancer of MRI has been demonstrated to be higher than that of mammography, MRI does not offer perfect sensitivity. Considering published sensitivity data and the stage distribution of the cancers detected (even in subsequent rounds of MR screening), women who undergo intensified surveillance including MR screening need to know that MR screening allows earlier detection than screening by conventional imaging and higher detection rates. However, *it cannot guarantee that all cancers are detected or that cancer is detected in time*. To date the best guarantee of avoiding breast cancer and breast cancer death and the only measure with evidence of proven mortality reduction is risk reduction mastectomy. In any surveillance program false negatives will occur. They can result from the inherent technological and biological limitations of MRI, patient factors, quality assurance failures, and human error.

False positives can also be due to these factors, and the fear of litigation over the consequence of missing a cancer may also be relevant.

The specificity of MRI is significantly lower than that of mammography in all studies to date, resulting in more recalls and biopsies. Recall rates for additional imaging ranged from 8% to 17% in the MRI screening studies; biopsy rates ranged from 3% to 15%. Furthermore several studies have not even mentioned the number of short-term follow-up examinations caused by MRI. Even though the availability of previous exams may be helpful and even though there is a hope for improved specificity in subsequent rounds, existing data have not shown a significant change in the accuracy, since the better specificity reported by at least two-thirds of authors was associated with somewhat lower sensitivity.

Even though many lesions detected by MRI can be found with a subsequent "second-look" ultrasound, a significant number of cancers (particularly early cancers) will be identified only on MRI (**Fig. 5.13**). Thus, all guidelines published to date recommend the facility to perform MRI-guided biopsy as an absolute essential to offering screening MRI. As MR-guided biopsy is time consuming, expensive and technically challenging, a high-quality regional service with specially trained and experienced personnel needs to be built up for such programs.

Recalls will inevitably lead to additional investigations, many of which will be negative for cancer. The knowledge of these women about their increased risk and the increased need for additional interventions and short-term follow-up have been shown to lead to anxiety.

High quality assurance and the recommendation for reading a sufficient number of studies may help to improve the known problems of the learning curve in MRI interpretation and to eventually achieve results comparable to those of the published studies.

Considering the fact that MRI screening also leads to the detection of numerous borderline lesions that range from LCIS to ADH and DCIS, the very sensitive detection of MRI very probably also leads to over-diagnosis and over-treatment, the side effects of which may be associated with any screening or diagnostic test. To date, no data exist on this subject.

For women at high risk, to date the advantages of earlier detection (even though not perfect) appear to justify the unavoidable side effects of imaging surveillance. However, high quality needs to be assured to maintain this fragile balance. Also, women should be adequately informed about advantages, limitations, and potential side effects of imaging surveillance to enable them to make their decision based on informed consent.

Preoperative MRI for Local Staging

The use of MRI for preoperative staging before breast-conserving therapy has been one of the first indications to be considered. Even though MRI has been confirmed as the most sensitive modality to detect small invasive cancers and even DCIS foci, the value of preoperative MRI is not clear.

Accuracy

Ample data from well-designed single institution studies, from multicenter studies, and from a large meta-analysis confirm that *DCE-MRI is the most sensitive method for assessment of tumor size, detection of multifocality, and multicentricity*.

In the mentioned studies MRI was able to detect additional invasive or in-situ breast cancer. Nonetheless, when compared with complete histopathologic assessment of all breast tissue, no imaging method is perfect, and a multicenter study in which this was investigated (Sardanelli et al. 2004) reported a sensitivity of 89% for MRI versus 72% for mammography for the detection of invasive foci and of only 40% for MRI and 37% for mammography concerning detection of DCIS. In almost all studies MRI and mammography proved to be complementary.

By far the largest incremental gain in sensitivity was reported for MRI in patients with histologically proven lobular breast cancer (which is understandable considering both the high sensitivity of MRI for invasive breast cancers and the limited sensitivity of mammography and ultrasound for lobular carcinomas in particular).

Studies which focused on the accuracy *of assessing size of DCIS and epithelial invasive cancer (EIC)* have shown that MRI (38–64% correct assessment) is more accurate than mammography (Schouten van der Velden et al. 2006, Kim et al. 2007, Van Goethem et al. 2007).

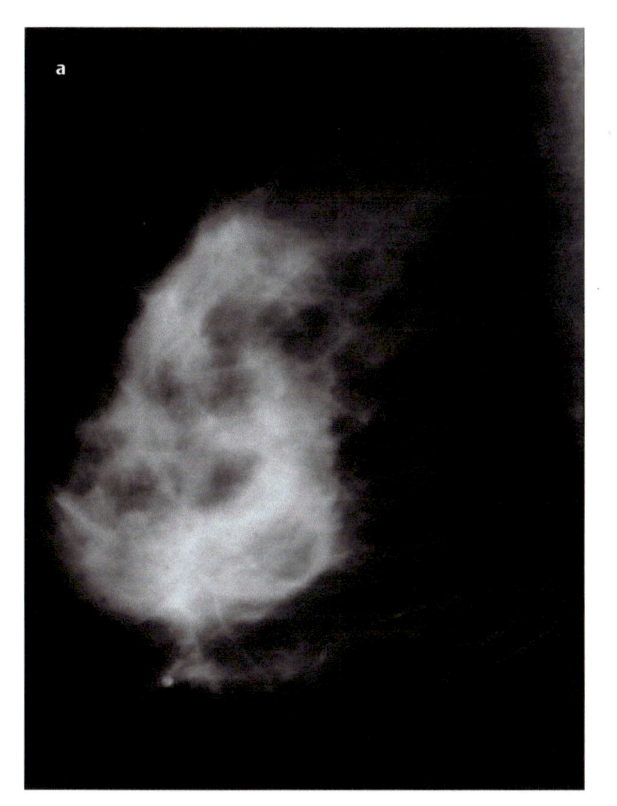

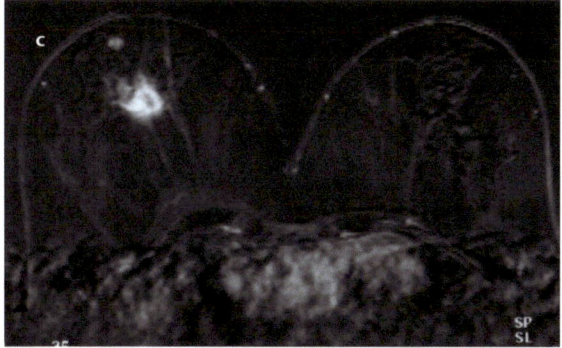

Patient Selection and Indications

Fig. 5.14a–c MRI performed for preoperative staging.

a Mammogram (mediolateral view): Dense tissue (ACR 3) is shown. The palpable breast cancer cannot be delineated within this tissue.

b Mammogram (craniocaudal view): The breast cancer is seen as an ill-defined mass posteriorly behind the nipple. On ultrasound the breast cancer was visualized as a hypoechoic, irregular, highly suspicious mass surrounded by homogeneous hyperechoic breast tissue. No further abnormality.

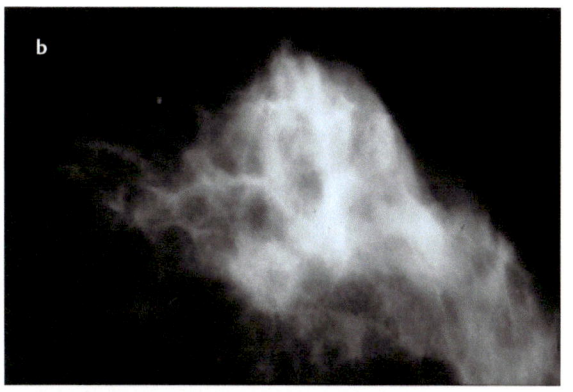

c The subtraction image demonstrates the early enhancing mass with ill-defined margins and highly suspicious rim enhancement. A second, round, early enhancing and slightly inhomogeneous 5-mm focus was noted ~1 cm behind the nipple.
Histology confirmed the invasive breast cancer and a second invasive focus, which without MRI would not have been detected. It remains unclear in the individual case whether detection of such small foci is of benefit, or whether radiation and systemic therapy might have achieved the same result with less extensive surgery.

However, over-estimates and underestimates ranging from 11% to 28% and from 17% to 28%, respectively, remain even with the use of MRI. Therefore, the addition of MRI may improve accuracy, which may be helpful for therapy planning in surgically difficult situations (close to the nipple or in cases where breast conservation may be difficult). This should, however, be decided by the interdisciplinary team. Overall, the best possible assessment of EIC will require close correlation of imaging and histopathology as the gold standard.

Finally, MRI has proved able to detect otherwise occult *contralateral malignancy* in about 3–4% of patients with breast cancer.

Unfortunately, only some of the foci detected by MRI prove to be malignant and thus represent false positive calls. Thus before any treatment decision (e.g., mastectomy) diligent histopathologic assessment of MR-detected lesions is crucial.

For those lesions that are visible by MRI alone, MR-guided histopathologic assessment is needed. Thus, when preoperative MRI is performed, availability of specialized equipment and highly specialized personnel is warranted and additional costs need to be covered. *The availability of biopsy capability is a prerequisite in all major guidelines concerning breast MRI* (see Chapter 7, pp. 188ff, 207ff and Chapter 8, pp. 216 and 222ff).

According to a large meta-analysis by Houssami et al. (2008) a correct therapeutic change with respect to the final histopathology (different surgical access, wider excision, excision of another focus in the same or contralateral breast) was reported in 12.8% of patients who underwent preoperative MRI (5.8% more extensive surgery, 7% mastectomies), but an incorrect change of therapy occurred in 6.6% of preoperatively examined cancers (5.5% more extensive surgery, 1.1% mastectomies) owing to changes detected by MRI that eventually proved benign (**Fig. 5.14**).

> It is important to understand that a correct decision with respect to final histopathology may not equate to improved outcome for this indication.

The reason is that it may not be necessary to excise every tiny focus of malignancy, since irradiation, adjuvant chemotherapy and anti-estrogen therapy also contribute to elimination of small and very small tumor foci.

To understand the importance of checking for final patient outcome the following should be remembered:
- Histopathology has always shown that multicentricity and multifocality are frequent findings (occurring in up to 50% of breast cancers). Nevertheless breast conservation was possible and proved equivalent to mastectomy in many past studies. (Moreover, breast conservation was based on clinical and mammographic assessment only.)
- Based on this knowledge it is unclear whether demonstration of multifocality or multicentricity beyond the previous capabilities is of true benefit to the patient and diligent analysis of true outcome, benefits, and advantages to the patient is of utmost importance when MRI is used as an additional method for this indication.

Patient Outcome

To date, evidence concerning patient outcome is still limited. Possible advantages to patients undergoing preoperative MRI could include the need for fewer re-excisions (clear margins at primary surgery), lower recurrence rate, lower rate of contralateral breast involvement in the years following treatment, and improved survival.

The first results addressing this issue come from prospective and retrospective single institution studies (Solin et al. 2008, Pengel et al. 2009) and from a large randomized multicenter study (COMICE) performed in Great Britain. As to number of re-excisions, the large randomized multicenter study found no difference between the MR and the non-MR groups. (One large single institution study [Pengel et al. 2009] reported some advantages for the MR group, which proved statistically significant for ductal invasive carcinomas).

With regard to the true benefit for rate of recurrence or frequency of contralateral malignancy, both the initial evaluation of the large randomized study (after 3 years' follow-up) and a large retrospective single institution study (Solin et al. 2008) found no difference between the MR and the non-MR groups after 8 years' follow-up.

Even though every study has its advantages and limitations, to date there exists no proof that preoperative MRI is of benefit to the average patient before breast conservation. This result does not exclude benefit for subgroups; neither does it exclude the possibility that with further improvement in preoperative histopathologic assessment or marking, a benefit might in the future be detected. However, to date it must be considered that benefit is not proven and preoperative MRI may lead to more aggressive surgery and possibly also a delay in treatment (Bleicher et al. 2009).

Present Recommendations

Considering the present state of affairs as described above, no general recommendation can be given for preoperative MRI in patients before breast conservation (e.g., for patients with dense breast tissue).

With regard to possible advantages in subgroups, however, the present guidelines support consideration of preoperative MRI in the following conditions:
- In patients at high risk (> 30% lifetime risk)
- For lobular invasive cancer of the index lesion, histologically proven (level III, strength)
- Discrepancy in tumor size greater than 1 cm between mammographic and sonographic findings with expected impact on treatment decision (Sardanelli et al. 2010: EUSOMA consensus)

To date, experience with the use of MRI in patients undergoing partial breast irradiation is very limited. Considering the differences in therapy compared with standard breast-conserving therapy, outcome will need to be investigated separately for this group of patients.

Problem-Solving after Breast-Conserving Therapy

Fortunately, today, breast-conserving therapy (BCT) has become the treatment of choice for the majority of newly diagnosed breast cancers. Classical BCT includes lumpectomy or quadrantectomy followed by radiation therapy. Whenever feasible and desired by the woman, it is performed to treat breast cancers less than 3 cm in size. Breast conservation also proves feasible in some breast cancers greater than 3 cm after neoadjuvant chemotherapy, if the cancer can be downstaged to a size that allows complete excision and a cosmetically acceptable result. For very early breast cancer, partial breast irradiation is evolving as a new treatment option.

Based on both risk of recurrence and increased risk of contralateral malignancy, yearly mammography and clinical examination is generally recommended. In dense breast tissue this is usually supplemented by ultrasound. Even though the prognostic impact of recurrence has been debated (some presume that recurrence may be an expression of an increased risk, but has no impact on overall survival; others disagree), a recent publication points out that early detection of recurrence or contralateral malignancy does improve relative survival from a second malignancy by between 27% and 47% (Houssami et al. 2009).

Unfortunately, diagnosis by clinical examination and conventional imaging may be impaired in some cases after breast conservation, since post-therapeutic changes and scarring may both mimic and obscure malignancy.

In these cases MRI appears to offer special advantages for the differentiation of scarring and malignancy. The reason is that in the vast majority of cases fresh granulation tissue is usually replaced by nonenhancing fibrotic scar tissue starting around 12 months after radiation therapy. Also, proliferative changes within surrounding breast tissue are then usually replaced by nonenhancing radiation fibrosis. This usually allows an excellent distinction of scarring and irradiated benign tissue from malignancy. Early after irradiation this may vary and—according to our own experience, which differs from that of some other authors—false positive calls due to fresh granulation tissue or enhancing fresh fat necrosis are more frequent within 12 months of irradiation than later on.

Accuracy

Accuracy data on BCT stem from several prospective single institution studies on patient cohorts of around 30 to 170 women. Recurrence vs. scarring is proven by histology or 1–2 year follow-up. Sensitivity for this indication usually exceeds 90–95%, while specificity ranges around 90%. According to our published experience of 169 cases (proven by histology or 2-year follow-up) a significant number of recurrences were detected by MRI only and the average size of MR-detected malignancy was smaller than that detected by conventional imaging with mammography and ultrasound (**Fig. 5.15**). (The case selection included consecutive cases after BCT with dense tissue and/or diagnostic problems [Viehweg et al. 1998].)

Depending on the study design, significant improvement in overall sensitivity and/or specificity has been reported in the published literature for the addition of MRI in diagnostically difficult cases. Accuracy data of MRI after BCT often exceed the results published for other indications. This may be explained by the usual lack of enhancement seen in irradiated breast tissue more than 12 months after irradiation.

In dense and severely scarred tissue, MRI may be the only modality that can detect or exclude small lesions. However, if a definite lesion or abnormality exists that can be targeted or requires histopathologic assessment; MRI should not be used to replace breast biopsy.

Recommended Use

Based on the existing experience, MRI should be considered after BCT in the following clinical situations:
- Inconclusive findings after clinical examination and conventional imaging
- Scar very close to the chest wall that cannot be imaged mammographically
- High risk of recurrence (close margins or multifocal disease at initial surgery, high family risk, or other individual risk factors such as ADH or lobular neoplasia grade 2–3)
- Initial breast cancer mammographically occult

Problem-Solving after Breast Reconstruction with or without Silicon Implant

Breast reconstruction is usually performed to achieve a cosmetically acceptable result when breast conservation has not been possible. Some breast reconstructions are performed with autologous flaps. Most are performed with implants, mostly silicone implants.

As usual for women with a history of breast cancer, imaging surveillance is recommended at yearly intervals. In patients with autologous flaps and saline implants mammography and ultrasound are possible and recommended. In women with silicone implants mammography is usually not possible, since the small amount of tissue that covers the implant cannot usually be mobilized and because silicone implants are usually not transparent. Thus, after reconstruction with a silicone implant the affected side is examined only clinically and by ultrasound.

Both clinical assessment and imaging may be compromised within the scar tissue and inconclusive findings may occur. In these patients, too, MRI may be very helpful.

Fresh granulation tissue usually regresses within about 6 months after surgery and is then replaced by nonenhancing (or slightly enhancing) scar tissue. Within such tissue residual tumor or recurrence that usually enhances is usually well detected by MRI. In patients with silicone implants the implant does not obscure abnormal enhancement.

In contrast to scarring after benign surgery, enhancing granulomatous tissue or fresh fat necrosis appears to be more frequent after flaps, mainly in the junction areas and around silicone implants. Small enhancing granulomas seen around implants may measure just a few millimeters in size and are mostly round lesions, whereas granulation tissue in patients with flaps may be more extended and usually has ill-circumscribed margins. Both may enhance fast (with or without washout) and may thus be the cause of a false positive call on MRI. To avoid unnecessary surgery for small enhancing nodules around implants, short-term follow-up should be considered after 3–4 months and then after 12 months, for example. Recurrences are expected to grow, while small enhancing granulomas usually persist.

Overall, however, MRI may prove extremely helpful to solve diagnostic problems in these patients, who in addition are at increased risk based on their individual history (**Fig. 5.16**).

5 Magnetic Resonance Imaging

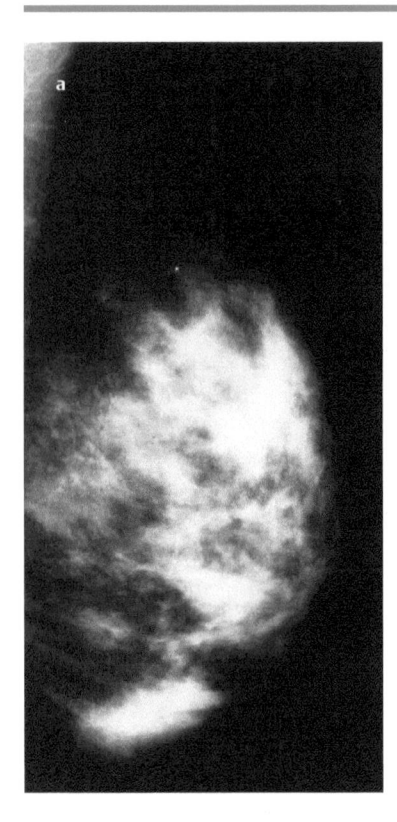

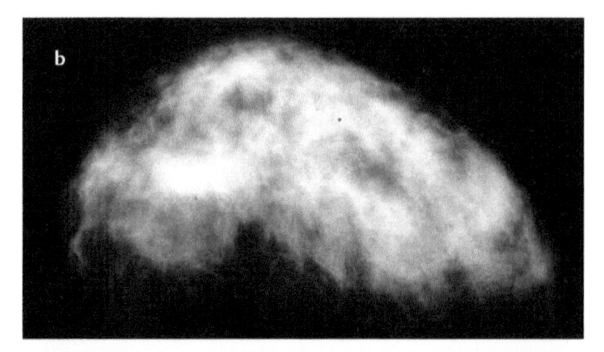

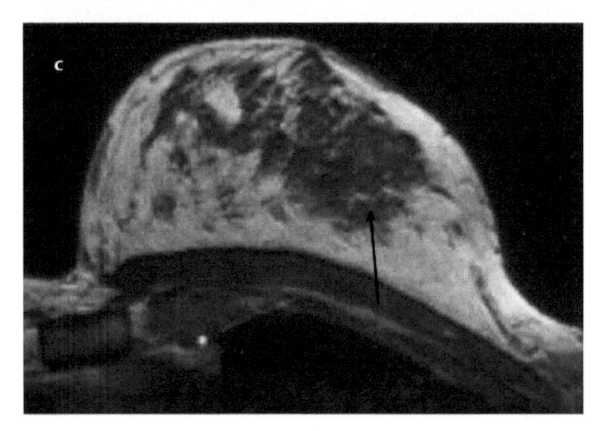

Fig. 5.15a–d This patient underwent MRI, since the initial breast cancer was mammographically occult. Mammographically and sonographically there was no sign of malignancy.

a Mammogram (mediolateral oblique view).
b Mammogram (craniocaudal view).
c,d On MRI a small plateau-type slightly irregular enhancing nodule was detected close to the scar (pre- and postcontrast images of the lesion are shown). MR-guided open biopsy confirmed a 5-mm invasive recurrence.

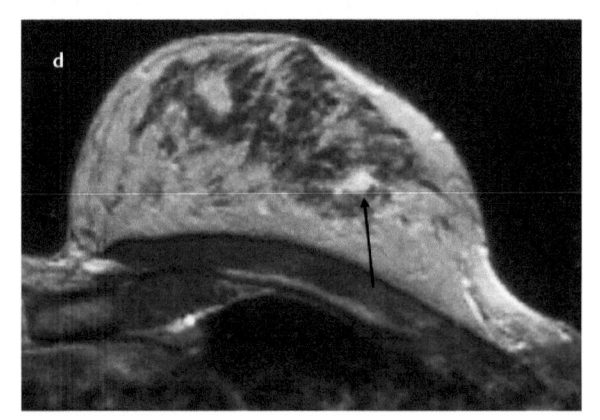

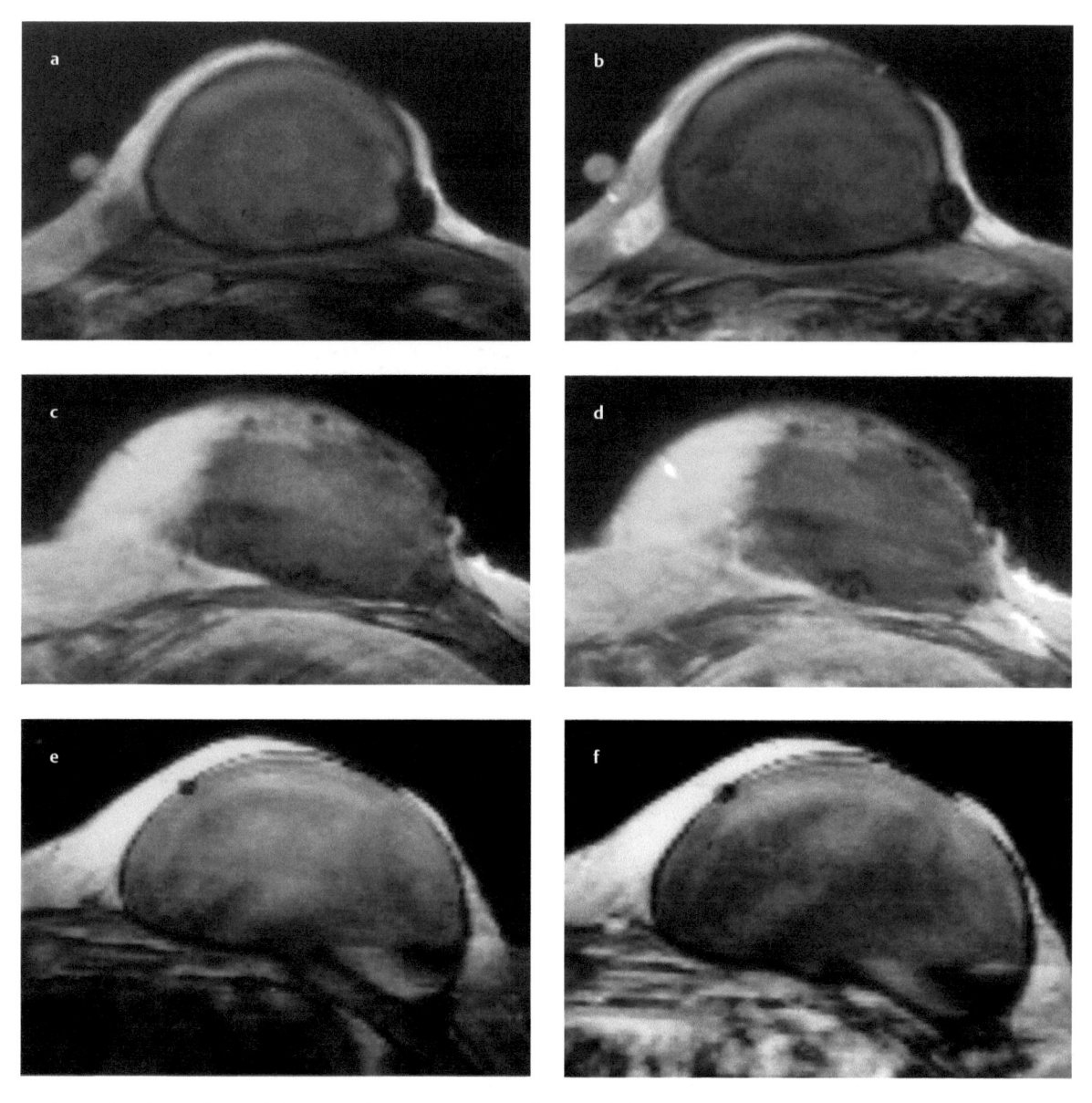

Fig. 5.16a–f Patient with a single lumen implant, reconstruction after extended breast cancer. The study simultaneously demonstrates the potential and limitations of imaging. The patient presented with a palpable nodule medial to the implant. The nodule was visible on ultrasound and MRI was performed preoperatively.

- **a,b** Pre- and postcontrast T1-weighted images of the palpable nodule (a capsule was attached to the skin to mark the palpable abnormality). The round but slightly irregular small mass enhanced strongly and was considered suspicious. *Histology*: An invasive ductal recurrence.
- **c,d** Pre- and postcontrast T1-weighted images of a more caudal slice. Incidentally another suspicious enhancing mass (located between the lower outer edge of the implant and the chest wall) was noted. This lesion, too, proved to be invasive ductal recurrence that was detected by MRI only.

Two years before, the same patient had undergone an MRI examination and indeed, in the area of the palpable mass, a tiny focal enhancement was seen in retrospect. The lesion was not identified prospectively since it was falsely considered to correspond to a vessel.

- **e,f** Pre- and postcontrast T1-weighted images in the area of the palpable nodule, examined 2 years prior to the study shown above (**a,b**).

Accuracy

Only few prospective studies exist on this topic. These studies report sensitivities > 90% and specificities ranging around 90% for conventional imaging with MRI and confirm a significant improvement in both specificity and sensitivity by the addition of MRI in patients with silicone implants (see **Fig. 13.6**). Good results are reported for diagnostic problems after autologous flaps. However, false positives appear to be somewhat more frequent with MRI. They are often caused by fat necrosis at the junction areas of the flaps.

Recommended Use

In patients with silicone implants or autologous flaps, MRI should be considered in the following situations:
- Inconclusive findings after clinical examination and conventional imaging
- Increased risk after silicone implant (close margin, multifocal disease)

No data exist that would support systematic MRI screening of these women.

Imaging the Augmented Breast and Implant Complications

The augmented breast can usually be adequately assessed by mammography (using special views) and ultrasound. For women with augmented breasts with usual risk profile no indication exists for MRI screening.

It should also be emphasized that silicone implants are not associated with any increased risk of breast cancer (Brinton et al. 1996, Friis et al. 2006).

Most diagnostic questions concerning the breast tissue surrounding the implant can be solved by mammography, ultrasound, and percutaneous breast biopsy, which in experienced hands is possible even with implants.

In rare cases, however, MRI may be helpful to solve diagnostic problems. These problems usually do not differ from those occurring in women without implants. If implant integrity needs to be assessed, MRI is the method of choice. For this indication contrast agent is not needed. Imaging technique has been described above.

MRI for assessment of breast implants is described in detail in Chapter 20.

Accuracy

According to a meta-analysis (Cher et al. 2001), the sensitivity of MRI for implant rupture was reported to be 78% and the specificity 91%. More recent publications usually report higher sensitivities of 80–90% with specificities ranging around 90%.

Recommended Use

In patients after augmentation mammoplasty using silicone implants, MRI is in general not necessary. It may be useful in selected cases, if a diagnostic question cannot be solved by conventional imaging and percutaneous biopsy.

In the case of a suspected implant complication, MRI is the most accurate imaging modality and is recommended to solve diagnostic problems.

Monitoring of Neoadjuvant Chemotherapy

Neoadjuvant chemotherapy (NAC) is used to reduce the size of a breast cancer before surgery with the goal of either making breast conservation possible or, in the case of inoperable breast cancer, making surgery possible. Even though breast conservation may eventually be possible in only some of the patients, NAC appears not to be associated with prognostic disadvantages. It also offers the opportunity to assess the response to chemotherapy in vivo.

DCE-MRI may be used:
- To monitor response, which appears possible after one or two cycles of chemotherapy, and
- To restage the breast before planning surgical therapy.

Special Issues in Patients undergoing Neoadjuvant Chemotherapy

Planning MRI

To allow optimum interpretation after NAC, it is generally recommended that a baseline MRI study be obtained before NAC. For monitoring it is recommended that DCE-MRI be performed 1–2 weeks after the second or third cycle and 2 weeks after the last cycle and before scheduled surgery.

Interpreting DCE-MRI

Image interpretation of DCE-MRI includes interpretation of changes in lesion morphology and the strength and dynamics of enhancement.

Absence of enhancement after NAC usually indicates complete response. It can, however, exclude neither residual DCIS/EIC nor residual nests of cells. Another good indicator of complete response is change of an enhancement curve from fast-rising enhancement (with or without washout) to delayed enhancement. Residual delayed enhancement at the site of the original tumor may be caused by residual dispersed nests of invasive tumor, by residual DCIS/EIC, or by granulation tissue. Thus, whenever possible, an attempt should be made to include such areas in the final excision.

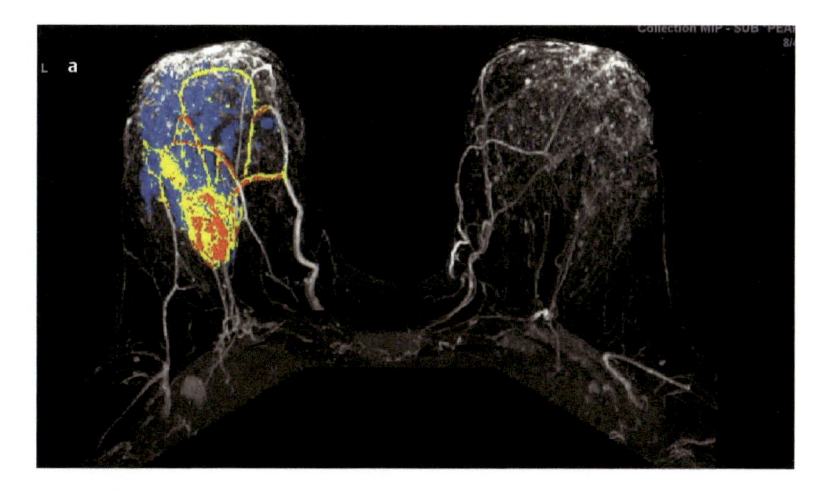

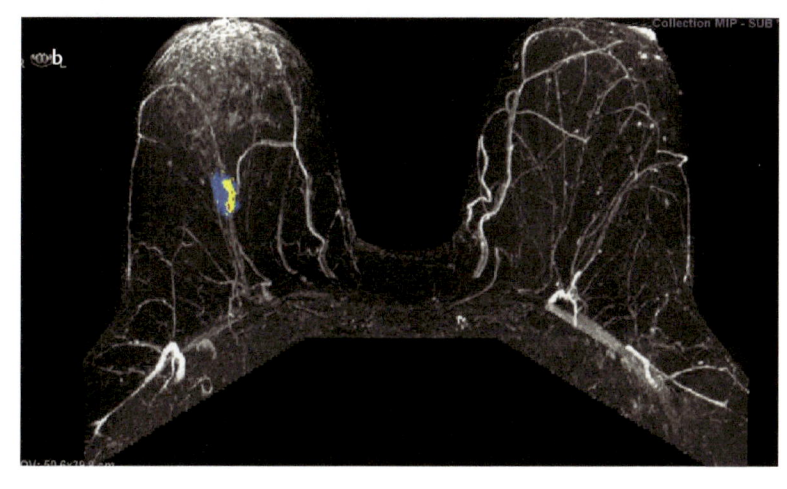

Fig. 5.17a,b Illustration of an excellent response of a grade III triple negative invasive ductal carcinoma to neoadjuvant chemotherapy.

a Pretreatment scan; 3D maximum intensity projection (MIP) postcontrast image. (In the axillary tail, part of a normal lymph node is seen.)

b Follow-up scan during treatment; 3D MIP postcontrast image. After two cycles of chemotherapy, the mass is already markedly reduced in size and the enhancement pattern is predominantly slow rising. On further follow-up the mass regressed completely. Pathology showed no residual tumor. All nodes were negative.
(CAD-generated colour map: red is rapid strong enhancement, and washout; blue is moderate enhancement, and plateau; yellow indicates slow rising enhancement.)

The *best chances for breast conservation* appear to exist if enhancement disappears.

Furthermore concentric shrinkage of the enhancing lesion identifies good candidates for breast conservation. Here residual enhancement often correlates with the residual disease.

The *worst chances for breast conservation* have been reported:
- In patients with persisting enhancement
- In patients with diffuse or fragmented or dendritic multifocal or multicentric enhancement after NAC (Nakamura et al. 2002)
- In patients who presented with nonmass lesions (Bahri et al. 2009). In the latter patients residual disease is often underestimated.

Figs. 5.17, 5.18, 5.19 show examples of different responses to NAC.

It may be useful to remember that an increased number of underestimates have been reported in patients who have been treated by NAC containing taxanes (Denis et al. 2004) and in patients treated with bevaizumab, an anti-angiogenic agent (Chen et al. 2008).

Quantitative measurement of lesion diameters for the assessment of response should follow RECIST (**Table 5.5**) (Therasse et al. 2000).

Accuracy and Use of DEC-MRI in monitoring

To date, MRI is not yet regularly used in patients undergoing NAC. One reason may be that the accuracy of DCE-MRI is not yet sufficiently convincing for this indication, even though most authors reported advantages over mammography and breast ultrasound.

So far, no multicenter study or systematic review has been published for this indication. The literature includes numerous small to intermediate-sized studies, which on average reported accurate assessment by DCE-MRI in 70% of the cases (Sardanelli et al. 2010). In the remaining cases under- or over-estimates occurred.

While data are still limited, increased evidence may be expected from a large ongoing multicenter study (American College of Radiology Imaging Network: ACRIN).

When analyzing studies of NAC it may be important to remember that presence of residual DCIS or EIC does not count when response is judged. (Even large areas

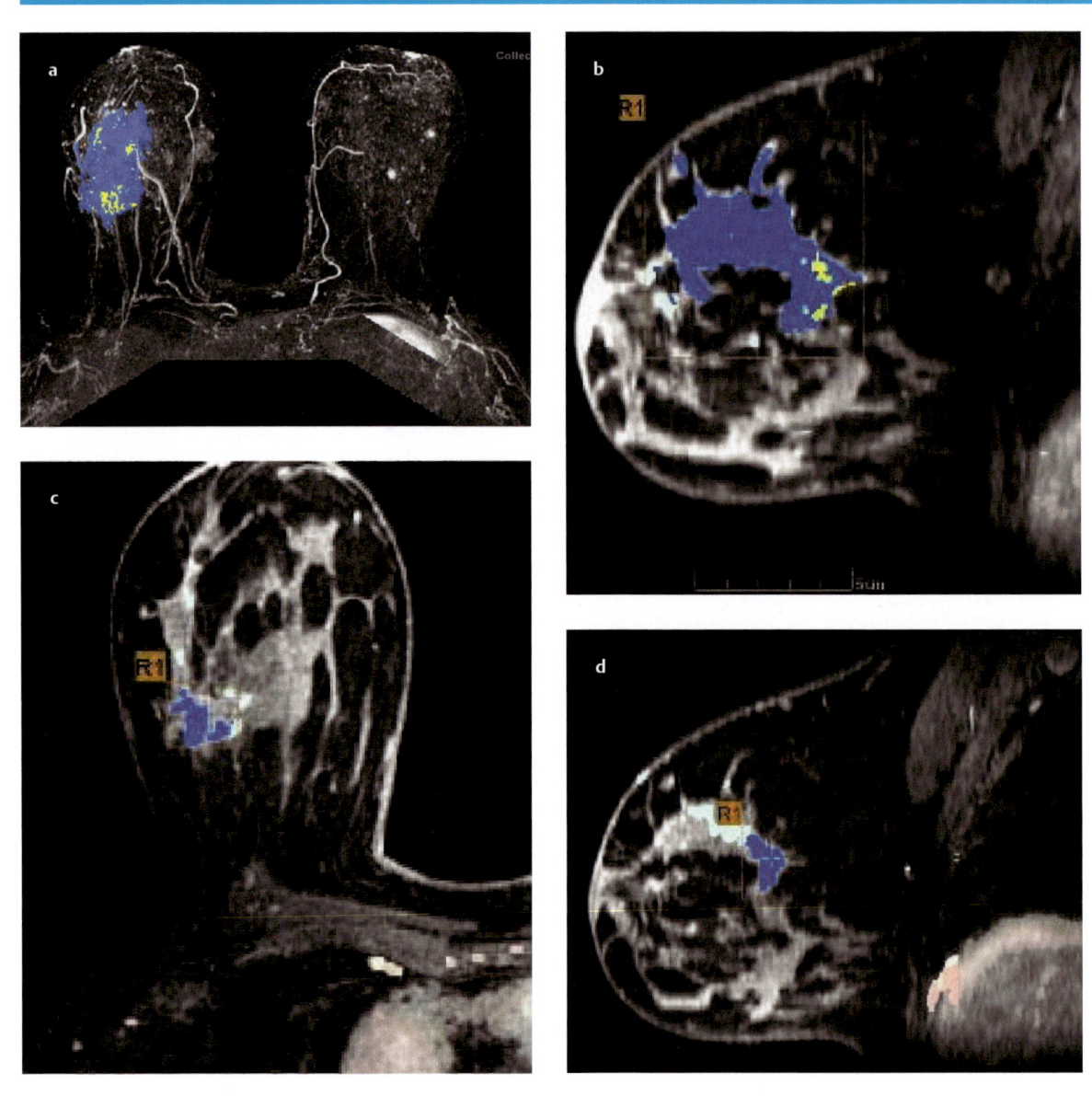

Fig. 5.18a–d Pre- and post-neoadjuvant chemotherapy (NAC). After-therapy MRI studies show fragmentation of tumor mass. Pathology after NAC was invasive lobular carcinoma and lobular carcinoma in situ, and there were multiple residual tumor foci separated by fibrous tissue. Total diameter of residual tumor 40 mm. Partial response.

a,b Before chemotherapy 3D MIP postcontrast transverse and sagittal reconstruction showing a large enhancing tumor in the upper outer quadrant of the right breast.

c,d The images after NAC show the tumor has fragmented with multiple small areas of residual slow-rising enhancement remaining.
(CAD-generated color map: red is rapid strong enhancement, and washout; blue is moderate enhancement, and plateau; yellow indicates slow rising enhancement.)

Patient Selection and Indications

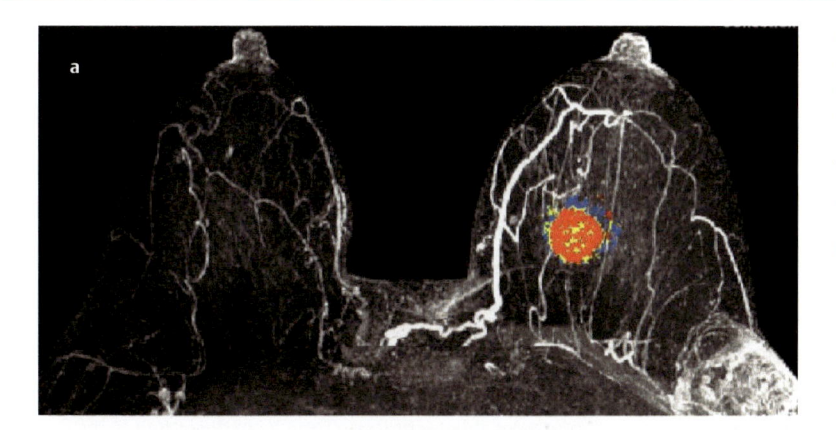

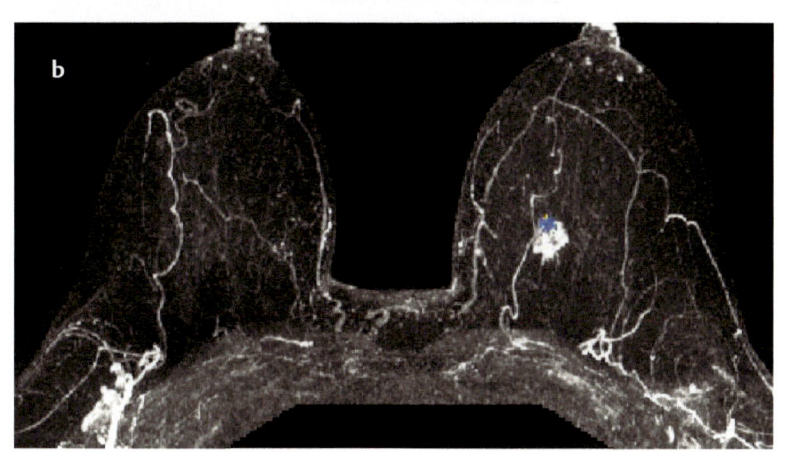

Fig. 5.19a,b Pre- and post-neoadjuvant chemotherapy MRI studies showing marked response with no enhancement on the post-treatment scan. Pathology showed fibrosis with no viable residual tumor cells.

a 3D MIP postcontrast image showing an enhancing tumor in the left breast.
b The tumor mass is considerably smaller and there is only a small area anteriorly of minimal slow-rising enhancement. (CAD generated color map: red is rapid strong enhancement, wash out, blue is moderate enhancement, and plateau, yellow indicates slow rising enhancement.)

Table 5.5 Definition of response evaluation criteria in solid tumors (RECIST), as agreed in 2000 (Therasse 2000) and updated in 2009 (Eisenhauer 2009)[a]

Classification of response	Response of target lesions	Further criteria requested to be fulfilled
Complete remission = CR	Complete disappearance of all target lesions	Complete disappearance of any sign of residual disease
Partial remission = PR	Sum of diameters reduced by ≥ 30%	No new lesion and no progression of nontarget lesions
Stable disease = SD	Neither PR nor PD	No new lesion and no progression of nontarget lesions
Progressive disease = PD	Either: sum of diameters increased by ≥ 20%	And: any change
	Or: any change	And: definite new lesion(s)

[a]According to RECIST guideline 1.1 it is recommended to choose five target lesions (two per organ), if present. Target lesions are those lesions which are chosen to be most appropriate for monitoring (mostly the largest lesions). The diameters of the target lesions are added and the sum of diameters is used for comparison. For target lymph nodes the shortest diameter is used. For all other solid target lesions the largest diameter is used.

of residual DCIS or EIC would be considered a complete response!). Irrespective of this issue, residual DCIS or EIC should always be excised.

Present Use

MRI is not yet generally used to monitor NAC. Unfortunately, when used for problem-solving, often no baseline study is available. Provided the use of proton spectroscopy or diffusion-weighted imaging can further improve its accuracy, MRI may play a more important role in the future. Advantages of MRI monitoring might include early detection of insufficient response to NAC, which might result in changing the patient's therapeutic regimen. Preoperative MRI after NAC might help to correctly increase the rate of breast-conserving surgery.

Response with Diffusion-Weighted MRI and Proton Spectroscopy

According to the latest research the additional use of diffusion-weighted MRI or proton spectroscopy may increase diagnostic accuracy. Early, accurate detection of nonresponse to chemotherapy could potentially allow an early change to second-line treatment and thus save the cost of ineffective treatment as well as sparing patients unnecessary toxicity and avoiding any delay in initiating effective treatment. For *diffusion-weighted MRI* (DWI) authors have successfully used gradient echo imaging (EPI) with a DWI pulse sequence (matrix = 128, FOV [mm] = 350.00, slice thickness = 5 mm, flip angle [deg] = 90.00, diffusion mode = SE, NSA = 1) with various diffusion weightings applied.

Apparent diffusion coefficient (ADC) maps are calculated automatically by software directly applied by the MR manufacturer's program, and must be evaluated on a dedicated workstation. Using the conventional MR images as a reference, regions of interest can be applied to suspicious lesions to calculate ADC values.

Care must be taken not to include areas which appear cystic or necrotic on conventional sequences to avoid error in ADC calculation.

Comparable techniques have been described in the literature (Pickles et al. 2006, Sharma et al. 2009).

Proton spectroscopy is currently also undergoing evaluation. Spectroscopic imaging using water/fat ratios, choline, and phosphorus have all been recently described. In patients with an elevated choline peak before NAC, a decrease in this peak appears to correlate with response to NAC. These studies all involve small patient numbers, and although this work shows promise in identifying patients who will not respond to chemotherapy, further large-scale studies are needed to validate these techniques for clinical use (Meisamy et al. 2004, Manton et al. 2006).

Figure 5.20 gives an example of the use of DWI for monitoring response to NAC.

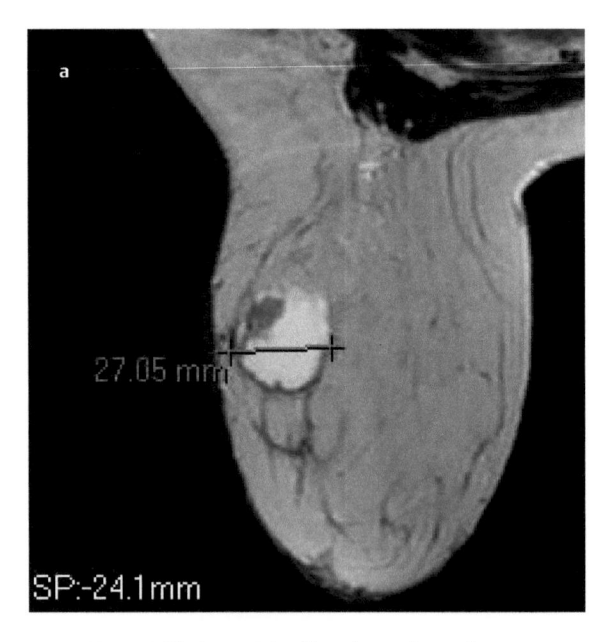

Fig. 5.20a–g Diffusion-weighted imaging and neoadjuvant chemotherapy. Before treatment there is a large 3-cm necrotic tumor in the left breast. The diffusion-weighted image (**c**) shows the importance of selecting the tumor nodule for analysis, which shows restricted diffusion only within the tumor and not in the necrotic cystic component.

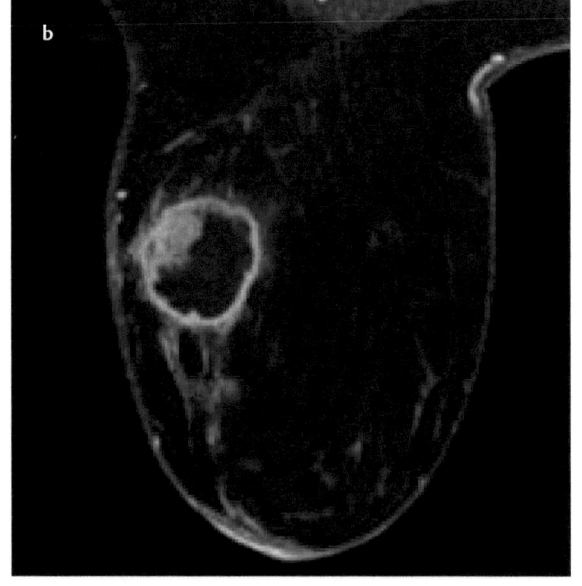

a T2-weighted image.
b Postcontrast subtraction image shows enhancing tumor versus nonenhancing necrosis.

Patient Selection and Indications

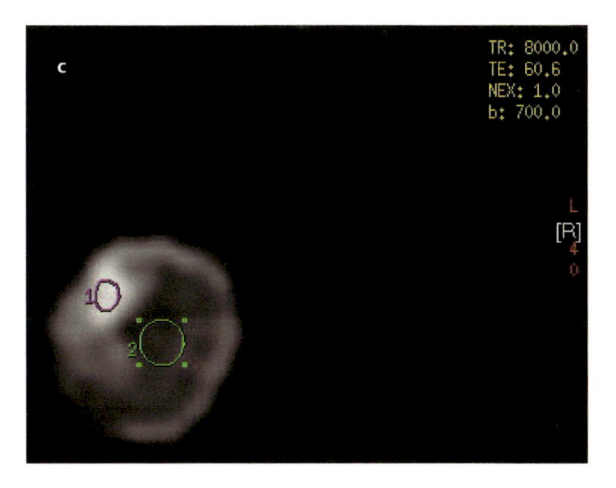

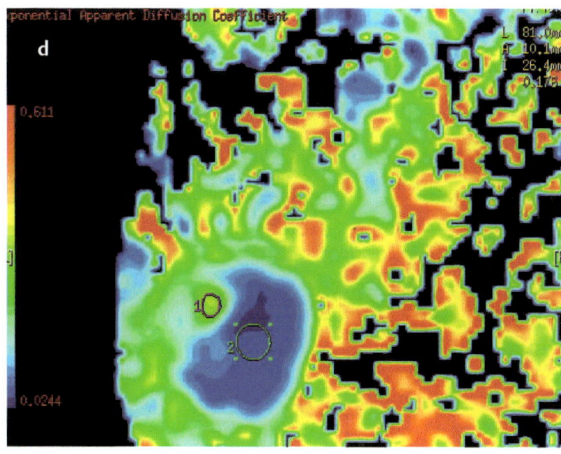

c Diffusion-weighted image.
d Exponential apparent diffusion coefficient map.
e Apparent diffusion coefficient map.
f,g After treatment the images show complete response to treatment. There are no residual areas of restricted diffusion.
f Diffusion-weighted image. **g** Exponential apparent diffusion coefficient.

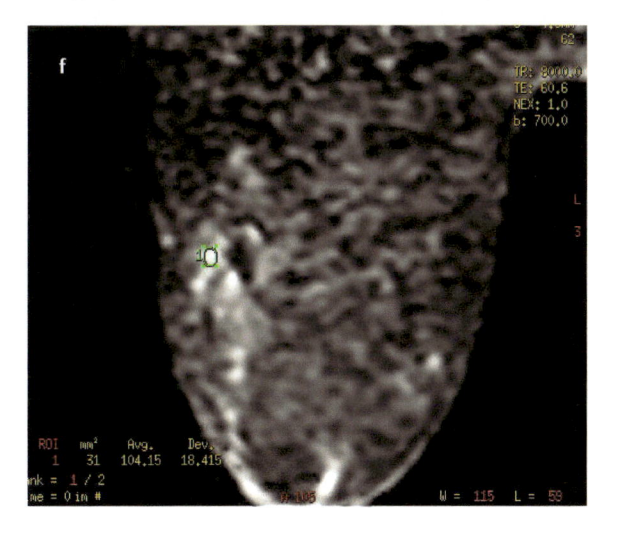

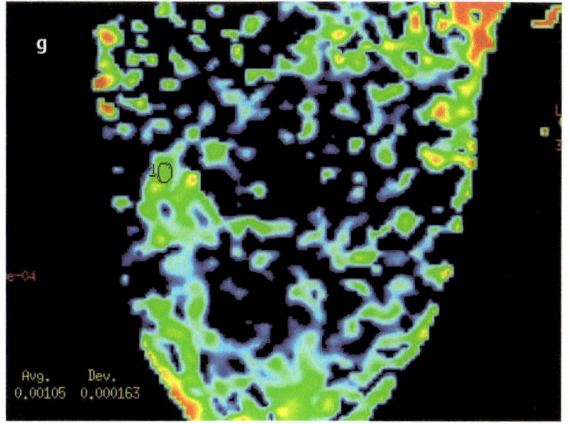

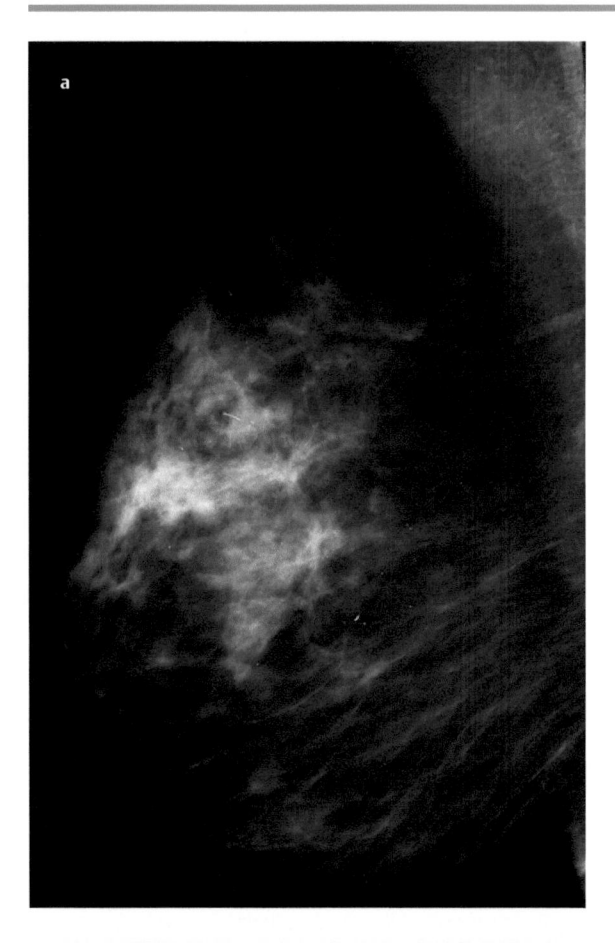

Fig. 5.21a–d In this patient a fine architectural distortion was noted (DD: radial lesion or malignancy) in the upper right breast on the mediolateral oblique view. The craniocaudal view revealed that it might be located medially.

Unfortunately the lesion could not be reproduced on further views. The lesion was not seen sonographically and could not be targeted stereotactically.
a   Mediolateral oblique view.
b   Craniocaudal view.
c   MRI precontrast scan.
d   MRI early subtraction image.
 On MRI a fine architectural distortion is imaged on the precontrast view. The lesion enhances strongly with contrast agent. The patient underwent MR-guided vacuum-assisted breast biopsy and subsequent surgery. *Histology* showed a 6-mm lobular carcinoma (pT1b G2).

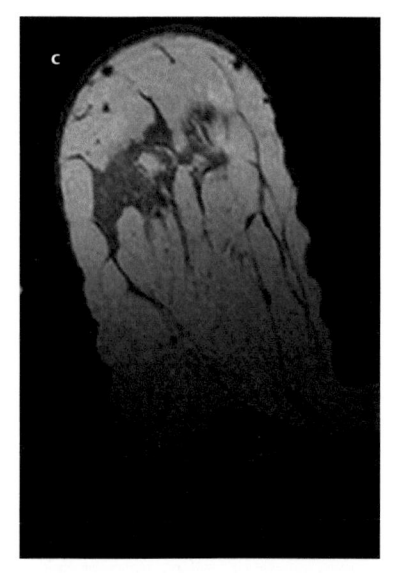

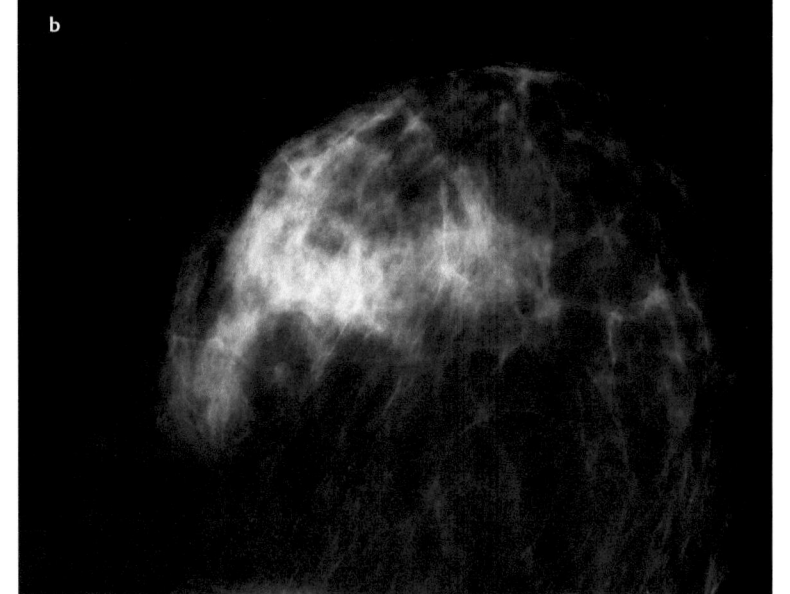

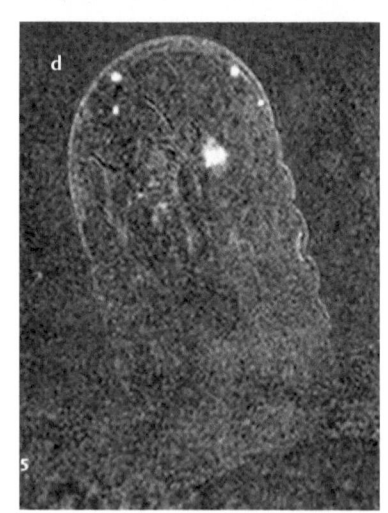

MRI to Solve Selected Diagnostic Problems

Given the availability of modern percutaneous breast biopsy methods, MRI is only rarely needed as an additional tool for problem-solving. Based on its average sensitivity of 90% and its average specificity of 70%, it cannot be used to replace percutaneous biopsy or other indicated histopathologic workup.

In some situations, however, MRI may be very helpful if highly experienced diagnosticians cannot solve the problem(s).

These situations may include:

- *Abnormality seen on one view only:* Some abnormalities are suspicious but still can be visualized neither on further mammographic views nor on ultrasound imaging. This may occur with architectural distortions, rarely, with a suspected mass in very dense or scarred tissue, or with lesions that are located very close to the chest wall. If in experienced hands it is impossible to target the suspected lesion and exclude or verify a true lesion, MRI—being the most sensitive imaging modality—should be the next in line. According to our own experience, MRI does allow definitive proof or exclusion of a lesion in the vast majority of such cases (**Fig. 5.21**). Further assessment of such lesions may, however, require MR guidance for histopathologic assessment.
- *Newly developing or increasing nipple retraction:* The differential diagnosis of this question usually includes malignancy (sometimes small lesions behind the nipple, sometimes intraductal disease) versus chronic inflammation. If mammography and ultrasound cannot show a lesion, this question may be extremely difficult to answer. Being the most sensitive imaging modality, MRI should be used to search for an underlying lesion, which then could be targeted using MR guidance. Since chronic inflammation in many cases causes only little to moderate enhancement, in the absence of a focal abnormality, MRI will often exclude malignancy with high certainty, justifying follow-up. The most difficult differential diagnosis concerns the approximately remaining 20% of cases in which MRI also shows diffuse enhancement. In these cases fanning either by core needle biopsy or open surgery might be considered.
- *Pathologic nipple discharge* (definition: see Chapter 3): In the absence of suspicious findings on conventional imaging, malignancy will eventually be verified in up to 10% of such cases. After mammography and ultrasound (which should include radial scanning following the ducts) galactography has usually been the next method applied. However, galactography often yields an unspecific result, and may not always be possible technically. Some publications have compared galactography and MRI, and report that the accuracy of MRI exceeded that of galactography, but while experience with MRI for this indication is still limited, galactography remains the method of choice. However, if galactography is not possible, MRI should be considered (Sardanelli et al. 2010).
- *Severe scarring:* In patients with severe scarring, assessment by conventional imaging may be strongly impaired. In these cases MRI is an excellent tool to distinguish fibrosed scarring from malignancy. Scars are usually fibrosed starting 4–6 months after surgery. Thus, the absence or presence of very little enhancement on MRI may be expected after this period. False positives may occur in areas of well-perfused granulation tissue and granulating fat necrosis. In diagnostically very difficult cases (e.g., in cases with uncertain removal of noncalcified lesions), MRI might be considered, if conventional imaging is inconclusive. A tumor that was missed at surgery may be recognized besides enhancing granulation tissue and fresh scarring based on its morphology and possibly based on its enhancement dynamics. For this indication, it may be better to perform MRI as soon after surgery as possible before fresh granulation tissue is fully developed. So in selected cases of fresh scarring the additional information from MRI may be useful. However the risk of false diagnoses increases (**Fig. 5.22**).
- *Multiple lesions:* Rarely, a patient presents with multiple indeterminate findings. Here MRI might be useful to decide which lesions may require histopathologic assessment, or to document and follow these lesions. At this point it should be emphasized that usual benign changes with multiple cysts or dense tissue can be solved by mammographic–sonographic assessment and do not require MRI.

Conclusion

To date the literature on the use of MRI for problem solving is limited. According to our own experience, a strict selection of suitable cases, which cannot be solved by highly experienced breast diagnosticians using state-of-the-art assessment, is crucial for good results. This selection helps to limit unnecessary false positive calls (which often may be caused by further lesions that are incidentally detected by MRI), while the chances of accurate problem-solving increase. Existing data confirm that with such strict selection MRI is helpful in difficult situations.

Application of MRI instead of percutaneous breast biopsy is not good practice. It risks false negative and false positive calls and is not recommended.

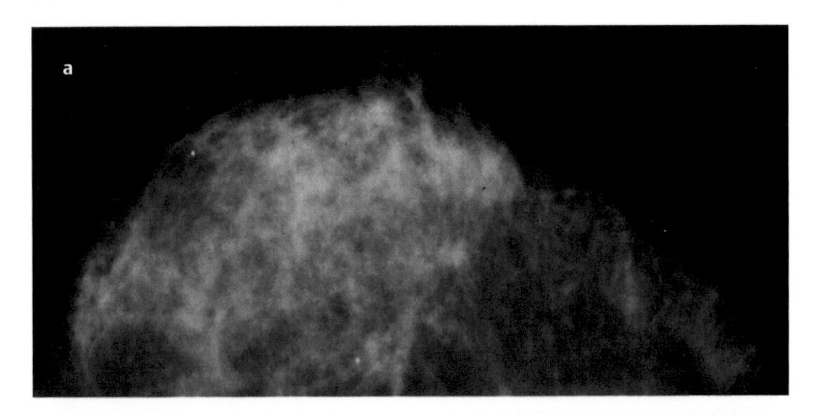

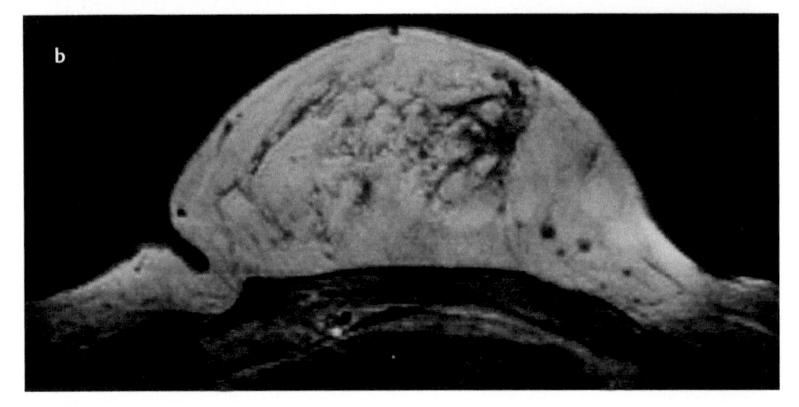

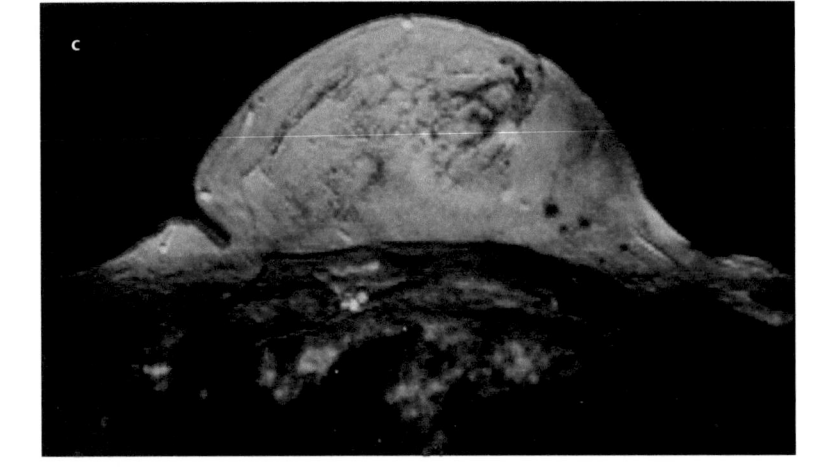

Fig. 5.22a–c In this patient, imaged after benign surgery, a small nodule was suspected within distorted scar tissue. This small nodule was not seen on the previous mammogram, but could not be reproduced on further views or detected by ultrasound.

a Mammogram (craniocaudal view).
b Precontrast scan.
c Postcontrast scan.
   A small enhancing nodule was confirmed, which could be excised after MR-guided preoperative wire marking. Histology confirmed a 5-mm invasive ductal carcinoma. (Reproduced with kind permission of Springer Science+Business Media from Heywang-Köbrunner SH, Beck R. Contrast-Enhanced MRI of the Breast. 2nd ed. Berlin: Springer; 1995: 186.)

Summary

Compared with conventional breast imaging, MRI provides different and often valuable information.

With variations depending on study design, patient selection, and interpretation guidelines the sensitivity of MRI is usually quite high (> 90%). Its specificity varies with indications, being usually lower than that of conventional breast imaging. Lesions that are detected only by MRI usually require availability of MR-guided interventions, preferably MR-guided percutaneous breast biopsy. Therefore MRI should not be performed unless these methods are available for workup of MR-detected lesions.

Considering the limitations of MRI (especially false negative and false positive calls), the technique should not be used without conventional imaging in women more than 30 years old. Hormonal influence (menstrual cycle or hormone replacement therapy) should be considered and MRI should in general be performed and interpreted together with conventional imaging.

To date MRI—being the most expensive imaging modality—should be restricted to acknowledged indications for which its benefits (high sensitivity) outweigh potential disadvantages (moderate specificity and difficult further assessment of MR-detected lesions).

Acknowledged indications include screening of women at high risk, preoperative staging of lobular carcinoma and high-risk patients, search for primary tumor, and diagnostic problems after breast-conserving surgery or insertion of silicone implants.

In selected cases MRI may also be useful for problem solving. Strict limitation to cases that cannot be solved by highly experienced breast radiologists is crucial.

References and Recommended Reading

History

Heywang SH, Bassermann R, Fenzl G, et al. MRI of the breast—histopathologic correlation. Eur J Radiol 1987;7(3):175–182

Heywang SH, Hahn D, Schmidt H, et al. MR imaging of the breast using gadolinium-DTPA. J Comput Assist Tomogr 1986;10(2):199–204

Heywang SH, Hilbertz T, Pruss E, et al. Dynamic contrast medium studies with flash sequences in nuclear magnetic resonance tomography of the breast. [Article in German] Digitale Bilddiagn 1988;8(1):7–13

Kaiser WA, Zeitler E. MR imaging of the breast: fast imaging sequences with and without Gd-DTPA. Preliminary observations. Radiology 1989;170(3 Pt 1):681–686

Pierce WB, Harms SE, Flamig DP, Griffey RH, Evans WP, Hagans JE. Three-dimensional gadolinium-enhanced MR imaging of the breast: pulse sequence with fat suppression and magnetization transfer contrast. Work in progress. Radiology 1991;181(3):757–763

MRI Technique

American College of Radiology. ACR practice guideline for the performance of magnetic resonance imaging (MRI) of the breast. In: Practice guidelines and technical standards. Reston, Va: American College of Radiology; 2008

Baltzer PA, Dietzel M. Breast lesions: diagnosis by using proton MR spectroscopy at 1.5 and 3.0 T—systematic review and meta-analysis. Radiology 2013, Mar 6 [Epub ahead of print]

Chen X, Li WL, Zhang YL, et al. Meta-analysis of quantitative diffusion-weighted MR imaging in the differential diagnosis of breast lesions. BMC Cancer 2010;10:693

Hefler L, Casselman J, Amaya B, et al. Follow-up of breast lesions detected by MRI not biopsied due to absent enhancement of contrast medium. Eur Radiol 2003;13(2):344–346

Heywang-Köbrunner SH, Haustein J, Pohl C, et al. Contrast-enhanced MR imaging of the breast: comparison of two different doses of gadopentetate dimeglumine. Radiology 1994;191(3):639–646

Heywang-Köbrunner SH, Wolf H-D, Deimling M, Kösling S, Höfer H, Spielmann RP. Misleading changes of the signal intensity on opposed-phase MRI after injection of contrast medium. J Comput Assist Tomogr 1996;20(2):173–178

Marini C, Iacconi C, Giannelli M, Cilotti A, Moretti M, Bartolozzi C. Quantitative diffusion-weighted MR imaging in the differential diagnosis of breast lesion. Eur Radiol 2007;17(10):2646–2655

Park MJ, Cha ES, Kang BJ, Ihn YK, Baik JH. The role of diffusion-weighted imaging and the apparent diffusion coefficient (ADC) values for breast tumors. Korean J Radiol 2007;8(5):390–396

Sardanelli F, Fausto A, Esseridou A, Di Leo G, Kirchin MA. Gadobenate dimeglumine as a contrast agent for dynamic breast magnetic resonance imaging: effect of higher initial enhancement thresholds on diagnostic performance. Invest Radiol 2008a;43(4):236–242

Sardanelli F, Fausto A, Podo F. MR spectroscopy of the breast. Radiol Med (Torino) 2008b;113(1):56–64

Shin HJ, Baek HM, Cha JH, Kim HH. Evaluation of breast cancer using proton MR spectroscopy: total choline peak integral and signal-to-noise ratio as prognostic indicators. AJR Am J Roentgenol. 2012;198(5):W488–W497

Wu LM, Hu JN, Gu HY, Hua J, Chen J, Xu JR. Can diffusion-weighted MR imaging and contrast-enhanced MR imaging precisely evaluate and predict pathological response to neoadjuvant chemotherapy in patients with breast cancer? Breast Cancer Res Treat 2012;135(1):17–28.

Guidelines and Consensus Statements

Albert US, Altland H, Duda V, et al. 2008 update of the guideline: early detection of breast cancer in Germany. J Cancer Res Clin Oncol 2009;135(3):339–354

American College of Radiology. ACR practice guideline for the performance of magnetic resonance imaging (MRI) of the breast. In: Practice guidelines and technical standards. Reston, VA: American College of Radiology; 2004

Flamm CR, Ziegler KM, Aronson N. Technology Evaluation Center assessment synopsis: use of magnetic resonance imaging to avoid a biopsy in women with suspicious primary breast lesions. J Am Coll Radiol 2005;2(6):485–487

Heywang-Köbrunner SH, Schreer I, Decker Th, Böcker W. Interdisciplinary consensus on the use and technique of vacuum-assisted stereotactic breast biopsy. Eur J Radiol 2003;47(3):232–236

Institute for Clinical Systems Improvement. Health care guideline: Diagnosis of breast disease. Available at: www.icsi.org

National Institute for Clinical Excellence. Familial breast cancer: the classification and care of women at risk of familial breast cancer in primary, secondary and tertiary care. London: National Institute for Clinical Excellence, Clinical Guideline 41; 2006: http://guidance.nice.org.uk/CG41

NCCN Clinical Practice Guidelines in Oncology. Breast cancer screening and diagnosis guidelines V.I 2008. Available at: www.nccn.org

Sardanelli F, Boetes C, Borisch B, et al. Magnetic resonance imaging of the breast: recommendations from the EUSOMA working group. Eur J Cancer 2010;46(8):1296–1316

Image Interpretation and Accuracy

American College of Radiology. ACR breast imaging reporting and data system (BIRADS): breast imaging atlas. Reston, Va: American College of Radiology; 2003

Baum F, Fischer U, Vosshenrich R, Grabbe E. Classification of hypervascularized lesions in CE MR imaging of the breast. Eur Radiol 2002;12(5):1087–1092

Eby PR, Demartini WB, Peacock S, Rosen EL, Lauro B, Lehman CD. Cancer yield of probably benign breast MR examinations. J Magn Reson Imaging 2007;26(4):950–955

Facius M, Renz DM, Neubauer H, et al. Characteristics of ductal carcinoma in situ in magnetic resonance imaging. Clin Imaging 2007;31(6):394–400

Gutierrez RL, DeMartini WB, Eby PR, Kurland BF, Peacock S, Lehman CD. BI-RADS lesion characteristics predict likelihood of malignancy in breast MRI for masses but not for nonmasslike enhancement. AJR Am J Roentgenol 2009;193(4):994–1000

Heywang-Köbrunner SH, Viehweg P, Heinig A, Küchler C. Contrast-enhanced MRI of the breast: accuracy, value, controversies, solutions. Eur J Radiol 1997;24(2):94–108

Heywang-Köbrunner SH, Bick U, Bradley WG Jr, et al. International investigation of breast MRI: results of a multicentre study (11 sites) concerning diagnostic parameters for contrast-enhanced MRI based on 519 histopathologically correlated lesions. Eur Radiol 2001;11(4):531–546

Ikeda DM, Hylton NM, Kinkel K, et al. Development, standardization, and testing of a lexicon for reporting contrast-enhanced breast magnetic resonance imaging studies. J Magn Reson Imaging 2001;13(6):889–895

Kinkel K, Helbich TH, Esserman LJ, et al. Dynamic high-spatial-resolution MR imaging of suspicious breast lesions: diagnostic criteria and interobserver variability. AJR Am J Roentgenol 2000;175(1):35–43

Kuhl CK, Schrading S, Bieling HB, et al. MRI for diagnosis of pure ductal carcinoma in situ: a prospective observational study. Lancet 2007;370(9586):485–492

Kuhl CK. The current status of breast MR imaging. Part I. Choice of technique, image interpretation, diagnostic accuracy, and transfer to clinical practice. Radiology 2007;244(2):356–378

Liberman L, Morris EA, Benton CL, Abramson AF, Dershaw DD. Probably benign lesions at breast magnetic resonance imaging: preliminary experience in high-risk women. Cancer 2003;98(2):377–388

Liberman L, Mason G, Morris EA, Dershaw DD. Does size matter? Positive predictive value of MRI-detected breast lesions as a function of lesion size. AJR Am J Roentgenol 2006;186(2):426–430

Medeiros LR, Duarte CS, Rosa DD, et al. Accuracy of magnetic resonance in suspicious breast lesions: a systematic quantitative review and meta-analysis. Breast Cancer Res Treat 2011;126(2):273–285

Peters NH, Borel Rinkes IH, Zuithoff NP, Mali WP, Moons KG, Peeters PH. Meta-analysis of MR imaging in the diagnosis of breast lesions. Radiology 2008;246(1):116–124

Rosen EL, Smith-Foley SA, DeMartini WB, Eby PR, Peacock S, Lehman CD. BI-RADS MRI enhancement characteristics of ductal carcinoma in situ. Breast J 2007;13(6):545–550

Sardanelli F, Giuseppetti GM, Panizza P, et al; Italian Trial for Breast MR in Multifocal/Multicentric Cancer. Sensitivity of MRI versus mammography for detecting foci of multifocal, multicentric breast cancer in Fatty and dense breasts using the whole-breast pathologic examination as a gold standard. AJR Am J Roentgenol 2004;183(4):1149–1157

Schnall MD, Blume J, Bluemke DA, et al. Diagnostic architectural and dynamic features at breast MR imaging: multicenter study. Radiology 2006;238(1):42–53

Viehweg P, Lampe D, Buchmann J, Heywang-Köbrunner SH. In situ and minimally invasive breast cancer: morphologic and kinetic features on contrast-enhanced MR imaging. MAGMA 2000;11(3):129–137

Wang LC, DeMartini WB, Partridge SC, Peacock S, Lehman CD. MRI-detected suspicious breast lesions: predictive values of kinetic features measured by computer-aided evaluation. AJR Am J Roentgenol 2009;193(3):826–831

Weinstein SP, Hanna LG, Gatsonis C, Schnall MD, Rosen MA, Lehman CD. Frequency of malignancy seen in probably benign lesions at contrast-enhanced breast MR imaging: findings from ACRIN 6667. Radiology 2010;255(3):731–737

Indications (See also Guidelines)

DeMartini W, Lehman C, Partridge S. Breast MRI for cancer detection and characterization: a review of evidence-based clinical applications. Acad Radiol 2008;15(4):408–416

Heywang-Köbrunner SH, Viehweg P, Heinig A, Küchler C. Contrast-enhanced MRI of the breast: accuracy, value, controversies, solutions. Eur J Radiol 1997;24(2):94–108

Kuhl CK. Current status of breast MR imaging. Part 2. Clinical applications. Radiology 2007;244(3):672–691

National Breast Cancer Centre. Magnetic Resonance Imaging for the Early Detection of Breast Cancer in Women at High Risk: a systematic review of the evidence. Camperdown, NSW: NBCC; 2006

Perlet C, Heinig A, Prat X, et al. Multicenter study for the evaluation of a dedicated biopsy device for MR-guided vacuum biopsy of the breast. Eur Radiol 2002;12(6):1463–1470

Sardanelli F, Boetes C, Borisch B, et al. Magnetic resonance imaging of the breast: recommendations from the EUSOMA working group. Eur J Cancer 2010;46(8):1296–1316

Swayampakula AK, Dillis C, Abraham J. Role of MRI in screening, diagnosis and management of breast cancer. Expert Rev Anticancer Ther 2008;8(5):811–817

Indications—Search for Primary Tumor

Buchanan CL, Morris EA, Dorn PL, Borgen PI, Van Zee KJ. Utility of breast magnetic resonance imaging in patients with occult primary breast cancer. Ann Surg Oncol 2005;12(12):1045–1053

Lieberman S, Sella T, Maly B, Sosna J, Uziely B, Sklair-Levy M. Breast magnetic resonance imaging characteristics in women with occult primary breast carcinoma. Isr Med Assoc J 2008;10(6):448–452

Obdeijn IM, Brouwers-Kuyper EM, Tilanus-Linthorst MM, Wiggers T, Oudkerk M. MR imaging-guided sonography followed by fine-needle aspiration cytology in occult carcinoma of the breast. AJR Am J Roentgenol 2000;174(4):1079–1084

Olson JA Jr, Morris EA, Van Zee KJ, Linehan DC, Borgen PI. Magnetic resonance imaging facilitates breast conservation for occult breast cancer. Ann Surg Oncol 2000;7(6):411–415

Varadhachary GR, Abbruzzese JL, Lenzi R. Diagnostic strategies for unknown primary cancer. Cancer 2004;100(9): 1776–1785

Indications—MRI Screening

Dall BJ, Gilbert F, Leach M, Wilson R. Technical guidelines for magnetic resonance imaging for the surveillance of women at increased risk of developing breast cancer (NHSBSP Publication No 68). Sheffield, UK: NHS Cancer Screening Programmes; 2009 http://www.rcrbreastgroup.com/Guidelines/Documents/HR_MRIsurveillanceNHSBSP.pdf

Kriege M, Brekelmans CT, Boetes C, et al; Magnetic Resonance Imaging Screening Study Group. Efficacy of MRI and mammography for breast-cancer screening in women with a familial or genetic predisposition. N Engl J Med 2004;351(5):427–437

Kuhl CK, Schrading S, Leutner CC, et al. Mammography, breast ultrasound, and magnetic resonance imaging for surveillance of women at high familial risk for breast cancer. J Clin Oncol 2005;23(33):8469–8476

Kuhl C, Weigel S, Schrading S, et al. Prospective multicenter cohort study to refine management recommendations for women at elevated familial risk of breast cancer: the EVA trial. J Clin Oncol 2010;28(9):1450–1457

Leach MO, Boggis CR, Dixon AK, et al; MARIBS study group. Screening with magnetic resonance imaging and mammography of a UK population at high familial risk of breast cancer: a prospective multicentre cohort study (MARIBS). Lancet 2005;365(9473):1769–1778

Lehman CD, Blume JD, Weatherall P, et al; International Breast MRI Consortium Working Group. Screening women at high risk for breast cancer with mammography and magnetic resonance imaging. Cancer 2005;103(9):1898–1905

Lord SJ, Lei W, Craft P, et al. A systematic review of the effectiveness of magnetic resonance imaging (MRI) as an addition to mammography and ultrasound in screening young women at high risk of breast cancer. Eur J Cancer 2007;43(13):1905–1917

National Institute for Clinical Excellence. Familial breast cancer: the classification and care of women at risk of familial breast cancer in primary, secondary and tertiary care. London: National Institute for Clinical Excellence Clinical Guideline 41; 2006 http://guidance.nice.org.uk/CG41

Passaperuma K, Warner E, Causer PA, et al. Long-term results of screening with magnetic resonance imaging in women with BRCA mutations. Br J Cancer 2012;107(1):24–30

Riedl CC, Ponhold L, Flöry D, et al. Magnetic resonance imaging of the breast improves detection of invasive cancer, preinvasive cancer, and premalignant lesions during surveillance of women at high risk for breast cancer. Clin Cancer Res 2007;13(20):6144–6152

Sardanelli F, Podo F, Santoro F, et al. Multicenter surveillance of women at high genetic breast cancer risk using mammography, ultrasonography, and contrast-enhanced magnetic resonance imaging (The High Breast Cancer Risk Italian 1 study). Final results. Invest Radiol 2011;46:94–105

Saslow D, Boetes C, Burke W, et al; American Cancer Society Breast Cancer Advisory Group. American Cancer Society guidelines for breast screening with MRI as an adjunct to mammography. CA Cancer J Clin 2007;57(2):75–89

Schmutzler RK, Rhiem K, Breuer P, et al. Outcome of a structured surveillance program in women with a familial predisposition for breast cancer. Eur J Cancer Prev 2006;15(6):483–489

Warner E, Plewes DB, Hill KAB, et al. Surveillance of BRCA1 and BRCA2 mutation carriers with magnetic resonance imaging, ultrasound, mammography, and clinical breast examination. JAMA 2004;292(11):1317–1325

Warner E, Messersmith H, Causer P, Eisen A, Shumak R, Plewes D. Systematic review: using magnetic resonance imaging to screen women at high risk for breast cancer. Ann Intern Med 2008;148(9):671–679

Indications—MRI for Staging

Bleicher RJ, Ciocca RM, Egleston BL, et al. Association of routine pretreatment magnetic resonance imaging with time to surgery, mastectomy rate, and margin status. J Am Coll Surg 2009;209(2):180–187, quiz 294–295

Brennan ME, Houssami N, Lord S, et al. Magnetic resonance imaging screening of the contralateral breast in women with newly diagnosed breast cancer: systematic review and meta-analysis of incremental cancer detection and impact on surgical management. J Clin Oncol 2009;27(33):5640–5649

Caramella T, Chapellier C, Ettore F, Raoust I, Chamorey E, Balu-Maestro C. Value of MRI in the surgical planning of invasive lobular breast carcinoma: a prospective and a retrospective study of 57 cases: comparison with physical examination, conventional imaging, and histology. Clin Imaging 2007;31(3):155–161

Fischer U, Kopka L, Grabbe E. Breast carcinoma: effect of preoperative contrast-enhanced MR imaging on the therapeutic approach. Radiology 1999;213(3):881–888

Godinez J, Gombos EC, Chikarmane SA, Griffin GK, Birdwell RL. Breast MRI in the evaluation of eligibility for accelerated partial breast irradiation. AJR Am J Roentgenol 2008;191(1):272–277

Hata T, Takahashi H, Watanabe K, et al. Magnetic resonance imaging for preoperative evaluation of breast cancer: a comparative study with mammography and ultrasonography. J Am Coll Surg 2004;199:173–174

Heywang-Köbrunner SH, Möhrling D, Nährig J. The role of MRI before breast conservation. Semin Breast Dis 2007;10(4):137–144

Hollingsworth AB, Stough RG, O'Dell CA, Brekke CE. Breast magnetic resonance imaging for preoperative locoregional staging. Am J Surg 2008;196(3):389–397

Houssami N, Ciatto S, Macaskill P, et al. Accuracy and surgical impact of magnetic resonance imaging in breast cancer staging: systematic review and meta-analysis in detection of multifocal and multicentric cancer. J Clin Oncol 2008;26(19):3248–3258

Hwang ES, Kinkel K, Esserman LJ, Lu Y, Weidner N, Hylton NM. Magnetic resonance imaging in patients diagnosed with ductal carcinoma-in-situ: value in the diagnosis of residual disease, occult invasion, and multicentricity. Ann Surg Oncol 2003;10(4):381–388

Kim JY, Cho N, Koo HR, et al. Unilateral breast cancer: screening of contralateral breast by using preoperative MR imaging reduces incidence of metachronous cancer. Radiology 2013, Jan 17 [Epub ahead of print]

Kim Y, Moon WK, Cho N, et al. MRI of the breast for the detection and assessment of the size of ductal carcinoma in situ. Korean J Radiol 2007;8(1):32–39

Lehman CD, Gatsonis C, Kuhl CK, et al; ACRIN Trial 6667 Investigators Group. MRI evaluation of the contralateral breast in women with recently diagnosed breast cancer. N Engl J Med 2007;356(13):1295–1303

Mann RM, Veltman J, Barentsz JO, Wobbes T, Blickman JG, Boetes C. The value of MRI compared to mammography in the assessment of tumour extent in invasive lobular carcinoma of the breast. Eur J Surg Oncol 2008;34(2):135–142

Pengel KE, Loo CE, Teertstra HJ, et al. The impact of preoperative MRI on breast-conserving surgery of invasive cancer: a comparative cohort study. Breast Cancer Res Treat 2009;116(1):161–169

Robertson C, Ragupathy SK, Boachie C, et al. Surveillance mammography for detecting ipsilateral breast tumour recurrence and metachronous contralateral breast cancer: a systematic review. Eur Radiol 2011;21(12):2484–2491

Sardanelli F, Giuseppetti GM, Panizza P, et al; Italian Trial for Breast MR in Multifocal/Multicentric Cancer. Sensitivity of MRI versus mammography for detecting foci of multifocal, multicentric breast cancer in fatty and dense breasts using the whole-breast pathologic examination as a gold standard. AJR Am J Roentgenol 2004;183(4):1149–1157

Schnall MD, Blume J, Bluemke DA, et al. MRI detection of distinct incidental cancer in women with primary breast cancer studied in IBMC 6883. J Surg Oncol 2005;92(1):32–38

Schouten van der Velden AP, Boetes C, Bult P, Wobbes T. The value of magnetic resonance imaging in diagnosis and size assessment of in situ and small invasive breast carcinoma. Am J Surg 2006;192(2):172–178

Solin LJ, Orel SG, Hwang WT, Harris EE, Schnall MD. Relationship of breast magnetic resonance imaging to outcome after breast-conservation treatment with radiation for women with early-stage invasive breast carcinoma or ductal carcinoma in situ. J Clin Oncol 2008;26(3):386–391

Tendulkar RD, Chellman-Jeffers M, Rybicki LA, et al. Preoperative breast magnetic resonance imaging in early breast cancer: implications for partial breast irradiation. Cancer 2009;115(8):1621–1630

Turnbull L, Brown S, Harvey I, et al. Comparative effectiveness of MRI in breast cancer (COMICE) trial: a randomised controlled trial. Lancet 2010;375(9714):563–571

Van Goethem M, Schelfout K, Dijckmans L, et al. MR mammography in the pre-operative staging of breast cancer in patients with dense breast tissue: comparison with mammography and ultrasound. Eur Radiol 2004;14(5):809–816

Van Goethem M, Schelfout K, Kersschot E, et al. MR mammography is useful in the preoperative locoregional staging of breast carcinomas with extensive intraductal component. Eur J Radiol 2007;62(2):273–282

Veronesi U, Cascinelli N, Mariani L, et al. Twenty-year follow-up of a randomized study comparing breast-conserving surgery with radical mastectomy for early breast cancer. N Engl J Med 2002;347(16):1227–1232

Indications—Problem-Solving after Breast Conservation or Silicon Implant

Belli P, Costantini M, Romani M, Marano P, Pastore G. Magnetic resonance imaging in breast cancer recurrence. Breast Cancer Res Treat 2002;73(3):223–235

Boné B, Aspelin P, Isberg B, Perbeck L, Veress B. Contrast-enhanced MR imaging of the breast in patients with breast implants after cancer surgery. Acta Radiol 1995;36(2):111–116

Drew PJ, Kerin MJ, Turnbull LW, et al. Routine screening for local recurrence following breast-conserving therapy for cancer with dynamic contrast-enhanced magnetic resonance imaging of the breast. Ann Surg Oncol 1998;5(3):265–270

Heinig A, Heywang-Köbrunner SH, Viehweg P, Lampe D, Buchmann J, Spielmann RP. Value of contrast medium magnetic resonance tomography of the breast in breast reconstruction with implant. Radiologe 1997;37(9):710–717 [Article in German]

Herborn CU, Marincek B, Erfmann D, et al. Breast augmentation and reconstructive surgery: MR imaging of implant rupture and malignancy. Eur Radiol 2002;12(9):2198–2206

Houssami N, Ciatto S, Martinelli F, Bonardi R, Duffy SW. Early detection of second breast cancers improves prognosis in breast cancer survivors. Ann Oncol 2009;20(9):1505–1510

Krämer S, Schulz-Wendtland R, Hagedorn K, Bautz W, Lang N. Magnetic resonance imaging in the diagnosis of local recurrences in breast cancer. Anticancer Res 1998;18(3C):2159–2161

Morakkabati N, Leutner CC, Schmiedel A, Schild HH, Kuhl CK. Breast MR imaging during or soon after radiation therapy. Radiology 2003;229(3):893–901

Preda L, Villa G, Rizzo S, et al. Magnetic resonance mammography in the evaluation of recurrence at the prior lumpectomy site after conservative surgery and radiotherapy. Breast Cancer Res 2006;8(5):R53

Viehweg P, Heinig A, Lampe D, Buchmann J, Heywang-Köbrunner SH. Retrospective analysis for evaluation of the value of contrast-enhanced MRI in patients treated with breast conservative therapy. MAGMA 1998;7(3):141–152

Indications—Implant Failure

Berg WA, Nguyen TK, Middleton MS, Soo MS, Pennello G, Brown SL. MR imaging of extracapsular silicone from breast implants: diagnostic pitfalls. AJR Am J Roentgenol 2002;178(2):465–472

Brinton LA, Malone KE, Coates RJ, et al. Breast enlargement and reduction: results from a breast cancer case-control study. Plast Reconstr Surg 1996;97(2):269–275

Caskey CI, Berg WA, Hamper UM, Sheth S, Chang BW, Anderson ND. Imaging spectrum of extracapsular silicone: correlation of US, MR imaging, mammographic, and histopathologic findings. Radiographics 1999;19(Spec No):S39–S51, quiz S261–S262

Cher DJ, Conwell JA, Mandel JS. MRI for detecting silicone breast implant rupture: meta-analysis and implications. Ann Plast Surg 2001;47(4):367–380

Friis S, Hölmich LR, McLaughlin JK, et al. Cancer risk among Danish women with cosmetic breast implants. Int J Cancer 2006;118(4):998–1003

Glynn C, Litherland J. Imaging breast augmentation and reconstruction. Br J Radiol 2008;81(967):587–595

Hölmich LR, Vejborg I, Conrad C, Sletting S, McLaughlin JK. The diagnosis of breast implant rupture: MRI findings compared with findings at explantation. Eur J Radiol 2005;53(2):213–225

Indications—Monitoring of Neoadjuvant Chemotherapy

Baek HM, Chen JH, Nie K, et al. Predicting pathologic response to neoadjuvant chemotherapy in breast cancer by using MR imaging and quantitative 1H MR spectroscopy. Radiology 2009;251(3):653–662

Bahri S, Chen JH, Mehta RS, et al. Residual breast cancer diagnosed by MRI in patients receiving neoadjuvant chemotherapy with and without bevacizumab. Ann Surg Oncol 2009;16(6):1619–1628

Belli P, Costantini M, Malaspina C, Magistrelli A, Latorre G, Bonomo L. MRI accuracy in residual disease evaluation in breast cancer patients treated with neoadjuvant chemotherapy. Clin Radiol 2006;61(11):946–953

Beresford M, Padhani AR, Goh V, Makris A. Imaging breast cancer response during neoadjuvant systemic therapy. Expert Rev Anticancer Ther 2005;5(5):893–905

Bhattacharyya M, Ryan D, Carpenter R, Vinnicombe S, Gallagher CJ. Using MRI to plan breast-conserving surgery following neoadjuvant chemotherapy for early breast cancer. Br J Cancer 2008;98(2):289–293

Chen JH, Feig B, Agrawal G, et al. MRI evaluation of pathologically complete response and residual tumors in breast cancer after neoadjuvant chemotherapy. Cancer 2008;112(1):17–26

Chen JH, Feig BA, Hsiang DJ, et al. Impact of MRI-evaluated neoadjuvant chemotherapy response on change of surgical recommendation in breast cancer. Ann Surg 2009;249(3):448–454

Denis F, Desbiez-Bourcier AV, Chapiron C, Arbion F, Body G, Brunereau L. Contrast enhanced magnetic resonance imaging underestimates residual disease following neoadjuvant docetaxel based chemotherapy for breast cancer. Eur J Surg Oncol 2004;30(10):1069–1076

Eisenhauer EA, Therasse P, Bogaerts J, et al. New response evaluation criteria in solid tumours: Revised RECIST guideline (version 1.1). Eur J Cancer 2009; 45(2) 228–247

Hattangadi J, Park C, Rembert J, et al. Breast stromal enhancement on MRI is associated with response to neoadjuvant chemotherapy. AJR Am J Roentgenol 2008;190(6):1630–1636

Kim HJ, Im YH, Han BK, et al. Accuracy of MRI for estimating residual tumor size after neoadjuvant chemotherapy in locally advanced breast cancer: relation to response patterns on MRI. Acta Oncol 2007;46(7):996–1003

Lobbes MB, Prevos R, Smidt M, et al. The role of magnetic resonance imaging in assessing residual disease and pathologic complete response in breast cancer patients receiving neoadjuvant chemotherapy: a systematic review. Insights Imaging 2013, Jan 29 [Epub ahead of print]

Manton DJ, Chaturvedi A, Hubbard A, et al. Neoadjuvant chemotherapy in breast cancer: early response prediction with quantitative MR imaging and spectroscopy. Br J Cancer 2006;94(3):427–435

Marinovich ML, Sardanelli F, Ciatto S, et al. Early prediction of pathologic response to neoadjuvant therapy in breast cancer: systematic review of the accuracy of MRI. Breast 2012;21(5):669–677

Meisamy S, Bolan PJ, Baker EH, et al. Neoadjuvant chemotherapy of locally advanced breast cancer: predicting response with in vivo (1)H MR spectroscopy—a pilot study at 4 T. Radiology 2004;233(2):424–431

Nakamura S, Kenjo H, Nishio T, Kazama T, Doi O, Suzuki K. Efficacy of 3D-MR mammography for breast conserving surgery after neoadjuvant chemotherapy. Breast Cancer 2002;9(1):15–19

Pickles MD, Gibbs P, Lowry M, Turnbull LW. Diffusion changes precede size reduction in neoadjuvant treatment of breast cancer. Magn Reson Imaging 2006;24(7):843–847

Schott AF, Roubidoux MA, Helvie MA, et al. Clinical and radiologic assessments to predict breast cancer pathologic complete response to neoadjuvant chemotherapy. Breast Cancer Res Treat 2005;92(3):231–238

Segara D, Krop IE, Garber JE, et al. Does MRI predict pathologic tumor response in women with breast cancer undergoing preoperative chemotherapy? J Surg Oncol 2007;96(6):474–480

Sharma U, Danishad KK, Seenu V, Jagannathan NR. Longitudinal study of the assessment by MRI and diffusion-weighted imaging of tumor response in patients with locally advanced breast cancer undergoing neoadjuvant chemotherapy. NMR Biomed 2009;22(1):104–113

Straver ME, van Adrichem JC, Rutgers EJ, et al. Neoadjuvant systemic therapy in patients with operable primary breast cancer: more benefits than breast-conserving therapy. [Article in Dutch] Ned Tijdschr Geneeskd 2008;152(46):2519–2525

Therasse P, Arbuck SG, Eisenhauer EA, et al. New guidelines to evaluate the response to treatment in solid tumors. J Natl Cancer Inst 2000;92(3):205–216

Uematsu T, Kasami M, Yuen S. Neoadjuvant chemotherapy for breast cancer: correlation between the baseline MR imaging findings and responses to therapy. Eur Radiol 2010;20(10):2315–2322

Yeh E, Slanetz P, Kopans DB, et al. Prospective comparison of mammography, sonography, and MRI in patients undergoing neoadjuvant chemotherapy for palpable breast cancer. AJR Am J Roentgenol 2005;184(3):868–877

Further Indications

Ballesio L, Maggi C, Savelli S, et al. Role of breast magnetic resonance imaging (MRI) in patients with unilateral nipple discharge: preliminary study. Radiol Med (Torino) 2008;113(2):249–264

Baum F, Fischer U, Füzesi L, Obenauer S, Vosshenrich R, Grabbe E. The radial scar in contrast media-enhanced MR mammography. Rofo 2000;172(10):817–823 [Article in German]

Buchberger W, DeKoekkoek-Doll P, Obrist P, Dünser M. Value of MR tomography in inconclusive mammography findings. Radiologe 1997;37(9):702–709 [Article in German]

Cilotti A, Iacconi C, Marini C, et al. Contrast-enhanced MR imaging in patients with BI-RADS 3–5 microcalcifications. Radiol Med (Torino) 2007;112(2):272–286

DeMartini W, Lehman C. A review of current evidence-based clinical applications for breast magnetic resonance imaging. Top Magn Reson Imaging 2008;19(3):143–150

Flamm CR, Ziegler KM, Aronson N. Technology Evaluation Center assessment synopsis: use of magnetic resonance imaging to avoid a biopsy in women with suspicious primary breast lesions. J Am Coll Radiol 2005;2(6):485–487

Gökalp G, Topal U. MR imaging in probably benign lesions (BI-RADS category 3) of the breast. Eur J Radiol 2006;57(3):436–444

Heywang-Köbrunner SH, Viehweg P, Heinig A, Küchler C. Contrast-enhanced MRI of the breast: accuracy, value, controversies, solutions. Eur J Radiol 1997;24(2):94–108

Hrung JM, Sonnad SS, Schwartz JS, Langlotz CP. Accuracy of MR imaging in the work-up of suspicious breast lesions: a diagnostic meta-analysis. Acad Radiol 1999;6(7):387–397

Morrogh M, Morris EA, Liberman L, Van Zee K, Cody HS III, King TA. MRI identifies otherwise occult disease in select patients with Paget disease of the nipple. J Am Coll Surg 2008;206(2):316–321

Moy L, Elias K, Patel V, et al. Is breast MRI helpful in the evaluation of inconclusive mammographic findings? AJR Am J Roentgenol 2009;193(4):986–993

Nakahara H, Namba K, Watanabe R, et al. A comparison of MR imaging, galactography and ultrasonography in patients with nipple discharge. Breast Cancer 2003;10(4):320–329

Orel SG, Reynolds C, Schnall MD, Solin LJ, Fraker DL, Sullivan DC. Breast carcinoma: MR imaging before re-excisional biopsy. Radiology 1997;205(2):429–436

Pediconi F, Catalano C, Occhiato R, et al. Breast lesion detection and characterization at contrast-enhanced MR mammography: gadobenate dimeglumine versus gadopentetate dimeglumine. Radiology 2005;237(1):45–56

Perfetto F, Fiorentino F, Urbano F, Silecchia R. Adjunctive diagnostic value of MRI in the breast radial scar. Radiol Med (Torino) 2009;114(5):757–770

Uematsu T, Yuen S, Kasami M, Uchida Y. Dynamic contrast-enhanced MR imaging in screening detected microcalcification lesions of the breast: is there any value? Breast Cancer Res Treat 2007;103(3):269–281

Zakhireh J, Gomez R, Esserman L. Converting evidence to practice: a guide for the clinical application of MRI for the screening and management of breast cancer. Eur J Cancer 2008;44(18):2742–2752

6 Emerging Technologies in Breast Imaging

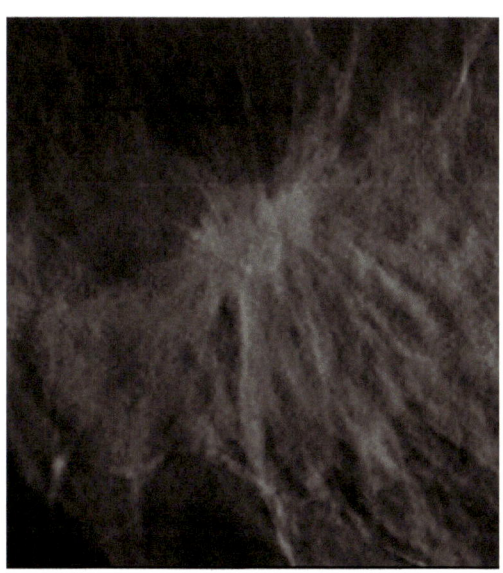

Introduction 178
Mammography 178
Digital Breast Tomosynthesis 178
Dual Energy Mammography (Spectral Mammography) 180
Contrast-Enhanced Digital Mammography 180

Ultrasound 180
Sonoelastography 181
Automated Whole Breast and 3D Ultrasound 181

Magnetic Resonance Imaging 181
Diffusion-Weighted imaging 181
Magnetic Resonance Elastography 182
Magnetic Resonance Spectroscopy 182

Nuclear Medicine 182
Breast-Specific Gamma Imaging 182
Positron Emission Mammography 182

References and Recommended Reading 183

6 Emerging Technologies in Breast Imaging

F. Kilburn-Toppin, S. Barter

Introduction

Breast imaging has undergone considerable evolution since the introduction of the mammogram over a quarter of a century ago. Breast imaging is continuously progressing as new modalities, and advances in applications of established modalities, are developed. Improved technologies have helped to individualize evaluation of breast lesions as well as treatment, improving efficacy while minimizing morbidity and mortality. Here we provide an overview of the latest developments in breast imaging, highlighting the evidence behind them and their potential future applications in breast imaging.

Mammography

Film mammography has been the gold standard for breast cancer screening for many years. However there are well-recognized limitations to this modality, most notably in the detection of cancers in women with radiographically dense breasts (Sree et al. 2011). There have been continuing efforts to improve this technology to overcome these problems, and the introduction of digital mammography has led to many benefits. These include more practical aspects, such as easier storage and transfer of images, as well as diagnostic benefits with increased cancer detection rates, particularly in younger women with denser breast tissue (Hall 2012).

Digital mammography has allowed the development of several derivative technologies including digital tomosynthesis and contrast-enhanced digital mammography (Helvie 2010).

Digital Breast Tomosynthesis

Digital breast tomosynthesis (DBT) provides three-dimensional (3D) information on breast tissue, with the premise of improving detection of lesions obscured by overlying dense breast tissue. The basic principle behind the technique involves rotating an X-ray tube through a limited arc angle while obtaining a series of exposures through a compressed breast. These raw projection image datasets are then reconstructed using specific algorithms into slices of variable thickness for the radiologist to view. Masses that may otherwise be obscured by superimposed breast tissue should be more easily visible in the thin-section reconstructed slice. Each exposure should be only a fraction of the dose used in conventional digital mammography, so that the overall dose is similar or just slightly higher than in conventional digital mammography. The potential benefits of tomosynthesis include superior detection of mammographic masses, thereby improving screening sensitivity. It also offers the possibility of a reduction in false positive recalls by allowing better characterization of detected lesions.

Recent research has demonstrated that DBT can more accurately assess breast cancer size and stage than conventional mammography (Förnvik et al. 2010). DBT has been shown to improve detection rate of cancers in women with dense breasts when using supplemental tomosynthesis in addition to standard digital mammography (**Fig. 6.1**) (Rafferty and Nicklason 2011) and has comparable sensitivity in the detection of noncalcified breast lesions when compared with digital mammography performed with additional views (Sumkin et al. 2011). Other studies have shown equal or even superior detection of calcifications when compared with conventional mammography, with the possibility of improved interpretation of calcific lesions (Kopans et al. 2011). The use of tomosynthesis when combined with digital mammography has been observed to reduce recall rates by up to 30%, with less of a reduction when used alone (**Fig. 6.2**) (Gur et al. 2009). The results of a small study suggest that the performance of DBT may be comparable to that of clinical mammographic spot views for breast mass characterization, implying that spot views may not be necessary when performing DBT and women may be spared from being recalled and exposed to increased radiation (Noroozian et al. 2012).

However, other studies have not demonstrated any convincing evidence that use of digital breast tomosynthesis alone or in combination with digital mammography results in a substantial improvement in sensitivity. A recent trial comparing two-view tomosynthesis with digital mammography demonstrated an improvement in detection of masses and calcification but only for readers with the least experience, with no differences in classification accuracy when comparing single-view tomosynthesis (Wallis et al. 2012). Research into the use of tomosynthesis in women with abnormal mammograms or clinical symptoms suggests that it can be used as an additional technique to mammography but, depending on patient selection, it is unlikely to detect a substantial number of additional cancers that would not have been detected by other methods (Teertstra et al. 2010).

There are other clinical considerations to take into account, including increased radiologist reading time for DBT images (Tingberg et al. 2011), although some studies have felt this increased time to be acceptable even in

Mammography

high-volume screening (Michell et al. 2009). And some studies have shown radiologist preference for DBT images (Andersson et al. 2008).

Computer-aided detection (CAD) may play a more significant role in DBT than in conventional mammography, given the increased number of images to view as well as the better visualization of lesion margins. CAD systems have been developed for DBT which in some instances have proved to be better than those for digital mammography systems (Chan et al. 2008). However, as with conventional mammography, CAD will remain a supplemental tool rather than a main reader.

Different proposals for utilizing DBT in clinical practice are being investigated. Large-scale clinical trials are currently under way. The first results from such trials and from ongoing screening trials report substantially improved detection rates and are thus quite promising (Svahn et al. 2012, Houssami and Skane 2013).

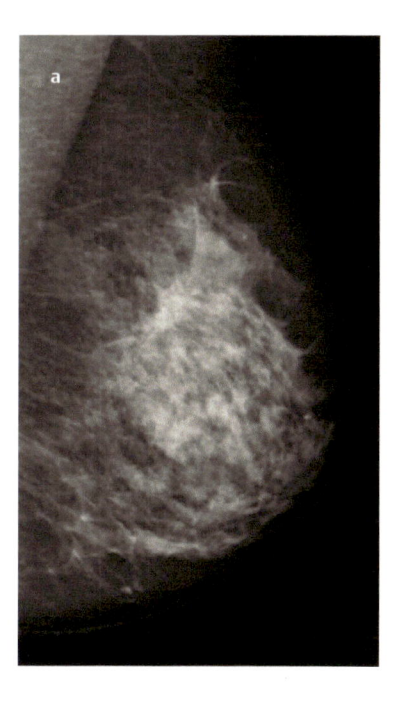

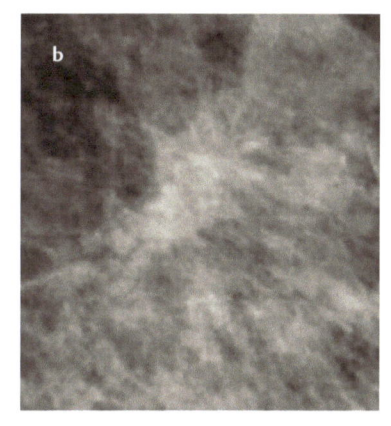

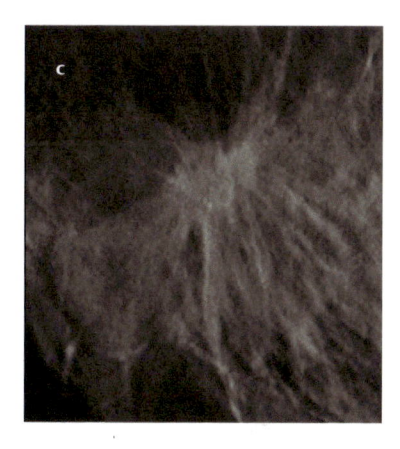

Fig. 6.1a–c

a Left mammogram (mediolateral oblique view) showing a dense breast with a possible area of distortion and asymmetry.
b A conventional magnification/paddle view demonstrates a probable area of distortion.
c The tomosynthesis clearly demonstrates a spiculate mass.
Images courtesy of Dr Matthew Wallis, Cambridge Breast Unit, Addenbrookes Hospital, UK.

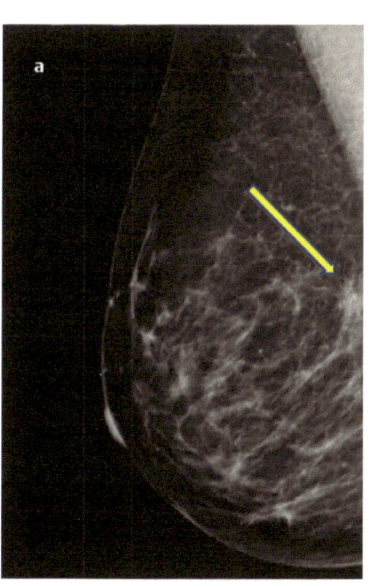

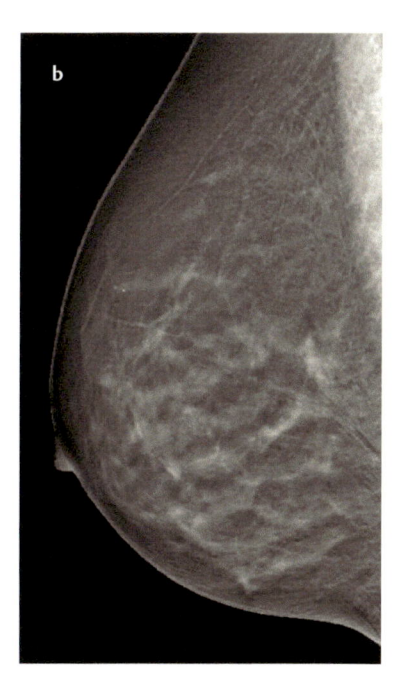

Fig. 6.2a,b

a Right mammogram (mediolateral oblique view) showing a possible spiculate mass posteriorly (arrow).
b The tomosynthesis view clearly demonstrates this was due to superimposition of glandular tissue.

Dual Energy Mammography (Spectral Mammography)

Dual energy or spectral mammography is being developed by some manufacturers. One technique exploits photon counting, whereby the pulses created by each photon emitted from the X-ray source are registered as they are absorbed in the X-ray sensor. A threshold is used to discriminate these pulses from the detector noise. The magnitude of each pulse is proportional to the energy of the photon. In spectral imaging an additional threshold is used to obtain information from high- and low-energy photons. Thus, the spectral imaging system generates one high-energy image and one low-energy image from each single exposure. These can be added into a normal mammogram (Fredenberg et al. 2010). The information in the two images can be used to distinguish between materials in the breast and also remove the contrast of, for instance, the glandular structures by subtraction.

There is also a possible clinical application of using a contrast agent, and subtracting pre- and postcontrast enhanced images to obtain clinical information (Schmitzberger et al. 2011) (see below).

An advantage of unenhanced spectral imaging using photon counting is that it is acquired in the same exposure as the normal mammographic view and therefore can be seen as a bonus to conventional mammography with no additional radiation burden to the patient. Therefore, in the large screening population, even if the benefit of spectral imaging is small, it is potentially beneficial.

Current research is focusing on breast density and using spectral imaging to characterize breast masses. Increased breast density is recognized as an independent risk factor for developing breast cancer. An objective and accurate measure of breast density is readily available with spectral imaging. It is expected that density measures will play an important role when investigating more personalized screening approaches. Potentially, spectral imaging will be able to characterize fluid-containing masses, that is, cysts in the breast, avoiding recall for simple cysts not clearly delineated on conventional mammography (Norell et al. 2012).

The evaluation of this technique is in its early stages but shows promise.

Contrast-Enhanced Digital Mammography

Another potential derivative of digital mammography is contrast-enhanced digital mammography (CEDM). This uses the advantages of contrast information on malignant neovascularity combined with anatomical information. Dynamic contrast-enhanced MRI is already routinely used for the assessment of tumor vascularity in specific patient groups, but despite its high sensitivity it has relatively low specificity and limitations in the detection of ductal carcinoma in situ. Contrast-enhanced MRI also has the associated issues of cost and patient acceptability. Two techniques of CEDM are available, both of which use iodinated contrast material and modified digital mammography units. The first method involves the temporal subtraction of images before and after contrast administration, allowing contrast curves to be obtained by a similar method to contrast-enhanced breast MRI. The method is limited both by potential motion misregistration artifacts as well as by imaging only a single projection at a time. The second spectral imaging dual energy technique makes use of different iodine k-edge X-ray absorption at high and low energies, and requires the use of a modified mammographic machine which can produce higher-energy images in addition to standard mammograms. This technique involves pairs of low- and high-energy images acquired after contrast administration being subtracted from each other, and has the benefit over temporal CEDM of allowing multiple views to be obtained.

Initial clinical results show that CEDM has better diagnostic accuracy than mammography alone or mammography with ultrasound (Dromain et al. 2011). Further research has shown that the addition of dynamic digital subtraction mammography to conventional mammography can significantly improve diagnostic quality, with increased sensitivity particularly pronounced in the women with dense breast tissue (Diekmann et al. 2011). Recent studies have demonstrated the benefit of combining tomosynthesis with CEDM, limiting the effect of surrounding soft tissue and achieving higher contrast between tumor and surrounding tissue (Schmitzberger et al. 2011).

The disadvantages of CEDM are the need for contrast medium and its potential adverse consequences, as well as the increased time, cost and radiation dose of the examination when compared with standard digital mammography. The lack of standardized diagnostic criteria and imaging protocols for CEDM has also been highlighted, which would need to be addressed before it is incorporated into mainstream imaging.

Ultrasound

Ultrasound is an invaluable tool for the detection, characterization, and image-guided biopsy of breast lesions. Although the Breast Imaging Reporting and Data System (BI-RADS) provides standardized ultrasound terminology to describe lesion features and subsequent investigation recommendations, the technique is still limited by the overlapping features of benign and malignant lesions as well as inter-operative variability. Various advancements in ultrasound technology have been developed in an attempt to overcome these limitations, including 3D ultrasound, automated ultrasound for overall breast views, and sonoelastography.

Sonoelastography

Sonoelastography was first introduced in 1991, and has been used in a clinical setting since 1997. It works on the basis that breast cancers tend to be stiff, whereas benign masses tend to be soft. Elastographic methods function by applying pressure to displace tissue, then monitoring the movement produced in the tissue. The rate of change in the amount of tissue displacement as a function of distance from the transducer is known as tissue strain. The strain data are converted into color images and superimposed on the standard B-mode images to create a mapped image of tissue stiffness.

Studies have shown that lesion stiffness detected with sonoelastography correlates with the malignant potential of the lesion, and has higher specificity than B-mode ultrasound in distinguishing benign from malignant masses. It has also been shown to potentially help reduce the number of biopsies with benign results (Yi et al. 2012). However, in hand-held techniques, the limitation of sonoelastography lies with the issue of inter-observer variability. The newly emerging technique of shear wave elastography (SWE) aims to substantially reduce operative dependence compared with standard static elastography.

In SWE an electronically generated acoustic impulse is produced which causes deformation of the tissues, leading to slow-moving lateral shear waves. The speed of propagation of the wave is proportional to the square root of the tissue's elastic modulus. Imaging of the propagation of shear waves allows measurement of the changes in velocity that occur when the waves pass through tissues of different stiffness.

This technique has been shown to be highly reproducible (Cosgrove et al. 2012). A recent multinational trial has shown very promising results, with the addition of shear wave elastography increasing the specificity of breast mass assessment. It has helped to identify the few malignancies among well-circumscribed lesions which would otherwise be assessed on ultrasound as low suspicion, and is suggested to allow the reduction of unnecessary biopsies of BI-RADS category 4a lesions (Berg et al. 2012).

Color Doppler is considered a useful adjunct to conventional ultrasound in differentiating benign from malignant masses, identifying features including both peripheral and central vascularity, and the presence of penetrating and branching vessels. A recent study has shown that the combined use of color Doppler with sonoelastography may increase diagnostic performance in distinguishing benign from malignant masses detected at ultrasound. The authors also suggest that simple follow-up can be recommended in lesions of low suspicion at ultrasound, when no stiffness or vascularity is seen.

Automated Whole Breast and 3D Ultrasound

New automated whole breast ultrasound (ABUS) machines have recently been developed. These allow the acquisition of a volume dataset of the whole breast in a standard manner, eliminating inter-observer variability and allowing more efficient use of time by radiologists interpreting the studies. Studies comparing ABUS and conventional hand-held ultrasound have shown that the automated breast scanner provides advantages of high diagnostic accuracy, better lesion size prediction, operator independence, and visualization of the whole breast (Lin et al. 2012). The automated systems are able to select individual diagnostic planes to provide 3D images, combining multiple different scan planes to allow the breast to be displayed as a volumetric image. This has the potential advantage of improved analysis of tumor margins and ductal structure, with a better appreciation of tumor volume, which is useful for monitoring patients undergoing neoadjuvant chemotherapy. The use of 3D ultrasound imaging may also help to differentiate benign from malignant lesions on the basis of their effect on surrounding tissue, with malignant lesions tending to invade adjacent parenchyma, causing a stellate appearance on 3D images. Recent research has demonstrated that automated 3D ultrasound is at least on a par, in terms of diagnostic accuracy, with standard hand-held ultrasound (Stöblen et al. 2011).

Potential future benefits include 3D US-guided techniques for breast biopsy and a computer-aided diagnosis system for the classification of breast masses in 3D ABUS images, which are currently being developed and show promising early results (Moon et al. 2011).

Magnetic Resonance Imaging

(See also Chapter 5.)

MRI now has an established role in the imaging of breast cancer following the development of surface coils, contrast agents, and faster imaging sequences. Although not used routinely for screening, contrast-enhanced MRI has shown benefit in select patient groups, including the screening of high-risk patients and to look for disease recurrence. New developments involving MR imaging technology have shown promising results.

Diffusion-Weighted Imaging

Diffusion-weighted imaging (DWI) is used for evaluating a wide variety of malignancies, providing functional information to complement MR anatomical information. When used in conjunction with apparent diffusion coefficient (ADC) mapping, DWI can aid in tumor detection and characterization. The use of DWI in breast imaging was introduced over 20 years ago, but only recently has it been shown that the average ADC value is higher for benign lesions than for malignant ones (Malayeri et al. 2011). Studies have shown that DWI may improve the diagnostic accuracy of conventional MRI, with ADC measurements used to differentiate benign from malignant breast masses (Sonmez et al. 2011). The difficulty lies in determining the optimum range of b-values for evaluation of breast malignancies, and recent studies have shown that the optimum ADC cutoff value for differentiating lesions is different for different b-values (Pereira et al. 2011). Research has shown promise in using DWI to determine tumor response to neoadjuvant chemotherapy, as well as predicting tumor response to treatment (Sharma et al. 2009, Park et al. 2010).

Magnetic Resonance Elastography

Magnetic resonance elastography is an experimental but developing technology which, similar to ultrasound elastography, obtains information about tissue stiffness for lesion characterization (Mariappan et al. 2010). Images are created using propagated shear waves in tissue to create quantitative maps of tissue stiffness. Shear waves with frequencies of 50–500 Hz are generated by an external driver, which is synchronized to the MR pulse sequence. This technology has been used clinically for the assessment of hepatic fibrosis, but is being investigated as a complementary technique to contrast-enhanced MRI of the breast and has shown promising results to increase diagnostic specificity (Sinkus et al. 2007).

Magnetic Resonance Spectroscopy

Magnetic resonance spectroscopy (MRS) is a technique used to assess metabolite levels of tissues in vivo, using equipment similar to that for standard MRI but with sequences for spectroscopic signal acquisition to measure the distribution of a particular metabolite in a volume of interest. Multiple studies have demonstrated that malignant lesions have higher levels of choline-containing compounds than their benign counterparts, and levels of upstream intermediates, primarily phosphocholine (pCho), are elevated in breast malignancy (Haddadin et al. 2009). MRS has been shown to further improve the specificity of MRI, as well as evaluating the response to breast cancer therapy (Bartella and Huang 2007). The use of 3 Tesla (3T) MRI to improve signal-to-noise ratio and the addition of quantitative analysis of choline levels has led to improved choline detection and more specific discrimination between benign and malignant lesions (Meisamy et al. 2005). Further work is still needed, however, before this technique becomes more widely used in a clinical setting.

Nuclear Medicine

Nuclear medicine is widely used in oncologic imaging, for diagnosis, planning of treatment, and assessment of treatment response (Tafreshi et al. 2010). Radiolabeled ligands are imaged using planar gamma cameras (scintigraphy) or single photon emission computed tomography (SPECT) systems to produce 3D images, and an idea of physiologic and functional response as well as anatomical information.

Breast-Specific Gamma Imaging

Technetium ($^{99}Tc^m$)-sestamibi is taken up by active mitochondria in breast malignancies; however, this technique has relatively poor sensitivity for small lesions owing to the absence of breast compression and the inability to have the detector near to the breast. Dedicated breast-specific gamma camera imaging (BSGI) systems have therefore been developed to overcome these problems, and allow detectors to be positioned on the breast with compression. This new technology has led to rejuvenated interest in scintimammography with promising preliminary results. Studies have shown increased sensitivity of BSGI detection of small tumors compared with standard gamma cameras (Brem et al. 2006), as well as similar sensitivity and better specificity than MRI in patients with equivocal mammograms. These results suggest that BSGI may play a future role in the imaging of patients with dense breasts, in whom mammogram sensitivity is reduced.

However, these studies have used standard dosages of the tracer. This leads to a much higher dosage than that needed for digital mammography. In a 40-year-old patient it has been estimated there is a 20- to 30-fold increased risk of radiation-induced breast cancer compared with digital mammography. Furthermore, by using tracers, a small but not negligible radiation dosage is also applied to the whole body including the ovaries (ICRP 1998, Hendrick 2010). The dosage to the ovaries ranges around 6–9 mGy, while the whole body equivalent dosage ranges around 6 mGy.

Whether the reported accuracy might be maintained with the use of a lower dose of tracer requires further investigation and possible developments in technology.

Before this method is considered for routine use or for any type of screening these issues need to be addressed.

Positron Emission Mammography

Positron emission tomography (PET) is used as an adjunct imaging tool for the detection and staging of breast cancer, and assessing response to treatment; however, it is limited by its sensitivity in the detection of small lesions (Fass 2008). Positron emission mammography (PEM) uses a similar principle to that of PET by using

¹⁸F-fludeoxyglucose (FDG) (fluorodeoxyglucose) to characterize malignant lesions, but has much improved spatial resolution since the detectors are placed directly on the breast, allowing gentle compression. This also has the benefit of allowing direct correlation with mammograms, and reconstructed 3D images. Results have shown high diagnostic accuracy for the detection of breast lesions, including ductal carcinoma in situ (Berg et al. 2006). Furthermore the development of new radiotracers to target cell proliferation, angiogenesis, and hypoxia, as well as estrogen receptors, offers promising advances in providing information on optimal therapeutic management and prognosis (Jordan and Brodie 2007).

The issues of radiation dose are the same as those described for scintimammography. Dose reduction studies will be need to be evaluated.

Summary

Technological advances in medical imaging such as digital breast tomosynthesis and sonoelastography are well under way, and have shown definite potential benefits in breast cancer detection and reduced recall rates. Other emerging technologies are still in more experimental stages, and further prospective trials to address appropriate patient selection and practical applications are needed prior to widespread clinical use. Ongoing research into new diagnostic technologies offers promising opportunities for the continued advancement of breast imaging.

References and Recommended Reading

Andersson I, Ikeda DM, Zackrisson S, et al. Breast tomosynthesis and digital mammography: a comparison of breast cancer visibility and BIRADS classification in a population of cancers with subtle mammographic findings. Eur Radiol 2008;18(12):2817–2825

Bartella L, Huang W. Proton (1H) MR spectroscopy of the breast. Radiographics 2007;27(Suppl 1):S241–S252

Berg WA, Weinberg IN, Narayanan D, et al; Positron Emission Mammography Working Group. High-resolution fluorodeoxyglucose positron emission tomography with compression ("positron emission mammography") is highly accurate in depicting primary breast cancer. Breast J 2006;12(4):309–323

Berg WA, Cosgrove DO, Doré CJ, et al; BE1 Investigators. Shear-wave elastography improves the specificity of breast US: the BE1 multinational study of 939 masses. Radiology 2012;262(2):435–449

Brem RF, Michener KH, Zawistowski G. Approaches to improving breast cancer diagnosis using a high resolution, breast specific gamma camera. Phys Med 2006;21 Suppl 1:17–19

Chan HP, Wei J, Zhang Y, et al. Computer-aided detection of masses in digital tomosynthesis mammography: comparison of three approaches. Med Phys 2008;35(9):4087–4095

Cosgrove DO, Berg WA, Doré CJ, et al; BE1 Study Group. Shear wave elastography for breast masses is highly reproducible. Eur Radiol 2012;22(5):1023–1032

Diekmann F, Freyer M, Diekmann S, et al. Evaluation of contrast-enhanced digital mammography. Eur J Radiol 2011;78(1):112–121

Dromain C, Thibault F, Muller S, et al. Dual-energy contrast-enhanced digital mammography: initial clinical results. Eur Radiol 2011;21(3):565–574

Fass L. Imaging and cancer: a review. Mol Oncol 2008;2(2):115–152

Förnvik D, Zackrisson S, Ljungberg O, et al. Breast tomosynthesis: accuracy of tumor measurement compared with digital mammography and ultrasonography. Acta Radiol 2010;51(3):240–247

Fredenberg E, Hemmendorff M, Cederström B, Aslund M, Danielsson M. Contrast-enhanced spectral mammography with a photon-counting detector. Med Phys 2010;37(5):2017–2029

Gur D, Abrams GS, Chough DM, et al. Digital breast tomosynthesis: observer performance study. AJR Am J Roentgenol 2009;193(2):586–591

Haddadin IS, McIntosh A, Meisamy S, et al. Metabolite quantification and high-field MRS in breast cancer. NMR Biomed 2009;22(1):65–76

Hall FM. Transition to digital mammography. Radiology 2012;262(1):374, author reply 374

Helvie MA. Digital mammography imaging: breast tomosynthesis and advanced applications. Radiol Clin North Am 2010;48(5):917–929

Hendrick RE. Radiation doses and cancer risks from breast imaging studies. Radiology 2010;257(1):246–253

Houssami N, Skaane P. Overview of the evidence on digital breast tomosynthesis in breast cancer detection. Breast 2013;22(2):101-108

ICRP [International Commission on Radiological Protection]. Radiation dose to patients from radiopharmaceuticals (addendum 2 to ICRP publication 53). Ann ICRP 1998;28(3):1–126

Jordan VC, Brodie AM. Development and evolution of therapies targeted to the estrogen receptor for the treatment and prevention of breast cancer. Steroids 2007;72(1):7–25

Kopans D, Gavenonis S, Halpern E, Moore R. Calcifications in the breast and digital breast tomosynthesis. Breast J 2011;17(6):638–644

Lin X, Wang J, Han F, Fu J, Li A. Analysis of eighty-one cases with breast lesions using automated breast volume scanner and comparison with handheld ultrasound. Eur J Radiol 2012;81(5):873–878

Malayeri AA, El Khouli RH, Zaheer A, et al. Principles and applications of diffusion-weighted imaging in cancer detection, staging, and treatment follow-up. Radiographics 2011;31(6):1773–1791

Mariappan YK, Glaser KJ, Ehman RL. Magnetic resonance elastography: a review. Clin Anat 2010;23(5):497–511

Meisamy S, Bolan PJ, Baker EH, et al. Adding in vivo quantitative 1H MR spectroscopy to improve diagnostic accuracy of breast MR imaging: preliminary results of observer performance study at 4.0 T. Radiology 2005;236(2):465–475

Michell M, Wasan R, Whelehan P, et al. Digital breast tomosynthesis: a comparison of the accuracy of digital breast tomosynthesis, two-dimensional digital mammography and two-dimensional screening mammography (film-screen). Breast Cancer Res 2009;11(Suppl 2):O1–O6, P1–P33

Moon WK, Shen YW, Huang CS, Chiang LR, Chang RF. Computer-aided diagnosis for the classification of breast masses in automated whole breast ultrasound images. Ultrasound Med Biol 2011;37(4):539–548

Norell B, Fredenberg E, Cederstrom B, Leifland K, Lundqvist M. Lesion characterization using spectral mammography. SPIE Medical Imaging Conference 8313 2012: Physics of Medical Imaging. San Diego, United States; 4–9 February 2012

Noroozian M, Hadjiiski L, Rahnama-Moghadam S, et al. Digital breast tomosynthesis is comparable to mammographic spot views for mass characterization. Radiology 2012;262(1):61–68

Park SH, Moon WK, Cho N, et al. Diffusion-weighted MR imaging: pretreatment prediction of response to neoadjuvant chemotherapy in patients with breast cancer. Radiology 2010;257(1):56–63

Pereira FP, Martins G, Carvalhaes de Oliveira RdeV. Diffusion magnetic resonance imaging of the breast. Magn Reson Imaging Clin N Am 2011;19(1):95–110

Rafferty E, Nicklason L. FFDM vs FFDM with tomosynthesis for women with radiographically dense breasts: an enriched retrospective reader study. Radiological Society of North America Annual Meeting 2011. Chicago, United States; 27 November–2 December 2011

Schmitzberger FF, Fallenberg EM, Lawaczeck R, et al. Development of low-dose photon-counting contrast-enhanced tomosynthesis with spectral imaging. Radiology 2011;259(2):558–564

Sharma U, Danishad KK, Seenu V, Jagannathan NR. Longitudinal study of the assessment by MRI and diffusion-weighted imaging of tumor response in patients with locally advanced breast cancer undergoing neoadjuvant chemotherapy. NMR Biomed 2009;22(1):104–113

Sinkus R, Siegmann K, Xydeas T, Tanter M, Claussen C, Fink M. MR elastography of breast lesions: understanding the solid/liquid duality can improve the specificity of contrast-enhanced MR mammography. Magn Reson Med 2007;58(6):1135–1144

Sonmez G, Cuce F, Mutlu H, et al. Value of diffusion-weighted MRI in the differentiation of benign and malign breast lesions. Wien Klin Wochenschr 2011;123(21-22):655–661

Sree SV, Ng EY, Acharya RU, Faust O. Breast imaging: a survey. World J Clin Oncol 2011;2(4):171–178

Stöblen F, Landt S, Stelkens-Gebhardt R, Sehouli J, Rezai M, Kümmel S. First evaluation of the diagnostic accuracy of an automated 3D ultrasound system in a breast screening setting. Anticancer Res 2011;31(8):2569–2574

Sumkin J, Ganott M, Bandos A. digital breast tomosynthesis vs supplemental diagnostic mammography images for the evaluation of noncalcified breast lesions. Radiological Society of North America Annual Meeting 2011. Chicago, United States; 27 November–2 December 2011

Svahn TM, Chakraborty DP, Ikeda D, et al. Breast tomosynthesis and digital mammography: a comparison of diagnostic accuracy. Br J Radiol 2012;85(1019):e1074–1082

Tafreshi NK, Kumar V, Morse DL, Gatenby RA. Molecular and functional imaging of breast cancer. Cancer Contr 2010;17(3):143–155

Teertstra HJ, Loo CE, van den Bosch MA, et al. Breast tomosynthesis in clinical practice: initial results. Eur Radiol 2010;20(1):16–24

Tingberg A, Förnvik D, Mattsson S, Svahn T, Timberg P, Zackrisson S. Breast cancer screening with tomosynthesis—initial experiences. Radiat Prot Dosimetry 2011;147(1-2):180–183

Wallis MG, Moa E, Zanca F, Leifland K, Danielsson M. Two-view and single-view tomosynthesis versus full-field digital mammography: high-resolution X-ray imaging observer study. Radiology 2012;262(3):788–796

Yi A, Cho N, Chang JM, Koo HR, La Yun B, Moon WK. Sonoelastography for 1,786 non-palpable breast masses: diagnostic value in the decision to biopsy. Eur Radiol 2012;22(5):1033–1040

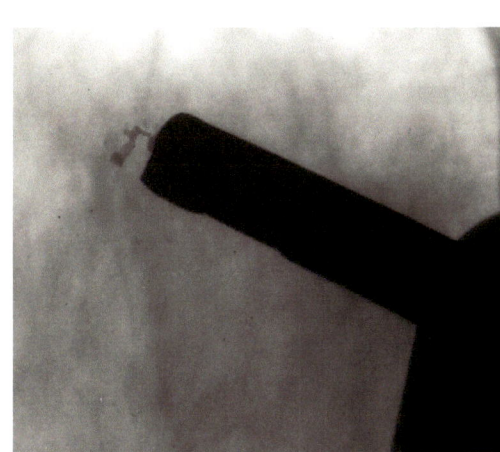

7 Imaging Assessment and Percutaneous Breast Biopsy

Purpose, Accuracy, Possibilities, and Limitations ⇢ 186
Purpose ⇢ 186
Measures Before Histopathologic Assessment ⇢ 186
Definitions ⇢ 187
Accuracy ⇢ 187
Possibilities, Limitations, Choice of Biopsy Method ⇢ 189
Patient Information, Patient Preparation, and Postbiopsy Care ⇢ 192

Techniques for Biopsy and Biopsy Guidance ⇢ 193
Fine Needle Aspiration ⇢ 193
Core Needle Biopsy ⇢ 194
Vacuum-Assisted Breast Biopsy ⇢ 195
Biopsy Under Ultrasound Guidance ⇢ 197
Stereotactic Biopsy ⇢ 203
MR-Guided Percutaneous Biopsy ⇢ 207
Handling the Biopsy Specimen ⇢ 210
Interpreting the Histopathologic Results ⇢ 210

References and Recommended Reading ⇢ 213

7 Imaging Assessment and Percutaneous Breast Biopsy

S. H. Heywang-Koebrunner, I. Schreer, S. Barter

Purpose, Accuracy, Possibilities, and Limitations

Purpose

Abnormalities may be detected either clinically or by imaging. Only some of these abnormalities are eventually proven to be malignant, whereas others eventually prove to be benign.

To correctly classify these abnormalities—that is, to find breast cancers as early as possible or exclude malignancy using the least invasive measures—international standards demand that any abnormality first undergoes state-of-the-art *imaging assessment*. If malignancy can reliably be excluded based on such assessment, no further measures are needed.

If this is not possible, *histopathologic assessment* must be considered. According to international guidelines, histopathologic assessment should wherever possible be performed using minimally invasive methods. European guidelines demand that at least 70% of histopathologic assessments be performed using minimally invasive methods, optimally more than 90%.

The goal is to avoid unnecessary diagnostic open surgery in cases that eventually prove to be benign. Owing to the smaller volume of tissue removed by minimally invasive procedures (percutaneous breast biopsy), morbidity is reduced. General anesthetic and associated perioperative risks (bleeding, infection, cardiac risks, etc.) can be avoided or reduced. Visible scarring and diagnostic problems due to imaging changes caused by scarring from open surgery are usually minimized with percutaneous breast biopsy.

In the case of malignancy, percutaneous breast biopsy allows optimal planning of the surgical and therapeutic approach for both the breast and the axilla. For this purpose it may be necessary to perform percutaneous breast biopsy in more than one location within the breast. It is proven that percutaneous breast biopsy allows a reduction in the number of surgical procedures needed, better cosmetic resulting from clear margins, fewer local recurrences, and overall better patient outcome.

Measures Before Histopathologic Assessment

State-of-the-art imaging assessment must be completed before biopsy of a lesion in question is considered (see Chapter 24).

If state-of-the-art imaging cannot exclude malignancy in the event of a clinically suspicious finding, or if it supports suspicion of malignancy of a lesion detected clinically, histopathologic assessment must be considered. The final classification should be based on the imaging findings, the clinical findings, and temporal changes (as gained from patient history and comparison with previous films).

Biopsy is usually indicated for any lesion classified as BI-RADS (*Breast Imaging Reporting and Data System*) *4a, 4b, 4c,* or *5*. (With this definition a well-circumscribed solid lesion that increases in size would usually be classified as BI-RADS 4a, for example, based on its temporal change.) For the category BI-RADS 3, biopsy should only rarely be considered (e.g., in a patient with a strong family history of breast cancer or in case of carcinophobia).

Before biopsy is considered, the *exact location of the lesion must be documented* (clockwise position, distance from the nipple). This is necessary to avoid any confusion of multiple lesions and to support preoperative localization when needed.

Ultrasound of the axilla should be performed before biopsy, whenever a lesion requiring histopathologic assessment is identified. Even though axillary ultrasound will mainly be needed in cases of proven malignancy, it is recommended that it be performed before percutaneous breast biopsy, because reactive changes of the lymph nodes after biopsy might be the cause of false positive findings. Fortunately, such problems appear to occur only rarely (Britton et al. 2009a, 2009b, 2010).

The *biopsy method and the optimum approach* need to be chosen and the *patient should be informed* about the recommended assessment, about the procedure, its advantages, and potential side effects. Contraindications and the necessity of changing any medication must be checked.

If more than one lesion is identified, *a concept should be made* as to what workup might be needed for each lesion and how further workup should proceed. Usually, histopathologic assessment should start with the lesion of highest suspicion. Again the exact location of each important lesion should be unequivocally documented.

Definitions

Percutaneous biopsy can be performed using a variety of biopsy techniques.

Fine needle aspiration (FNA) allows sampling of cells, which are then cytologically analyzed. For fine needle aspiration a thin needle (e.g., 21 gauge) is used.

Core needle biopsy (CNB) yields larger tissue samples, which are analyzed histologically. Usually 3 to 10 tissue cores (each 20 mm long, 2 mm in diameter) are acquired using 14-gauge (or thicker) needles, which are shot into the lesion by means of a high-speed firing mechanism. Tissue acquisition is either performed by repeated needle insertion into the breast or by using a 13-gauge (or thicker) coaxial system, through which the needle is reinserted into the lesion.

Vacuum-assisted breast biopsy (VABB) is a method that allows harvesting even larger amounts of tissue. The vacuum needle is inserted into the lesion once. Then tissue is suctioned into the needle, cut off, and transported to the back end of the needle, where it is picked off. While the needle stays in place this is repeated, for example, 12 times or more, and tissue is acquired from all directions around the clock by rotating the needle around its axis. That way, with a single needle insertion, a contiguous volume of tissue (diameter ~15 mm) is acquired for histopathologic analysis, while the fluid from bleeding is simultaneously suctioned out of the cavity.

Accuracy

Fine Needle Biopsy

Fine needle aspiration biopsy (FNAB) was the first method applied for percutaneous biopsy of breast abnormalities. Initially it was used for supplementary evaluation of palpable abnormalities together with mammography (so-called triple diagnosis). FNAB has also come to be applied to the workup of nonpalpable mammographically or sonographically detected lesions. Swedish research groups initiated these applications (Azavedo et al. 1989) and thus inaugurated modern percutaneous breast biopsy. These groups still have the largest experience with FNAB. They have reported a sensitivity of up to 100% and specificity of 96–100% under stereotactic guidance. A critical issue in interpreting literature data is whether nondiagnostic aspirations enter into the calculation. Another critical issue concerns whether the accuracy data of FNAB have been adjusted by correlation with imaging. Discrepancies between benign results of FNAB and imaging have mostly been considered as an indication for further workup, usually by surgical biopsy, and have therefore been counted as a true positive call. This mode of evaluation may yield unrealistically high accuracy data.

Also the very high accuracy reported have been achieved only in highly specialized facilities with experienced radiologists and cytopathologists with on-site availability of cytologic evaluation. Other authors have been unable to reproduce these results in wider use of the technique (Cytology Sub-Group of the National Coordinating Committee for Breast Screening Pathology NHS Breast Screening Programme 1992, Pisano et al. 1998), and published results from other groups vary between 53% and 90% for sensitivity (average of complete sensitivity for stereotactic fine needle aspiration 83%, for ultrasound [US]-guided fine needle aspiration 95%) and 91% and 100% for specificity (average 98%). Complete sensitivity is based on the true positive rate, if atypia and suspicious and malignant findings are considered true positive.

Core Needle Biopsy

In contrast to aspiration cytology, CNB obtains cores of tissue and thus permits histologic diagnosis. It also permits receptor analysis. US-guided CNB can today be considered the method of choice for histopathologic assessment of the large number of mass lesions visible by ultrasound. Based on comparative studies, both a large needle size (14 gauge) and a sufficient number of cores (usually more than three cores) are considered prerequisites for high accuracy (Liberman et al. 1994, Brenner et al. 1996, Fishman et al. 2003, Schulz-Wendtland et al. 2003, de Lucena et al. 2007).

Accuracy data of CNB are available from preoperative studies and from large series of patient examinations. With few exceptions, sensitivity of all studies ranges from 92% to 99% with a specificity of 100% (Fahrbach et al. 2006, El-Sayed et al. 2008, Bruening et al. 2010).

Studies reporting sensitivity data for masses, architectural distortions, and microcalcifications have shown a higher sensitivity for masses (> 97%) than for microcalcifications (85–95%) or for architectural distortion (Mainiero et al. 1996, Liberman et al. 1997, Meyer et al. 1998, Lee et al. 1999). The sensitivity of CNB is higher under US guidance than under stereotactic guidance (Britton 1999).

Most of the reported accuracy data refer to sensitivities obtained after correlation with imaging, so that a negative result of CNB is considered a true positive call if re-biopsy was initiated based on a discrepant correlation with imaging.

To avoid a false negative diagnosis and delayed treatment, strict adherence to standards is essential. This includes selection of the appropriate indications, standardized acquisition of sufficient tissue, critical imaging check of correct sampling, and systematic correlation of imaging and histopathology of CNB. Uncertain correlations and B3–5a lesions should be discussed in an interdisciplinary team. Only compatible results should be accepted. For lesions with uncertain correlation re-biopsy needs to be considered.

In contrast to FNB, CNB allows immunohistochemistry to be performed on the tissue obtained, which may be helpful for improved distinction of difficult lesions.

Furthermore, immunohistochemistry yields information on the receptor status, which may be very important for very small invasive cancers, which may be completely removed intact, at least in some cases, by CNB.

A correct final classification of lesions containing cellular atypia is usually not possible by CNB, and upgrade rates range around 40–50% in the literature (Houssami et al. 2007, Jackman et al. 2002, Fahrbach et al. 2006). Standard practice is that when cellular atypia is present in the histologic specimen, surgical biopsy will be necessary.

Vacuum-Assisted Breast Biopsy

Vacuum-assisted breast biopsy (VABB) was introduced in 1996 by F. Burbank and S. H. Parker (Burbank et al. 1996). We were able to introduce the method in Europe and to develop MR-guided VABB.

Today, an increasing number of data from single and multicenter studies exist on the accuracy of stereotactic VABB, including an updated systematic review on this technique (Yu et al. 2010) and another review in which VABB and CNB are compared (Fahrbach et al. 2006). Our own experience is based on several thousand cases performed at our institutions, on a multicenter study conducted by us, and on evaluation of the introduction of VABB in our screening program (Kettritz et al. 2004, Heywang-Köbrunner et al. 2010).

All existing data confirm that VABB achieves excellent accuracy. Yu et al. (2010) reported a sensitivity of 98.1% and a specificity of 99.9%. Fahrbach et al. (2006) confirmed excellent sensitivity for both VABB (98%) and CNB (97.4%). The rate of technical failure and of nondiagnostic biopsies was higher for CNB than for VABB. However, as shown by the data published by Fahrbach et al., the cases included were not comparable: the lesions examined by VABB were much smaller, contained a significantly higher proportion of microcalcifications, and eventually proved to consist of earlier lesions than those examined by CNB, with 60% versus 34%, respectively, of the cancers proving to be ductal carcinoma in situ (DCIS). So, even though the reported sensitivities of CNB and VABB appear to be equal, those obtained by VABB were for earlier and more demanding lesions. With increasing experience and further optimization of equipment, this result appears to hold true.

Overall, false negative findings of VABB are rare (up to 2%). Strict adherence to quality assurance, including close correlation of histopathology and imaging, is necessary for VABB, as it is for the other minimally invasive biopsy methods. Based on our experience the systematic acquisition of a sufficient volume of tissue helps avoid false negative biopsies. We recommend acquiring at least 12 cores with a 10-gauge vacuum needle or an equivalent volume, preferably even more. With a larger tissue volume, sampling error can be reduced; tissue shift due to needle insertion or application of local anesthetic can be even better compensated for. Complete removal of the area in question and visibility of a well-centered cavity further enhance the reliability of imaging–histopathology correlation.

One special advantage of VABB has been its much lower rate of underestimated high-risk lesions. (Fahrbach reported 20% underestimates of atypical ductal hyperplasia by VABB vs. 38% by CNB). Similar results have been reported by other authors, too. The rate of incorrect classifications of DCIS (upgraded to invasive carcinoma) has been reported to range around 11% (Jackman et al. 2002, Kettritz et al. 2004, Fahrbach et al. 2006, Margenthaler et al. 2006 Houssami et al. 2007b, Eby et al. 2009, Heywang-Köbrunner et al. 2010).

Even though small lesion size, mammographically complete removal of the lesion, low suspicion on mammography, and fewer than three foci of atypia detected within the cores indicate a lower probability of an underestimate, so far no sufficiently reliable combination or algorithm exists that would allow such lesions to be managed conservatively and avoid surgery. Exceptions may be made for elderly patients or patients in whom surgery is contraindicated due to co-morbidities.

Very good results have also been reported for VABB under sonographic guidance (Sohn et al. 2007, Schueller et al. 2008, Heywang-Köbrunner et al. 2009). Since most lesions which can be reliably visualized and assessed under ultrasound guidance are amenable to core biopsy, VABB is only needed occasionally. Its use has been described for very small lesions, for suspected papillary lesions, or changes within scarring. Owing to the inability of ultrasound to detect fine microcalcifications or to exactly assess their morphology or distribution, we do not recommend using US-guided VABB for assessing microcalcifications without an associated mass.

VABB is particularly well suited for the assessment of MR-detected lesions. As most MR systems will not permit continuous monitoring during the biopsy procedure, compensation of possible tissue shift, removal of bleeding, and the acquisition of sufficient tissue afforded by the use of VABB proves quite valuable. Acquisition of sufficient tissue and visibility of a well-centered cavity prove quite helpful for imaging correlation with histopathology, which otherwise may be quite demanding. There are challenges correlating histopathology with enhancing lesions detected by MR: specimen imaging is not an option (as the specimen does not enhance with contrast agent), a high proportion of indeterminate-appearing benign changes may enhance, and there may be a high proportion of early malignancy or borderline lesions among those lesions visible by MR only.

While only limited numbers of cases have been published for MR-guided CNB, it has today mainly been replaced by MR-guided VABB for the above-mentioned reasons.

For MR-guided VABB published experience to date includes more than 2,000 examinations. The published experience includes several larger series (Heywang-Köbrunner et al. 1999, Liberman et al. 2005, Fischer et al.

2009, Han et al. 2008, Malhaire et al. 2010) and one multicenter study with 517 cases (Perlet et al. 2006). With few exceptions the technical success rate ranged around 96–98%. Discordant biopsies were reported on average in 3.5% of cases with few cancers missed. The rate of malignancy reported ranged around 30%, of which 44% proved to be DCIS. The upgrade rates to DCIS or invasive disease were reported to range around 18%. Thus the overall reported results are similar to those of stereotactic biopsy of mammographic lesions.

Today, MR-guided VABB can be considered a reliable and reproducible technique for MR-detected lesions. It is, however, quite expensive and has so far mainly been performed by highly experienced teams.

Possibilities, Limitations, Choice of Biopsy Method

Histopathologic assessment is needed for any lesion or change that cannot unequivocally be classified as benign when based on the above-described standard imaging assessment.

Based on the preceding imaging assessment and the assumed underlying pathology, both the method of guidance and the method of biopsy (fine needle biopsy, core needle biopsy, vacuum-assisted breast biopsy, or open biopsy) need to be chosen. When choosing the method of guidance, preference should be given to the *simplest and usually best tolerated technique that allows visualization and reliable targeting of the lesion*. In an individual case the choice may depend on the type of lesion, lesion location, breast configuration, on the patient (risk factors, scoliosis, etc.), on the availability of equipment, and on expertise.

- *Imaging guidance* serves to insert the needle into the lesion, to guide it to different areas within the lesion, to verify and document correct needle position, or to adjust needle position during the intervention. It is mandatory for nonpalpable lesions.
- *Imaging guidance improves the accuracy of percutaneous biopsy* of palpable lesions by directing the needle into the lesion or into favorable areas within the lesion (avoiding nondiagnostic biopsies of necrotic areas).

> Imaging guidance of nonpalpable lesions should in general be performed sonographically for lesions visible by ultrasound, and stereotactically for mammographically visible lesions.

We strongly recommend using stereotaxis on systems with a digital receiver and with automated needle guidance. This reduces procedure time and decreases calculation or handling errors, and errors caused by patient motion. Overall, stereotaxis is a well-established method. However, the risk of a targeting error appears to be slightly higher with stereotactic guidance than with sonographic guidance.

If a lesion is visible equally well by both methods, US guidance should be preferred. In experienced hands it offers excellent accuracy; being the fastest technique it is usually best tolerated by the patient. It is also associated with the lowest cost.

For areas of mammographic microcalcifications, US guidance should be used if the microcalcifications are associated with a mass that is visible by ultrasound. In this situation US guidance may allow the biopsy to enter into areas with the highest probability of containing invasive malignancy. (This is important since it will influence the surgical management of the axilla.) Stereotactic guidance is the method of choice for biopsy of lesions that consist solely of microcalcifications. Limited accuracy of targeting and increased risk of sampling error (with DCIS) could compromise reliability of US-guided biopsy.

If a lesion is visible only by MRI, MR guidance is indispensible to target the biopsy of the correct area. Considering the high number of additional lesions detected and visualized by MRI alone, and the significant proportion of benign pathologic changes among these lesions, most guidelines stipulate that MR-guided biopsy is warranted if MRI is offered to a patient.

It is important to perform a "second look" ultrasound before proceeding to breast biopsy. Knowing the exact position of the lesion on MRI, it is possible in retrospect to identify and thus target the lesion, using US guidance in some cases. Since US-guided biopsy is the simpler and better tolerated method it should be preferred to MR-guided biopsy. According to our experience retrospective identification by ultrasound is possible in about 30% of cases. The percentage may increase if the quality of the initial ultrasound is low.

Percutaneous biopsy of lesions that are detected and visible only by MRI is desirable for several reasons:
- Open surgery of benign MR-detected lesions can often be avoided. (In most series one out of three or four lesions detected by MRI alone proves to be malignant.)
- Logistic problems due to difficult timing of MR localization procedure and surgery can be reduced.
- Since enhancing lesions cannot usually be visualized in a specimen MRI, specimen radiograph, or sonogram, uncertainties concerning correct excision of lesions visualized only by MRI may remain after surgery. Image-guided percutaneous removal can help to solve this problem, since reduction or removal of the enhancing lesion may be directly visualized after MR-guided VABB.

Currently, experience with percutaneous MR-guided CNB has been reported by a few authors. Being a complicated procedure that is hampered by the inability to monitor the biopsy without major image artifacts, it has not been recommended for lesions less than 1 cm in size. Tissue shift during biopsy might go undetected. Furthermore, with CNB only small amounts of tissue are removed, local anesthetic and hematoma due to the biopsy may impair visualization, and assessment of correct tissue acquisition is uncertain. MR-guided VABB overcomes these issues.

In contrast to MR-guided CNB, significant published data, including data from a large multicenter study, exist for MR-guided VABB. Reproducibility and excellent accuracy (comparable to that of stereotactic VABB) have been proven in experienced hands. However, this method is currently the most complicated, time-consuming, and costly among the percutaneous breast biopsy techniques. Major cost factors include the need for MR-compatible biopsy probes, the significant MR time required, and the need for highly trained personnel, plus special biopsy coils and software for needle guidance.

- *Fine needle biopsy* allows only cytologic analysis of cells. Histology or immune staining is not possible with FNAB. It also requires a cytopathologist with considerable expertise and close cooperation of a highly experienced team.

  Fine needle aspiration requires the least expensive materials. Limitations in the use of fine needle aspiration include the limited reliability of a negative diagnosis, the inability to differentiate invasive from in-situ carcinoma, a high rate of cellular atypia requiring surgical biopsy, and a high insufficient sampling rate. The last may be reduced by the presence of a cytopathologist at the time the fine needle aspiration is performed to evaluate the specimen for adequacy of cells retrieved. (This, however, increases the costs and is often logistically difficult.)

  Owing to the limited specificity of a positive result (91–100%) a cytologic diagnosis of malignancy is, in most countries, not accepted for decisions on important therapeutic measures (such as mastectomy, neoadjuvant chemotherapy, axillary dissection). Considering the very variable published sensitivity (ranging from 50% to 100%) caution is necessary if a negative cytologic finding is used to avoid surgical biopsy.

  However, some entities do exist where a cytologic diagnosis may be considered reliable. They include diagnosis of malignant involvement of a lymph node and diagnosis of a fibroadenoma.

- *Core needle biopsy* is the method of choice for the vast majority of lesions that can be approached under US guidance. With sufficient experience, even small carcinomas presenting as a sonographic mass or architectural distortion can be correctly targeted and verified by US-guided CNB.

  CNB may also be used under stereotactic guidance. For workup of microcalcifications, CNB has a limited reliability, even if up to 10 cores are taken. For microcalcifications and—in our experience—for small masses that are not visible by ultrasound, VABB has become the method of choice. We do not recommend using CNB for lesions visible by MRI only.

  To reduce potential errors that may occur with CNB, systematic correlation of the histopathologic result with the imaging findings is always required, preferably by multidisciplinary discussion. CNB is highly reliable if a specific histologic diagnosis is possible, which is compatible with the imaging findings: for example, a carcinoma, a benign intramammary lymph node, or a fibroadenoma. Caution is necessary with unspecific benign findings (such as diffuse benign changes). Repeat percutaneous biopsy or open surgical biopsy should be considered for unspecific findings that may not fully explain the imaging abnormality, for discrepant imaging findings, and for all lesions containing atypias. It is recommended that lesions with uncertain correlation, those with discrepant findings, and all lesions belonging to the B3 category are discussed by an interdisciplinary team.

In experienced hands the accuracy of US-guided CNB is excellent for masses upward of 5 mm diameter in size. Therefore US-guided CNB is the method of choice for the large number of mass lesions which can be visualized only by ultrasound. Those masses that can be visualized only by mammography need to be assessed stereotactically. The accuracy of stereotactic CNB of small masses may be compromised by lesion shift due to local anesthesia or bleeding. Such lesion shift may go undetected, since local anesthesia and bleeding may obscure visibility of the masses.

CNB of microcalcifications is less accurate than CNB of masses (Brenner et al. 1996, Liberman et al. 1994, 1997, Meyer et al. 1998, Jackman et al. 1999). Depending upon tissue resistance to the motion of the needle, the amount of deflection of the needle from its intended course can make it difficult to retrieve calcifications. With repetitive biopsy puncturing, the site usually becomes increasingly hemorrhagic, limiting the value of further punctures. Finally, it is important to understand that microcalcifications are often located adjacent to malignant cells, but not within these cells. This means that acquisition of a sufficient amount of tissue around the microcalcifications may be crucial. Generally, diagnostic accuracy increases with the increasing number of cores that contain microcalcifications. However, acquisition of cores with microcalcifications still may not guarantee the correct diagnosis of DCIS by the pathologist.

The value of CNB for the workup of architectural distortions is limited, since only the positive diagnosis of malignancy is reliable. An unspecific benign diagnosis (e.g., fibrosis or ductal hyperplasia) has to be considered discrepant. The benign diagnosis of a radial scar may be compatible but is unreliable, since associated DCIS or tubular carcinoma has been reported in up to 25% of radial scars. Because malignancy associated with radial scars is mostly located in the periphery of the lesion, it may not be adequately sampled by CNB. However, a positive finding may be very helpful and can support treatment decisions.

Overall, in experienced hands, excellent accuracy can be achieved by CNB. With the appropriate selection and systematic imaging–histopathology correlation accuracy comparable to that of surgical biopsy can be achieved.

- *Vacuum-assisted breast biopsy* is the latest method of percutaneous biopsy. It appears to have the highest accuracy. Its superiority is meanwhile generally accepted for histopathologic assessment of microcalcifications. However, it also offers advantages for sampling of small masses and even for architectural distortions. VABB is, however, associated with the highest costs.

VABB allows acquisition of a significantly larger volume of tissue than CNB and it allows compensation of moderate tissue shift due to needle insertion or bleeding. Also, by removing a visible part of the lesion and by creating a cavity it provides an additional countercheck of correct sampling.

These factors are considered highly important for percutaneous breast biopsy under stereotactic or MR guidance. While early cancers, DCIS, and borderline lesions are most frequently detected by mammography or MRI, CNB under stereotactic or MR guidance for these lesions has been limited by an increased risk of sampling error, and by targeting error due to the inability to continuously monitor the lesion during the procedure.

Increasing data prove an excellent accuracy of VABB under stereotactic guidance. Thus, currently VABB allows reliable tissue diagnosis in an increasing number of small and early lesions, avoiding open surgery.

Several guidelines recommend stereotactic VABB as the method of choice for the assessment of microcalcifications without associated mass. We have observed similar advantages for the assessment of those small masses or architectural distortions that cannot be approached under US guidance.

For the same reasons *VABB appears to be the method of choice for percutaneous breast biopsy of MR-detected lesions*. Today, MR-guided VABB has largely replaced MR-guided CNB (Warren and Hayes 2000, Perlet et al. 2006, Heywang-Köbrunner et al. 2007).

As mentioned above, the vast majority of lesions visible by ultrasound are masses for which US-guided CNB is well established as the standard biopsy method. In selected cases *US-guided VABB* may be considered. These may include very small lesions suggestive of papilloma, very small lesions, or changes within scarred tissue—if acquisition of a larger volume of tissue or complete removal of the lesion may help avoid open biopsy of an otherwise noncompatible unspecific benign change or of a probably benign BI-RADS 3 lesion.

Irrespective of the high accuracy that may be achieved with VABB, errors can never be excluded. So, close imaging–histopathology correlation remains necessary to assess whether the lesion in question has been correctly targeted and sampled, and whether the obtained result may be representative for the complete area or finding in question. All lesions with uncertain correlation and all lesions belonging to the histopathologic B3 or 4 categories should be discussed in an interdisciplinary conference.

Even though diagnostic *open biopsy* should be replaced by percutaneous breast biopsy if possible, no guideline demands that 100% of diagnostic biopsies be performed using minimally invasive methods. Although percutaneous breast biopsy is usually associated with fewer side effects than open biopsy, there may be contraindications to this technique such as patient-associated problems, the position of the lesion, or technical issues. Diffuse or regional changes of large areas of breast tissue may not be appropriate for percutaneous breast biopsy.

If in an individual case open biopsy may be more appropriate, the best solution for the patient should always be chosen.

Indication for Percutaneous Breast Biopsy

Before any decision is made to perform tissue sampling, imaging workup must be completed. It is important to remember that biopsy should not be used to replace adequate imaging workup.

There are several indications for percutaneous biopsy:

- The most frequent and cost-effective use of percutaneous needle biopsy procedures is in eliminating the need for surgical biopsy. In women with indeterminate lesions (BI-RADS category 4), it may be possible to make a definite diagnosis of a benign entity, thus possibly sparing the patient surgical biopsy.
- Percutaneous tissue sampling may be used for selected patients for whom short-term mammographic follow-up is recommended for probably benign lesions (BI-RADS category 3) but who cannot be relied on to return for follow-up or are too anxious to wait.
- When women have lesions that are highly suspicious for carcinoma (BI-RADS category 5) and for whom a two-stage surgical approach is planned (diagnostic surgical biopsy followed by a second therapeutic surgical procedure at a different date), needle biopsy can eliminate the initial surgery. A preoperative diagnosis of invasive malignancy is also useful for treatment planning of the axilla and when discussing further treatment options with the patient and her family.
- Finally, in the patient with a probable or proven carcinoma in whom more than one lesion is present, the ability to prove or exclude the presence of multiple foci of cancer will influence surgical management. In the same setting, the ability to prove that only one worrisome area is malignant allows the surgeon and patient to plan for breast conservation.

Contraindications

Contraindications to percutaneous breast biopsy are few. They include:

- Allergy to local anesthetic. (In most cases, however, an appropriate local anesthetic can be found by dermatological testing.) Inability of an individual patient to cooperate during the biopsy may make it impossible to perform.
- Adequate precautions should be taken if a patient has a history of an underlying medical condition whereby higher risk of side effects may be anticipated (e.g., diabetes, cardiac arrhythmia, patients with artificial cardiac valves for which antibiotic prophylaxis has been recommended, patients with seizures, with high blood pressure, etc.).
- Anticoagulation is a relative contraindication. Anticoagulation with coumarin should be replaced by anticoagulation with a short-acting substance such as heparin. This switch usually has to be monitored by the patient's internist. Provided the other coagulation parameters are normal, percutaneous breast biopsy can usually be performed with INR (international normalized ratio) values of 1.6 or lower.

  Whenever possible, aspirin or comparable agents (inhibitors of platelet aggregation such as Plavix or Ticlopidin) should be discontinued for up to 8 days before and after the procedure.

  Heparin should be discontinued on the day of biopsy (and if possible for another 2–3 days). The switch back to coumarin or inhibitors of platelet aggregation is usually recommended after biopsy results are available and surgery is unnecessary.
- In some patients stereotactic biopsy may be impossible if the breast is too thin once compressed to accommodate a biopsy needle (i.e., the distance between the needle acquisition chamber and the needle tip is greater than the thickness of the compressed breast), or if a lesion is in a thin area of the breast. In most of these cases novel short needles may help solve the problem. Also, lesions that are high in the axillary tail or near the chest wall may not be imageable using the stereotactic unit, making it impossible to perform stereotactic procedures in these women.

Complications

Major complications are rare (Kettritz et al. 2004, Bruening et al. 2010). Most complications concern hemorrhage, rarely infection. Mild complications such as pain, hematomas requiring no surgical treatment, or bruising are common and may be slightly more frequent and more pronounced with VABB than with CNB. Severe hemorrhage or infection requiring surgical treatment is uncommon.

The overall rate of complications and their degree, however, appears to be well below that of surgical biopsy.

- In sonographically guided biopsies, pneumothorax is a possible complication if the needle penetrates the chest wall. This is a rare complication, but because sonographically guided biopsy is performed without a guidance mechanism that could prevent needle deviation toward the chest wall, the operator must choose an approach parallel to the chest wall and always visualize the complete needle path within the sonographic slice to avoid potentially puncturing the pleura. Because the chest wall is out of the field of view in most stereotactic biopsies, and because the needle is guided by a rigid mechanism, the needle cannot penetrate the chest wall during these procedures.
- When a stereotactic biopsy is done with a patient sitting using an add-on unit, there is the possibility of vasovagal reaction. When the patient is prone on a stereotactic table or reclining using an add-on unit, or supine during a sonographically guided procedure, these reactions are very rare.
- Possible side effects of local anesthetics, although rare (allergy, cardiac arrhythmia, rarely seizures), need to be considered, particularly in patients with cardiac disease, and the maximum dose must be strictly observed.
- Pain may occur during the procedure if insufficient local anesthetic was used and this should be avoided. Very rarely, patients do not respond to local anesthetic or react very late. In these patients sufficient time may be needed between application of local anesthetic and biopsy (sometimes up to 20 min). Patients who do not respond to local anesthetic may not be suitable for percutaneous CNB or VABB.
- Some pain may be reported after biopsy. Strong or long-lasting pain (more than 1–2 weeks) is quite rare.
- For many women undergoing these procedures, anxiety about the possibility of a breast cancer diagnosis can be debilitating, compromising their ability to return to normal activities on the day of the procedure.

Patient Information, Patient Preparation, and Postbiopsy Care

Informed consent should be obtained before a procedure is performed. The patient should be aware of the possible complications, limitations, and risks of the procedure. She should understand how the procedure will be performed and what she will experience during it.

For patients who are on medications that compromise coagulation (anticoagulation or pain medication containing aspirin) these have to be adapted as described above. A switch from coumarin or inhibitors of platelet aggregation (such as aspirin, Plavix or Ticlopidin) to heparin usually needs to be monitored by the patient's internist, who should also be consulted concerning the risks to the patient associated with discontinuation of the initial medication. As mentioned above, heparin should be discontinued on the day of the procedure (and if possible for another 2–3 days). The time span for discontinuing heparin medication will depend on the patient's underlying disease and the resulting risks and the type of biopsy performed, and should be agreed locally after discussions with the hematology department. (In our experience a somewhat longer discontinuation is desirable for VABB as compared with CNB or FNAB.)

For FNB or CNB it does not appear necessary to check the patient's coagulation profile unless abnormalities are expected from the patient's history (e.g., during/after coumarin therapy, chemotherapy, known coagulation defects). For VABB differing opinions exist. The need for prophylactic antibiotics should be discussed with the internist responsible for individual patients with cardiac valvular prostheses.

At the end of the procedure, hemostasis is established and an appropriate dressing applied to the breast. After percutaneous biopsy, the patient should avoid analgesics containing aspirin and other drugs that can compromise coagulation for 5 days after biopsy. Vigorous exercise, unnecessary manipulation of the breast, and hot bathing should also be avoided during the first 5–8 days after biopsy. The patient should be given written postbiopsy instructions; it is helpful to review these orally with the patient. These should include when to remove the dressing, how the results will be received, and what signs of possible complications to look for.

Techniques for Biopsy and Biopsy Guidance

Fine Needle Aspiration

Fine needle aspiration is performed by placing a small needle, 21–23 gauge, within the suspicious lesion, with the needle tip near the far edge of the lesion (**Fig. 7.1**). After applying negative pressure, the needle is moved within the lesion, fanning throughout the volume of the mass and applying a corkscrew movement to the needle. Usually 5–10 thrusts within the mass are performed during each pass. If cellular material or blood is seen within the needle hub, the needle is removed. It is customary to perform the aspiration at least three to five times.

The specimen can be placed on slides or directly injected into preservative. If slides are used, training is needed to spread the material on the slides correctly, or the specimen may not be interpretable.

Cytologic analysis may be also performed on specimens obtained at cyst aspiration. Aspiration of a cyst containing solid elements that could be malignant or cyst fluid that contains blood should be sent for cytologic analysis. For this sampling, the needle tip should be positioned within the center of the cyst and as much fluid as possible removed from the cyst. The specimen is prepared as for fine needle aspiration. If no solid material is obtained (only cyst fluid), no slides can be prepared, and the fluid is placed directly into preservative, or as recommended by the individual cytopathologist.

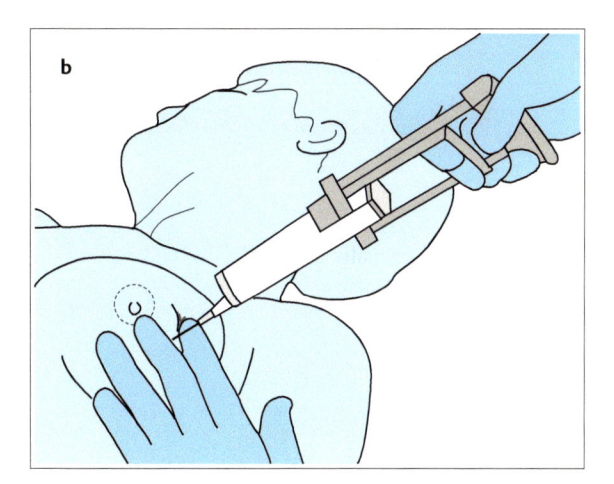

Fig. 7.1a,b

a Equipment for fine needle aspiration. A small-gauge needle can be attached to tubing and a 10-mL syringe. This makes it possible for a second set of hands to be used to apply negative pressure while the physician performing the biopsy holds the ultrasound transducer and moves the needle. The specimen can placed on slides or in fixative.

b Alternatively, the Cameco handle can be used. The handle enables negative pressure to be created without the need for another set of hands.

7 Imaging Assessment and Percutaneous Breast Biopsy

Core Needle Biopsy

Core biopsies are commonly performed using needles of 14 gauge. They allow specimens to be obtained that can be analyzed histopathologically (**Fig. 7.2**). Apart from the usual H&E (hematoxylin and eosin) staining, further staining (to analyze for hormone receptors, receptors for Her2neu, etc.) is usually possible from the obtained material.

A cutting needle is fired into the breast lesion, and a core of tissue is removed (**Fig. 7.2c**). The needle is removed after each biopsy and must be reinserted for another biopsy to be performed.

Gun-needle biopsy probes, usually paired with 14-gauge needles, are the most widely used type of biopsy probe for these procedures.

Studies have demonstrated that the cutting needle size in gun-needle systems should be at least 14 gauge (Nath et al. 1995). Smaller needles result in smaller diagnostic tissue specimens. The larger needle size does not result in a greater complication rate and does not significantly impact on the cost of performing these procedures. These systems are available in "long throw" and "short throw" configurations, describing the length the needle moves during the biopsy. Long throw systems move the needle at least 20 mm; short throw systems move the needle less than 15 mm. The long throw configuration is more effective in obtaining a diagnostic specimen. Since accuracy appears to correlate with the number of cores taken, it is generally recommended that three or more cores should be obtained (depending on the indication and the type of lesion) (Liberman et al. 1997, Schulz-Wendtland et al. 2003, Leifland et al. 2004).

A coaxial system is useful for easier reintroduction of the needle, as multiple cores can be acquired. Core needle biopsy allows removal of noncontiguous cores from the targeted site and is very well suited for biopsy of mass lesions. For small masses exact targeting is crucial. Since bleeding may push the lesion away from the needle and impair the diagnostic quality of the tissue for the pathologist, precise targeting of the very first core is quite important. Further cores should be acquired from different areas within the lesion to decrease the risk of sampling error. An attempt should always be made to obtain samples from both the center and the periphery of the lesion. It is known that sensitivity increases with the number of good cores. However, when the acquired cores become hemorrhagic their diagnostic value decreases and the biopsy should be stopped.

A careful assessment to ensure a representative biopsy has been obtained is always needed. Unspecific or uncertain correlation of results should lead to repeat biopsy (mostly VABB or open biopsy). VABB is today considered the method of choice for areas of microcalcifications, unless on ultrasound there is an associated mass, in which case US-guided CNB targeting the mass is indicated. The mass is likely to represent the invasive part of the lesion (if malignant) and therefore US-guided biopsy is preferred in this instance. In cases with very small masses core needle biopsy may be able to remove most or rarely all of the mass (5% or less of cases). In case of malignancy this could pose a problem, if excision of the area in question is planned or indicated subsequently. Also, bleeding may obscure a small lesion after biopsy.

To avoid these problems *clip marking* should be considered for small lesions that are visualized only

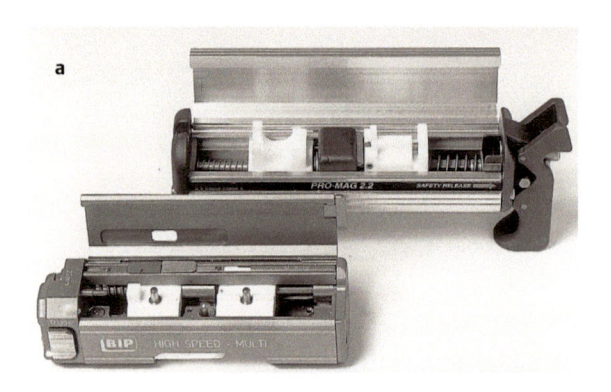

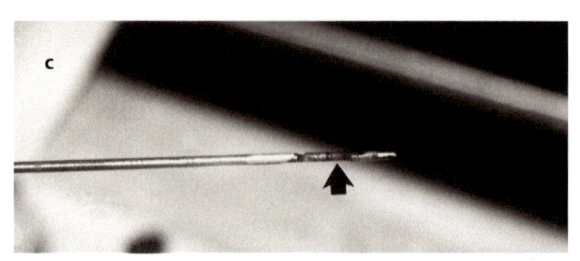

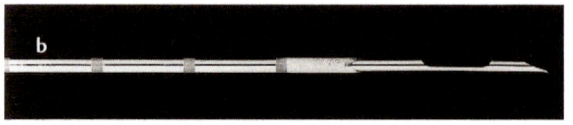

Fig. 7.2a–c

a Biopsy guns that use a spring mechanism to advance inner and outer parts of a needle at high speed.
b Trucut needle for obtaining a tissue core: the inner needle has a notch, which traps the tissue as the inner needle is advanced. The outer needle closes over it, cutting and trapping the tissue core.
c After the gun is fired and tissue is obtained, the needle is removed from the breast. Note that tissue fills the acquisition chamber of the biopsy needle (arrow).

by ultrasound. The clip will remain as a marker in the breast, whereas postbiopsy changes often last only a few days and, therefore, cannot be used for localization if re-excision is necessary. Correct position of the clip must be checked and documented by postbiopsy imaging.

Vacuum-Assisted Breast Biopsy

Careful planning of the approach is needed to ensure the needle is placed in the lesion in such a way that it is centered at the acquisition chamber.

Fig. 7.3 demonstrates how a typical vacuum system works. The chamber is opened. Tissue is then suctioned into the needle through the chamber (which is located on the side of the probe). Next, tissue is cut off by a rotating knife. Then, by means of a second vacuum, the tissue is transported within the needle to its far end, where it can be removed from the probe (**Fig. 7.4a,b**). By repeating the procedure and by turning the needle around its axis, multiple tissue cores can be acquired from adjacent sites through a single probe insertion. That way, focal areas of up to 15 mm diameter can be removed. With the standard systems blood is also removed by continuous suction. Despite some differences in design among the various manufacturers, the principle (continuous suction, avoidance of hematoma, ample tissue acquisition) is the same for the standard systems. Based on this principle, compensation can be made for potential errors caused by needle deviation, lesion shift due to hemorrhage, or local anesthetic. Sampling error is reduced, and direct visualization of representative biopsy is possible by demonstrating removal of the entire imaging abnormality or a major part of it on postbiopsy imaging. The cores obtained should be imaged to verify the presence of calcification in the specimens obtained.

Even though removal of an imaging abnormality is certainly the best proof of representative biopsy, it must be emphasized that so far no percutaneous biopsy method may be considered therapeutic in case of a malignant lesion or definitive in the diagnosis of atypical ductal hyperplasia (ADH). Imaging alone cannot reliably assess the full extent of malignancy or detect residual microscopic disease.

Therefore, surgical excision remains necessary in all cases where percutaneous biopsy yields a diagnosis of malignancy or ADH. For other borderline lesions (B3 category), an individual decision by the interdisciplinary team is necessary.

To avoid problems in subsequently localizing the biopsy site, placement of a localizing clip or other marker is recommended unless there is an adjacent landmark which makes it possible to unequivocally locate the site subsequently (**Fig. 7.5**). This can be done by deploying a clip through one of the larger probes—for example, 11 gauge—or by inserting a clip with its own introduction system. The clip will remain as a marker in the breast,

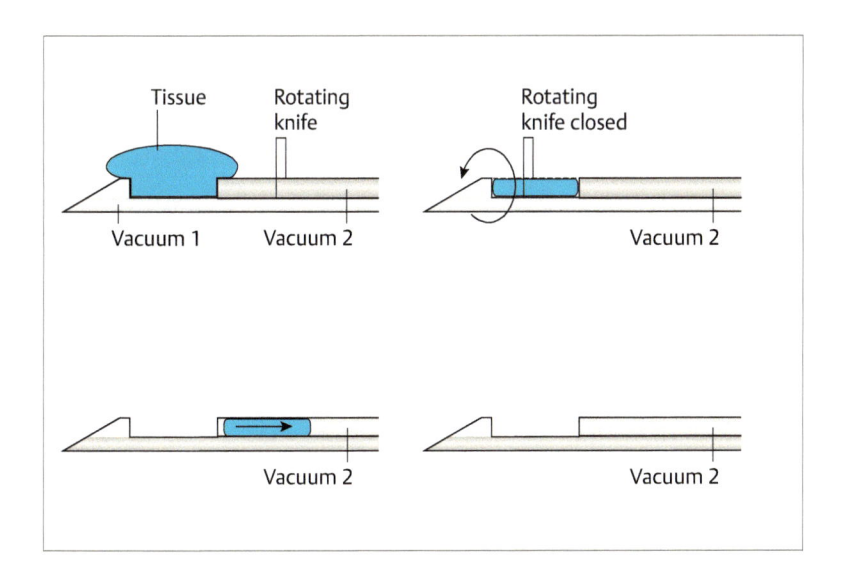

Fig. 7.3 The principle of vacuum biopsy is shown: The first image illustrates placement of the probe into the lesion. The acquisition chamber at the side of the probe is opened and tissue is suctioned into the probe by means of vacuum 1.

The second image shows the closing of the acquisition chamber by moving the rotating knife forward. Thus a core is cut off. Before the core is transported back and while the acquisition chamber is still closed, the needle can be turned around its axis so that the next core can be acquired from a different direction.
The third image shows that by means of vacuum 2 the core can be pulled back to the far end of the probe, where it can be taken off by a forceps. (During this procedure only the parts within the probe move. The probe itself remains in the lesion throughout the procedure).
The fourth image shows that, while the first core is transported to the far end of the needle, the acquisition chamber opens and the next core can be acquired. By repeating this procedure and turning the probe stepwise around the clock, lesions can be removed.

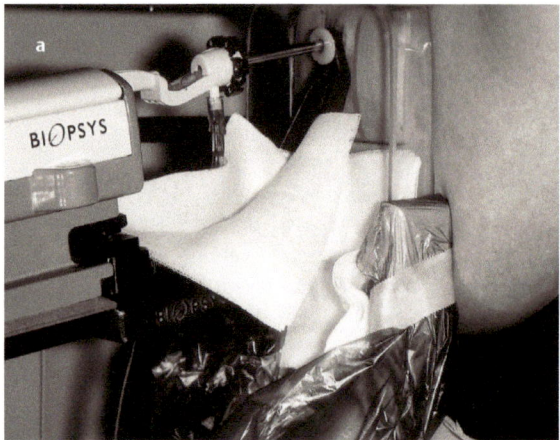

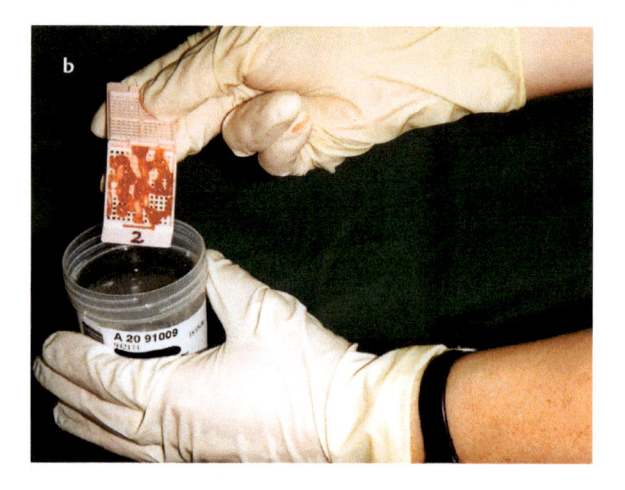

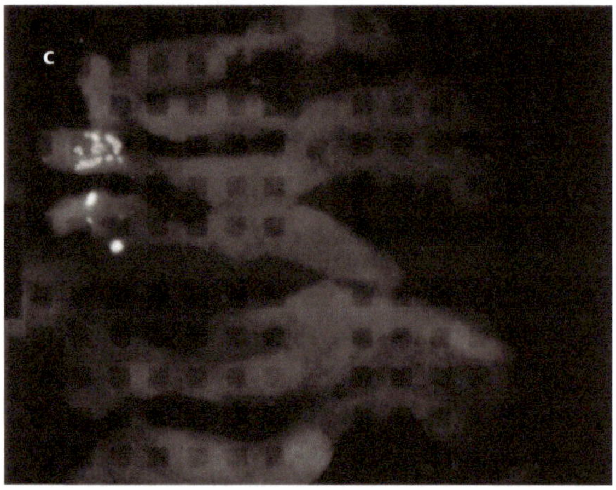

7 Imaging Assessment and Percutaneous Breast Biopsy

Fig. 7.4a–c Specimen acquisition with vacuum-suction biopsy.
a This image shows the needle in place during a procedure. A specimen is visible in the acquisition chamber where it can be taken off.
b Part of the specimen is shown. It is arranged in a sieve-like box and put into formalin. Further specimens are aranged in boxes (not shown).
c The specimen radiograph shows the specimens in the box.

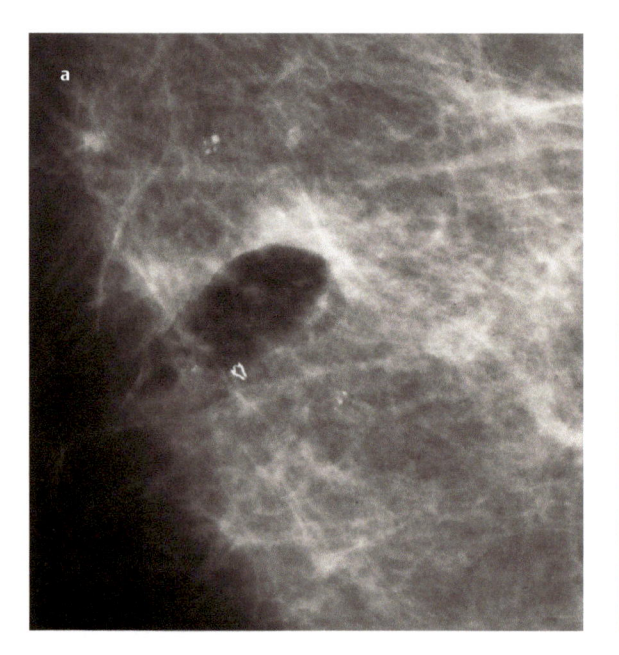

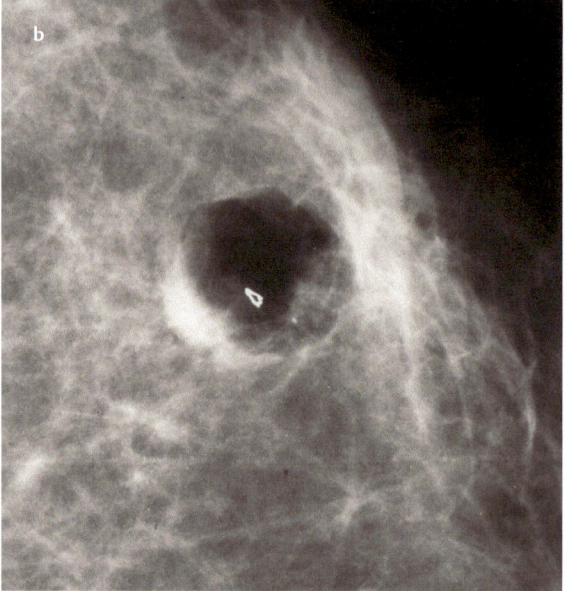

Fig. 7.5a,b Localizing clip. A stereotactic biopsy was performed of a lesion that was removed completely with an 11-gauge vacuum suction biopsy probe. A clip is placed at the biopsy site so that it can be readily localised if a repeat biopsy or surgical excision is subsequently required. On a mammogram done immediately after the biopsy, the clip is shown to be in the wall of the cavity created by the biopsy on both the mediolateral and craniocaudal views.

while postbiopsy changes often last only a few days and, therefore, cannot be used for localization if re-excision is necessary. Correct positioning of the clip must be checked by postbiopsy imaging. This is especially important when a clip is placed under mammographic guidance (i.e. in the compressed breast), because in some cases the clip might be displaced because of the "accordian effect." (Because the breast is compressed in one direction, when the clip is placed, displacement of the clip of 5–10 mm can result in a dislocation of several centimeters from the biopsy site after compression is released. This movement of the clip with relaxation of the tissue, which may be unpredictable while placing the clip, is called the "accordian effect.")

Postbiopsy imaging serves to countercheck and document correct location of the biopsy site and the clip and to assess the extent of removal of the imaging abnormality. Since the biopsy site and the number of radiographic abnormalities removed are usually more evident after VABB, compared with CNB, errors can be minimized, thus increasing reliability of the subsequent imaging–histopathology correlation.

Biopsy Under Ultrasound Guidance

Biopsies performed with US guidance (**Figs. 7.6, 7.7, 7.8, 7.9, 7.10, 7.11**) are appropriate for any lesion that can reproducibly be visualized by ultrasound. Because calcifications are not reliably seen sonographically, this technique is usually not appropriate for the biopsy of calcifications without an associated mass. It is, however, very useful to assess all cases of microcalcifications for which percutaneous biopsy is considered, to check for an associated mass. If an associated mass is detected, US-guided biopsy may allow the diagnosis of areas of invasion —which is helpful for further planning of subsequent surgery. US-guided biopsy is often faster to perform than stereotactic biopsies. Also, the supine position is usually much better tolerated than the prone or reclining position (or sometimes upright position) used with stereotactic biopsy.

This also applies to lesions near the chest wall and in areas that are difficult to position in the field of view of stereotactic systems. However, care must be taken not to violate the chest wall.

Ultrasound is also useful for biopsy guidance in the axilla, which can be done using FNAB or 14–20 gauge CNB.

Special care should be taken not to violate the larger vessels of the axilla, which are visible by ultrasound. The goal is to avoid the rare complication of a significant hematoma, which might compress the brachial plexus.

For US-guided breast biopsy no equipment is needed other than the usual ultrasound equipment and high-resolution linear-array transducers. Larger transducers (> 5 cm) may be very useful for targeting deeply located lesions, as they will allow visualization of the complete needle path even with a flat approach. We do not recommend using biopsy devices that are attached laterally to the transducer. They do not allow adequate tracking of the flexible and movable breast tissue during needle insertion, and usually encourage needle angulation toward the chest wall, which should always be avoided.

For the biopsy, the patient should be positioned as for ultrasound examination, depending on the lesion location (in the medial or lateral quadrants). Although an infinite number of approaches can be used, it is important to select an approach in which the lesion is well visualized and which, after needle insertion, allows angulation of the tip of the needle away from the chest wall. Usually lesions in the lateral quadrants, and in the 6 or 12 o'clock position, can easily be approached laterally. Lesions in the medial quadrants can sometimes be reached laterally, mostly caudally. Rarely, a medial approach is the only one feasible. If possible, attempts should be made to avoid approaching the lesion from the décolleté (for cosmetic reasons).

Some investigators seem to believe that "women do not feel pain within the breast" and therefore advocate that deep local anesthetic is not necessary. Even though perception of pain in the breast may vary between women and in differing areas of the breast, there is no anatomical or pathophysiological substance for this belief.

> Core needle biopsy and vacuum-assisted breast biopsy should never be performed without superficial and deep local anesthetic!

Performing a biopsy with as little pain as possible is a matter of respect for patients. We therefore appeal to all investigators to observe this recommendation, even

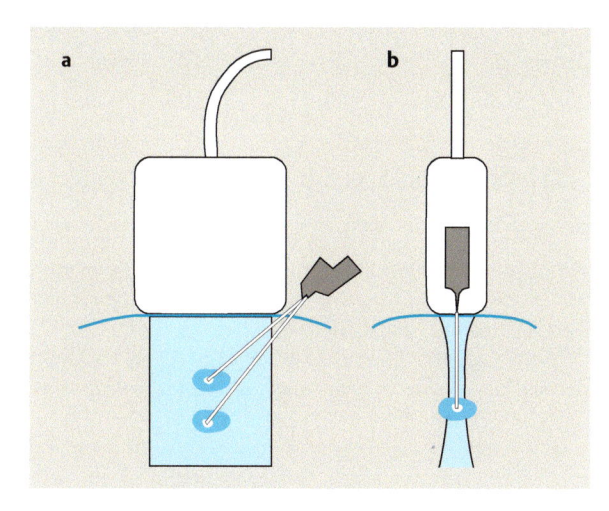

Fig. 7.6a,b Schematic diagram of ultrasound-guided biopsy (from Löfgren et al. 1990).
a The needle is advanced toward the lesion under the transducer within the plane of the ultrasound beam. Thus its entire length is visible. Anterior view.
b Lateral view, that is, in the direction of the biopsy.

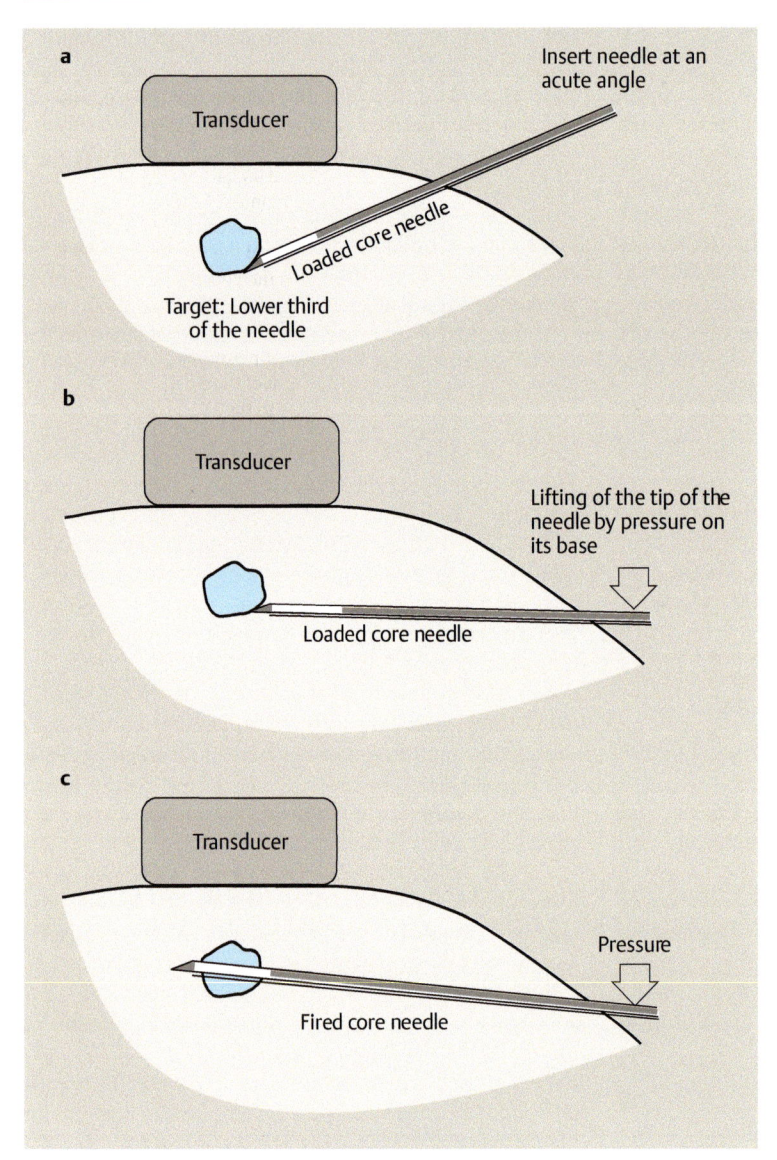

Fig. 7.7a–c Procedure for ultrasound-guided needle biopsy:

a The needle is held at an acute angle to the surface of the breast. The needle points at the lower third of the lesion.
b Pressing on the base of the needle lifts the tip of the needle upward.
c This prevents injury to the chest wall when the device is fired.

though percutaneous breast biopsy with local anesthetic is more time-consuming and may require more skill.

Any anesthetic used for US-guided breast biopsy must be purged of air, since air compromises sonographic imaging. First a small superficial infiltration of local anesthetic (LA) is made at the anticipated point of needle entry. Small aliquots of LA are introduced along the needle path. Deep LA should be applied on the proximal side of the lesion and underneath before entering the lesion. Then, depending on the size of the area to be biopsied, it may be useful to apply LA along the needle path or by fanning. Considering that the fired needle will often extend beyond the lesion, sufficient LA should also be deposited distal to the anticipated biopsy site.

Application of LA into the lesion may be necessary only for very extended lesions.

Special care should be taken to apply sufficient LA for lesions close to the nipple.

The injection of LA has to be done under sonographic visualization to place it optimally and to avoid violation of the chest wall during this step, and to stop injection if the LA threatens to obscure the lesion.

When approaching the lesion, the needle should always be imaged in the long axis and the following should be observed:
- The needle needs to be exactly aligned with the plane of the transducer. Otherwise part of the needle will not lie within the imaging plane. The image must, therefore, show the needle and the lesion in one plane. The focus of the ultrasound beam should be at the level of the lesion and the needle tip, otherwise the slice thickness of the B-mode image may be too thick.

Techniques for Biopsy and Biopsy Guidance

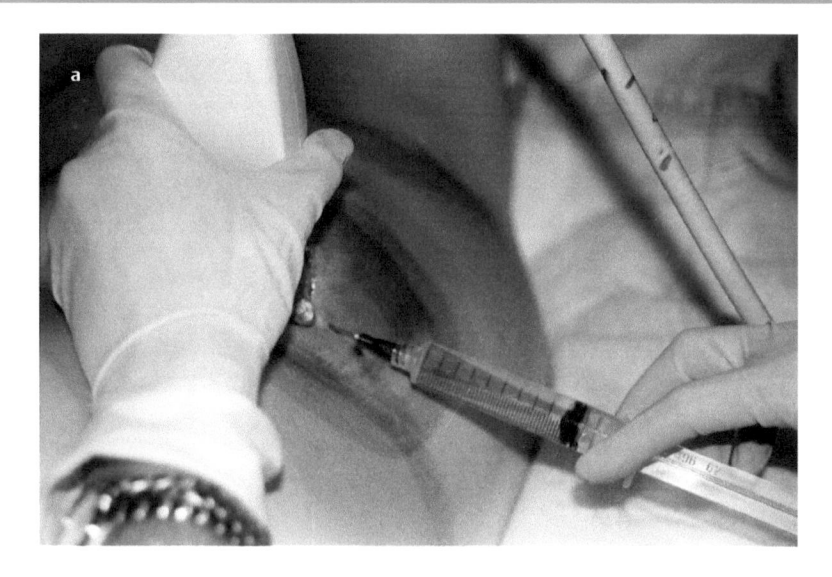

Fig. 7.8a,b Sonographically guided core biopsy.

- **a** After the skin has been cleaned and sterile gel or alcohol used as coupling agent for the transducer, anesthetic is injected under sonographic visualization.
- **b** The skin has been cut with a scalpel to ease entry of the cutting needle. The needle is then introduced along the long axis of the transducer. Alignment of the needle with the long axis of the transducer permits visualization of the length of the needle so it can be guided into the appropriate position.

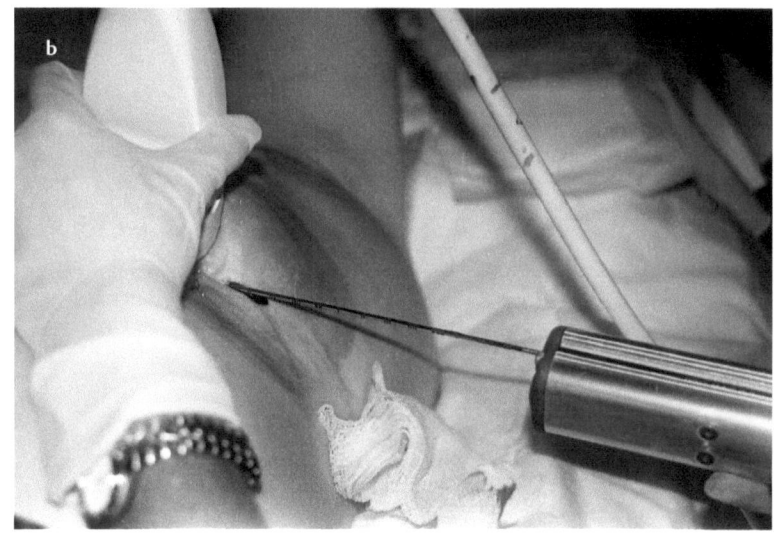

Such an image may give the perception that the needle passes through the lesion, while in reality it passes in front of or behind it because it is only imaged in the same (thick) slice.
- Imaging of the needle tip is of utmost importance. Only visualization of the needle tip allows avoidance of complications (e.g. inadvertent puncture of the chest wall).
- The biopsy should always be performed using a path that is as parallel to the chest wall as possible. There are two advantages to this:
  - Aiming the needle parallel to the chest wall minimizes the danger of injuries. This can be done by choosing a longer, but flat, approach to deeply located lesions. First the needle should target at the deep lateral border of the lesion. The needle thus acts as a fulcrum to pick up the lesion (see **Figs. 7.6, 7.7, 7.8, 7.9**). Then the end of the needle is pressed down to lift the tip of the needle upward, that is, away from the chest wall, before firing.
  - The needle is more readily visible since the ultrasound beam is reflected back to the transducer and not away from it. This makes it possible to image the entire length of the needle (see **Figs. 7.6, 7.7, 7.8, 7.9, 7.10**).

Never fire a gun with the needle pointing toward the chest wall!

For CNB and VABB a small skin cut should be made to facilitate introduction of the needle. For FNAB the needle should be positioned within the mass near its far wall before negative pressure is applied. As described before, the needle will then be moved back and forth within the mass, fanning out within the mass (5–10 thrusts), dur-

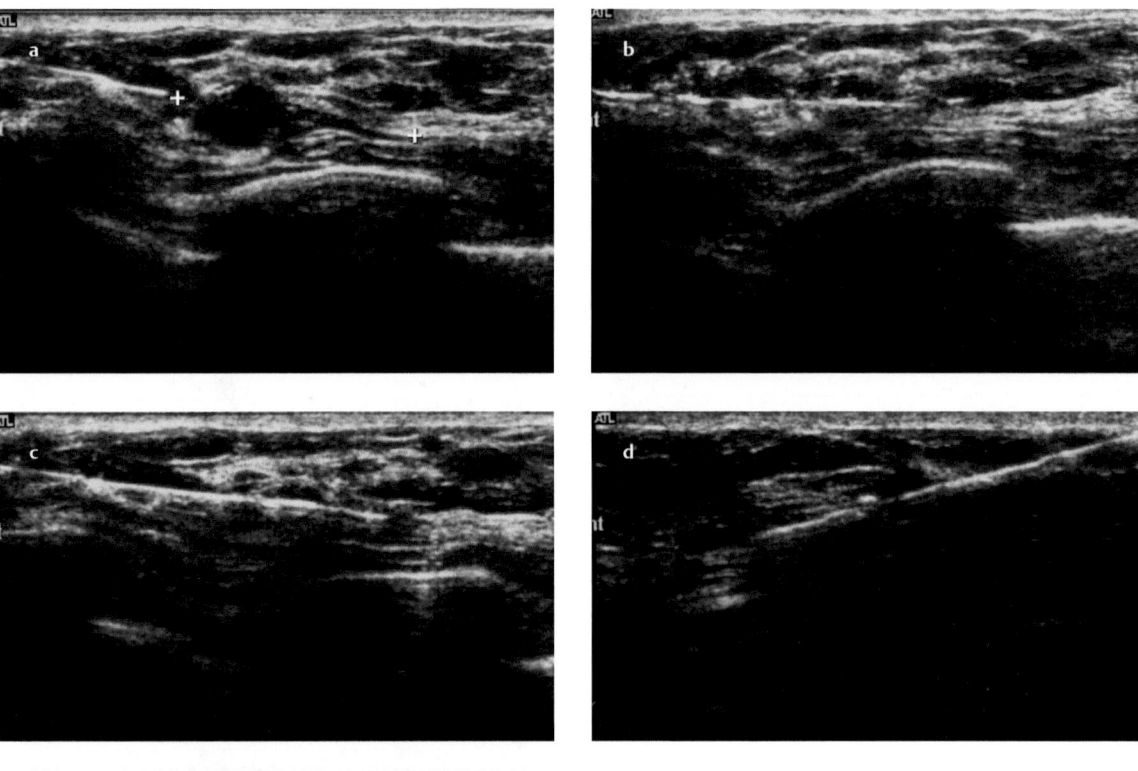

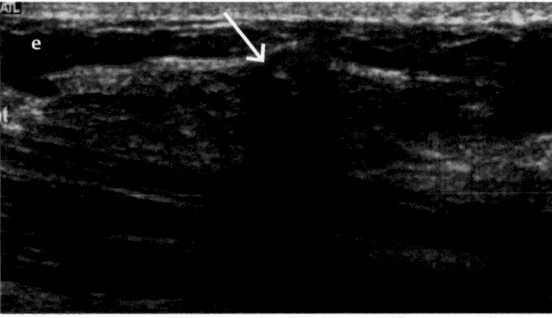

7 Imaging Assessment and Percutaneous Breast Biopsy

Fig. 7.9a–e

a–c An indeterminate mass, 1 cm in size. *Histology* revealed a 1-cm invasive ductal carcinoma. **a** First, the coaxial system or the biopsy needle is placed at the lateral (optimally the lateral lower) border of the lesion. Before firing, the angulation must be adapted parallel to the chest wall and should be seen in full length to ensure that the tip is included in the ultrasound slice. **b** After firing again the complete needle should be visualized in full length. On this image the back and middle end of the needle is seen sharply. However, the tip is slightly indistinct, indicating that the tip may extend beyond the imaged slice. There is still no danger, since the angulation is exactly parallel to the chest wall. **c** When the needle is imaged in full length it correctly extends beyond the lesion, since the acquisition window starts approximately 8 mm from the tip of the needle.

d,e A lesion 7 cm in size in another patient. *Histology* revealed an invasive ductal carcinoma. **d** Most guidelines require that the needle is shown in full length before and after firing. The image demonstrates the ideal needle position. The needle penetrates the lesion and is seen in full length, and courses parallel to the chest wall (**d**). If any doubts exist the transducer can be turned and an orthogonal image may be obtained (**e**). This image demonstrates an exactly centered biopsy needle. Such a countercheck may be useful for small lesions, since partial volume might give the impression that a needle coursing directly in front of or behind the lesion would correctly penetrate the lesion. Such a false impression may be enhanced if the image is not correctly focused (since the slice thickness increased outside the focal zone), or if very small lesions are imaged with transducers of moderate focusing capability.

Techniques for Biopsy and Biopsy Guidance

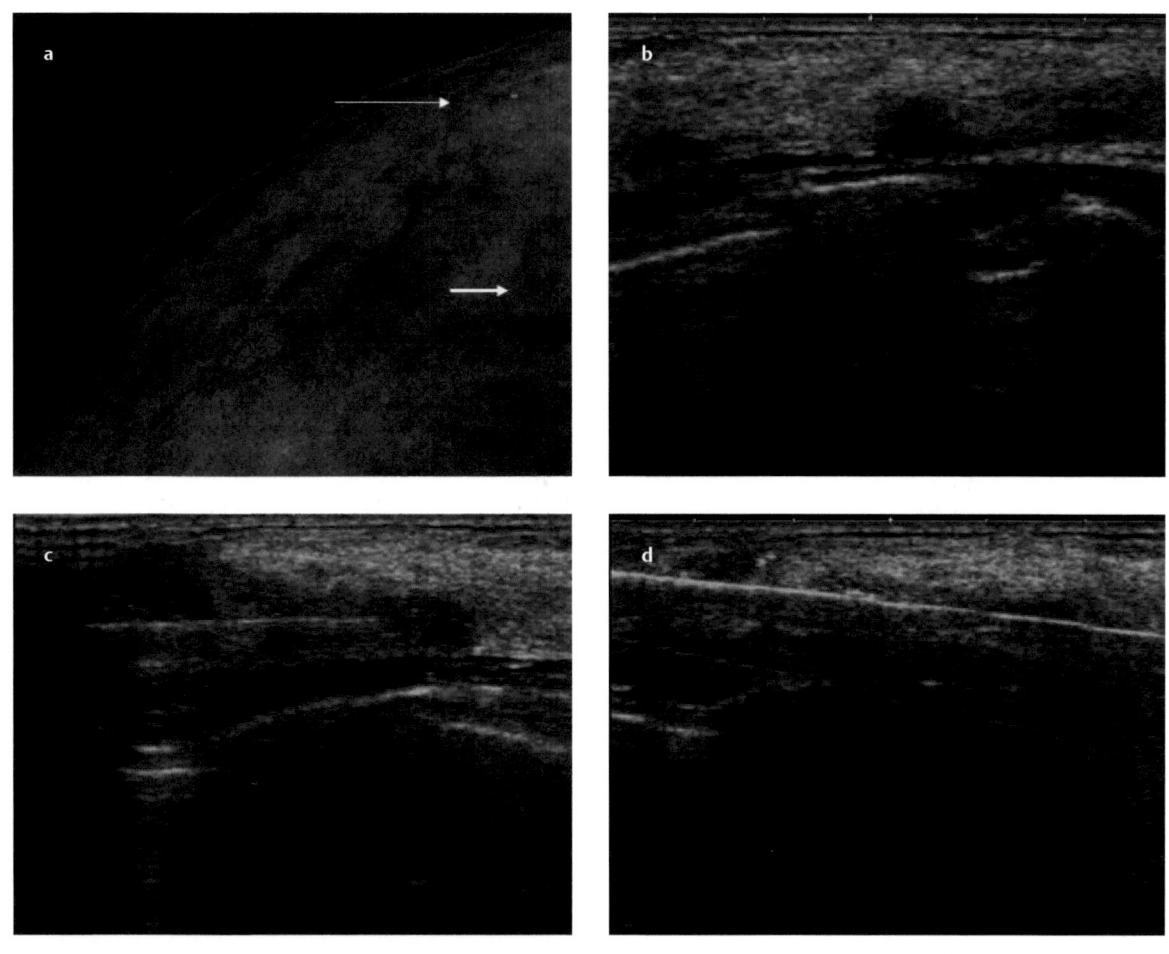

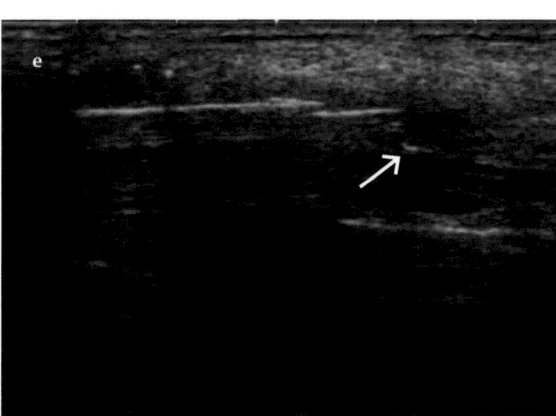

Fig. 7.10a–g To countercheck correlation with mammography, specimen radiography of the acquired cores is an option (to check for microcalcifications). Furthermore the biopsy site may be marked with a clip and a postinterventional mammogram may be considered.

a In this 38-year-old patient with a positive family history (mother and grandmother had breast cancer before age 45 and at age 55, respectively) mammography showed one suspicious group of around eight microcalcifications (smaller thick arrow), some very fine dispersed microcalcifications throughout the tissue, and another single microcalcification laterally on this mammogram (longer arrow). No clinical abnormality was detected.
b Ultrasound demonstrated a small nodule (5 mm) in the upper outer quadrant. However, the correlation with the mammographic finding was uncertain.
c Assessment started with a core needle biopsy (CNB) of the sonographic finding (prefire image).
d Postfire image of ultrasound-guided CNB, after which a clip was deposited exactly through the coaxial system.
e A clip (arrow) has then been deposited at the biopsy site.

Fig. 7.10 f,g ▷

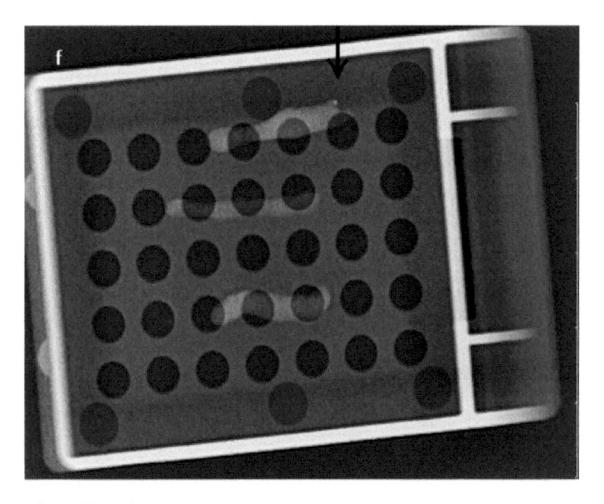

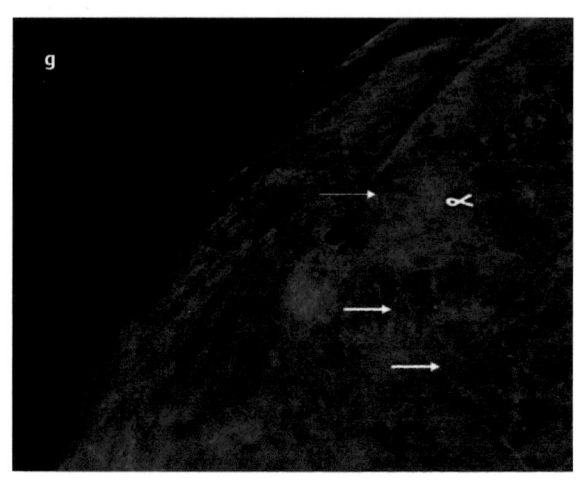

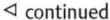

◁ continued
- **f** To countercheck whether the finding might correlate with the suspicious group of microcalcifications, specimen radiography was performed, which demonstrated one single microcalcification within one of the three acquired specimens. Retrospectively this microcalcification might correspond to the single microcalcification laterally (compare **a** and **f**).
- **g** A postprocedural mammogram (here an XCC view is shown that is slightly rolled compared with (**a**) demonstrating that the clip is placed approximately 1.7 cm from the suspicious group of microcalcifications. Comparing the pre- and postprocedural mammograms, one microcalcification of a tiny group of microcalcifications has been removed.

Histology of the CNB yielded a small invasive ductal breast cancer surrounded by ductal carcinoma in situ (DCIS). Excision (after marking of the clip and the suspicious microcalcifications medial to the clip) verified the invasive breast cancer and an adjacent area of altogether 12 cm of cribriform DCIS grade 2 medial to the invasive carcinoma.

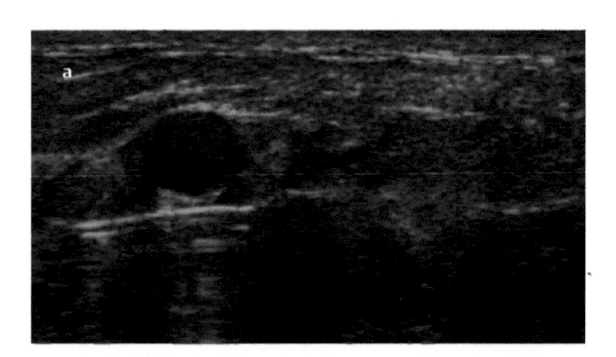

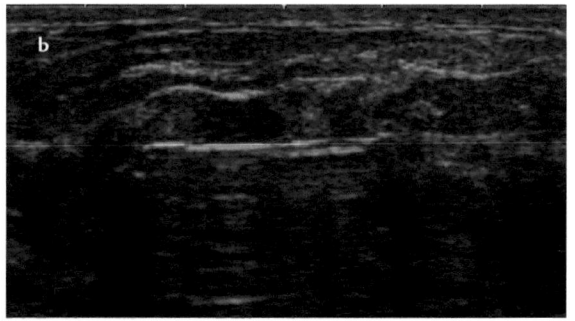

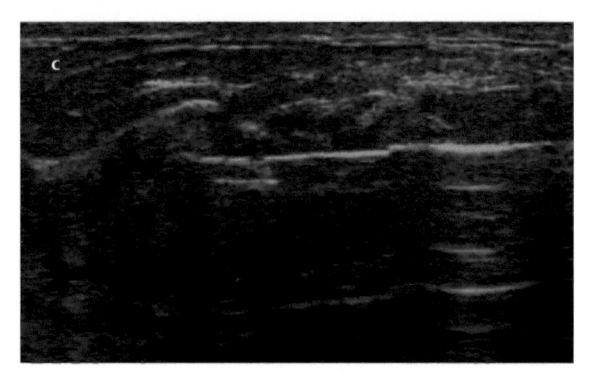

Fig. 7.11a–c Ultrasound (US)-guided vacuum-assisted breast biopsy (VABB).

US-guided breast biopsy may be chosen to assess lesions, for which (owing to the smaller volume of tissue obtained from standard core needle biopsy) sampling error may occur or which may not yield a sufficiently reliable diagnosis (e.g., within scarred tissue or for suspected papillary lesions). Re-excision might be recommended by the pathologist unless the lesion is at least largely removed. In this case a papillary lesion was suspected owing to the complex internal echo structure of the lesion.
- **a** For US-guided VABB the needle is placed underneath the lesion. Otherwise the thick needle would obscure the tissue underneath the lesion. The acquisition window thus faces the more superficial layers and tissue acquisition can be exactly monitored during the procedure.
- **b** Image taken after several specimens had been acquired; the lesion is already partly removed. This was achieved by acquiring cores and moving the acquisition window stepwise between the 8 o'clock and 2 o'clock positions.
- **c** Sonographically the lesion has been removed.
Histology yielded a benign adenoma. Follow-up ultrasound showed no residual lesion.

ing aspiration. This has to be repeated four or five times. For CNB the tip of the needle is placed at the deep lateral border of the lesion and the needle is fired, so that it will travel parallel to or away from the chest wall. Using 14-gauge needles, four to six good specimens should be obtained. Further cores are taken by re-targeting at different areas within the lesion. If a VABB probe is used (which is not fired into the breast), the probe is positioned underneath the deep margin of the lesion or in the deeper third of the lesion (**Fig. 7.11**), performing a similar "fulcrum motion" as described for core needle positioning. If the probe is positioned too superficial in relation to the lesion, it will be obscured by acoustic shadowing from the probe.

Image recording for US-guided breast biopsy should first include exact documentation of the position of the lesion in the breast in two orthogonal projections before biopsy. The exact lesion position should be reported, indicating its clockwise position, its distance to the nipple and distance underneath the skin. The chosen approach should also be documented on the on the ultrasound image. Next the complete needle should be imaged in its prebiopsy and in its postbiopsy positions. Visualization of the complete needle path is crucial to be sure that the needle courses within the imaged slice. If this is not the case incorrect placement of the needle tip (e.g., in a location too close to the chest wall) cannot be excluded.

In some very small lesions orthogonal imaging of the needle may help to countercheck and unequivocally document that the lesion was penetrated by the needle.

Film and specimen labeling should include the date of the procedure, the side and location of the lesion within the breast, the name of the facility where the biopsy was done, the name of the patient, the patient's date of birth and, if desired, a patient-identifying number and the name or identification of the physician performing the procedure.

If biopsies are taken from more than one lesion, special care is necessary to exactly document the location of each lesion, to exactly label image documentation, and to label separate pathology boxes containing the specimens from each lesion.

At the end of the procedure, the breast is compressed until adequate hemostasis is assured. The site of needle introduction should then be dressed appropriately. The patient should be instructed as to how she will receive the results of her biopsy, and how she should care for herself after the procedure (see pp. 192–193).

Stereotactic Biopsy

Stereotaxis (**Figs. 7.12, 7.13, 7.14**) localizes the lesion through triangulation. Angled views make it possible to calculate the position of the lesion as defined in its location on a horizontal (x) axis, vertical (y) axis, and depth (z) axis (see **Fig. 7.12**).

Several configurations of stereotactic equipment are available:
- Add-on units which can be attached to mammographic machines can be used to convert these machines to stereotactic biopsy units. When these are used, the patient is usually biopsied in a sitting position and must remain motionless in position during the procedure. This can sometimes be difficult. Motion may compromise the examination. Maintaining this position may cause considerable discomfort in the patient's neck, back, and shoulders. Since the procedure may be partly visible to the patient, the possibility of fainting needs to be considered. Owing to the unstable position of the sitting patient who has a needle in her breast, this situation may be difficult to handle. There is minimal space available within the confines of the equipment used to actually perform the biopsy and, because of the size of most needle-guns, VABB may not be possible with some of the add-on units. However, this set-up is the least expensive configuration for stereotactic equipment. In rare cases accessibility of lesions near the chest wall or in the axilla in the field of view of an add-on unit may be better than with prone tables.
- Couches are now available which allow the patient to recline in the decubitus position, using mammography equipment and an add-on unit, which avoids some of the disadvantages outlined above. To reduce imaging and waiting time (which is necessary for accurate biopsy without patient motion and for maximum of patient comfort and minimum complications), digital mammographic units are important for any type of stereotactic percutaneous biopsy and should be a prerequisite today for stereotactic VABB.
- Dedicated prone tables position the patient face-down with the breast protuding through a hole in the table in compression (**Fig. 7.13**). A mammographic unit is positioned under the table. The patient is less likely to move and is unlikely to faint with this equipment. There is a large amount of space for the physician to perform the biopsy. Some women may experience pain in their neck, back, or shoulders with this type of equipment. For many patients, however, psychological stress during the procedure is reduced, since they cannot see the procedure and the biopsy equipment.
- Stereotactic biopsies are appropriate for any lesions that can be seen mammographically and that cannot be approached using US guidance. Because microcalcifications are not reliably seen with sonography, biopsy of microcalcifications should be done under stereotactic guidance. As noted above, lesions too close to the chest wall, or lesions in breasts that are too thin under compression to contain the biopsy probe, cannot undergo stereotactic CNB or VABB. If US-guided biopsy is not possible either, open biopsy after wire localization (e.g., placing the wire so that the lesion

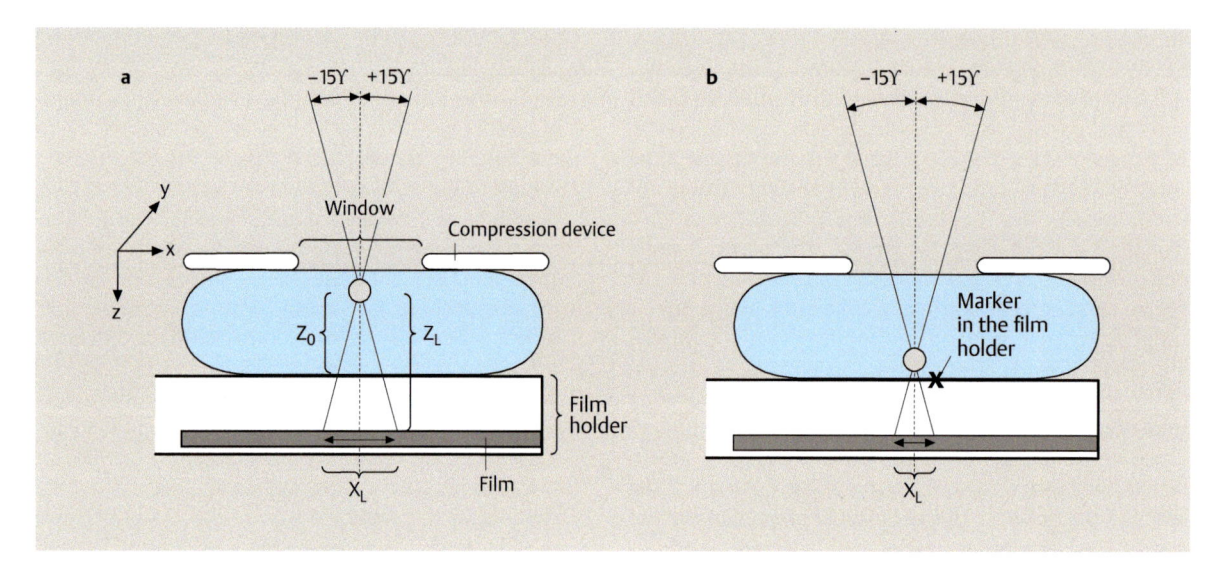

Fig. 7.12a,b Principle of depth localization

a First, the breast is compressed with a fenestrated compression plate. The opening needs to be precisely above the lesion to be sampled. Spot compression views are obtained by tilting the X-ray tube +15° and −15° from the midline.

b Lesions closer to the film (**b**) will appear with less of a shift (X_L) on the film than lesions farther from the film (**a**). The mammography unit can calculate the depth of the lesion from the parallax shift of the lesion (X_L). The depth of the lesion (Z_L) is calculated using the following formula:

$$\frac{X_L}{2} = Z_L \cdot \tan 15° \quad \text{or} \quad Z_L = \frac{X_{L2}}{2 \cdot \tan 15°}$$

The formula can be adapted accordingly to determine the depth of the lesion with respect to the film holder. To do so, a reference point on the film holder is used and the formula is changed accordingly. This reference point is also used as a reference point for the lateral shift, since the film cassette is also moved manually between the +15 and −15 views to avoid exposing it twice.

is between the wire and chest wall) may have to be considered. Since some vendors offer special probes for very small breasts, this problem has significantly decreased.

During stereotactic biopsy, a scout film without tube angulation is first obtained to document accurate positioning of the target in the field of view. Then the stereotactic pair is obtained by moving the X-ray tube along the horizontal axis; lesions will move to the right and left on these images (**Fig. 7.14a**). The amount of movement depends on the distance of the lesion from the image receiver. From this movement the distance between lesion and image receiver is calculated by the stereotactic unit. If the lesion is too close to the right or left side of the scout film, it will not appear on one of the stereotactic pairs and calculation of the lesion coordinates is not possible. Therefore, when positioning the patient, an attempt should be made to image the target as close as possible to the center of the scout.

After the stereotactic pair has been obtained, a cursor is placed over the identical site of interest on the two chosen stereotactic views. Based on these cursor positions the unit calculates the coordinates of the lesion. Great care is needed to identify exactly the same structure. If this is not possible (multiple similar calcifications, architectural distortion, which is imaged differently on different views), biopsy might be attempted in a different plane of compression, or percutaneous biopsy may not be possible using stereotaxis. In such rare cases open biopsy after wire localization should be considered unless the lesion is visible by ultrasound. (In contrast to percutaneous biopsy, wire localization can be performed using manual localization or using a grid combined with manual localization in the second plane.)

Percutaneous breast biopsy should not be performed if the same structure cannot unequivocally be identified, since errors identifying the same structure on the stereotactic views will cause miscalculation of the lesion location. To recognize errors identifying the target, we recommend always counterchecking the calculated needle position with the position of the lesion in the two mammographic planes of the original mammogram. It is important to remember that (the center of) the lesion

Techniques for Biopsy and Biopsy Guidance

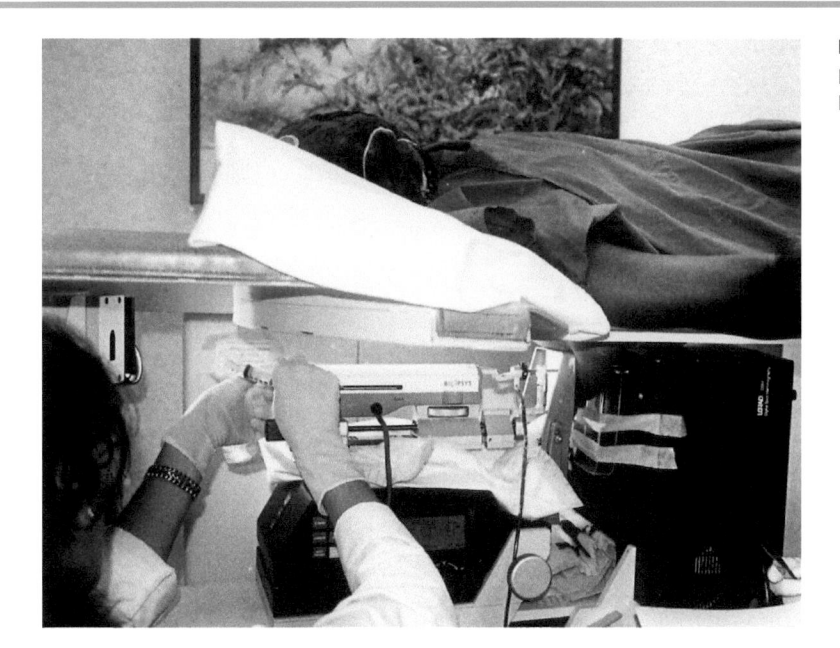

Fig. 7.13 This image shows the patient position on a prone table during a procedure.

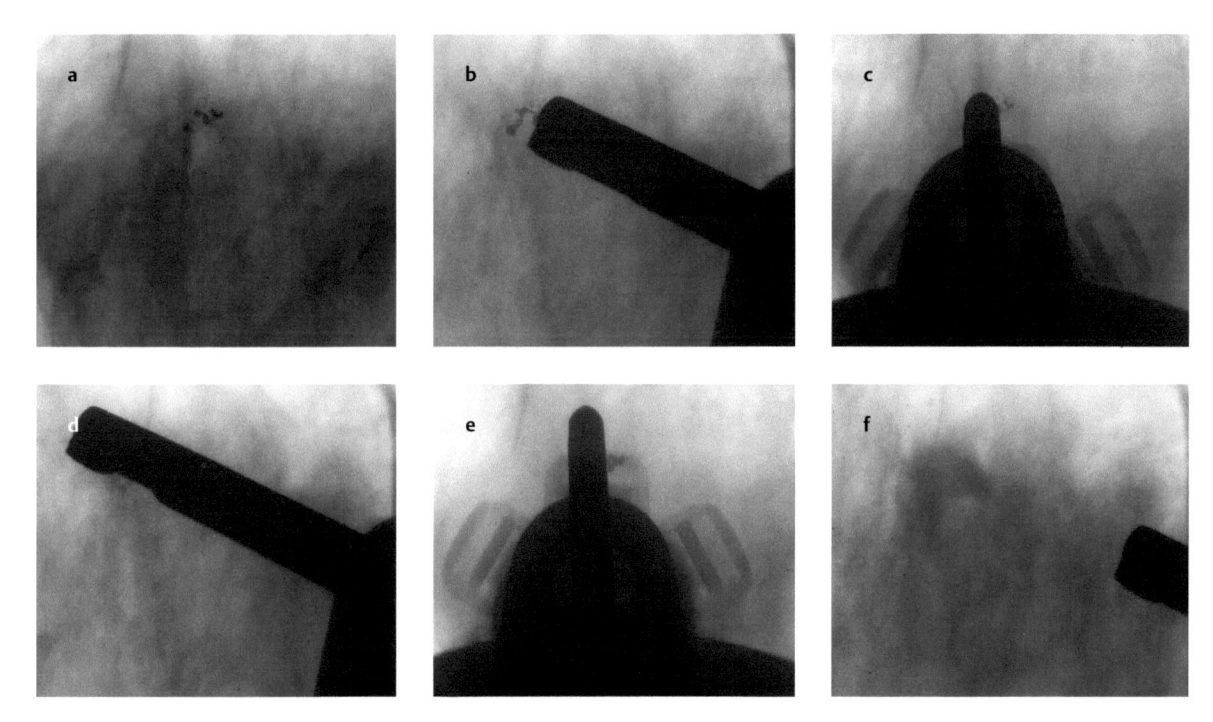

Fig. 7.14a–f Images taken during a vacuum biopsy are shown.

a The scout view shows an indeterminate group of microcalcifications. From the three views (−15°, 0°, and +15°) the 0° and the −15° views were selected for planning the procedure.
b After planning, the needle, which is not yet fired, is introduced to the calculated "prefire" position. Its correct position is checked on this −15° view.
c Correct "prefire" position is also confirmed on the 0° view.
d,e After the needle is fired into the lesion, needle position is once more checked on the −15° and 0° views.
f After withdrawing the needle, no more microcalcifications are visible at the biopsy site.
Histology revealed ductal carcinoma in situ, which was confirmed after re-excision.

205

should be located at the center of the acquisition chamber of the biopsy probe (see **Fig. 7.3**).

The depth of needle insertion (as calculated by the unit) always has to be adapted to the type of needle or probe and the center of the acquisition chamber with respect to the needle or probe tip (**Fig. 7.14b,c**). This latter distance varies with the chosen type of biopsy needle. It should also be known to the interventionist when counterchecking the calculated coordinates.

During the procedure the needle position is checked by stereotactic views before and after firing the needle into the lesion. These views are important to recognize possible lesion shift due to needle insertion or bleeding and thus allow for a correction if necessary. Ideally the lesion should be exactly placed at the tip of the needle before firing and at the acquisition window of the needle after firing.

When planning the approach it should be borne in mind that there is a dead space between the tip of the needle and the acquisition window, which measures up to 10 mm. Therefore, when planning the approach the lesion should not be positioned distally in the breast. In such a position the needle tip might breach the skin at the far side of the breast and the lesion may be pushed ahead by the needle.

Before core biopsy needles or vacuum probes are introduced into the breast, a small cut (5 mm) is made in the skin after local anesthetic has been injected intracutaneously. Deep local anesthesia is also necessary for core biopsy, but it must be remembered that ample local anesthetic may obscure mass lesions and cause lesion shift. If VABB is performed, a minimal volume of local anesthetic (2 mL) can be applied along the anticipated needle path. After the needle is fired into the lesion the major part of local anesthetic (usually up to 20 mL lidocaine 1% or equivalent medication) is then injected in the tissues surrounding the acquisition window, because then the tissue is fixed by the probe itself. Minor shifts will be compensated by suction.

After correct needle placement is achieved and documented and after sufficient local anesthetic has been applied, VABB can start. We recommend performing the complete VABB without interruption by acquiring at least 12 cores (usually 18–24 cores) using 11-gauge needles (or an equivalent volume of tissue using 8 G or 9 G needles).

After biopsy has been performed the needle is withdrawn and another stereotactic pair is obtained (before releasing the compression). This pair of images serves to countercheck that tissue was acquired from the area in question.

When microcalcifications are the object of biopsy, specimen radiography is necessary to confirm that the microcalcifications of concern have been obtained and to show their location within the cores to the pathologist for direct correlation (**Fig. 7.4c**). When CNB is performed, the specimen radiograph(s) should be taken during the biopsy procedure, so more samples can be taken if necessary. Owing to the excellent accuracy of VABB (which normally allows removal of a representative volume of tissue containing microcalcifications), it is usually sufficient to obtain just one specimen radiograph at the end of the VABB procedure.

CNB should be continued until calcifications are obtained or until tissue becomes so hemorrhagic that continued biopsy fails to obtain any useful tissue. In the latter case interdisciplinary imaging–histopathology correlation will decide whether the biopsy may be considered representative.

VABB allows removal of the majority or even all imaging-detected abnormality. If possible we attempt to remove small lesions completely, since complete sampling will allow the highest possible reliability of a negative diagnosis (irrespective of whether the final histopathologic result is specific or unspecific). It must, however, be understood that complete excision of the radiologic abnormality to date does not eliminate the need for therapeutic surgery in case of malignancy. Since malignancy may occur adjacent to B3 or B4 lesions, complete excision of the visible abnormality cannot exclude histopathologic underestimates. The need for excision versus follow-up remains a decision taken at the interdisciplinary conference and with diligent imaging–histopathology correlation.

Specimen radiography should be performed using magnification mammography or dedicated specimen radiography units. It is indicated for all lesions containing microcalcifications. For the specimen radiograph of cores the lowest kVp and mAs settings on the unit should be used as the initial settings. Specimen radiographs should be kept as part of the medical record. The pathologist may appreciate a copy of the specimen radiograph.

In case of a mass lesion it may only be possible to countercheck that the hematoma (or cavity) is exactly centered in the previous location of the lesion.

If the lesion has been completely removed or if a mass lesion is obscured by significant hematoma, placement of a *marker clip* should be considered.

After biopsy has been completed we recommend obtaining mammograms using two orthogonal views. These serve to demonstrate correct sampling and correct positioning of the marker. In contrast to stereotactic views, projection error is excluded and an overview of the complete breast is given. The orthogonal views are also helpful for subsequent surgical planning if needed.

In most cases we perform this two-view mammogram directly after the procedure, while the breast is still anesthetized. If there has been significant bleeding during the procedure, this final documentation can also be obtained some days later.

As with US-guided biopsy, at the end of the procedure pressure should be held over the biopsy site to obtain hemostasis, the patient should have an appropriate dressing applied, and she should be given instruction on how to care for her breast after the biopsy and how she will receive the results.

If biopsies are taken from more than one lesion, special care is necessary to label each lesion precisely. Since VABB usually requires more local anesthetic than CNB and since both prone and upright positions may be difficult to tolerate for the patient (as usually needed for stereotactic procedures), stereotactic biopsy of more than one lesion during one session requires careful consideration.

MR-Guided Percutaneous Biopsy

When a lesion is identified by breast MRI, before MR-guided biopsy is considered, a second-look ultrasound examination should always be performed to confirm that the lesion is only visible by MRI. A diligent selection of MR indications, adequate consideration of hormonal influence, and sufficient experience with the interpretation of MRI and conventional imaging helps maintain a sensible ratio of malignant to benign biopsies (**Fig. 7.15**).

Whenever possible, MR-guided VABB should be timed according to the menstrual cycle. Influence from hormone replacement therapy should be avoided if possible by either discontinuing it for 4 weeks or (according to our experience) limiting it to estrogens only or tibulone.

MR-guided biopsy should be performed only using dedicated equipment (biopsy coil and targeting software) and MR-compatible VABB probes.

The vast majority of biopsy systems today allow fixation of the breast and guidance of a coaxial system (or the biopsy needle) into the lesion by using a guidance system, on which the coaxial system or needle is mounted.

In the literature, only few biopsies have been described as freehand biopsies, which in principle are only possible in magnets allowing open access to the patient during the procedure and using so-called navigation tracker systems. Such systems guide needle introduction by infrared or ultrasound and allow real-time monitoring.

The following paragraphs describe a standard procedure, as it is performed with the commonly used types of equipment (with this equipment the breast is fixed by compression and biopsy is performed through the compression plate using either a so-called "post and pillar system" or a grid with perforated holes):

- Before biopsy the patient has to be positioned prone on the MR table that is equipped with the biopsy coil. Positioning should consider the anticipated location of the lesion and the limited areas of access. The breast is then fixed by moderate compression. Too strong compression may alter enhancement by reducing perfusion (Hefler et al. 2003). The fiducial marker(s), which serve to calibrate the guidance system, need to be placed as required for the chosen biopsy coil.
- After moving the patient table into the bore, the dynamic series including pre- and postcontrast 3D images of the fixed breast are acquired, and 3D subtraction sets are calculated. Then the fiducial marker and the lesion need to be identified on the obtained images. Their position is usually entered into the targeting software by clicking the tip of the fiducial marker and the center of the lesion. Thereafter, the parameters that need to be transferred to the guidance unit are calculated by the software.
- With the MR table moved out of the bore, the MR-compatible coaxial system is mounted on the guidance system.
- Next the calculated parameters need to be set on the guidance unit to allow introduction of the coaxial system into the lesion. For post-and-pillar systems the parameters usually indicate the shift that needs to be set on the guidance system in three dimensions (foot–head; anterior–posterior; and depth of needle insertion into the breast depending on the chosen needle angulation). These parameters are calculated with respect to a "zero-position" that is also identified by the location of the fiducial marker(s). The calculated parameters that need to be set on the biopsy device will vary with the chosen angle of access and with the dimensions of the coaxial and the biopsy system (distance of the acquisition window from the needle tip, dimensions of the acquisition window, and the position where the needle is mounted on the guidance device). For grid systems (which allow only horizontal needle insertion without angulation), the software indicates the hole through which the needle has to be inserted
- The depth of needle insertion is usually set manually after the other parameters have been transferred to the guidance unit. This is necessary, since, when setting this parameter, the needle will be introduced into the breast.
- Before the coaxial system is advanced to the lesion, a small amount of local anesthetic is administered in the skin and in the anticipated path of the needle to the calculated depth of needle insertion.
- Then the coaxial system can be advanced to the calculated position. Usually the cutting needle of the coaxial system is then exchanged by an MR-visible core at the center of the acquisition window or the tip of the anticipated biopsy probe (as defined by the vendor).
- The patient is moved back into the bore and imaging counterchecks the correct position of the coaxial system. In case of significant lesion shift (during introduction of the needle or local anesthetic), in case of patient motion, or in case of a calculation error, retargeting or adjustment of the depth of insertion may be needed. Corrections of the needle position are performed with the biopsy table moved out of the bore. Significant manipulations need to be followed by re-imaging that is performed with the patient table moved back into the bore.

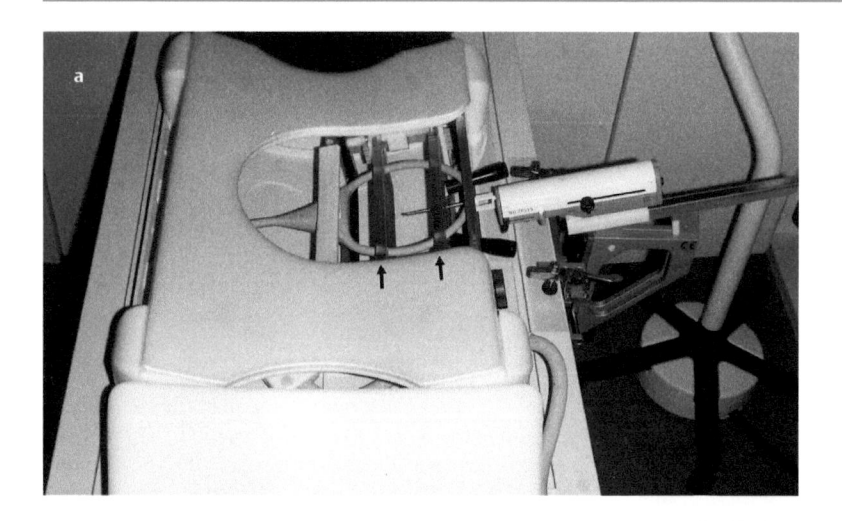

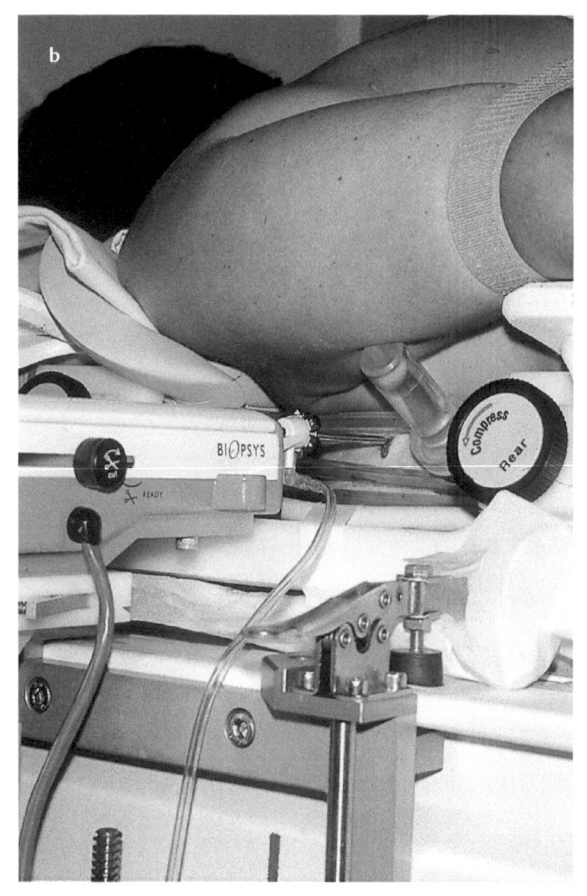

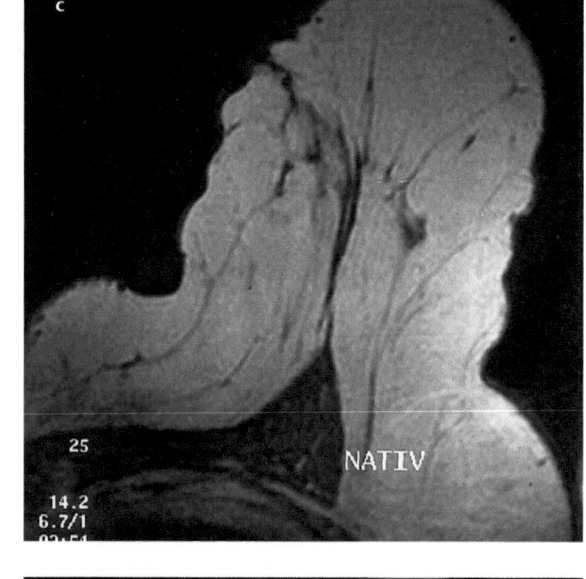

7 Imaging Assessment and Percutaneous Breast Biopsy

Fig. 7.15a–g

a Equipment for MR-guided localization, core needle, or vacuum biopsy. The housing of the biopsy coil is placed on the MR table. The patient has to lie prone on this housing, and the pendant breast will be moderately compressed between the two compression plates (arrows). A ring coil is inserted between the bars of the compression plates. With her breast fixed, the patient has to lie still on this biopsy device throughout the procedure. For imaging she is moved into the bore; for biopsy she is moved out of the magnet. Based on

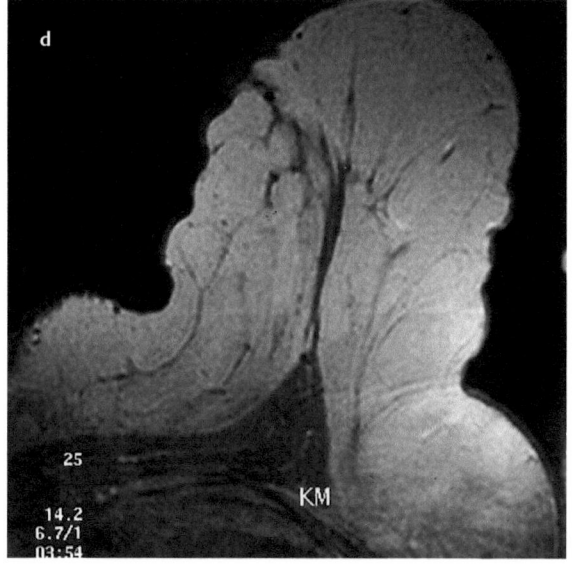

Techniques for Biopsy and Biopsy Guidance

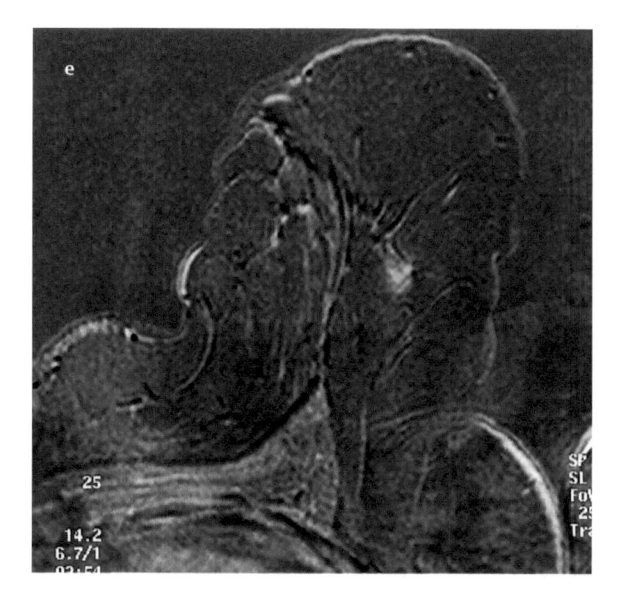

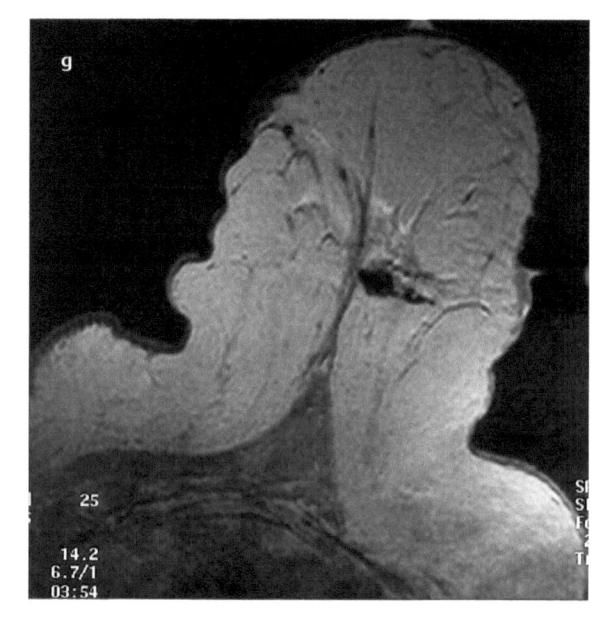

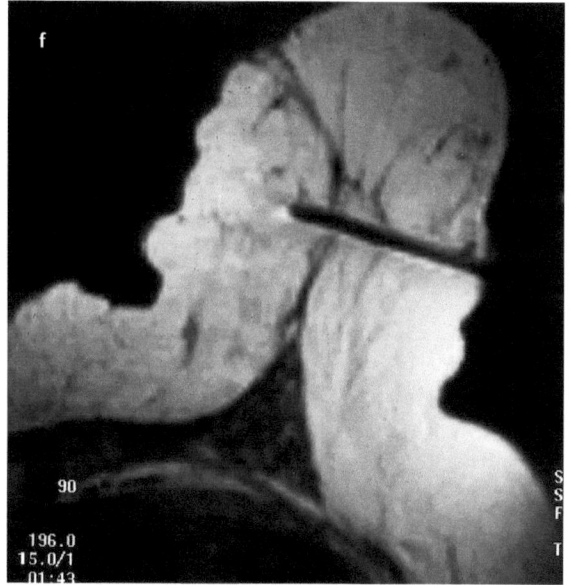

the MR images, the transverse slice that contains the lesion can be identified. This is aligned with the aiming device that supports the biopsy gun. The height and depth of needle insertion is also determined from the transverse MR images and transferred to the aiming device. That way, by setting the aiming device to the calculated coordinates, the lesion will be pierced by the biopsy probe and centered exactly at the acquisition window of the probe.
b Close-up images of an MR-guided vacuum biopsy. The patient lies prone on the biopsy coil. The vacuum biopsy probe is inserted into the patient's breast after the bars of the compression plate have been spread by a spacer.
c–g Representative images of an MR-guided vacuum biopsy. In this patient MRI was performed because of impaired assessment after breast-conserving therapy, as a result of overlying tissue (other slices) and scarring. A small enhancing focus was detected by MRI, which in retrospect could be reproduced on only one mammographic view.
c Precontrast MR image of the lesion.
d Postcontrast MR image. The lesion enhances and becomes almost isointense to fat.
e Subtraction image of the lesion.
f Based on the imaging coordinates of the lesion, first, a thin MR-compatible substitute needle was inserted to the calculated position and checked by MRI. Then its correct position, which was shown here, was confirmed (to have the lesion at the acquisition chamber of the probe, the probe has to reach beyond the lesion). Then the patient was moved away from the magnet. The substitute needle was exchanged for the vacuum device, and vacuum biopsy was performed at the calculated position. (Today MR-compatible coaxial systems are available and used instead of a substitute needle.)
g Finally, correct removal is checked. This image shows that the cavity is in the exact place where the lesion had initially been. *Histology*: Ductal carcinoma G2.

- After correct placement of the coaxial system is verified, the patient table is again moved out of the bore, the MR-visible core is withdrawn from the coaxial system and the biopsy needle is introduced through the coaxial system without moving the coaxial system.
- All coaxial systems are constructed to harbor the corresponding biopsy needle in such a way that the biopsy needle is exactly placed in the lesion when the coaxial tube ends at the lesion. So VABB is performed blindly through the coaxial system relying on the correct position of the coaxial system.
- Before biopsy is started, sufficient local anesthesia should be given surrounding the anticipated area of biopsy. We recommend administering 4–5 mL of lidocaine 1% in four sites around the biopsy site (altogether 20 mL of local anesthetic). Alternatively, local anesthetic may be administered through the biopsy needle. According to our experience this may be less effective than the former method. (Maximum dosage of local anesthetic and possible contraindications must be considered.)
- We strongly recommend acquiring at least 12 cores of 10-gauge thickness (preferably more) or an equivalent volume of tissue using thicker probes. We usually acquire 18–24 cores. With a sufficient amount of removed tissue minor tissue shift is well compensated for, sampling error is reduced, and reduction or removal of the lesion in question, or its replacement by a visible and correctly centered cavity, can usually be verified by subsequent imaging.

If several lesions are biopsied or require biopsy special attention to correct labeling is necessary.

Considering the duration of the procedure (which is performed in prone position) and the maximum recommended dosage of local anesthetic, we advise against performing MR-VABB of more than one location during one session.

To obtain reproducible results, the procedure should follow the agreed recommendations of quality assurance (Heywang-Köbrunner et al. 2009).

Handling the Biopsy Specimen

If the needle is removed from the breast and reinserted, care should be taken not to place the needle in preservative and reintroduce it into the breast (**Fig. 7.14**). For fine needle aspirations, a new needle should be used for each aspiration. If cores are undergoing specimen radiography, they should be kept moist with saline until they are placed in preservative so that drying artifact does not compromise the ability of the pathologist to make a diagnosis. The specimens should then be placed in fixative solution immediately. Before fixation the specimen should be arranged straight. Multiple cores should be arranged parallel.

The tissue fixation protocol should be based on a standard procedure agreed between the involved departments.

The specimen containers must be labeled correctly (patient name, date of birth, ID number, name of institution, date of biopsy, right or left breast, number of the lesion—if several lesions are biopsied).

The pathologist should be supplied with adequate clinical information to interpret the specimen. The location of the biopsied lesion always has to be clearly indicated. The lesion should be described (lesion type and size) and the suspected diagnosis and BI-RADS category should be included in the lesion description.

If the biopsy was of calcifications, the pathologist should be provided with the specimen radiograph or a copy. Any pertinent clinical history should also be provided.

The pathologist should examine cores at four or five levels. If the microcalcifications in question are not identified in these levels but are present on the specimen X-ray, further levels are necessary. Radiography of the paraffin blocks may be helpful. If problems identifying the microcalcifications remain, the blocks have to be worked up completely.

Pathologists should be aware that microcalcifications below 100 μm in size are usually not visible on the mammogram. Thus, smaller microcalcifications usually do not correlate with a mammographically visible cluster.

If histopathology cannot identify a correlation with the imaging abnormality, further levels of the cores have to be analyzed by the pathologist. In difficult cases complete histopathologic workup of the acquired tissue is necessary.

Interpreting the Histopathologic Results

A pivotal step in the successful application of these biopsy procedures to patient care is the correlation of the biopsy results with the imaging pattern of the targeted lesion and concordance should always be checked very diligently. Ideally, this should be performed in regular interdisciplinary conferences with an experienced team including at least the interventionist and the specialized pathologist. For optimum recommendations in borderline lesions (B3, B4) and for adequate preoperative planning and information transfer, a larger interdisciplinary team (including also the surgeon, the radiation oncologist and/or gynecologist) is desirable.

To improve communication and systematic analysis of each lesion recommended classifications should be used by radiologists and by the pathologists.

For the radiologic classification of lesions after completed imaging assessment, the BI-RADS nomenclature should be used (see Chapter 3).

For classification of cytology, the following classification (Perry et al. 2006) should be used:
- C1: Inadequate for diagnosis
- C2: Benign epithelial cells
- C3: Atypia, probably benign
- C4: Suspicious of malignancy
- C5: Malignant

For percutaneous breast biopsy using CNB or VABB pathologists should classify lesions according to the European Guidelines (Perry et al. 2006), as follows:
- B1a: Unsatisfactory (e.g., insufficient tissue because of a technical problem etc.).
- B1b: Normal tissue. If normal or fatty tissue is the result of a needle biopsy, very diligent correlation is needed to determine whether this histopathologic finding explains the imaging finding and may thus be representative.
- B2: Benign lesion. Benign lesions include fibroadenomas, papillomas, adenosis tumors, cysts, sclerosing adenosis, and fibrocystic or inflammatory changes. Whereas tumorous B2 lesions may well explain a mammographic or sonographic mass, diligent correlation is necessary for histopathologic changes that may not explain the imaging finding.
    - *For all B1 and B2 lesions exact imaging–histopathology correlation is crucial to determine whether biopsy is representative and compatible with imaging.*
- B3: Benign lesion of uncertain malignant potential. This category includes lesions which are known to show histologic heterogeneity and have an increased risk of associated malignancy or of developing into a higher-grade lesion. On average 25–35% of subsequent surgical biopsies prove to be malignant after diagnosis of a B3 lesion at needle biopsy.
- B4: Benign lesion of unknown biological potential with changes suspicious of malignancy. Diagnosis of malignancy may not be possible based on the obtained material, even though malignancy is suspected. Such situations may occur if a small volume of tissue is available, if artifacts (poor fixation, drying of cores, blood) exist, if only few malignant cells are present (very early lesions), or in case of a finding that may be difficult to distinguish with the usual H&E staining. To achieve a final diagnosis special staining (immunohistochemistry) may be necessary; possibly further levels may help. In all other cases repeat biopsy (e.g., VABB) or surgical biopsy is necessary. On average 66% of surgical biopsies after diagnosis of a B4 lesion at needle biopsy will prove malignancy.
- B5: Malignant. Accuracy of this diagnosis is usually very high (> 99.5% according to the European guidelines). Thus therapeutic decisions can be safely based on such a diagnosis. The subcategory B5a indicates a ductal carcinoma in situ (or a nonobligatory precursor of an invasive breast cancer). The subcategory B5b stands for invasive breast cancer. The category B5c includes other malignancies of the breast.

A diagnosis of malignancy that is classified as B5 and based on the histology of percutaneous breast biopsy that was performed following the above-mentioned standards may be considered reliable in > 99.9% of cases. In case of doubt, the pathologist should classify the lesion as B4 (suspicious of malignancy). Usually, after additional immunohistology or after excision of residual changes the lesion can be classified as benign or malignant.

Lesions classified as B3 should always be discussed in the interdisciplinary conference. The presence of such a lesion may indicate that even though the lesion is classified as a benign entity, the patient may be at increased risk of developing a malignancy in the future. If left in the breast, the lesion could develop into a higher-grade lesion (such as a DCIS or invasive breast cancer). Such lesions could also already be associated with higher grade changes, which—due to the small volume of tissue obtained by percutaneous breast biopsy—might not have been sampled. This risk varies with the histology of the lesion, the chosen method of biopsy, the volume of tissue sampled, and the approximate percentage of tissue sampled.

If complete removal of the imaging abnormality is possible at percutaneous biopsy, the risk of missing an associated malignancy can be reduced, but cannot be eliminated. Therefore the optimum recommendation (which may imply intensified follow-up or re-excision) should be given individually to the patient after diligent consideration of the following information in an interdisciplinary conference:
- Imaging before and after the intervention and specimen radiography should be correlated with histopathology to assess whether biopsy is representative and whether the initial question posed by imaging was solved. (For example, the question is not solved if lobular intraepithelial atypia grade 1 is detected incidentally, while there is no explanation on histopathology for a mass or area of microcalcifications seen on imaging.)
- Based on the estimated extent of the lesion, the volume of sampled tissue, and the histopathologic type of B3 lesion (based on standard H&E or special staining as indicated), the probability of presence of a higher-grade lesion (i.e., the probability of associated malignancy) should be considered.
- Based on this information and other risk factors (individual history or family history), the risk of cancer at the biopsy site or in other locations of the same or contralateral breast should be estimated.
- Based on the type of lesion (incidental or associated with a defined imaging finding) and the type of sur-

rounding tissue it should be considered whether monitoring is possible.
- Finally, other risk factors and patient age need to be considered to avoid treating a lesion that may not lead to death during the anticipated life span of the patient.
- Any decision may be associated with a risk of either over- or undertreatment. To allow the best possible decision, treatment recommendations for B3 and B4 lesions should always be discussed by an interdisciplinary team, based on all available information, and should consider the continuously growing evidence from the literature.

When checking for concordance, the type of biopsy (its reliability depending on the type of lesion), the accuracy of the individual radiologist (audit), and the success of the biopsy procedure (adequacy of the specimens, volume of tissue acquired with respect to the expected extent of the abnormality, certainty or proof of correct needle placement or tissue acquisition, presence of hemorrhage) need to be taken into account.

For lesions that are BI-RADS category 5 and have benign histopathologies, the need for re-biopsy should be strongly considered. Although some entities, such as focal fibrosis and scar, can have a spiculated pattern, re-biopsy may be appropriate to be certain that carcinoma is not present.

Proof of complete removal of the imaging abnormality by VABB, however, does increase certainty, but care must be taken not to miss a residual soft tissue mass that might be obscured by postbiopsy changes.

Nonspecific findings at CNB must be reviewed very critically if the imaging finding concerns a mass. A mass on imaging may be compatible with a fibroadenoma, a papilloma, or an intrammamary lymph node, and, rarely, with an adenosis tumor or localized granuloma or fat necrosis. The size of the abnormality on imaging and histopathology should be correlated. However, nonspecific or diffuse benign changes do not explain a mass on imaging.

If percutaneous breast biopsy was performed because of an architectural distortion, nonspecific benign changes cannot be considered compatible with imaging. In general, architectural changes which are not caused by malignancy may be explained by scarring, by a focal area of fat necrosis, or by radial sclerosing lesions. Since the latter may be associated with malignancy (DCIS, tubular or lobular carcinoma) in its periphery, sufficient sampling may be crucial. Whether complete sampling by VABB may be sufficient to avoid open surgery is presently being discussed and should be decided individually in the interdisciplinary conference.

If biopsy was performed for microcalcifications and the microcalcifications are removed at biopsy and correlated at histopathology, the result may be considered representative. If only a major part of the microcalcifications is sampled, it is important to assess whether the most suspicious calcifications were sampled and to countercheck whether the changes on imaging are explained by the histopathology. Larger areas of microcalcifications may consist of histopathologically inhomogeneous tissue. It must be remembered that DCIS or malignancy may be located within or adjacent to areas of microcalcifications. Thus the amount of tissue sampled around microcalcifications may be as important as the degree of suspicion on imaging and its correlation with the histopathologic benign change. The presence of microcalcifications in the tissue specimen increases the probability of correct sampling, but cannot be considered sufficient proof in doubtful cases.

If biopsy was performed for microcalcifications but specimen radiography does not show any microcalcifications or microcalcifications of the appropriate size or morphology, a benign diagnosis may still be compatible—if removal of the microcalcifications from the breast is proven on the two-view postbiopsy mammograms and if all the acquired tissue is completely worked up by histopathology. The microcalcifications may have been washed out with the blood. Since cells are not washed out, the final diagnosis will probably be compatible. It is not necessary to filter blood, but care should always be taken that the biopsy probe is completely empty before tissue undergoes specimen radiography and goes to pathology.

If the specimen radiograph shows suspicious microcalcifications but microcalcifications or microcalcifications of the appropriate size are not detected by histopathology, a benign diagnosis may still be compatible, if the complete tissue was worked up by histopathology and no malignancy was detected. In this rare case microcalcifications may have fallen out of the specimens during cutting and processing. Cells indicating malignancy would not be lost during processing.

When correlating percutaneous biopsy of diffuse changes, critical counterchecking is needed to decide whether the obtained tissue may be representative and can explain the underlying changes, or whether further measures such as open biopsy need to be considered.

Whenever doubts concerning the correlation between imaging and histopathology remain, re-biopsy (using the same or a different approach) or surgical excision should be considered or (in case of low suspicion) follow-up may be justified. A biopsy that failed should always lead to re-biopsy unless the indication changes (lesion not reproducible).

After percutaneous breast biopsy we usually recommend one follow-up by imaging 6 months later. This serves to verify the result. Furthermore it will allow detection of scarring after biopsy, which on follow-up might cause confusion or even re-biopsy.

References and Recommended Reading

Guidelines and Consensus Statements

ACR Practice. Guideline for the performance of stereotactically guided breast interventional procedures. American College of Radiology; 2009. Available at: http://www.acr.org

ACR Practice. Guideline for the performance of ultrasound guided percutaneous breast interventional procedures. American College of Radiology; 2009. Available at: http://www.acr.org

Albert US, Altland H, Duda V, et al. 2008 update of the guideline: early detection of breast cancer in Germany. J Cancer Res Clin Oncol 2009;135(3):339–354

Heywang-Köbrunner SH, Schreer I, Decker Th, Böcker W. Interdisciplinary consensus on the use and technique of vacuum-assisted stereotactic breast biopsy. Eur J Radiol 2003;47(3):232–236

Heywang-Köbrunner SH, Sinnatamby R, Lebeau A, Lebrecht A, Britton PD, Schreer I; Consensus Group. Interdisciplinary consensus on the uses and technique of MR-guided vacuum-assisted breast biopsy (VAB): results of a European consensus meeting. Eur J Radiol 2009;72(2):289–294

International Breast Cancer Consensus Conference. Image-detected breast cancer: state of the art diagnosis and treatment. J Am Coll Surg 2001;193(3):297–302

Perry N, Broeders M, de Wolf C, Toernberg S, Holland R, von Karsa L, Eds. European guidelines for quality assurance in breast screening and diagnosis. Luxembourg: Office for Official Publications of the European Communities; 2006: 221-56

Other Publications

Azavedo E, Svane G, Auer G. Stereotactic fine-needle biopsy in 2594 mammographically detected non-palpable lesions. Lancet 1989;1(8646):1033–1036

Brenner RJ, Fajardo L, Fisher PR, et al. Percutaneous core biopsy of the breast: effect of operator experience and number of samples on diagnostic accuracy. AJR Am J Roentgenol 1996;166(2):341–346

Britton PD. Fine needle aspiration or core biopsy. Breast 1999;8:1–4

Britton PD, McCann J. Needle biopsy in the NHS Breast Screening Programme 1996/97: How much and how accurate? Breast 1999;8:5–11

Britton PD, Goud A, Godward S, et al. Use of ultrasound-guided axillary node core biopsy in staging of early breast cancer. Eur Radiol 2009a;19(3):561–569

Britton PD, Provenzano E, Barter S, et al. Ultrasound guided percutaneous axillary lymph node core biopsy: how often is the sentinel lymph node being biopsied? Breast 2009b;18(1):13–16

Britton P, Moyle P, Benson JR, et al. Ultrasound of the axilla: where to look for the sentinel lymph node. Clin Radiol 2010;65(5):373–376

Bruening W, Fontanarosa J, Tipton K, Treadwell JR, Launders J, Schoelles K. Systematic review: comparative effectiveness of core-needle and open surgical biopsy to diagnose breast lesions. Ann Intern Med 2010;152(4):238–246

Burbank F, Parker SH, Fogarty TJ. Stereotactic breast biopsy: improved tissue harvesting with the Mammotome. Am Surg 1996;62(9):738–744

Cytology Sub-Group of the National Coordinating Committee for Breast Screening Pathology NHS Breast Screening Programme. Guidelines for cytology procedures and reporting in breast cancer screening. Sheffield: NHSBSP (Issue 22); 1992

de Lucena CE, Dos Santos Júnior JL, de Lima Resende CA, do Amaral VF, de Almeida Barra A, Reis JH. Ultrasound-guided core needle biopsy of breast masses: How many cores are necessary to diagnose cancer? J Clin Ultrasound 2007;35(7):363–366

Dillon MF, McDermott EW, Hill AD, O'Doherty A, O'Higgins N, Quinn CM. Predictive value of breast lesions of "uncertain malignant potential" and "suspicious for malignancy" determined by needle core biopsy. Ann Surg Oncol 2007;14(2):704–711

Eby PR, Ochsner JE, DeMartini WB, Allison KH, Peacock S, Lehman CD. Frequency and upgrade rates of atypical ductal hyperplasia diagnosed at stereotactic vacuum-assisted breast biopsy: 9-versus 11-gauge. AJR Am J Roentgenol 2009;192(1):229–234

El-Sayed ME, Rakha EA, Reed J, Lee AH, Evans AJ, Ellis IO. Audit of performance of needle core biopsy diagnoses of screen detected breast lesions. Eur J Cancer 2008;44(17):2580–2586

Fahrbach K, Sledge I, Cella C, Linz H, Ross SD. A comparison of the accuracy of two minimally invasive breast biopsy methods: a systematic literature review and meta-analysis. Arch Gynecol Obstet 2006;274(2):63–73

Fischer U, Schwethelm L, Baum FT, Luftner-Nagel S, Teubner J. Effort, accuracy and histology of MR-guided vacuum biopsy of suspicious breast lesions—retrospective evaluation after 389 interventions. [Article in German] Rofo 2009;181(8):774–781

Fishman JE, Milikowski C, Ramsinghani R, Velasquez MV, Aviram G. US-guided core-needle biopsy of the breast: how many specimens are necessary? Radiology 2003;226(3):779–782

Han BK, Schnall MD, Orel SG, Rosen M. Outcome of MRI-guided breast biopsy. AJR Am J Roentgenol 2008;191(6):1798–1804

Hefler L, Casselman J, Amaya B, et al. Follow-up of breast lesions detected by MRI not biopsied due to absent enhancement of contrast medium. Eur Radiol 2003;13(2):344–346

Heywang-Köbrunner SH, Heinig A, Schaumlöffel U, et al. MR-guided percutaneous excisional and incisional biopsy of breast lesions. Eur Radiol 1999;9(8):1656–1665

Heywang-Köbrunner SH, Heinig A, Pickuth D, Alberich T, Spielmann RP. Interventional MRI of the breast: lesion localisation and biopsy. Eur Radiol 2000;10(1):36–45

Heywang-Köbrunner SH, Möhrling D, Nährig J. The role of MRI before breast conservation. Semin Breast Dis 2007;10(4):137–144

Heywang-Köbrunner SH, Heinig A, Hellerhoff K, Holzhausen HJ, Nährig J. Use of ultrasound-guided percutaneous vacuum-assisted breast biopsy for selected difficult indications. Breast J 2009;15(4):348–356

Heywang-Köbrunner SH, Nährig J, Hacker A, Sedlacek S, Höfler H. B3 lesions: radiological assessment and multi-disciplinary aspects. Breast Care 2010;4:1–9

Houssami N, Ciatto S, Bilous M, Vezzosi V, Bianchi S. Borderline breast core needle histology: predictive values for malignancy in lesions of uncertain malignant potential (B3). Br J Cancer 2007a;96(8):1253–1257

Houssami N, Ciatto S, Ellis I, Ambrogetti D. Underestimation of malignancy of breast core-needle biopsy: concepts and precise overall and category-specific estimates. Cancer 2007b;109(3):487–495

Jackman RJ, Nowels KW, Rodriguez-Soto J, Marzoni FA Jr, Finkelstein SI, Shepard MJ. Stereotactic, automated, large-core needle biopsy of nonpalpable breast lesions: false-negative and histologic underestimation rates after long-term follow-up. Radiology 1999;210(3):799–805

Jackman RJ, Birdwell RL, Ikeda DM. Atypical ductal hyperplasia: can some lesions be defined as probably benign after stereotactic 11-gauge vacuum-assisted biopsy, eliminating the recommendation for surgical excision? Radiology 2002;224(2):548–554

Jackman RJ, Marzoni FA Jr, Rosenberg J. False-negative diagnoses at stereotactic vacuum-assisted needle breast biopsy: long-term follow-up of 1,280 lesions and review of the literature. AJR Am J Roentgenol 2009;192(2):341–351

Jang M, Cho N, Moon WK, Park JS, Seong MH, Park IA. Underestimation of atypical ductal hyperplasia at sonographically guided core biopsy of the breast. AJR Am J Roentgenol 2008;191(5):1347–1351

Johnson NB, Collins LC. Update on percutaneous needle biopsy of nonmalignant breast lesions. Adv Anat Pathol 2009;16(4):183–195

Kettritz U, Rotter K, Schreer I, et al. Stereotactic vacuum-assisted breast biopsy in 2874 patients: a multicenter study. Cancer 2004;100(2):245–251

Kohr JR, Eby PR, Allison KH, et al. Risk of upgrade of atypical ductal hyperplasia after stereotactic breast biopsy: effects of number of foci and complete removal of calcifications. Radiology 2010;255(3):723–730

Lee AH, Denley HE, Pinder SE, et al; Nottingham Breast Team. Excision biopsy findings of patients with breast needle core biopsies reported as suspicious of malignancy (B4) or lesion of uncertain malignant potential (B3). Histopathology 2003;42(4):331–336

Lee CH, Philpotts LE, Horvath LJ, Tocino I. Follow-up of breast lesions diagnosed as benign with stereotactic core-needle biopsy: frequency of mammographic change and false-negative rate. Radiology 1999;212(1):189–194

Leifland K, Lundquist H, Lagerstedt U, Svane G. Stereotactic core needle biopsy in non-palpable breast lesions. What number is needed? Acta Radiol 2004;45(2):142–147

Liberman L, Evans WP III, Dershaw DD, et al. Radiography of microcalcifications in stereotaxic mammary core biopsy specimens. Radiology 1994;190(1):223–225

Liberman L, Dershaw DD, Glassman JR, et al. Analysis of cancers not diagnosed at stereotactic core breast biopsy. Radiology 1997;203(1):151–157

Liberman L, Bracero N, Morris E, Thornton C, Dershaw DD. MRI-guided 9-gauge vacuum-assisted breast biopsy: initial clinical experience. AJR Am J Roentgenol 2005;185(1):183–193

Linda A, Zuiani C, Bazzocchi M, Furlan A, Londero V. Borderline breast lesions diagnosed at core needle biopsy: can magnetic resonance mammography rule out associated malignancy? Preliminary results based on 79 surgically excised lesions. Breast 2008;17(2):125–131

Löfgren M, Andersson I, Lindholm K. Stereotactic fine-needle aspiration for cytologic diagnosis of nonpalpable breast lesions. AJR Am J Roentgenol 1990;154(6):1191–1195

Londero V, Zuiani C, Linda A, Vianello E, Furlan A, Bazzocchi M. Lobular neoplasia: core needle breast biopsy underestimation of malignancy in relation to radiologic and pathologic features. Breast 2008;17(6):623–630

Mainiero MB, Philpotts LE, Lee CH, Lange RC, Carter D, Tocino I. Stereotaxic core needle biopsy of breast microcalcifications: correlation of target accuracy and diagnosis with lesion size. Radiology 1996;198(3):665–669

Malhaire C, El Khoury C, Thibault F, et al. Vacuum-assisted biopsies under MR guidance: results of 72 procedures. Eur Radiol 2010;20(7):1554–1562

Margenthaler JA, Duke D, Monsees BS, Barton PT, Clark C, Dietz JR. Correlation between core biopsy and excisional biopsy in breast high-risk lesions. Am J Surg 2006;192(4):534–537

Melotti MK, Berg WA. Core needle breast biopsy in patients undergoing anticoagulation therapy: preliminary results. AJR Am J Roentgenol 2000;174(1):245–249

Meyer JE, Smith DN, Lester SC, et al. Large-needle core biopsy: nonmalignant breast abnormalities evaluated with surgical excision or repeat core biopsy. Radiology 1998;206(3):717–720

Nath ME, Robinson TM, Tobon H, Chough DM, Sumkin JH. Automated large-core needle biopsy of surgically removed breast lesions: comparison of samples obtained with 14-, 16-, and 18-gauge needles. Radiology 1995;197(3):739–742

Parker SH, Burbank F, Jackman RJ, et al. Percutaneous large-core breast biopsy: a multi-institutional study. Radiology 1994;193(2):359–364

Perlet C, Heywang-Kobrunner SH, Heinig A, et al. Magnetic resonance-guided, vacuum-assisted breast biopsy: results from a European multicenter study of 538 lesions. Cancer 2006;106(5):982–990

Perry N, Broeders M, de Wolf C, Toernberg S, Holland R, von Karsa L, Eds. European guidelines for quality assurance in breast screening an diagnosis. Luxembourg: Office for Official Publications of the European Communities; 2006: 221-56

Pisano ED, Fajardo LL, Tsimikas J, et al. Rate of insufficient samples for fine-needle aspiration for nonpalpable breast lesions in a multicenter clinical trial: The Radiologic Diagnostic Oncology Group 5 Study. The RDOG5 investigators. Cancer 1998;82(4):679–688

Plantade R, Hammou JC, Gerard F, et al. Ultrasound-guided vacuum-assisted biopsy: review of 382 cases. [Article in French] J Radiol 2005;86(9 Pt 1):1003–1015

Rakha EA, Lee AH, Jenkins JA, Murphy AE, Hamilton LJ, Ellis IO. Characterization and outcome of breast needle core biopsy diagnoses of lesions of uncertain malignant potential (B3) in abnormalities detected by mammographic screening. Int J Cancer 2011;129(6):1417–1424

Schueller G, Schueller-Weidekamm C, Helbich TH. Accuracy of ultrasound-guided, large-core needle breast biopsy. Eur Radiol 2008;18(9):1761–1773

Schulz-Wendtland R, Aichinger U, Krämer S, et al. Sonographical breast biopsy: how many core biopsy specimens are needed?. [Article in German] Rofo 2003;175(1):94–98

Sohn V, Arthurs Z, Herbert G, et al. Atypical ductal hyperplasia: improved accuracy with the 11-gauge vacuum-assisted versus the 14-gauge core biopsy needle. Ann Surg Oncol 2007;14(9):2497–2501

Warren RM, Hayes C; Advisory Group of MARIBS. Localization of breast lesions shown only on MRI—a review for the UK Study of MRI Screening for Breast Cancer. Br J Radiol 2000;73(866):123–132

Yu YH, Liang C, Yuan XZ. Diagnostic value of vacuum-assisted breast biopsy for breast carcinoma: a meta-analysis and systematic review. Breast Cancer Res Treat 2010;120(2):469–479

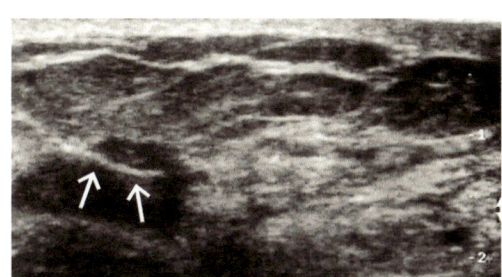

8 Preoperative Localization

Purpose, Definition, Indications, and Side Effects → 216
Purpose → 216
Definition → 216
Indication → 216
Side Effects → 216

Methods and Technique → 217
Mammographically Guided Localization Techniques → 217
Ultrasound-Guided Localization → 221
MR-Guided Localization → 222
CT-guided Localization → 222
Galactographically Guided Localization → 222

Materials for Lesion Localization → 222

Problems and Their Solutions → 227

References and Recommended Reading → 228

8 Preoperative Localization

I. Schreer, S. H. Heywang-Koebrunner, S. Barter

Purpose, Definition, Indications, and Side Effects

Purpose

The increasing use of screening mammography has resulted in an increased rate of detection of clinically occult disease. Lesions requiring surgical excision that are detected only by diagnostic imaging studies—that is, nonpalpable lesions—must be localized for the surgeon. Nonpalpable lesions can be localized under mammographic or ultrasound guidance or, less frequently, under computed tomographic (CT) or magnetic resonance (MR) guidance.

For image-guided localization those modalities that clearly show the lesion should be chosen. When several modalities fulfill this requirement, the modality that allows the fastest and easiest approach should be chosen.

There are several mammographically guided preoperative localization methods. They differ with respect to their technical requirements, the time required, their precision, and thus their accuracy.

Lesions that can be unequivocally identified by sonography can also be localized under sonographic guidance. On the whole, to achieve precision for ultrasound (US)-guided localization requires as much experience as does mammographically guided localization. US-guided localization can usually be performed more quickly than mammographic localization by experienced personnel.

Lesions that are detected only by contrast-enhanced MRI must be localized using contrast-enhanced MRI or CT. The latter can be performed with acceptable accuracy (deviation from the target < 10 mm) with the patient supine, similarly to the standard CT-guided biopsy of other organs. However, CT-guided breast biopsy is associated with a significantly higher radiation dose than mammography. Also, small lesions may be quite difficult to detect owing to the lower contrast of the CT contrast agents compared with MR contrast agents. CT-guided wire marking may be needed, however, to localize lesions in areas of the breast that cannot be reached by MR guidance.

Owing to breathing artifacts and the lower resolution we do not recommend performing MR-guided localization procedures in the supine position.

Special so-called "biopsy" coils are now available. They allow MR-guided percutaneous biopsy or MR-guided localization with an excellent accuracy. International guidelines stipulate that both equipment and expertise for MR-guided localization (optimally for MR-guided percutaneous breast biopsy too) should be available whenever MRI is offered.

Definition

Preoperative localization refers to marking a nonpalpable lesion detected in a diagnostic imaging study for subsequent excision.

Indication

Any nonpalpable lesion requiring excision detected by mammography, sonography, or MRI must be preoperatively localized and marked for the surgeon. Reliable excision and histologic examination of nonpalpable lesions can be performed only after such lesions have been correctly marked. Preoperative localization also enables the surgeon to excise a lesion with the removal of a minimal volume of breast tissue, minimizing postsurgical deformity.

In the case of extended lesions, placement of several wires may be necessary to optimally support the surgeon's attempt to excise as much as necessary with the best possible cosmetic result. The best way of marking should be agreed with the surgeon and the result of a marking procedure must be communicated in the written report and documented on postprocedural images.

Additional foci which are remote from the main focus require additional wires, which may also be marked at the distal end with tapes of different color. To allow the best possible oncological and cosmetic result it is recommended that any surgical planning is preceded by diagnostic percutaneous breast biopsy to avoid unnecessary removal of benign lesions.

Neoadjuvant chemotherapy has been established as a widely accepted method for down-staging and possibly allowing breast conservation. Some patients respond excellently and the tumor may shrink fast. In these cases placement of one or several marker clips after the first few cycles of chemotherapy may be necessary to assure that after completion of chemotherapy the tumor bed can still be identified and correctly excised by the surgeon.

Side Effects

The following side effects are possible:
- Pain
- Bleeding
- Vasovagal reaction

- Allergy to local anesthetic (if applied)
- Chest wall injury
- Movement of a wire may need to be considered, if wire is placed long before the anticipated surgery
- The risk of infection might need to be considered if a wire is placed for several days, which is extremely uncommon

The major pain perceived by the patient is felt during insertion of the needle through the skin itself. Advancing the needle or wire through the breast or injecting contrast solution (dye or carbon) is mostly less painful. The compression required in mammographically guided localization is also generally well tolerated, even with the needle in place. This assumes, of course, that the examiner proceeds gently. Since perception of pain may differ greatly between patients, application of local anesthetic is recommended.

Bleeding is a problem only when an artery is inadvertently injured during localization. If this occurs, firm compression has to be applied for a sufficient period of time (~10 min).

The physician must always be prepared for vasovagal reactions since individual tolerance to the introduction of a needle into the breast varies greatly.

In patients with a known allergy to local anesthetic the procedure is usually possible without local anesthesia, or a topical anesthetic may be considered. These patients usually know which local anesthetic can be used instead. If uncertainty exists, skin testing should be considered for future procedures.

Chest wall injury is a rare complication of localization procedures since, for lesions which are very close to the chest wall, the needle and wire may be placed anterior to the lesion, while the surgeon is advised to excise the area between the wire and the chest wall.

Nevertheless, chest wall injury and pneumothorax need to be considered as rare possible complications. Chest wall injury may occur with US-guided wire marking, if the needle is not fully visualized within the slice. It may even occur with stereotactic or MR-guided procedures, if the needle bends within very hard tissue. Since needles for marking are much thinner than needles used for percutaneous breast biopsy, and since needle introduction is not continuously monitored, the possibility of chest wall injury should be kept in mind before applying too much force. For MR-guided wire marking (MR-compatible material is softer than the usual steel) bending of needles has been observed by the authors. We therefore recommend that thin needles are not used for MR-guided wire marking.

Finally, after the needle is correctly placed, the wire should be advanced only until the anchor opens (usually ~10–15 mm). Thereafter, the wire must be kept in place while the needle is withdrawn over the wire; otherwise the wire might advance beyond the target and eventually could even advance beyond the breast. Moving of long-standing wires has been described.

Wires with a large curve should not be placed too close to the chest wall or too close to implants to avoid potential damage.

If it is necessary to place a wire on the day before surgery, it should be checked that the wire is not located too close to the chest wall. Also a wire system should be chosen that does not tend to move (based on its type of anchoring).

Methods and Technique

Mammographically Guided Localization Techniques

Before any preoperative localization, the radiologist should review the imaging studies to be certain that a lesion exists and requires excision. If a lesion is seen only on mammography, an additional 90° lateral view may be very helpful to determine the exact lesion position (see **Fig. 3.33**).

Although lesions seen only on one view can be localized with stereotactic technique, an effort should be made to assess a lesion fully on two orthogonal views before scheduling needle localization. For this purpose it is recommended that a mediolateral or lateromedial view be obtained to supplement the craniocaudal and mediolateral oblique views. The true lateral view gives a better sense of the depth of the lesion in the breast and thus helps to improve orientation.

Because the patient needs to cooperate during the localization procedure, she should not be premedicated.

Localizing Lesions Using a Perforated or Marked Compression Plate

Depending on the position of the lesion and the chosen method of access, a craniocaudal, caudocranial, mediolateral, or lateromedial view is obtained using a perforated Plexiglas compression plate (**Fig. 8.1**) or a fenestrated compression plate with alphanumeric markings along its edge. The needle is to be inserted through the perforated or fenestrated compression plate and perpendicular to it. An initial image is taken with the patient's breast in compression between the localization plate and the receiver plate. On this film the lesion must be imaged within the fenestration. The patient is held in compression while the image is acquired and checked. The point of needle insertion on the skin is chosen according to the coordinates of the lesion with reference to the markings. The skin over the lesion is cleansed, local anesthetic applied and the needle is inserted into the breast, parallel to the chest wall. It is inserted beyond a depth calculated on the second orthogonal view, or as deep as possible if

8 Preoperative Localization

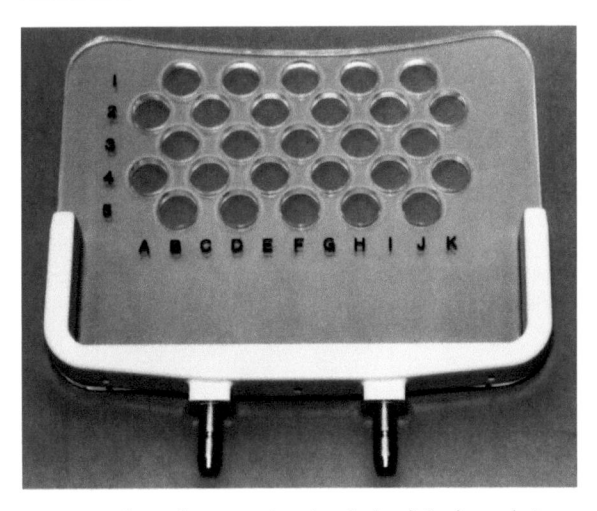

Fig. 8.1 Perforated compression plate for localizing breast lesions.

this depth cannot be exactly determined on the initial view. The needle should pass far enough through the lesion so that its tip will still penetrate the lesion after compression is removed and the breast relaxes. Next, a mammogram in the second orthogonal imaging plane is obtained. After this, image compression on the breast is maintained. Based on this image, the depth of needle insertion is adjusted, if necessary. Once the needle is in the correct position, the wire is deployed (or a marker solution injected). Correct needle insertion or correct placement and distribution of the marker solution is then also documented in two planes before the patient is sent to the operating room.

The advantage of this method is that it can easily be performed even by minimally experienced personnel and without expensive equipment. Because the approach is parallel to the chest wall, patients should never develop a pneumothorax.

The most relevant disadvantage is that perforated or fenestrated plates are not regularly offered by some vendors. If so desired, an approach that approximates the probable surgical one can usually be achieved by careful selection of the initial plane of compression that is decisive for the direction of needle insertion. Although the surgeon can approach a localized lesion independent of the position of the wire, some prefer to follow the path of the wire for the excision.

Stereotactic Localization

The accuracy that can be achieved with this procedure is comparable to that using a perforated compression plate, provided sufficient experience of possible pitfalls exists and the procedure is performed diligently. This is due to various hazards (see below) and the failure to readjust the needle depth on a second, orthogonal view before final deployment. The procedure is the same as in a stereotactic biopsy (see pp. 204–205). Once the correct position of the needle is verified, a marker wire is placed (or a contrast solution injected). The needle usually just acts as a guide for the wire and needs to be removed before releasing the compression on the breast. If the needle is to stay in place, an appropriate opening in the needle holder is necessary to allow the needle to be detached. First the needle is placed in the same manner as for stereotactic percutaneous biopsy. After the wire is placed, the proper position is first documented in the usual stereotactic views (+ 15° and − 15°). After compression is released a two-view mammogram consisting of a cranocaudal and a 90° lateral view needs to be performed to document correct wire placement and allow optimum orientation for the surgeon (**Fig. 8.2a–e**). This is important because, particularly in dense breasts, tissue elasticity can cause the tip of the needle to lie above the lesion, not readily apparent in the stereotactic views. A positioning error of a few millimeters in a compressed breast can correspond to a large positioning error (> 1 cm) in the relaxed breast.

To minimize the upward displacement of the needle that often occurs as a result of tissue elasticity, the needle may be placed 3–6 mm deeper than the calculated target point. This compensates for tissue elasticity, and once compression is relieved, the needle will usually lie at the desired location.

For localization, the stereotactic method is comparable to localization procedures using a perforated compression plate. The major importance of stereotaxis is its use for percutaneous biopsy.

The following special problems can occur in stereotactic needle localization:

Owing to the geometry of stereotaxis, slight deviations in the position of the needle in the targeting or documentation views can correspond to a significant deviation in depth localization. Localization errors can occur if the patient moves (in nondigital systems significant time may elapse for development of the localization views and for depth determination), or if the targets chosen on the +15° and −15° stereotactic views prove not to be identical. This may occur with ill-defined lesions, for which it is difficult to identify the same structure on the +15° and −15° views or with multiple microcalcifications showing minimal pleomorphism.

Even with the tip of the needle in the correct position, inserting the marker wire will usually push the denser breast tissue forward a few millimeters. The resulting positioning error in the compressed breast can result in a final positioning error in the relaxed breast of over 1 cm.

To minimize these problems, the following steps are recommended:
- Exercise extreme care in selecting the target point and in verifying it in the + 15° and − 15° views.
- Switch to another localization method if identical target points cannot be clearly located on the compression views.
- Always advance the needle a few millimeters deeper than the target point to compensate for tissue elasticity.

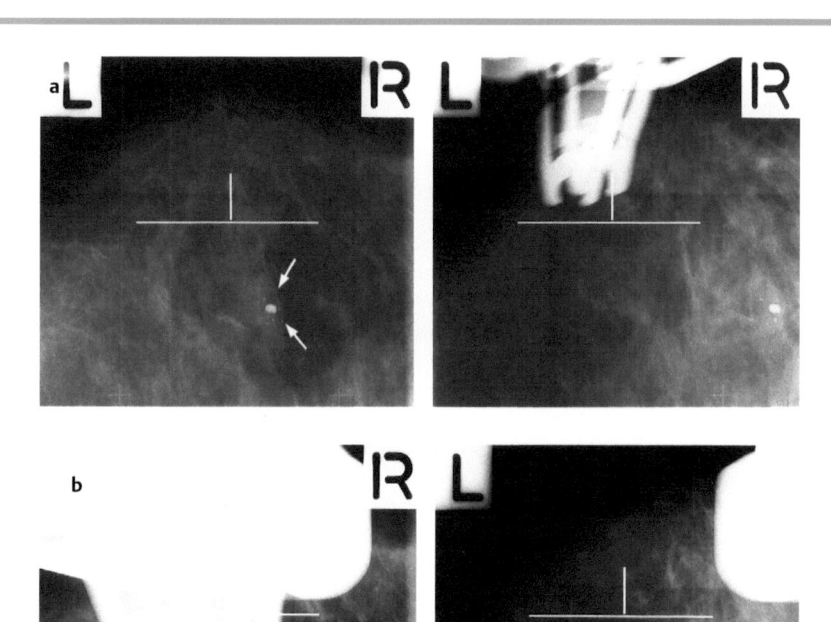

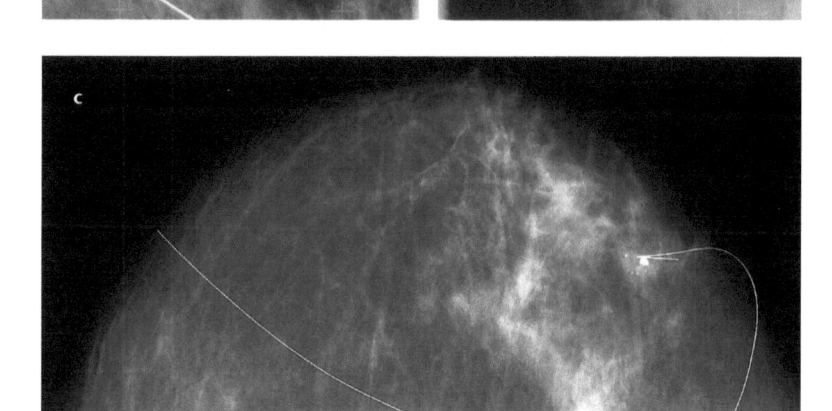

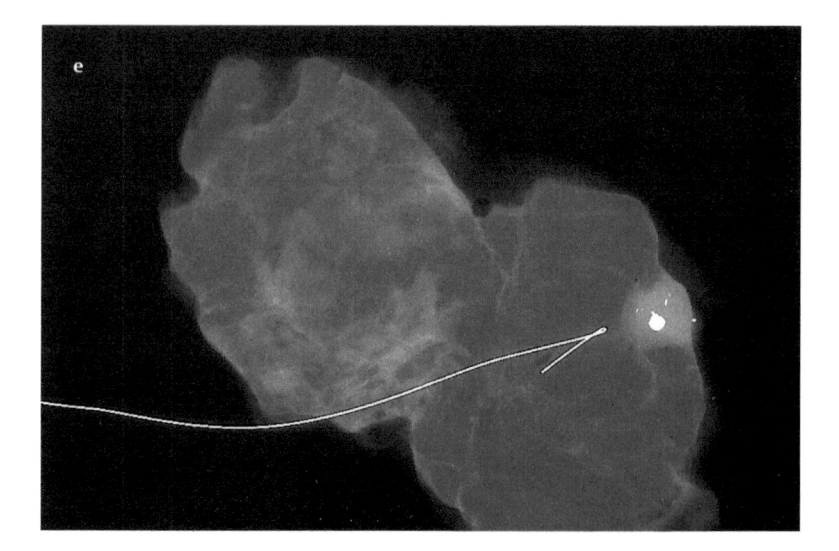

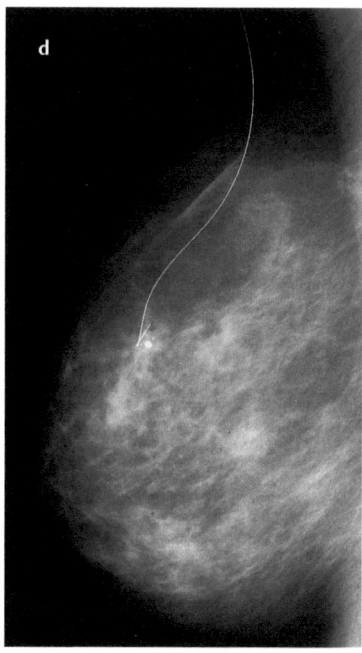

Fig. 8.2a–e

a Two partial views with the tube tilted −15° and +15° reveal a small focal lesion requiring localization or biopsy.
b Demonstrating the tip of the needle in the center of the focal lesion.
c,d Documentation view demonstrating correct positioning of the localization wire.
e Specimen radiography. Today—unlike n this case—preoperative marking mainly concerns proven cancers or B3 lesions unless a patient refuses preoperative percutaneous breast biopsy.

8 Preoperative Localization

- Always verify the final result in two perpendicular planes.
- Always (with this method) use localization needles that can be repositioned in case of an unsatisfactory position.

Manual Localization

Manual localization was the first and is the simplest method of advancing a needle to a lesion under mammographic guidance. In most institutions, it has been replaced by the grid or the stereotactic technique, since an approach parallel to the chest wall is preferred. In the hands of an experienced radiologist it may, however, allow a fast approach to superficial lesions and to lesions which may be difficult to localize by the standard methods (retroareolar lesions).

The advantages are the simplicity and the fact that the point of entry lies directly anterior to the lesion, which often corresponds to the approach preferred by the surgeon.

Disadvantages are that, in the case of deeply situated lesions, it may not be as precise as localizing with add-on devices. Thus, corrections will be necessary in a certain percentage of lesions, and it requires more practice and skill in three-dimensional visualization than other methods of localization. Finally, the axis of the needle is perpendicular to the chest wall, increasing the risk of injury to the chest wall when a lesion is located posteriorly.

Procedure

Fig. 8.3 shows how the point of entry on the skin is selected based on the mammograms and how the depth of the lesion is measured. When transferring the coordinates of

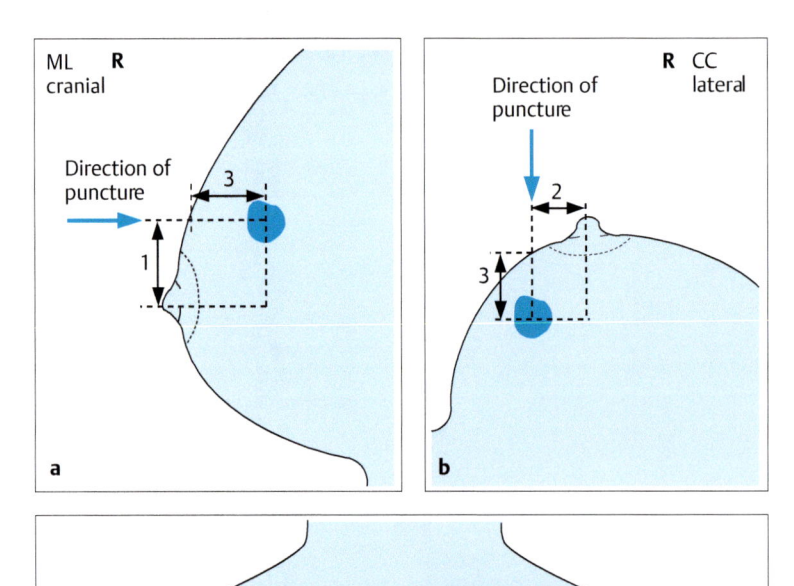

Fig. 8.3a–c Schematic diagram of manual localization: The coordinates of the lesion in the horizontal (CC view) and vertical (ML view) direction (**a**, **b**) with reference to the nipple are marked on the skin of the breast (**c**) and the depth of the lesion from the skin surface is measured.

Methods and Technique

the lesion with respect to the nipple, the assistant must be careful to hold the breast in the same position as it was in the original mediolateral view. When inserting the needle, the physician places his or her other hand around the tissue into which the needle is to be inserted. This minimizes the risk of injury to the chest wall and brings the breast into a shape similar to that on the mediolateral view. The position of the needle is then verified in mammograms in two planes (craniocaudal and 90° mediolateral) and corrected if necessary. After verification of the correct needle position, a contrast solution is injected or a wire is placed through the needle.

Ultrasound-Guided Localization

US-guided localization requires that the lesion is visible on ultrasound. This means that it usually cannot be used for microcalcifications, yet it is very effective in localizing focal lesions. The procedure is similar to US-guided percutaneous biopsy (see pp. 197–203). Instead of aspirating or performing a core biopsy, the radiologist deploys a marker wire through the needle. Contrast solutions are not generally used in US-guided localization. Sonographic verification of the correct needle position is mandatory (**Fig. 8.4**). We also recommend taking post-localization

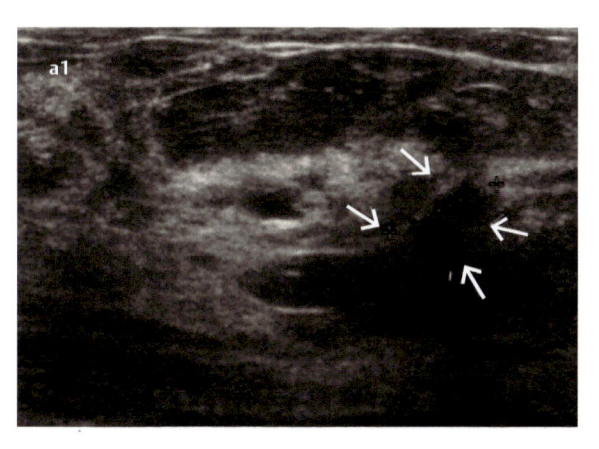

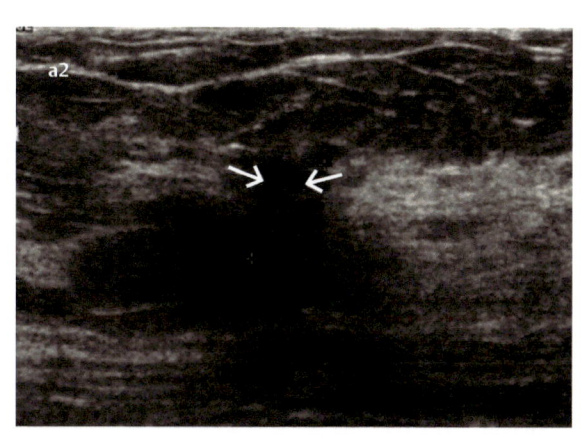

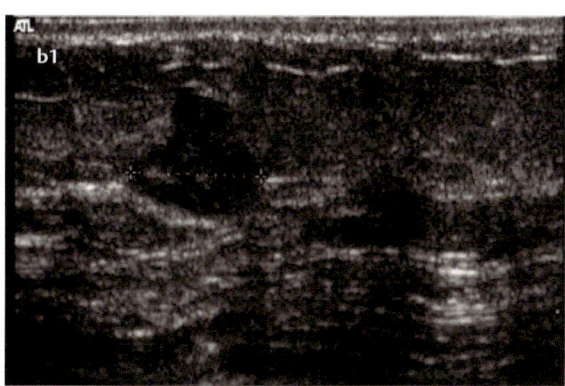

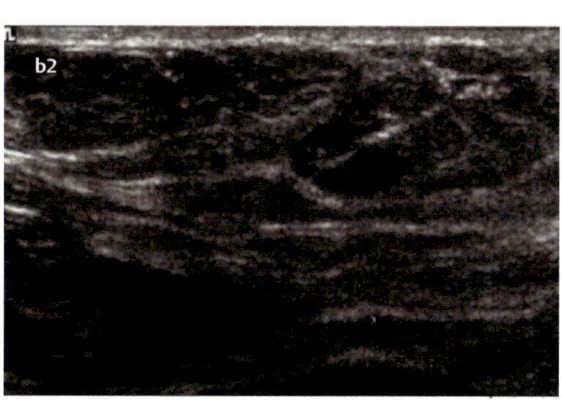

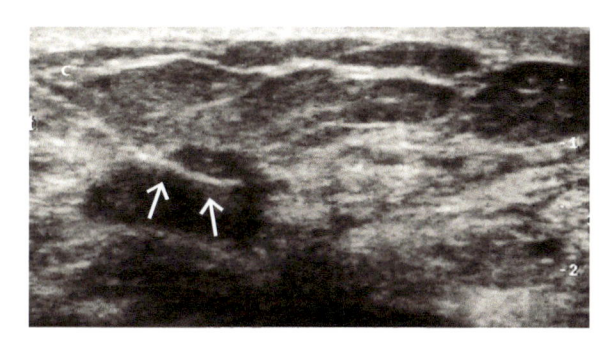

Fig. 8.4a–c Correct positioning of the wire after ultrasound-guided localization.

a One of the two curved arms of a marking wire.
b The tip of the wire just outside the localization needle.
c Documentation of the definite wire position within the tumor. The arrows point to the wire.

mammograms in two views so that the surgeon can see the relationship of the needle to the lesion accurately.

The advantage of US-guided localization over other methods of localization is that it takes the least amount of time. A disadvantage is that visualization of small or pre-invasive lesions may be uncertain or impossible. Furthermore, it may sometimes be difficult to identify the lesion in a subsequent specimen sonogram.

MR-Guided Localization

If a lesion is detected by MRI and cannot be visualized by mammography or ultrasound, it must be preoperatively marked using contrast-enhanced MRI or (rarely, if this approach is impossible) contrast-enhanced CT.

When a lesion is detected by MRI and a subsequent "second look" ultrasound examination unequivocally demonstrates the lesion, then US-guided localization by a physician experienced in both sonography and MRI is recommended. Owing to respiratory motion, identification of small MR-detected lesions using an MRI unit without a special biopsy coil may be difficult.

Precise preoperative marking (and localization for core biopsy) is possible through the use of special "biopsy" or "localization" coils. Various devices for MR-guided localization are available. The exact procedure may vary with the device. However, with most devices the patient lies prone, while the breast is fixed and moderately compressed by a compression device with integrated imaging coil. Imaging is performed and the lesion coordinates are calculated with respect to a fiducial marker that is usually integrated in the compression device. Using dedicated software, the coordinates can usually be transferred to an aiming device that supports the coaxial localization system. Imaging checks are performed after needle insertion before and after deploying the wire.

As for all other localization procedures it is recommended that medial lesions are approached medially and lateral lesions laterally. Other approaches do not necessarily provide the access needed by the surgeon.

After excision a specimen radiograph or a specimen sonogram may be performed in an attempt to check for the MR-detected lesion.

Fig. 8.5 shows the typical arrangement of a MR-guided biopsy coil and demonstrates the marking of an area that contained a multicentric carcinoma.

CT-Guided Localization

Owing to the higher radiation dose and the high dose of contrast agent required for CT identification of MR-detected lesions, CT guidance should be chosen only if MR guidance is impossible. With most breast biopsy coils the area of tissue that is located medially close to the chest wall cannot be approached from medially. For such indications CT-guided marking may be quite helpful.

It may also be helpful in cases with multiple or bilateral lesions, since most biopsy coils will not allow simultaneous access to one breast from both sides or to both breasts.

Fig. 8.6 demonstrates the principle of CT marking.

Galactographically Guided Localization

If a lesion is detected only at galactography, it might be marked by one or (in the case of a larger area) more clips immediately (**Fig. 8.7**). The clip(s) may later be used as landmarks for planning the surgical access and can be targeted for an additional wire marking at any time.

If this is not possible, repeat galactography will be required for preoperative localization of the lesion.

> Whenever an involved duct or ductal system can be identified sonographically, US-guided biopsy or marking is indicated instead of galactographically guided localization.

Technique

Several options for galactographically guided localization are available:
1. After galactography (see Chapter 3, pp. 85–90) in the craniocaudal and mediolateral planes, the galactographic findings are localized using standard mammographic localization techniques (i.e., manually, using a perforated plate, or by means of stereotaxis).
2. If only a single duct is involved, the duct may be galactographically visualized and delineated immediately preoperatively using a combination of contrast medium and Patent Blue. The blue-dyed ductal system must be excised immediately after instillation of contrast medium.

Materials for Lesion Localization

The selection of localization materials depends on the interval between localization and surgery. Usually, localization is performed shortly before surgery.

In this case, some physicians elected to use low-cost dye marking with Patent Blue immediately preoperatively. Having verified correct needle position, the radiologist injects 0.2–0.3 mL of blue dye, such as methylene blue or patent blue, after which the surgeon removes the blue-stained parenchymal tissue. For mammographically guided localization, the radiologist adds 0.2–0.3 mL of a nonionic radiographic contrast medium. This is necessary for subsequent documentation of proper dispersion

Materials for Lesion Localization

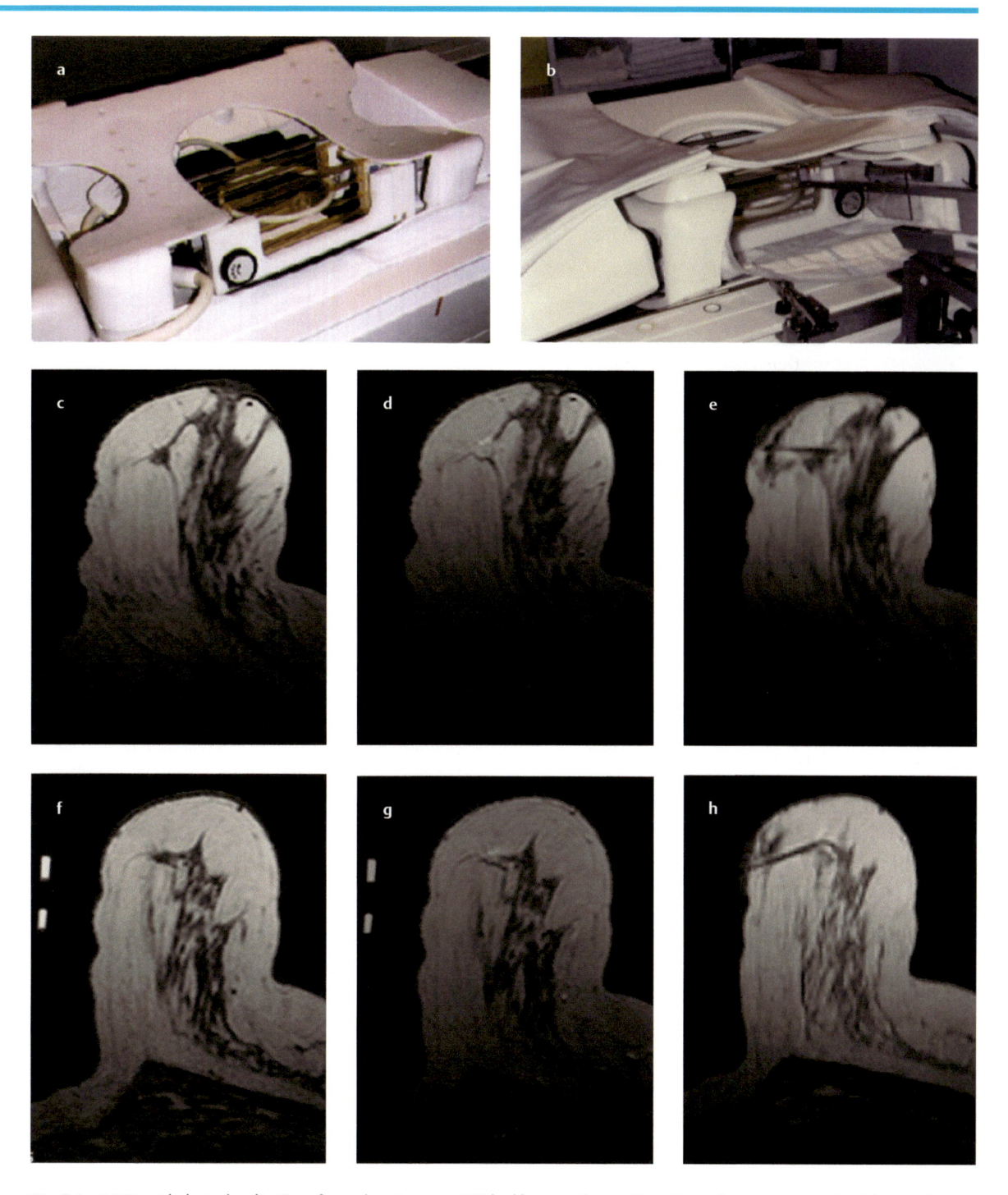

Fig. 8.5a–i MR-guided wire localization of an enhancing area. MRI had been performed based on a discrete suspected architectural distortion visible mammographically on one view only. There were no findings on further mammographic or sonographic assessment. MRI exhibited several enhancing foci within in the left breast medially. MR-guided wire marking was undertaken at the cranial and at the caudal border of the area.

a,b The breast biopsy coil is shown. The compression plates consist of bars, which hold the breast. The breast can be accessed medially or laterally between the bars. The aiming device is attached on the side of the anticipated approach. (Access to the breast medially is possible from underneath the patient support using a long needle holder on the aiming device.)

c–e The most cranial lesion is shown: precontrast image (**c**), postcontrast image (**d**) and image showing the wire in place (**e**).

f–h The most caudal lesion is shown: precontrast image (**f**), postcontrast image (**g**) and image showing the wire in place (**h**).

8 Preoperative Localization

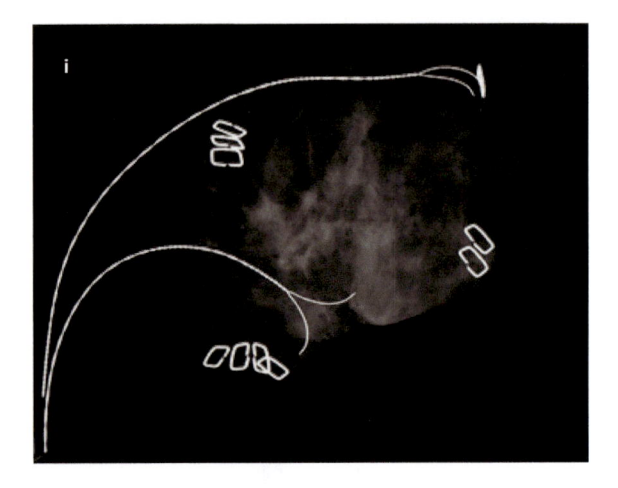

◁ continued

i The specimen radiograph shows the suspicious area with the two marking wires. Clips mark the anterior, lateral and cranial borders of the specimen.

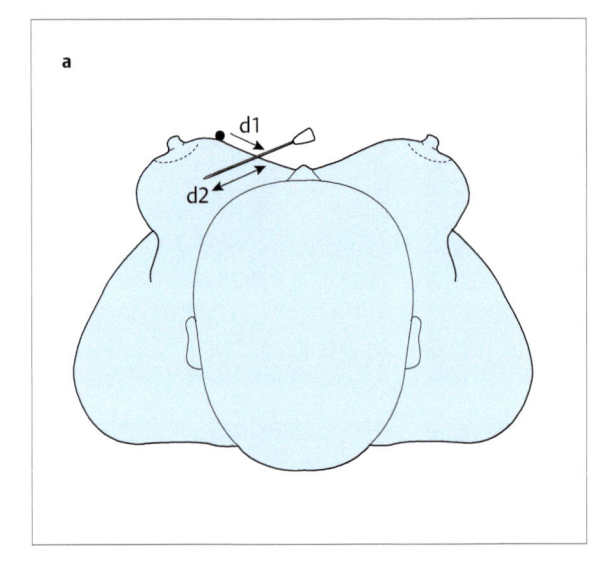

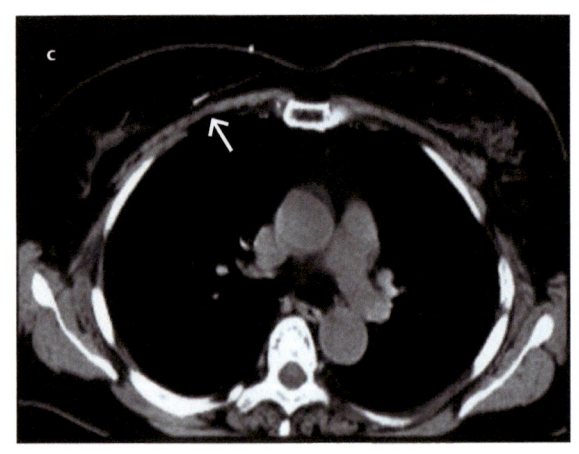

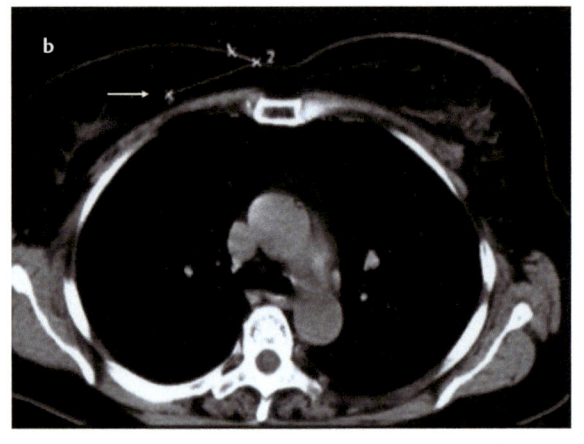

Fig. 8.6a–c The principle of CT-guided wire marking is shown on a small MR-detected nodule. The nodule was located in the area of the dead space (2–3 cm of tissue adjacent to the chest wall medially) which cannot be approached using our MR biopsy coil.

a CT-guided wire marking is performed similarly to other CT-guided punctures. A wire which is positioned parallel to the sternum is attached to the skin. It will be imaged on all transverse slices and can thus be used as a fiducial marker. After the lesion is identified, an approach is planned that allows puncturing the lesion with an access parallel to the chest wall. Based on the flat approach the entry point into the skin is defined as the point in the slice that contains the lesion, where the anticipated needle path crosses the skin. Next the distance of this entry point from the wire (d1) is measured in this slice. This distance is transferred to the skin. Then the needle is angled to follow the anticipated path within the slice. The correct angulation needs to be counterchecked during stepwise needle insertion. The depth of needle insertion corresponds to d2.

b In this case a tiny MR-detected lesion medially in the right breast had to be identified by comparing the indispensible precontrast and postcontrast slices (using 3 mL 60% CT contrast agent per kg body weight). The measurements for the anticipated approach were taken.

c One of the curved branches of the tip of the wire is shown coursing through the lesion. The wire that courses from the skin to the lesion is partly contained in the imaged slice. It is therefore only faintly seen (arrow).

Materials for Lesion Localization

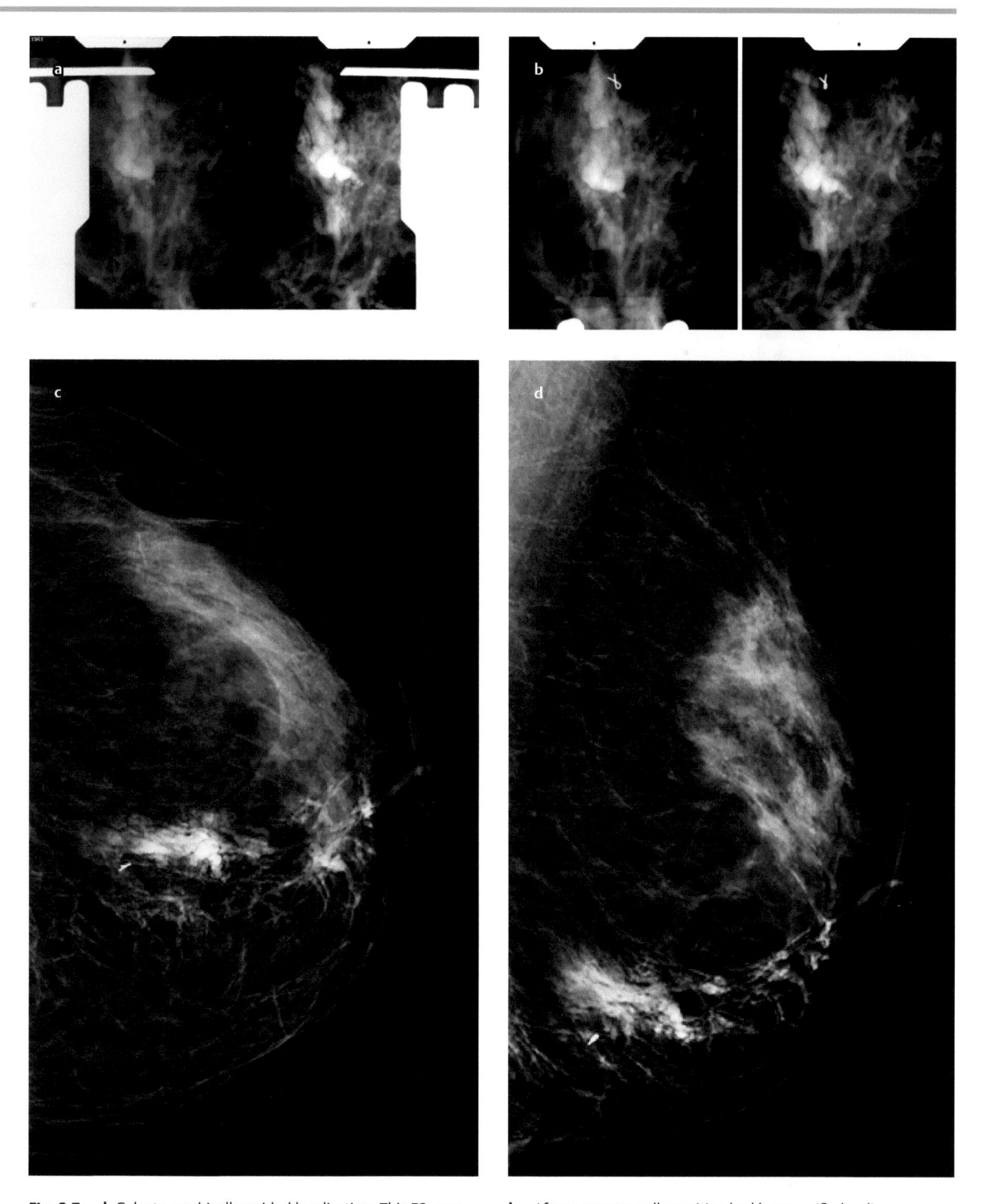

Fig. 8.7a–d Galactographically guided localization. This 53-year-old patient presented with a history of spontaneous nipple discharge for 3 months. Galactography revealed a segment with dilated ducts and small filling defects. Since the segment was considered too large to enable the problem to be solved by percutaneous biopsy alone, immediate clip marking of the posterior extent of the segment was undertaken.

a Stereotactic views after introduction of the coaxial needle. One point at the base of the segment was chosen as target.

b After correct needle position had been verified a clip was deposited through the needle and clip position was confirmed on two stereotactic views.

c The CC view after galactographic marking shows the clip centrally at the basis of the segment.

d To allow subsequent surgical planning the second plane is an orthogonal ML view. It shows the clip at the caudal posterior end of the contrasted segment.

8 Preoperative Localization

of the contrast solution on the two-view mammogram obtained after localization is complete.

It is important to perform the surgery as quickly as possible after injecting the blue solution because within a few hours the solution can diffuse throughout large areas of the breast or even the entire breast, rendering precise localization impossible. If the interval between administration of the contrast solution and surgery cannot be limited to a few hours, the radiologist should choose a different localization procedure. Further disadvantages are that diffusion renders it impossible for the pathologist to identify the exact injection site. Also, the dye may follow tissue planes and thus will not be able to precisely mark the lesion in some cases. Finally, contrast allergies or severe allergies to patent blue, although rare, have been known to occur. Thus, dye marking has mostly been replaced by wire marking.

Another simple procedure is to use a carbon solution for marking the lesion. The advantage of carbon is that it does not diffuse. Therefore, this can be done several days preoperatively since the carbon remains at the injection site until the surgeon removes it along with the lesion. However, even though inert and harmless, carbon solution is not approved in some countries (e.g., the United States) for use in the breast.

This method has mainly been used for CT- and MR-guided localization since in these cases it is often difficult to coordinate the scheduling of the examination and surgery.

The sterile carbon solution, which can be prepared by most pharmacies (4 g of activated charcoal in 100 mL of 0.9% saline solution), is injected into the center of the lesion to be excised or directly proximal to it. Approximately 1–1.5 mL of solution has to be injected to achieve sufficient dispersion and visualization. For mammographically guided localization, 0.2–0.3 mL of nonionic radiographic contrast medium should be added to the solution for subsequent image documentation of correct dispersion. Then, a fine line of carbon extending all the way to the skin is injected as the needle is withdrawn, which permits the surgeon to locate the lesion after the needle or wire has been removed. A particular advantage of this method is that the carbon also enables the pathologist to locate the injection site in the specimen. However, carbon may also follow tissue planes. Since it does not diffuse, it may be difficult to find if the path to the skin is lost. Finally, thick injection needles should be used with carbon, since carbon may obstruct the needle. Owing to the logistic difficulties and lack of approval by some regulating authorities, carbon is only rarely used today.

The technique of radio-guided occult lesion localization (ROLL) has been also been described. ROLL involves an injection of small amount of radioactive tracer into the center of the lesion under sonographic or mammographic control by the radiologist. Surgeons identify the lesion as a hot spot by using a hand-held gamma probe intraoperatively, allowing accurate lesion localization and removal with minimal excision of healthy tissue. As a result, this technique enables a good cosmetic outcome.

More recently there have been several studies describing the use of dual radioisotopes in the localization of early breast cancer and sentinel lymph nodes and this technique is gaining popularity. The advantages of this technique when combined with the injection of Patent Blue dye are that it allows the breast lesion and sentinel node to be readily identified and it reduces the risks associated with wire insertion. It is a safe and easy procedure. A recent study (Thind et al. 2011) reported 100% lesion localization with 94.8% negative clearance margin and 100% sentinel node localization. Difficult and complex cases may still require a wire and, since radioactivity decreases with time, this technique is best suited to localizations where surgery is to be performed on the same day.

Currently, localization wires are mostly used for preoperative marking (**Fig. 8.8**). They have the advantage of being more flexible and better anchored in the tissue. This minimizes the risk of wire migration.

There are various types of localization wires. Their tenacity of fixation varies with their design and the type of breast tissue involved. Dislocation can occur particularly in soft fatty tissue. In rare cases, wires have been observed to migrate distally. This usually occurs only in wires whose form predisposes them to migrate in a certain direction, such as a simple L-shaped hookwire. Marker wires which have one or more curved arms after being deployed are nondirectional. Another advantage of these wires is that they can be withdrawn or retracted through the needle, making it possible to correct the position of the needle.

Regardless of the wire chosen, the physician should ensure that the needle through which the wire is advanced is sufficiently stiff (it should not be too thin and flexible) because otherwise it can deviate considerably in dense tissue. This may seriously compromise the

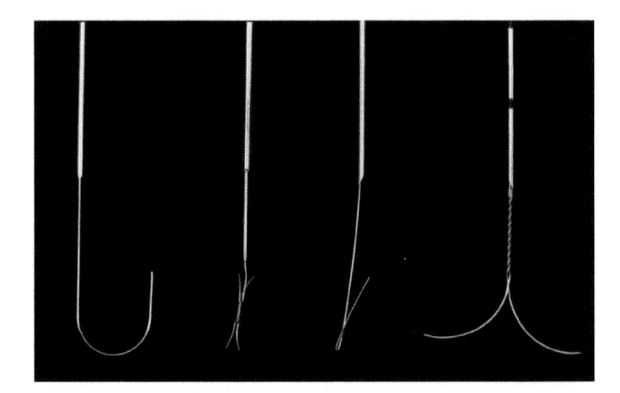

Fig. 8.8 Various localization wires.

accuracy of localization. Rarely, chest wall injury might occur. An adequate length of wire should extend beyond the skin and be securely taped to it to avoid retraction of the wire and its subsequent loss. During surgery, if the surgeon is dissecting along the length of the wire, he or she should be careful not to transect it. It may then retract into the breast and be very difficult to locate. Some wires consisting of twisted metal threads are difficult to transect, which helps avoid this problem.

Instead of a wire which protrudes through the skin and might (if long-standing) become a source of infection, clip-marking is another option. Clip-marking is usually chosen to mark an area or lesion for which the necessity of surgery is uncertain or for which the date of surgery is much later or unknown, and is also used in patients undergoing neoadjuvant chemotherapy to ensure the tumor bed is marked when there is excellent response. If on imaging during the chemotherapy cycles the visible lesion has been noted to shrink significantly and might even disappear after completion of chemotherapy, clip-marking should be considered (**Fig. 8.9**). Depositing one or several clips will always allow identification of the tumor bed. Since regression of the imaging abnormality can never exclude microscopic or diffusely growing residual or ductal carcinoma in situ (DCIS), excision of the tumor bed is considered state of the art.

Thus, clip-marking is used after percutaneous biopsy if a small lesion (whose nature is usually unknown) is completely or partly removed at biopsy, or if a small lesion might be obscured by postinterventional changes. Under such circumstances identification of the lesion might be impaired, if surgery later on turns out to be necessary.

When choosing the type of clip, its visibility on mammography, ultrasound, or MRI should be counterchecked depending on the imaging modality chosen for clip deposition and the imaging methods available to the surgeon. All clips are readily visible on mammography. According to our experience, however, ultrasound visibility varies markedly with different types of metal clips. Some clips are surrounded by a gel capsule to increase sonographic visibility, but this decreases with time and may disappear after 1–2 weeks. Good visibility on ultrasound may allow the surgeon identify the clip by intraoperative ultrasound imaging during surgery making an additional preoperative (stereotactic wire) marking of the clip unnecessary. Visibility of MR-compatible clips on MRI may be quite difficult, since the signal void of small metal clips may be difficult to distinguish from other signal voids caused by air bubbles. Use of non–MR-compatible material must be avoided, since it is not approved for use in the magnetic field.

Problems and Their Solutions

All methods require documentation of the final position of the localization wire or the contrast solution. This means that after mammographically guided localization, the position of the needle should be documented in two mammographic planes (craniocaudal and mediolateral). If the wire is improperly positioned but the distance between the tumor and the tip of the wire is still acceptable (i.e., does not exceed 10 mm), the radiologist may describe to the surgeon the exact position of the lesion in the image with respect to the tip of the wire. Large areas undergoing excision should have their margins marked with more than one wire. Multiple lesions require additional localization of distant lesions.

The exact position of the wire (or contrast solution) also has to be documented in MR-guided and US-guided localization. If the surgeon asks for more help, an additional two-view mammogram may be helpful.

Imaging documentation and a written report that explains the procedure should accompany the patient so that all necessary information is available to the surgeon

If improper positioning occurs, the necessary corrections should also be directly discussed with the surgeon, assuming of course that the deviation is within accept-

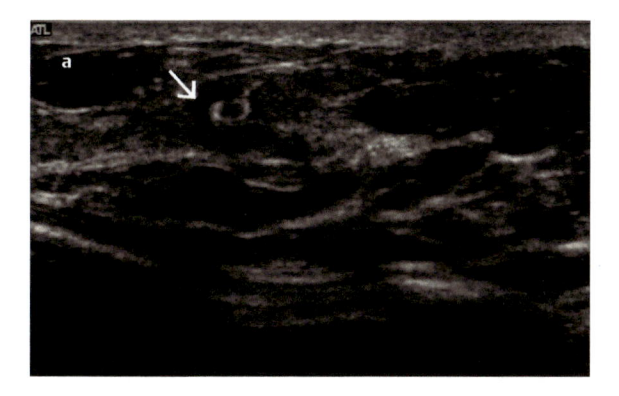

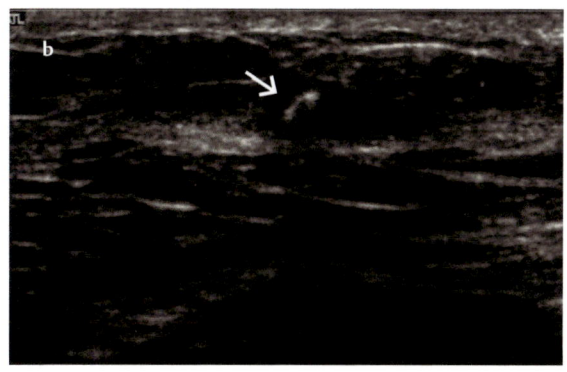

Fig. 8.9a,b Clip marking in a 35-year-old patient who had excellent response to neoadjuvant chemotherapy. After four cycles of chemotherapy only a small residue of the initial ductal carcinoma of 2.8 cm was seen (**a**). After needle localization a small ring-shaped clip was deposited in the area of the hypoechoic residue (**b**).

able limits. Sufficient experience and thorough discussion of the results are essential. It should be remembered that it is not always easy for the surgeon to find the contrast solution or marker wire, particularly in large breasts. Perioperative or intraoperative dislocation of the wire may occur. Close cooperation between radiologist and surgeon is essential for effective management—that is, removal of the suspicious lesion with the smallest possible volume of breast tissue.

Correct excision of microcalcifications and nonpalpable lesions detected at mammography should also be documented by specimen radiography. Correct excision of lesions detected only at sonography may be counter-checked by specimen sonography.

Even though correct preoperative localization may support complete excision of malignancy with the best possible cosmetic result, there are known limitations:

- In spite of correct preoperative localization, nonpalpable lesions may be missed at surgery. This has been described to occur even in good centers, on average in 2–3% of cases. The most likely reason for such misses may be wire displacement directly before or during surgery.
- Partial excision of nonpalpable lesions may occur in spite of correct, state-of-the-art preoperative localization of the imaging abnormality. One reason may be that only a limited number of markers can be set. The breast is a flexible organ and anatomy changes between the position assumed during imaging and during surgery. Therefore, exact marking of the three-dimensional extent of large lesions is generally difficult. The other, probably even more important, reason is that DCIS and microscopic disease, which do not correspond to palpable abnormalities either, may partly be occult to imaging.

The best recommendations which can be given for the above problems include:

- Correct information to the patient concerning limitations of imaging, localization procedures, and surgery.
- Whenever preoperative histology is available of the leading and other lesions, surgical planning can be optimized. A better outcome of patients treated according to these standards is proven.
- Exact orientation of all excised specimens (marking of three sides, e.g., lateral, upper, and anterior side pointing to the nipple) and close communication of the radiologist and the surgeon before and during surgery (considering all available imaging information).
- If a lesion is missed or partly included, additional imaging may be considered. Mammographic check for residual microcalcifications is possible (with moderate compression) starting about 1 week after the initial surgery. MRI may be the best method to check for residual mass lesions.
- Before re-excision the preoperative and postoperative imaging and histopathologic information should be discussed in a multidisciplinary conference.

Summary

The increasing use of mammography has resulted in an increased rate of detection of clinically occult lesions. Whenever surgery is necessary, these lesions must be marked for the surgeon to ensure that they can be effectively removed. Several methods are available. Accepted methods involve use of a perforated or marked compression plate, stereotaxis, or manual localization in selected cases.

Focal lesions with correlating sonographic findings or focal lesions detected only at ultrasound can be quickly and reliably marked using US-guided localization.

MR-guided localization techniques permit accurate marking of lesions that are detected only at MRI and require excision.

CT-guided localization after administration of contrast remains an alternative for marking nonpalpable MR-detected lesions that are also visible by contrast-enhanced CT but not by conventional imaging. It is faster and easier than MR-guided localization without a dedicated biopsy coil.

Owing to the significant radiation dose and the lower accuracy, CT-guided localization should, however, in the future be replaced by MR-guided localization using dedicated coils.

The choice between needle marking, wire marking with various marker wires, or marking with carbon or methylene blue depends on the time interval between localization and surgery, the conditions under which the patient must be transported to the operating room, and the surgeon's preferences.

References and Recommended Reading

Albert US, Altland H, Duda V, et al. 2008 update of the guideline: early detection of breast cancer in Germany. J Cancer Res Clin Oncol 2009;135(3):339–354

American College of Radiology. ACR Practice Guideline for the performance of stereotactically guided breast interventional procedures. American College of Radiology; Revised 2009: http://www.acr.org/SecondaryMainMenuCategories/quality_safety/guidelines/breast.aspx

American College of Radiology. ACR Practice Guideline for the performance of ultrasound guided percutaneous breast interventional procedures. American College of Radiology; Revised 2009: http://www.acr.org/SecondaryMainMenuCategories/quality_safety/guidelines/breast.aspx

Graham RA, Homer MJ, Sigler CJ, et al. The efficacy of specimen radiography in evaluating the surgical margins of impalpable breast carcinoma. AJR Am J Roentgenol 1994;162(1):33–36

Helvie MA, Ikeda DM, Adler DD. Localization and needle aspiration of breast lesions: complications in 370 cases. AJR Am J Roentgenol 1991;157(4):711–714

Heywang-Köbrunner SH, Heinig A, Pickuth D, Alberich T, Spielmann RP. Interventional MRI of the breast: lesion localisation and biopsy. Eur Radiol 2000;10(1):36–45

Homer MJ, Smith TJ, Safaii H. Prebiopsy needle localization. Methods, problems, and expected results. Radiol Clin North Am 1992;30(1):139–153

Lampe D, Hefler L, Alberich T, et al. The clinical value of preoperative wire localization of breast lesions by magnetic resonance imaging—a multicenter study. Breast Cancer Res Treat 2002;75(2):175–179

Perlet C, Heywang-Kobrunner SH, Heinig A, et al. Magnetic resonance-guided, vacuum-assisted breast biopsy: results from a European multicenter study of 538 lesions. Cancer 2006;106(5):982–990

Perry N, Broeders M, de Wolf C, Toernberg S, Holland R, von Karsa L, Eds. European guidelines for quality assurance in breast cancer screening and diagnosis. Luxembourg: Office for Official Publications of the European Communities; 2006

Thind CR, Tan S, Desmond S, et al. SNOLL. Sentinel node and occult (impalpable) lesion localization in breast cancer. Clin Radiol 2011;66(9):833–839

Warren RM, Hayes C; Advisory Group of MARIBS. Localization of breast lesions shown only on MRI—a review for the UK Study of MRI Screening for Breast Cancer. Br J Radiol 2000;73(866):123–132

II Appearance

9 The Normal Breast

Anatomy 234

The Adolescent Female Breast 235
Histology 235
Clinical Examination 235
Mammography 235
Sonography 235

The Mature Female Breast 235
Histology 235
Clinical Examination 235
Mammography 236
Sonography 237
Magnetic Resonance Imaging 237

Breast Density and Changes with Age 241
Histology 241
Clinical Examination 241
Mammography 241
Sonography 241
Magnetic Resonance Imaging 242

Variants of Normal Findings 242
Definition 242
Anisomastia 242
Macromastia 242
Accessory Breast Tissue (Polymastia) 244
Inverted Nipple 244

Pregnancy and Lactation 246
Histology 246
Clinical Examination 246
Mammography 246
Sonography 246
Magnetic Resonance Imaging 246

Breast Response with Hormone Replacement Therapy 248
Mammography 248
Sonography 248
Magnetic Resonance Imaging 248
Percutaneous Biopsy 248

References and Recommended Reading 252

9 The Normal Breast

S. H. Heywang-Koebrunner, I. Schreer, S. Barter

Anatomy

The mammary gland consists of 15 to 20 lobes with varying numbers of ducts and lobules. These structures are surrounded by collagenous connective tissue or stromal tissue. A lobule comprises around 30 terminal branches (acini or ductules) that form the parenchymal part of the lobule. Acini and terminal ducts are surrounded by loose mesenchyma. The lobule with its terminal branches, its short intralobular and longer extralobular duct form the terminal ductulobular unit (**Fig. 9.1**). All terminal ducts open into a lactiferous duct that runs toward the nipple. The 15 to 20 main lactiferous ducts open in the nipple (**Fig. 9.1**).

The body of the gland is imbedded in fatty tissue. It is supplied by a network of blood and lymph vessels and is supported in the subcutaneous fatty tissue by connective tissue structures known as Cooper ligaments. These ligaments arise from the stromal tissue of the body of the gland and insert into the prepectoral fascia and the skin. The body of the gland, which can vary greatly in form, size, and composition, converges toward the nipple, is generally symmetrical, and is particularly pronounced in the upper outer quadrants.

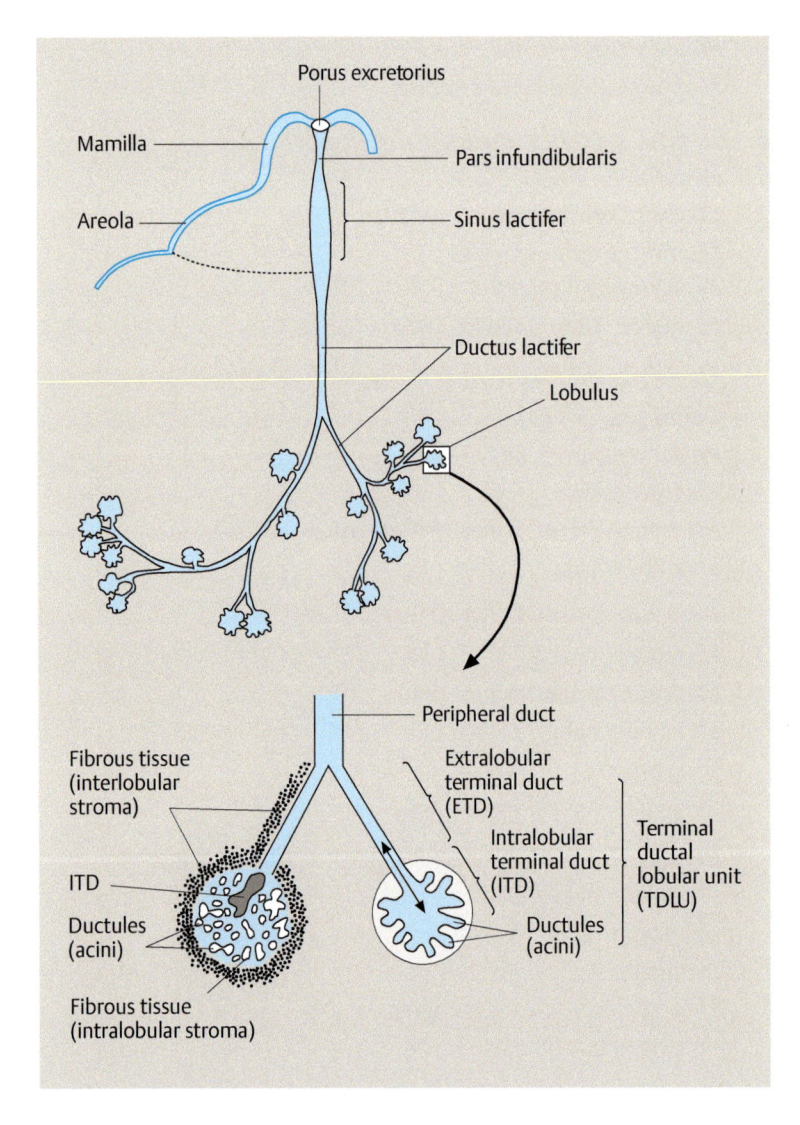

Fig. 9.1 Schematic diagram and terminology of the lactiferous duct system.

The Adolescent Female Breast

Histology

Histologically, the prepubescent breast consists of lactiferous ducts with adventitial alveoli comprising primarily connective tissue and small amounts of fatty tissue. During puberty, the ducts increase in length, and the terminal alveoli increase in number. These later develop into lobules. Ductal growth triggers mesenchymal metaplasia and formation of connective tissue.

Clinical Examination

On palpation the breast is uniformly firm while the glandular tissue may commonly feel somewhat nodular. However, the usual nodularity of breast tissue should be uniform, elastic, and mobile.

Mammography

The developing glandular body initially appears as a small nodule, later as a small treelike glandular structure. The lactiferous ducts and connective tissue appear as a homogeneously dense, milky structure surrounded by a narrow layer of subcutaneous fatty tissue. Substructures are not usually discernible with the exception of some vessels and Cooper ligaments within the subcutaneous tissue.

> None of the European or American guidelines recommends mammography in adolescents. Malignancy is very rare in adolescence and sonography is the investigation of choice. If an abnormality is confirmed by ultrasound examination, percutaneous breast biopsy is preferable to mammography, which in the adolescent patient is of limited value.
>
> High mammary density results in a dense, homogeneous, opaque zone which is difficult to interpret. Furthermore, the risk of radiation-induced malignant changes is much higher in the young glandular breast than beyond the age of 40.

Sonography

The immature glandular tissue is initially relatively hypoechoic. The nodule of glandular tissue may appear as a hypoechoic nodule and should not be confused with a tumor (**Fig. 9.2**). Even the developed glandular body is still relatively hypoechoic in adolescence and cannot always be distinguished from the surrounding hypoechoic fat. The echogenicity of the glandular tissue increases with maturity. However, local differences in the maturity of breast tissue can occur, producing alternating areas of predominantly hypoechoic or predominantly hyperechoic glandular tissue (**Fig. 9.3**).

The Mature Female Breast

Histology

Under the influence of estrogen, progesterone, prolactin, somatotropin, adrenocorticotropin, and corticoids, the ductal system becomes increasingly branched. A treelike glandular structure with glandular lobules develops. This process of growth and differentiation continues until about age 30 years. The highest proportion of lobules is located far from the nipple along the periphery, particularly in the upper outer quadrant.

Clinical Examination

Physical examination of the normal female breast can vary considerably. Large, fatty breasts generally have a soft consistency. In some cases, however, even fatty breasts will be firm and nodular on palpation. Glandular tissue with a high proportion of parenchymal or connective tissue usually feels firm. Generally, there will be less glandular tissue in the inner half of the breast than in the outer half. Therefore, the breast is generally firmer in the upper outer quadrant owing to the increased proportion

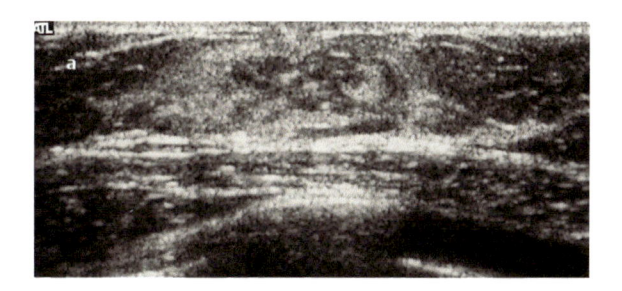

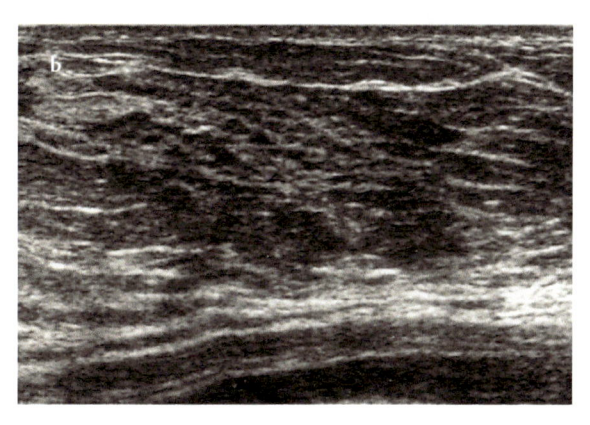

Fig. 9.2a,b Immature glandular tissue.
a An 8-year-old girl with precocious puberty: A small, palpable painful tumor was the reason for consultation. On ultrasound examination a triangular bud of breast tissue explains the clinical finding. No further diagnostic steps are needed.
b Mostly echogenic parenchyma of a 16-year-old adolescent girl.

9 The Normal Breast

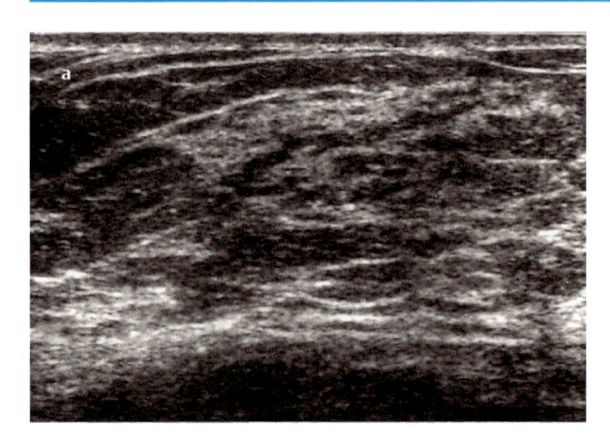

Fig. 9.3a,b Sonography of the adolescent breast.
a The subcutaneous layer of fat seen here is narrow, as in many adolescent breasts. The glandular tissue is still relatively hypoechoic and thus more difficult to differentiate from the subcutaneous fat than in an adult breast.
b Diagram for **Fig. 9.3a**.

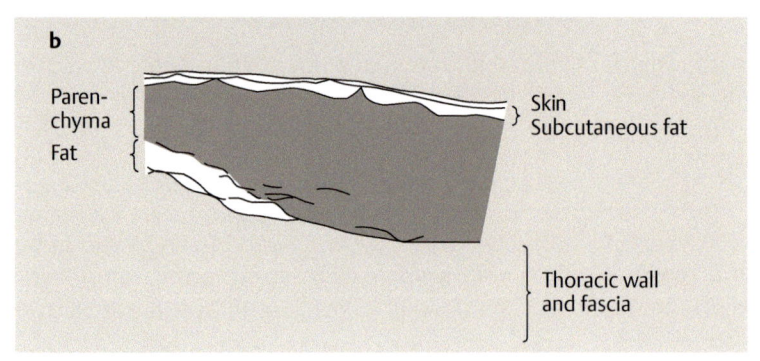

of parenchymal tissue in this region. If fibrocystic changes develop, the uniformly soft-to-firm consistency of the breasts may change from a finely granular to coarsely nodular pattern on palpation.

The glandular tissue undergoes cyclical fluctuations, which may become apparent to the woman in the second half of the menstrual cycle as increased tissue tension or pain and enlargement of the breasts. This is due to the cyclical swelling of the lobular tissue. Temporary enlargement of the acini also occurs. For this reason, the glandular tissue of the breast in the second half of the cycle and especially immediately prior to menstruation will usually be firmer, more sensitive to pressure, and more painful.

Mammography

Normal glandular tissue (**Fig. 9.4**) will appear as a summation image of all microscopic parenchymal and connective tissue structures, that is, it will produce a homogeneous mammographic appearance. This homogeneous pattern will be interspersed with islands of fatty tissue appearing as round or curved radiolucencies in a wide variety of individual configurations. Often, increased opacity corresponding to the physiologic distribution of parenchymal tissue will be seen in the upper outer quadrants.

Cooper ligaments appear in the mammogram as curved to linear densities. They extend from the cone of breast tissue through the fatty tissue to the skin. Depending on the specific composition of the breast, the glandular, connective, and fatty tissues, and the ligaments can be distinguished more or less clearly. Generally, Cooper ligaments are most prominent in the subcutaneous fatty tissue along the superior margin of the parenchyma on the oblique or mediolateral mammogram and in the prepectoral space.

The lactiferous duct system will not be visualized except for the large lactiferous ducts converging in the retroareolar region, where they are visible as bandlike structures.

The density of the parenchyma may vary with the menstrual cycle. It may be denser in the premenstrual phase than in the postmenstrual phase. This means that the mammographic appearance of the parenchyma may vary both in terms of its structure and with respect to the phase of the menstrual cycle.

Parenchymal structures are always more easily discerned and their regular arrangement converging at the nipple more easily demonstrated when fatty tissue is present. Where less fatty tissue is interspersed, the parenchymal structures tend to blend into a homogeneous pattern of density that can hide small pathologic lesions. Owing to premenstrual pain with resulting diminished compressibility of the glandular tissue and increased premenstrual density, routine mammography should—if possible—be performed in the postmenstrual phase of the cycle.

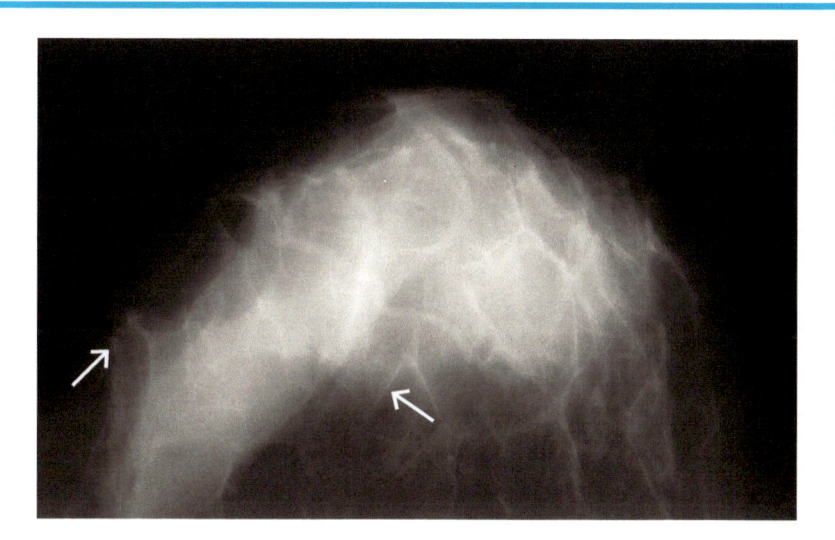

Fig. 9.4 Normal glandular tissue appears as a milky density. Cooper ligaments appear as fine arcs or stripes of increased density (arrow).

Sonography

(See **Fig. 9.5**.)

Glandular tissue generally appears hyperechoic, although its sonographic appearance may vary from moderately to highly echogenic. Surrounding or interspersed fat is hypoechoic. Rotating the transducer will usually identify these interspersed fat lobules as oblong hypoechoic areas to be distinguished from hypoechoic tumors. Sometimes a connection between the fat lobules and the subcutaneous fatty tissue allows their identification. Also, fat lobules are usually very elastic and can easily be compressed. Depending on the imaging plane, hypoechoic tubular or punctate structures traversing the glandular parenchyma will occasionally be visible. These structures are arranged regularly in the tissue and probably correspond to small ductal structures with periductal fibrosis or small foci of adenosis. Such findings represent a normal variant and do not require further workup. The examiner should verify that the layer of fatty tissue surrounding the body of the gland is completely intact and unchanged.

Cooper ligaments are hyperechoic and permeate the layer of fatty tissue, appearing as fine linear structures. Owing to their orientation (almost parallel to the direction of sound propagation), Cooper ligaments can produce acoustic shadows that occur when the sound is reflected away from the transducer. These acoustic shadows can be recognized by the fact that they originate from Cooper ligaments. They can generally be eliminated by compression and do not represent a pathologic finding.

The skin itself appears as a hyperechoic line or, depending on the resolution of the transducer, as a double contour whose thickness generally does not exceed 3 mm except at the areola. Since the retroareolar ducts run nearly parallel to the direction of sound propagation and periductal fibrosis is frequently present, the sound waves will often be reflected away from the transducer or absorbed behind the nipple. The acoustic shadow ("nipple shadow") thus produced does not represent a pathologic finding but is a normal structure that can vary. This nipple shadow may impair visualization of the retroareolar region.

Magnetic Resonance Imaging

(See **Fig. 9.6**.)

MRI is not necessary for imaging the normal breast. However, normal breast tissue will often be incidentally visualized on MR images, or normal tissue will be described after a suspected pathologic change has been ruled out.

In T1-weighted spoiled-gradient echo sequences (FLASH, T1 FFE, and SP GRASS), fat has moderate signal intensity, whereas all glandular and ductal structures and fibrous connective tissue (with Cooper ligaments) are visualized with low signal intensity. After intravenous injection of the contrast medium, glandular, fatty, and connective tissue do not normally enhance, that is, these structures appear identical in precontrast and postcontrast images. Only vascular structures can be traced through the images as small, enhancing, wormlike structures or punctate cross-sections of high signal intensity. Contrast enhancement of the nipple itself occurs in about 50% of all patients and should not be regarded as pathologic in the absence of suggestive clinical findings. Occasionally, a milky or patchy diffuse enhancement, sometimes even focal enhancement, can appear in normal glandular tissue. This enhancement is probably due to hormonal changes and usually occurs in young patients with active glandular tissue or in postmenopausal patients receiving hormone therapy (particularly

9 The Normal Breast

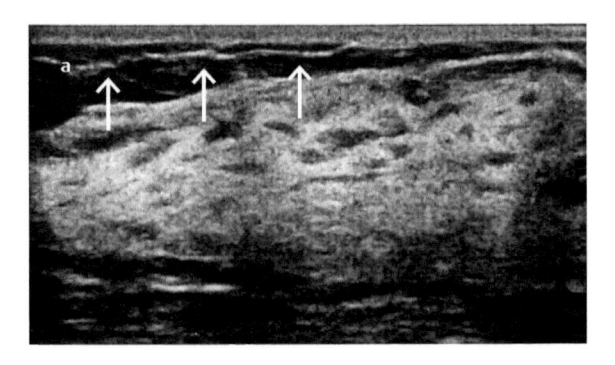

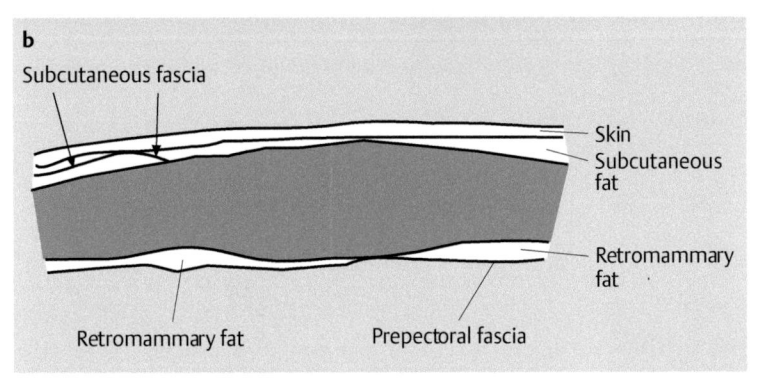

Fig. 9.5a–j Sonography of the adult breast. Significant individual variations can occur both in the relative proportion of hyperechoic glandular versus hypoechoic fatty tissue and in the echogenicity of the glandular tissue itself.

a Breast with dense hyperechoic glandular tissue surrounded by a narrow layer of fat. The subcutaneous fascia is only partially visible (arrows). The prepectoral fascia is readily discernible.
b Diagram for **Fig. 9.5a**.
c In this breast, the hyperechoic glandular tissue is permeated with extremely regular tubular hypoechoic structures. This image also represents a normal finding. The hypoechoic structures probably correspond to small ductal structures with periductal fibrosis or small foci of adenosis. Subcutaneous and retromammary fat are visible as wide and very narrow hypoechoic strips. The subcutaneous fascia (arrows) is partly visible as a fine line of more distinct echoes.

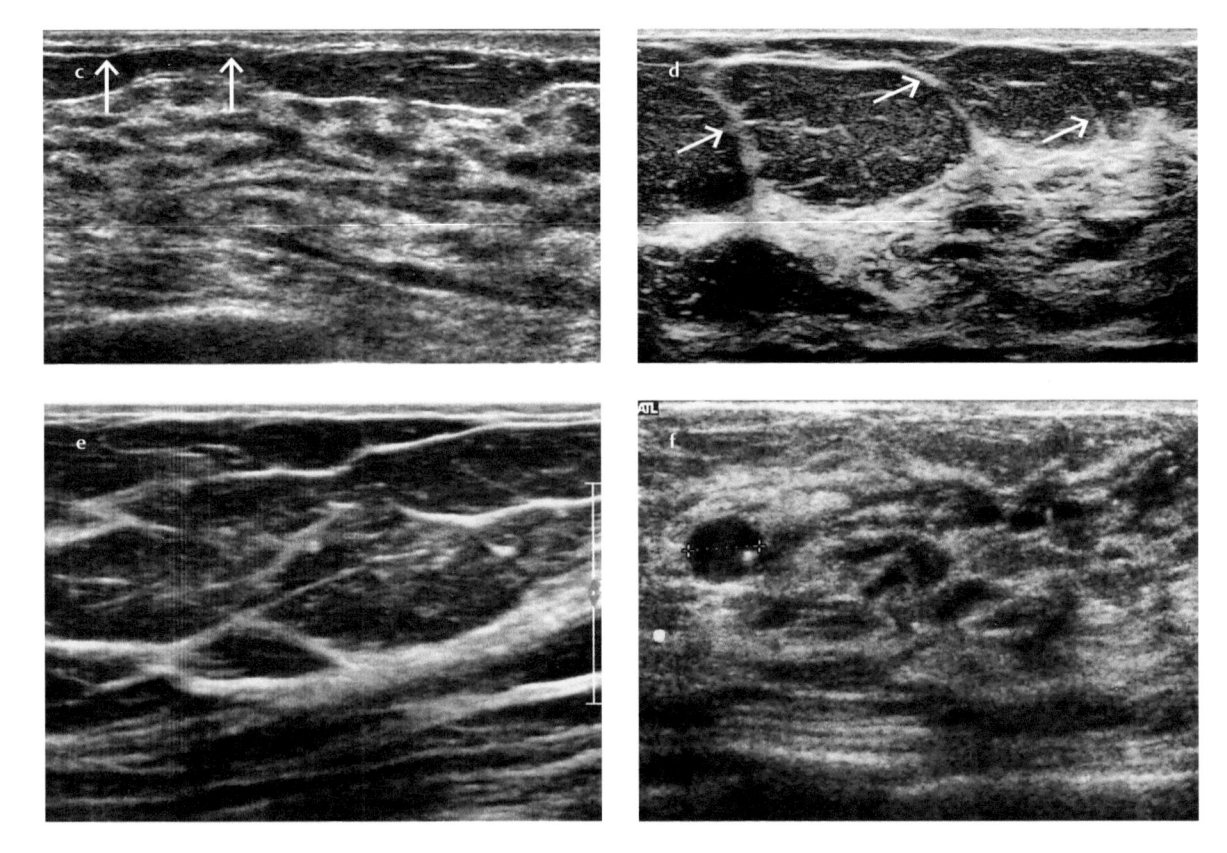

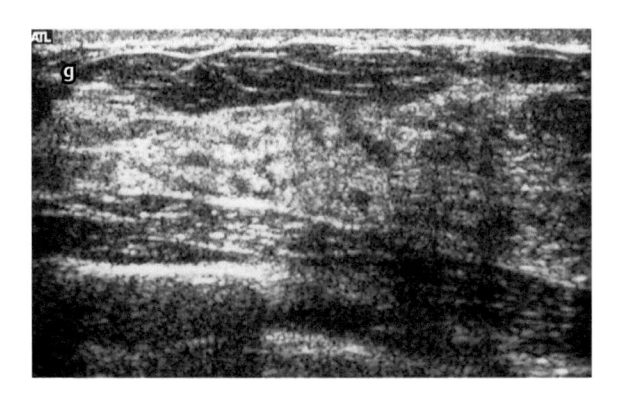

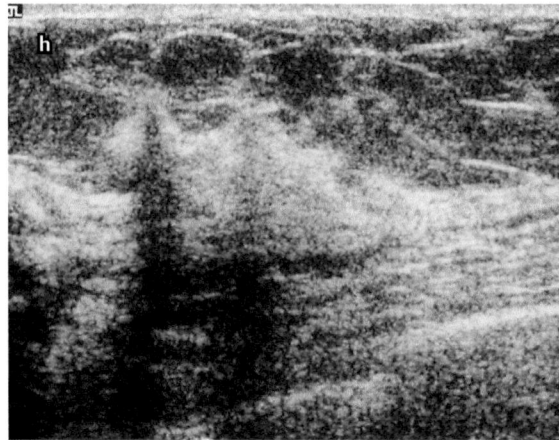

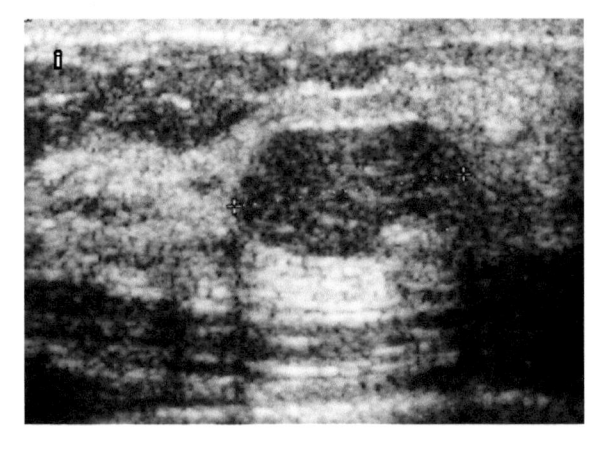

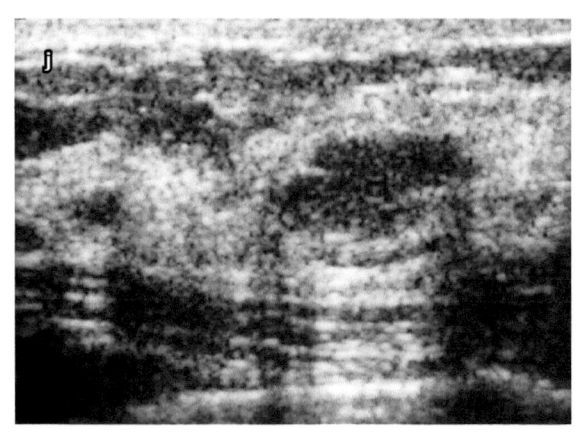

- **d** This partially involuted breast contains typical hypoechoic fatty tissue in addition to a smaller amount of remaining hyperechoic glandular tissue. Permeating this fatty tissue are thin hyperechoic ligamentous structures, corresponding to fine Cooper ligaments inserting into the skin (arrows).
- **e** Extremely fatty breasts appear hypoechoic on sonography. The hypoechoic fat is traversed only by thin hyperechoic linear ligamentous structures.
- **f** Benign changes with some duct ectasia surrounded by echogenic fibrous tissue. Some microcalcifications are visualized in the ducts and within one tiny hypoechoic cyst, which contains a small hyperechoic calcification at its posterior wall.
- **g** Dense hyperechoic breast tissue is shown with regularly interspersed hypoechoic tubular structures corresponding to small areas of ductal fibrosis or adenosis.
- **h** Prominent shadowing produced by Cooper ligaments. Owing to their angulation the ultrasound beam is reflected away from the transducer, which results in shadowing. With compression the ligaments assume more transverse orientation and the shadowing resolves.
- **i,j** Interspersed fat lobules may simulate a tumor. During compression (j) the "mass" totally flattens, which is typical of fat lobules.

9 The Normal Breast

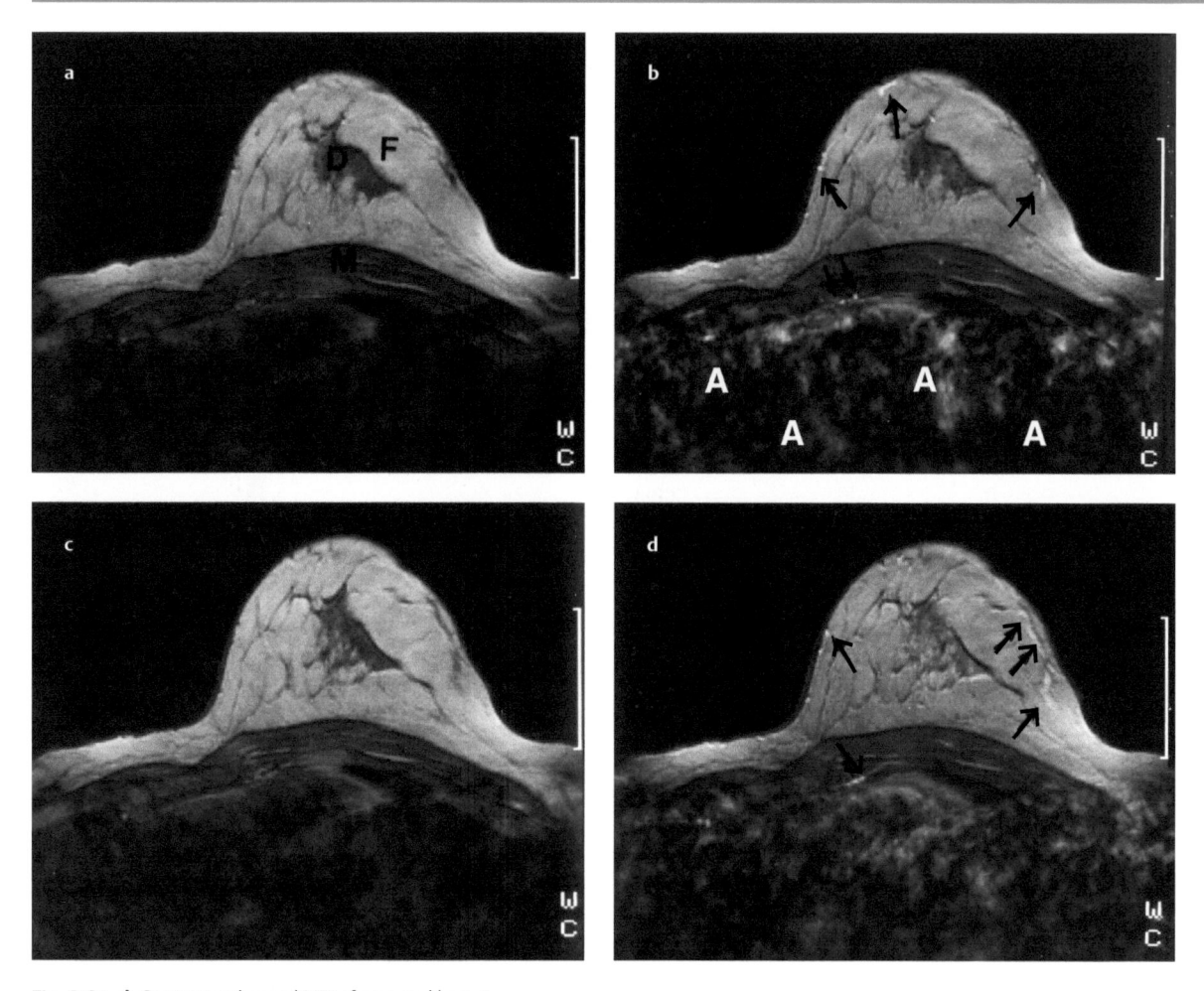

Fig. 9.6a–d Contrast-enhanced MRI of a normal breast.

a On the T1-weighted transverse slice of the breast (FLASH 3D), glandular and connective tissue (D) are visualized with low signal intensity, as is muscle (M). Fat (F) shows moderate signal intensity.

b After administration of contrast, normal glandular tissue and fatty tissue enhance slightly only at the beginning of the menstrual cycle (between the 6th and 16th days) and in the postmenstrual phase. This means that the signal intensity hardly changes at all in comparison with the plain image (**a**). Only the band of artifacts caused by blood flowing through the heart (A) significantly increases in signal intensity, as do the vessels (arrow), which can be traced through the images after contrast application as winding or punctiform structures of high signal intensity.

c,d In the second half of the menstrual cycle, slight to intense diffuse or nodular enhancement patterns are often seen in normal glandular tissue. **c** Comparable image of the same breast as in **Fig. 9.6a** in the second half of the cycle before application of contrast. **d** After application of contrast in the second half of the cycle, moderate diffuse enhancement may be seen (arrows indicate vascular structures).

where preparations with high progesterone content are used). The enhancing areas usually correspond to areas consisting of cellular tissue (like adenosis), which may be surrounded by dense fibrosis. Most areas of normal enhancement are transient and more pronounced before and during menstruation. Since this enhancement can interfere with the exclusion of malignancy, and can lead to false positive findings, we recommend performing contrast-enhanced MRI between day 7 and day 15 (or 17) of the menstrual cycle (depending on the length of the menstrual cycle), wherever possible.

Breast Density and Changes with Age

Histology

As ovarian function decreases, involution of the glandular body sets in. Lactiferous ducts, lobules, and parenchyma become atrophic, and fatty and fibrous tissue dominate. Often ectasia of the large excretory ducts occurs.

Clinical Examination

The findings of the clinical examination vary considerably, depending on the extent of the parenchymal involution, the presence of structural changes due to benign breast disorders, and the extent of fibrosis.

Mammography

The formerly dense epithelial and mesenchymal parts of the glandular tissue that absorb radiation are replaced with fat as involution progresses. The body of the gland itself becomes considerably more radiolucent and fibrous tissue, vascular structures, and remaining glandular lobules become more readily discernible, as do the large retroareolar ectatic lactiferous ducts (**Fig. 9.7**).

Involution begins in the inner half of the breast and involves the upper outer quadrant and the retroareolar region later. Thus, mammography in the older woman will mostly reveal residual glandular tissue primarily in the retroareolar region and in the upper outer quadrant. In addition to the described changes with age there are large differences in both overall breast density and the distribution of glandular or fibrous versus fatty tissue between individuals. Hormone replacement therapy may cause increased or persisting breast density, even in elderly women. Antiestrogen therapy may often lead to decreased breast density. Involution improves the visualization of the breast. In a completely involuted fatty breast, the sensitivity of mammography approaches 98%. However, in the very dense breast it may drop below 50%.

As sensitivity of mammography varies with the overall amount of dense breast tissue, the American College of Radiology demands that mammographic reporting include a description of the amount of dense tissue visible on mammography. The amount of dense tissue in a mammogram is thus classified as:
- ACR (category) 1: almost entirely fatty breast tissue
- ACR (category) 2: scattered fibroglandular densities
- ACR (category) 3: heterogeneously dense (51–75% dense tissue)
- ACR (category) 4: heterogeneously dense (> 75% dense tissue) to extremely dense

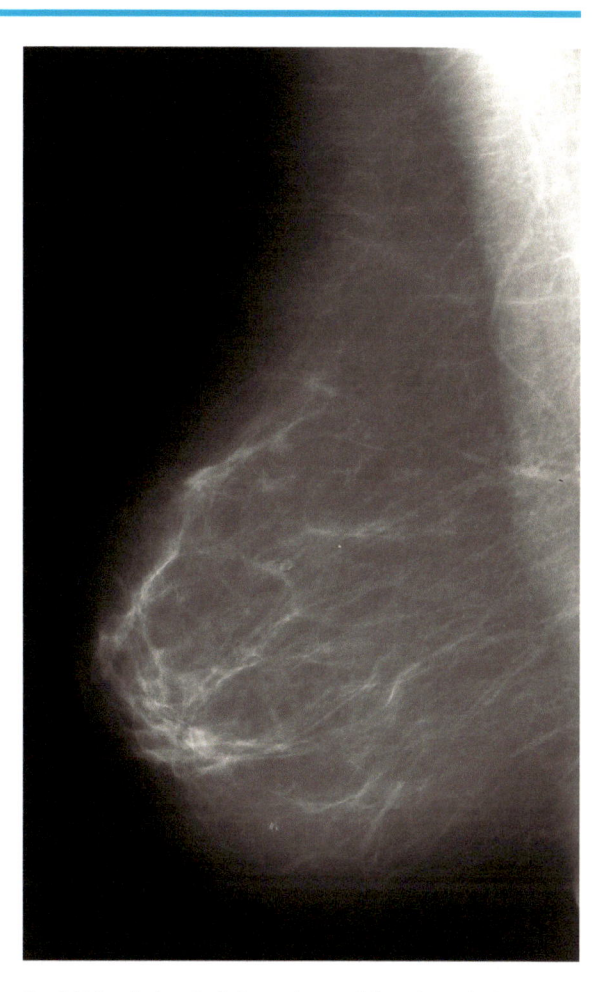

Fig. 9.7 Involution. Radiolucent breast delineating only Cooper ligaments, few glandular and ductal as well as vascular structures (mediolateral oblique view).

Sonography

The fatty involuted breast appears hypoechoic on sonographic examination (see **Fig. 9.5e**). Only remaining islands of hyperechoic connective tissue and Cooper ligaments traverse the hypoechoic fatty tissue. Residual parenchyma generally appears as moderately echogenic islands in hypoechoic fat.

Over 90% of breast carcinomas are hypoechoic (similar to fatty tissue). Only some breast carcinomas have a distinctive posterior acoustic shadow or a hyperechoic peripheral rim. This compromises the sensitivity of ultrasonography in the fatty breast. Islands of fatty tissue with or without posterior shadowing due to fibrous septa can also be mistaken for tumors. To avoid both false positive and false negative calls the sonogram should generally be read in conjunction with mammography.

With the excellent sensitivity of mammography applied to the involuted breast, sonography is not necessary for detecting or excluding malignancy. However, it is indicated for evaluating breast masses, since sonography is reliable for the differentiation of simple cysts from solid masses, even in the fatty breast.

In dense breast tissue ultrasound is able to detect mammographically occult tumors. Therefore its complimentary use in difficult to assess breast tissue may be quite helpful.

Magnetic Resonance Imaging

In MR images, fatty tissue has high signal intensity before and after intravenous administration of contrast medium, whereas residual parenchyma and connective tissue structures have low signal intensity. When imaged during the recommended time frame in the menstrual cycle and without influence of hormonal replacement therapy, glandular tissue usually enhances only mildly after iintravenous application of contrast agent. Slight diffuse and symmetric enhancement may be seen in some patients with glandular tissue. The enhancement curve is usually progressive. Connective tissue usually exhibits no or very low enhancement.

Rarely active adenosis or hyperplastic changes may cause strong, asymmetric or focal enhancement with a progressive or even plateau-type enhancement curve. Whereas symmetric moderate enhancement may impair sensitivity of MRI for small or in-situ malignancy, the latter changes, which may occur even in normal breast tissue, may cause false positive calls and additional workup.

Owing to the high sensitivity of mammography, contrast-enhanced MRI is not generally needed in the fatty breast.

In dense tissue MRI may in appropriate indications (see Chapter 5) add valuable information. However, because of the added risk of false positive calls MRI is not recommended for screening of women at normal or low risk. It is recommended for screening of women at high risk (> 30% in Europe; > 20% United States). For moderate risk, insufficient data exist. MRI may be helpful to solve rare diagnostic problems that cannot be solved by percutaneous breast biopsy and state-of-the-art standard breast imaging.

Variants of Normal Findings

Definition

Breasts may vary considerably with respect to size, shape, consistency and distribution of glandular, connective and fatty tissue components. The following conditions are regarded as variants:

- Anisomastia
- Macromastia
- Accessory breast tissue (e.g., ectopic breast tissue in the axillary tail or axilla)
- Inverted nipple

Anisomastia

Clinical Examination

The most frequent abnormality is asymmetry in breast size (anisomastia). Depending on the severity of this condition, which can vary greatly, the difference in size will be more or less apparent upon visual inspection. The difference in palpable findings between the two breasts can vary accordingly. Patients will typically have long been aware of the asymmetry and, apart from cyclical fluctuations, no significant changes will be observed over time. This distinguishes anisomastia from pathologic asymmetry in size, such as can occur in the presence of benign masses (cysts, fibroadenomas, or phyllodes tumor) or when the consistency of one breast gradually changes as a result of a disseminated malignant process. When this is accompanied by retraction and loss of volume, which is highly suggestive of scirrhous breast cancer, malignancy must be considered highly probable until proven otherwise.

Asymmetry must always be assessed carefully because it may be the presenting sign of malignancy.

Mammography

Mammography will reveal asymmetric parenchymal distribution correlating with the clinical and anatomic asymmetry (**Fig. 9.8**).

Macromastia

Clinical Examination

Macromastia is a condition in which breast volume exceeds the physiologic value by 50%, that is, when the weight of the breast exceeds 600 g. Macromastia occurs most frequently during puberty, sometimes during pregnancy, and may occur during the perimenopause. A significant increase in breast size can accompany general obesity as increased fatty deposits are found in the breast. The same differences in tissue consistency are encountered as in normal patients. However, increased breast size can render clinical examination of deeper-lying tissue difficult or even impossible.

Fig. 9.8a–d Glandular tissue in the axillary tail and ectopic glandular tissue (**Fig. 9.8b–d** from Heywang-Köbrunner 1996). ▷

a Glandular tissue in the axillary tail will generally have the same structure as glandular tissue within the breast. In the presence of regular architecture, mammography at usual follow-up intervals will generally be sufficient (negative sonography supports this diagnosis).

Variants of Normal Findings

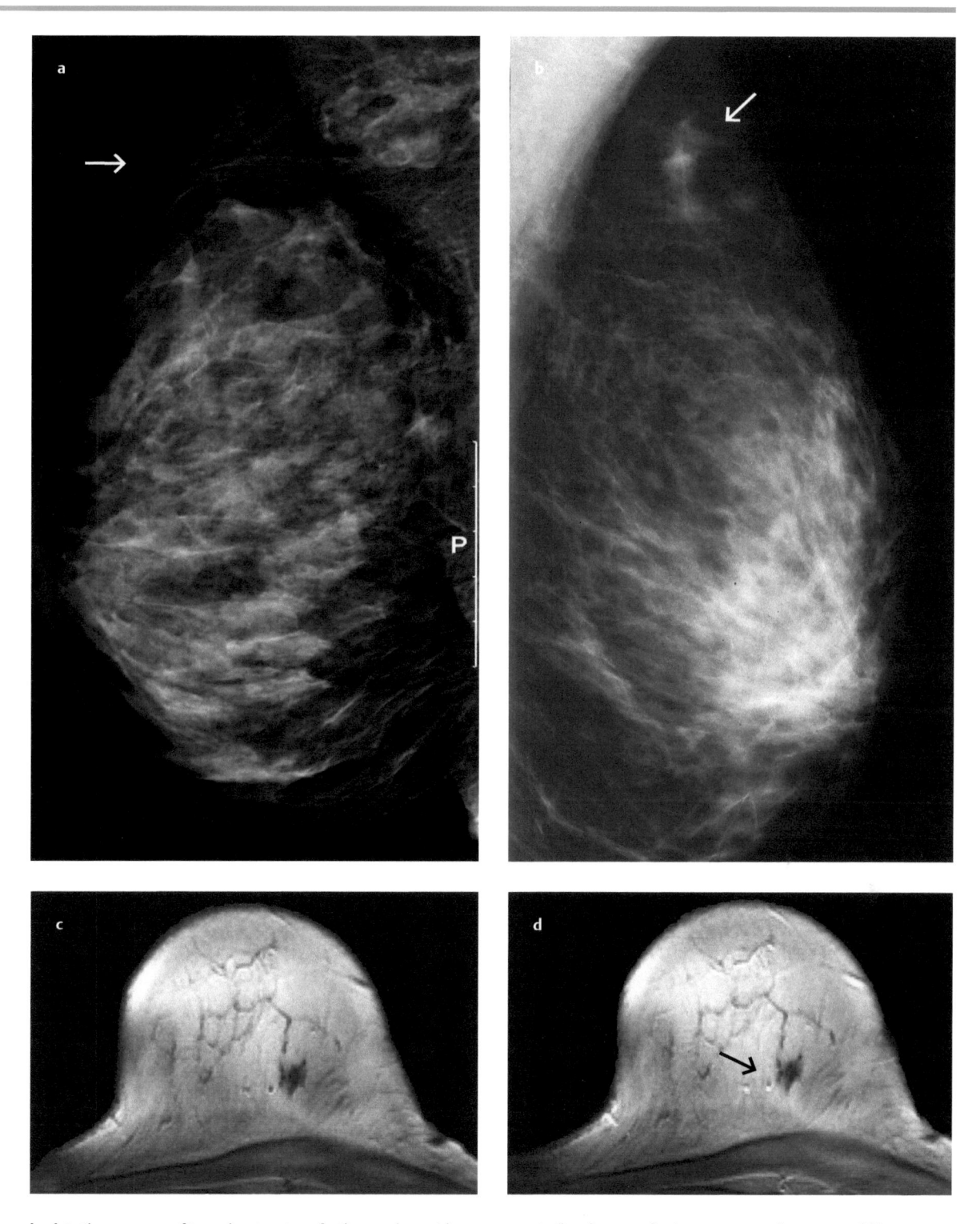

b–d In the presence of irregular structure, further workup with MRI or needle core biopsy is appropriate. **b** Irregularly shaped tissue is visualized in the axillary tail. Its eccentric location did not allow its visualization in other imaging planes. It could not be identified sonographically.
c Transverse MR section through the lesion prior to administration of contrast medium. **d** The same slice after intravenous injection of Gd-DTPA.

In the absence of enhancement, malignancy could be excluded with a high degree of certainty. Follow-up examinations over 4 years showed a slight decrease in density. The finding is compatible with residual asymmetric glandular or benign breast tissue.

Mammography

Depending on the tissue composition, the mammographic appearance will vary between radiolucent in fatty breasts to radiopaque in breasts with a high proportion of glandular and connective tissue. Whereas mammography can achieve close to 100% sensitivity in detecting pathologic changes in the fatty breast, the sensitivity of mammography in dense and voluminous tissue is significantly reduced.

Sonography

The diagnostic value of sonography is often limited, particularly in very large breasts. It is difficult and often even impossible to image the entire glandular tissue. Furthermore, acoustic shadows and limited sound penetration may not permit sufficient visualization of the deeper-lying tissue. For this reason, sonography in large breasts should be used exclusively to assess focal findings.

Accessory Breast Tissue (Polymastia)

Circumscribed development of glandular parenchyma in the axilla is the most common site of accessory breast tissue. This tissue is either completely separate from the rest of the parenchyma (Fig. 9.8) or connected with the parenchymal tissue in the axillary tail. Glandular tissue extending far into the axillary tail can occur on one or both sides. Since breast cancer can also occur in ectopic glandular tissue, this tissue should always be carefully examined.

Supernumerary mammary glands are found along the milk line (mamma accessoria) and may or may not have an associated nipple (mamma aberrata). Polythelia refers to the presence of supernumerary nipples without mammary tissue.

Clinical Examination

Palpation will reveal what appears to be a soft tumor in the axilla, which may be isolated or adjacent to the glandular tissue in the axillary tail or at other locations. Sometimes the patient will report tenderness and fluctuations in size related to her menstrual cycle. Swelling may also occur during pregnancy and lactation.

Mammography

Corresponding parenchymal densities can be visualized mammographically with an oblique view in the axillary tail or in the axilla on an axillary view (Fig. 9.8a,b). The criteria for assessment are the same as those for glandular tissue within the breast.

Sonography and Magnetic Resonance Imaging

Sonography also visualizes the asymmetric configuration of normal or mastopathic glandular tissue. The same applies to MRI (Fig. 9.8c,d), with normal tissue and benign proliferative breast disorders normally exhibiting low or little enhancement with progressive enhancement dynamics.

Owing to its high sensitivity in detecting malignancy, MRI may be used for differential diagnostic problems caused by asymmetric tissue.

Inverted Nipple

(See Fig. 9.9.)

Clinical Examination

Unilateral or bilateral inverted nipples may represent normal variants. It is important to establish that the inversion has been present since birth or is long-standing (unchanged for years). Recently occurring retraction and/or inversion can be the result of chronic inflammatory or malignant processes. Therefore, careful history is required to determine the need for further investigation of this finding.

Mammography

Depending on the projection, the inverted nipple can appear as a round, smooth-contoured mass mammographically. However, in most cases, the skin will be clearly seen to dip into this mass. The risk of confusing this condition with a lesion is minimal if the examiner is familiar with the clinical findings. Failure to image the nipple in profile may result in a false mammographic picture of nipple inversion.

Sonography

The inverted nipple itself can appear as a hypoechoic nodule with or without an acoustic shadow. Here, too, the risk of confusion is minimal if one knows the clinical findings and is familiar with the typical sonographic findings.

Magnetic Resonance Imaging

In MR imaging studies, the examiner should bear in mind that the normal inverted nipple can enhance.

Variants of Normal Findings

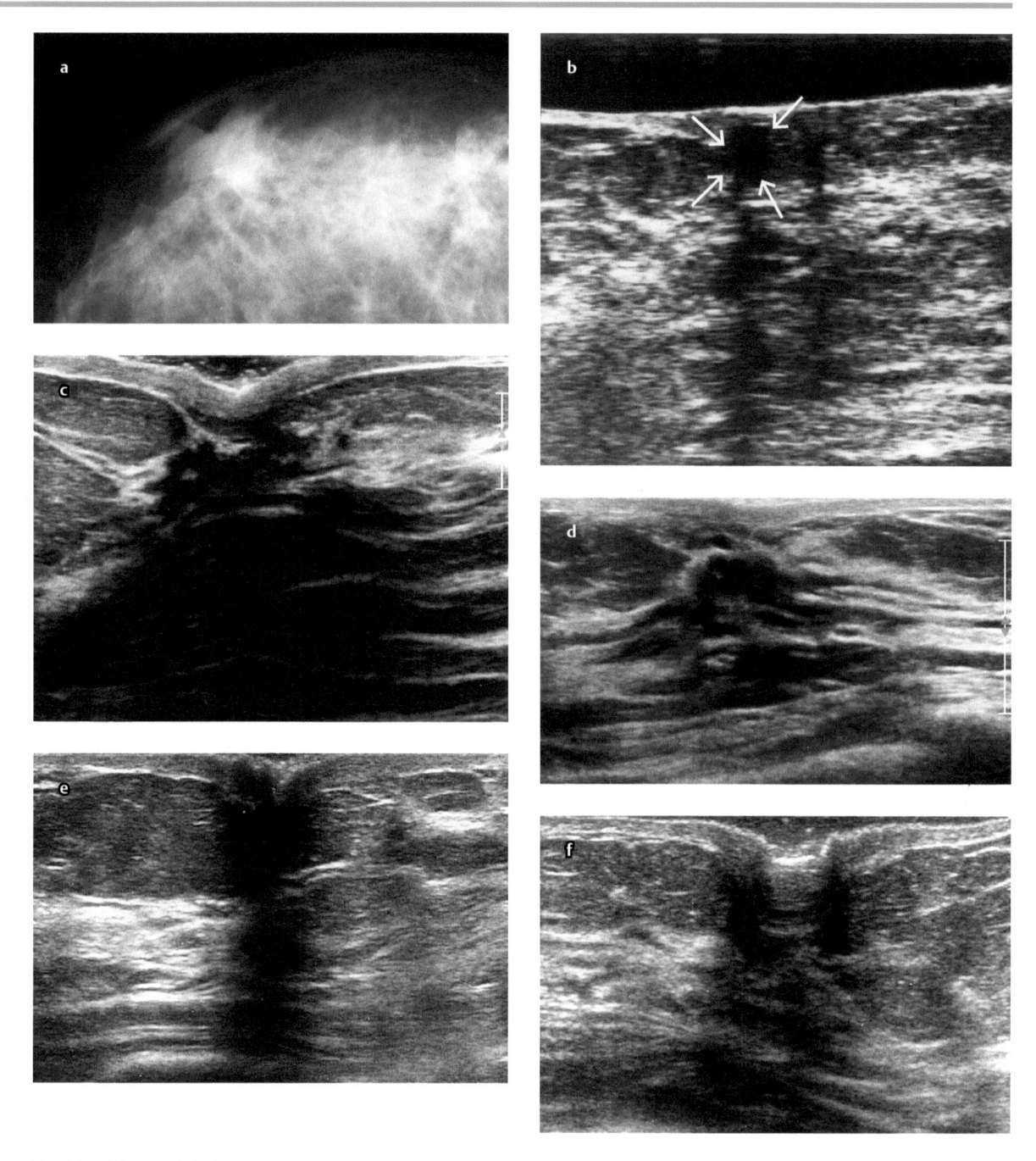

Fig. 9.9a–f Inverted nipple.

a,b Mammographically, the inverted nipple typically appears as a funnel-shaped density (**a**) or a mass (**b**).
c Sonographically the inverted nipple should be investigated with enough gel to enable evaluation of the tissue posterior to the structures of the nipple–areolar complex.
d The inverted nipple is visible as a hypoechoic nodule.
e,f Sonographically the inverted nipple can produce a pronounced nipple shadow (**e**) that can be overcome with the use of enough additional gel and smooth compression (**f**).

Pregnancy and Lactation

Histology

During pregnancy, proliferative changes occur, with lobular hyperplasia, hyperemia, and fluid retention in breast tissue. Lactogenesis, the milk synthesis in the glandular cell, begins in the second half of pregnancy. Toward the end of pregnancy, the alveoli begin to secrete and parenchyma largely displaces the stromal tissue.

Clinical Examination

During pregnancy, the breast increases in size and acquires a firmer consistency, accompanied by hyperpigmentation of the areola and nipple and by prominent veins. The firmer consistency of the breast makes palpation more difficult.

The proliferative stimulation can cause existing fibroadenomas to increase rapidly in size, typically leading to smooth-contoured, mobile, and round or oval palpable findings with a firmer consistency than that of the surrounding glandular tissue. Nevertheless malignancy, which can occur during pregnancy, needs to be excluded with great care.

Milk retention can develop during lactation. This can lead to focal thickening, inflammation, or formation of a galactocele (see **Fig. 11.4a,b**, p. 284).

Mammography

(See **Fig. 9.10a**.)

Mammographically, the body of the gland appears very dense with heterogeneously coarse, nodular, confluent densities and minimal fatty tissue. This severely limits the diagnostic value of mammography. If clinical examination and mammography become necessary during the nursing period, the examination should be performed after breast-feeding or pumping since the breast then has a softer consistency and is less radiodense. Screening mammography is usually not performed during pregnancy or lactation. It should be delayed for approximately 3 months after the cessation of lactation to allow the breast density to decrease. Diagnostic mammography may be indicated during pregnancy or lactation if clinical suspicion exists. Although mass lesions may not be discernible because of the increased radiodensity of the breast tissue, microcalcifications typical of malignancy can be detected even in extremely dense breasts.

When mammography is performed during pregnancy, the abdomen should be shielded with lead aprons despite the fact that most of the extremely soft radiation will be absorbed in soft tissues of the abdomen and almost no radiation will reach the fetus.

In common with any X-ray examination in pregnancy, mammography should not be performed without a well-founded indication.

Whenever a diagnostic problem occurs during pregnancy, the risk of radiation must be weighed against the risk of delaying detection of malignancy. In general, the latter risk by far exceeds the former and mammography should be performed with adequate shielding, since with shielding no significant radiation will reach the uterus.

If mammography has been performed without shielding (e.g., if the pregnancy was unknown), the patient may be informed that, even without shielding, only a minimal dose will reach the uterus. If mammography was performed during the first 10 days of pregnancy (pre-implantation phase), she can be informed that any radiation reaching the uterus could lead to abortion but not to malformation. After day 10, it may be wise to inform the local radiation protection authority and document the radiation dose. In general, the radiation dose of mammography and the risk that the extremely soft radiation might reach the uterus will still be calculated to be so low that therapeutic abortion will not be recommended by the local radiation protection authority.

Sonography

(See **Fig. 9.10b,c**.)

In light of the limited diagnostic value of mammography during pregnancy and lactation, sonography is extremely helpful in evaluating palpable findings. Sonography should therefore be used first. If ultrasound imaging reveals a cyst, or fibroadenoma, mammography will not be necessary.

Normally, the echogenicity of the breast tissue decreases somewhat during pregnancy and lactation. The echo pattern generally appears homogeneous and finely granular. Particularly in late pregnancy and lactation, the distended lactiferous ducts are discernible as tubular, extremely hypoechoic or anechoic structures (**Fig. 9.10c**).

Magnetic Resonance Imaging

MRI is usually not indicated during pregnancy and lactation since strong generalized contrast enhancement is expected in the engorged breast tissue and therefore identification of malignant processes would be difficult.

Pregnancy and Lactation

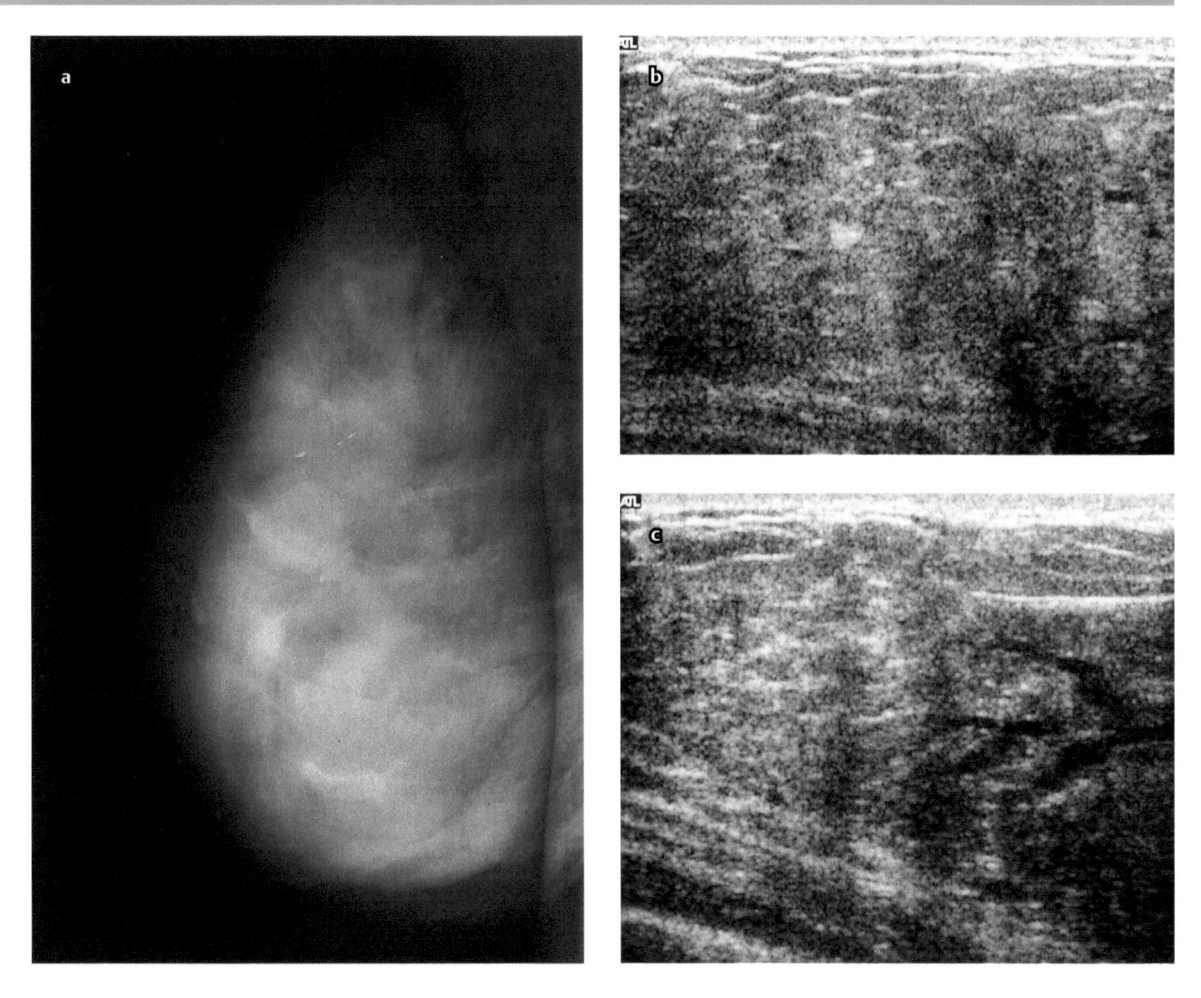

Fig. 9.10a–c Lactating breast.

a–c Pregnant patient with an uncertain palpable abnormality in her right breast, which eventually proved to be benign. **a** Mammography reveals an extremely dense, heterogeneous, coarse, nodular parenchymal structure. Suspicious microcalcifications are thus ruled out. However, mammographic evaluation of masses is impaired. Thus, ultrasound is indispensable. In this case, no abnormality was seen and the benign daignosis was confirmed by follow-up. The recommendation for short-term follow-up versus histopathological assessment in such cases depends on the degree of clinical suspicion, which has to be dilligently considered.

b,c During lactation most of the glandular tissue shows a fine granular hypoechoic pattern. Expanded ducts may also be visible (**c**).

Breast Response with Hormone Replacement Therapy

The number of women receiving hormone replacement therapy (HRT), either for relief of menopausal symptoms or as prophylaxis against osteoporosis and cardiovascular disease, has increased in several countries. Even though its use decreased in the United States after publication of the WHI study (Women's Health Initiative), the use of HRT varies widely from country to country. The value of HRT for cardio-protection has been shown to be of little value in several recent long-term large studies.

As a result of the hormonal proliferation stimulus, breast size may increase in some of these women, occasionally accompanied by a sensation of fullness and breast pain.

Hormone replacement has an impact on the mammographic image:
- A generalized increase in the extent and density of partially involuted parenchyma is possible. Sometimes the breasts may even respond differently, leading to a more prominent change in one breast than the other.
- In older women, single or multiple cysts, fibroadenomas, and other benign breast changes can develop in one or both breasts.
- Cysts and fibroadenomas can enlarge and simulate a malignant process.
- After breast-conserving treatment of a mammary carcinoma, the extent and density of the parenchyma of the healthy breast can increase unilaterally since the irradiated fibrosed breast tissue generally does not respond to hormones.

The degree of increased density and development of masses appears to be more pronounced for HRT with estrogen–progesterone combinations than for estrogen alone.

Discontinuing HRT generally leads to involution of the proliferative parenchymal effects.

Mammography

(See **Fig. 9.11**.)

Where previous mammograms are available for comparison, the examiner may observe a unilateral or bilateral increase in the extent and density of the parenchyma due to HRT in about 30% of cases. This increase can be diffuse or patchy and may change the overall structure.

In some women the increase in density can be so profound that mammographic interpretation is impaired. With HRT use, new cysts and fibroadenomas can develop or existing ones can increase in size, representing an exception to the rule that any new occurrence or increase in size of a focal lesion in a postmenopausal patient represents a sign of malignancy. Thus, particular care is necessary in further diagnostic workup of increasing densities. Multiple or single cysts or fibroadenomas can develop bilaterally or unilaterally and increasing evidence exists that HRT has a negative effect on the accuracy of mammography (and breast diagnostics in general, see below), at least in some patients.

Sonography

Sonography is an important diagnostic procedure in assessing mammographically dense parenchyma and as an adjunct in diagnosing probably benign focal findings detected mammographically. The glandular tissue under hormone stimulation will generally appear homogeneous and moderately hyperechoic. However, variations such as those seen in benign breast disease (increasing visualization of hypoechoic ductal structures, increased shadowing, and growth of cysts or fibroadenomas) are possible.

If a simple cyst is diagnosed sonographically, no further workup will be required. Solid focal lesions that are not definitely benign mammographically and sonographically should usually be biopsied to assess for malignancy. If a change is suspected to represent a process due to hormonal stimulation, the patient may be given the option of discontinuing hormones for 2 or 3 months, following which the breast should be re-imaged to determine if the lesion has regressed. If the change is suspicious or the patient is concerned, histopathologic assessment should be performed.

Magnetic Resonance Imaging

MRI is not indicated for diagnosing changes occurring with HRT. The resulting proliferative changes can be expected to enhance with MR contrast agents, impairing both detection and exclusion of malignancy.

According to the authors' experience, HRT using estrogens only rarely causes diagnostic problems with MRI; the same is true for HRT using tibolone. However, with increasing dosage of progesterone, an increasing number of patients with diffuse, sometimes patchy, and even focal enhancement is seen and diagnostic accuracy may be severely impaired. Therefore, we recommend discontinuing progesterone formulations of HRT for at least 4 weeks prior to breast MRI, whenever possible (Heywang-Köbrunner et al. 2010).

Percutaneous Biopsy

This method should be used to diagnose any finding or change for which malignancy cannot be excluded. According to international data, histopathologic assessment is more frequent among hormone users than women who do not use hormones.

Breast Response with Hormone Replacement Therapy

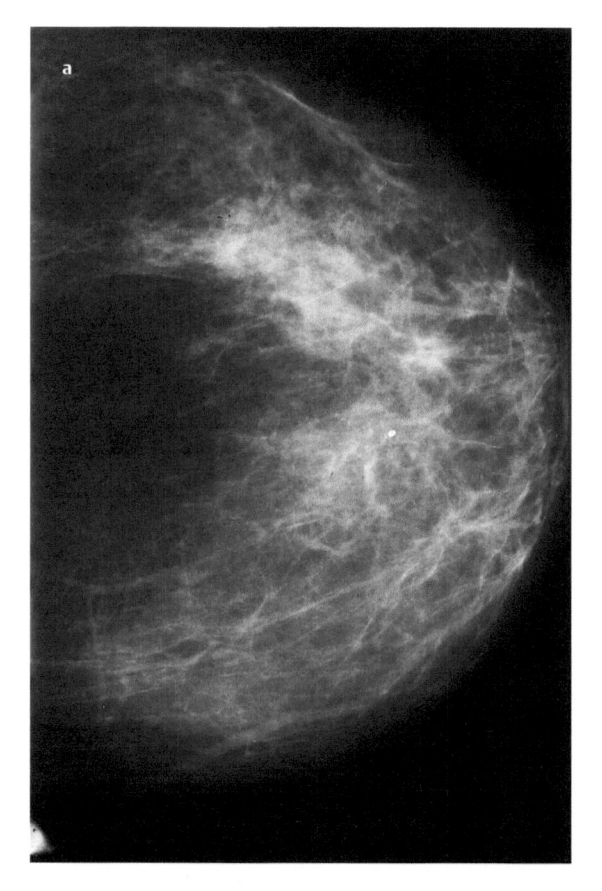

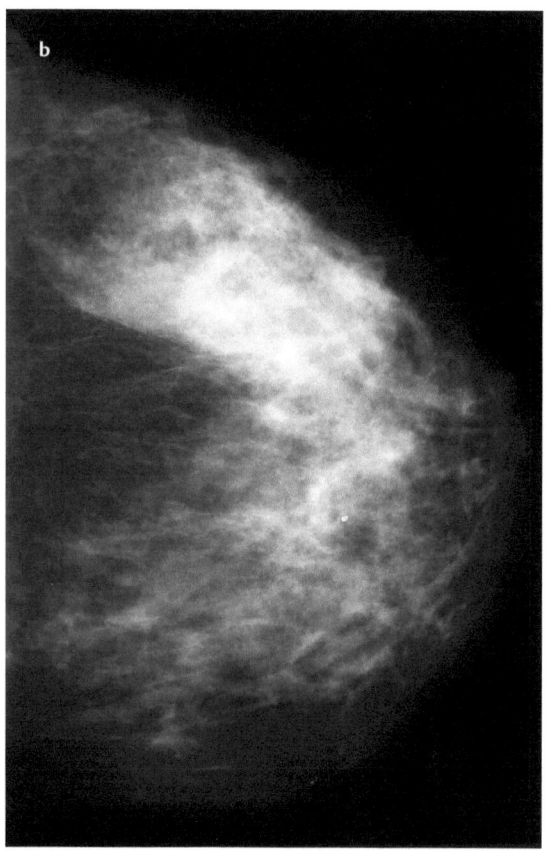

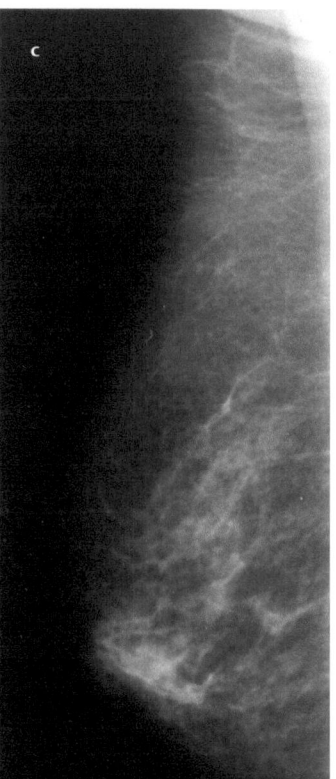

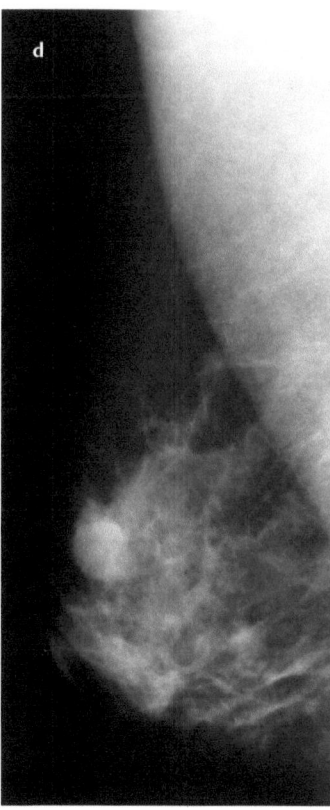

Fig. 9.11a–g

a,b Changes under hormone replacement therapy (HRT).
a Normal, partially involuted breast in a 59-year-old patient.
b After 12 months of hormone replacement, the patient complained of a sensation of fullness and breast enlargement. Mammography reveals extensive generalized nodular proliferation of glandular tissue. Mammographic evaluation is impaired under HRT compared with before.
c,d In some patients new masses may develop during HRT. **c** Baseline mammogram before hormone replacement therapy in a 66-year-old patient. **d** Two years later. The patient has been on HRT for 6 months. Note that there is a proliferation of glandular tissue in the breast. The mass in the upper breast was shown to be a simple cyst on sonography.

Fig. 9.11e–g ▷

9 The Normal Breast

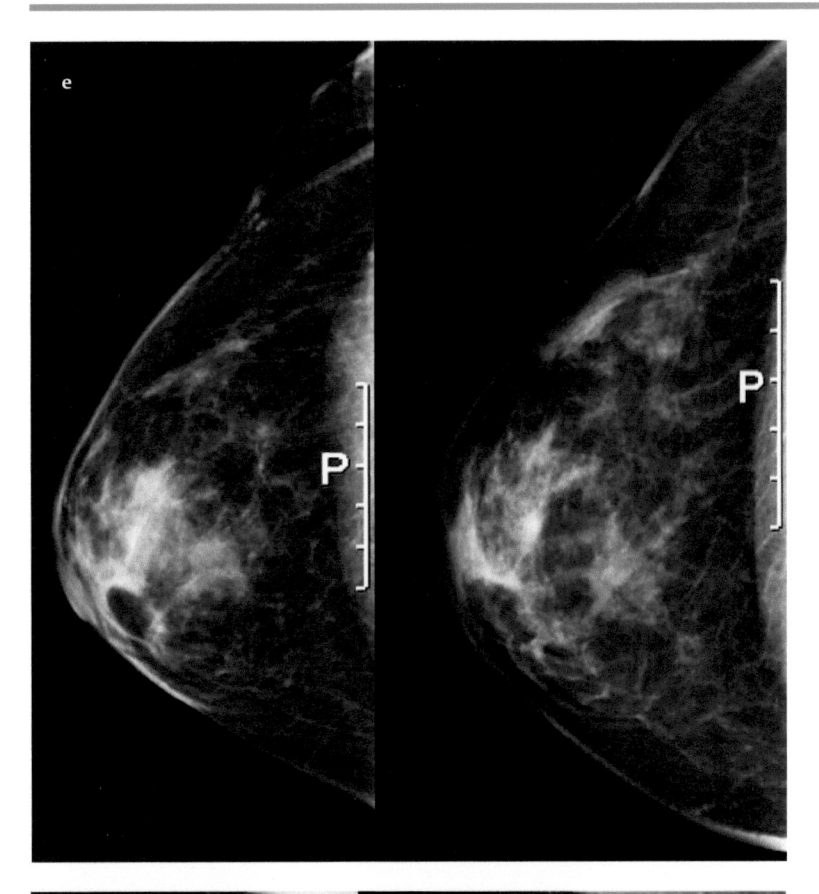

◁ continued

e Mammography (craniocaudal views) in 2008 (left) and 3 years later after implantation of a progesterone-containing intrauterine device (IUD) (right).

f Oblique projections, 2008 (left) and 2011 (right).

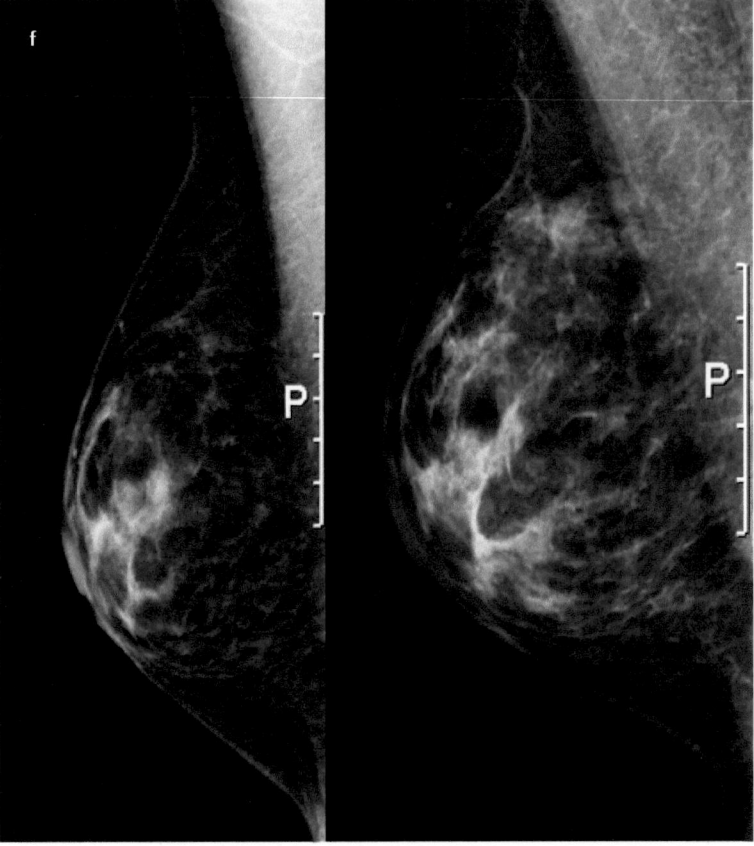

Breast Response with Hormone Replacement Therapy

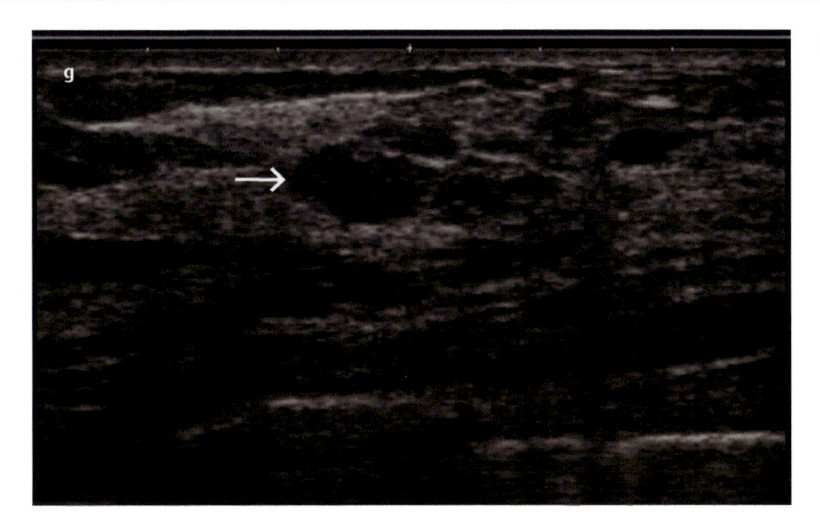

g Ultrasound examination after implantation of a progesterone-containing IUD in 2011 demonstrates an oval, ill-defined hypoechoic mass in an area of a palpable increased nodularity. *Core needle biopsy*: Focal adenosis.

Summary

Mammography is the primary method to screen asymptomatic women aged 50–70 years. Based on a somewhat lower effect of mammography screening at age 40–50, national recommendations concerning mammography screening of this age group diverge.

In the presence of clinical findings or increased risk, sonography provides complementary information and is the main additional method of investigation. Even though limitations of mammography in dense tissue are known (decreased sensitivity, increased rate of interval cancers), insufficient evidence exists to recommend sonographic screening on a population basis. Also, to date insufficient experience exists concerning the quality assurance that would be needed for sonographic screening.

The physician should verify the clinical absence of:

- Palpable pathologic findings
- Asymmetry
- Skin or nipple retraction
- Pathologic discharge

In diagnostic imaging studies, special attention should be given to:

- Uniform and thin skin thickness
- Visualization of fine Cooper ligaments
- Visualization of an undisturbed subcutaneous and retromammary layer of fat
- Symmetric distribution of the body of the gland
- Regular configuration of ductal structures converging at the nipple

Furthermore, imaging studies serve to verify the absence of:

- Masses and densities
- Architectural distortion
- Suspicious microcalcifications

In patients at risk and in symptomatic patients sonography is complementary to mammography and should be considered for the assessment of the dense breast at intermediate risk and for the assessment of abnormalities. In patients at high risk MRI is the recommended screening method starting at age 25 or 5–10 years before the youngest family member developed breast cancer. In the high-risk group, yearly MRI should be combined with yearly mammography after age 30.

In the presence of uncertain palpable and mammographic findings, ultrasound examination can provide additional information. Sonography is indicated as the first diagnostic imaging procedure in symptomatic women less than 40 years old. Mammography should be added unless malignancy can definitely be excluded.

Comparison with the contralateral breast is important both in light of the immense variety in size, arrangement, and density of the parenchyma among patients, and because clinical, mammographic, and sonographic detection of abnormalities will depend on the recognition of sometimes subtle structural abnormalities.

Comparison with previous diagnostic imaging studies (where available) should be attempted if possible.

Asymmetry and polymastia are congenital conditions that will generally be identified with a careful history. The examiner must exclude significant changes that are not due to hormonal influences (i.e., pregnancy or menstrual cycle). If the breast examination is normal (revealing only increased glandular tissue, but no change in consistency, and no retraction) and mammographic appearance is normal (composition corresponds to normal glandular tissue), then it is highly probable that the condition represents a normal variant.

In the presence of uncertain densities, further diagnostic studies (mammography, sonography, or percutaneous biopsy and rarely MRI) are indicated (see also Chapter 22).

Congenital inverted nipple is another normal variant which cannot be confused with a mass if the examiner is aware of the history and physical examination. This condition should be distinguished from recently occurring nipple inversion. Here, particular care should be taken to exclude malignancy.

Pregnancy and lactation: During this time the size, consistency, and radiographic density of the breast increase, which may compromise clinical and imaging assessment. Uncertain findings that cannot be clarified as being benign at clinical or ultrasound examination require mammography, which can be performed with adequate shielding, even during pregnancy. During lactation the mammogram should be taken directly after breast-feeding to decrease overall breast density. MRI is not indicated.

Knowledge of the effects of hormone replacement therapy (HRT) is extremely important for interpreting diagnostic imaging studies. This underscores the value of taking a thorough history.

HRT can produce significant parenchymal changes, which can include an increase in the amount and density of parenchymal tissue, and a new occurrence or an increase in the size of focal densities. Mammographic evaluation is limited instead of improved with increasing patient age and breast involution. The additional information from sonography may be helpful in older women undergoing HRT. Percutaneous or excision biopsy may be indicated for further workup of focal findings during HRT.

References and Recommended Reading

Albert US, Altland H, Duda V, et al. 2008 update of the guideline: early detection of breast cancer in Germany. J Cancer Res Clin Oncol 2009;135(3):339–354

Berg WA, Blume JD, Cormack JB, et al; ACRIN 6666 Investigators. Combined screening with ultrasound and mammography vs mammography alone in women at elevated risk of breast cancer. JAMA 2008;299(18):2151–2163

Boyd NF, Guo H, Martin LJ, et al. Mammographic breast density and the risk and detection of breast cancer. N Engl J Med 2007;356:297–300

Brenner RJ. Asymmetric densities of the breast: strategies for imaging evaluation. Semin Roentgenol 2001;36(3):201–216

D'Orsi CJ, Bassett LW, Berg WA, et al. BI-RADS: Mammography, 4th edition. In: D'Orsi CJ, Mendelson EB, Ikeda DM et al., Eds: Breast Imaging Reporting and Data System: ACR BI-RADS – Breast imaging atlas. Reston, Va: American College of Radiology; 2003

Greendale GA, Reboussin BA, Sie A, et al; Postmenopausal Estrogen/Progestin Interventions (PEPI) Investigators. Effects of estrogen and estrogen-progestin on mammographic parenchymal density. Ann Intern Med 1999;130(4 Pt 1):262–269

Heywang-Köbrunner SH, Beck R. Contrast-enhanced MRI of the Breast. 2nd ed. Berlin, New York, Heidelberg: Springer 1996

Heywang-Köbrunner SH, Hacker A, Sedlacek S. Contrast-enhanced MRI of the breast for staging and early detection: where do we need it? Geb Fra. 2010;70(3):184–193

Ikeda DM, Hylton NM, Kuhl CK, et al. BI-RADS: Magnetic Resonance Imaging 1st edition. In: D'Orsi CJ, Mendelson EB, Ikeda DM et al., Eds: Breast Imaging Reporting and Data System: ACR BI-RADS – Breast imaging atlas. Reston, VA: American College of Radiology; 2003

Kavanagh AM, Mitchell H, Giles GG. Hormone replacement therapy and accuracy of mammographic screening. Lancet 2000;355(9200):270–274

Laya MB, Gallagher JC, Schreiman JS, Larson EB, Watson P, Weinstein L. Effect of postmenopausal hormonal replacement therapy on mammographic density and parenchymal pattern. Radiology 1995;196(2):433–437

Laya MB, Larson EB, Taplin SH, White E. Effect of estrogen replacement therapy on the specificity and sensitivity of screening mammography. J Natl Cancer Inst 1996;88(10):643–649

Litherland JC, Stallard S, Hole D, Cordiner C. The effect of hormone replacement therapy on the sensitivity of screening mammograms. Clin Radiol 1999;54(5):285–288

Lundström E, Wilczek B, von Palffy Z, Söderqvist G, von Schoultz B. Mammographic breast density during hormone replacement therapy: differences according to treatment. Am J Obstet Gynecol 1999;181(2):348–352

Mandelson MT, Oestreicher N, Porter PL, et al. Breast density as a predictor of mammographic detection: comparison of interval- and screen-detected cancers. J Natl Cancer Inst 2000;92(13):1081–1087

Marugg RC, van der Mooren MJ, Hendriks JH, Rolland R, Ruijs SH. Mammographic changes in postmenopausal women on hormonal replacement therapy. Eur Radiol 1997;7(5):749–755

Mendelson EB, Baum JK, Berg WA, et al. BI-RADS: Ultrasound, 1st edition. In: D'Orsi CJ, Mendelson EB, Ikeda DM et al., Eds: Breast Imaging Reporting and Data System: ACR

BI-RADS – Breast imaging atlas. Reston, Va: American College of Radiology; 2003

Sardanelli F, Boetes C, Borisch B, et al. Magnetic resonance imaging of the breast: recommendations from the EUSOMA working group. Eur J Cancer 2010;46(8):1296–1316

Shetty MK, Watson AB. Sonographic evaluation of focal asymmetric density of the breast. Ultrasound Q 2002;18(2):115–121

Sterns EE, Zee B. Mammographic density changes in perimenopausal and postmenopausal women: is effect of hormone replacement therapy predictable? Breast Cancer Res Treat 2000;59(2):125–132

Stomper PC, Van Voorhis BJ, Ravnikar VA, Meyer JE. Mammographic changes associated with postmenopausal hormone replacement therapy: a longitudinal study. Radiology 1990;174(2):487–490

10 Benign Breast Disorders

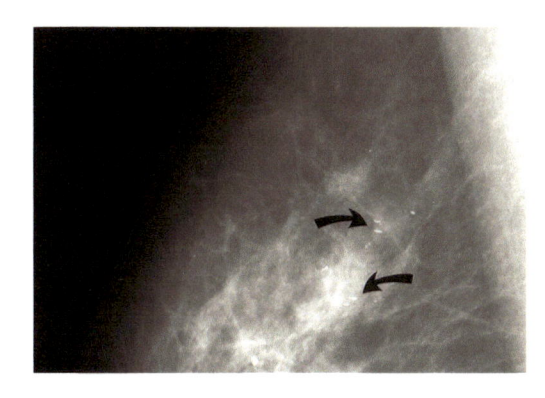

Definition ⇢ *256*
Pathogenesis ⇢ *256*
Incidence ⇢ *256*
Histopathology ⇢ *256*
Clinical Findings ⇢ *258*
Mammographic Density and Risk ⇢ *258*
Diagnostic Strategy and Objectives ⇢ *260*
Mammography ⇢ *261*
Sonography ⇢ *266*
Magnetic Resonance Imaging ⇢ *268*
Percutaneous Biopsy ⇢ *272*

References and Recommended Reading ⇢ *273*

10 Benign Breast Disorders

S. H. Heywang-Koebrunner, I. Schreer, S. Barter, J. Naehrig

Definition

In contrast to the age-related physiologic changes in the mammary gland, benign breast disorders involve qualitative and quantitative tissue transformation that differs from the age-related "norm," for which no exact definition exists. Mostly, these changes become apparent prior to and during menopause. The distinctions between normal findings, variations, and fibrocystic changes are blurred, as are the distinctions between individual types of these disorders.

Pathogenesis

The causes of benign breast disorders are probably partly inherited and thus may lie in the patient's genes. Some are due to hormonal imbalances and the interactions of several hormones (estrogens, progesterone, prolactin, androgens, thyroxine, and insulin), and the individually defined response to these factors may trigger the following mechanisms:
- Hormonally induced secretion (with retention of the secretions), development of duct ectasia, cysts, and sometimes reactive inflammatory changes and fibrosis
- Endocrine-stimulated proliferation of the ductal and lobular epithelium with development of various patterns and degrees of epithelial and myoepithelial proliferations in the form of adenosis, epithelial hyperplasia, and epithelial metaplasia

Incidence

Data on the frequency of benign breast disorders vary considerably, depending on the study group. According to statistics, the frequency of benign disorders lies between 50% and 70% for all types and is around 30% for types with epithelial proliferation.

Diagnosis of a benign breast disorder is significant for three reasons:
1. Even a benign disorder can be accompanied by clinical symptoms (such as pain or palpable findings) that frighten patients and can arouse clinical suspicion of malignancy.
2. Benign disorders are generally characterized by increased radiodensity, occasionally microcalcifications, and often nodular or firm palpable findings. Both mammographic density and the presence of multiple microcalcifications may interfere with the detection of malignancy. Furthermore, focal benign changes may mimic malignancy. Therefore the diagnostic accuracy may be limited in comparison with fatty breasts.
3. Most cases of benign breast disorder (~70%) *do not have an increased risk of cancer* in comparison with the normal population. A portion of these cases (~25%) show an increased risk of cancer (by a factor of 1.5–2). From 3% to 5% of cases of benign disorder are associated with an increased risk of cancer (by a factor of 4–5).

Histopathology

Normal Anatomy and Benign Breast Disorders

Normal constituents of breast parenchyma include (1) fat, (2) fibrous tissue, containing (3) ducts—that is, lactiferous ducts, segmental ducts, subsegmental ducts, interlobular ducts, and terminal ductal lobular units (TDLUs) including acini/lobules.

TDLUs are surrounded by interlobular stroma. The ducts are contained within the extralobular stroma, which is rich in collagenous and elastic fibers. The glandular epithelium of the ducts and the lobular system is a bilayer of basal myoepithelium and luminal glandular epithelium.

Breast disorders may result from epithelial and myoepithelial proliferations, either intraluminal (e.g., ductal epithelial hyperplasia, fibroadenoma) or extraluminal (e.g., adenosis). Any component may grow larger during benign changes or proliferative processes, often involving more than one constituent of normal tissue. Epithelial change occurs through hormonal influence—that is, secretion during lactation—but may occur as a localized response, for example pseudolactational changes.

The most common benign changes of the breast are summarized under the term fibrocystic change ("mastopathia"). It is a common finding and regarded as a physiologic phenomenon rather than a disease (Hutter 1985). Fibrocystic changes include formation of cysts, fibrosis, and lobular and ductal epithelial hyperplasia including adenosis. Cysts may be the result of the unfolding of lobules (Wellings and Alpers 1984), often associated with aprocrine metaplasia. Cysts often rupture ("complicated cyst"), causing inflammation and fibrosis.

Microcalcifications are a common finding in benign processes and belong to the entity of mastopathy. They are most often associated with cysts, adenosis, and periductal (obliterating) mastitis. The last may also be called plasma cell mastitis, which is an old clinical term for periductal elongated calcifications. Nowadays this term is rarely used by pathologists.

Most benign epithelial proliferations comprise a proliferation of both types of epithelia, that is, luminal cells and basal myoepithelial cells, of which one may dominate. Benign processes result in structural changes in breast parenchyma at microscopic and often macroscopic levels. The various histomorphologic processes are more or less mirrored by changes in breast imaging; however, many histopathologic changes result in unspecific radiologic features.

Several of these benign proliferations have to be considered a neoplastic process harboring gene mutations of limited significance, for example apocrine adenosis, fibroadenoma, or ductal papilloma. The disorders can involve the entire mammary gland or can be focal; they present as more limited entities such as fibroadenoma or adenosis or can form a complex with numerous histologic components. In postmenopausal women involution continues to influence histomorphology and imaging features, which may involve normal breast parenchyma and benign processes, for example adenosis. Finally, various non-neoplastic benign processes—such as fibrocystic change, sterile or nonsterile inflammation, cyst rupture, and fat necrosis—add to the broad morphologic spectrum of breast pathology and imaging.

Cysts

Both *microcysts* (measuring 1–2 mm in diameter) and *macrocysts* can form in the breast. Cysts may be solitary, multiple, or multiloculated (see Chapter 11). Microcysts develop in the acini. They may form conglomerates or may grow into to macrocysts involving adjacent ductules. The appearance of cysts is specifically associated with the histologic finding of focal apocrine metaplasia of acinar/ductular epithelia. The content may be clear, but owing to (sterile) chronic inflammation, rupture and hemorrhage it is often colored, which gives the macroscopic impression of the characteristic "blue domed cysts" on cut surfaces. Cysts may contain microcalcifications (and macrocalcifications). Ruptured cysts may disappear over time or may cause focal inflammation and fibrosis (complicated cyst).

Adenosis

Adenosis is of clinical/radiologic significance for two reasons:
1. It is associated with microcalcifications, and accounts for up to 50% of all microcalcifications.
2. It rarely presents as a (benign) tumorous lesion.

Adenosis refers to morphologically heterogeneous processes involving acini and terminal ducts (TDLUs), which increase in size.

The patterns of adenosis include dilation and/or proliferation of TDLUs as well as apocrine metaplasia. Adenosis may be unilateral or bilateral, unifocal, multifocal, or generalized. The changes generally occur at the microscopic level but macroscopic lesions may develop, especially in sclerosing adenosis (i.e., adenosis tumor) and microglandular adenosis. In postmenoausal women adenosis undergoes involution at the same time to uninvolved lobules. However, in some women the breast tissue does not involute. Adenosis variants are often associated with microcalcifications and include blunt duct adenosis (synonym: columnar cell metaplasia/columnar cell hyperplasia), sclerosing adenosis, and apocrine adenosis. Admixtures of the various forms are quite common. Microcalcifications can be isolated or clustered and are typically small, lamellar/rounded, monomorphous or slightly polymorphous, and mostly consist of calcium phosphate, calcium oxalate can be polyhedral and more polymorphous and is found mainly in benign apocrine lesions, i.e., apocrine adenosis.

Adenosis is frequently associated with other benign breast disorders. It can also occur in fibroadenomas ("complex fibroadenomas"), in papillomas or in ductal adenomas. Adenosis can be colonized by neoplastic lesions, especially by lobular neoplasia (LN), comprising atypical lobular hyperplasia (ALH) and lobular carcinoma in situ (LCIS).

The relative risk of malignancy is increased by a factor of 1.5–2.

Microglandular adenosis is a rare, peculiar variant of adenosis, closely resembling invasive tubular carcinoma owing to its infiltrative ("pseudoinvasive") pattern of growth and its lack of myoepithelial cells. It often presents as unifocal tumor, occasionally diffusely involving the breast.

Radial Scar

Radial scar (synonym: complex sclerosing lesion) is another tumorous breast lesion. Radial scar in a pure form is completely benign and the term refers to a lesion that simulates both macroscopically and mammographically the patterns of low-grade invasive carcinoma—that is, invasive tubular carcinoma, invasive ductal carcinoma grade 1, and even invasive lobular carcinoma. Radial scar is characteristically associated with epithelial proliferations such as benign ductal papilloma and usual ductal hyperplasia (UDH), but it can also be associated with atypical proliferations, namely atypical ductal hyperplasia, less often lobular LN, and even invasive carcinoma, most often of a low-grade type. The distribution and extent of any component of an individual lesion can be quite heterogeneous. Therefore, radial scars are included in the group of lesions of uncertain malignant potential (see Chapter 14).

Diffuse Fibrosis

Benign changes may be associated with diffuse fibrosis of all or of parts of the breast tissue. Areas of fibrosis are palpable as induration. Mammographically, fibrosis results in increased density. Sonographically, diffuse fibrosis with interspersed cellular components and ducts will mostly present as echogenic tissue. Sometimes increased periductal fibrosis will decrease echogenicity along ductal structures. Dense fibrosis may absorb or deflect the ultrasound beam and thus leads to shadowing. On magnetic resonance imaging (MRI) fibrosis does not enhance.

Focal Fibrosis

Focal fibrosis is a proliferation of mammary stromal tissue that may be associated with focal parenchymal atrophy and causes induration. The mean focus size measures 1–3 cm in diameter. Mammography shows increased density without microcalcifications.

Clinical Findings

- Benign breast disorders can be completely *asymptomatic*.
- They can cause pain (*mastodynia*).
  - Breast pain due to a benign disorder will typically be more pronounced in the premenstrual phase (i.e., premenstrual tension or sensitivity to touch).
  - The pain is usually bilateral, but sometimes more pronounced on one side. Rarely, it may be unilateral. Most often it will occur as generalized pain in the upper outer quadrants. Localized pain that is not due to a cyst is not typical of benign breast disease.
- In some cases, *discharge* may accompany benign breast disease. This will usually occur *bilaterally* and involve several excretory ducts. The discharge is usually clear or amber colored, occasionally yellowish green or greenish black.
- The palpable findings in the presence of a benign breast disorder can vary greatly from patient to patient.

Typical findings in the presence of a benign breast disease include:
- The tissue has a *firmer consistency*.
- Palpation reveals *fine to coarse nodular* changes.
- The firmer consistency and nodular transformation are more often *symmetrical* and particularly pronounced in the upper outer quadrants—"lumpy breasts."
- *Cysts* are usually palpable as round, elastic lumps. Deeper-lying cysts or cysts that are not completely filled may not be palpable.

Some benign breast disorders can also be associated with *unilaterally firmer consistency* or *formation of focal lumps*. With focal findings, it can be difficult or even impossible to distinguish the disorder from a malignant process. In such cases further diagnostic workup (diagnostic imaging, percutaneous biopsy, or perhaps excisional biopsy) is indicated.

Mammographic Density and Risk

Mammographic density is caused by glandular tissue and by stromal components such as fibrosis or interstitial water contents. Increased density is often associated with benign changes. While density decreases with age, large inter-individual variations exist.

Increased density may obscure those breast cancers that present as masses without microcalcifications, and thus may interfere with the detection of breast cancer.

However, since the initial description of density patterns in mammography, a prognostic impact has been suggested (Byrne et al. 1995). Today, data from large studies prove that increased mammographic density is associated with an increased risk of malignancy (McCormack and dos Santos Silva 2006, Boyd et al. 2007, Kerlikowske 2007). Based on these data the risk appears to increase continuously from fatty breast tissue (ACR1) to breast tissue with scattered fibroglandular elements (ACR2) to heterogeneously dense (ACR3) and very dense breast tissue (ACR4) from an odds ratio of 1 to approximately 4.7.

According to the screening data presented by Kerlekowske (**Table 10.1**), only 8% of all women aged 40–69 presented with predominantly fatty breast tissue (ACR1) and 9% with extremely dense tissue (ACR4). This suggests that the majority of women aged over 40 will have odds ratios for their risk of breast cancer ranging around 2–3 (Boyd et al. 2007, Kerlikowske 2007). (With these models the majority of women at age 50–69 will have an odds ratio of 2–3.)

Interestingly, an increased risk of breast cancer has been confirmed based on data from the Danish screening program. However, breast cancer detected in dense breast tissue may be fatal in a lower percentage of cases, on average (Olsen et al. 2009).

Compared with other risk factors mammographic density has proven to be a significant risk indicator for the occurrence of breast cancer (see Chapter 1). As a risk factor it appears to be at least as strong as many other risk factors, except for high family risk (*BRCA1* or *BRCA2* carrier) or high individual risk (after cancer in childhood, after mantle field irradiation or after personal history of breast cancer before age 50), which exceed the prognostic impact of mammographic density. Also, it may be (together with age-related insufficiently visible lobular involution [Ghosh et al. 2010]) at least as important as most of the presently investigated genetic polymorphisms (see Chapter 1).

Mammographic density itself appears to be determined by various factors, too. The main factor may be genetic predisposition, which at present is estimated to

Table 10.1 Breast density and risk of breast cancer: the age-related frequency of different types of breast density, their associated risk of breast cancer, and their risk of being detected as interval cancer

Age (years)	Density	Frequency among women of that age range (%)	Risk of breast cancer (no./1,000 women)	Risk of having a breast cancer detected as interval cancer (no./1,000)
40–49	ACR1	5	1.1	0.1
	ACR2	36	2.2	0.4
	ACR3	46	3.4	0.9
	ACR4	13	4.0	1.5
50–59	ACR1	8	1.6	0.1
	ACR2	45	4.0	0.6
	ACR3	40	5.8	1.3
	ACR4	7	6.4	2.2
60–69	ACR1	12	2.8	0.4
	ACR2	51	6.0	1.0
	ACR3	33	8.1	1.7
	ACR4	4	8.3	3.0
All: 40–69	ACR1	8	1.7	0.2
	ACR2	43	3.8	0.6
	ACR3	41	5.4	1.2
	ACR4	9	5.9	2.1

Source: From the Breast Cancer Surveillance Consortium (Kerlikowske 2007).

make up around 65% of the impact (Becker and Kaaks 2009, Boyd et al. 2009). Possibly many of the genetic polymorphisms which appear to contribute to the multifactorial genesis of most breast cancers may be associated with both an increased risk of breast cancer and increased mammographic density (Dumas and Diorio 2010, Lindström et al. 2011, Peng et al. 2011).

Other factors influencing breast density include patient age, menopausal status, body mass index (which has a counteracting effect, i.e., increased body mass index leads to decreased mammographic density but increases the risk of breast cancer), influence from endogenous hormones or hormone intake, and lifestyle (age at birth of first child, number of children, weight at birth, possible nutritional factors). Although hormones (mainly the combination of estrogen and synthetic progestin, prolactin) are known to increase mammographic density and to increase breast cancer risk, the exact risk of hormone-related increased density is not yet clear (Becker and Kaaks 2009, Lowry et al. 2011, Pearce et al. 2012).

Athough mammographic breast density appears to be a promising risk indicator, its prospective use is not as easy or as straightforward as it might appear at first sight. Mammographic density varies with the technique used (tube, filtering, image receiver, compression thickness, positioning, etc.). Two-dimensional information concerning density distribution in the mammogram may not correctly reflect the density distribution in the 3D volume. Visual evaluations (such as the classifications of Boyd or Kerlikowske) appear to be associated with significant inter-observer variability (Kerlikowske et al. 1998, Ciatto et al. 2005, Kopans 2008). Automated programs promise a better reproducibility. Prospective testing, optimization of the accuracy and adaptation for the logistically feasible routine use of automated programs remain topics of ongoing research (Chopier et al. 2008, Stone et al. 2010, Kallenberg et al. 2011).

This explains why risk assessment schemes that integrate breast density so far have proved only moderately predictive (Barlow et al. 2006, Tice et al. 2008). Also, to date it is not yet clear which options for surveillance should be offered to women at intermediate risk. The use and efficiency of additional methods for this purpose such as sonography or MRI are not yet tested. Limitations concerning nationwide quality assurance and the presumed significant additional rate of histopathologic assessments have so far prevented the use of other modalities for the screening of asymptomatic women (see Chapters 4 and 23). Whether mammography screening at shorter intervals or novel developments such as tomosynthesis might improve the outcome in women with dense tissue is not yet known.

Thus, so far mammographic density has not been integrated into the concept of national screening programs or international recommendations. Its use as a risk indicator remains, however, a promising topic of ongoing research.

Diagnostic Strategy and Objectives

Classification

Benign breast disorders can only be classified histologically. Palpation, mammography (structural changes, radiodensity, microcalcifications), or sonography (hyperechoic glandular tissue with or without cysts or dilated ductal structures) can be suggestive of a benign breast disease, but cannot prove it.

Risk of Malignancy

Since there is insufficient correlation among mammographic, sonographic, or MRI findings and cellular proliferations or the degree of cellular atypia present, it is not possible to assess the individual risk of carcinoma based on diagnostic imaging studies. This means that suspicious findings will have to undergo biopsy.

The value and reproducibility of mammographic density as a prospective risk indicator (which might help to individualize screening recommendations for asymptomatic women) are being evaluated and may gain increasing importance.

It is a general rule that the majority of histopathologically verified benign breast disorders (70–80%) are associated with no risk or only a low risk of carcinoma.

Screening and Diagnosis in Patients with Benign Changes

The change in consistency, nodularity, sometimes pain, nipple discharge, and the change in symptoms limits the diagnostic accuracy of the clinical examination in patients with benign breast disorders in comparison with patients with fatty breasts.

Mammographic evaluation may be impaired by increased density, since dense tissue may obscure breast cancers that do not contain typical microcalcifications or are otherwise visible because of some surrounding fat or bulging or retraction of normal structures. Furthermore, benign changes (cysts, focal asymmetry, nodular changes or microcalcifications) may mimic malignancy. These changes will compromise sensitivity and specificity of diagnostic and screening mammography (van Gils et al. 1998, Evans 2002, Kerlikowske 2007, Olsen et al. 2009, Britton et al. 2012).

Diagnostic problems may be further increased by hormonal influences (increased density during the luteal phase, increased nodularity, changing cysts and nodularity) during the menstrual cycle or in women receiving hormonal replacement therapy (HRT).

For the combined use of estrogen plus progesterone (sequential or nonsequential) as HRT, an increased risk of breast cancer, an increase in mammographic density (in up to 30% of the treated women), an increase in interval cancers, and a significantly increased rate of false positive calls (factor 1.5–2) have been reported from large databases (Banks et al. 2004, McCormack and dos Santos Silva 2006, Tamimi et al. 2007, Boyd et al. 2011). A high false positive rate has also been reported in women treated with estrogens, if injected, whereas dermally or orally applied estrogens appear to increase false positive rates only slightly. No increased false positive rate (even a slight decrease) has been reported for tibolone (Njor et al. 2011). Negative effects of HRT on diagnostic accuracy are observed in HRT users, but seem to persist for several years (Banks et al. 2004).

Irrespective of potential diagnostic problems, which may occur more frequently in patients with benign changes and in patients who use certain types of HRT, and which affect both clinical evaluation and mammography, to date there is no alternative to mammography. Owing to its very good specificity in the screening situation and its capability of detecting at least a significant proportion of breast cancers at an early stage, mammography is still the best available screening test and an indispensable tool for evaluating symptoms in women above age 40 years.

Whenever possible, mammography should not be performed during the luteal phase of the menstrual cycle. In our experience the best time to perform mammography is (as for MRI) about week 2 of the menstrual cycle. During that time the breast tissue appears to be most readily compressible and exhibits the lowest density. Thus, the best possible accuracy and least pain may be expected.

To date mammography remains the only recommended screening test, even in women with dense breast tissue. Whether other tests might be recommended for additional systematic screening of certain groups of asymptomatic women is being investigated. For high-risk screening the combination of MRI and mammography has been widely accepted (see Chapters 5 and 23).

At present, additional diagnostic methods are not routinely indicated in the presence of typical findings of benign breast disease in women without an increased risk or without mammographically or clinically suggestive findings.

If clinical examination reveals suspicious findings (i.e., palpable findings, uncertain palpable asymmetry, or atypical discharge), mammography is indicated as the first step in imaging workup in women age 40 years and above. Below age 40 the probability of breast cancer is lower and the accuracy of mammography is often impaired by dense tissue. Therefore, diagnostic workup below age 40 should usually start with ultrasonography, but needs to be complemented by mammography or (in the very young patient, i.e., < 30) by histopathologic assessment, unless malignancy can definitely be excluded (e.g., by visualization of a cyst).

Mammography can detect a carcinoma at the site of the palpable findings, or at another unexpected location, by revealing a typical density or typical microcalcifications. The absence of microcalcifications or densities typical of malignancy in radiodense tissue does not exclude a malignancy suspected on the basis of clinical findings.

Therefore, in the presence of clinically suggestive or indeterminate findings, sonography is indicated. Ultrasonography is particularly helpful when it can identify a simple cyst as the cause of uncertain palpable findings, uncertain mammographic densities, or asymmetry. In some patients with probably benign palpable changes, sonography may be able to support the diagnosis of a benign change and help rule out malignancy, for example if the palpable change correlates with elastic homogeneously echogenic tissue or if a mobile and elastic nodule in a young patient exhibits the typical sonographic features of a fibroadenoma. Aside from this, most palpable carcinomas in radiodense tissue are also discernible as hypoechoic masses. In these cases sonography may be used to guide biopsy.

If imaging by mammography and ultrasound cannot exclude malignancy, percutaneous biopsy is the next most important diagnostic step and the most valuable alternative to open biopsy in the diagnosis of probably benign palpable findings or changes detected at mammography.

Open biopsy is indicated as a diagnostic and therapeutic method if percutaneous biopsy does not appear appropriate (e.g., if percutaneous biopsy is not possible in a certain patient or in certain lesions such as diffuse or barely palpable findings without imaging correlations), if percutaneous biopsy yielded a borderline lesion (atypical hyperplasia), or if the results of the existing diagnostic studies or of imaging versus percutaneous biopsy are contradictory.

Mammography

The mammographic appearance of benign breast disease (**Fig. 10.1**) is characterized by the following features:
- Structural changes and/or increased density in the parenchyma
- Calcifications

These changes can occur individually or in combination.

Structural Changes and/or Increased Density

These changes include:
- Coarsened structure
- Finely to coarsely nodular densities, usually relatively uniform, often found along the tree-shaped structure of the mammary gland
- Areas of increased density or generalized increased density

- In some cases the structures appear indistinct and not readily discernible
- Fibrosis and/or secondary inflammatory processes can produce random and irregular densities

Structural changes or densities are suggestive of a benign breast disorder, although they are not conclusive.

Distribution Pattern

Benign changes are *typically generalized and symmetric*. When this is the case, the findings are characteristic of benign breast disorders and cannot usually be confused with changes typical of malignancy. However, in the presence of generalized and symmetric benign changes, detection or exclusion of carcinomas without microcalcifications is more difficult because they may easily be obscured by the surrounding dense tissue.

Atypical Distribution

Diagnostic problems occur with increased density, architectural distortion, or even a smooth or irregular mass:
- Asymmetric location or distribution of tissue change (focal asymmetry, global asymmetry, microcalcifications (**Fig. 10.1e–g**).
- Nodular, irregular, or spiculated masses can occur in certain benign breast diseases and characteristically also in the rare tumorous form of sclerosing adenosis

Note:
- Irregular foci of benign breast disease and radial scars will often produce palpable findings smaller and less pronounced than the findings expected with a carcinoma of comparable size.
- Radial scars may produce an architectural distortion with a "starlike" pattern. The center should be small. It may be dense ("white star") or lucent ("dark star"). Although the probability of malignancy is higher in architectural distortions presenting with a dense center than in those with a lucent center, imaging often cannot rule out malignancy (lobular, tubular, or sometimes ductal invasive carcinoma or ductal carcinoma in situ [DCIS]) with sufficient reliability. Ultrasound may be able to visualize the architectural distortion and guide biopsy, but cannot rule out malignancy. On MRI, absent enhancement supports a benign diagnosis. However, exceptions (nonenhancing DCIS, tubular or lobular carcinoma) are known to exist. Therefore histopathologic assessment of architectural distortions is usually indicated.

Cysts can produce sharply defined round shadows, semicircular discernible shadows, or poorly discernible densities (when obscured by superimposition). They may merely contribute to a nonspecific increase in density, or they may not be visible at all.

10 Benign Breast Disorders

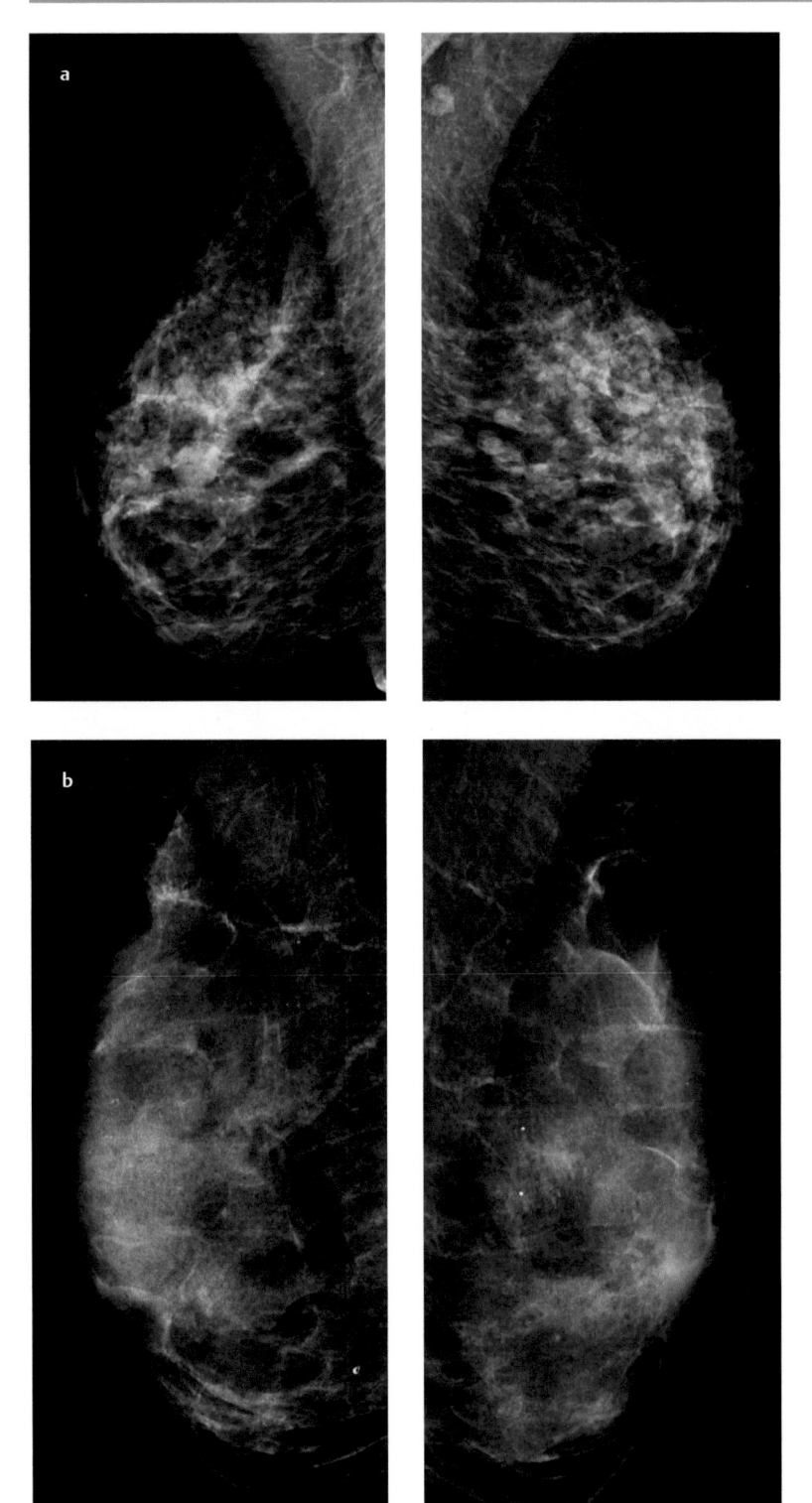

Fig. 10.1a–i

a Nodular parenchymal pattern in predominantly dense breasts (ACR3) with multiple disseminated calcifications.

b This patient presents with very dense breast tissue (ACR4). The breast tissue contains disseminated single calcifications and asymmetrically distributed very fine further microcalcifications. The latter (which are more pronounced in the far upper outer quadrant of the right breast) can be seen in more detail in **Fig. 10.1c3**.

c Patterns of microcalcifications are shown: c1 shows disseminated microcalcifications of varying sizes and shapes. These microcalcifications were symmetrically distributed in both breasts. c2 shows an asymmetric area of not completely monomorphic microcalcifications. As the area was asymmetric and contained some calcifications arranged in a pattern, suggesting ductal calcification, VABB was performed, which confirmed sclerosing adenosis. c3 shows very fine, barely visible microcalcifications which are asymmetrically more densely packed in the extreme right upper outer quadrant of this patient's right breast. The very fine granular appearance and monomorphic appearance rules in benign changes.

Mammography

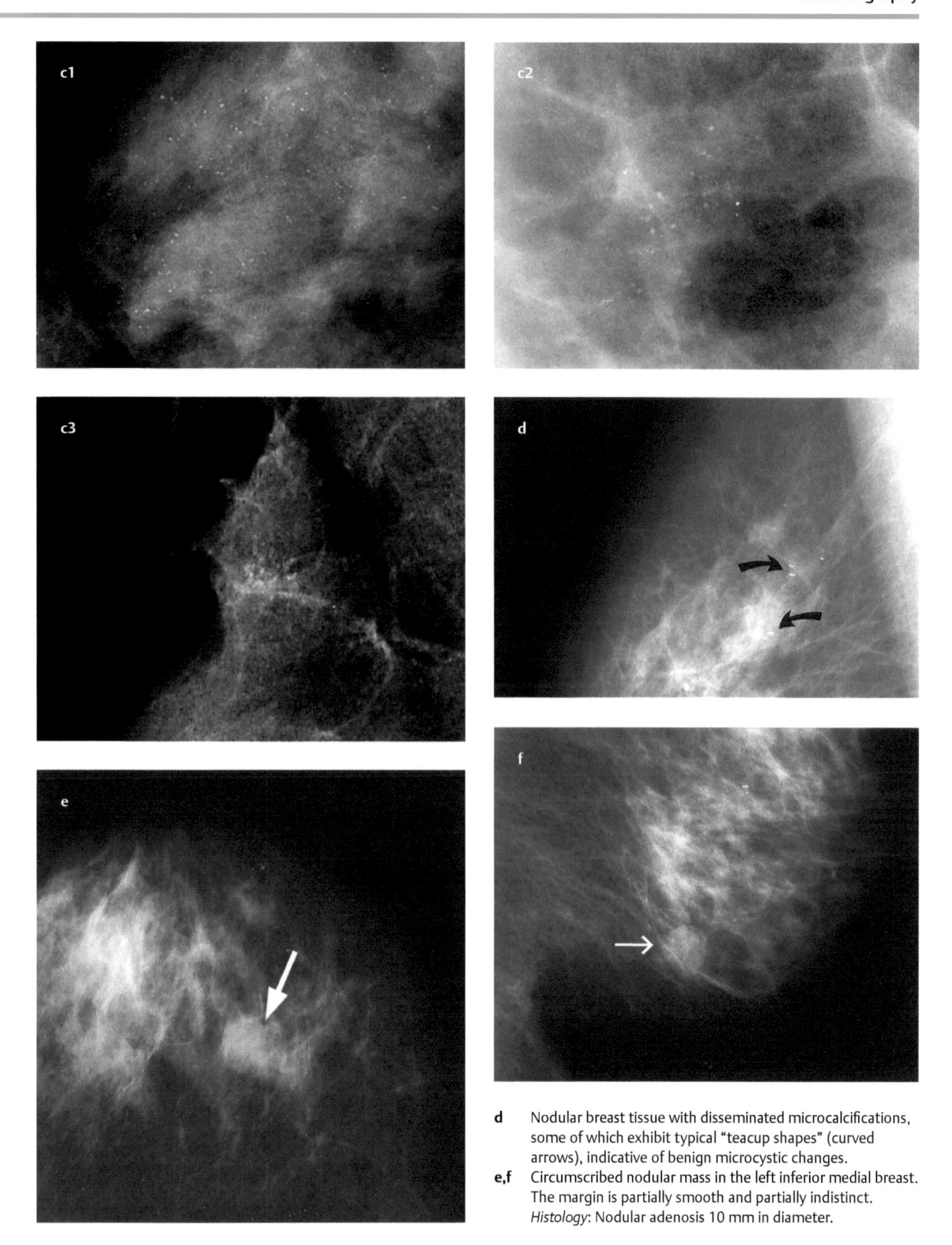

d Nodular breast tissue with disseminated microcalcifications, some of which exhibit typical "teacup shapes" (curved arrows), indicative of benign microcystic changes.
e,f Circumscribed nodular mass in the left inferior medial breast. The margin is partially smooth and partially indistinct.
Histology: Nodular adenosis 10 mm in diameter.

Fig. 10.1g–i ▷

◁ continued

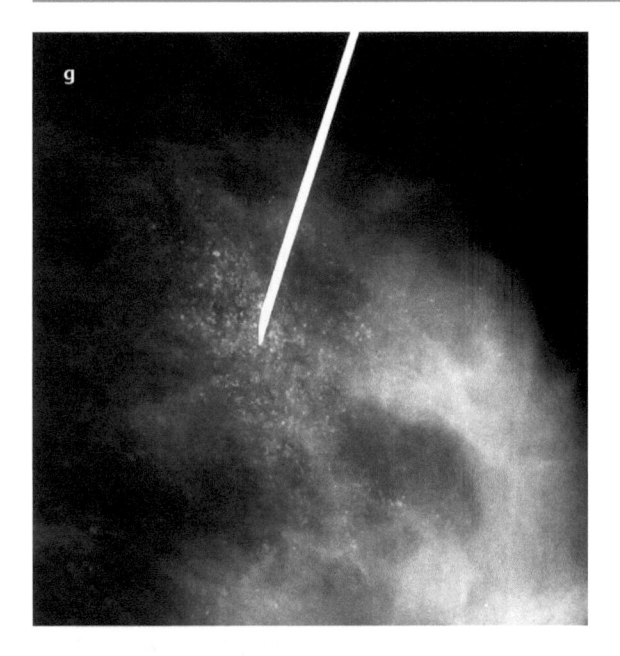

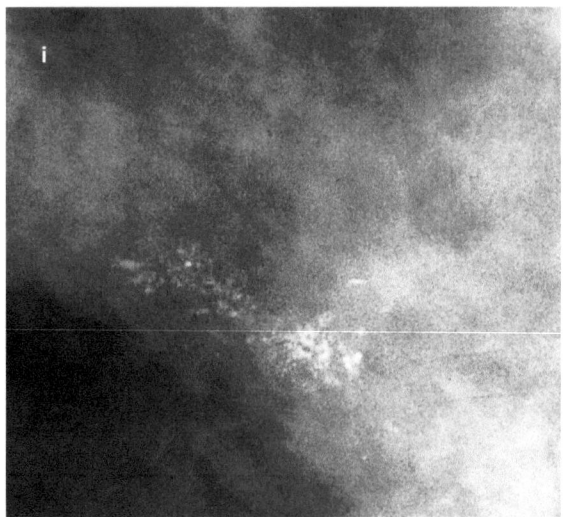

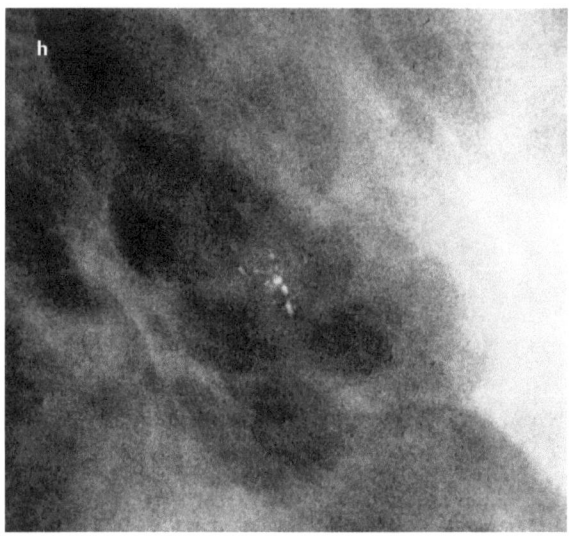

g–i Some microcalcifications that occur with benign changes raise suspicion owing to their regional, segmental, or even ductlike distribution. Even casting microcalcifications may occur in benign disease. If one of these patterns is seen or suspected, workup is indicated. **g** There are multiple, uniformly distributed, relatively round, monomorphic and punctate microcalcifications. Histopathologic assessment was performed because of their asymmetric unilateral distribution and a planned liver transplant. *Histologic examination* revealed simple fibrocystic benign breast disease with psammomatous calcifications. Although morphology of the calcifications appears benign, workup is justified by their regional (possibly even segmental) distribution. **h** Magnification mammography reveals a tiny cluster consisting of round and two or three linear microcalcifications arranged in a linear pattern. *Histology*: Focal fibrocystic breast disease with calcified intraductal and intralobular calcific deposits. **i** Magnification mammography shows a long cluster of round, linear, and polymorphic microcalcifications. *Histology*: Focal fibrous breast disease with multiple fine microcalcifications.

Diagnosing cysts and differentiating cysts from solid masses is a task for sonography (see also Chapter 11).

Significance of Changes in Structure and Density

Whereas focal and asymmetrical densities or structural changes can simulate a carcinoma at mammography and clinical examination, generalized changes can make detection of malignant processes difficult as a result of generally increased radiodensity.

There is no correlation between the extent of structural changes or increased radiodensity and the degree of cellular proliferation or atypia. As a result, it is not possible to correlate mammographically detected structural changes and changes in density with the possible risk of carcinoma.

If an asymmetric density is seen on one view only, comparison with the other view (or additional views) should allow determination of whether the density might just be caused by superimposition. Inclusion of fat lobules and undisturbed tissue lines together with the absence of a palpable abnormality may support the diagnosis of a benign asymmetry. Considering that asymmetric tissue is a frequent finding, mammographic analysis should precede further evaluation in patients without clinical symptoms. Due to the high frequency of benign asymmetry, it will not be possible to recall all patients with some asymmetry.

Ultrasonography may help to exclude a mass that is hidden within or causes the asymmetry.

If doubts persist, percutaneous biopsy (which in the case of larger areas may be fanning with core needle biopsy) should be considered. MRI may be helpful but carries the risk of false positive calls. MRI should not be carried out if the patient is on HRT.

Calcifications

Microcalcifications frequently occur in benign breast disorders. They exhibit a broad range of variation with respect to their morphology and pattern of distribution. They can be the result of calcified secretions. Necrotic cells shed into intraductal or intralobular spaces can calcify, and calcifications can occur in the stroma. Accordingly, they may be found diffusely disseminated, arranged in a lobular pattern, or without any clear pattern of distribution.

Spectrometry has revealed these structures to consist primarily of calcium phosphates in addition to compounds involving other elements.

The following forms are *typical of benign breast disorders*.

- *Isolated*, generally round *calcifications*.
- *Scattered punctate microcalcifications*, generally occurring symmetrically. These occur in many benign breast disorders and particularly often with sclerosing adenosis.
- *Milk of calcium in microcysts*. These correspond to the typical teacup-shaped calcifications described by Lanyi. They represent small "lakes" of milk of calcium in cystic distended lobules. The milk of calcium contains extremely fine suspended particles of calcium not resolved on the mammogram. This accumulation of calcified milk in a distended microcystic structure appears as one "calcification."

  In the craniocaudal view, these individual "calcifications" appear as lakes of calcified milk, generally round, sometimes faceted, and frequently of different size. Their margins are often indistinct or amorphous. They are nonspecific and can vary in density. The lobular arrangement of these deposits can be assessed only when some of these calcifications lie close together in small flowerlike or rosettelike clusters.

  In the mediolateral 90° view, the characteristic sedimentation of extremely fine particles in the calcified milk produces a characteristic sign: The inferior border of the small lake that appears to be a calcification is arc shaped and shows a horizontal surface produced by sedimentation. This surface corresponds to the fluid–fluid level of sedimented milk of calcium (**Fig. 10.1d**).

  Intense compression can cause the calcium salt precipitates to well up so that the fluid–fluid level appears to form a superior dome.

  These so-called "teacups" often occur bilaterally, but can also be observed unilaterally or asymmetrically. The typical teacup sign can usually only be demonstrated in some of the calcifications.

  Where the typical teacup sign can be demonstrated and other changes typical of malignancy (casting or pleomorphic microcalcifications, or suggestive densities) are absent, the examiner can diagnose a benign breast disorder.

- *Clusters of microcalcifications following a lobular pattern*. These may be isolated or multifocal. The calcifications lie closely clustered together in a small area corresponding to the size of a normal or hypertrophic lobule (1–5 mm). At mammography, this will appear like a morula or rosette. Several lobules may be involved.

- *Atypical distribution pattern*. Despite certain variations in the size of the individual calcifications, the individual calcifications within a cluster appear round and monomorphic. Such clusters occur primarily in the presence of cystic and sclerosing adenosis.

Unfortunately, aside from these typical benign calcifications, benign breast disorders can also involve indeterminate and, occasionally, even suspicious calcifications.

Indeterminate microcalcifications that can occur in benign breast disorders include the following forms:

- Ill-defined and amorphous calcifications with slight to pronounced pleomorphism

- Microcalcifications appearing in an isolated area that are asymmetrical with the contralateral side and not clearly benign
- Clusters of microcalcifications that are not clearly arranged in a monomorphic lobular pattern

Suspicious calcifications may rarely also occur in benign breast disorders. These appear as:
- Casting, rodlike, V-shaped, or Y-shaped, or
- Coarsely granular and pleomorphic
- They may even be arranged in a segmental configuration, and/or follow the ductal structures, indistinguishable from microcalcifications associated with malignancy and therefore necessitating biopsy

Indeterminate calcifications and, rarely, suspicious calcifications may also be associated with benign breast disease. This is just an expression of the fact that benign transformation can affect both the lobules and the ductal system. Calcifications can occur in a typically benign "lobular" configuration but also in a ductal configuration, simulating a malignant process, albeit less frequently. In sclerosing adenosis, myothelial and connective tissue proliferation can lead to deformity of the lobules. This can explain the greater polymorphism of the individual calcifications detected in sclerosing adenosis and individual rodlike microcalcifications.

Importance of Microcalcifications in Benign Breast Disorders

On the whole, indeterminate and suspicious *microcalcifications occur more frequently in benign proliferative disorders* than in nonproliferative breast disorders. Microcalcifications associated with benign breast disorders nevertheless *do not permit an assessment of the risk of malignancy of the underlying breast disease* in a specific case.

In the presence of *calcifications typical of benign breast disorders*, routine screening (at intervals depending on the patient's general risk and her age) is all that is needed. Biopsy should not be performed. The examiner should verify that these benign calcifications are not accompanied by additional microcalcifications or calcification clusters typical of malignancy.

Suspicious microcalcifications require biopsy for histologic examination. Where nonspecific microcalcifications are present, the physician may elect to perform further workup (i.e., needle core biopsy, vacuum-assisted biopsy, or excisional biopsy). Rarely, follow-up imaging studies will be needed. This decision should be made on the basis of the analysis of the microcalcifications, clinical examination, and patient history data (see also Chapter 24). It should be pointed out that newly developing or increasing microcalcifications may be indicative of a developing malignancy. Therefore these microcalcifications should be analyzed with great caution and—unless they are typically benign—the threshold for histopathologic assessment (or at least short-term follow-up) should be lower.

Sonography

At sonography (**Fig. 10.2a–e**), benign breast disorders are typically characterized by the following features:
- *The mammary gland is homogeneously hyperechoic* (a frequent finding).
- Cysts are frequently encountered. They may appear in various sizes and can be diagnosed once they reach about 2 mm in diameter.
- *Ectatic ducts* (occasionally present).
- *Regular hypoechoic structures* (generally tubular, less frequently nodular) extending throughout the

▷

Fig. 10.2a–h

a–f Sonographic appearance of changes in benign breast disorders.
a Benign breast disorders will often appear homogeneously hyperechoic at sonography. This tissue can be visualized well by ultrasound. However, even this image cannot exclude a carcinoma in situ or very small carcinoma if one is suspected (e.g., in the presence of mammographically suspicious microcalcifications).
b Less frequently, extremely regular hypoechoic tubular structures will be discernible within the hyperechoic benign tissue. These most likely correspond to ductal or lobular structures in the presence of periductal fibrosis or adenosis. This image is relatively characteristic of a benign breast disorder, but can render it difficult to detect or exclude small carcinomas.
c Sometimes single or multiple nodular hypoechoic structures (arrows) that do not correspond to fat lobules will appear within hyperechoic benign tissue (see **Fig. 9.5g**). These most likely represent focal areas of adenosis or fibroadenomas. These focal findings often render differential diagnosis difficult and would, if biopsied, lead to an unacceptably high biopsy rate. Therefore, we tend to follow these lesions by sonography if they are small, do not clearly correlate with mammographic or clinical findings, and lack sonographic signs of malignancy (acoustic shadow, hyperechoic halo, and so forth). The shadowing on the left side of this image (double arrow) disappeared with different angulation of the ultrasound transducer, and thus was also compatible with benign changes.
d Another example of a benign hypoechoic nodule is shown, which proved to correspond to a focal area of adenosis and papillomatosis at CNB.
e In some cases, acoustic shadows (arrows) can occur in benign tissue. These probably correspond to areas of increased fibrosis; variable shadows are nonspecific, particularly when they disappear under compression or when the transducer is moved. Constant shadows, as shown here, may occur in the presence of extensive focal fibrous breast disease or proliferative disorders, but have also been reported with small carcinomas and DCIS. Thus, constant shadowing may impair sonographic assessment and reliability of the diagnosis.

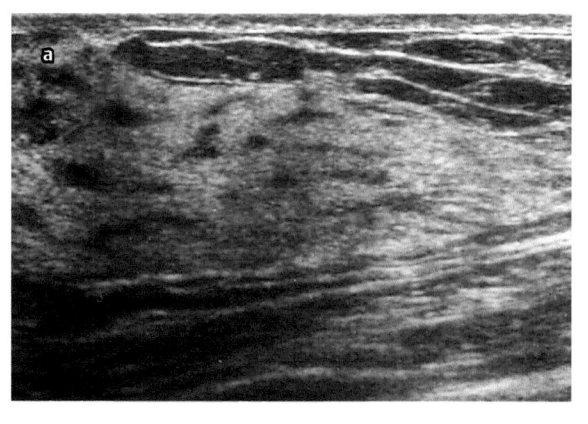

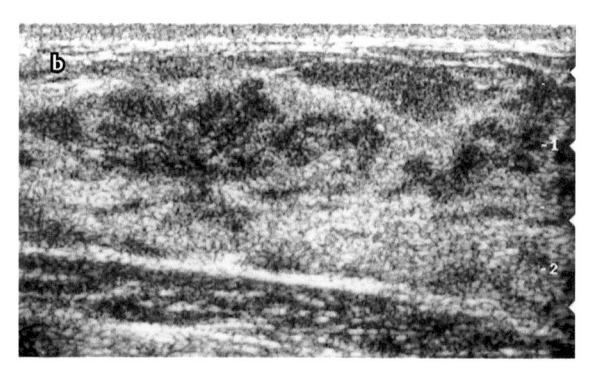

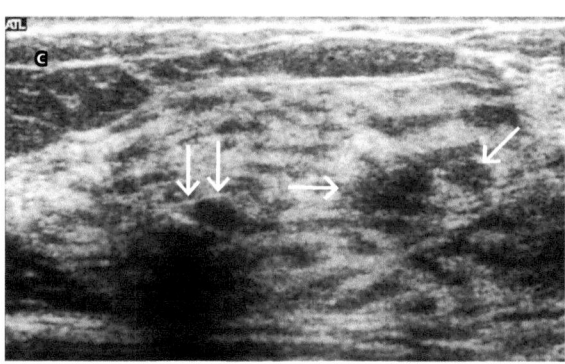

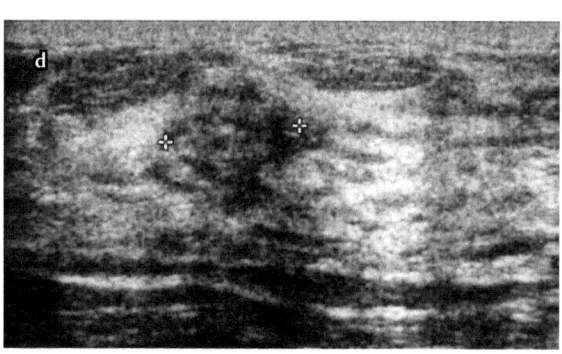

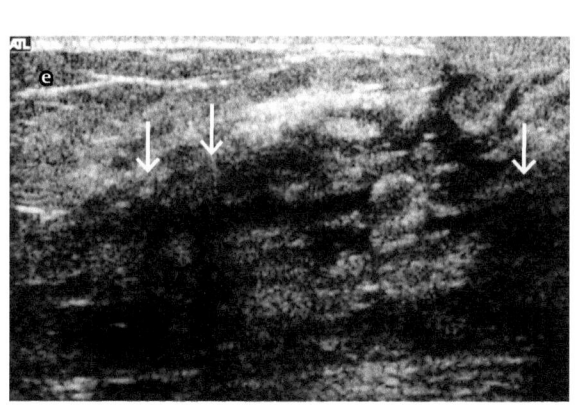

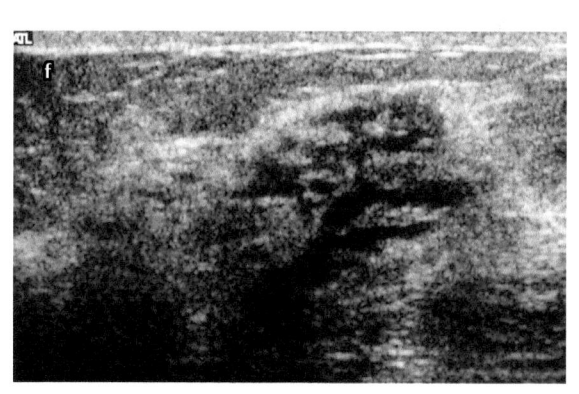

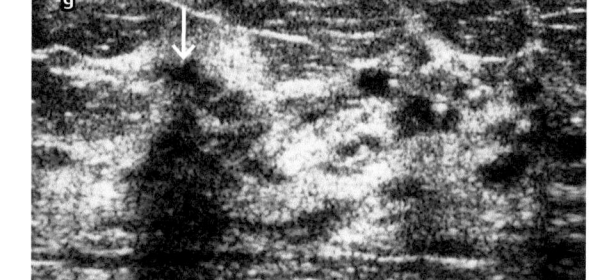

e,f Distinct acoustic shadowing (arrow) may occur with extensive focal fibrous breast disease. The suspicious area corresponded to a suggestive palpable finding (in a radiodense breast), histologically confirmed to be extensive focal fibrous breast disease.
g Severe fibrocystic changes. In this case, with mammographically very dense tissue, persistent shadowing arose from dense fibrous tissue (proven by core needle biopsy and follow-up).

mammary gland. These hypoechoic structures that follow the ductal system most likely correspond to periductal fibrosis or to foci of adenosis. Where such a regular overall structure is present, there is a high probability that these changes are benign.
- *The mammary gland* is partially or entirely homogeneously *hypoechoic*. This finding is rare. Differentiation between hypoechoic areas of breast disease and fat is significantly more difficult here, and the capability to discern hypoechoic tumors is greatly reduced.

Less Reliable Changes

The following focal changes may also be due to just benign breast disorders:
- *Hypoechoic foci*. These are generally irregular, less frequently round, and circumscribed. They can appear as isolated foci, in which case they have to be considered suspicious. They can also occur as multiple foci. Histologically, they may correspond to foci of adenosis, foci of benign proliferative disorders, or areas of focal fibrosis (this usually is accompanied by an acoustic shadow). The tumorous form of sclerosing adenosis can also appear as a hypoechoic focus. Hypoechoic foci resulting from benign breast disorders usually do not show a hyperechoic rim (which is typical of malignancy). Also, they rarely exhibit posterior shadowing like some carcinomas. However, carcinomas (and small carcinomas in particular) can vary considerably, and a reliable differentiation of benign and malignant hypoechoic foci or acoustic shadows is not generally possible. Thus hypoechoic foci, in particular single foci, should be considered suspicious until proven otherwise.
- *Acoustic shadows with or without hypoechoic focal findings*. Shadows can occur at multiple locations or in an isolated area. If shadows arise from Cooper ligaments, they can usually be eliminated by applying the transducer at a slightly different angle or by applying the transducer with more compression. Furthermore, shadowing may occur in the presence of diffusely proliferative fibrosis or focal fibrosis within the tissue. Often, tumorous sclerosing adenosis or radial scar will appear as a hypoechoic focus with an acoustic shadow or as an isolated acoustic shadow. Isolated shadowing usually requires histopathologic assessment, which in most cases is possible using ultrasound-guided core needle biopsy.

Purpose

Sonography is not recommended as a screening tool in asymptomatic women (Heywang-Köbrunner et al. 2008, Lee et al. 2010). However, in symptomatic women and in women with mammographic abnormalities sonography may provide valuable additional information (Stavros et al. 1995, Skaane and Engedal 1998, Dennis et al. 2001, Soo et al. 2001, Graf et al. 2004, Mendelson 2004, Mainiero et al. 2005, Nothacker et al. 2009,).

Identifying cysts as the cause of a palpable abnormality or of a mammographic density allows malignancy to be excluded and unnecessary biopsy to be avoided.

A malignant process in homogeneously hyperechoic benign tissue is improbable. Since carcinomas are generally hypoechoic and are easily discernible in such tissue, sonography is often helpful as an adjunctive imaging modality in patients with homogeneously hyperechoic tissue. However, in the presence of clinical or mammographic suspicion (such as microcalcifications or a definitely suspicious palpable finding), *sonography alone cannot exclude malignancy* even in homogeneously hyperechoic tissue. This is because some carcinomas in situ and some rare diffusely growing malignancies also appear hyperechoic and thus may escape detection by sonography.

The following applies in the presence of a heterogeneous or hypoechoic pattern:
- The capability of sonography to exclude a malignant process is reduced in the presence of a *hypoechoic mammary gland with a benign disorder* (rare).
- *Excluding a malignant process is not possible with certainty in the presence of sonographically heterogeneous breast tissue* (with hypoechoic foci and/or multiple acoustic shadows). Close correlation with clinical and mammographic findings is required.
- *Areas with acoustic shadows or a hypoechoic mass with and without acoustic shadows*—if reproducible—require further workup. Depending on the specific suspicion, mammographic findings, and clinical examination, further workup may include ultrasound-guided core needle biopsy, excisional biopsy or sonographic follow-up (in the case of benign-appearing or very small hypechoic area).

Magnetic Resonance Imaging

Glandular tissue and benign breast presents with low signal intensity on T1-weighted MR images and with variable, mostly low to intermediate signal on T2-weighted MR images, as opposed to fatty tissue (**Fig. 10.3a–h**).

After contrast injection:
- *Most benign breast disorders (70–75%) enhance only slightly, if at all* (**Fig. 10.3a,b** and **Fig. 9.8a–d**). Most of these cases involve nonproliferative disorders (such as increased fibrosis of benign breast tissue with or without cysts)
- Contrast enhancement occurs in 20–30% of benign breast disorders. It is more common in young women and hormonally active tissue. The *pattern of enhancement can vary greatly*. The following patterns can occur:

- Diffuse milky enhancement: Diffuse enhancement is an enhancement over a wide area (for example, the entire breast or the upper outer quadrant) without an abrupt transition from surrounding tissue
- Diffuse nodular, confluent enhancement (**Fig. 10.3c,d**)
- Focal enhancement with irregular contours, or focal nodular enhancement (**Fig. 10.3g,h**)

Benign breast disorders without cellular hyperplasia or proliferation usually exhibit continuous enhancement. Enhancement (mostly continuous, sometimes plateau-type) can occur infrequently in nonproliferative disorders where they involve inflammatory reactions (galactophoritis), when adenosis or significant hyperplastic changes are present, or sometimes under hormonal stimulation (see below). Proliferative breast disorders usually enhance (with a continuous or plateau-type enhancement curve). However, there is no correlation of enhancement in benign changes and presence of atypias.

Effects of the Menstrual Cycle

Enhancement due to breast disorders is often inconstant and varies during the menstrual cycle. Since enhancement due to breast disorders is often more pronounced in the second half of the cycle and since some of such enhancing areas disappear after menstruation, it is recommended that the MRI examination be performed between the 7th and 14th days of the menstrual cycle whenever possible.

Predictive Value

Whether the degree of proliferation in breast disorders correlates with the extent or speed of contrast enhancement is controversial. Our experience has shown that, particularly with respect to the important distinction between proliferative breast disorders with and without atypia, no reliable correlation with the extent or speed of contrast enhancement exists. Also, so far no data exist as to whether enhancement within benign changes might be associated with any increased risk of breast cancer

Advantages and Disadvantages

Contrast-enhanced MRI has advantages and disadvantages for the differential diagnosis of changes due to benign breast disorders (Heywang-Köbrunner et al. 1997, Zakhireh et al. 2008, Moy et al. 2010):
- Because of its high sensitivity for invasive carcinomas, absence of contrast enhancement (as occurs in ~70% of benign breast disorders) is a highly reliable sign of the absence of an invasive carcinoma. (Rare exceptions, however, have been encountered.)
- In the presence of nonenhancing benign breast disorders, nonpalpable carcinomas (or focal carcinomas) can be detected even in radiodense or irregularly structured tissue. This has proven valuable for screening of women at high risk and for visualization of tumor extent or multicentricity before breast conservation in the selected groups of women for whom it is presently recommended (women with lobular breast cancer, women at high risk who develop breast cancer, and women whose breast cancers exhibited a very different size on mammography compared with sonography) (Sardanelli et al. 2010).
- In those cases of difficult diagnostic problems that cannot be solved by mammography, sonography, and percutaneous biopsy, MRI may be attempted. In those cases with absent enhancement, MRI will be useful to help exclude malignancy or define the area of highest suspicion for subsequent biopsy (see also Chapter 5)
- Presence of a generalized diffuse or patchy pattern of enhancement limits the capability of MRI to detect or exclude a carcinoma. Focal enhancement resulting from benign breast disorders cannot be reliably distinguished from focal carcinomas and thus may lead to false positive results.

Relevance for Differential Diagnosis

Previously mentioned disadvantages pertain primarily to the impaired assessment of those benign breast disorders with generalized enhancement. Furthermore, focal areas of enhancement may cause false positive calls. In light of this, we *do not recommend using contrast-enhanced MRI for every form of benign breast disorder* or *unselectively* in radiodense tissue, but recommend *limiting its use to special cases* that cannot be resolved otherwise.

Contrast-enhanced MRI is not recommended in the following situations:
- Follow-up examination of known enhancing breast disorders (i.e., known from previous diagnostic studies).
- Differentiation between inflammatory and malignant changes (both enhance allowing no reliable distinction).
- In patients undergoing hormone therapy (generally with preparations containing intermediate or high dosages of gestagen) who complain of tension (nonspecific enhancement will often impair diagnostic accuracy).
- In asymptomatic patients with dense breast tissue. The majority of these patients are below the age of 40 years. Here, frequently occult fibroadenomas or areas of adenosis will be detected (nonspecific enhancement may be encountered in around 1 of 5 cases) leading to expensive workup, while the chance of detecting a malignancy is low, since the prevalence of malignancy

10 Benign Breast Disorders

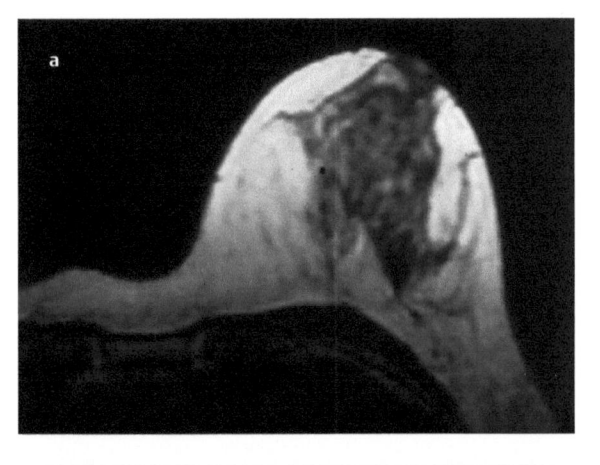

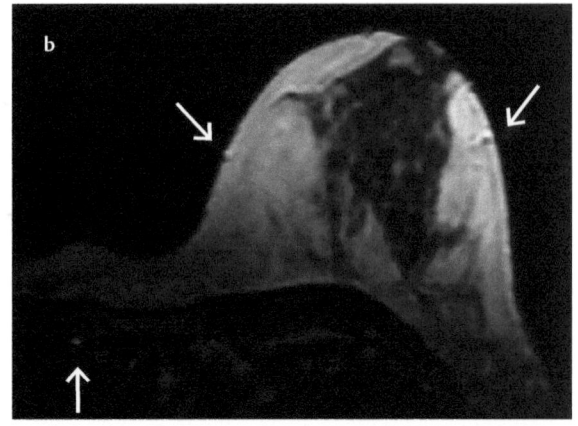

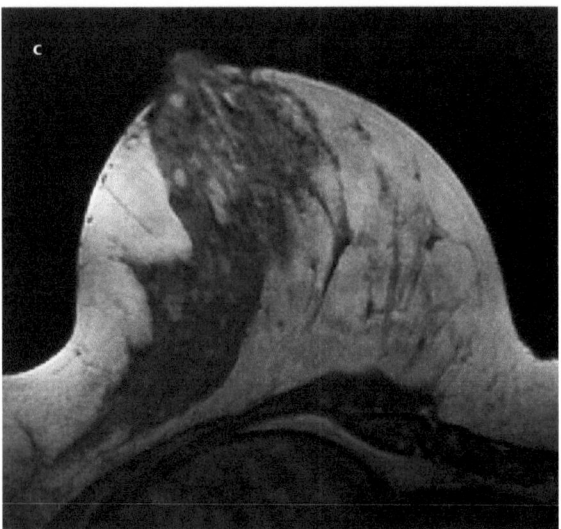

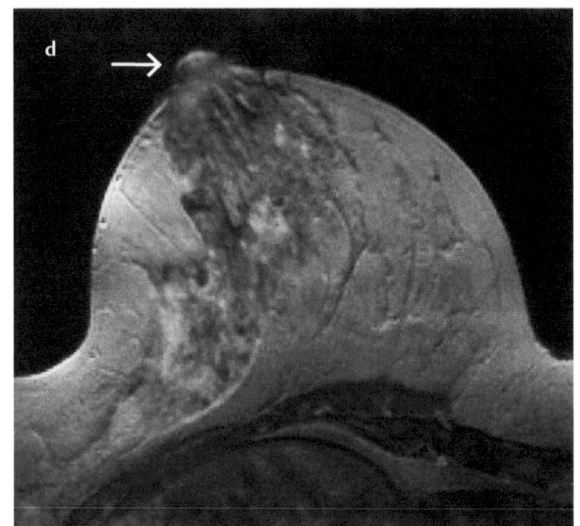

Fig. 10.3a–h MRI appearance of benign breast disorders.

a,b Most benign breast disorders (70–75%) enhance only slightly with Gd-DTPA. **a** Representative slice (FLASH 3D) before contrast administration. **b** The same slice after injection of Gd-DTPA.
Glandular tissue and fat show no significant changes in signal intensity; only vascular structures enhance (arrows). MRI examination was performed as an adjunct to mammography to verify the absence of a carcinoma in radiodense tissue after a contralateral carcinoma was detected.

c,d 25% to 30% of all benign breast disorders demonstrate a diffuse milky to nodular pattern of enhancement (these disorders usually involve adenosis, proliferation, or atypia).
c Representative slice before injection of contrast medium. MRI was performed because of impaired mammographic assessment in the presence of radiodense breast tissue, diffusely disseminated microcalcifications, and a family history of malignancy. **d** The same slice after injection of Gd-DTPA. A confluent patchy pattern of progressive contrast enhancement is demonstrated in the glandular tissue. This finding is compatible with benign breast disease, but the capability to exclude malignancy is limited.
The nipple itself (arrow) enhances in approximately 50% of all patients. In the absence of clinical suspicion this represents a normal finding.

e–h Occasionally, mammography and MRI (sometimes only MRI) will reveal a benign focal breast disorder. Focal fibrous breast disease will not enhance (see **Fig. 9.8a–d**). In a benign proliferative breast disorder, the focus can enhance significantly, which represents a suspicious MRI finding.

e,f Mammographically suspicious indistinct lesion on the craniocaudal and mediolateral preoperative localization images.

g Slice through the suspicious lesion before contrast injection (MR examination was part of a study protocol).

h After injection of Gd-DTPA, the indistinct focal lesion enhances rapidly and early, behaving in the same manner as a malignant lesion on MRI. *Histologic examination* revealed mildly proliferative benign focal breast disease accompanied by a pronounced but unspecific inflammatory reaction.

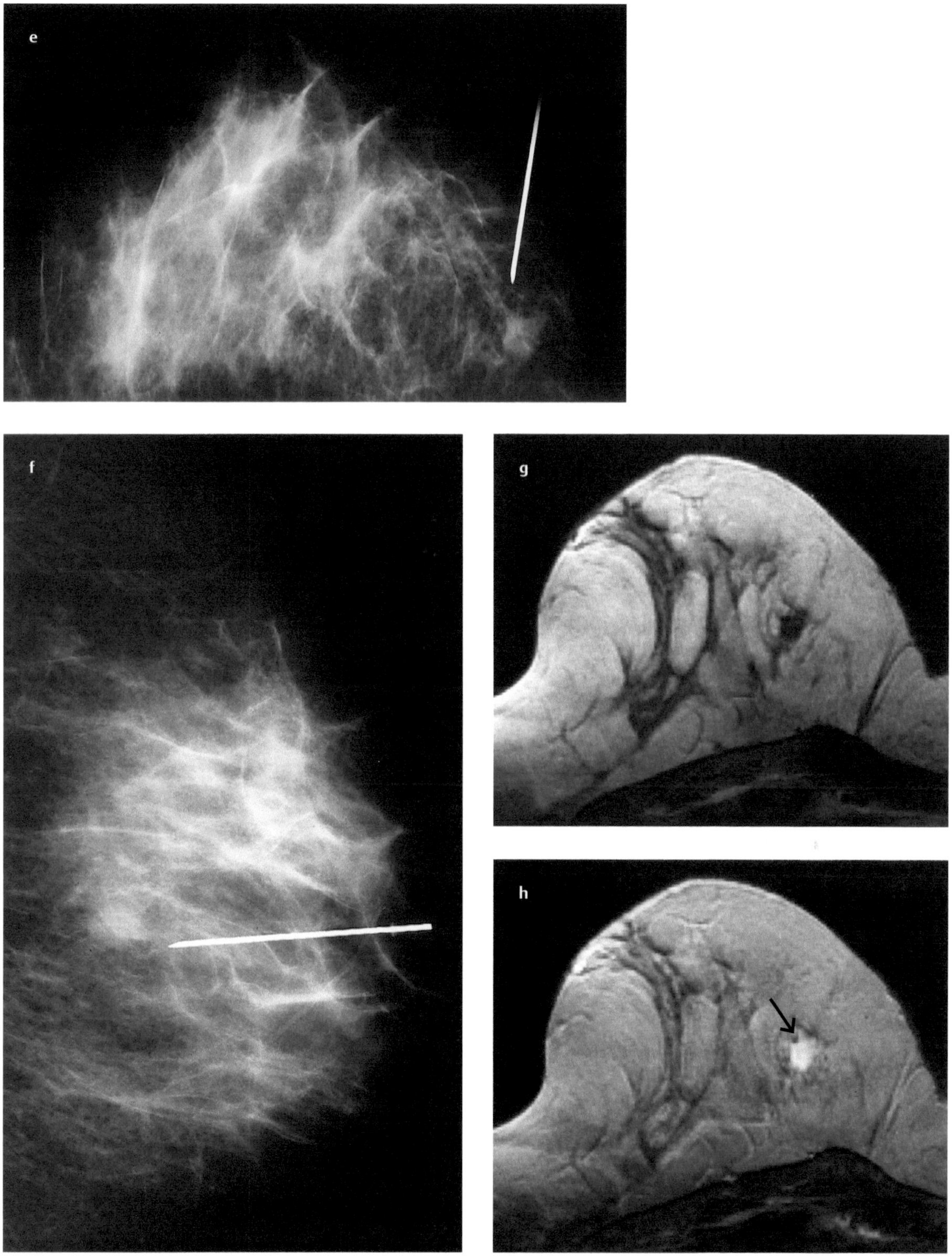
e
f
g
h

is low in unselected patient populations. (About 3 in 1,000 patients or < 1 per 1,000 for patients below 40).

MRI is not suitable for further differentiation between uncharacteristic microcalcifications (Cilotti et al. 2007, Uematsu et al. 2007). Data in the literature concerning sensitivity of contrast MRI for carcinomas in situ vary significantly (from about 40% to 90%) (Sardanelli et al. 2004, Kuhl et al. 2007, Rosen et al. 2007). The variations may be explained by patient preselection and by the chosen gold standard. Since benign disorders with microcalcifications may often be associated with uncharacteristic enhancement (the enhancement type that is frequently seen in DCIS, too), MRI will not be useful to avoid biopsy.

Contrast-enhanced MRI, however, may be helpful for the following indications:
- Screening of women at high risk
- In radiodense tissue searching for a primary tumor in patients with a carcinoma of unknown primary tumor (CUP syndrome)
- Staging in radiodense tissue to exclude additional foci or a contralateral malignancy (only in selected cases before conservative treatment of a small breast carcinoma—see above and Chapter 5)
- In selected cases with radiodense tissue with uncharacteristic disturbed architecture or asymmetry, in patients with severe scarring, in radiodense tissue in the presence of (multiple) contradictory findings, in patients with nipple retraction of unknown origin or nipple discharge—if the problem cannot be solved by conventional imaging and percutaneous breast biopsy

Percutaneous Biopsy

Whenever malignancy cannot be excluded, histopathologic assessment is mandatory.
- For lesions that can be visualized and targeted by ultrasound (e.g., most masses), ultrasound-guided core needle biopsy is the standard method for further assessment. Fine needle biopsy should be used only by highly experienced examiners and interdisciplinary teams.
- For the workup of indeterminate or suspicious microcalcifications or for those small masses that cannot be visualized and targeted by ultrasound, vacuum-assisted breast biopsy (VABB) is the method of choice.
- In the case of small focal asymmetries or for architectural distortions VABB may also help avoid open biopsy.
- Close correlation of imaging and histopathology and discussion of all discrepant cases and B3 lesions is necessary to avoid false negative calls.
- Heterogeneous changes in benign breast disorders and diffuse changes of large areas limit the accuracy of percutaneous breast biopsy. In these cases open biopsy may be preferable to percutaneous biopsy, from which only a small part of the area in question may be assessed.
- Great care is necessary when assessing clinical changes without definite imaging correlation. Depending on the imaging presentation, open biopsy, fanning by core needle biopsy (which requires acquisition of many cores under local anesthesia), or short-term follow-up may be considered as options.

Summary

Histologically, benign breast disorders encompass a broad spectrum of tissue changes. We differentiate the following types according to their prognosis:
- Benign nonproliferative breast disorders (70% of all benign disorders) without an increased risk of carcinoma
- Benign proliferative breast disorders without cellular atypia (~25% of all benign disorders) with a slightly increased risk of carcinoma (by a factor of 1.5–2)
- Benign proliferative breast disorders with cellular atypia (4–5% of all benign disorders) with an increased risk of carcinoma (by a factor of 5)

Mammographic density may be an evolving indicator of risk. Owing to limitations of reproducibility and logistic limitations concerning its use and the lack of widely agreed further diagnostic or therapeutic options for the individual patient, this risk factor has not yet been applied.

Otherwise diagnostic imaging studies do not permit reliable assessment of risk or a correlation with the histopathologic presence or absence of atypias.

Clinical signs of benign breast disorders can include pain, palpable findings, and, rarely, discharge.

The primary *mammographic signs* are increased density and microcalcifications, sometimes asymmetry, masses or architectural distortion.

Sonography may reveal hyperechoic tissue texture. Often cysts can be identified. Hypoechoic structures or acoustic shadows may also be found presenting as diffuse change of all or major parts of the breast tissue or even as focal change. The former will impair diagnostic evaluation and may be difficult to distinguish from diffusely growing malignancy. The latter can mimic malignancy and usually requires histopathologic assessment.

On *MRI examination*, nonproliferative disorders usually enhance only slightly, while contrast enhancement can vary greatly in adenosis and proliferative benign disorders (uptake can vary equally in proliferative changes with and without atypia).

Depending on the extent of the benign changes, findings in all modalities may overlap with changes associated with preinvasive and early invasive carcinomas.

Diffuse benign changes are usually recognizable as such but can often *limit visualization of malignancy*. *Focal changes* usually differ qualitatively and quantitatively from surrounding benign tissue. Such changes require careful workup. In general diagnostic imaging studies are unable to reliably distinguish these changes from malignant processes. Therefore focal changes frequently lead to false positive findings and necessitate percutaneous or open biopsy of benign changes.

Clinical examination and mammography are the methods of choice for assessing benign breast disorders detected by screening, and they are fully adequate for this purpose. In the presence of *questionable or suggestive mammographic or clinical findings, adjunctive procedures* are indicated for the following reasons:

To minimize the number of excisional biopsies of benign findings

To improve early detection of malignancy where the risk of malignancy is high and visualization is limited

In the presence of indeterminate focal findings, adjunctive sonography is recommended as a first step of the workup. Biopsy should follow in all cases where carcinoma is not excluded with reasonable certainty.

Contrast-enhanced MRI may be helpful in selected cases that cannot be adequately solved by mammography, sonography, and percutaneous breast biopsy.

Open biopsy remains the most reliable method for assessing borderline lesions (e.g., benign breast changes with atypias), or for contradictory findings. In the case of malignancy, it will constitute the first therapeutic measure as well.

References and Recommended Reading

Banks E, Reeves G, Beral V, et al. Impact of use of hormone replacement therapy on false positive recall in the NHS breast screening programme: results from the Million Women Study. BMJ 2004;328(7451):1291–1292

Barlow WE, White E, Ballard-Barbash R, et al. Prospective breast cancer risk prediction model for women undergoing screening mammography. J Natl Cancer Inst 2006;98(17):1204–1214

Becker S, Kaaks R. Exogenous and endogenous hormones, mammographic density and breast cancer risk: can mammographic density be considered an intermediate marker of risk? Recent Results Cancer Res 2009;181:135–157

Berg WA, Blume JD, Cormack JB, et al; ACRIN 6666 Investigators. Combined screening with ultrasound and mammography vs mammography alone in women at elevated risk of breast cancer. JAMA 2008;299(18):2151–2163

Boyd NF, Guo H, Martin LJ, et al. Mammographic density and the risk and detection of breast cancer. N Engl J Med 2007;356(3):227–236

Boyd NF, Martin LJ, Rommens JM, et al. Mammographic density: a heritable risk factor for breast cancer. Methods Mol Biol 2009;472:343–360

Boyd NF, Melnichouk O, Martin LJ, et al. Mammographic density, response to hormones, and breast cancer risk. J Clin Oncol 2011;29(22):2985–2992

Britton P, Warwick J, Wallis MG, et al. Measuring the accuracy of diagnostic imaging in symptomatic breast patients: team and individual performance. Br J Radiol 2012;85(1012):415–422

Byrne C, Schairer C, Wolfe J, et al. Mammographic features and breast cancer risk: effects with time, age, and menopause status. J Natl Cancer Inst 1995;87(21):1622–1629

Chopier J, Gibeault M, Salem C, Marsault C, Thomassin Naggara I. How to measure breast density? [Article in French]. J Radiol 2008;89(9 Pt 2):1151–1155

Ciatto S, Houssami N, Apruzzese A, et al. Categorizing breast mammographic density: intra- and interobserver reproducibility of BI-RADS density categories. Breast 2005;14(4):269–275

Cilotti A, Iacconi C, Marini C, et al. Contrast-enhanced MR imaging in patients with BI-RADS 3-5 microcalcifications. Radiol Med (Torino) 2007;112(2):272–286

Consensus Meeting. Is "fibrocystic disease" of the breast precancerous? Arch Pathol Lab Med 1986;110(3):171–173

Dennis MA, Parker SH, Klaus AJ, Stavros AT, Kaske TI, Clark SB. Breast biopsy avoidance: the value of normal mammograms and normal sonograms in the setting of a palpable lump. Radiology 2001;219(1):186–191

Dumas I, Diorio C. Polymorphisms in genes involved in the estrogen pathway and mammographic density. BMC Cancer 2010;10:636

Dupont WD, Page DL. Risk factors for breast cancer in women with proliferative breast disease. N Engl J Med 1985;312(3):146–151

Dupont WD, Page DL. Relative risk of breast cancer varies with time since diagnosis of atypical hyperplasia. Hum Pathol 1989;20(8):723–725

Evans A. Hormone replacement therapy and mammographic screening. Clin Radiol 2002;57(7):563–564

Ghosh K, Vachon CM, Pankratz VS, et al. Independent association of lobular involution and mammographic breast density with breast cancer risk. J Natl Cancer Inst 2010;102(22):1716–1723

Graf O, Helbich TH, Fuchsjaeger MH, et al. Follow-up of palpable circumscribed noncalcified solid breast masses at mammography and US: can biopsy be averted? Radiology 2004;233(3):850–856

Heywang-Köbrunner SH, Schreer I, Heindel W, Katalinic A. Imaging studies for the early detection of breast cancer. Dtsch Arztebl Int 2008;105(31–32):541–547

Heywang-Köbrunner SH, Viehweg P, Heinig A, Küchler C. Contrast-enhanced MRI of the breast: accuracy, value, controversies, solutions. Eur J Radiol 1997;24(2):94–108

Hutter RV. Goodbye to "fibrocystic disease". N Engl J Med 1985;312(3):179–181

Kallenberg MG, Lokate M, van Gils CH, Karssemeijer N. Automatic breast density segmentation: an integration of different approaches. Phys Med Biol 2011;56(9):2715–2729

Kerlikowske K. The mammogram that cried Wolfe. N Engl J Med. 2007;356(3):297–300. Comment on N Engl. J Med 2007;356(3):227–236

Kerlikowske K, Grady D, Barclay J, et al. Variability and accuracy in mammographic interpretation using the American College of Radiology Breast Imaging Reporting and Data System. J Natl Cancer Inst 1998;90(23):1801–1809

Kopans DB. Basic physics and doubts about relationship between mammographically determined tissue density and breast cancer risk. Radiology 2008;246(2):348–353

Kuhl CK, Schrading S, Bieling HB, et al. MRI for diagnosis of pure ductal carcinoma in situ: a prospective observational study. Lancet 2007;370(9586):485–492

Lanyi M. Diagnostik und Differentialdiagnostik der Mammaverkalkung. Berlin: Springer; 1986

Lee CH, Dershaw DD, Kopans D, et al. Breast cancer screening with imaging: recommendations from the Society of Breast Imaging and the ACR on the use of mammography, breast MRI, breast ultrasound, and other technologies for the detection of clinically occult breast cancer. J Am Coll Radiol 2010;7(1):18–27

Linden SS, Sickles EA. Sedimented calcium in benign breast cysts: the full spectrum of mammographic presentations. AJR Am J Roentgenol 1989;152(5):967–971

Lindström S, Vachon CM, Li J, et al. Common variants in ZNF365 are associated with both mammographic density and breast cancer risk. Nat Genet 2011;43(3):185–187

Lowry SJ, Aiello Bowles EJ, Anderson ML, Buist DS. Predictors of breast density change after hormone therapy cessation: results from a randomized trial. Cancer Epidemiol Biomarkers Prev 2011;20(10):2309–2312

McCormack VA, dos Santos Silva I. Breast density and parenchymal patterns as markers of breast cancer risk: a meta-analysis. Cancer Epidemiol Biomarkers Prev 2006;15(6):1159–1169

Mainiero MB, Goldkamp A, Lazarus E, et al. Characterization of breast masses with sonography: can biopsy of some solid masses be deferred? J Ultrasound Med. 2005;24(2):161–167

Mendelson EB. Problem-solving ultrasound. Radiol Clin North Am 2004;42(5):909–918, vii

Moy L, Elias K, Patel V, et al. Is breast MRI helpful in the evaluation of inconclusive mammographic findings? AJR Am J Roentgenol 2009;193(4):986–993

Müller-Schimpfle M, Ohmenhaüser K, Stoll P, Dietz K, Claussen CD. Menstrual cycle and age: influence on parenchymal contrast medium enhancement in MR imaging of the breast. Radiology 1997;203(1):145–149

Njor SH, Hallas J, Schwartz W, Lynge E, Pedersen AT. Type of hormone therapy and risk of misclassification at mammography screening. Menopause 2011;18(2):171–177

Nothacker M, Duda V, Hahn M, et al. Early detection of breast cancer: benefits and risks of supplemental breast ultrasound in asymptomatic women with mammographically dense breast tissue. A systematic review. BMC Cancer 2009;9:335–344

Olsen AH, Bihrmann K, Jensen MB, Vejborg I, Lynge E. Breast density and outcome of mammography screening: a cohort study. Br J Cancer 2009;100(7):1205–1208

Pearce MS, Tennant PW, Mann KD, et al. Lifecourse predictors of mammographic density: the Newcastle Thousand Families Cohort Study. Breast Cancer Res Treat 2012;131(1):187–195

Peng S, Lü B, Ruan W, Zhu Y, Sheng H, Lai M. Genetic polymorphisms and breast cancer risk: evidence from meta-analyses, pooled analyses, and genome-wide association studies. Breast Cancer Res Treat 2011;127(2):309–324

Rosen EL, Smith-Foley SA, DeMartini WB, Eby PR, Peacock S, Lehman CD. BI-RADS MRI enhancement characteristics of ductal carcinoma in situ. Breast J 2007;13(6):545–550

Sardanelli F, Giuseppetti GM, Panizza P, et al; Italian Trial for Breast MR in Multifocal/Multicentric Cancer. Sensitivity of MRI versus mammography for detecting foci of multifocal, multicentric breast cancer in fatty and dense breasts using the whole-breast pathologic examination as a gold standard. AJR Am J Roentgenol 2004;183(4):1149–1157

Sardanelli F, Boetes C, Borisch B, et al. Magnetic resonance imaging of the breast: recommendations from the EUSOMA working group. Eur J Cancer 2010;46(8):1296–1316

Skaane P, Engedal K. Analysis of sonographic features in the differentiation of fibroadenoma and invasive ductal carcinoma. AJR Am J Roentgenol 1998;170(1):109–114

Soo MS, Rosen EL, Baker JA, Vo TT, Boyd BA. Negative predictive value of sonography with mammography in patients with palpable breast lesions. AJR Am J Roentgenol 2001;177(5):1167–1170

Stavros AT, Thickman D, Rapp CL, Dennis MA, Parker SH, Sisney GA. Solid breast nodules: use of sonography to distinguish between benign and malignant lesions. Radiology 1995;196(1):123–134

Stone J, Ding J, Warren RM, Duffy SW, Hopper JL. Using mammographic density to predict breast cancer risk: dense area or percentage dense area. Breast Cancer Res 2010;12(6):R97

Tamimi RM, Byrne C, Colditz GA, Hankinson SE. Endogenous hormone levels, mammographic density, and subsequent risk of breast cancer in postmenopausal women. J Natl Cancer Inst 2007;99(15):1178–1187

Tice JA, Cummings SR, Smith-Bindman R, Ichikawa L, Barlow WE, Kerlikowske K. Using clinical factors and mammographic breast density to estimate breast cancer risk: development and validation of a new predictive model. Ann Intern Med 2008;148(5):337–347

Uematsu T, Yuen S, Kasami M, Uchida Y. Dynamic contrast-enhanced MR imaging in screening detected microcalcification lesions of the breast: is there any value? Breast Cancer Res Treat 2007;103(3):269–281

van Gils CH, Otten JD, Verbeek AL, Hendriks JH, Holland R. Effect of mammographic breast density on breast cancer screening performance: a study in Nijmegen, the Netherlands. J Epidemiol Community Health 1998;52(4):267–271

Wellings SR, Alpers CE. Subgross pathologic features and incidence of radial scars in the breast. Hum Pathol 1984;15(5):475–479

Young KC, Wallis MG, Blanks RG, Moss SM. Influence of number of views and mammographic film density on the detection of invasive cancers: results from the NHS Breast Screening Programme. Br J Radiol 1997;70(833):482–488

Zakhireh J, Gomez R, Esserman L. Converting evidence to practice: a guide for the clinical application of MRI for the screening and management of breast cancer. Eur J Cancer 2008;44(18):2742–2752

11 Cysts

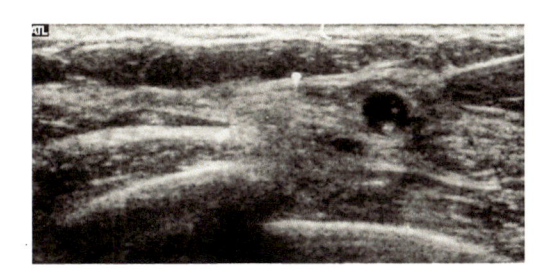

Histology → 276
Definition → 276

Medical History and Clinical Findings → 276

Breast Examination → 276

Objectives of Diagnostic Studies → 276

Diagnostic Strategy → 278
Sonography → 278
Aspiration of the Cyst → 281
Pneumocystography → 282
Mammography → 282
Magnetic Resonance Imaging → 282

Galactoceles and Oil Cysts → 284
Definitions → 284

References and Recommended Reading → 286

11 Cysts
I. Schreer, S. H. Heywang-Koebrunner, S. Barter

Cysts are by far the most common mass in the female breast. Approximately half of all women aged 30 to 40 years and older develop fibrocystic changes in the breast that manifest themselves in single or multiple cysts of varying sizes. Larger cysts occur in 20–25% of all women. Simple cysts are benign lesions.

Cysts become clinically important when the patient presents with pain, or when palpable findings require further diagnostic studies to determine if they are benign or malignant. Asymptomatic cysts may also be initially detected by mammography or sonography.

Cysts can simulate tumors—particularly if they are not well defined or if their borders are indistinct—and conceal malignancy.

Histology

Cysts are locally distended peripheral ductal segments filled with fluid. They usually occur in the terminal ductal lobular units and are associated with fibrocystic changes in the breast. While simple cysts are always benign, "complicated cysts" can sometimes harbor malignancy.

Definition

Simple cysts consist of two layers of cells, an inner layer of epithelial cells and an outer layer of myoepithelial cells. They are benign processes that are not associated with an increased risk of cancer.

The term "complicated cysts" refers collectively to cysts or conglomerate cysts detected in imaging studies or by clinical examination that are complicated by inflammation or bleeding or contain neoplastic tissue changes in their wall or lumen. In the widest sense of the term, these include cavities containing hemorrhage and necrotic carcinomas.

Simple cysts are usually lined with linear epithelium surrounded by a layer of compressed connective tissue. Like the surrounding fibrocystic disease, the cyst wall can exhibit various forms of epithelial hyperplasia, sometimes even atypia. The risk of malignant degeneration depends only on the cellular changes of the underlying fibrocystic alterations. Simple cysts themselves are not premalignant lesions.

Complicated cysts have a heterogeneous origin, occurring in either preformed cavities (lactiferous ducts or cysts) or in cavities resulting from necrosis or bleeding. Inflammatory changes in cysts occur in retention cysts or in the presence of chronic mastitis. Cystic cavities can also develop in centrally necrotic tumors, or they can occur as a result of secretion and recurrent bleeding, as in intraductal papillomas and papillary carcinomas.

Medical History and Clinical Findings

Cysts can be totally asymptomatic. As they become larger, they manifest themselves as palpable findings, sometimes associated with breast pain.

Cysts are typically seen to develop acutely. They may wax and wane. However, based on the patient's history, it is mostly impossible to distinguish a suddenly developed cyst from a slowly developed lesion (e.g., carcinoma) that has just been noticed by the patient.

Generally, cysts will first appear after the age of 30 or 40, occurring with peak frequency in premenopausal and perimenopausal women between the ages of 40 and 45.

In women under 40 and especially under 30, fibroadenomas tend to occur more frequently than cysts; after 40, the opposite is true. Since the risk of cancer is also higher in this age group, special care should be taken to exclude the possibility of breast cancer in these patients.

Breast Examination

Cysts are generally palpable as smooth-contoured, mobile masses. Most frequently, they are firm and somewhat compressible. However, they can also manifest themselves as hard masses. Distinguishing a cyst from a malignant growth can be difficult, particularly in the presence of conglomerate cysts and surrounding inflammation. Since some malignancies are relatively smooth contoured and mobile, further diagnostic studies are always indicated in the presence of a clinical diagnosis of suspected breast cysts.

Objectives of Diagnostic Studies

1. To differentiate between simple cysts and noncystic changes, such as benign tumors or breast cancer (the most important diagnosis to be excluded).
2. To distinguish simple cysts from other cystic masses. These include complicated cysts accompanied by inflammation, papilloma, or proliferative changes, as well as cystic carcinomas (mural cancer growing into a cyst and carcinomas with central necrosis that can have the appearance of a cystic mass) (**Fig. 11.1**).

If a simple cyst is confirmed, further diagnostic studies will not be necessary. In the presence of complicated cysts or solid masses, further studies are essential, and if necessary the mass should be biopsied.

Objectives of Diagnostic Studies

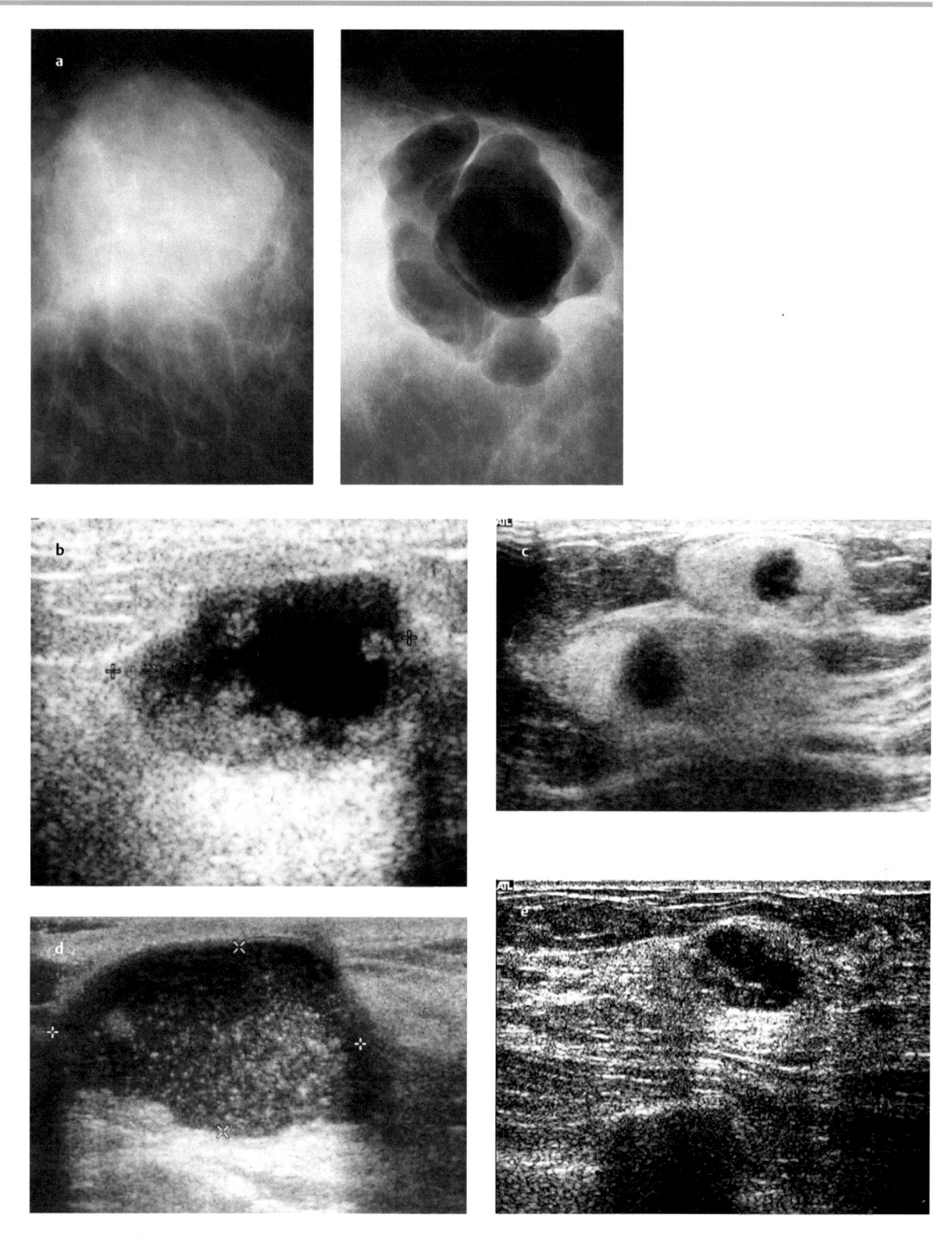

Fig. 11.1a–g Differential diagnosis of cystic lesions.

a,b Round, posteriorly ill-defined mass. The left image (**a**) shows the initial mammographic appearance. The right image demonstrates the lesion on mammography after aspiration of the necrotic contents and air filling (pneumocystography). Pneumocystography is no longer used today, but in this case it illustrates nicely the many septations and the irregular inner surface of this complex cystic mass. The sonographic image (**b**) reveals nodular structures projecting into the cyst. *Histology*: Intracystic papillary carcinoma. Note that, because of the necrotic contents, cytology may even be negative.

Fig. 11.1f,g ▷

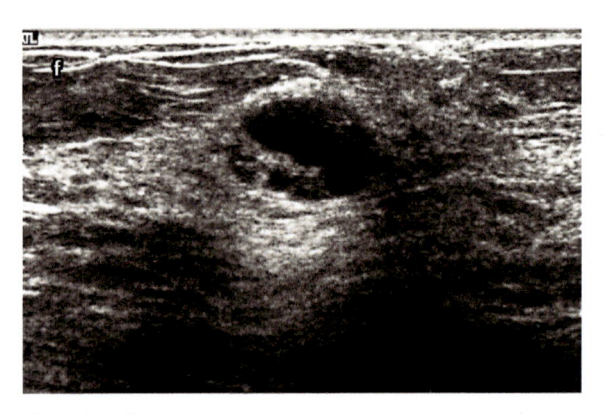

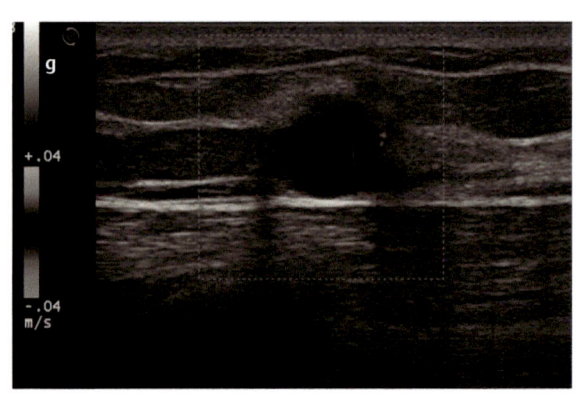

◁ continued

c Two roundish, very hypoechoic lesions surrounded by broad echogenic rims correspond to fresh hematomas due to coumarin treatment.
d Organizing postsurgical hematoma.
e,f This complex lesion (**e**) (image without compounding) is much better delineated using spatial compounding (**f**). It corresponded to an old post-treatment hematoma.
g This nearly anechoic lesion with posterior enhancement, but not clearly delineated, was a mucinous carcinoma on histology.

Diagnostic Strategy

Sonography is the method of choice for diagnosing cysts.

In women under 40, sonography should be the initial imaging study in the workup of a palpable lump. If it confirms that the mass is a cyst, the workup is completed. If the cyst is painful and conservative treatment does not lead to sufficient resolution of symptoms, aspiration may be considered for symptomatic relief. However, aspiration is not generally recommended. The reason is that, after the pressure is relieved, new cysts may develop or the initial cyst may recur. The patient should be informed and understand that the cyst is a symptom of a benign change. The cyst itself is not associated with an increased risk of breast cancer.

If the diagnosis of a cyst is equivocal sonographically, aspiration should be attempted. If aspiration is not possible, further assessment (usually core needle biopsy; in special cases vacuum-assisted breast biopsy [VABB] and rarely surgery) should be considered as the next step, since the lesion then probably represents a solid or complex cystic mass (see Chapter 4).

We consider VABB if the lesion is very small or situated in scarred tissue, or if a papillary lesion is suspected, since—in the case of a completely removed benign papilloma (classified as B3 lesion) or probably benign fibrotic tissue (classified as B1)—the need for a subsequent diagnostic excision may be averted (Heywang-Köbrunner et al. 2010).

In patients beyond age 40 the combined use of mammography and sonography should be considered in symptomatic women. This is recommended since the risk of malignancy increases beyond age 40. Changes (including development of a cyst) may rarely be associated with an adjacent malignancy that might be occult to ultrasound. Also, depending on the individual risk, mammography screening may be indicated, since beyond age 40 the incidence of malignancy rises.

In patients with frequently recurring masses, a repeat mammogram is not necessary if a recent mammogram is available and the new lump is proven to be a cyst based on the sonogram.

When mammographic and sonographic findings are consistent with a cyst, and malignancy is excluded in the remaining breast tissue as well, the workup is complete. If the lesion is solid, the diagnostic workup of solid masses is followed (see Chapter 24). If the diagnosis of a cyst is equivocal, and aspiration is attempted, the further workup will depend on the result of aspiration (see pp. 187–190)

In cases with large equivocal cysts it may be useful to perform ultrasound-guided aspiration first and then proceed with mammography. After cyst aspiration the mammogram may be less painful. Also, after eliminating superimposition by the cyst, mammographic density will decrease, which may improve mammographic assessment.

Sonography

(See **Fig. 11.2**.)

Unit Settings / Examination Technique

Optimum unit settings are particularly important in diagnosing cysts. If the gain is set too low, solid hypoechoic processes can appear anechoic, which can lead to serious diagnostic errors.

Diagnostic Strategy

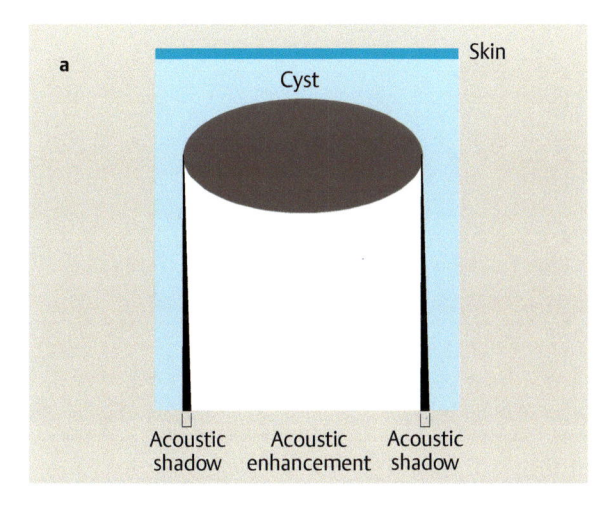

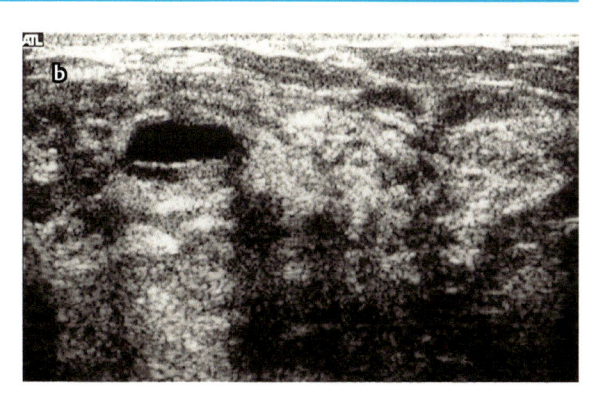

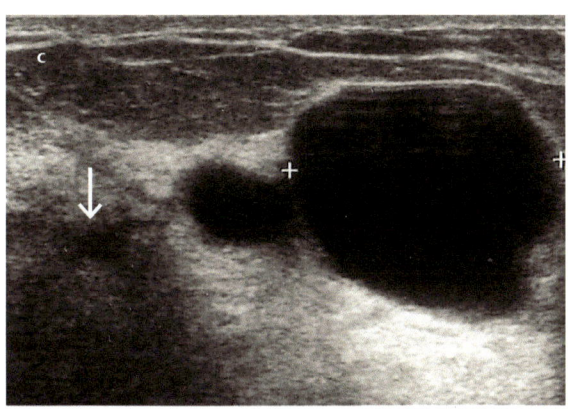

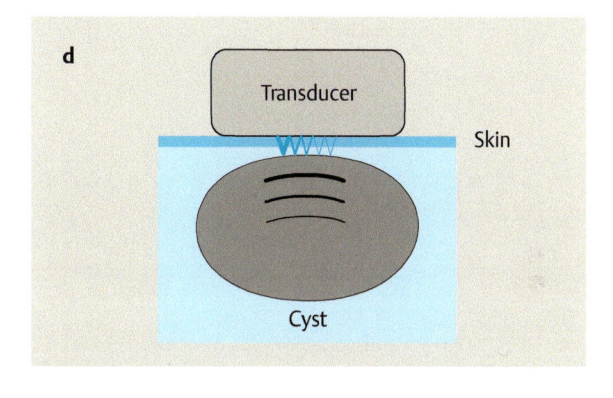

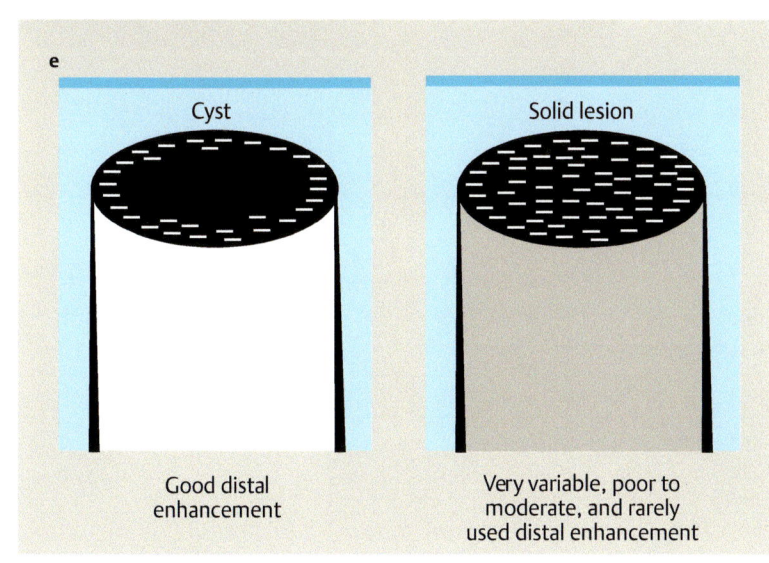

Fig. 11.2a–m Sonographic appearance of cysts.

a Schematic drawing of a typical cyst: The typical cyst is anechoic with pronounced distal enhancement. Fine lateral acoustic shadowing can occur at the margins.
b Sonographic image of a small cyst that mammography was unable to detect in dense tissue (see **Fig. 11.3a–d**).
c Sonographic image of a large cyst and a partly imaged cyst on the left. Another extremely small cyst, only partially visible in this imaging plane, is suspected (arrow).
d Reverberation echo occurring at the wall of the cyst: Echoes are repeatedly reflected between the transducer and the anterior wall of the cyst. The ultrasound system registers echoes that are reflected twice (or several times) as if they came from twice (or several times) as deep in the tissue.
e In genuine cysts, increasing the gain produces echoes beginning at the periphery, that is, the cyst appears to "fill in" from the periphery.

Fig. 11.2f–m ▷

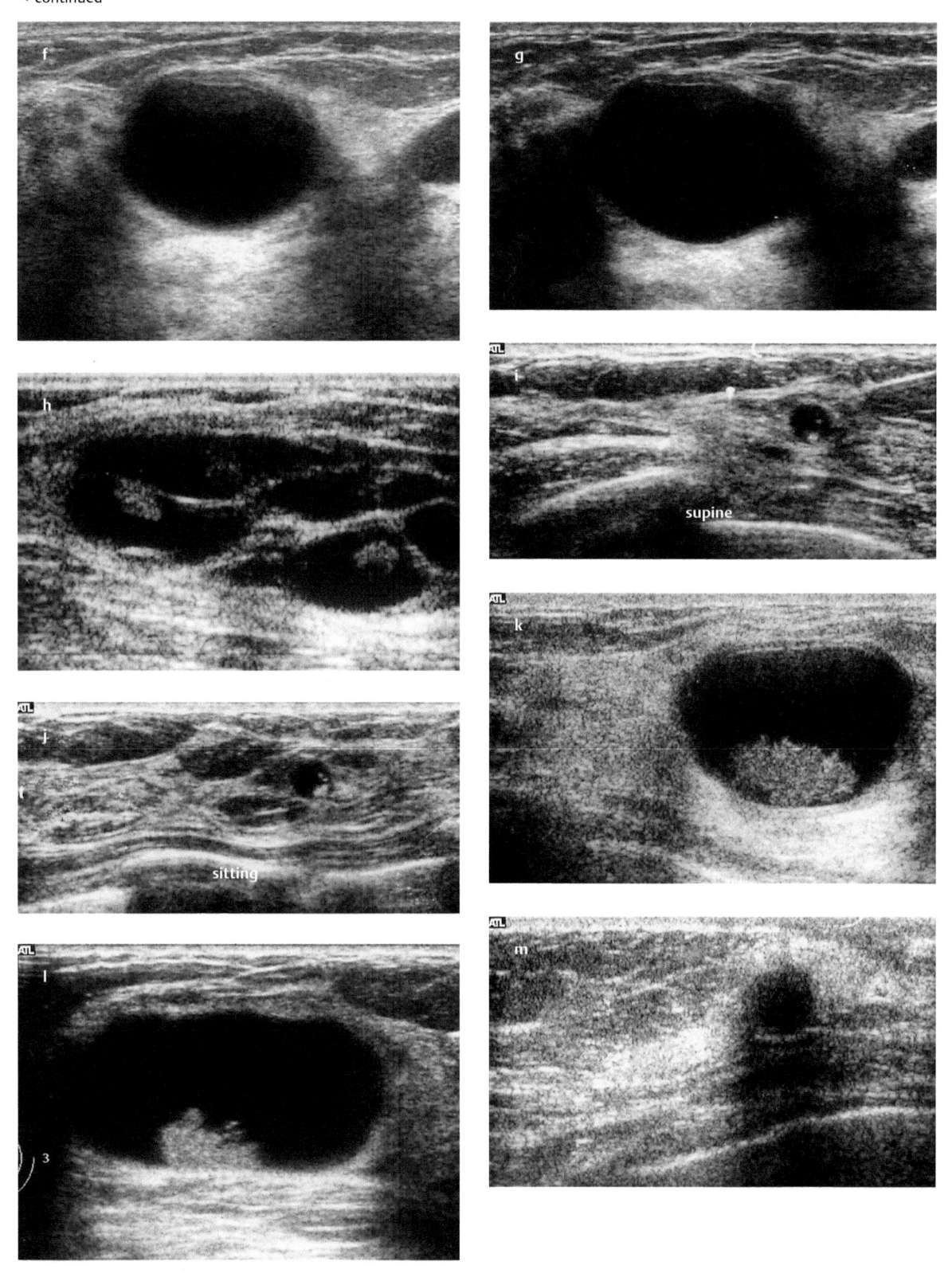

11 Cysts

◁ continued

f Cyst visualized with increased gain. The echoes fill in from the periphery of the cyst, but a few reverberation echoes are visible in the cyst near the transducer as well. The echoes that fill in from the periphery of the cyst make it appear to shrink (cf. **Fig. 11.1g**).
g The same cyst with reduced gain. No echoes are seen in the cyst. However, distal enhancement remains readily visible.
h Septa in the cyst can be visualized by rotating and angling the transducer accordingly. In this case multiple intracystic, roundish, echogenic lesions were visible corresponding to small papillomas.

i,j Small intracystic particles can be proven to be mobile by additional investigation in the sitting position: Supine (**i**); sitting (**j**).
k Intracystic debris may be indistinguishable from solid lesions. In this case, too, it could be distinguished from a real solid lesion by compressing and observing movement.
l This image demonstrates intracystic echoes caused by a real intracystic lesion. *Histology*: papillary hyperplasia.
m Calcified cysts are ill defined and hypoechoic and show sound attenuation.

In case of doubt, the following simple technique can be helpful (**Fig. 11.2e–g**). Gradually increase the gain on the unit until the echoes in the lesion begin to appear:
- Typically, cysts will fill with echoes from the periphery, whereas echoes in solid structures will simultaneously increase at different places within the mass.
- Occasionally, reverberation echoes will also be visible in cysts. They are more prominent in the upper part of the cyst adjacent to its leading wall and are parallel to the transducer. (Reverberation echoes are artifacts and do not represent tissue in the cyst.)

Turning and tilting the transducer can visualize the entire length of septa, making it possible to distinguish them from intracystic processes (**Fig. 11.2h**). Changing the patient's position and repeating the examination can be helpful in identifying sedimentation, which layers in the dependent portion of the cyst appearing as hypoechoic material on its floor.

Typical Appearance

(See **Fig. 11.2a–g**.)
The simple cyst is characterized by its smooth thin wall, absence of internal echoes, and distal enhancement. The walls of the cyst are smooth. Fine acoustic shadowing can extend from the lateral walls.

Unusual Features

If an acoustic shadow, which does not correspond to a fine side-wall shadow and cannot be explained by a mammographically visible large calcification, appears to arise from the wall of the cyst, the possibility of malignancy in, or directly adjacent to, the wall of the cyst must be considered.

If the contents of the cyst are not completely anechoic or if adequate acoustic enhancement is not present behind the cyst, it does not meet the criteria for a simple cyst. Some simple cysts of the breast may not appear as such on ultrasound examination.

If echoes are detected within the cyst, the examiner should above all consider the following questions:
- Can sedimentation, blood clots, or septa be identified?
- Does the cyst contain a tumorous process?
- Does the image not show a cyst at all, but a solid process?

In such cases the major differential diagnostic considerations include:
- High-protein, inflamed, or blood-filled cysts (**Fig. 11.3a,b**)
- Intracystic papillomas (see also **Figs. 14.6** and **14.7**) or malignancies that partially or completely fill the cyst
- Extremely hypoechoic benign tumors such as fibroadenomas
- Some malignancies, particularly a medullary carcinoma, which can occasionally appear very hypoechoic (**Figs. 11.2k** and **11.1a,b**)

Diagnostic Accuracy

When due care is exercised, sonography is highly accurate in diagnosing cysts. Depending on the sonography unit and transducer, even very small cysts measuring 1–2 mm in diameter can be identified and diagnosed. However, only typical findings should be classified as cysts. If any doubt remains, further diagnostic studies are indicated.

In the case of very small cysts (which due to partial volume effect may sometimes be difficult to diagnose with certainty), or if a suspected cyst does not meet all criteria for a cyst (some high-resolution ultrasound units tend to display echoes in many cysts), follow-up sonography might be considered to avoid biopsy of too many benign lesions.

Aspiration of the Cyst

Aspirating the cyst is the next step if sonography fails to reveal typical cyst findings or if the cyst is to be decompressed to relieve symptoms.

If, sonographically, the needle tip proves to be within the lesion and aspiration is unsuccessful, a solid tumor must be suspected (differential diagnosis, see Chapter 24).

Cysts may contain clear, yellowish, greenish, brownish or even black-tainted fluid, sometimes with increased protein content or with hemoglobin breakdown products. There is some controversy over whether all aspirated fluids need to be submitted to cytology. The vast majority of the findings from these cytologic examinations are negative, while numerous indeterminate findings due to necrotic material may cause unnecessary further workup. Furthermore, the cytologic examination of cysts with a mural carcinoma or necrotic tumor is frequently unreliable because the contents of such cystic lesions often just contain necrotic cells from which malignancy cannot be diagnosed.

If the clinical or imaging findings, or the fluid aspirated, are not consistent with a simple cyst (e.g., green or yellow fluid), cytologic examination must be performed. The usual cytology of a cyst is apocrine metaplasia.

However, when imaging findings show a solid lesion in a cyst or suggest that it corresponds to a necrotic mass, a negative cytology should never dissuade the physician from a biopsy.

If blood is present in the contents of the cyst, then the possibility of an intracystic papilloma or cancer should be considered in addition to possible iatrogenic introduction of blood. In the presence of inconclusive sonographic findings, or findings suggesting malignancy, a biopsy is indicated to verify the diagnosis.

If cytologic examination reveals atypical cells or groups of papillary cells, further workup of the cyst (which will usually fill up again) is necessary. The same applies if an intracystic tumor has been verified sonographically.

For some pathologists the differentiation of various papillary lesions may be difficult, with the small volume of tissue obtained with percutaneous biopsy procedures. In this setting VABB (which should attempt to remove the entire lesion) or surgical excision of these lesions is desirable because papillary lesions represent the majority of intracystic masses. If these diagnoses are readily made by consulting pathologists on the basis of percutaneous biopsy procedures, they should be performed when histologic assessment of these lesions is needed. However, because there is sometimes difficulty in establishing an exact diagnosis at pathology, the assessment of such lesions in general and in each individual case must be agreed by the interdisciplinary team.

Pneumocystography

Pneumocystography (**Fig. 11.1a** and **11.3b**) can be performed through the aspiration needle following aspiration of the cyst (see Chapter 3, pp. 92–93 for examination technique). In current clinical practice it is, however, rarely needed. The combination of attempted cyst aspiration followed by percutaneous breast biopsy has largely replaced pneumocystography and promises higher accuracy.

Typical Appearance

Typically, a simple cyst is oval or round, with a smooth thin wall. In the presence of inflammation, the wall may appear thickened but the inner wall will not usually show any irregularities. Papillomas, carcinomas of the wall of the cyst, and necrotic carcinomas can be identified as solid irregularities in the wall (**Figs. 11.1a,b**). Any deviation from the usual finding of a thin-walled cyst requires further assessment (at least core needle biopsy).

Indications

The high accuracy of sonography has largely eliminated the use of pneumocystography.

The diagnostic value or indication for diagnostic pneumocystography is a matter of controversy. Some investigators use it therapeutically, since it may have a favorable effect on involution of the cyst (prevents refilling and improves adhesion due to the pressure exerted by the air, which is gradually resorbed).

Mammography

(See **Fig. 11.3**.)

Cysts surrounded by fatty tissue usually appear as round or oval, well-circumscribed masses on the mammogram.

If they are partially or completely surrounded by breast parenchyma, the cysts can appear as a nonspecific mass or as a smooth-contoured or partially obscured mass. They may also be invisible when completely surrounded by dense parenchyma. Owing to compression of adjacent fat, cysts can sometimes have a partial or complete halo sign. When a mass that may be a cyst is palpable, it is helpful to place a radiographic skin marker over the mass to help to identify it on the mammogram. The mass may appear indistinct if the cyst is inflamed. It may also be indistinct after previous infections. Unless acute inflammation exists and therapy resolves the symptoms, further assessment (sonography, possibly aspiration or needle biopsy) should be considered.

A thin, semicircular calcification may appear in the wall of a cystic process (such as a calcified oil cyst, calcified sebaceous cyst, or calcified simple cyst) or along the periphery (semicircular-appearing level of milk of calcium). In rare cases, calcification of the wall can be due to bleeding into cysts. Particular care should be taken to exclude a small intracystic tumor via sonography.

Magnetic Resonance Imaging

Indication and Diagnostic Accuracy

Diagnosis or exclusion of cysts is not an indication for breast magnetic resonance imaging (MRI). However, if a contrast-enhanced MRI study conducted for other reasons reveals cysts, malignant growths in simple cysts can be easily excluded by the absence of enhancement.

Examination Technique

In contrast to what some regard as standard practice, we see hardly any need for using T2-weighted images. On these images, cysts typically exhibit extremely high and homogeneous signal intensity. To exclude safely other smooth-contoured lesions with high water content (such as mucinous carcinoma or a phyllodes tumor) that can have a similar appearance, a T2-weighted multiecho sequence or the usual T1-weighted pulse sequence before and after intravenous injection of a contrast medium will be required anyway and is more important.

Typical Appearance

In the customary T1-weighted pulse sequence before and after intravenous contrast-medium injection, simple cysts have the following MRI appearance: in the precontrast T1-weighted image, they typically exhibit a smooth contour and extremely low signal intensity. If the cyst contains old blood products (especially methemoglobin), the contents of the cyst can have a high signal intensity, or rarely a fluid level on the T1-weighted image. Its signal on the T2-weighted image may be low in these cases. The decisive criterion is the enhancement behavior. If the lesion enhances, it is not compatible with a cyst but must

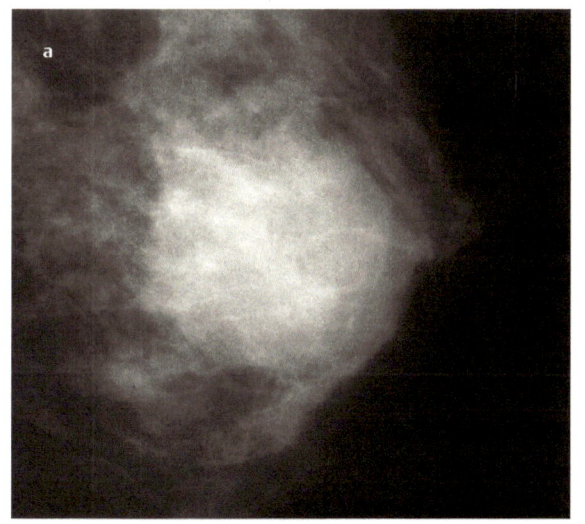

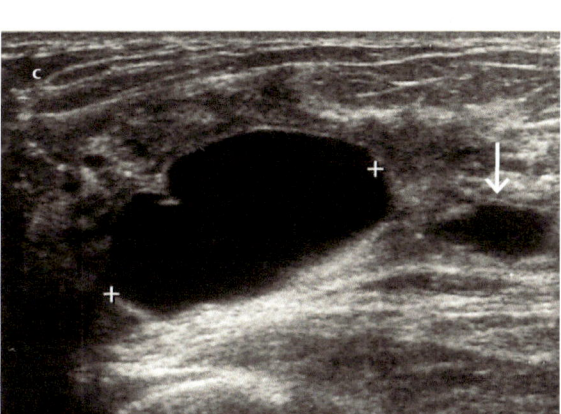

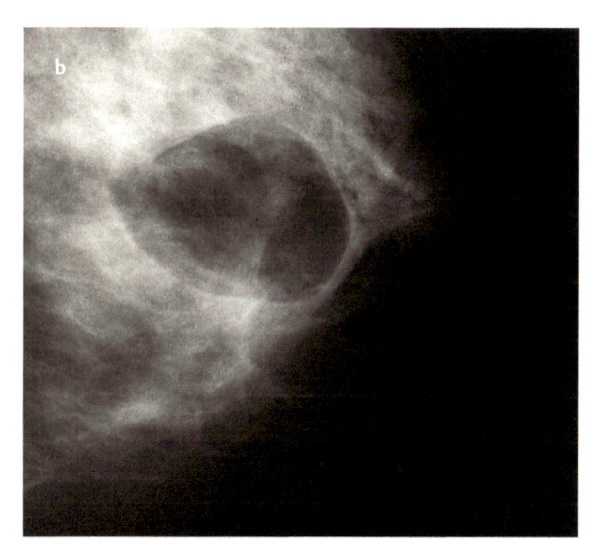

Fig. 11.3a–c Mammographic appearance of cysts.
a Painful mass, not entirely anechoic in the sonographic image. Suspected cyst (DD: centrally necrotic tumor), ill defined on the mammogram.
b Pneumocystography reveals smooth inner contour of the wall. Surgery followed aggravation of symptoms. *Histology*: Inflamed cysts.
c Sonographic image of the large cyst with excellent posterior enhancement. Another smaller cyst (arrow) is shown adjacent to it. The posterior enhancement of this second cyst is less obvious because of its smaller size and possibly some proteinaceous contents. Also, sometimes, the posterior enhancement is not well seen when a cyst is close to the posterior fascia.

11 Cysts

represent a solid mass. Enhancement of walls without focal thickening is a sign of inflammation or mastopathic changes.

Papillomas and carcinomas in the wall of the cyst generally appear as an irregularity in the contour of the wall with moderate to intense contrast enhancement.

Galactoceles and Oil Cysts

Definitions

A *galactocele* is a single or multichambered, milk-filled retention cyst. Galactoceles develop during pregnancy or lactation, and in newborns and infants, due to disturbed absorption of the so-called witch's milk (infantile galactoceles).

On mammography, galactoceles appear as follows (**Fig. 11.4a**):
- They can be hidden in dense glandular tissue, or can appear as round or oval masses (similar to a cyst). They may be of fatty rather than water density.
- A typical but infrequent sign is an oil–fluid level in the 90° lateral mammogram. The fluid surface appears as a horizontal border between the transparent fatty and nonfatty fluid.

On sonography, galactoceles appear as follows:
- Like cysts, they are single or multichambered, mostly well-circumscribed masses.
- Depending on the consistency of the milk in the galactocele, the contents can be anechoic or hypoechoic, homogeneous or inhomogeneous (**Fig. 11.4b**). Good distal enhancement can be present, as can attenuation (**Fig. 11.4b**).

An *oil cyst* is a cystic mass that contains oily necrotic material. Oil cysts are usually associated with a history of previous trauma or surgery. Some galactoceles may turn into oil cysts. Clinically, oil cysts are usually palpable as nonmobile masses mostly located within tissue thickening. They are, therefore, often a reason for concern.

On mammography oil cysts appear as follows (**Fig. 11.5a,b**):
- They are visible as a radiolucent mass with smooth internal margins. The mass may also appear as a conglomerate of radiolucent masses with smooth internal margins with or without smooth septations.
- The mass is surrounded by a capsule, which is always smooth, may be thickened, and may blend with the surrounding tissues.
- Typical eggshell-like calcifications may develop in the capsule.

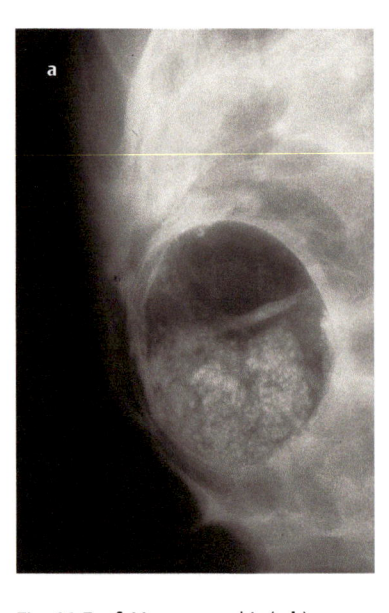

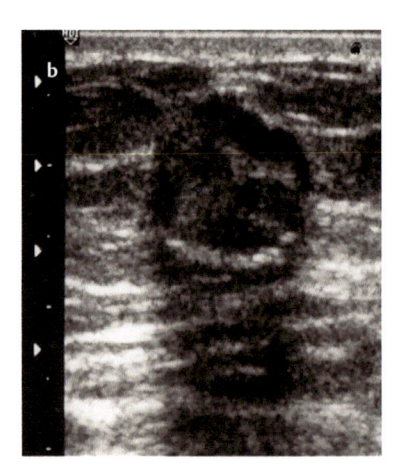

Fig. 11.4a,b Galactocele.
a Clinically smooth-contoured mass 4 months after nursing. Mammography reveals a large, oval, smooth-contoured radiolucent area ~3 cm in diameter. The lucent area is probably air that has entered the galactocele via the lactiferous ducts. The contents of the galactocele are coarsely granular and partly calcified, compatible with a saponifying galactocele.
b This galactocele in a different patient was not apparent on the mammogram. Sonographically it has the appearance of a complex mass.

Fig. 11.5a–f Mammographic (**a,b**), sonographic (**c,d**) and MRI (**e,f**) delineation of oil cysts.
a Mammography. Status 1-year post reduction mammoplasty. Two oil cysts are visualized as sharply outlined, radiolucent lesions in the scar region (arrows).
b Mammography 12 months later. Both oil cysts are now surrounded by pleomorphic, linear, or ringlike calcifications, partially forming an eggshell-like pattern. Despite the pleomorphism of some of the individual calcifications, the finding itself is characteristic.
c,d Sonographically oil cysts show a complex structure with or without calcification and can be reliably detemined in conjunction with the mammographic image.
e,f The oil cyst presents as an oval mass in T1-weighted imaging with a low-intensity rim and high-intensity (fat) content. After contrast application (**f**) no contrast enhancement is visible, but some oil cysts may show a discrete rim enhancement.

Galactoceles and Oil Cysts

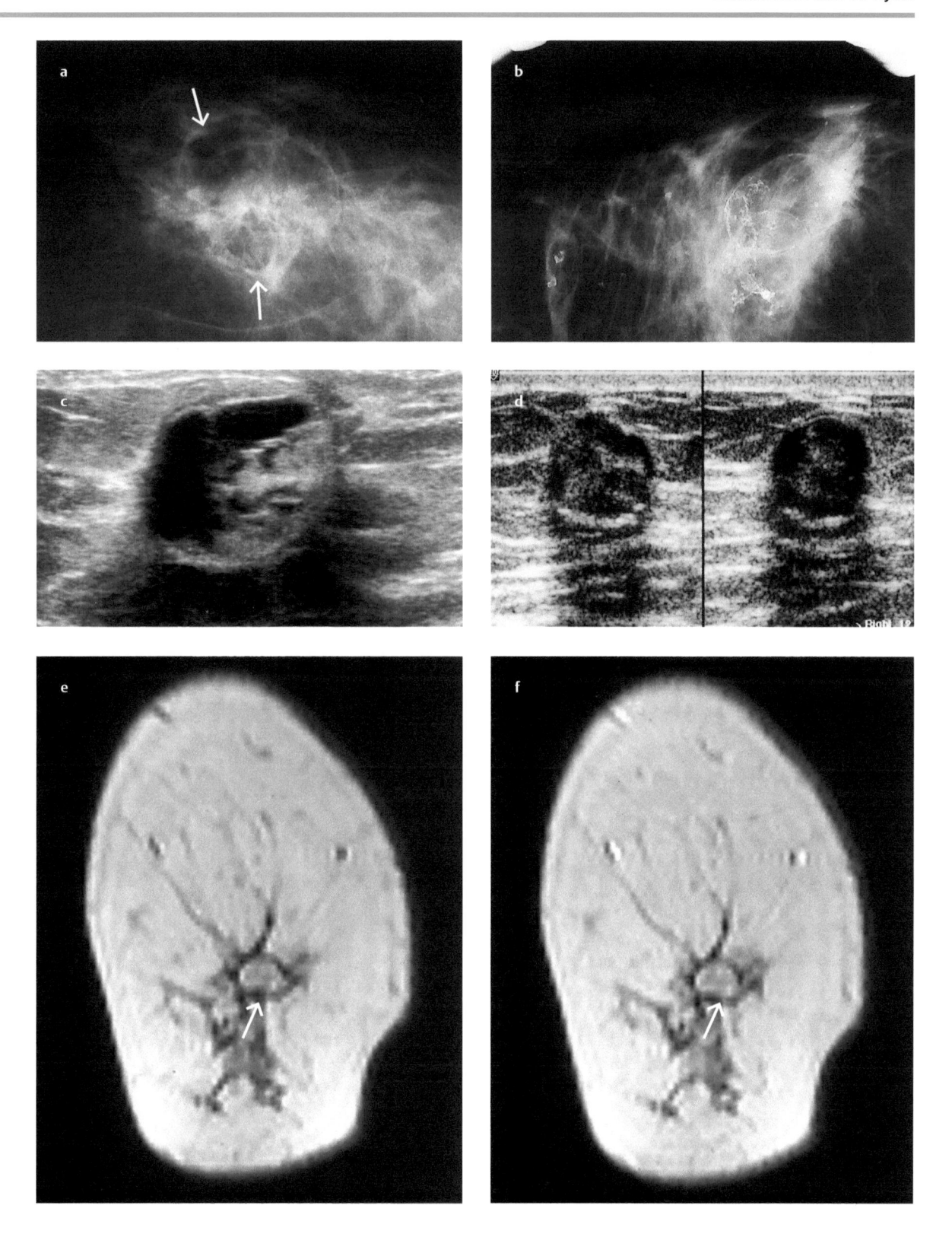

The above-described appearance is typical and requires no further workup, even if clinical findings may appear suspicious, or if it has been sonographically classified as an interdeterminate complex mass. Sometimes newly emerging calcifications may appear indeterminate to suspicious until they assume their characteristic eggshell-like appearance.

On sonography oil cysts may appear as follows (**Fig. 11.5c,d**):
- Relatively smoothly outlined hypoechoic lesions.
- Rarely as echogenic lesions (**Fig. 11.5c,d**).
- Sometimes they can contain echogenic material mimicking an intracystic tumor. This sonographic appearance can be due to the necrotic material and fibrin.
- The transmitted sound distal to the oil cyst can be unchanged, enhanced, or attenuated. Distal acoustic shadowing can be caused by sound-absorbing components within the necrotic contents, such as blood, or by calcifications in the wall of the oil cyst (**Fig. 11.5c,d**).

Although at least some of the sonographic features by themselves could be considered worrisome, no further workup is necessary whenever mammography shows a typical appearance.

On MRI (**Fig. 11.5e,f**) the oily content is identified by its high signal intensity on all pulse sequences (except fat-saturated pulse sequences). The internal wall is smooth. The capsule may enhance moderately with contrast agent. In the presence of a typical mammographic appearance this should not be interpreted as a sign of malignancy unless a definite nodule or mass is visualized within or beside the capsule.

In summary, mammography has to be considered the leading method for the diagnosis of oil cysts.

Summary
Sonography is the method of choice for the diagnosis of cysts. This method usually permits differentiation between simple and complicated cysts, which is crucial for further management.

Simple cysts appear as smooth-contoured, thin-walled anechoic masses with distal acoustic enhancement.

If the sonographic findings cannot be definitively categorized as simple cysts, the next step is aspiration of the cyst. Complex cystic lesions, however, require histopathologic assessment, usually core needle biopsy. Surgical biopsy or (for small lesions that can be removed) vacuum-assisted breast biopsy may be needed. Mammography is performed to further characterize the mass, if it is not a cyst, and to exclude malignancy in the rest of the breast.

Mammography is therefore indicated as the initial workup for a palpable mass in all symptomatic patients over the age of 40 years. In patients under 40, the workup should begin with sonography and needs to be complemented by mammography, unless sonography proves, for example, that the palpable mass is a simple cyst. In very young patients at low risk, aspiration or core needle biopsy may precede a mammogram.

Indications for biopsy include:
- Malignancy is suspected or cannot safely be excluded, as is the case when solid findings remain after aspiration, or when suspicious microcalcifications or other suspicious findings are detected close to the cyst or at another site.
- Sonographic or cytologic studies demonstrate or suggest the presence of intracystic proliferation.
- Blood is present in the contents of the cyst, unless it is felt to be iatrogenic.

References and Recommended Reading

Beer GM, Kompatscher P, Hergan K. Diagnosis of breast tumors after breast reduction. Aesthet Plast Surg 1996;20(5):391–397

Bilgen IG, Ustun EE, Memis A. Fat necrosis of the breast: clinical, mammographic and sonographic features. Eur J Radiol 2001;39(2):92–99

Carvajal J, Patiño JH. Mammographic findings after breast augmentation with autologous fat injection. Aesthet Surg J 2008;28(2):153–162

Del Vecchio DA, Bucky LP. Breast augmentation using preexpansion and autologous fat transplantation: a clinical radiographic study. Plast Reconstr Surg 2011;127(6):2441–2450

Dyreborg U, Blichert-Toft M, Boegh L, Kiaer H. Needle puncture followed by pneumocystography of palpable breast cysts. A controlled clinical trial. Acta Radiol Diagn (Stockh) 1985;26(3):277–281

Eidelman Y, Liebling RW, Buchbinder S, Strauch B, Goldstein RD. Mammography in the evaluation of masses in breasts reconstructed with TRAM flaps. Ann Plast Surg 1998;41(3):229–233

Gómez A, Mata JM, Donoso L, Rams A. Galactocele: three distinctive radiographic appearances. Radiology 1986;158(1):43–44

Haagensen CD. Diseases of the breast. 2nd ed. Philadelphia, PA: Saunders; 1986

Harvey JA, Moran RE, Maurer EJ, DeAngelis GA. Sonographic features of mammary oil cysts. J Ultrasound Med 1997;16(11):719–724

Heywang-Köbrunner SH, Beck R. Contrast-enhanced MRI of the breast. 2nd ed. Berlin, New York, Heidelberg: Springer; 1996

Heywang-Köbrunner SH, Nährig J, Hacker A, Sedlacek S, Höfler H. B3 lesions: radiological assessment and multi-disciplinary aspects. Breast Care (Basel) 2010;5(4):209–217

Hogge JP, Zuurbier RA, de Paredes ES. Mammography of autologous myocutaneous flaps. Radiographics 1999;19(Spec No.):S63–S72

Ikeda DM, Helvie MA, Adler DD, Schwindt LA, Chang AE, Rebner M. The role of fine-needle aspiration and pneumocystography in the treatment of impalpable breast cysts. AJR Am J Roentgenol 1992;158(6):1239–1241

Jackson VP. The role of US in breast imaging. Radiology 1990;177(2):305–311

Khaleghian R. Breast cysts: pitfalls in sonographic diagnosis. Australas Radiol 1993;37(2):192–194

Lee JM, Georgian-Smith D, Gazelle GS, et al. Detecting non palpable recurrent breast cancer: the role of routine mammographic screening of transverse rectus abdominis myocutaneous flap reconstructions. Radiology 2008;248(2):398–405

Mandrekas AD, Assimakopoulos GI, Mastorakos DP, Pantzalis K. Fat necrosis following breast reduction. Br J Plast Surg 1994;47(8):560–562

Ruch M, Brade J, Schoeber C, et al. Long-term follow-up-findings in mammography and ultrasound after intraoperative radiotherapy (IORT) for breast cancer. Breast 2009;18(5):327–334

Sabate JM, Clotet M, Torrubia S, et al. Radiologic evaluation of breast disorders related to pregnancy and lactation. Radiographics 2007;27(Suppl 1):S101–S124

Salvador R, Salvador M, Jimenez JA, Martinez M, Casas L. Galactocele of the breast: radiologic and ultrasonographic findings. Br J Radiol 1990;63(746):140–142

Sickles EA, Vogelaar PW. Fluid level in a galactocele seen on lateral projection mammogram with horizontal beam. Breast Dis 1981;7:32–33

Soo MS, Kornguth PJ, Hertzberg BS. Fat necrosis in the breast: sonographic features. Radiology 1998;206(1):261–269

Venta LA, Dudiak CM, Salomon CG, Flisak ME. Sonographic evaluation of the breast. Radiographics 1994;14(1):29–50

12 Benign Tumors and Tumorlike Masses

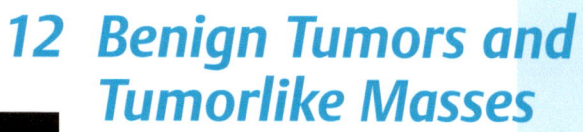

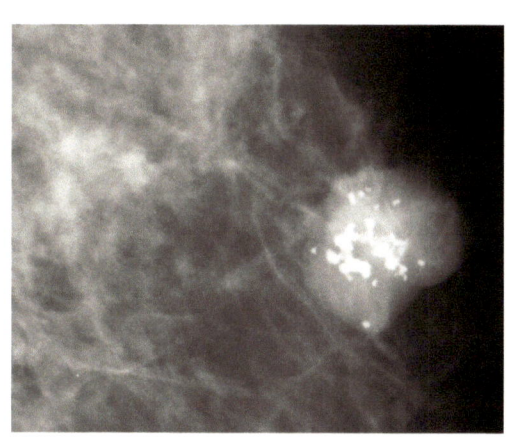

Hamartoma or Adenofibrolipoma → 290

Cowden Syndrome → 292

Fibroepithelial Mixed Tumors → 292
Fibroadenoma, Adenofibroma, Juvenile or Giant Fibroadenoma → 292
Papilloma → 306
Lipoma → 306

Rare Benign Tumors → 306
Leiomyoma, Neurofibroma, Neurilemmoma, Benign Spindle Cell Tumor (Myofibroblastoma), Chondroma, Osteoma → 306
Angiomas → 308
Granular Cell Tumor (Myoblastoma) → 309
Pseudoangiomatous Stromal Hyperplasia → 309

Benign Fibroses → 310
Focal Fibrous Disease or Fibrosis Mammae → 310
Amyloidosis of the Breast → 310
Steatocystoma Multiplex → 310
Intramammary Lymph Nodes → 310

References and Recommended Reading → 312

12 Benign Tumors and Tumorlike Masses

S. H. Heywang-Koebrunner, I. Schreer, S. Barter

Hamartoma or Adenofibrolipoma

The hamartoma of the breast is an abnormal collection of tissues that are normally found within the breast. It is surrounded by a pseudocapsule of compressed fat.

Histology

Hamartomas are demarcated from the surrounding tissue by a pseudocapsule of compressed fat and not by a connective tissue capsule. They are composed of the same elements as normal breast parenchyma. Hamartomas present as collections of parenchymal tissue (adenolipomas) and rarely as myoid hamartomas with smooth muscles, parenchyma, and fatty tissue. Hamartomas are benign. Malignancy is found no more frequently in hamartomas than in the respective breast parenchyma.

Clinical Findings

Hamartomas are usually nonpalpable, but like lipomas can present as soft, smoothly delineated mobile tumors. Rarely their consistency may be increased if they contain larger amounts of dense fibrous tissue. They are often only found mammographically.

Diagnostic Strategy

The diagnosis is usually made on mammography. A mammographically pathognomonic image, which is to be expected in the majority of the hamartomas, does not require further evaluation.

A mammographically atypical manifestation may undergo further evaluation by sonography.

A needle biopsy will only demonstrate normal breast tissue. The diagnosis of a hamartoma can be established only in an interdisciplinary conference by correlating the imaging and pathologic findings, ensuring that all are compatible with the diagnosis.

Mammography

Most hamartomas are definitively diagnosed by mammography (**Fig. 12.1a**). The following mammographic findings are pathognomonic:
- A smoothly demarcated mass that contains fat and soft tissue density comingled in varying amounts
- Smooth demarcation of the mass and a thin pseudocapsule seen in its entirety or in part
- The classic description of the pattern is that of a piece of "cut sausage"

If these findings are present, no further evaluation is indicated. Suspicious findings, such as microcalcifications, within a mammographically diagnosed hamartoma, of course, require clarification.

The mammographic finding is atypical if fat lobules cannot be identified due to inadequate fat content or if the nodule is not well demarcated. Features not distinctive enough to allow the diagnosis of a hamartoma must be differentiated from other causes of asymmetric glandular tissue.

Sonography

A mammographically unequivocal finding does not require sonography. If a mammographically suspected hamartoma is partially obscured by dense tissue, supplementary sonography might be helpful.

The sonographic diagnosis of a hamartoma (**Fig. 12.1b**), which should be made together with mammography, is based on the following findings:
- A smooth margin of the entire nodule with or without delicate acoustic shadows at the lateral wall
- Hypoechoic, smoothly marginated fat islands can be identified within the nodule
- The nodule must be compressible and easily moveable

Although some rare hamartomas may be firm, this is not typical, and therefore firm consistency on palpation should lead to further evaluation, usually core biopsy and histopathologic assessment.

Percutaneous Biopsy

Biopsy supports the exclusion of malignancy by demonstrating that components of the mass are that of normal breast tissue. The diagnosis of a "hamartoma" can only be established in an interdisciplinary conference if histology exhibits normal tissue, while the imaging findings are compatible. Certainty (in difficult cases with high amounts of dense tissue) may increase with increasing tissue volume. A definite diagnosis is also possible by excisional biopsy, which is only rarely needed.

Magnetic resonance imaging (MRI) is unnecessary for diagnosis of a hamartoma.

Hamartoma or Adenofibrolipoma

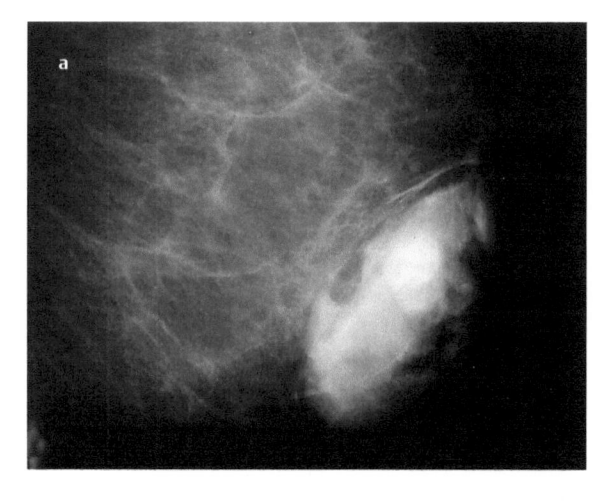

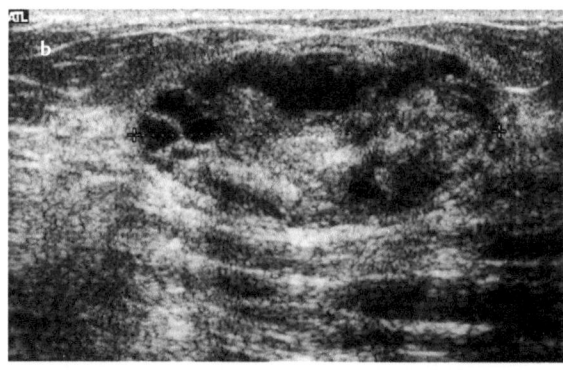

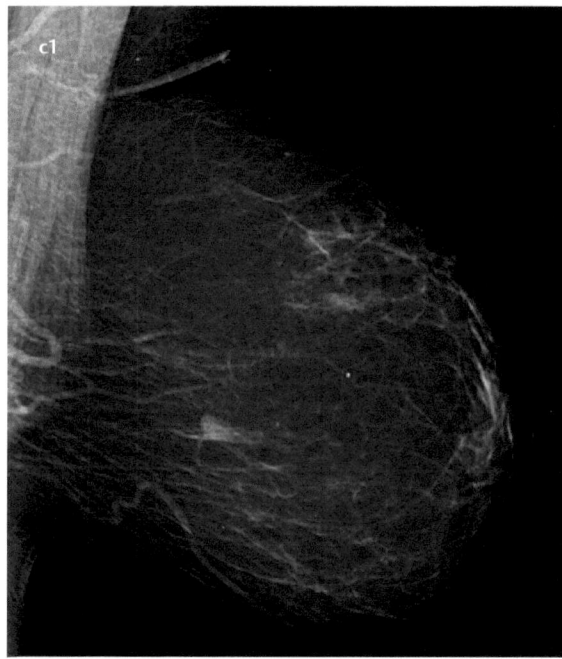

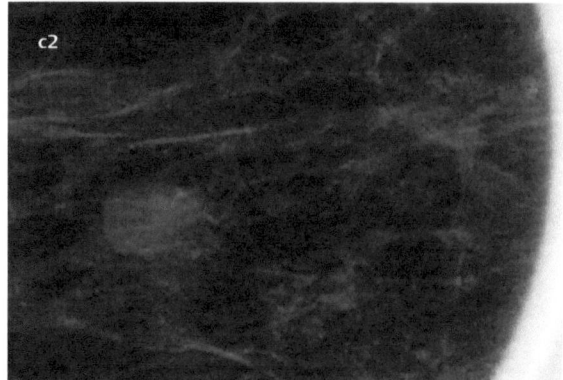

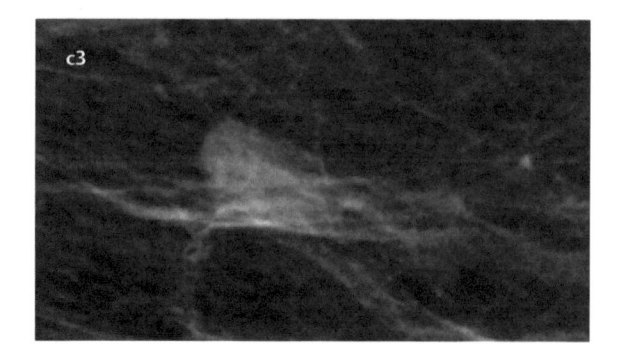

Fig. 12.1a–c Hamartoma.

a Mammography. The density of the hamartoma is variable, incorporating areas of fatty and soft tissue, surrounded by a thin pseudocapsule.

b Fat-containing lobules are sonographically hypoechoic. They are separated by hyperechoic septa of connective tissue and surrounded by a pseudocapsule, which is best seen distally. Good compressibility supports the diagnosis. The characteristic image shown here is sonographically not always as impressive. If the mammographic finding is typical, sonography is not necessary.

c Some hamartomas show atypical features and thus cannot be diagnosed by imaging: In this patient an oval lesion was detected on the screening mammogram. On additional views the lesion was not completely well circumscribed. Since the lesion was not visible on ultrasound imaging, vacuum-assisted breast biopsy was performed. After complete removal of the mammographic lesion, a diagnosis of a hamartoma was made based on imaging findings and histopathology.

12 Benign Tumors and Tumorlike Masses

Cowden Syndrome

Cowden syndrome is a very rare autosomal dominant genetic syndrome (PTEN germline mutation), which is characterized by multiple hamartomas in the body (gastrointestinal tract, genitourinary tract, central nervous system, skin, breast, and thyroid). Women with Cowden syndrome may present with multiple hamartomas, fibroadenomas, or adenomas in the breast. In male family members gynecomastia has been described. Recognition or exclusion of the syndrome (by a geneticist) is important, since these women are at high risk of being affected by breast cancer. They are also at increased risk of thyroid and endometrial cancer. Thus if Cowden syndrome is confirmed by a geneticist, both adequate counseling and surveillance, as suggested by international guidelines for women at high risk, is recommended (Sabaté et al. 2006, Cao et al. 2011).

Fibroepithelial Mixed Tumors

Fibroadenoma, Adenofibroma, Juvenile or Giant Fibroadenoma

The fibroadenoma is by far the most common tumor of the breast. It is important to know that the fibroadenoma occurs in all age groups, but that it is predominantly a lesion found in young women, even during puberty and adolescence. Fibroadenomas are hormone-induced hyperplastic tumors of the lobular connective tissue with the highest incidence between the ages of 25 and 35 years.

Because the incidence of fibroadenomas decreases after the age of 40 years, while that of carcinomas increases, a well-circumscribed malignancy, which is always a possibility, should be even more strongly considered if a smoothly marginated, solid lesion is newly discovered in a woman above the age of 40.

The fibroadenoma is a benign tumor. Only in rare instances (0.1–0.3%) are carcinomas, which are predominantly in situ, located within a fibroadenoma in any otherwise normal mammary tissue (Dupont et al. 1994).

Most fibroadenomas (~80%) show a smooth, round, or oval contour. Variations of the pattern, however, are not unusual. Certain malignancies can present as lesions that are similar in appearance.

The diagnostic relevance of the fibroadenoma rests on differentiating it from smoothly marginated malignant tumors.

Histology

Fibroadenoma

The fibroadenoma is a benign fibroepithelial mixed tumor, surrounded by a pseudocapsule and generally exhibiting an oval, round, or lobulated shape with a smooth surface.

Fibroadenomas are usually found in young women as solitary tumors about 1–3 cm in size.

Depending on the arrangement of the stromal and epithelial components, they are histologically divided into intracanalicular and pericanalicular tumors. This differentiation is clinically and prognostically irrelevant and also plays a secondary role in determining its presentation on imaging. Only minor differences in calcification pattern have been described.

Types characterized by edematous stroma correspond radiographically to "young" fibroadenomas.

They predominantly occur in young women and under hormonal stimulation, corresponding to fibroadenomas in the growth phase. They frequently show a high proportion of loose, edematous and mucopolysaccharide-containing stroma, and generally are well vascularized. The edematous stroma can compress the epithelial components. In addition, some fibroadenomas have hypercellular, adenomatous components. The "young" fibroadenoma is usually soft and easily compressible.

Focal or total sclerosis of the stroma occurs in "older fibroadenomas," which are predominantly diagnosed in older patients during or after menopause.

Sometimes extremely large fibroadenomas occur. These so-called giant fibroadenomas are more frequent before the age of 20 years. They have a strong growth tendency and must be differentiated histologically from a phyllodes tumor. All fibroadenomas are benign tumors. Irrespective of their speed of growth, all have a good prognosis and are adequately treated with simple excision.

Adenoma

Adenomas of the breast are rare, benign, usually solitary, and well-differentiated neoplasms characterized by a dominant ductulobular component and very scarce stroma. Adenomas are subject to hormonal regulation during pregnancy and lactation, and are further subclassified into tubular, lactating, ductal adenomas, and a few unusual types. Lactating adenomas frequently present as a palpable mass during the last months of pregnancy or during breast-feeding (see **Fig. 12.4i**). Their diagnosis is established by core needle biopsy. They mostly regress after lactation. If this is not the case, treatment by prolactin antagonists may be indicated (Cao et al. 2011). Adenomas are indistinguishable from fibroadenomas on imaging. Their imaging features will be presented together with the fibroadenomas (see **Fig. 12.4h**).

History

Fibroadenomas are often detected as a palpable finding but are also found mammographically. They rarely cause secretion. They can grow, decrease in size, or remain stationary through hormonal interaction.

Clinical Findings

Like the juvenile fibroadenoma, the "young" adult fibroadenoma feels smoothly marginated, elastic, and easily moveable on palpation. Some fibroadenomas may cause localized pain. "Old" fibroadenomas can be very firm on palpation. Since a few smoothly marginated malignant lesions can be soft on palpation, diagnostic clarification is necessary for all noncystic nodules.

Diagnostic Strategy

Mammography

Image Presentation: Soft-tissue Density

The mammographic manifestations of the fibroadenoma are as follows (**Fig. 12.2a–h**):
- It usually presents as circumscribed, oval, lobulated, or round mass (**Fig. 12.2a–h**).
- Characteristically, it is sharply demarcated from the surrounding structures or accompanied by a halo (**Fig. 12.2b**).

The halo is a radiolucent border frequently seen around smoothly marginated lesions.

According to Sickles (Sickles 1994) a round or oval nodule is called "circumscribed" if it is sharply outlined and more than 75% of its circumference is not obscured by adjacent isodense fibroglandular tissue.

If a round or oval nodule is well circumscribed, with or without a halo, it can be assumed to represent a benign tumor, generally a fibroadenoma, with a probability exceeding 98%.

If a distinct margin is not observed on the standard mammographic views, a magnification view may be helpful to improve visualization of the lesion's contour (see **Fig. 3.23d,e**).

However, not all fibroadenomas are well defined (**Fig. 12.2d,e**; see also **Fig. 12.5a–d**, and **Fig. 12.6a–d**):
- If a fibroadenoma is partially surrounded or obscured by dense parenchyma, its presence might only be suggested by a semiconvex density. If a fibroadenoma is completely surrounded by dense parenchyma, it may be totally obscured.
- Older fibroadenomas can shrink and become irregular or indistinct, causing differential diagnostic problems (**Fig. 12.2e**).
- The *juvenile or giant fibroadenoma* is mammographically indistinguishable from other hypercellular fibroadenomas. Since it is mainly found in juvenile patients, it is often obscured by dense parenchyma. Because of its rapid growth, it can be rather large at the time of presentation (**Fig. 12.3a–c**).
- The adenoma may present on mammography like a typical fibroadenoma (**Fig. 12.4h**). Some adenomas (predominantly those in older patients) may be ill defined, similar to a malignancy.

Image Presentation: Calcifications

Old fibroadenomas may partially calcify. The following types of dystrophic calcifications can be seen in fibroadenomas:
- A calcification completely or almost completely occupying the fibroadenoma is pathognomonic. A surrounding soft tissue density can be present, but not always (**Fig. 12.2a,f**).
- Coarse, popcornlike, or bizarre calcifications (> 2 mm) are also pathognomonic (**Fig. 12.2a,f and i**).
- Evolving calcifications in a fibroadenoma can be rather indeterminate and include (**Fig. 12.2h and j–n**):
  - punctate calcifications
  - linear calcifications and
  - granular, pleomorphic calcifications.

If such evolving monomorphous calcifications are found within a circumscribed soft tissue density (see definition) or in an oval grouping, or if at least one additional shell-like calcification is present, the finding mammographically is highly consistent with a fibroadenoma. (Calcifications of the fibroadenomatous stroma characteristically begin along the periphery.) Otherwise evolving and uncharacteristic calcifications may require biopsy for diagnosis (**Fig. 12.2j, l and m**).

Calcification Pattern in Various Subtypes

There seem to be minor differences in the calcification pattern of the *pericanalicular and intracanalicular fibroadenomas*, according to their different histologic compositions (**Fig. 12.2g,h**) (Lanyi 1986, Travade et al. 1995).

Evolving calcifications in the pericanalicular fibroadenoma begin frequently in the lactiferous ducts, and consequently can be linear, Y-shaped, or V-shaped like the branching calcifications observed in comedo carcinomas.

In contrast, the calcifications in the intracanalicular fibroadenoma, which has its epithelium usually compressed and atrophied by the myxoid stroma, are more often round or punctate.

While both of these calcification patterns can be explained by the histologic findings, they are not specific. Unless additional mammographic findings characteristic of a fibroadenoma are present (circumscribed and smoothly outlined soft tissue density or additional characteristic coarse calcifications), a reliable differentiation from malignant calcifications may be impossible.

12 Benign Tumors and Tumorlike Masses

1 Oval, well-circumscribed lesion without superimposition
A

2 Dense tissue partially obscured by surrounding tissue
B

3 Fibroadenoma obscured by dense tissue
B: sonographically guided

4 Lesion with indistinct outline or irregular contour
C

5 Lobulated lesion
B

6 Round lesion
B

7 Typical calcifications in a round, oval, or lobulated lesion
A

8 Typical calcifications, surrounding lesion undetectable
A

9 Typical calcifications, surrounded by a lesion indistinct in outline and not quite regular
C

10 Diff. diagn: Necrotic calcifications in a carcinoma surrounded by large lesion characteristic of a malignancy
C

11 Calcifications suggestive of a fibroadenoma within a smoothly outlined lesion
A

12 Calcification as in 11 and surrounding lesion not visualized
B

13 Calcification as in 11 and surrounded by an irregularly outlined or ill-defined soft tissue density
C

14 Atypical calcifications within an entirely smoothly outlined soft tissue density
C

15 Atypical calcifications without soft tissue density
C

16 Atypical calcifications within a not entirely smoothly outlined soft tissue density
C

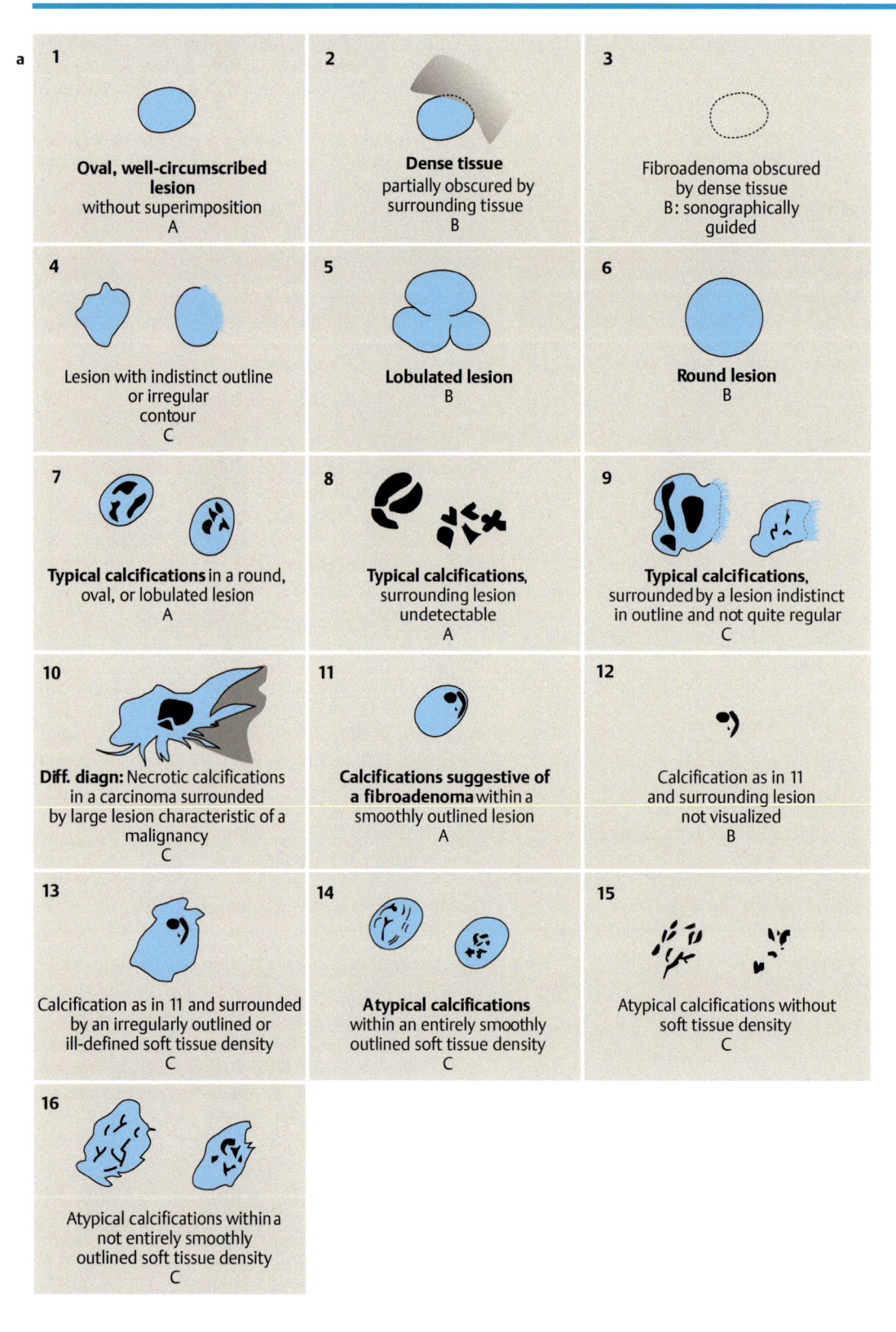

Fig. 12.2a–n Fibroadenoma.

a After a complete mammographic workup, mammographic appearance of fibroadenomas with the conventional therapeutic recommendation:

A = Follow-up adequate
B = Follow-up or biopsy
C = Biopsy.

Fibroepithelial Mixed Tumors

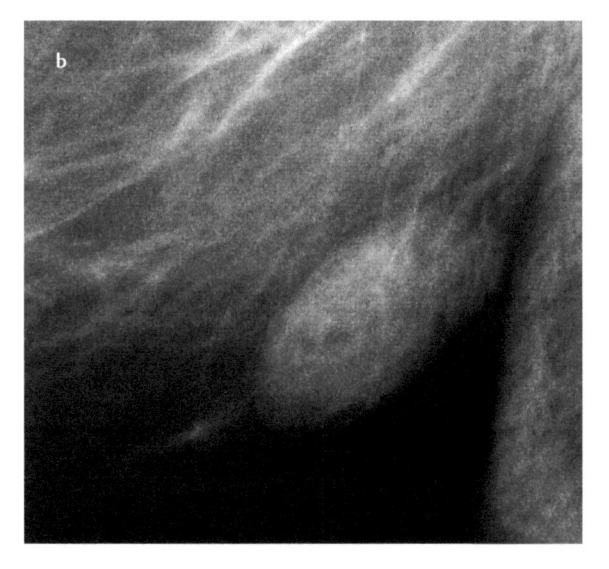

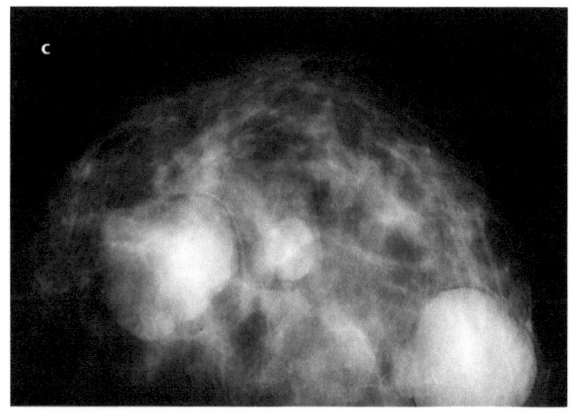

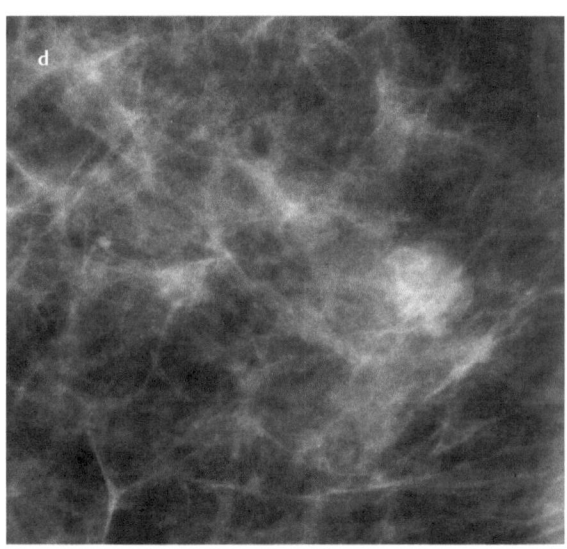

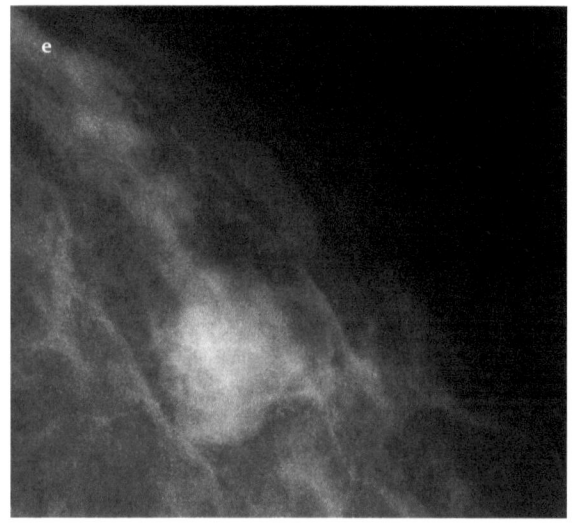

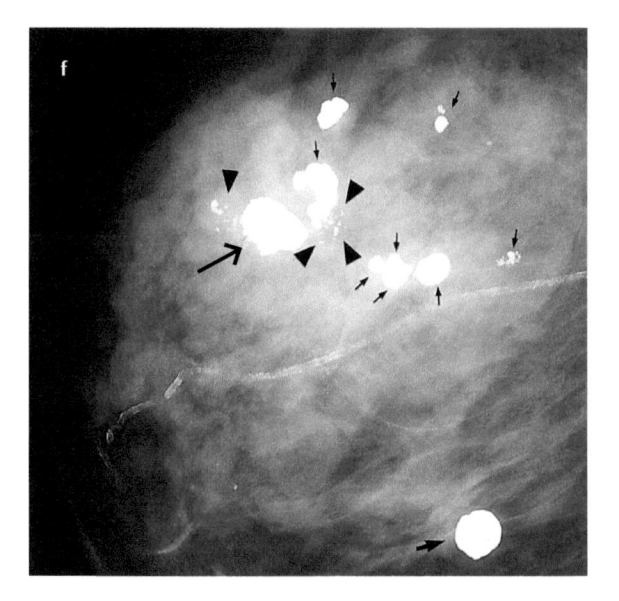

b Mammographically entirely smoothly outlined lesion (removed upon patient's request). *Histology*: Myxoid fibroadenoma.
c Young patient with multiple, smoothly outlined lesions with typical gentle lobulations.
d Round mass. About 60% of its margin is smoothly outlined while 40% of its margin is obscured by overlying and adjacent breast tissue. (*Sonography*, see **Fig. 12.4e**.) Fibroadenoma verified by CNB.
e Nodular lesion, not entirely smoothly outlined, detected by screening mammography. *Histology*: Predominantly fibrotic fibroadenoma.
f In addition to fibroadenomas with typical coarse calcifications (arrows), fibroadenomas with small and partially bizarre calcifications (arrowheads) are present. The corresponding (and, because of fibrotic changes, indistinctly outlined) soft tissue densities are only partially seen in the surrounding soft tissues.

Fig. 12.2g–n ▷

12 Benign Tumors and Tumorlike Masses

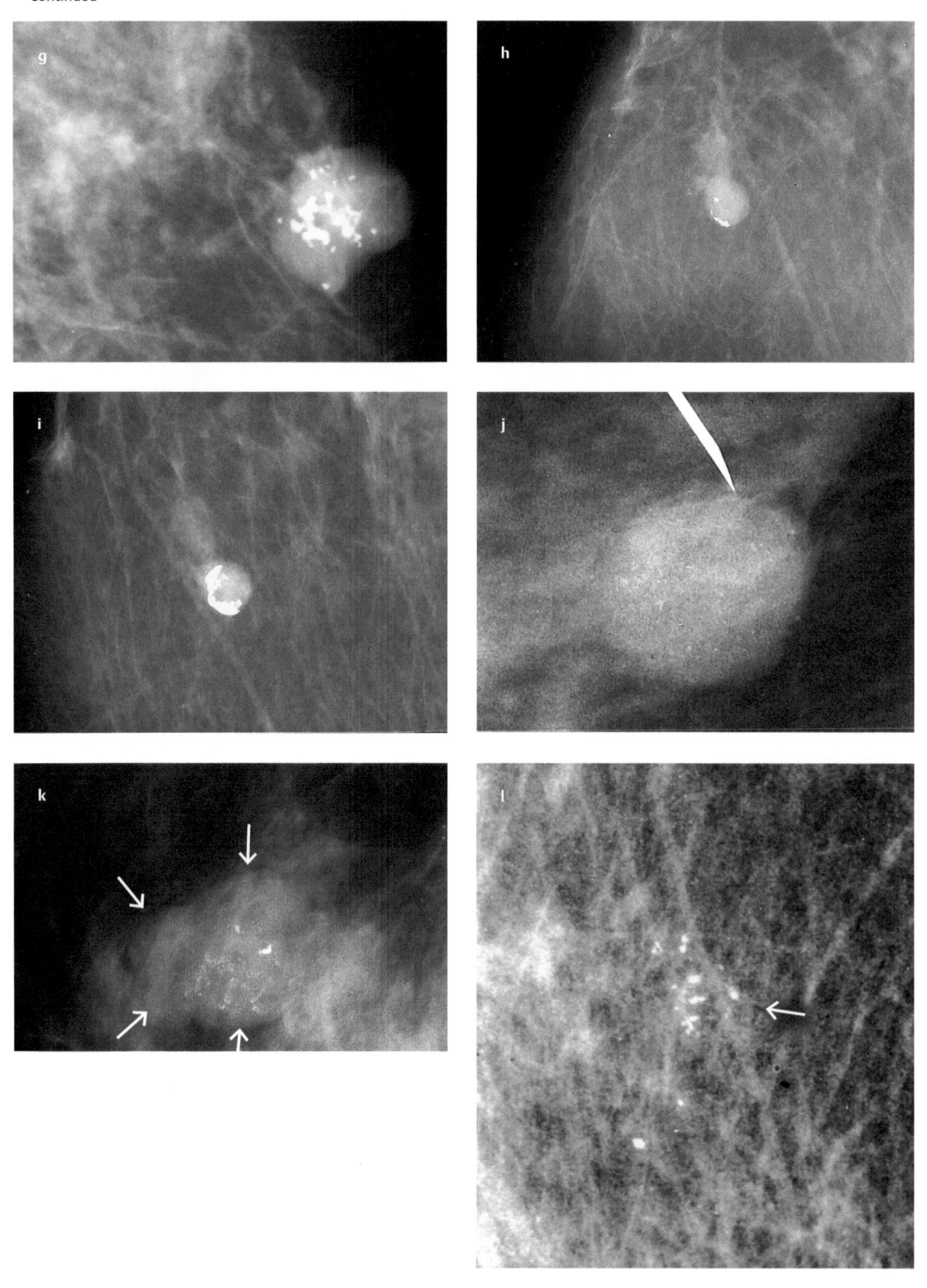

◁ continued

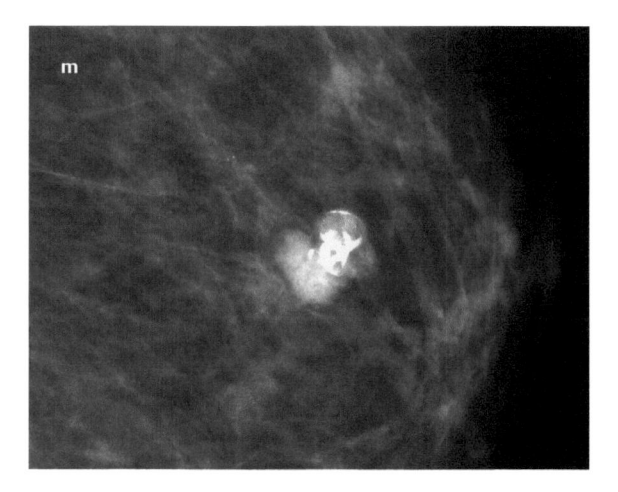

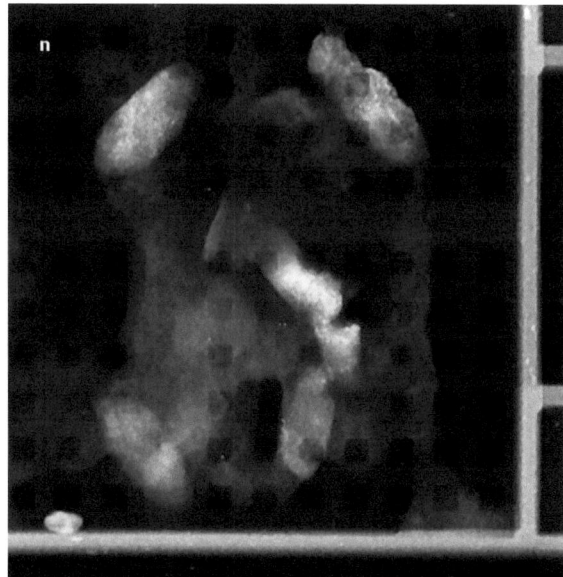

g Typical coarse bizarre calcifications are seen in this lobulated fibroadenoma.

h,i Often calcifications of the fibroadenomatous stroma begin along the periphery. Such eggshell-type calcifications are characteristic. They may increase with time. The second nodular lesion probably corresponds to a fibrosed fibroadenoma with somewhat irregular contours. It did not change for years.

j Round to oval localized density with many delicate, punctate calcifications. Although fine microcalcifications may occur in fibroadenomas, further workup is considered necessary to rule out other causes such as low-grade ductal carcinoma in situ. *Histology*: Intracanalicular fibroadenoma.

k Lobulated but sharply outlined localized density (arrows) with multiple most delicate, occasionally also linearly arranged, calcifications (as well as coarse calcifications) requiring further workup. *Histology*: Pericanalicular fibroadenoma.

l In some fibroadenomas the mass itself may be obscured by dense tissue. In some old fibroadenomas the mass may disappear and only the calcifications persist. Only if these calcifications are characteristic (see **Fig. 12.2f–i**) is the diagnosis of a fibroadenoma obvious. In this case biopsy was recommended because of indeterminate microcalcifications, which also included some elongated shapes.

m,n Adjacent to a typical fibroadenoma there is an oval well-circumscribed mass (**m**). Its increased density is due to numerous very fine microcalcifications, which are better visualized on the specimen radiograph of the vacuum biopsy cores (**n**). In spite of its smooth margin and the halo, biopsy was performed because of the very fine microcalcifications. *Histology*: Non-high-grade ductal carcinoma in situ.

Adenomas, too, may develop microcalcifications. These appear to be mostly punctate, densely packed, and sometimes irregular (Soo et al. 2000).

Accuracy

- If mammographically characteristic calcifications are found, the diagnosis of a fibroadenoma can be established with a high degree of certainty. Further evaluation is unnecessary.
- In the presence of a mammographically smooth border (circumscribed nodule, see definition on p. 293), a benign mass can be assumed with a 98% certainty, usually a fibroadenoma.
- If multiple, well-circumscribed oval masses are present, the probability of dealing with benign entities increases further.
- Considering the high prevalence of benign cysts and fibroadenomas (which is much higher than that of malignancy), for asymptomatic women without increased risk in the screening situation, usual screening is generally considered justified, if multiple, well-circumscribed masses are seen or if a single, oval, well-circumscribed mass of low density is seen (assuming that this may be an involuting fibroadenoma or a cyst).
- In women at risk or in symptomatic women, histopathologic assessment should be considered for newly diagnosed single masses. In cases with very low suspicion and low risk (based on family history and patient age) short-term follow-up may be an adequate option if all clinical and imaging findings (mammography and sonography) support the diagnosis of a benign lesion.

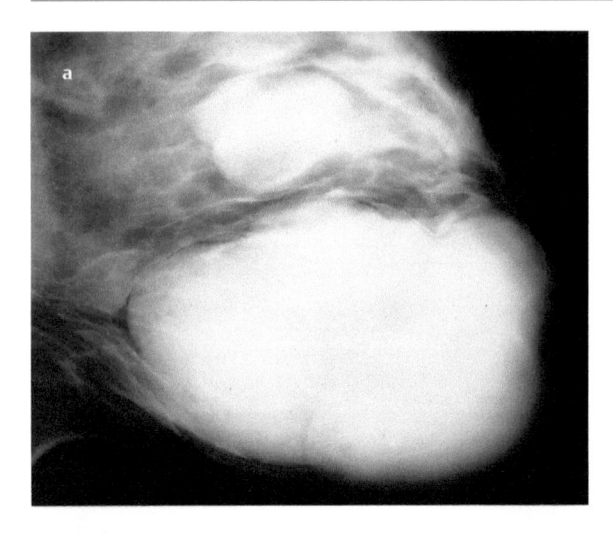

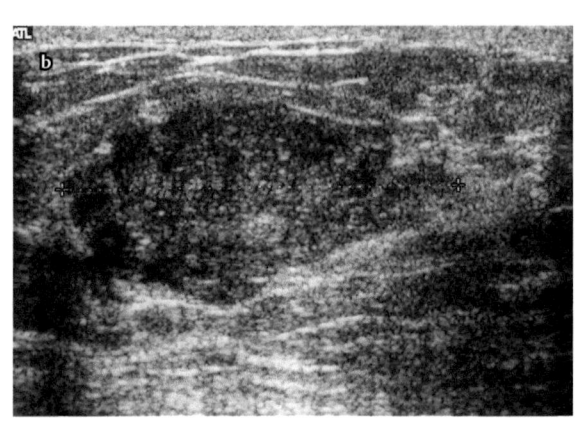

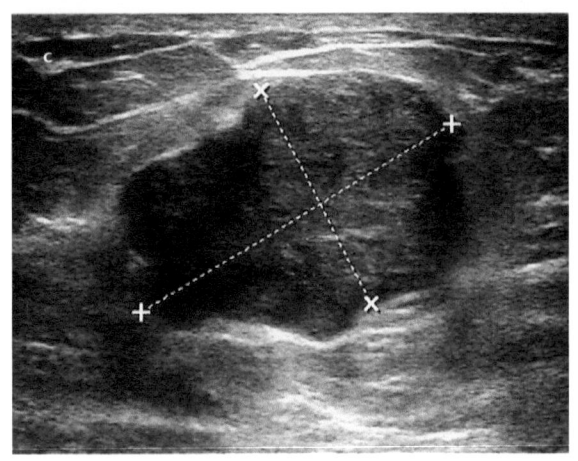

Fig. 12.3a–c Specific manifestations of fibroadenomas. Juvenile fibroadenoma in a 19-year-old patient.

a A larger and a smaller macrolobulated fibroadenoma with smooth outline. The outline of the smaller fibroadenoma is partially obscured by dense parenchyma. The rapidly growing juvenile fibroadenomas characteristically do not contain any calcifications.

b,c Sonographically, the juvenile fibroadenomas characteristically exhibit a homogeneous internal structure but can be heterogeneous. They are characteristically smooth in outline, show good sound transmission, and are easily compressible. The sound transmission is moderate, the internal structure seems somewhat heterogeneous. Two years' follow-up showed no change. With spatial compounding (**c**), the typical macro-lobulated contour is much better visible and the texture appears to be more homogeneous. Posterior shadowing decreases with compounding.

- Follow-up imaging is indicated at 6, 12, and 24 months to assess stability.
- In women at high risk, percutaneous breast biopsy is indicated for any newly diagnosed mass including well-circumscribed lesions. This takes into account that in these families well-circumscribed breast cancers (predominantly medullary type cancers, which may imitate fibroadenomas completely) are more frequent.
- Any (well-circumscribed) solid lesion that develops newly or increases in size should undergo histopathologic assessment.
- For the remaining variants (which do not exhibit well-circumscribed margins as defined above), accuracy is decreased. Depending on the imaging features, history, and clinical findings, follow-up mammography may be adequate. Otherwise, the evaluation should continue with percutaneous biopsy.
- If multiple nodular densities are present (which increases the probability of dealing with benign entities) follow-up imaging at 6, 12 and 24 months may be a option. In the rare case of multiple indeterminate findings (which may occur with "old" fibrosed fibroadenomas), MRI may be helpful—in the case of nonenhancing fibrosed fibroadenomas it may help exclude malignancy, or it may indicate which lesion(s) is/are of the highest suspicion and should be biopsied.
- Because of the higher risk of malignancy, biopsy in the case of equivocal findings should be generously used in women above the age of 40 years. Percutaneous biopsy is always appropriate if the lesion has an indistinct border, contains suspicious calcifications, or has enlarged on serial mammography.
- Excisional biopsy is recommended if the lesion has increased in size after core biopsy or, rarely, if the lesion is very painful. (Small deeply located lesions might also be removed by vacuum-assisted breast biopsy [VABB], but recurrence has been described.) For superficial fibroadenomas and for fibroadenomas close to the nipple, excision may remain the least traumatic and most elegant way of treatment.

Sonography

Indications

Sonography is indicated in the diagnostic evaluation of presumed fibroadenomas if a cyst needs to be distinguished from a noncystic (i.e, solid) lesion or if a questionable palpable finding in a mammographically dense breast requires further evaluation.

Sonography may be helpful to support the diagnosis of a benign mass if mammography shows no sign of malignancy, for example if a benign-appearing mass is partly obscured by overlying tissue.

In very young patients without increased risk the diagnosis of a benign mass may also be possible without mammography. Thus, in the absence of any criteria of malignancy by sonography and mammography (where indicated) ultrasound imaging can avert biopsy in selected solid lesions that fulfill all criteria of benignity (see below). In these cases short-term follow-up—usually at 6, 12 and at least 24 months—is recommended to document stability.

In all other cases and in cases for which growth is suspected or documented, the diagnosis should be established by percutaneous breast biopsy.

Image Presentation

The following sonographic features are characteristic of a benign lesion, usually a fibroadenoma (Stavros et al. 1995, 2003, Skaane and Engedal 1998) (**Fig. 12.4a,b**):
- A completely smooth contour with or without a delicate lateral boundary echo, which should optimally be surrounded by a thin hyperechoic pseudocapsule (the strongest indicator of a benign lesion)
- Homogeneous good sound transmission
- The nodule should be oval with its long axis oriented parallel to the transducer and its horizontal diameter should exceed the vertical diameter by a factor of at least 1.5
- In our experience it should be readily mobile and elastic
- Uniform internal echoes may also be observed in many fibroadenomas
- Finally, some fibroadenomas consist of several oval adjacent parts and thus form a macro-lobulated, well-circumscribed mass, which—if all other characteristics of a benign entity are fulfilled—may also be quite reliably diagnosed as such

In contrast to these typical sonographic features, which are primarily found in young fibroadenomas with high water content, two-thirds of fibroadenomas show the *following variations* (**Figs. 12.4c–e,g, 12.5b, 12.6b**):
- A macro-lobulated nodule is suggestive but not diagnostic of a fibroadenoma.
- A round configuration can be primarily found in small fibroadenomas (**Fig. 12.6b**), but other lesions, including malignant lesions, can have an identical pattern.
- Some fibroadenomas are not sonographically detectable. They are isoechoic with the surrounding tissue.

The following findings develop with increasing fibrosis within a fibroadenoma:
- Contour irregularities
- Heterogeneous internal echoes
- Formation of a complete or partial acoustic shadow behind the lesion
- Impaired compressibility

Fibroadenomas with the above-mentioned sonographic features cannot be differentiated from malignancies.
- Calcifications in a fibroadenoma often cause acoustic shadowing. With increasing size of the calcification, the acoustic shadowing often arises from a well-recognized echogenic structure (**Fig. 12.4g**). Though shadowing is in general atypical for a benign tumor, it is not significant when mammographically the mass contains calcifications that are typical of a fibroadenoma.

Accuracy

If all features mentioned above as being sonographically typical for a benign lesion are present, which is the case in only 20–30% of fibroadenomas, the diagnosis of a fibroadenoma can be made with reasonable certainty (> 95%) (Stavros et al. 1995, 2003, Skaane and Engedal 1998). Any sonographic or mammographic features of malignancy must be absent and mammography should be performed in all cases except in very young women without increased risk before a benign lesion (probably a fibroadenoma) may be assumed and short-term follow-up is recommended.

The following approach is recommended:
- Follow-up examinations (at intervals of 6 months) are justified if the sonographic features are characteristic of a fibroadenoma (compressible, easily moveable nodule with a smooth contour and homogeneous internal structure, as well as acoustic enhancement or unchanged posterior acoustic intensity) and if there is no clinical or mammographic evidence of malignancy in a young woman (under the age of 30 years). In symptomatic women above age 30 an additional mammogram should be performed for evaluation of any newly detected mass.
- For newly discovered findings above age 30, and in all women at increased risk, needle biopsy should be considered for further confirmation.
- Since malignancies may occasionally have findings resembling those of a fibroadenoma, a sonographic presentation typical of a fibroadenoma does not eliminate the possibility of a malignancy.

12 Benign Tumors and Tumorlike Masses

a

Fibroadenomas are characteristically seen as oval, smoothly outlined lesions with homogeneous internal structure and good to moderate acoustic enhancement:

1 A delicate hyperechoic capsule is another important sign of a benign tumor such as a fibroadenoma

2 Less frequent: Lobulated forms

3 Round form, diff. diagn.: malignancy!

4 With increasing fibrotic changes, heterogeneity of the internal structures, irregularities of the contours, and partial acoustic shadowing can occur. The compressibility of these fibroadenomas is generally poor

5 Within calcified fibroadenomas, large acoustic shadows can be seen, sometimes arising behind hyperechoic structures

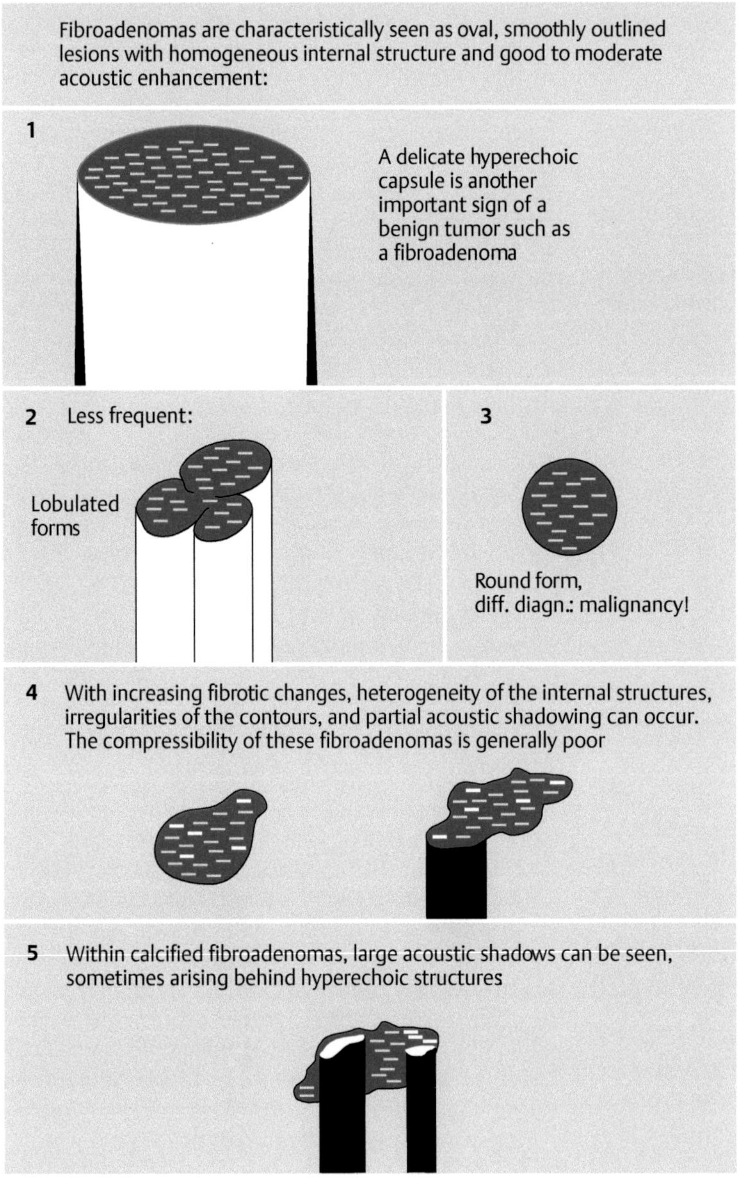

Fig. 12.4a–i Sonographically characteristic appearance of fibroadenomas.

a Diagrammatic scheme.
b A typical fibroadenoma is shown: Smooth margins; faint, very delicate capsule; homogenous echo texture. The ratio of the longitudinal and transverse diameters exceeds 1.5, and the long axis is parallel to the transducer.
c Smoothly outlined fibroadenoma. The heterogeneous internal echo structures and the variable sound transmission are uncharacteristic.
d Atypical presentation of a fibroadenoma: No hyperechoic capsule is seen, the texture is not homogeneous, and the form only partly macro-lobulated: fibrosed fibroadenoma on histology.
e Fibroadenoma with irregular outline and heterogeneous internal structure. This finding is sonographically not distinguishable from a malignancy. Fibroadenoma proven by CNB.
f The fibrosed fibroadenoma shown here (arrows) is markedly sound absorbing. Consequently, it has a strong acoustic shadow and cannot be sonographically distinguished from a malignancy.
g This fibroadenoma is very hypoechoic and macro-lobulated and the mammographically visible calcifications are seen as hyperechoic internal structures.
h This nodule looks like a fibroadenoma and *histologically* turned out to be a tubular adenoma.
i This multinodular tumor was diagnosed during pregnancy. It corresponded to a palpable, soft mass. *Core biopsy* yielded a lactating adenoma.

Fibroepithelial Mixed Tumors

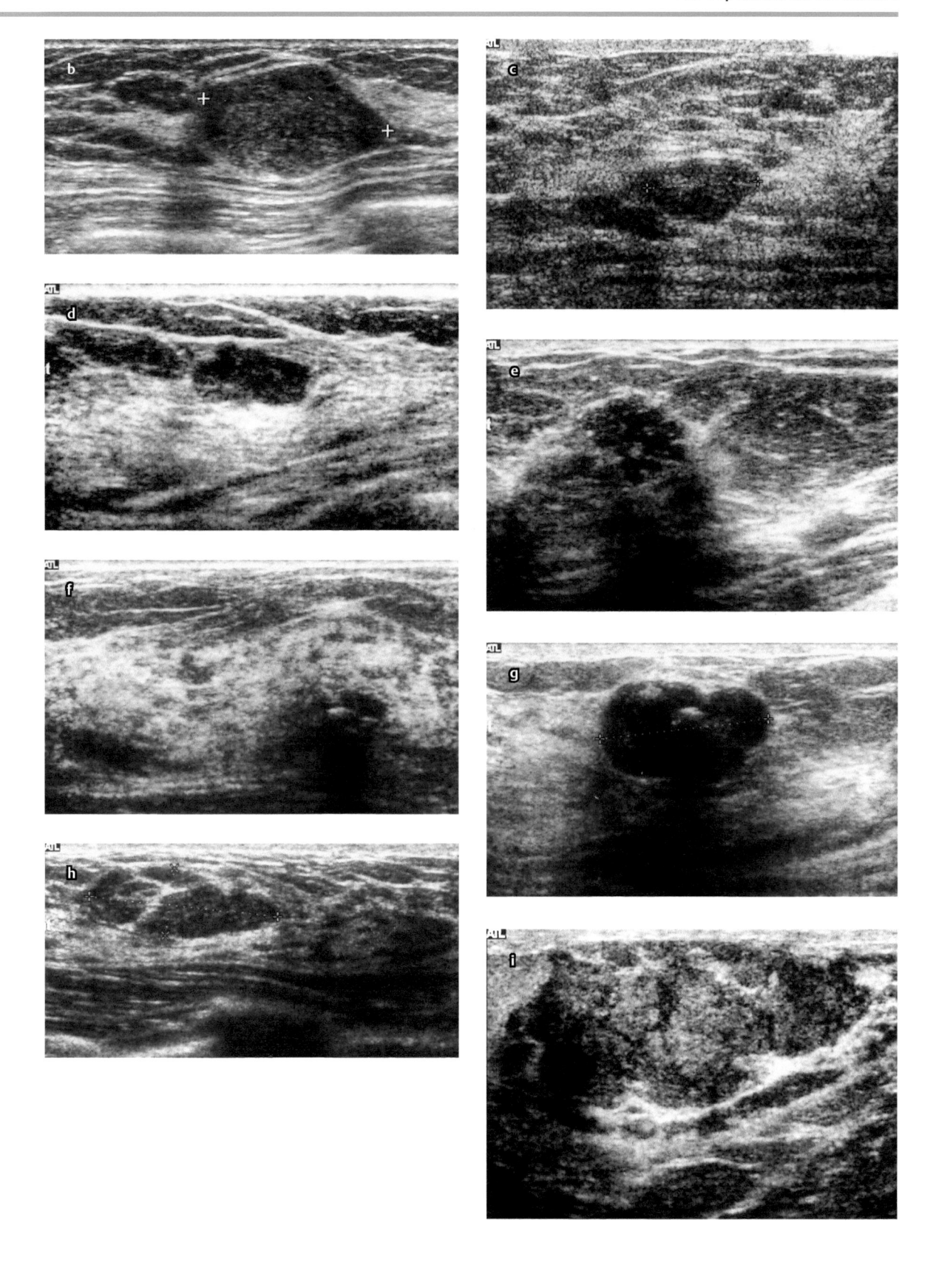

12 Benign Tumors and Tumorlike Masses

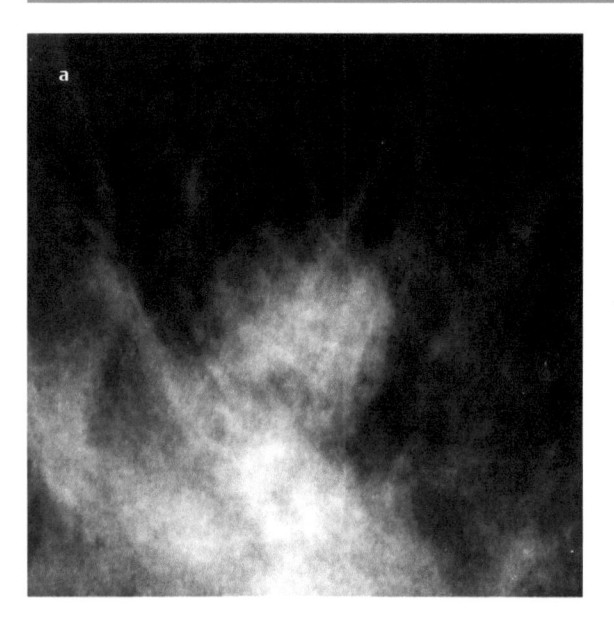

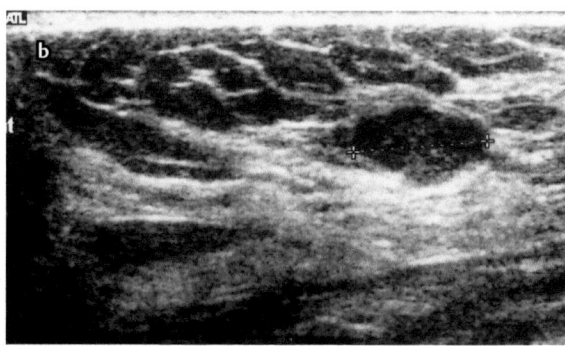

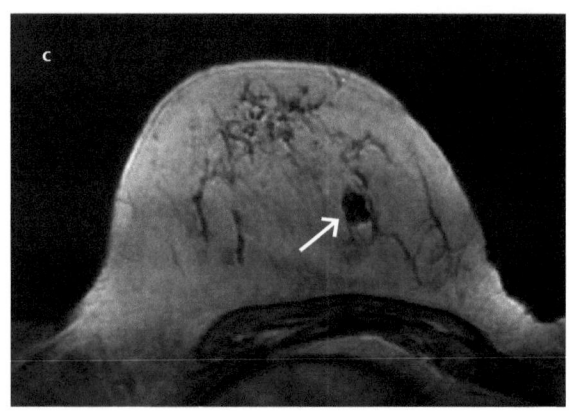

Fig. 12.5a–d Imaging of an "old" fibroadenoma.
a Sclerosed fibroadenomas are often not entirely smoothly outlined mammographically, as illustrated here.
b Sonographically the contour is regular and macro-lobulated, but the internal structures are heterogeneous.
c Magnetic resonance imaging (FLASH-3D) before contrast enhancement. The fibroadenoma is seen within the surrounding fat as a nodular, not entirely smoothly outlined lesion of low signal intensity (arrow).
d There is very little contrast enhancement of the tumor, which excludes a malignancy with a high degree of certainty (this can be confirmed by stable mammographic and clinical findings over a 3-year period).

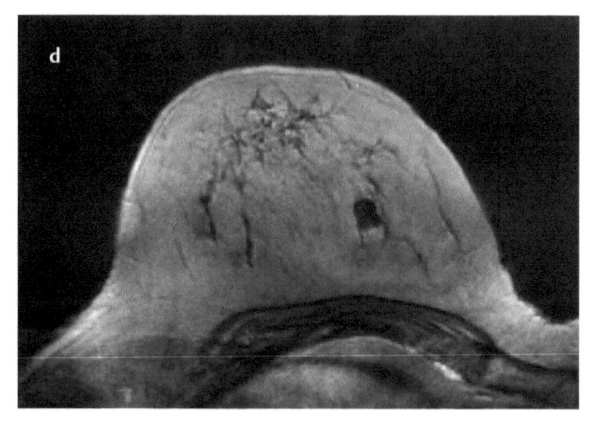

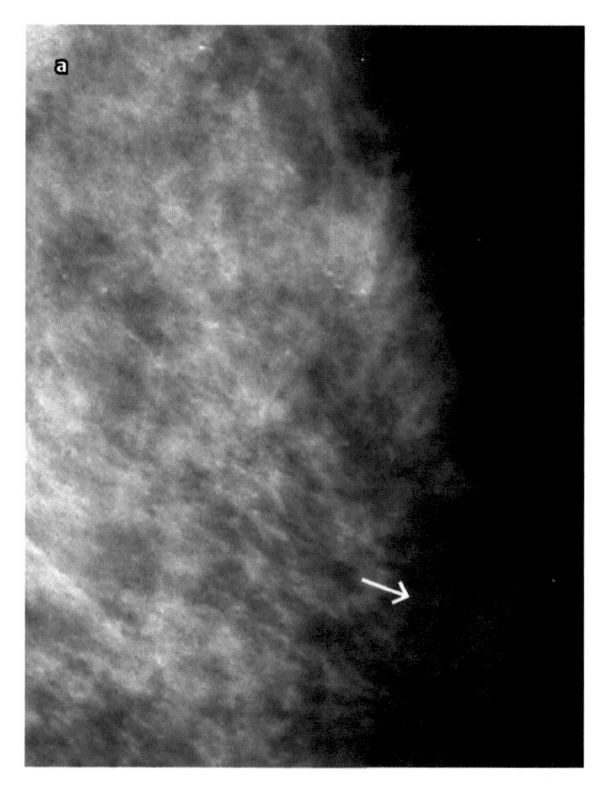

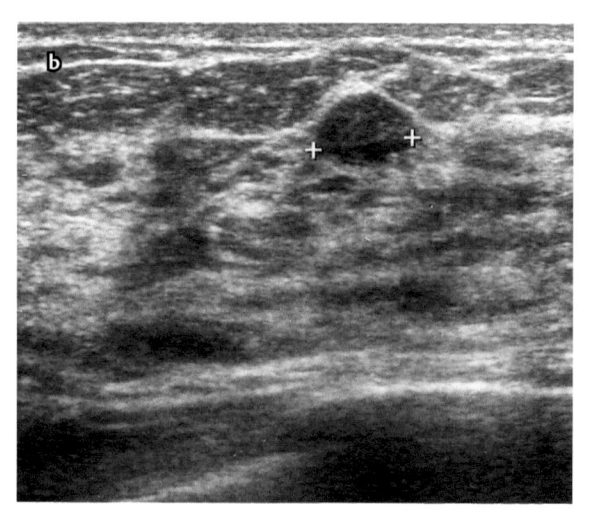

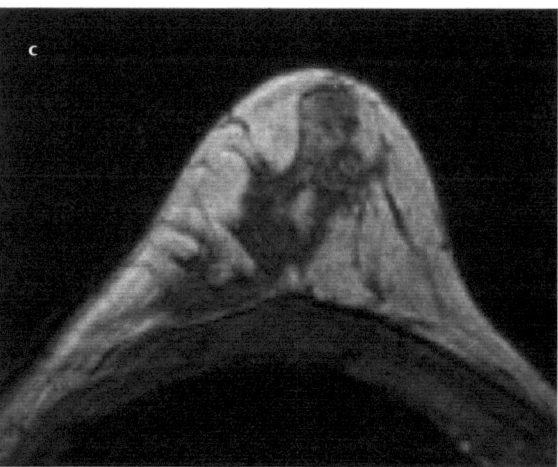

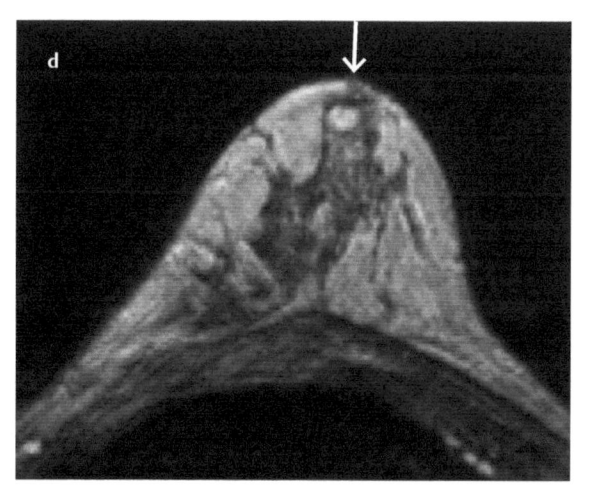

Fig. 12.6a–d Imaging of the nonfibrosed fibroadenoma. Since most nonfibrosed fibroadenomas show definite contrast enhancement and are consequently not distinguishable from a smoothly outlined fibroadenoma, core biopsy should be preferred rather than MRI as the most cost-effective method to evaluate a suspected fibroadenoma.

a   This patient presented with a mammographically very dense nodular breast. There was a hard mobile mass at the 12 o'clock position, 2–3 cm from the nipple, which can barely be discerned in the very dense nodular breast tissue (a section of the area in question is shown).

b   Sonographically a round solid lesion without enhanced through transmission is shown and was considered indeterminate. Magnetic resonance imaging (MRI) was performed because of a positive family history of breast cancer.

c,d   MRI before (**c**) and after (**d**) intravenous injection of contrast medium. The nodule exhibits typical, but not diagnostic, MRI appearances of a "young" fibroadenoma—a smooth outline and intense enhancement. *Histology*: Nonfibrosed intracanalicular fibroadenoma.

For *deviations from the typical image presentation*, the following applies:
- Even if the sonographic features are atypical, follow-up examinations are adequate as long as the mammographic diagnosis is unequivocal on the basis of typical calcifications or the nodule is known not to have changed for several years. This implies a fibroadenoma with a high degree of certainty.
- If mammographic and sonographic findings are atypical, biopsy should be considered.

Percutaneous Biopsy

Percutaneous biopsy is a proven and cost-effective method of establishing the diagnosis of a fibroadenoma if an adequate amount of tissue has been obtained. The vast majority of fibroadenomas are reliably diagnosed by percutaneous biopsy.

The diagnosis of sclerosed fibroadenomas may be more difficult. If, in spite of correct targeting, the histopathologic diagnosis is difficult, the interdisciplinary conference will have to decide whether the benign diagnosis is compatible (based on sparse or mainly fibrotic tissue) or whether re-biopsy (using core needle biopsy, VABB, or even surgical biopsy) or short-term follow-up at 4–6, 12, and 24 months should be recommended. Also, for some very cellular variants definite distinction from phyllodes tumor may not be possible based on needle biopsy. For such rare cases the pathologist may recommend surgical biopsy. However, the vast majority of fibroadenomas can be reliably assessed by percutaneous breast biopsy alone.

Magnetic Resonance Imaging

Image Presentation

The MRI appearance depends on the composition of the fibroadenoma:
- *Sclerosed fibroadenomas* (**Fig. 12.5a–d**) do not enhance, or enhance only minimally following injection of Gd-DTPA. Since only a few, rare, nonenhancing mucinous carcinomas have been described, it may be useful generally to perform an additional T2-weighted sequence. Because of their high water content, mucinous carcinomas have high signal intensity on T2-weighted images. Fibrosed fibroadenomas, on the contrary, will display low signal intensity on T1- and T2-weighted images.
- *Edematous and hypercellular young fibroadenomas*, however, show strong (sometimes very strong) mostly plateau-type or progressive enhancement of Gd-DTPA (**Fig. 12.6a–d**). The smooth contours, oval shape, or gentle lobulations combined with visualization of low signal intensity septations will support the diagnosis of a benign lesion. Although slow enhancement, as well as a smooth contour, is indicative of a fibroadenoma, a malignancy cannot be excluded with certainty. The reason is that some well-circumscribed malignancies also exhibit progressive or plateau-type enhancement (papillary, medullary carcinoma, some ductal carcinomas, and ductal carcinomas in situ).

Owing to the described overlapping appearance of some benign and malignant tumors, MRI is not recommended for further assessment of masses that can be diagnosed by percutaneous breast biopsy, which usually has a higher reliability. Also—unlike MRI—it is not associated with the risk of incidentally detecting further benign entities in the same or contralateral breast that would cause additional unnecessary workup.
- Only in the rare case of multiple suspected lesions (including fibrosed fibroadenomas) might MRI be useful for excluding malignancy or guiding biopsy to the most suspicious lesion(s).
- If a small lesion that is compatible with a fibroadenoma is detected only by MRI in an asymptomatic patient, we recommend a countercheck by mammography and retrospective sonography. If no sign of malignancy exists and the lesion is not visible by ultrasound in retrospect, follow-up may be considered instead of MR-guided biopsy if the patient is at low risk (e.g., repeat MRI after 4 and 12 months). The recommendation for follow-up is justified by the low probability of such a lesion being malignant. If there are any doubts or if the patient is at high risk, MR-guided biopsy of the lesion, which is visible only on MRI, should be considered.

It should be pointed out that a peripheral enhancement, irregular contours, or an early washout of contrast agent, if present, would be atypical for a fibroadenoma. This finding should lead to further workup (biopsy).

Accuracy

The high sensitivity of MRI in the detection of young enhancing fibroadenomas and other benign entities and the inadequate specificity in differentiating them from circumscribed malignancies is problematic. Therefore MRI is not recommended for the workup of suspected fibroadenomas or indeterminate masses.

Percutaneous biopsy is most appropriate and the generally recommended next step for evaluating clinically, mammographically, or sonographically suspected fibroadenomas.

In rare cases with multiple lesions MRI may provide valuable additional information to plan further assessment. Fibrosed fibroadenomas and nonenhancing cysts may be entities that can be correctly diagnosed by MRI.

Diagnostic Goals

The most important role of imaging in the diagnosis of fibroadenoma consists of differentiating it from well-circumscribed malignancies with similar findings. In addition to the well-circumscribed ductal carcinoma, this includes medullary and papillary carcinomas, lymphomas, sarcomas, and metastases. The phyllodes tumors can also have a similar pattern. All these tumors can occasionally be completely well circumscribed, even surrounded by a mammographically detectable halo (see p. 293 for significance of the halo).

The excision of all circumscribed or round lesions, performed as a safety measure to find a rare circumscribed malignancy, does not appear to be in the best interests of the patient and cannot be justified. Responsible use of imaging may allow avoidance of histopathologic assessment in cases with a low or very low risk of malignancy. If the latter is uncertain, percutaneous breast biopsy is the next step, which in the vast majority will allow a reliable diagnosis.

Overview of the Diagnostic Strategy

- The typically calcified fibroadenoma is mammographically pathognomonic. Additional evaluation or follow-up examinations are not necessary.
- Mammographically well-circumscribed solid masses (see definition, p. 293), which are primarily fibroadenomas, are benign in 98% of cases. In this situation follow-up mammography at intervals of 6, 12, 24, and 36 months is appropriate.
- The remaining solitary, circumscribed nonpalpable, and most likely benign lesions that do not entirely fulfill the above-mentioned criteria may be subjected to percutaneous or excisional biopsy.
- Because of the characteristic doubling rates of breast carcinomas and the rather slow growth rates of some circumscribed malignancies, the intervals of follow-up examinations should not be less than 6 months. The follow-up period should not be less than 3 years, and the current examination should be compared with the initial and not with the most recent examination.
- When masses do not contain calcifications, sonography should be used to differentiate between a cyst and a solid tumor, as well as to characterize palpable lesions that are obscured by mammographically dense tissue.
- Sonography cannot achieve a definitive differentiation of mammographically indeterminate noncystic masses from malignancy.
- A lesion seen only sonographically and exhibiting the typical features of a fibroadenoma may be followed up at regular intervals or undergo a percutaneous biopsy if neither the patient's history nor clinical and mammographic findings reveal evidence of malignancy.
- For further evaluation of a suspected fibroadenoma that has been newly discovered and appears clinically and mammographically benign but does not fulfill all criteria of a benign lesion, percutaneous biopsy is appropriate. If biopsy reveals a fibroadenoma, an excisional biopsy is not necessary.
- If a small sclerosed fibroadenoma is not amenable to percutaneous needle biopsy, or if the lesions are multiple, MRI (contrast-enhanced MRI combined with T2-weighted pulse sequence) can be obtained.
- Increasing size of a circumscribed tumor or suspected malignancy (irregular contour, suspected calcifications) is an indication for biopsy.

Summary

The most important role of the diagnostic methods used to distinguish a fibroadenoma is to establish the definitive differentiation, if possible, from the rare circumscribed malignancies and the avoidance of high rates of excisional biopsies exclusively performed for diagnostic purposes.

The mammographically pathognomonic finding of a calcified fibroadenoma unfortunately comprises only a small proportion of the fibroadenomas. The typical mammographic finding is the well-circumscribed nodule (see definition, p. 293), with or without halo. Its risk of malignancy is less than 2%. In asymptomatic women at low risk who undergo screening mammography, further assessment is not usually recommended if multiple well-circumscribed masses are present. The probability of malignancy of such masses (which mostly represent cysts or fibroadenomas) is quite low. Also the presence of multiple masses further decreases the probability of malignancy.

Sonography serves to distinguish fibroadenomas from cysts and to demonstrate fibroadenomas that are mammographically obscured by dense tissue. If the sonographic solid lesion corresponds to a newly detected finding, confirmation of the presumed diagnosis by percutaneous biopsy is recommended.

Exceptions and variations of the typical mammographic and sonographic findings are common. They require further evaluation, which can be achieved by follow-up examinations, usually percutaneous biopsy. If (rarely) there are contraindications to percutaneous breast biopsy, or if multiple lesions are present, MRI may be considered.

Based on their smooth contour and absence of significant enhancement fibrosed fibroadenomas can be diagnosed by MRI quite reliably.

If multiple well-circumscribed masses exist, MRI may be useful to document sizes and identify lesions with atypical morphology or enhancement pattern that should undergo biopsy.

When a lesion is being followed, the follow-up examinations should be done initially at 6 months and then at intervals of 12 months for a total of at least 2–3 years. If any suspicion arises, for example, if the lesion increases in size, excisional biopsy should be considered.

Papilloma

Papillomas belong to the group of fibroepithelial tumors of the breast. They represent 1–1.5% of breast tumors.

While most papillomas are benign tumors, there is a low association with malignancy.

When diagnosed histopathologically from small amounts of tissue there is a low risk that a higher-grade lesion is missed or that a higher-grade lesion may develop in this location sometime in the future. For this reason papillary lesions are today considered as B3 lesions or benign lesions of uncertain malignant potential. These lesions are discussed in Chapter 14.

Lipoma

Lipomas are benign tumors composed of fat. They may be palpable lesions or a dominant area of fat within the breast, usually surrounded by a thin capsule.

Differentiation: Lipomatous metaplasias of the connective tissue may appear with advancing age. They are a manifestation of lipomatous atrophy of the breast parenchyma. Occasionally, these lipomatous structures are incorrectly termed lipomas but do not correspond to real ones.

Tumors, which are largely but not completely composed of fat and surrounded by a pseudocapsule, may be found in the breast as well. These are adeno-(fibro)-lipomas or hamartomas and not true lipomas.

Clinical Findings

Clinically, lipomas appear as soft, smoothly outlined tumors, but can be firm, smoothly outlined, and moveable. They might only be seen mammographically.

Diagnostic Strategy

Mammography is the most important method for diagnosing the lipoma. Definitive diagnosis and reliable exclusion of a malignancy can be achieved for all lipomas by mammography.

Mammography

(See **Fig. 12.7**.)

Lipomas are positively diagnosed mammographically:
- The fat density of the nodule is pathognomonic, exclusively comprising fat lobules, which are traversed by thin connective tissue septa.
- The delicate connective tissue capsule is seen completely or partially around the nodule. This mammographic appearance is so characteristic that further evaluation is superfluous.

Sonography, MRI, and needle biopsy are not indicated in the diagnostic investigation of the lipoma.

Rare Benign Tumors

The following rare benign tumors of the breast are briefly discussed:
1. Leiomyoma, neurofibroma, neurilemmoma, benign spindle cell tumor, chondroma, osteoma
2. Angioma
3. Granulosa cell tumor
4. Pseudoangiomatous stromal hyperplasia

Leiomyoma, Neurofibroma, Neurilemmoma, Benign Spindle Cell Tumor (Myofibroblastoma), Chondroma, Osteoma

(See **Figs. 12.8** and **12.9**.)

These benign tumors are very rare.

The leiomyoma arises from the smooth muscles of the vessels, nipple region, and ductal structures.

The neurofibroma, as well as the rare neurilemmoma, derives from the sheath of the peripheral nerves. It usually is located intracutaneously (see Chapter 21), less frequently subcutaneously.

The extremely rare benign spindle cell tumor originates from the mesenchymal cells, similar to the mesenchymal origin of the metaplastic chondroma and osteoma.

Epithelial and dermoid cysts are found more frequently in the cutaneous or subcutaneous connective and lipomatous tissues.

According to their histologic growth pattern, these tumors are seen as smoothly outlined, oval to round structures. Except for their frequent subcutaneous location, there are no further criteria that distinguish these tumors from fibroadenomas or other smoothly outlined lesions. Only chondromas and osteomas can have characterizing matrix calcifications that might resemble bizarre fibroadenomatous calcifications.

Because of their unspecific appearance, the final diagnosis cannot be made by diagnostic imaging. The diagnostic approach is the same as that applied to other masses with a nodular pattern (e.g., fibroadenoma). The diagnosis of benignity is possible for those rare benign tumors that are well circumscribed or fat containing on mammography. Specific diagnosis is only possible histologically.

Percutaneous breast biopsy is able to yield the correct diagnosis for some of the above changes based on H&E (hematoxylin and eosin) staining and immunostaining. If core biopsy does not make a specific diagnosis, follow-up is justified provided the imaging is clearly benign and compatible with the histopathologic findings.

Rare Benign Tumors

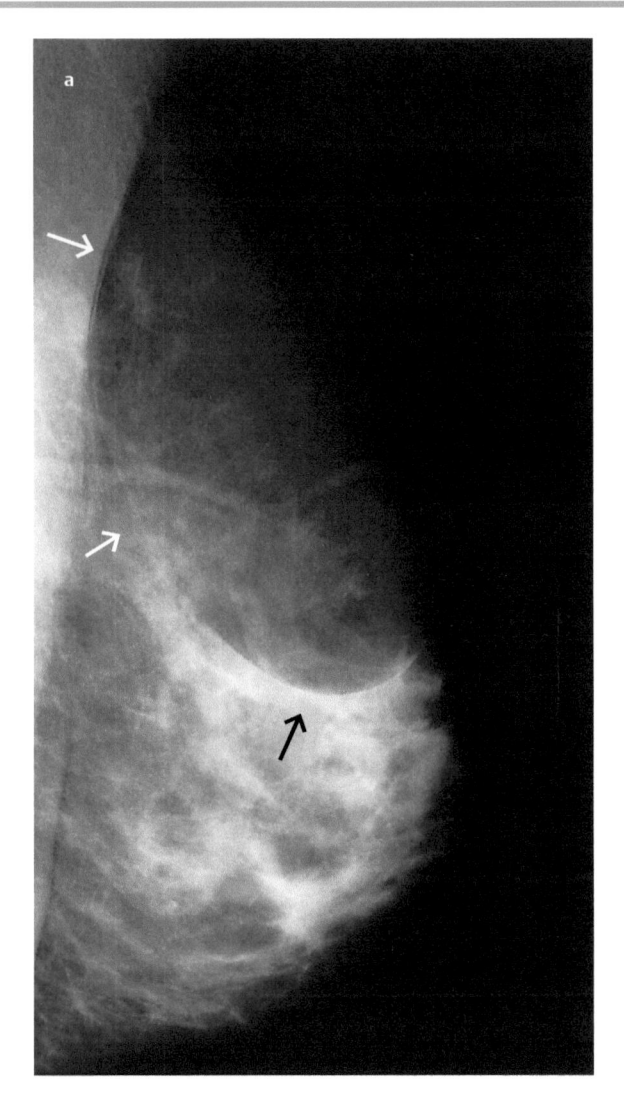

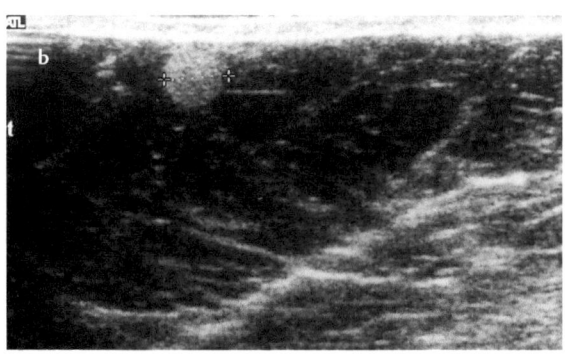

Fig. 12.7a–d Lipoma.

a Lipoma is visualized as a smoothly outlined nodule of fat density and a delicate capsule of fibrous tissue. (The subtle densities observed in a pure lipoma should correspond to superimposed parenchyma.) This unequivocally benign finding is not an indication for a biopsy.

b Typical subcutaneous lipoma: Homogeneously hyperechoic round lesion.

c Another example of an intramammary lipoma corresponding to a typical palpable, smooth, elastic, well-defined lump.

d This male patient was worried about a palpable lump at the inframammary fold at the chest wall 4 cm caudal to the nipple. The lesion was clinically suspected to correspond to a lipoma, as proven by the characteristic sonographic finding.

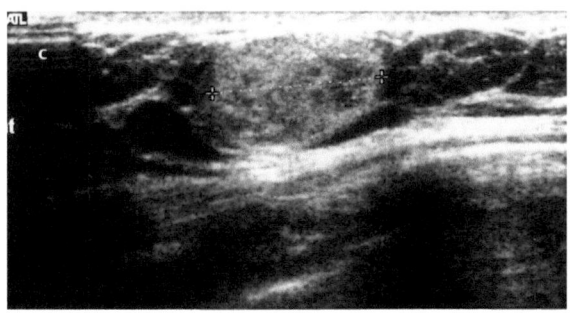

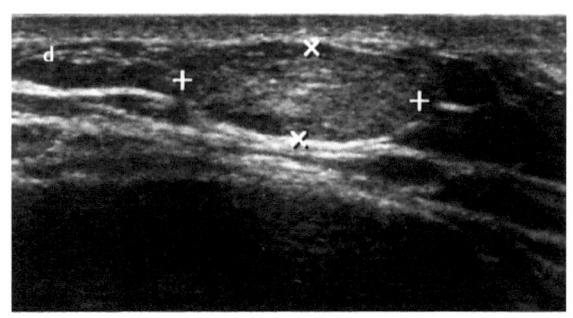

12 Benign Tumors and Tumorlike Masses

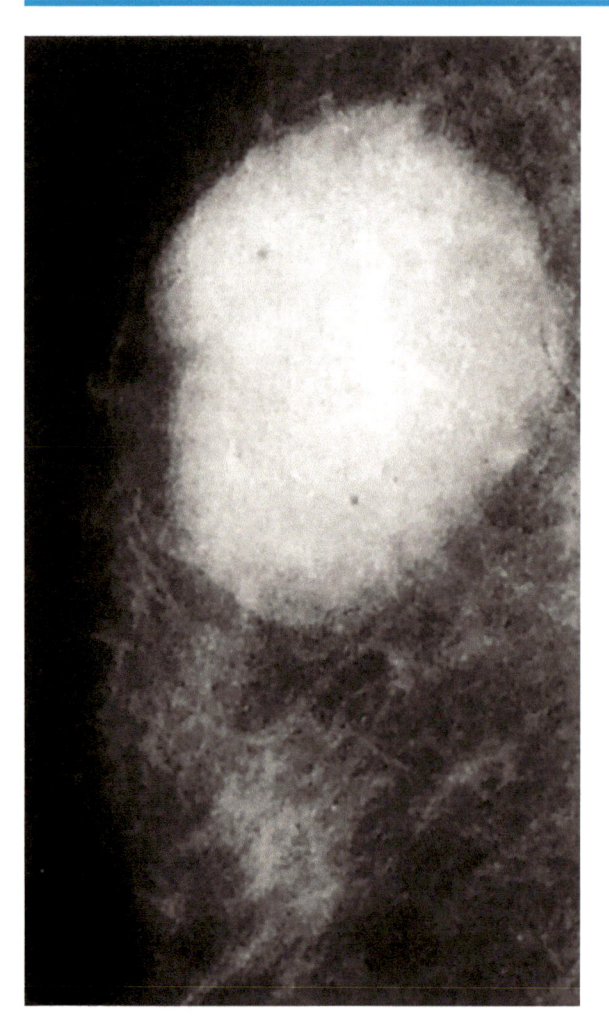

Fig. 12.8 This painless, easily moveable breast nodule in a 58-year-old man was found to be a leiomyoma (from Barth 1994). The mammographic pattern is nonspecific. *Histology:* Leiomyoma.

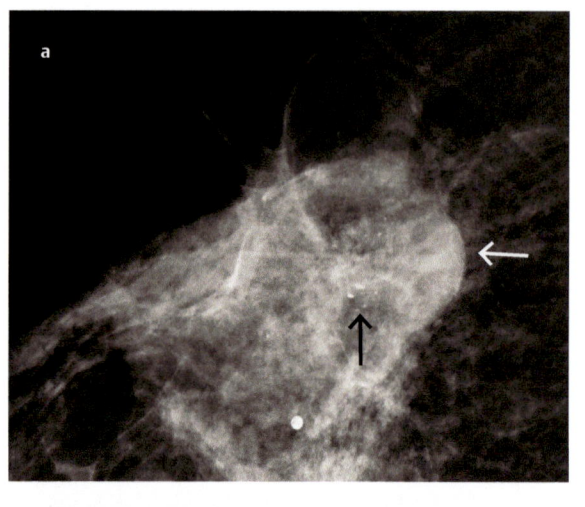

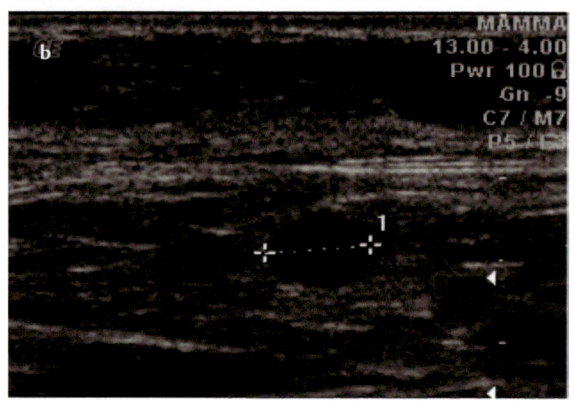

Fig. 12.9a,b Myofibroblastoma.
a An oval mass partly obscured by dense tissue is shown at the posterior border of the glandular tissue. There are also some "teacup" calcifications of superimposed benign microcystic changes (section of mediolateral oblique view).
b Sonography confirms a well-circumscribed oval mass with slight posterior enhancement. Utrasound-guided biopsy verified a myofibroblastoma. Follow-up was recommended.

Angiomas

Intramammary angiomas that are not in the skin or in the subcutaneous tissues are rare. They encompass:
- Various forms of hemangioma, the angiolipoma, the lymphangioma, and angiomatosis

These tumors are benign. Hemangioma, angiolipoma, and angiomatosis are well vascularized. *Clinically*, they are inconspicuous, unless intracutaneous or subcutaneous. They can cause the sensation of tension or pain, grow slowly or thrombose, and then become painful. Subcutaneous angiomas may appear bluish through the overlying skin and can even grow into the skin. If they are palpable, they feel soft and spongelike.

Most hemangiomas are smoothly marginated and oval to lobulated. An indistinct outline is rare.

Mammographically, most hemangiomas have a density similar to glandular tissue, are well circumscribed, lobulated or oval, and are thus indistinguishable from fibroadenomas. The occurrence of round calcifications (small phleboliths) has been described as typical but appears to occur rarely. Often they are located subcutaneously, sometimes intracutaneously (Mesurolle et al. 2008). Owing to their benign appearance, the majority of hemangiomas do not undergo biopsy and are thus not diagnosed as such. In rare cases with indistinct margins core needle biopsy will usually yield the correct diagnosis.

Lymphangiomas, angiolipomas—which always contain lipomatous inclusions—and angiomatoses often grow in a lobulated and permeative fashion, with corresponding image presentation. Rarely, round calcifications can occur in angiomas. Most will not undergo histopathologic assessment owing to their benign appearance (containing fat inclusion) and because of the absence of change (mostly since childhood).

The sonographic pattern of benign vascular lesions is variable. Hemangiomas may be hyper-, iso- or hypoechoic depending on the size and arrangement of vessels and connective tissue. Most present as a well-circumscribed oval or lobulated mass (Mesurolle et al. 2008).

Typical clinical presentation of an intracutaneous or subcutaneous hemangioma, angioma, or lymphangioma obviates the diagnostic biopsy. If percutaneous breast biopsy is performed because of a somewhat indistinct margin, the diagnosis reliably excludes a breast cancer. Since angiosarcoma is a very rare lesion anyway, the negative predictive value of the diagnosis obtained at percutaneous breast biopsy is expected to be very high and follow-up can be justified.

Increasing size of a vascular lesion should usually be an indication for excision, since the differentiation from an angiosarcoma may otherwise be difficult.

Granular Cell Tumor (Myoblastoma)

(See **Fig. 12.10**.)

The granular cell tumor is a rare benign neurogenic mesenchymal tumor, derived from Schwann cells and histologically recognized by an eosinophilic granular cytoplasm. It may occur at any age. It may appear as a well-circumscribed mass or more often as an ill-defined or even spiculated mass.

Mammographically and sonographically, it may exhibit features of a well-circumscribed benign-appearing mass, or of an ill-circumscribed irregular or often spiculated mass resembling a carcinoma macroscopically. Very rarely it may infiltrate and retract the skin. Mammographically it is not calcified; sonographically it may exhibit posterior shadowing.

The few granular cell tumors for which MR appearance has been published exhibited signs indistinguishable from breast cancers (strong masslike enhancement, rim enhancement in one case) (B. Allgayer 1995, pers. comm., Hoess et al. 1998, Kohashi et al. 1999, Irshad et al. 2008). The diagnosis can be suspected at core needle biopsy and may further be confirmed by immunostaining.

Excision should be recommended for tumors with locally infiltrative growth pattern. Recurrence has been described after inadequate excision and very rarely has a malignant granular cell tumor with metastases been mentioned in the literature (Feder et al. 1999).

Pseudoangiomatous Stromal Hyperplasia

Pseudoangiomatous stromal hyperplasia (PASH) mostly manifests as a microscopic change without any clinical or image correlate. However, its spectrum ranges from incidental microscopic changes to nonpalpable and palpable masses and diffuse changes.

Histologically, PASH is characterized by pseudovascular slitlike spaces, which are acellular or lined by spindle cells. There may be myofibroblastic proliferation of the stroma.

Clinically, PASH is usually asymptomatic. It may be palpable as a painless mobile mass. Very rarely, rapid growth of a nodular PASH has been reported (Cohen et al. 1996, Polger et al. 1996, Lakhani 2012, Mercado et al. 2004, Salvador et al. 2004, Irshad et al. 2008, Jaunoo et al. 2011).

On imaging non-masslike growing PASH has no specific features and usually cannot be distinguished from other benign changes.

Mammographically nodular PASH is imaged as a well-circumscribed mass, mostly with smooth borders. Sometimes margins are ill defined or obscured.

Sonographically nodular PASH is mostly imaged as a well-circumscribed hypoechoic or heterogeneous mass with increased, indifferent or decreased posterior enhancement (**Fig. 12.11a,b**).

Lacelike reticular areas and cystic changes have been described in the literature (Mercado et al. 2004, Salvador et al. 2004, Irshad et al. 2008).

PASH is not a specific finding when diagnosed at core needle biopsy. Interdisciplinary correlation has to ensure that the growth pattern at histology and the imaging findings are compatible. Where the findings are compatible, follow-up (or excision in the case of a growing lesion) may be considered.

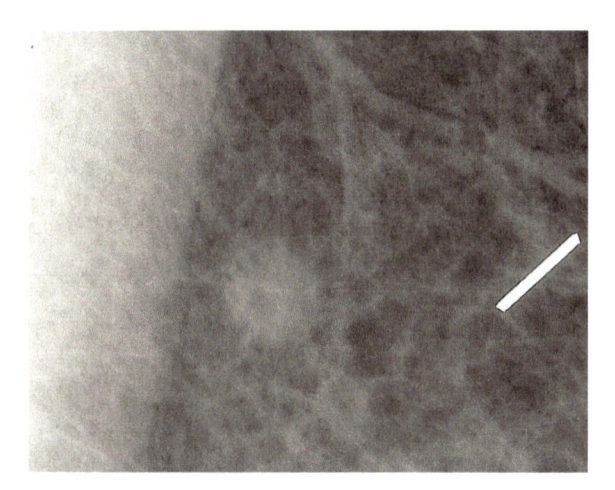

Fig. 12.10 Mammographically indistinctly outlined nodular lesion, right upper quadrant. This indistinctness prompted a diagnostic excision. *Histology*: Granular cell tumor.

12 Benign Tumors and Tumorlike Masses

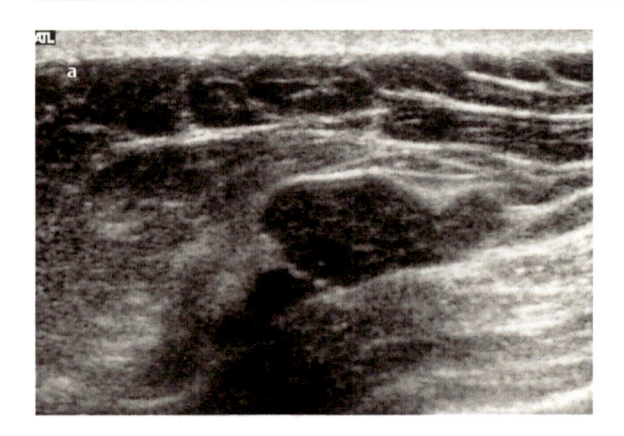

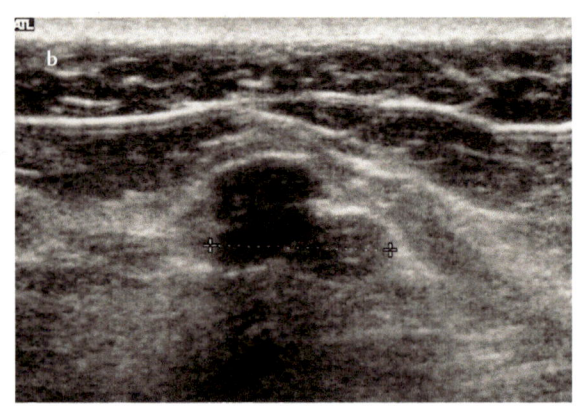

Fig. 12.11a,b Radial and anti-radial ultrasound scan of a pseudoangiomatous stromal hyperplasia, detected as a soft nodule in the upper inner quadrant of the breast.

Benign Fibroses

The benign fibroses include diabetic mastopathy and focal fibrosis.

Diabetic mastopathy is a rare disease. It is reported to occur in patients with insulin-dependent diabetes and is probably caused by some type of vasculitis. It is discussed in Chapter 13.

Fibromatosis (extra-abdominal desmoid) is a very rare tumorous lesion. It does not metastasize, but grows locally infiltrative and tends to recur. Therefore it is considered a semi-malignant tumor. It is discussed in Chapter 18.

Focal Fibrous Disease or Fibrosis Mammae

Focal fibrous disease is found in young women. It is a circumscribed fibrous proliferation of the mammary stroma associated with regional atrophy of the surrounding parenchyma. The average size is 1–3 cm, and it is observed in biopsies with an incidence of 4–8%.

Focal fibrosis may correspond to a focal palpable asymmetry or may just be detected by imaging. Imaging presentations are very variable:
- Mammographically, focal fibrous disease can appear as a sharply outlined mass, as a lobulated nodule, or as an irregularly outlined mass (Revelon et al. 2000, Goel et al. 2005).
- Sonographically focal fibrosis may be hypo- or isoechoic to fat. Fibrosis may cause acoustic shadowing.
- MRI of focal fibrosis shows no enhancement and can therefore be distinguished from malignancy.

Percutaneous biopsy shows the presence of abundant fibrosis, which is a nonspecific finding. Owing to the nonspecific nature of such a histopathologic finding, close correlation of imaging and histopathology and critical analysis is needed to ascertain whether such a finding is acceptable and malignancy can be excluded with sufficient confidence based on the available material. With a larger sample, confidence in the diagnosis will increase. However, great caution is necessary with the interpretation of findings from core needle biopsy.

Amyloidosis of the Breast

Amyloidosis is characterized by deposition of amyloid in various organs. In the breast various findings have been reported (Röcken et al. 2002, Sabaté et al. 2005, 2008, Cao et al. 2011). Amyloidosis may present as a palpable or mammographic mass. Reported mammographic findings include irregular mass, asymmetry, or even clustered microcalcifications. On ultrasound imaging a hypo- or hyperechoic mass may be seen. Histologically amyloid is visualized by polarized light and proven by Congo red staining.

Steatocystoma Multiplex

Steatocystoma multiplex is a rare autosomal dominant disorder, which is characterized by hamartomatous malformation of the pilosebaceous ducts (Cao et al. 2011). This results in multiple subcutaneous oil cysts, which are visualized as subcutaneous fatty masses. They may or may not calcify. They are typical and do not require further assessment.

Intramammary Lymph Nodes

(See **Fig. 12.12**.)

Definition

Intramammary lymph nodes are located within the breast, that is, between the parenchyma and connective tissue of the breast. Lymph nodes in the axillary extension of the breast are considered intramammary if they

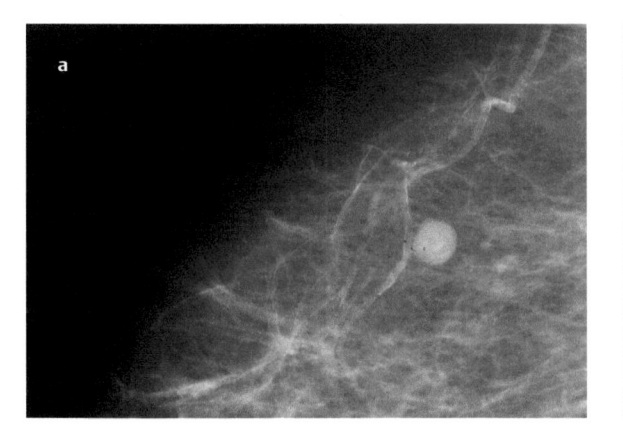

Fig. 12.12a–c
a Mammographic screening detected a well-defined mass measuring 10 mm.
b,c Sonographically it corresponded to a roundish hypoechogenic lesion, which by fine needle aspiration biopsy (c) proved to be a lymph node.

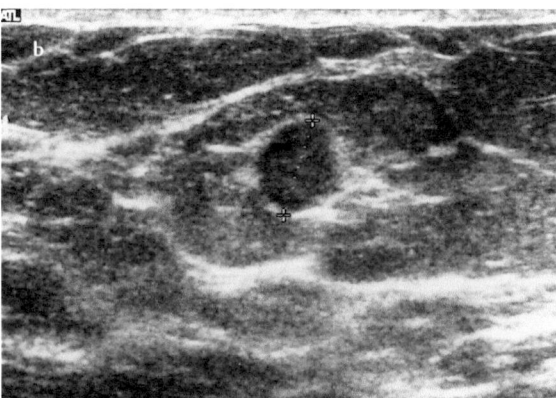

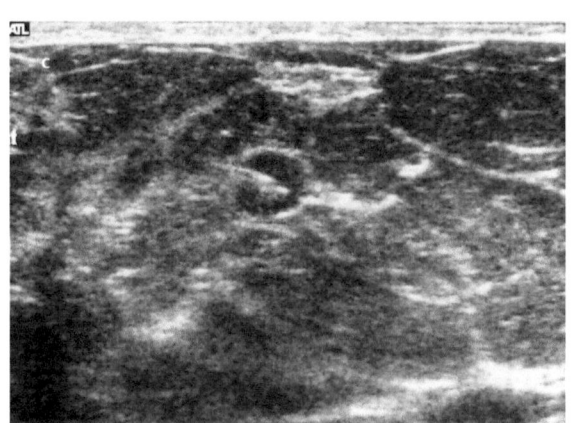

are located anterior to the pectoral muscle. Lymph nodes that project behind the anterior border of the pectoral muscle in two planes, or lymph nodes that project in this region and are visualized only in this plane, are assigned to the axilla unless proven otherwise.

Prevalence

Intramammary lymph nodes are frequently seen by mammography. Small intramammary lymph nodes are often not visualized because of their small size and insufficient density, particularly within mammographically dense parenchyma.

Purpose

In the *asymptomatic patient*, the intramammary lymph node is considered a *normal structure*. The correct diagnostic identification—often achievable on the basis of the image presentation—is important, to avoid unnecessary biopsies.

The pathology and imaging presentations of intramammary lymph nodes have an identical spectrum to that of axillary lymph nodes.

If an underlying malignant condition is present, the intramammary lymph nodes may contain metastatic deposits. Macroscopic metastatic involvement causes the mammographically typical nodal morphology to disappear. Microscopic involvement is undetectable by imaging. Lymph nodes affected by inflammatory changes may also lose their typical imaging appearance and may thus require further assessment for differentiation from other benign or malignant masses.

Histology

Histologically, intramammary nodes are not different from other lymph nodes.

Clinical Findings

Clinically, the intramammary lymph node is generally not noticed. On occasion, superficially located lymph nodes can be palpable as soft, mobile, discretely palpable masses.

Diagnostic Strategy and Goals

The goal of the diagnostic workup should be:
- The correct recognition of a lymph node in asymptomatic patients, to avoid unnecessary biopsies
- The detection of macroscopically involved intramammary lymph nodes (contour, density, hilus) in patients with a known carcinoma

Imaging

The imaging morphology of normal lymph nodes and of lymph nodes with benign and malignant changes is described in Chapter 17. The imaging morphology of intramammary lymph nodes is identical to that of axillary lymph nodes (**Fig. 12.12a,b**).

Masses which exhibit the typical features of a benign lymph node (see Chapter 17) can be considered benign and should not undergo histopathologic assessment or short-term follow-up.

Percutaneous Biopsy

A mass which might correspond to an intramammary lymph node but on imaging does not show the typical characteristics of a benign or normal lymph node requires further workup.

Cytology or core needle biopsy is capable of diagnosing a benign lymph node. Malignant involvement can be detected by needle biopsy in most (but not all) of involved lymph nodes.

In patients with ipsilateral breast cancer, correlation of imaging and histopathology is necessary to decide whether the result of a benign lymph node is compatible with imaging. Since sampling by cytology or core needle biopsy allows assessment of less than 10% of the lymph node tissue, these methods may not be able to exclude microscopic involvement.

In some cases VABB may be performed for a small indeterminate mass and will eventually yield the diagnosis of a lymph node. This diagnosis will usually be able to explain the imaging findings. Reliable detection of microscopic disease may be expected if the lymph node is removed at VABB.

In patients with ipsilateral breast cancer, percutaneous breast biopsy of indeterminate masses or inclusion of a suspected lymph node that is located within the path of lymphatic drainage may be considered when planning therapeutic surgery.

> **Summary**
>
> Intramammary lymph nodes are frequent normal findings and only some are detected by imaging methods. If the findings are typical, the correct diagnosis can be made in the majority of intramammary lymph nodes. Sonography and MRI are generally not indicated for further evaluation of intramammary lymph nodes.

References and Recommended Reading

Azzopardi JG, Salm R. Ductal adenoma of the breast: a lesion which can mimic carcinoma. J Pathol 1984;144(1):15–23

Barth V. Mammographie: Intensivkurs für Fortgeschrittene. Stuttgart: Enke; 1994

Bauer BS, Jones KM, Talbot CW. Mammary masses in the adolescent female. Surg Gynecol Obstet 1987;165(1):63–65

Bongiorno MR, Doukaki S, Aricò M. Neurofibromatosis of the nipple-areolar area: a case series. J Med Case Reports 2010;4:22

Brinck U, Fischer U, Korabiowska M, Jutrowski M, Schauer A, Grabbe E. The variability of fibroadenoma in contrast-enhanced dynamic MR mammography. AJR Am J Roentgenol 1997;168(5):1331–1334

Cao MM, Hoyt AC, Bassett LW. Mammographic signs of systemic disease. Radiographics 2011;31(4):1085–1100

Cohen MA, Morris EA, Rosen PP, Dershaw DD, Liberman L, Abramson AF. Pseudoangiomatous stromal hyperplasia: mammographic, sonographic, and clinical patterns. Radiology 1996;198(1):117–120

Dragoumis D, Atmatzidis S, Chatzimavroudis G, Lakis S, Panagiotopoulou K, Atmatzidis K. Benign spindle cell tumor not otherwise specified (NOS) in a male breast. Int J Surg Pathol 2010;18(6):575–579

Dupont WD, Page DL, Parl FF, et al. Long-term risk of breast cancer in women with fibroadenoma. N Engl J Med 1994;331(1):10–15

Engin G, Acunaş G, Acunaş B. Granulomatous mastitis: gray-scale and color Doppler sonographic findings. J Clin Ultrasound 1999;27(3):101–106

Feder JM, de Paredes ES, Hogge JP, Wilken JJ. Unusual breast lesions: radiologic–pathologic correlation. Radiographics 1999;19(Spec No):S11–S26, quiz S260

Goel NB, Knight TE, Pandey S, Riddick-Young M, de Paredes ES, Trivedi A. Fibrous lesions of the breast: imaging-pathologic correlation. Radiographics 2005;25(6):1547–1559

Hertel BF, Zaloudek C, Kempson RL. Breast adenomas. Cancer 1976;37(6):2891–2905

Heywang-Köbrunner SH, Beck R. Contrast-enhanced MRI of the breast. Heidelberg, New York: Springer; 1996

Hochman MG, Orel SG, Powell CM, Schnall MD, Reynolds CA, White LN. Fibroadenomas: MR imaging appearances with radiologic-histopathologic correlation. Radiology 1997;204(1):123–129

References and Recommended Reading

Hoess C, Freitag K, Kolben M, et al. FDG PET evaluation of granular cell tumor of the breast. J Nucl Med 1998;39(8):1398–1401

Irshad A, Ackerman SJ, Pope TL, Moses CK, Rumboldt T, Panzegrau B. Rare breast lesions: correlation of imaging and histologic features with WHO classification. Radiographics 2008;28(5):1399–1414

Jaunoo SS, Thrush S, Dunn P. Pseudoangiomatous stromal hyperplasia (PASH): a brief review. Int J Surg 2011;9(1):20–22

Jozefczyk MA, Rosen PP. Vascular tumors of the breast. II. Perilobular hemangiomas and hemangiomas. Am J Surg Pathol 1985;9(7):491–503

Kohashi T, Kataoka T, Haruta R, et al. Granular cell tumor of the breast: report of a case. Hiroshima J Med Sci 1999;48(1):31–33

Krishnan MM, Krishnan R. An unusual breast lump: neurilemmoma. Aust N Z J Surg 1982;52(6):612–613

Lakhani SR, Ellis IO, Schnitt SJ, Tan PH, van der Vijver MJ, eds. WHO classification of tumours of the breast. 2012.

Lanyi M. Diagnostik und Differentialdiagnostik der Mammaverkalkungen. Berlin: Springer; 1986

Mercado CL, Naidrich SA, Hamele-Bena D, Fineberg SA, Buchbinder SS. Pseudoangiomatous stromal hyperplasia of the breast: sonographic features with histopathologic correlation. Breast J 2004;10(5):427–432

Mesurolle B, Sygal V, Lalonde L, et al. Sonographic and mammographic appearances of breast hemangioma. AJR Am J Roentgenol 2008;191(1):W17-22

Minami S, Matsuo S, Azuma T, et al. Parenchymal leiomyoma of the breast: a case report with special reference to magnetic resonance imaging findings and an update review of literature. Breast Cancer 2011;18(3):231–236

Polger MR, Denison CM, Lester S, Meyer JE. Pseudoangiomatous stromal hyperplasia: mammographic and sonographic appearances. AJR Am J Roentgenol 1996;166(2):349–352

Porter GJ, Evans AJ, Lee AH, Hamilton LJ, James JJ. Unusual benign breast lesions. Clin Radiol 2006;61(7):562–569

Revelon G, Sherman ME, Gatewood OM, Brem RF. Focal fibrosis of the breast: imaging characteristics and histopathologic correlation. Radiology 2000;216(1):255–259

Röcken C, Kronsbein H, Sletten K, Roessner A, Bässler R. Amyloidosis of the breast. Virchows Arch 2002;440(5):527–535

Rosen PP. Vascular tumors of the breast. III. Angiomatosis. Am J Surg Pathol 1985;9(9):652–658

Sabaté JM, Clotet M, Gómez A, De Las Heras P, Torrubia S, Salinas T. Radiologic evaluation of uncommon inflammatory and reactive breast disorders. Radiographics 2005;25(2):411–424

Sabaté JM, Gómez A, Torrubia S, et al. Evaluation of breast involvement in relation to Cowden syndrome: a radiological and clinicopathological study of patients with PTEN germ-line mutations. Eur Radiol 2006;16(3):702–706

Sabaté JM, Clotet M, Torrubia S, et al. Localized amyloidosis of the breast associated with invasive lobular carcinoma. Br J Radiol 2008;81(970):e252–e254

Salvador R, Lirola JL, Domínguez R, López M, Risueño N. Pseudo-angiomatous stromal hyperplasia presenting as a breast mass: imaging findings in three patients. Breast 2004;13(5):431–435

Sickles EA. Nonpalpable, circumscribed, noncalcified solid breast masses: likelihood of malignancy based on lesion size and age of patient. Radiology 1994;192(2):439–442

Skaane P, Engedal K. Analysis of sonographic features in the differentiation of fibroadenoma and invasive ductal carcinoma. AJR Am J Roentgenol 1998;170(1):109–114

Soo MS, Dash N, Bentley R, Lee LH, Nathan G. Tubular adenomas of the breast: imaging findings with histologic correlation. AJR Am J Roentgenol 2000;174(3):757–761

Stavros AT, Thickman D, Rapp CL, Dennis MA, Parker SH, Sisney GA. Solid breast nodules: use of sonography to distinguish between benign and malignant lesions. Radiology 1995;196(1):123–134

Stavros AT, Rapp CL, Parker SH. Breast ultrasound. Philadelphia, PA: Lippincott, Williams and Wilkins; 2003

Toker C, Tang CK, Whitely JF, Berkheiser SW, Rachman R. Benign spindle cell breast tumor. Cancer 1981;48(7):1615–1622

Tomaszewski JE, Brooks JS, Hicks D, Livolsi VA. Diabetic mastopathy: a distinctive clinicopathologic entity. Hum Pathol 1992;23(7):780–786

Travade A, Isnard A, Gimbergues H. Imagerie de la pathologie mammaire. Paris: Masson; 1995

Viehweg P, Heywang-Köbrunner SH, Bayer U, Friedrich T, Spielmann RP. Simulation of breast carcinoma by diabetic mastopathy. [Article in German] Rofo 1996;164(6):519–521

13 Inflammatory Conditions

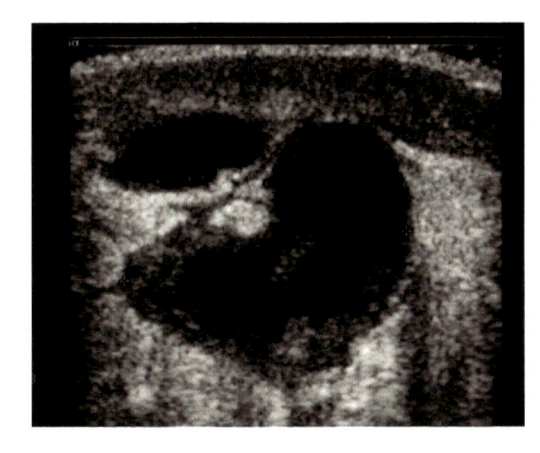

Mastitis → *316*
Etiology → *316*
Clinical Findings → *316*
Diagnostic Strategy and Goals → *317*

Abscesses and Fistulas → *321*
Histology → *321*
Clinical Findings → *321*
Diagnostic Strategy → *321*

Granulomatous Conditions → *327*
Histologic and Microbiological Confirmation → *327*
Clinical Findings → *327*
Diagnostic Strategy → *328*

References and Recommended Reading → *335*

13 Inflammatory Conditions

I. Schreer, S. H. Heywang-Koebrunner, S. Barter

In the last few decades, the etiologic and pathologic spectrum of the various inflammatory breast conditions has changed, with the decreasing incidence of bacterial puerperal mastitis. Today, chronic inflammatory conditions that are unrelated to gravidity or delivery are in the foreground of the clinical and radiologic diagnostic evaluation of these disorders.

Mastitis is frequently associated with an inflammatory pseudotumor (infiltration, abscess, granuloma). This can imitate malignancy, particularly an inflammatory carcinoma.

Pathogenetic and clinical criteria distinguish:
- Puerperal mastitis
- Nonpuerperal mastitis (bacterial, purulent and granulomatous types)
- Specific granulomatous mastitis
- Mycoses and parasitic infestations

Mastitis

Etiology

Acute puerperal mastitis occurs during pregnancy and lactation. It is bacterial in origin and develops through infection of the lactiferous ducts and lymphatic clefts during nursing, primarily in the presence of galactostasis.

If the therapy is inadequate, the acute mastitis can change into a subacute or chronic mastitis, causing abscesses or fistulous tracts.

Acute Nonspecific Mastitis

Outside lactation and the postoperative period, acute mastitides are rare. They can be caused by:
- Infection of distended subareolar lactiferous ducts = subareolar abscess formation—this can be precipitated by squamous metaplasia and hyperplasia of the subareolar lactiferous ducts, resulting in obstruction, secretory retention, and infection
- Infection originating from the skin of the breast or areola (infection of sebaceous or sweat glands, infection from cosmetic piercing)
- Infection in the presence of secretion and/or duct ectasia
- Hematogenous bacterial (or mycotic) spread, a rare occurrence
- Other rare causes

Subacute and Chronic Mastitis

Any acute mastitis can evolve into a subacute or chronic mastitis, usually after inadequate therapy. In some cases, abscesses or fistulas may occur. They can be quite resistant to therapy and might persist or recur.

Chronic nonbacterial mastitis is often incorrectly called "plasma cell mastitis," though plasma cells are found neither frequently nor invariably, and pathologically it is a chronic granulomatous mastitis. It usually occurs in older women and is mostly bilateral. It is caused by secretory retention due to duct ectasia, leading to pressure atrophy of the epithelium and diffusion of the secretion into the periductal connective tissue. It progresses to galactophoritis and to total ductal obliteration. Fibrosis and retraction of the parenchyma and nipple may develop.

Prevalence and Purpose

Aside from puerperal mastitis, acute and subacute mastitides are rare. Consequently, the diagnosis of a nonpuerperal acute or subacute mastitis must be carefully assessed. In particular, inflammatory carcinoma must be excluded. If nipple or parenchymal retraction develops or parenchymal thickening is palpable, differentiation from a diffusely growing carcinoma is necessary.

Clinical Findings

Acute Mastitis

Acute mastitis presents as:
- Pain
- Erythema
- Swelling, and
- Hyperthermia of the breast

The thickened skin can resemble a peau d'orange and might be fixed. In addition, the axillary lymph nodes may be swollen and painful. Together with an elevated sedimentation rate, leukocytosis, and systemic symptoms, the diagnosis of the typical acute mastitis can be made on the basis of these findings, without further diagnostic tests, and the appropriate therapy (antibiotics, incision, and drainage) can be instituted.

It is important to monitor therapy. Atypical findings, no association with pregnancy, lactation, or surgery, and inadequate resolution are an indication to proceed with diagnostic tests to exclude inflammatory carcinoma.

Subacute and Chronic Mastitides

Depending on their manifestation, they can:
- Be unnoticed or associated with minimal inflammatory changes
- Lead to chronic retracting changes such as nipple retraction or diffuse density—symmetric presentation supports a "plasma cell mastitis" and is generally not indicative of a malignancy
- Lead to thickening and erythema of the skin
- Progress to a more or less circumscribed palpable finding with or without erythema and/or hyperthermia
- Be due to chronic fistulous tracts and abscess formation

It is important to exclude an inflammatory or diffusely spreading carcinoma by observing the clinical course and by proceeding with supplemental diagnostic evaluation.

Diagnostic Strategy and Goals

Acute Mastitis

- Imaging (usually sonography) can detect abscesses that need surgical intervention. This not only allows early intervention but also informs the surgeon of the extent of the abscess cavity.
- Through follow-up examinations (usually sonography) obtained at short intervals, the therapeutic response can be evaluated objectively and therapeutic failure recognized early.
- Further evaluation by imaging (usually mammography, sonography, and biopsy) is absolutely necessary if the therapeutic response is not adequate to rule out malignancy.

Subacute or Chronic Mastitis

- Imaging can be used to determine preoperatively the extent of fistulas and abscesses.
- Imaging and histologic evaluation is absolutely necessary to exclude diffusely spreading or inflammatory carcinoma.

Mammography

Mammography should be used in cases of acute mastitis that show no therapeutic response or have equivocal sonographic findings.

Mammographically, acute mastitis is characterized by (**Fig. 13.1**):
- Skin thickening, which is often pronounced in the caudal region of the breast and around the areola
- Diffusely increased density and edema-related impaired structural delineation, characteristically pronounced around and beneath the areola
- Edema-related linear to reticular thickening of the entire connective tissue, including Cooper ligaments
- Possible formation of abscesses, mostly seen as ill-defined masses

Despite the characteristic periareolar and subareolar increased density seen in acute mastitis, there are no findings pathognomonic of acute mastitis that exclude a malignancy in the absence of any therapeutic response.

Mammography is important for detecting or excluding any microcalcifications suggestive of malignancy. If such calcifications are present, an inflammatory carcinoma should be strongly suspected. Biopsy should then target the area of suspicious microcalcifications. If a mass is seen by sonography or mammography, biopsy should target the mass. Absent mammographic microcalcifications and absence of a detectable mass do not exclude a malignancy, since no reliable differentiating findings exist between inflammatory carcinoma without microcalcifications and mastitis.

The subacute or chronic diffuse mastitis (**Fig. 13.2**) can be present mammographically as follows:
- Skin thickening
- Reticular densities in the subcutaneous or prepectoral
- Diffuse or localized increase in density
- Unilateral increased breast density
- Retraction of ligaments and/or nipple
- Obvious scar formation and fistulous tracts (elongated structures of increased density), sometimes inclusion of air
- It may also be barely or not visualized at all in dense parenchyma

Chronic mastitis can cause mammographically characteristic calcifications (**Fig. 13.2e**) (so-called "plasma cell mastitis"). These calcifications are intraductal, in the wall of the lactiferous duct (intramural), and periductal.

Pathognomonic are:
- Coarse, elongated calcifications (measuring several millimeters)
- Elongated calcifications with central radiolucency
- Round calcifications with or without radiolucency
- The orientation of the coarse elongated intraductal and periductal calcifications, which follows the ductal structures (as seen with malignant intraductal calcifications)

While these described calcifications are pathognomonic, differentiation from intraductal carcinoma may be uncertain if the calcifications are small and delicate. This happens only occasionally. Calcifications may also be absent.

13 Inflammatory Conditions

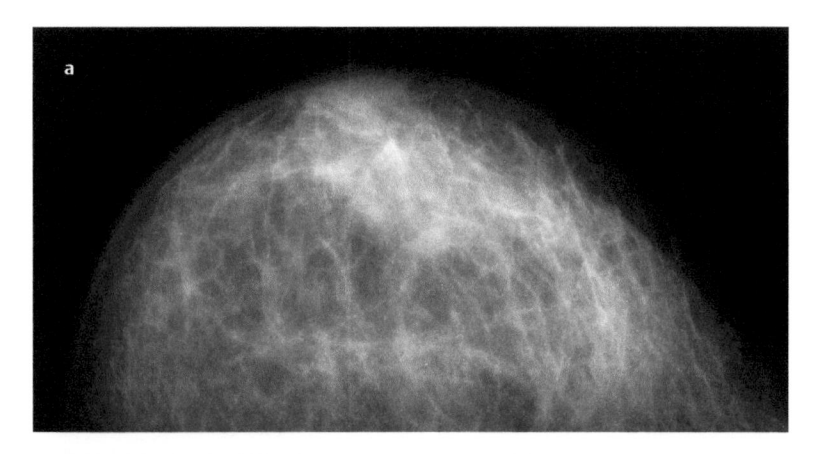

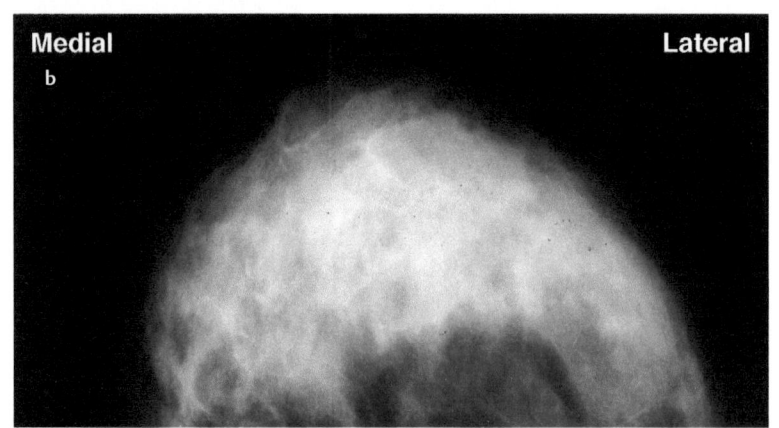

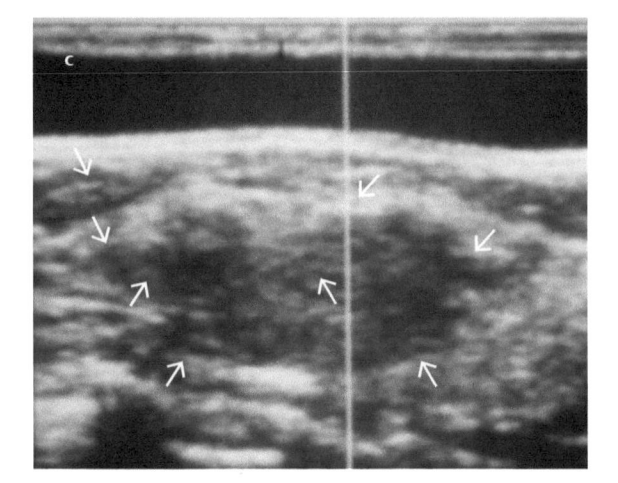

Fig. 13.1a–c Acute mastitis.

- **a** Mammographically, acute mastitis presents with diffuse skin thickening, coarsened septa, and indistinct structures, most pronounced in the retroareolar region.
- **b** This focal mastitis was detected as palpable density. Left, medial; right, lateral. Mammographically, the medially located inflamed region is not separable from the adjacent dense parenchyma. The only finding is an unusually radiodense upper inner quadrant (in comparison with the usual distribution of more radiodense tissue in the upper outer quadrant).
- **c** Sonographically (arrows), the inflamed region is swollen and hypoechoic. The narrowed subcutaneous space shows increased echogenicity. Skin thickening is not yet apparent. *Histology*: Focal mastitis.

Moreover, chronic mastitis (so-called "plasma cell mastitis") can present as (**Fig. 13.2a**):
- Diffusely increased density
- Linear or reticular accentuation in the lipomatous tissue (reactive fibrous strands)
- Retractions (in the parenchyma, thickening and shortening of Cooper ligaments)
- Nipple retraction

The presence of characteristic calcifications is pathognomonic. Since it is possible to have a carcinoma within a plasma cell mastitis, further evaluation is indicated, even in the presence of calcifications, if an additional suspected mass, architectural distortion, increasing nipple retraction, or suspicious microcalcifications exist. The distinction between malignant and chronic inflammatory masses and retractions can be extremely difficult or impossible. However, imaging can direct biopsy to the area(s) of highest suspicion.

Sonography

Acute mastitis is sonographically characterized (**Fig. 13.1c**) by:
- Skin thickening
- Increased echogenicity in the subcutaneous space and poor separation between subcutaneous space and parenchyma
- Decreased echogenicity in the parenchyma (sometimes)
- Acoustic shadowing in the parenchyma (minimal to moderate in degree)
- Detection of dilated ducts (anechoic to hypoechoic) in cases of retained secretion. They are often indistinct in outline because of inflammatory reaction. Echoes might be seen within the ducts because of the high protein content of the inflammatory exudate.
- Possible detection of confluent hypoechoic cavities
- Possible detection of large hypoechoic abscesses

For acute mastitis, sonography is used to evaluate the therapeutic success, above all in the detection or exclusion of large abscesses that usually have to undergo surgical therapy, as well as for preoperative assessment of the extent of the inflammatory process.

For subacute and chronic mastitis, sonography (**Fig. 13.2b**) can:
- Detect dilated ducts (which, however, can also be present as a manifestation of benign changes)
- Visualize fistulas and abscesses as hypoechoic or anechoic cavities or interconnected cavities

Subacute and chronic mastitis can—depending on stage and extension—cause:
- Skin thickening (usually slight and sometimes absent)
- Structural changes in the parenchyma
- Dilated ductal structures with hypoechoic (rarely anechoic) content
- Acoustic shadowing (with increasing fibrosis)
- Hypoechoic structures (through local fibrosis or granulomas) and
- Possible fistulas or abscesses (rare)

The exclusion of a malignancy is generally not possible by sonography. However, it may be very helpful for assessing the extent of abscess formation, for monitoring response to therapy, and for guiding percutaneous or surgical biopsy and therapeutic interventions.

Magnetic Resonance Imaging

Inflammatory changes show (depending on the activity) contrast enhancement:
- Moderate to strong combined with any type of enhancement dynamics (washout, plateau-type or progressive), but sometimes rapid or delayed (during the acute stage)
- Mostly progressive or plateau-type moderate (subacute to chronic)
- Minimal to moderate progressive (chronic stage with minimal activity) (**Fig. 13.2c,d**)

Abscesses are imaged as nonenhancing cavities surrounded by an enhancing wall.

Diffuse mastitic changes generally cause a diffuse enhancement of the entire parenchyma, often most pronounced in the subareolar region.

Since the enhancement in inflammatory processes, even when considering degree and rate of enhancement, is no different from the variable enhancement in malignancies, magnetic resonance imaging (MRI) is not suitable for the differential diagnosis between inflammatory and malignant changes.

Biopsy Methods

The response to antibiotic therapy determines the further approach to inflammatory processes.

If inadequate response of inflammatory changes to antibiotic therapy suggests a malignancy, excisional biopsy with sampling of the skin overlying the suspicious region is indicated. This should exclude a malignancy (inflammatory carcinoma, lymphoma, leukemia) as the cause of diffuse changes.

13 Inflammatory Conditions

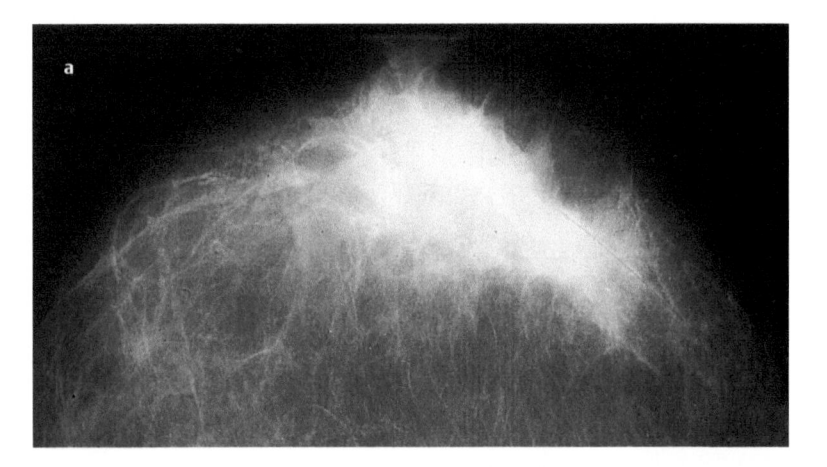

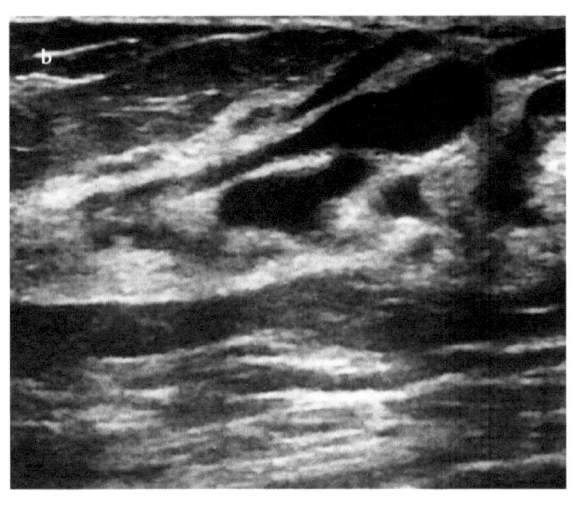

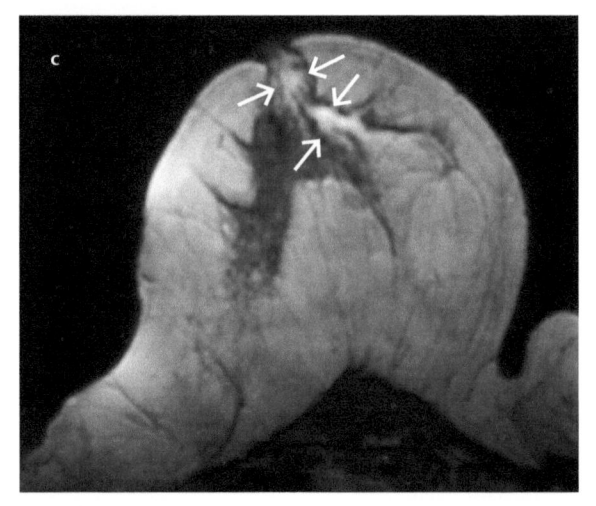

Fig. 13.2a–e Chronic mastitis.

a–d Patient with mammographically indeterminate density detected by screening mammography. No signs of acute inflammation.

a With chronic mastitis, architectural distortion and masses can develop secondary to increasing fibrosis. Mammographically, differentiation from a diffusely growing carcinoma is extremely difficult at this stage. The clinical changes (palpation) were discrete in comparison with the mammographic findings, suggesting that it is not a diffusely growing carcinoma.

b Furthermore, the sonographically dilated ductal structures (arrows) suggest a so-called chronic comedomastitis caused by retained secretion. However, sonographically, ductal carcinoma in situ might mimic this presentation.

c The magnetic resonance image before administration of Gd-DTPA shows dilated ducts of high signal intensity (arrows). The remaining low signal parenchyma exhibits the same irregular structure that is apparent mammographically.

d After administration of Gd-DTPA, the entire visualized parenchyma fails to show any appreciable enhancement. *Diagnosis*: "Burnt-out" comedomastitis with fibrosis, no evidence of malignancy.

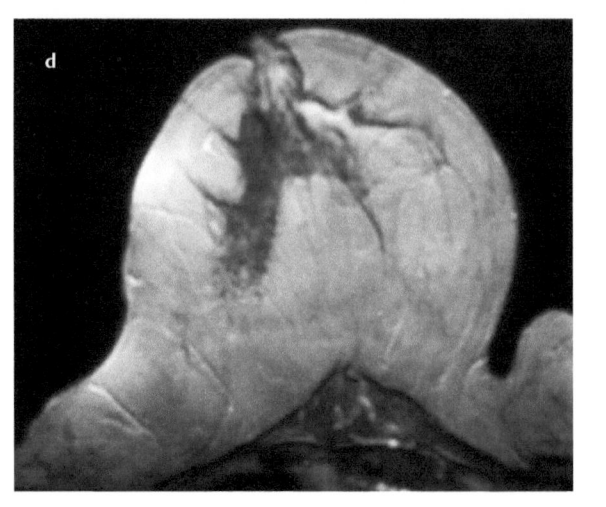

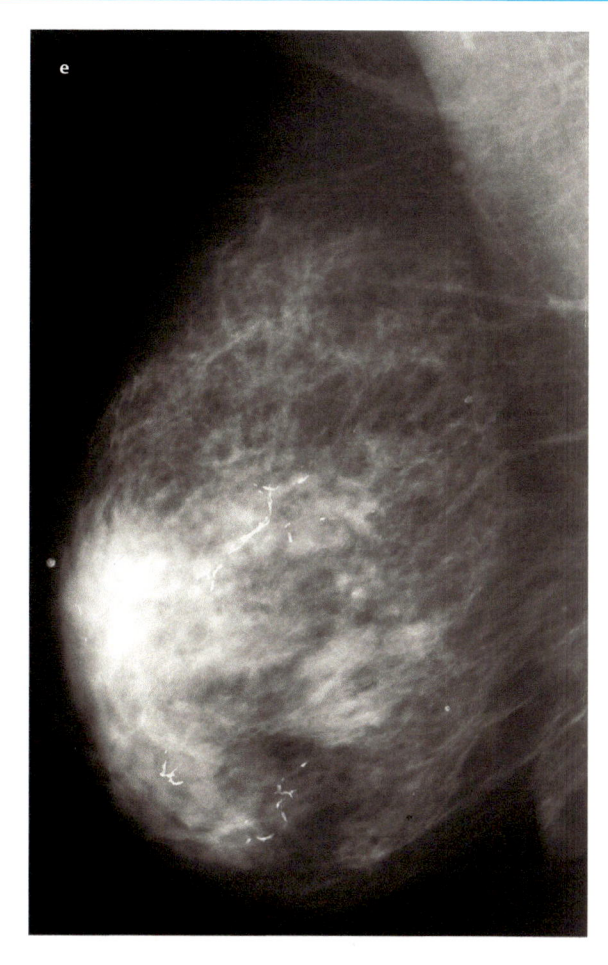

e Periductal calcifications that develop in context with a so-called "plasma-cell mastitis" generally have a characteristic pattern. The individual calcification is coarse and relatively large, needlelike, or round, occasionally with central radiolucency. Corresponding to their periductal and intraductal location, the typical calcifications of the so-called "plasma-cell mastitis" follow the orientation of the ductal structures.

Abscesses and Fistulas

Abscesses can be formed:
- On the basis of an acute or chronic mastitis, also following a galactophoritis
- From a local infection; also following infections of, for example, the Montgomery glands, sweat glands, and so forth
- Through direct extension (arising from pleural or chest wall abscesses)

The causes to be considered are:
- Bacterial infections
- Tuberculosis (actinomycosis, syphilis)
- Fungal infections
- Parasitoses, such as echinococcal cysts, which are mentioned here as an extreme rarity

Histology

An abscess is a pus-filled uniloculated or multiloculated cavity surrounded by a so-called abscess capsule, consisting of granulation tissue with inflammatory cells and fibroblasts. Abscess cavities are usually round or oval, ill-defined, and often surrounded by inflammatory edema.

Inflammatory processes with a subacute or chronic course can develop fistulas. The fistulous system consists of necrotic, often branching tracts containing pus and necrotic material, which are surrounded by granulation tissue. Air may be contained within fistulas.

Clinical Findings

Most abscesses are:
- Palpable as localized, often fixed mass sometimes with fluctuation, and
- Can have thickening and fixation of the overlying skin

The typical inflammatory changes are:
- Skin discoloration over the abscess (bluish-red)
- Hyperthermia
- Pain

Rarely:
- These typical inflammatory changes can be absent or minimally present (e.g., tuberculous "cold abscess").
- Such inflammatory changes can be imitated by a carcinoma with inflammatory component.

Fistulas are generally diagnosed as:
- Tracts with openings on the skin or nipple
- Having transient (or constant) purulent drainage

The tissue surrounding the fistulous tracts is generally diffusely indurated and may—depending on the activity of the inflammation—exhibit inflammatory changes (skin discoloration, erythema, pain).

Diagnostic Strategy

(See **Fig. 13.3**.)

A clinically obvious diagnosis does not require mammography.
- During the acute phase of a clinically evident abscess, mammography should be avoided because of the associated discomfort.
- Sonography is appropriate to determine:
  - Whether the abscess has one or several loculations
  - Whether the abscess has an even larger solid component and
  - The extent of fistulization

13 Inflammatory Conditions

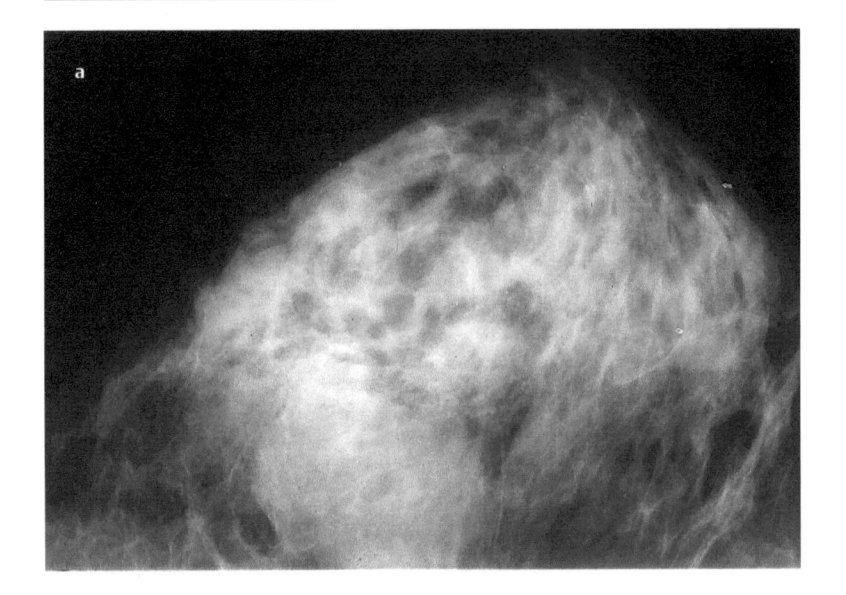

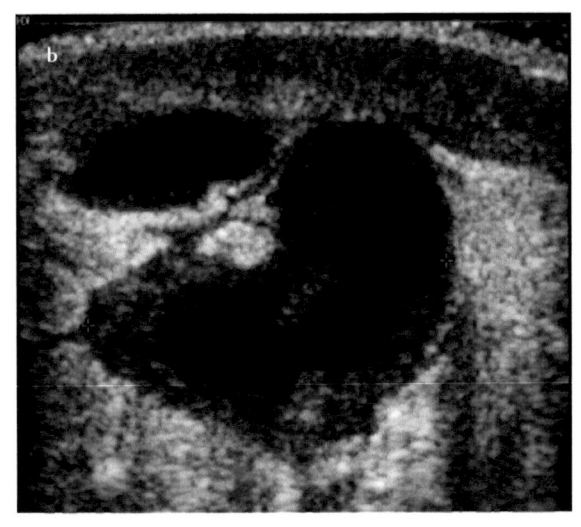

Fig. 13.3a–i Abscess
a Mammographically (mediolateral view), the abscess is visualized as an oval, indistinctly outlined mass.
b Sonographically, two anechoic, partly complex ill-defined masses with increased sound transmission represented two adjacent abscesses.

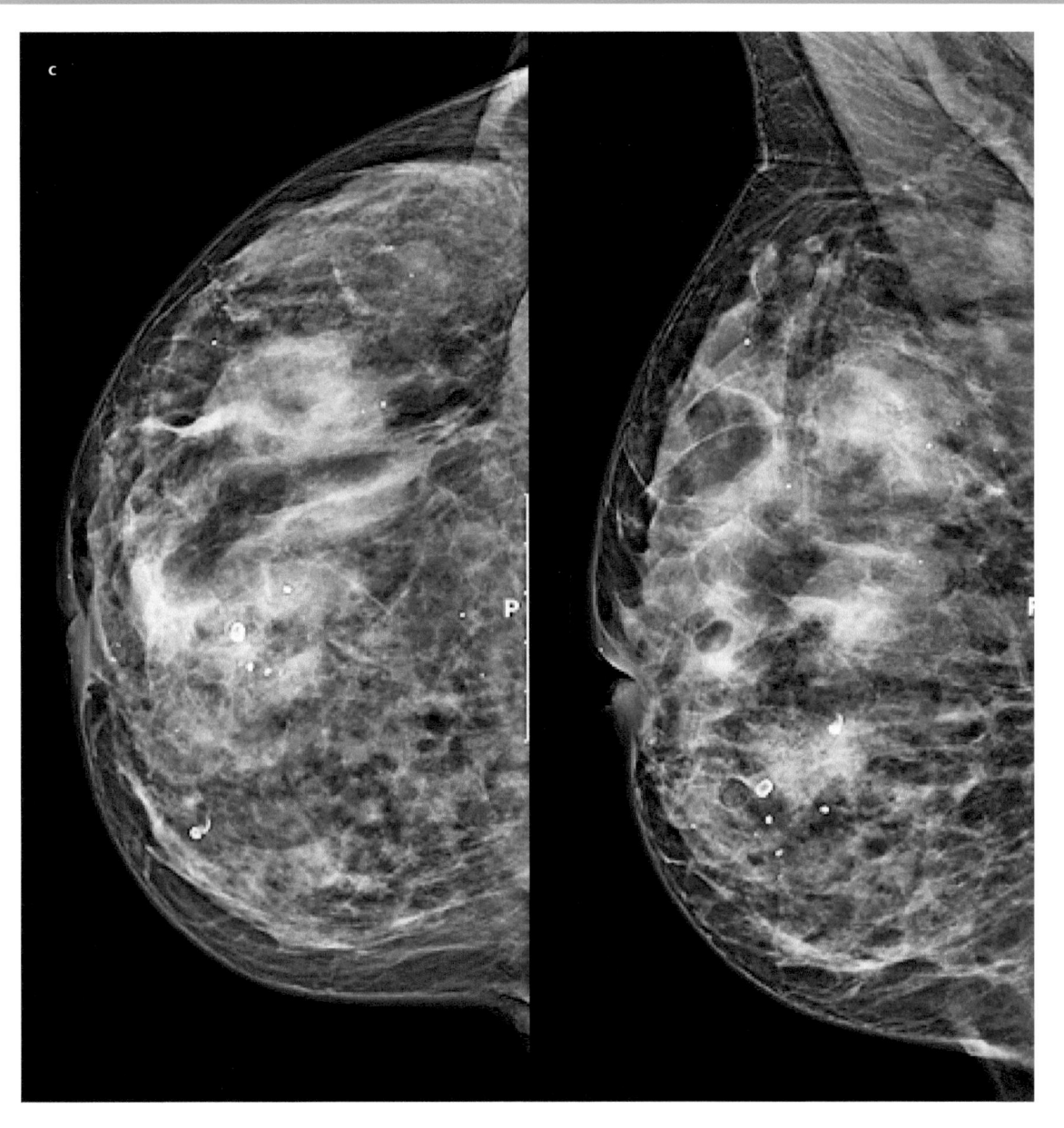

c,d Patient with recurrent (bilateral) subacute abscesses and inflammation. The patient again presented with a newly palpable mass in the right upper inner quadrant, which is barely recognized within the moderately dense breast tissue in the upper inner quadrant (arrows). The microcalcifications (**d**) far laterally and posterior were unchanged for many years and have therefore not been further assessed. They may correspond to calcified ductal debris due to chronic inflammation. Nipple retraction is also seen and is explained by fibrotic changes due to chronic inflammation.

Fig. 13.3d–i ▷

◁ continued

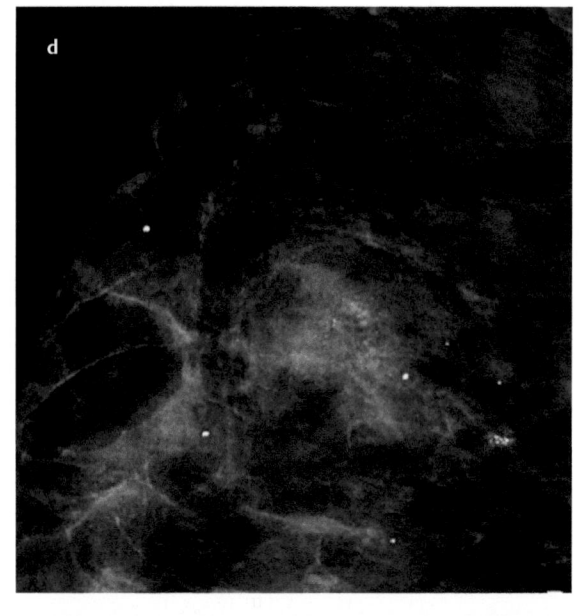

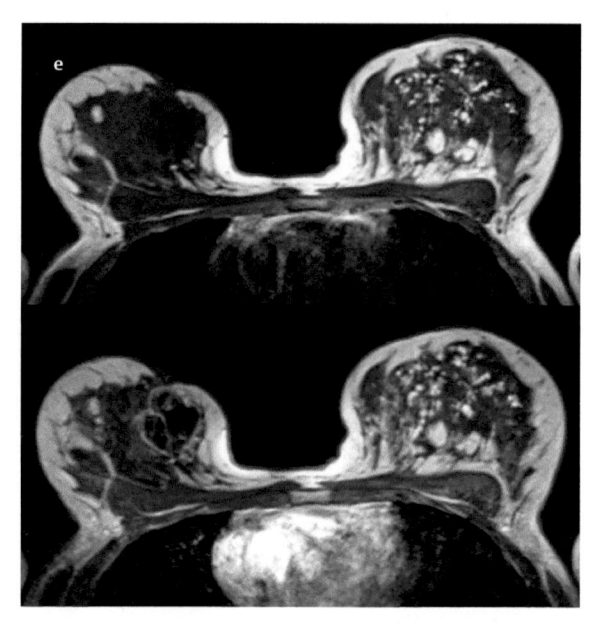

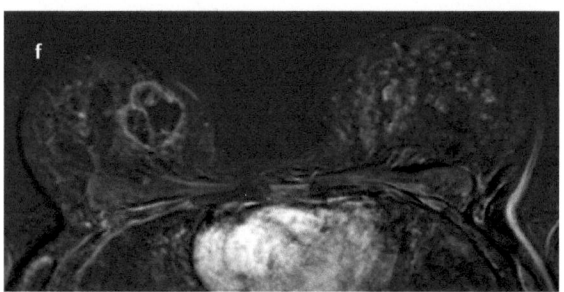

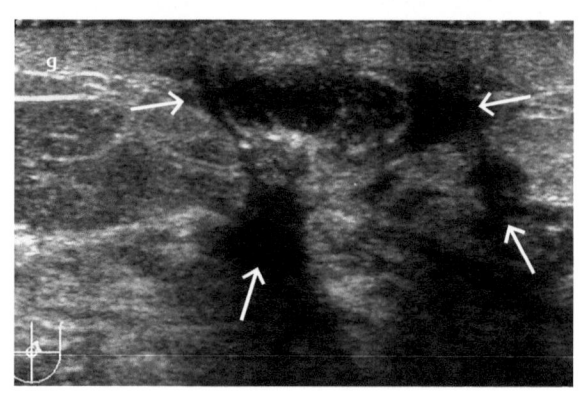

e,f Representative precontrast, postcontrast, and subtraction images. On the precontrast image (**e**) mucous material is retained in the ducts (mainly on the left) and exhibits bright signal. On the postcontrast and subtraction (**e, f**) images slight patchy enhancement compatible with chronic inflammatory changes is seen in both breasts. Furthermore, on the right early enhancement is seen in the wall and septations of the medially located abscess. Due to insufficient response to antibiotics, therapeutic excision was necessary, proving unspecific chronic granulomatous and inflammatory changes.

g Further ultrasound images of acute abscess: There is marked skin thickening with loss of the normal structure of the subcutaneous fascia and fat layer, replaced by diffuse echo scattering. One superficial oval complex lesion is visible (long arrows) and further irregular, hypoechoic, ill-defined masses in the deeper tissue layer. All lesions corresponded to abscesses.

Abscesses and Fistulas

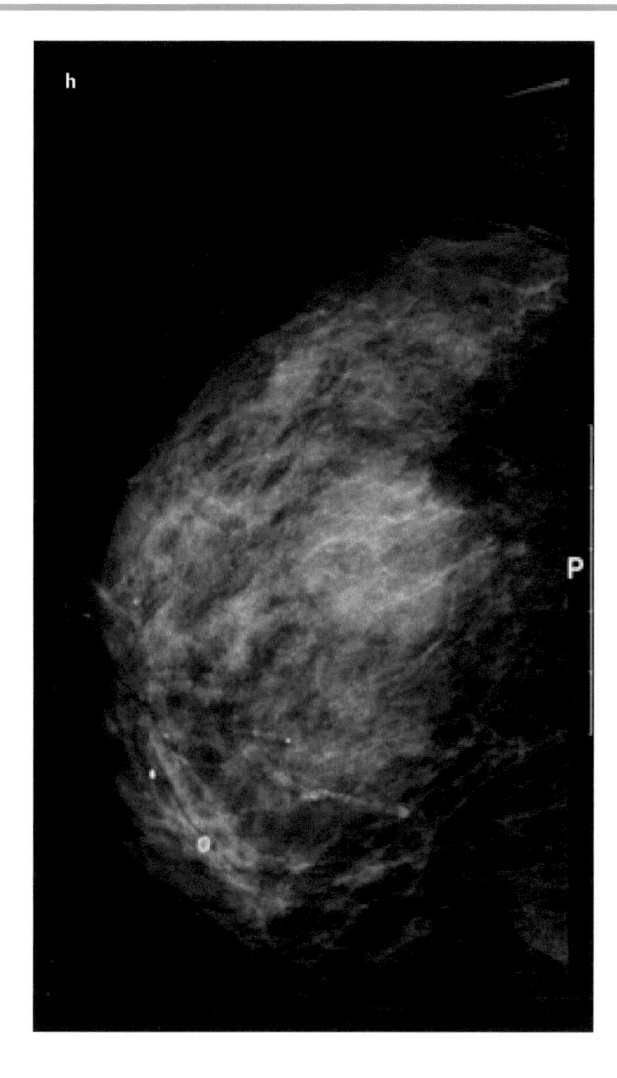

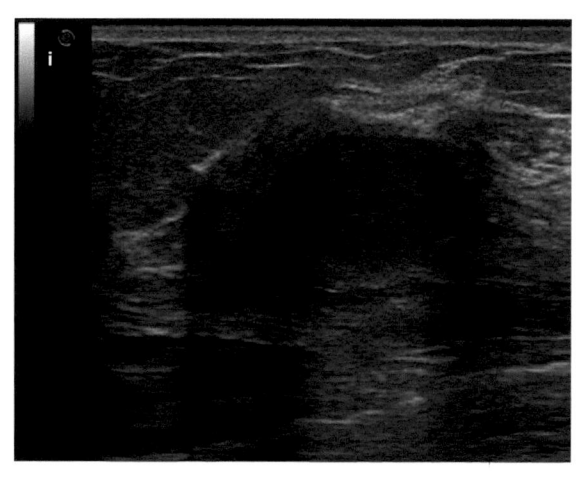

h,i In this asymptomatic screening patient an ill-defined mass was noted on mammography (**h**). The mass was palpable within very nodular breast tissue. On sonography (**i**) it corresponded to a complex ill-defined oval lesion with both posterior shadowing and enhanced sound transmission. Ultrasound-guided biopsy, which yielded necrotic material, was considered possibly nonrepresentative (since necrosis may also occur in malignancy); therefore ultrasound-guided vacuum-assisted biopsy was performed and yielded chronic inflammatory disease.

Depending on the clinical findings, sonographic findings and size of the abscess, the clinician will select:
- Antibiotic therapy (e.g., multiple small abscesses)
- Aspiration
- Sonographically guided percutaneous drainage
- Incision and drainage
- Excision

Conservative therapy is monitored by:
- Sonography as the method of choice
- Mammography for clarifying remaining uncertainty in clinically confusing situations where the possibility of malignancy is suspected

Diagnostic uncertainties, which may occur in the subacute or chronic stage, and recurrent abscesses and fistulas should be further evaluated by:
- Mammography to detect malignancy, if present
- Mammography and sonography to assist the preoperative assessment of the extent of the inflammatory process

Since imaging generally cannot exclude a malignancy, in the presence of uncharacteristic inflammatory processes, excision is unavoidable for diagnostic—and often also for therapeutic—reasons in most cases.

Sonography

Sonographically, an abscess appears as follows (**Fig. 13.3b,g,h**):
- The lesion is hypoechoic, generally round to oval in shape.
- The outline is smooth or irregular.
- The sound transmission is good to moderate.
- The central internal echoes found in the mature abscess are generally regular, but sedimentations—moveable echoes—or septations can occur. Individual, very strong echoes that rise with positional changes are suggestive of gas bubbles.
- Most abscesses are surrounded by edematous, hypoechoic tissue.

Fistulous tracts can be followed as hypoechoic, serpiginous tubular structures within an indurated area. However, sometimes fistulas may be difficult to visualize.

Value

Sonography is the method of choice for evaluating the extent and morphology of abscesses and fistulas and to monitor the therapeutic response. It can be used to guide percutaneous drainage.

Mammography

(See **Fig. 13.3a**.)
- An abscess is generally seen as a round, not entirely smoothly outlined, space-occupying lesion.
- Characteristically, an abscess exhibits an ill-defined, indistinct demarcation caused by the surrounding edema. Also characteristically, but not always present, there is an edematous, ill-defined increase in overall density that is most pronounced around the lesion extending to the subareolar region.
- In dense parenchyma, an abscess may be seen only as a nonspecific increase in density, or may not be noted at all.
- In addition, increased reticular markings and skin thickening may be observed.
- Occasionally, air collections or air–fluid levels are present, with the latter seen only in the mediolateral projection.

Fistulas are not mammographically visualized unless they contain air or are injected with contrast material. The fistulous segments that contain air (rarely observed with compression) can be seen as hypodense serpiginous structures.

Most fistulous inflammatory conditions are revealed only through ill-defined densities caused by thickening of the surrounding tissues. In dense parenchyma, this might only be seen as asymmetry or not at all.

Depending on the activity and extent of the inflammation, the same findings observed with an abscess—such as edematous changes, thickened Cooper ligaments, and skin thickening—might suggest the presence of a neoplastic process.

Value

If the diagnosis is unclear, mammography can be used as a supplemental examination. Indistinct demarcation from the surrounding tissue due to edema as well as subareolar extension of the edema due to inflammation suggests an inflammatory process. There are no criteria that can reliably exclude a malignancy.

If suspicious calcifications are seen in the area in question or elsewhere in the breast, a malignancy must be considered.

Magnetic Resonance Imaging

Contrast-enhanced MRI can be used in selected cases in which findings were difficult to evaluate mammographically and sonographically (e.g., after multiple injections of silicone and wax or for monitoring of large involved areas), for the preoperative evaluation of the extent of the abscess and fistulous formation:
- MRI visualizes abscesses (**Fig. 13.3e,f**) as round or irregularly outlined fluid-filled cavities, with variable signal intensity and without enhancement.
- Abscesses are generally surrounded by a thin, internally smooth capsule, which shows intense and early enhancement.
- The inflammatory edematous tissue around an abscess usually enhances with Gd-DTPA; enhancement is delayed and of moderate intensity.

Percutaneous Biopsy

If the therapy is successful, percutaneous biopsy is unnecessary, and if it is unsuccessful, it is superfluous since these cases require surgical intervention. In indeterminate cases, where malignancy has to be excluded, it may be considered. When inflammation is suspected care should be taken to provide material for aerobic and anaerobic bacterial analysis.

Percutaneous Drainage

This can be performed under sonographic guidance. In multiloculated abscesses, surgical drainage may be preferable.

> **Summary**
>
> Most abscesses and fistulas can be correctly diagnosed clinically. Sonography is the method of choice for the morphologic evaluation of the degree of liquefication and extent, and for monitoring the therapeutic response.
>
> Mammography is indicated in diagnostically unclear cases. Ill-defined, indistinct transition to the surrounding tissue and ill-defined subareolar densities mammographically favor the diagnosis of inflammation. Suspicious calcifications can reveal a coexistent carcinoma, a centrally necrotic or inflammatory carcinoma, which may mimic an inflammation or abscess.
>
> In general, a clinically suspected malignancy cannot be reliably excluded. If the therapeutic response is inadequate, an excision is diagnostically and therapeutically indicated.

Granulomatous Conditions

Granulomas are an additional manifestation of inflammatory processes and can be seen in a variety of diseases. The most important granulomatous conditions encountered in the breast are:
- Foreign body granulomas (including granulomas around deposits of wax and silicone)
- Tuberculosis
- Sarcoidosis
- Rare fungal infections
- Rare parasitic infestations (cysticercosis)
- Autoimmune diseases such as rheumatoid arthritis, Wegener granulomatosis, giant cell arteritis, polyarteritis nodosa, lupus erythematosus, scleroderma (see also skin lesions), dermatmyositis, and Churg–Strauss syndrome
- Diabetic mastopathy or fibrosis. This is a rare disease and histologically corresponds to granulomatous mastitis and lobulitis. It is reported to occur in patients with insulin-dependent diabetes, mostly in patients under the age of 40 years (Tomaszewski et al. 1992). Presenting as palpable breast masses and asymmetric mammographic densities, it can mimic a malignancy and poses a diagnostic problem. Such palpable masses can recur in different regions of the breast.

The diagnosis of granulomas or rare granulomatous mastitis may be suspected on the basis of the history, palpatory findings, and clinical course. A rare involvement of the breast should be considered in patients afflicted with one of the generalized granulomatous conditions. Since no distinguishing criteria exist, a malignancy (carcinoma, lymphoma) should be excluded first because of its considerably higher incidence.

Histologic and Microbiological Confirmation

Foreign body granulomas are histologically diagnosed. Their underlying causes range from talcum and sutures to deposits of wax and silicone (see also Chapter 20) and they can be recognized histologically.

Histologically, foreign body granulomas mostly have a rounded lobulated contour. In their initial stage, they consist of highly vascularized granulomatous tissue with round cellular infiltrates and giant cells. The inflammatory process may resolve, replacing the granulation tissue with dense scar tissues containing foreign body material.

The diagnosis of *tuberculosis or another infectious granulomatous disease*, such as a fungal infection or parasitosis, is made histologically. The causative agent can be positively identified only by microbiologic examination.

Sarcoidosis is diagnosed histopathologically on the basis of characteristic granulomas. A positive Kveim test supports the diagnosis of sarcoidosis.

The diagnosis of an *autoimmune disease* of the breast, such as Wegener granulomatosis, giant cell arteriitis, or polyarteriitis nodosa, has to be made histologically, supported by the clinical presentation (in the case of multiorgan involvement) and specific laboratory tests.

Diabetic mastopathy is a unifocal or multifocal fibrosis associated with lymphoid lobulitis or perivasculitis. These changes are attributed to autoimmune reaction to diabetogenic abnormal matrix accumulation.

Clinical Findings

Foreign body granulomas are characteristically found in scars. They are seen as small, barely moveable nodules, without erythema or pain. They are often indistinguishable from small recurrences within scars.

Foreign body granulomas around large silicone and wax deposits (following injection for breast augmentation or after rupture of a prosthesis) are palpable as barely moveable nodules.

A sterile inflammation or a secondary infection with formation of abscesses and fistulas can develop many years after silicone or wax injection (see also Chapter 20).

The findings of *tuberculous mastitis* include:
- A so-called cold abscess formation: Fluctuating nodule, with or without skin thickening, characteristically with or without some coloration of the skin, usually without hyperthermia. Induration and fistulae may be another presentation
- Mastitis through extension of pleuritis
- Involvement of the breast with one or multiple large and small granulomatous foci

Granulomatous lesions may be palpable as barely moveable nodules, with or without fixation of the overlying skin. Rarely, such a mass may arise from an involved (tuberculous) intramammary lymph node.

Diffuse extension leads to a poorly defined induration, with or without skin thickening or fixation, as seen with a diffusely spreading carcinoma.

Other cases of rare inflammatory disease such as *sarcoidosis, mycobacterial or fungal infections or other rare granulomatous changes* of the breast may resemble findings seen in tuberculosis. Overall, singular and multiple lesions, as well as diffuse spread may occur, which clinically cannot be differentiated from a carcinoma.

Filariasis (a tropical disease) may in its early stage present like an acute infection (mass, reddening and thickening of the skin). Later the parasites may calcify and can thus be visible as wormlike calcified structures on mammography.

Most *autoimmune diseases* present with bilateral palpable or nonpalpable lymph node enlargement. Masses, which may or may not be palpable, may present with concomitant inflammatory changes, sometimes even with involvement of the overlying skin (thickening, abscess formation, ulceration, or fistula). Such changes have been reported with sarcoidosis and Wegener granulomatosis.

Churg–Strauss syndrome has been reported to occur with increased global breast density and skin thickening.

Scleroderma may be generalized or circumscribed. The circumscribed variant may present as a circumscribed area with skin thickening and moderate reddish coloration limited to the involved skin. This benign entity (also named "morphea") appears to sometimes occur in patients after radiation therapy (Seale et al. 2008, Clark and Wechter 2010). As with other autoimmune diseases circumscribed scleroderma is diagnosed histologically.

Some autoimmune disease may cause calcifications of the skin or subcutaneous tissues.

Diabetic mastopathy presents as newly developed palpable breast mass(es) or induration(s) that cannot be distinguished from malignancies.

Diagnostic Strategy

Foreign body granulomas in scars may be clinically suspected on the basis of their localization, postoperative development, and stable size. In cases that are difficult to differentiate from malignancy, the following should be considered:

- Imaging, primarily mammography, is indicated to exclude suspicious microcalcifications as a sign of malignancy within the area of question or at another site.
- Differentiation between scar granuloma and recurrence is usually possible by contrast-enhanced MRI for those granulomas that are completely fibrosed. Most recurrences enhance strongly or at least moderately. Rarely, low or insignificant enhancement has been reported for skin recurrence.
- In those cases with persisting enhancement in granulomatous scar tissue, differentiation of a granuloma from a carcinoma or recurrence within the scar may be difficult with any imaging modality, including MRI. New development, increasing size, or clinical suspicion makes histopathologic assessment obligatory. Stable small size or a clinically suspected granuloma justify short-term follow-up examinations.

Infectious granulomas as well as granulomas caused by *sarcoidosis* and *autoimmune disease* are generally indistinguishable from malignancy by clinical or imaging criteria. Even a palpable breast nodule that develops in a patient with known tuberculosis, sarcoidosis, and so forth, must first be assumed to be a carcinoma rather than a rare manifestation of the underlying disease.

The diagnosis can be established by percutaneous biopsy, supplemented by additional evaluation (microbiology, blood tests, and clinical findings).

In patients with suspected *diabetic mastopathy* imaging will often be unable to provide definite differentiation between diabetic mastopathy and carcinoma. Suspicious calcifications, however, would tend to rule out a diabetic mastopathy. In insulin-dependent diabetics with recurrent suspicious nodules, the possibility of a diabetic mastopathy should be considered. The diagnosis may be confirmed by percutaneous biopsy. Since the findings may also resolve, aggressive surgery should be avoided.

Mammography

Granulomas within scarring:
- Might not be visualized within the increased density of the scar
- Might be apparent as more or less sharply delineated nodular density (**Fig. 13.4a,b**)
- Dystrophic calcifications might develop as part of the scar formation but are rarely seen in granulomas. Other types of microcalcifications (pleomorphic microcalcifications, and fine microcalcifications) may be indicative of malignancy and may require further assessment (see also **Fig. 19.4n,o**).
- Characteristic shell-like calcifications often form around silicone and wax deposits.

Neither lack of visualization nor evidence of well-defined borders allows mammographic differentiation from a carcinoma with sufficient certainty. It is therefore necessary to proceed with histopathologic assessment of a clinically suggestive abnormality regardless of the mammographic appearance.

The most important tasks of mammography are the detection of a possible carcinoma within the scar (e.g., by suspicious microcalcifications) and the preoperative exclusion of a carcinoma at a separate site.

Old granulomas around silicone and wax deposits are positively identified by their shell-like calcifications. The superimposition of masses and calcifications can interfere with mammographic evaluation and, consequently, limit the ability to detect carcinoma in breasts with multiple silicone or wax injections (see Chapter 20).

Inflammatory granulomas may present as one (or several) mass(es). Such masses are mostly ill circumscribed with indistinct margins. Sometimes the margins may be obscured by surrounding dense tissue. The overlying skin may be involved. Rarely, fistulas may be visible by inclusion of air. Chronic granulomas may exhibit calcifications. Mostly these are dystrophic calcifications. Other types of calcifications may require further assessment. Mammography may help detect malignancy anywhere in the breast. It is, however, generally not able to distinguish inflammatory densities or masses from malignancy. Therefore histopathologic assessment is usually necessary to confirm the diagnosis.

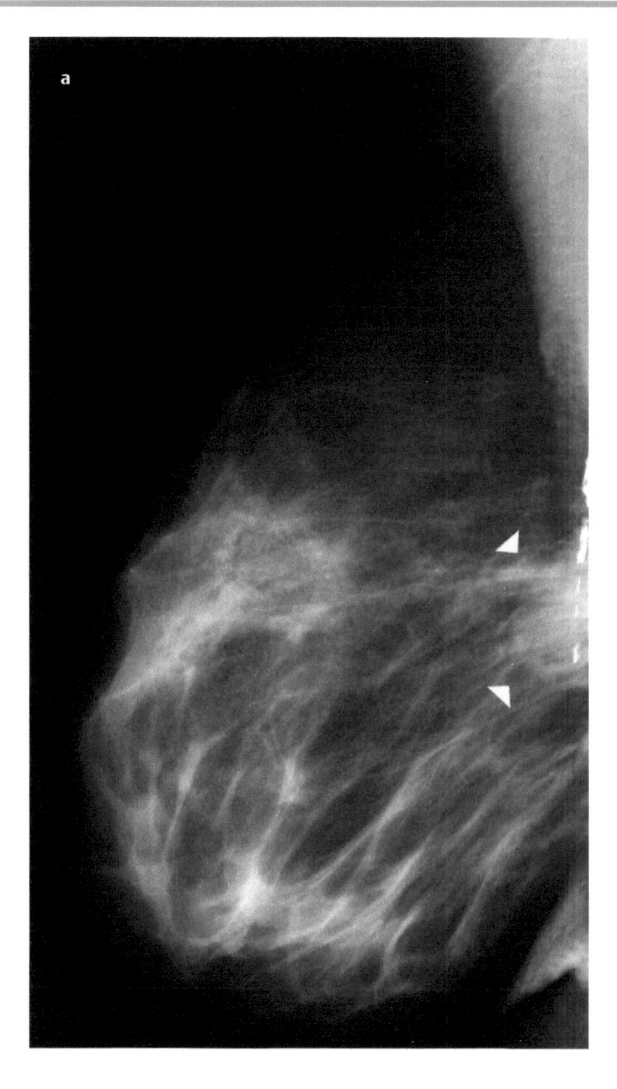

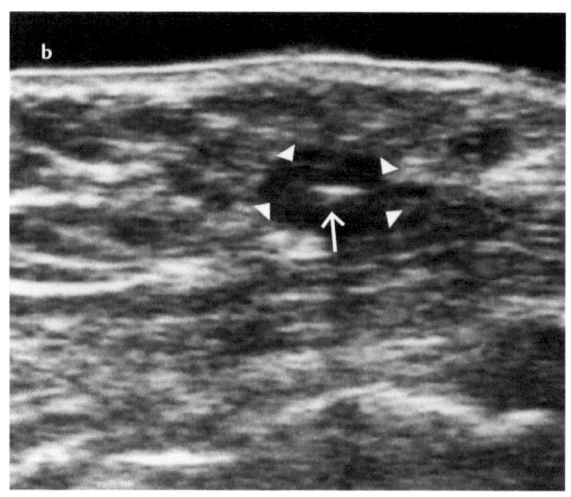

Fig. 13.4a,b Scar granuloma due to a long-standing ventriculoperitoneal shunt, situated subcutaneously and medially in the breast.

a Mammographically, an indistinctly outlined density (arrow heads) is seen, traversed by calcified shunt material. Its mammographic size corresponds to the palpable finding.

b Sonographically, the palpable lesion (arrow heads) is hypoechoic, traversed by the shunt material that appears as an echogenic structure (arrow). *Histology*: Scar granuloma.

Depending on the type of disease, unilateral or bilateral lymphadenopathy may be visualized. Enlarged lymph nodes may or may not have a visible hilum. Lymph nodes in patients with tuberculosis or fungal disease may contain calcifications (see also Chapter 17).

Wormlike calcifications may be seen and represent rare parasites, which may calcify.

In patients with *autoimmune disease* (**Fig. 13.5**) or *sarcoidosis*, bilateral lymph node enlargement is a frequent finding. In patients with *rheumatoid arthritis* gold deposits (caused by previously administered intravenous gold salt therapy) may be visible in the lymph nodes as fine elongated sharp densities resembling microcalcifications (see also **Fig. 17.8**).

Sarcoidosis and *Wegener granulomatosis* may present with mammographically visible breast masses. Skin involvement, ulceration, and fistulas are possible.

In patients with lupus erythematosus fine curvilinear subcutaneous calcifications resembling calcifications of fat necrosis have been described (Georgian-Smith et al. 2002, Kim et al. 2004). In scleroderma, skin thickening and subcutaneous calcifications have been described. Dermatomyositis may be associated with bizarre and densely packed subcutaneous calcifications (Feder et al. 1999, Cao et al. 2011).

Based on current knowledge, the mammographic spectrum of *diabetic mastopathy* encompasses radiodense tissue as seen with mastopathy, indeterminate masses, or asymmetries and ill-defined nodules with spiculation. Retraction is also possible. A mammographic differentiation from a carcinoma is generally not possible and percutaneous biopsy will usually be needed (see **Fig. 13.7**) (Thorncroft et al. 2007).

13 Inflammatory Conditions

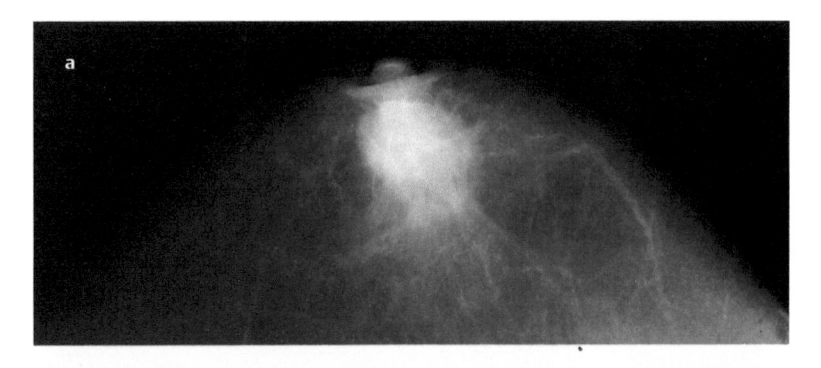

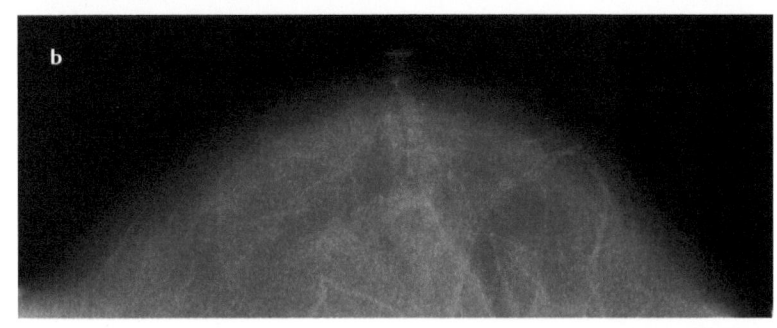

Fig. 13.5a–d Wegener granulomatosis.
- **a** Craniocaudal mammographic view of a patient with known Wegener granulomatosis. The diagnosis was confirmed by fine needle aspiration.
- **b** The patient underwent immunosuppressive therapy. The follow-up examination 3 years later is unremarkable. (Image reproduced courtesy of H. K. Deiniger.)
- **c,d** This 54-year-old patient had recurrent ulcerating granulomatous abscesses caused by Wegener granulomatosis, which regressed after high-dose immunosuppressive therapy. After dose reduction a new sonographically detected nodule appeared. **c** Mammography (performed to exclude underlying malignancy) shows retractive scarring behind the nipple which includes some air (white arrow) within persisting fistulae. The new nodule is only faintly seen as an oval mass (black arrows).

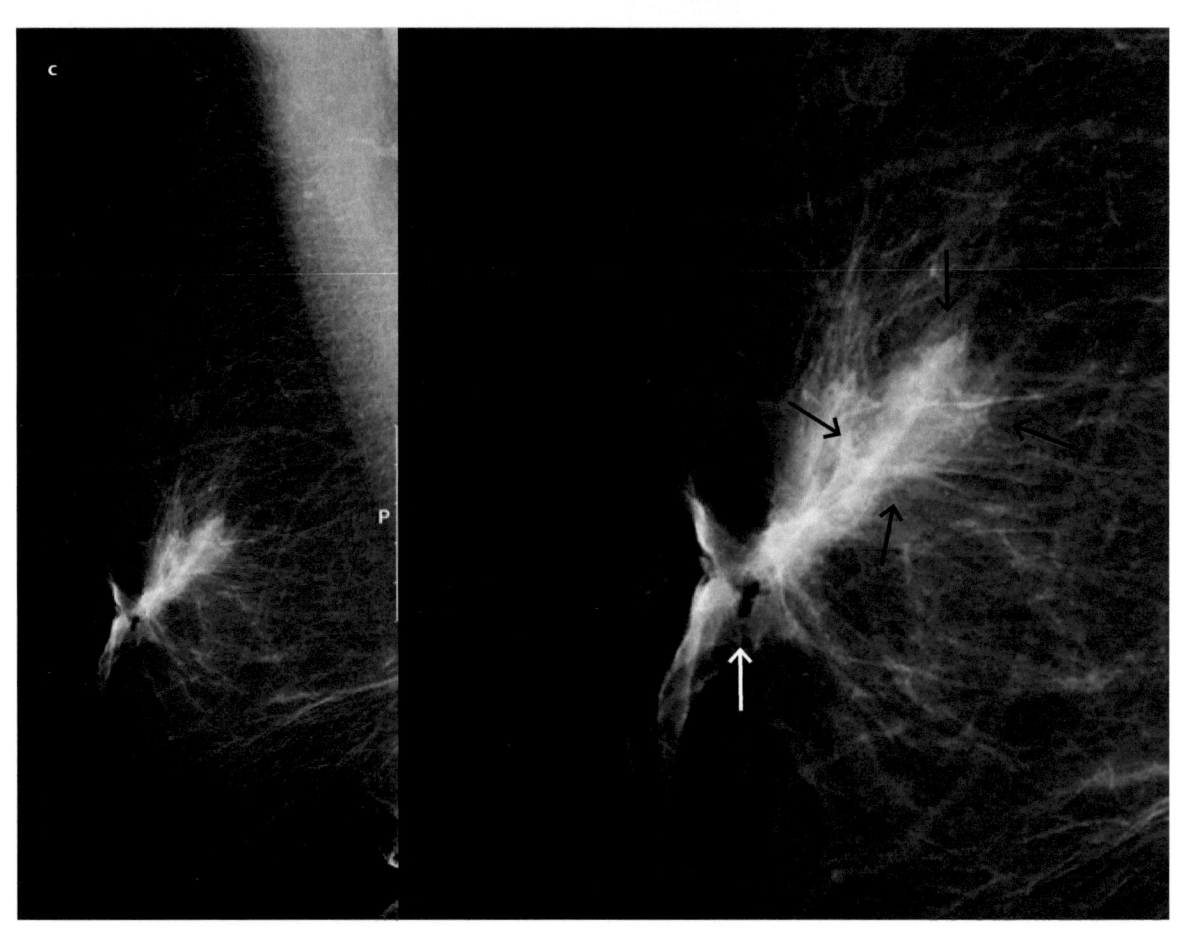

Granulomatous Conditions

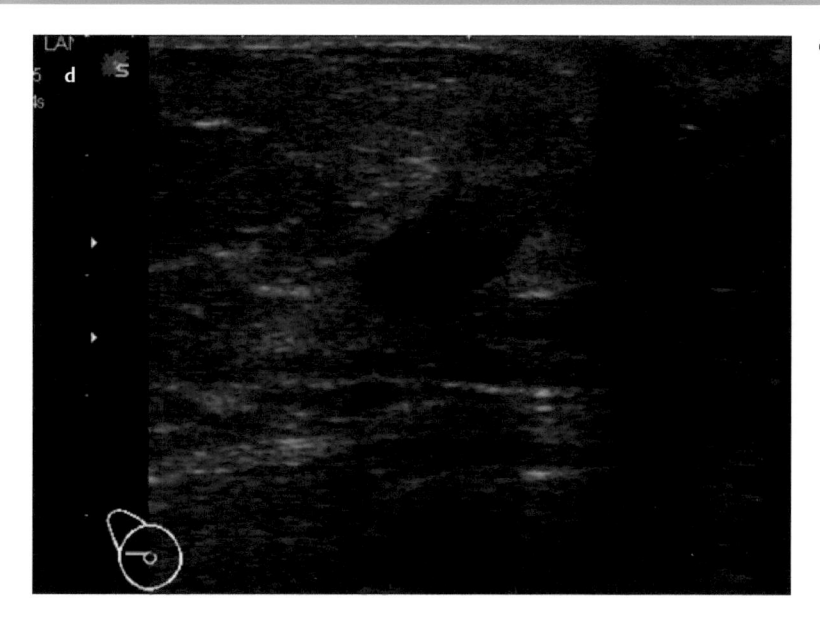

d Sonography demonstrates shadowing from the fibrous scarring behind the nipple. The new nodule is shown as a very hypoechoic oval mass.

Sonography

Scar granulomas (see **Fig. 13.4b**) are visualized sonographically as either well-circumscribed or irregular small nodules that are mostly hypoechoic with or without distal acoustic shadowing. They cannot be reliably differentiated from a small carcinoma within the scar.

Silicone granulomas (**Fig. 13.6a**) are visualized sonographically as:
- Hyperechoic masses with marked acoustic attenuation. A thin, crescentic hyperechoic rim may appear on the side close to the transducer if the granuloma is calcified.
- Characteristically, the acoustic shadow within and distal to the lesion contains clearly identifiable echoes that decrease with increasing distance from the transducer (so-called snowstorm pattern).

Despite these characteristic features, differentiation from a carcinoma can be difficult in an individual case. Multiple silicone or wax deposits may considerably compromise the evaluation because of marked attenuation phenomena.

Diabetic mastopathy (**Fig. 13.7**) is known to present sonographically with dense acoustic shadowing posterior to the region of concern (Garstin et al. 1991, Viehweg et al. 1996, Thorncroft et al. 2007, Hovanessian Larsen et al. 2009).

The remaining inflammatory granulomatous diseases, such as *tuberculosis, fungal infections, parasitosis, sarcoidosis,* and *autoimmune diseases,* have been reported only anecdotally. A sonographic separation from a carcinoma cannot be expected.

Magnetic Resonance Imaging

Scar granulomas as well as granulomas around small silicone leaks (**Fig. 13.6b–e**) show:
- An intense and early contrast enhancement in the early and inflammatory–granulating stage
- A moderate and delayed contrast enhancement, with increasing fibrosis, and
- No contrast enhancement, with complete fibrosis
- The MRI-demonstrated contour is generally round and nodular, with a more or less sharp outline

Due to absence of enhancement, a fibrotic granuloma can be easily distinguished from a carcinoma or scar recurrence. This is not applicable to the nonfibrotic granulomas, since these are mostly well perfused and may exhibit progressive or plateau-type moderate or even strong enhancement.

Silicone and *wax granulomas* after injection of contrast medium (see also Chapter 20):
- Can enhance peripherally or throughout due to a chronic granulating inflammation and are then indistinguishable from abscesses or malignancies
- Do not enhance in the fibrotic stage

Since no contrast enhancement can be expected in the majority of these cases (Yang et al. 1996, Wang et al. 2002, Khedher et al. 2011) contrast-enhanced MRI is advantageous as a supplemental examination to exclude a malignancy, especially in view of the limited evaluation after silicone and wax injections by other methods.

In women who have undergone polyacrylamide injections, granulomatous reactions and abscesses appear to lead more often to severe complications. MRI may not be

13 Inflammatory Conditions

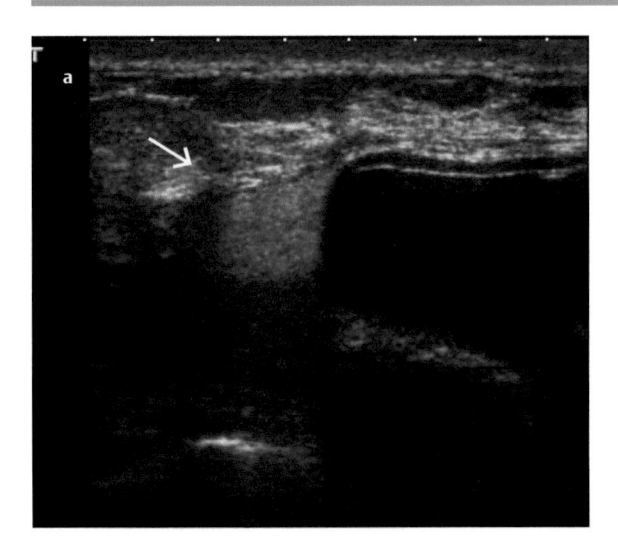

Fig. 13.6a–f Silicone granuloma

a–c A 50-year-old patient, 10 years after augmentation mammoplasty, who for 6 months had a palpable finding adjacent to the prosthesis. **a** Sonographically, the palpable lesion is seen as a hyperechoic mass probably due to many interfaces between silicone and breast tissue (arrow). The echoes decrease distally supporting the presence of a silicone granuloma. **b** Magnetic resonance imaging (MRI) delineates a fairly well circumscribed mass of low signal intensity medial to the prosthesis (arrow heads) in the region of the palpable finding (arrows). **c** After administration of Gd-DTPA, the palpable lesion fails to show any appreciable enhancement. (A special pulse sequence for the detection of silicone outside the prosthesis was not employed at that time). *Histology*: Fibrosed granuloma with silicone inclusion.

d,e A 54-year-old patient; 2-year status after reconstruction mammoplasty. A small low signal mass was discovered adjacent to the double-lumen prosthesis (**d**). The small nodule shows strong and early enhancement after administration of Gd-DTPA (**e**). This nodule discovered by MRI was followed up after 3 months and thereafter every 6 months, without evidence of any growth. Subsequent follow-up confirmed the diagnosis of silicone granuloma.

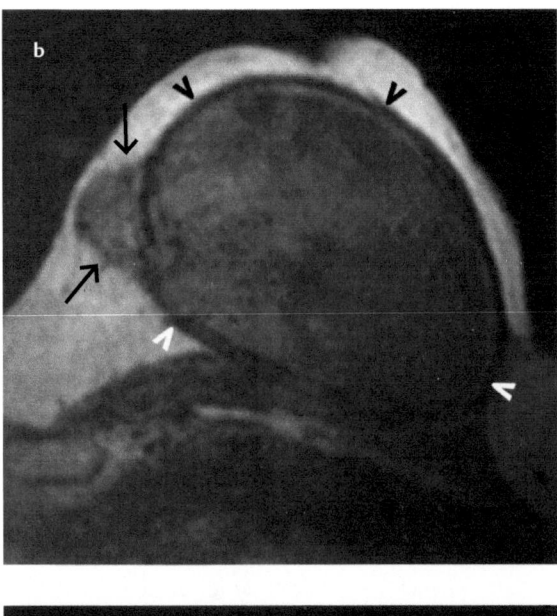

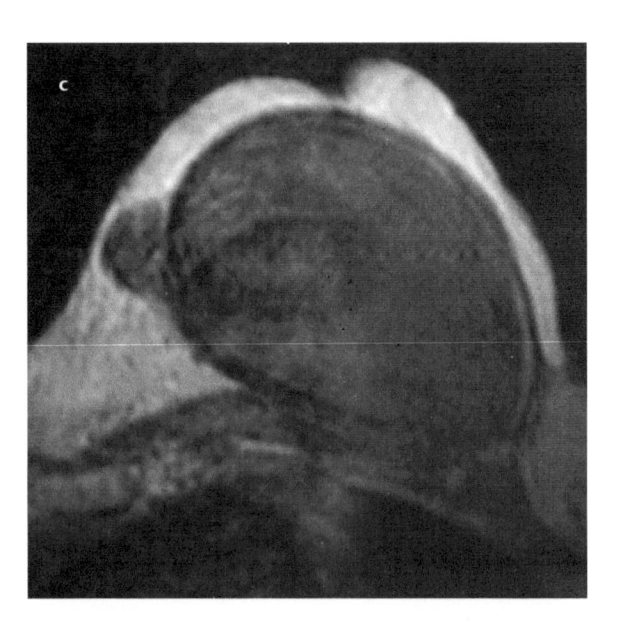

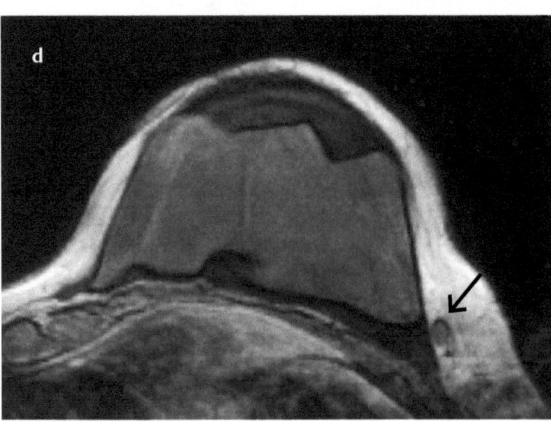

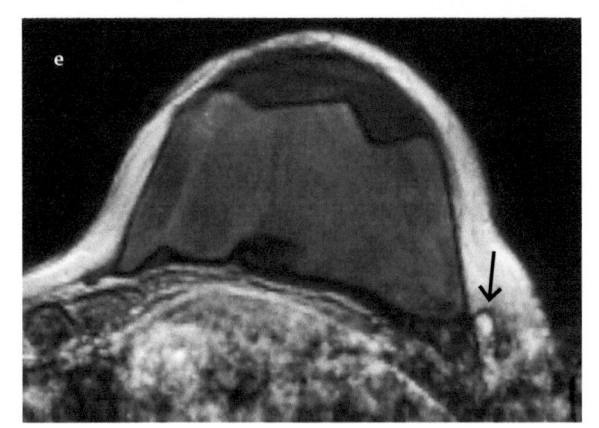

Granulomatous Conditions

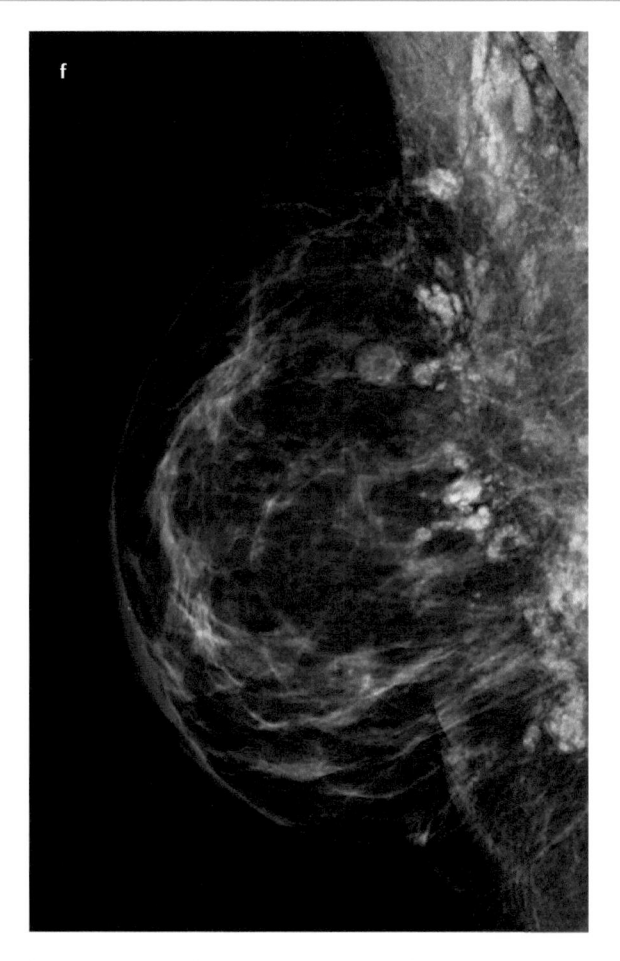

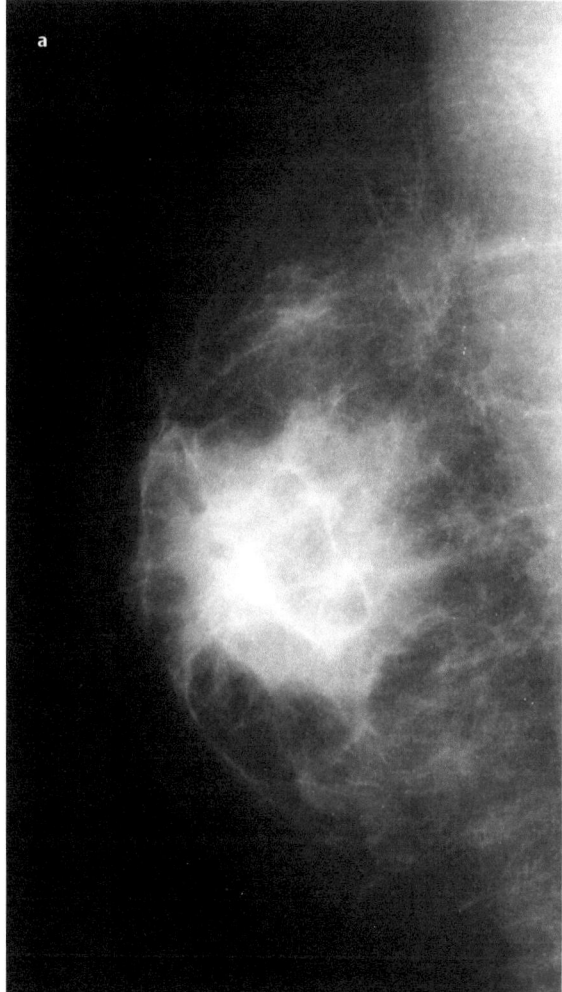

f Patient with multiple silicone deposits in the breast tissue, in the draining lymphatics and lymph nodes after removal of a ruptured silicone implant.

Fig. 13.7a,b Diabetic mastopathy, 39-year-old patient with juvenile diabetes.
a Mammographically and clinically very suspicious spiculated central mass.
b Sonographically, the lesion is hypoechoic with moderate sound attenuation and ill-defined margins.
Histology: Fibrosis with signs of inflammation. A follow-up visit a year later was arranged because of similar finding in the contralateral breast. Magnetic resonance imaging (MRI) showed intense enhancement. Suspecting a diabetic mastopathy, a core biopsy was obtained and the patient observed. The mammographic and clinical findings and MRI contrast enhancement resolved within 1 year.

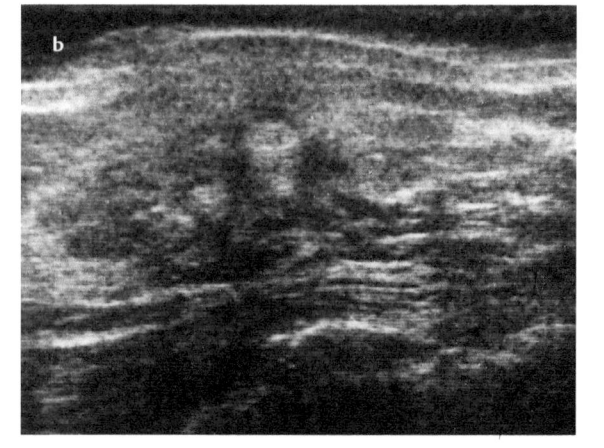

able to distinguish between inflammatory granulomas and malignancy, but may be helpful in depicting the full extent of the injections and of inflammatory complications (Lui et al. 2008).

Granulomas along silicone implants may be induced by silicone that escaped in small amounts through leakage or frank rupture (silicone granulomas), but can also be caused by suture material or talcum.

Except for the few granulomas with only negligible enhancement, most show enhancement (Heinig et al. 1997).

- In cases that arouse clinical or mammographic suspicion, the excision of enhancing granulomas is unavoidable. In our experience, follow-up examinations of nonenhancing granulomas can be justified.
- According to our experience, MRI may be very sensitive for demonstrating small enhancing granulomas. In order to refrain from unnecessary biopsies of diminutive granulomas we would recommend short-term follow-up of smoothly marginated small nodules that are incidentally discovered by MRI directly adjacent to the implant and are otherwise inconspicuous. To avoid missing a small malignancy we would, however, recommend following up such lesions, for example, at 4 and 12 months. We found that granulomas, in contrast to carcinomas, do not increase in size.

The MRI features of the rare granulomatous conditions, such as *tuberculosis, fungal infections, parasitosis, sarcoidosis*, and *autoimmune disease*, have been only sporadically reported.

According to current experience, granulomatous changes enhance with variable enhancement dynamics ranging from progressive to plateau-type to (less frequently) washout. Neither enhancement dynamics nor morphology (of diffuse or focal) granulating lesions allows a definite differentiation from carcinomas by contrast-enhanced MRI.

This also applies to the present experience concerning *diabetic mastopathy*. In one case examined by us (Viehweg et al. 1996), intense plateau-type enhancement was found in an irregularly outlined area corresponding to a suggestive palpable finding. This regressed within a year. The strong enhancement can be explained on the basis of an inflammatory process. However, in the acute stage, MRI does not offer any distinguishing feature from a malignancy. Other authors (Wong et al. 2002), who probably examined subacute stages, reported unspecific enhancement. In general, however, MRI will not be able to avert histopathologic assessment.

Percutaneous Biopsy

Occasionally, the diagnosis of a *scar granuloma* may be hampered by severe fibrosis and result in difficulty in obtaining an adequate amount of material. However, in most cases percutaneous needle biopsy will be valuable in differentiating a scar from a carcinoma.

The diagnosis of most *granulomatous inflammations* is possible from needle biopsy. In cases of bacterial or fungal infection and in the case of autoimmune disease, additional microbiological testing and specific blood tests can complement the required information.

> **Summary**
>
> *Scar granulomas* appear clinically as small nodules in the region of the scar and can be suspected by history and clinical course. Mammographically (nodular density) and sonographically (hypoechoic nodule, with or without acoustic shadowing), differentiation from a malignancy cannot be achieved. In cases of clinical suspicion, biopsy of the usually superficially located lesions is therefore the method of choice. A suspected scar granuloma following multiple surgeries can be further evaluated by contrast-enhanced MRI to avoid further surgical interventions for diagnostic purposes. Granulomas that are fibrosed and do not enhance can mostly be distinguished from malignancies.
>
> *Granulomas around silicone or wax deposits*, usually after cosmetic injections, can calcify. Because of the increased density and the multiple superimposed calcifications, the mammographic evaluation of these breasts is compromised. The same applies to the sonographic evaluation. Since contrast-enhanced MRI shows no enhancement in two-thirds of patients, MRI appears to be suitable as supplemental method for excluding and detecting malignancies.
>
> Large silicone granulomas are sonographically characterized as hyperechoic to hypoechoic masses with acoustic shadowing that exhibits a snowstorm pattern.
>
> MRI is highly sensitive in detecting diminutive silicone granulomas around breast prostheses. These granulomas can often be differentiated from small malignancies solely by absent growth over time.
>
> *Granulomatous diseases of the breast* can be found as extremely rare manifestations of tuberculosis, fungal infections, parasitosis, sarcoidosis, or autoimmune diseases. In insulin-dependent patients with suspected or previously diagnosed diabetic mastopathy, core needle biopsy may help avoid unnecessary biopsy. However, close interdisciplinary correlation will always be necessary to ensure representative biopsy and exclude malignancy.

References and Recommended Reading

Afridi SP, Memon A, Shafiq-ur-Rahman, Memon A. Granulomatous mastitis: a case series. J Coll Physicians Surg Pak 2010;20(6):365–368

Al-Marri MR, Aref E, Omar AJ. Mammographic features of isolated tuberculous mastitis. Saudi Med J 2005;26(4):646–650

Bastarrika G, Pina L, Vivas I, Elorz M, San Julian M, Alberro JA. Calcified filariasis of the breast: report of four cases. Eur Radiol 2001;11(7):1195–1197

Blohmer JU, Bollmann R, Chaoui R, Kürten A, Lau HU. Nonpuerperal mastitis in real time and color Doppler ultrasound. [Article in German] Geburtshilfe Frauenheilkd 1994;54(3):161–16

Boarki K, Labib M. Imaging findings in idiopathic lobular granulomattous mastitis, case report and review of literature. Gulf J Oncolog 2010;7:46–52

Clark CJ, Wechter D. Morphea of the breast—an uncommon cause of breast erythema. Am J Surg 2010;200(1):173–176

Cao MM, Hoyt AC, Bassett LW. Mammographic signs of systemic disease. Radiographics 2011;31(4):1085–1100

Deininger HK. Wegener granulomatosis of the breast. Radiology 1985;154(1):59–60

Feder JM, de Paredes ES, Hogge JP, Wilken JJ. Unusual breast lesions: radiologic–pathologic correlation. Radiographics 1999;19(Spec No):S11–S26, quiz S260

Garstin WIH, Kaufman Z, Michell MJ, Baum M. Fibrous mastopathy in insulin dependent diabetics. Clin Radiol 1991;44(2):89–91

Georgian-Smith D, Lawton TJ, Moe RE, Couser WG. Lupus mastitis: radiologic and pathologic features. AJR Am J Roentgenol 2002;178(5):1233–1235

Heinig A, Heywang-Köbrunner SH, Viehweg P, Lampe D, Buchmann J, Spielmann RP. Value of contrast medium magnetic resonance tomography of the breast in breast reconstruction with implant. [Article in German] Radiologe 1997;37(9):710–717

Heywang-Köbrunner SH, Beck R. Contrast-enhanced MRI of the breast. Heidelberg; New York: Springer; 1996

Hovanessian Larsen LJ, Peyvandi B, Klipfel N, Grant E, Iyengar G. Granulomatous lobular mastitis: imaging, diagnosis, and treatment. AJR Am J Roentgenol 2009;193(2):574–581

Irshad A, Ackerman SJ, Pope TL, Moses CK, Rumboldt T, Panzegrau B. Rare breast lesions: correlation of imaging and histologic features with WHO classification. Radiographics 2008;28(5):1399–1414

Jordan JM, Rowe WT, Allen NB. Wegener's granulomatosis involving the breast. Report of three cases and review of the literature. Am J Med 1987;83(1):159–164

Khedher NB, David J, Trop I, Drouin S, Peloquin L, Lalonde L. Imaging findings of breast augmentation with injected hydrophilic polyacrylamide gel: patient reports and literature review. Eur J Radiol 2011;78(1):104–111

Kim SM, Park JM, Moon WK. Dystrophic breast calcifications in patients with collagen diseases. Clin Imaging 2004;28(1):6–9

Lui CY, Ho CM, Iu PP, et al. Evaluation of MRI findings after polyacrylamide gel injection for breast augmentation. AJR Am J Roentgenol 2008;191(3):677–688

Mirsaeidi SM, Masjedi MR, Mansouri SD, Velayati AA. Tuberculosis of the breast: report of 4 clinical cases and literature review. East Mediterr Health J 2007;13(3):670–676

Panzacchi R, Gallo C, Fois F, et al. Primary sarcoidosis of the breast: case description and review of the literature. Pathologica 2010;102(3):104–107

Sakr AA, Fawzy RK, Fadaly G, Baky MA. Mammographic and sonographic features of tuberculous mastitis. Eur J Radiol 2004;51(1):54–60

Seale M, Koh W, Henderson M, Drummond R, Cawson J. Imaging surveillance of the breast in a patient diagnosed with scleroderma after breast-conserving surgery and radiotherapy. Breast J 2008;14(4):379–381

Seymour EQ. Blastomycosis of the breast. AJR Am J Roentgenol 1982;139(4):822–823

Surendrababu NR, Thomas E, Rajinikanth J, Keshava SN. Breast filariasis: real-time sonographic imaging of the filarial dance. J Clin Ultrasound 2008;36(9):567–569

Stigers KB, King JG, Davey DD, Stelling CB. Abnormalities of the breast caused by biopsy: spectrum of mammographic findings. AJR Am J Roentgenol 1991;156(2):287–291

Thorncroft K, Forsyth L, Desmond S, Audisio RA. The diagnosis and management of diabetic mastopathy. Breast J 2007;13(6):607–613

Tomaszewski JE, Brooks JS, Hicks D, Livolsi VA. Diabetic mastopathy: a distinctive clinicopathologic entity. Hum Pathol 1992;23(7):780–786

Viehweg P, Heywang-Köbrunner SH, Bayer U, Friedrich T, Spielmann RP. Simulation of breast carcinoma by diabetic mastopathy. Article in German] Rofo 1996;164(6):519–521

Wang J, Shih TT, Li YW, Chang KJ, Huang HY. Magnetic resonance imaging characteristics of paraffinomas and siliconomas after mammoplasty. J Formos Med Assoc 2002;101(2):117–123

Wong KT, Tse GM, Yang WT. Ultrasound and MR imaging of diabetic mastopathy. Clin Radiol 2002;57(8):730–735

Yang WT, Suen M, Ho WS, Metreweli C. Paraffinomas of the breast: mammographic, ultrasonographic and radiographic appearances with clinical and histopathological correlation. Clin Radiol 1996;51(2):130–133

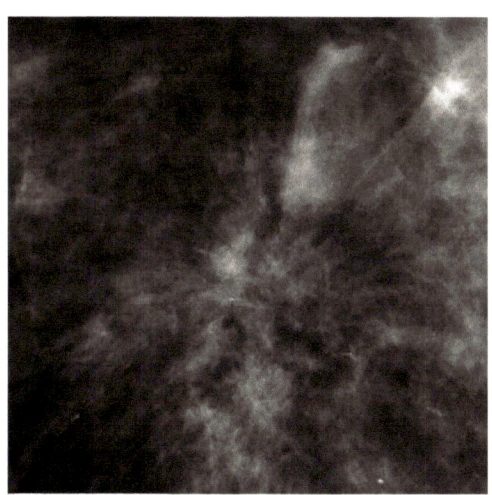

14 Lesions of Uncertain Malignant Potential (B3 Lesions)

Definition → *338*
Rationale for Diagnostic Strategy and Therapeutic Recommendations for B3 Lesions → *338*
Diagnostic Strategy and Management → *339*
Prevalence of Lesions of Uncertain Malignant Potential, Imaging and Overall Risk → *339*

Atypical Intraductal Epithelial Proliferations → *340*
Atypical Ductal Hyperplasia → *340*
Flat Epithelial Atypia and Columnar Cell Lesions with Atypia → *341*
Atypical Lobular Hyperplasia, Lobular Carcinoma in Situ (and Pleomorphic-Type LCIS) → *345*

Radial Scars → *346*

Papillary Lesions → *348*

Fibroepithelial Lesions of Uncertain Malignant Potential → *356*
Other B3 Lesions → *360*

References and Recommended Reading → *361*

14 Lesions of Uncertain Malignant Potential (B3 Lesions)

S. Barter, S. H. Heywang-Koebrunner, F. Kilburn-Toppin, J. Naehrig

Definition

The term "lesions of uncertain malignant potential" (B3 lesions) was coined by the Coordinating Group for Breast Screening Pathology (NHS Breast Screening Programme) in Great Britain in 2001 and by the European Working Group on Breast Screening Pathology (Amendoeira et al. 2006) to characterize specific lesions encountered in core needle biopsies (CNBs).

It includes a wide variety of histopathologic diagnoses that are by convention considered as benign lesions. However, for these entities the diagnosis should be considered only provisional, since:
- The lesion may be incompletely removed or sampled by the biopsy, and
- It harbors a certain risk of upgrade in the final diagnosis after surgical excision because of the possible association with malignant lesions

"Lesions of uncertain malignant potential" (B3 lesions) thus may qualify as risk indicators for malignancy, or as nonobligatory precursors of malignancy, or as lesions which may be heterogeneous in nature and where (even when correctly performed) CNB or vacuum-assisted breast biopsy (VABB) sampling may miss a more sinister area.

Lesions of uncertain malignant potential include the following main entities:
- Atypical intraductal and intralobular epithelial proliferations (for nomenclature and abbreviations, see also Chapter 15, **Table 15.1**, p. 367):
  - Atypical epithelial proliferation of ductal type/ Atypical ductal hyperplasia (ADH)
  - Flat epithelial atypia (FEA) (identical to Columnar cell change with atypia and Columnar cell hyperplasia with atypia)
  - Atypical lobular hyperplasia (ALH)
  - Lobular carcinoma in situ (LCIS); the pleomorphic type with its subtypes macroacinar, necrotic, pleomorphic and signet cell constitute a special category of lobular neoplasia (LN), which is associated with invasive malignancy in a higher percentage of cases. According to the EU guidelines it is currently categorized as a B5 lesion in percutaneous breast biopsy specimens. It is therefore discussed in Chapter 15
- Radial scars or sclerosing lesions (RSLs)
- Papillary lesions
- Fibroepithelial lesions such as phyllodes tumors and cellular fibroepithelial lesions in which a phyllodes tumor cannot be excluded
- Miscellaneous entities such as mucocele-like lesions, difficult to classify atypical epithelial and stromal spindle cell proliferations, vascular lesions, etc.

The risk that a B3 lesion is already associated with a higher-grade lesion or that the B3 lesion might develop into a higher-grade lesion varies with the type of lesion and its extent, with the mode of diagnosis (CNB vs. VABB), with complete (or incomplete) removal, with other risk factors of the patient, and with patient age.

In this chapter, histopathology, imaging appearances, and risk of associated malignancy of these lesions will be discussed.

Rationale for Diagnostic Strategy and Therapeutic Recommendations for B3 Lesions

In contrast to excision biopsy, only a small volume of tissue is available from needle biopsies. Therefore close correlation of imaging and histopathology is needed for all needle biopsies to decide whether the biopsy specimen is representative and adequately explains the imaging findings.

A nonrepresentative result may occur if the lesion is missed owing to a targeting error. It may also be caused by a sampling error, which may occur in lesions composed of inhomogeneous tissue or in which small nests of tumor cells are surrounded by large amounts of benign glandular tissue without significant atypias or even acellular fibrotic tissue. The biopsy may be correctly taken from the lesion but the acquired tissue does not represent the most concerning area within this lesion and may lead to a false negative result.

For lesions of uncertain malignant potential this problem is of particular concern, as a B3 area of pathology may occur within or in the periphery of higher-grade lesions such as ductal carcinoma in situ (DCIS) or invasive breast cancer.

B3 lesions may also function as a "nonobligate precursors of malignancy," that is, they may have the potential to develop into DCIS or invasive carcinoma. The risk of progression to invasive cancer and/or threatening the patient's life is, however, much lower than it is for DCIS.

Finally, some of these lesions are considered to be a "risk indicator," signifying an increased probability that the patient will develop a breast cancer in either the ipsilateral or contralateral breast at some time in the future.

Considering the low but significant rate of malignancy within the lesion or adjacent tissue, excisional biopsy needs to be considered for a significant number of B3 lesions. Recommending excisional biopsy in all such cases reduces the risk of missing occult malignancy. However, it will also correspond to overtreatment in a significant number of women and possibly even overtreatment with a questionable effect. Overtreatment concerns those women who (during their remaining lifetime) would not develop malignancy or, strictly speaking, a life-threatening (metastasizing) breast cancer. B3 lesions are also associated with an increased rate of breast cancer in other locations of the same or contralateral breast and, considering that a newly developing DCIS or invasive carcinoma might in many cases still be detected at an early stage, excision of all B3 lesions might have only a minor effect on preventing breast cancer or decreasing breast cancer mortality. Thus, today, depending on the histology, imaging, lesion extent and degree of sampling or removal and individual risk factors, both excision and follow-up should be considered for individual B3 lesions and patients.

Diagnostic Strategy and Management

Considering the pros and cons of existing treatment options and the limited prediction of the individual course, the management of these lesions has become a significant clinical problem. This problem has been increasing with the widespread use of diagnostic imaging and mammographic screening, since a significant number of B3 lesions are detected by screening.

Because of the diagnostic challenges, international guidelines strongly recommend that all needle biopsies yielding a B3 pathology classification are discussed in a multidisciplinary meeting. Attempts should be made to tailor treatment to each individual case, taking into account factors including the size and extent of the lesions, the risk of malignant change, and the probability of representative sampling of the lesion, as well as individual patient risk factors (Heywang-Köbrunner et al. 2003, 2009, Silverstein 2003, Amendoeira et al. 2006, Albert et al. 2009).

As to lesion type, B3 lesions of high risk include atypical ductal hyperplasia (ADH), papillary lesions with atypical features (and the pleomorphic type of LCIS, which, if diagnosed at percutaneous biopsy, is currently classified as a B5 lesion). Intermediate risk may be associated with classic LCIS or flat epithelial atypia (FEA), low to intermediate risk with atypical lobular hyperplasia (ALH), and low risk with radial scars or sclerosing lesions (RSLs), phyllodes tumors, and papillary lesions without atypical features.

For high-risk lesions, excision should in general be recommended. Rare exceptions might include very small lesions in patients with limited life expectancy or high risk of surgery. For B3 lesions of intermediate or low risk, excision or follow-up might be considered. Options for management range from surgical excision to VABB and excision or simply increased surveillance.

In spite of its low risk of malignancy, phyllodes tumor is usually excised, since even benign phylloid tumors mostly grow quite fast (leading to cosmetic problems and clinical symptoms) and tend to recur.

To develop an optimum treatment plan for the patient the following aspects should be considered:
- Type of the highest grade lesion and estimated risk of malignancy based on histopathology
- Imaging findings before, during, after biopsy and specimen imaging (Is the biopsy representative, is it compatible with the suspected histopathology, is the diagnostic question solved?)
- Estimated extent (What is the estimated extent based on imaging findings and on the analysis of the available histopathologically assessed tissue? What is the estimated reliability of imaging and histopathology?)
- Percentage of sampling, estimated percentage of removal (Is the lesion homogeneous? Is it multifocal? Is there risk of missing a higher-grade lesion?)
- Individual risk factors of the patient (personal or family history of breast cancer)
- Patient age (risk for remaining lifetime and risk factors limiting the patient's life expectancy)
- Risk of considered treatment (for the individual patient)
- Possibilities of surveillance (reliability of imaging as to detection of associated or developing malignancy)

Options for management or treatment include individualized imaging surveillance (usually yearly mammography, which may be complemented by ultrasound or rarely by MRI), chemoprevention using antiestrogen treatment, and surgical excision. Currently there are no definitive management guidelines.

Further research into predictive and prognostic factors may allow better assessment of individual patient risk, and allow better adaptation of treatment options to strike the balance between avoidance of overtreatment and risk of malignant change.

Prevalence of Lesions of Uncertain Malignant Potential, Imaging and Overall Risk

Lesions of uncertain malignant potential may coexist with other benign or malignant changes. The epithelial proliferations belonging to the B3 category are frequently detected incidentally during a biopsy that is performed to assess a different lesion. Many B3 lesions are detected due to histopathologic assessment of screen-detected microcalcifications.

The reported prevalence of B3 lesions among percutaneous breast biopsies ranges between 3% and 10% (Lee et al. 2003, Kettritz et al. 2004, Fahrbach et al. 2006, Dillon et al. 2007, Houssami et al. 2007b, El-Sayed et al. 2008, Heywang-Köbrunner et al. 2010a,b). With increasing use of mammographic screening and VABB, an increased detection rate of B3 lesions has been observed (Liberman 2002, Lee et al. 2003).

Some B3 lesions may also be detected on ultrasound. From the assessment of mammographically detected B3 lesions, it is known that about 50–60% are associated with some sonographic findings (Heywang-Köbrunner et al. 2010a, 2010b). B3 lesions with sonographic changes include papillary lesions and phyllodes tumors, some of the radial sclerosing lesions, and unspecific hypoechoic areas that may be associated with benign changes that contain atypia or lobular neoplasia. B3 lesions detected by ultrasound are fewer than those detected by mammography, owing to the generally lower sensitivity of ultrasound for small lesions and in particular to the limited detection of microcalcifications. The vast majority of mammographically detected lesions that are visible by ultrasound will undergo ultrasound-guided CNB (Heywang-Köbrunner et al. 2010a,b).

Few reports exist on the use of magnetic resonance imaging (MRI) for B3 lesions and the evidence is mixed. In larger biopsy series of MR-detected lesions the proportion of B3 lesions ranges from around 6% to 14.5% (Liberman et al. 2005, Perlet et al. 2006, Han et al. 2008, Fischer et al. 2009, Johnson and Collins 2009, Heywang-Köbrunner et al. 2010a, 2010b, Malhaire et al. 2010). Currently MRI is not used routinely for the assessment of B3 lesions, and studies have reported a high rate of false positive biopsies; however, ongoing research in this area may lead to more widespread use of MRI for lesion differentiation (Perlet et al. 2006, Port et al. 2007, Han et al. 2008, Linda et al. 2008, Fischer et al. 2009, Johnson and Collins 2009, Malhaire et al. 2010).

Whenever percutaneous breast biopsy yields a B3 lesion, the risk of missing an associated malignancy is assessed by combining (1) the risk associated with the given histopathologic entity, (2) its radiologic features, and (3) the probability of representative sampling of the lesion. The latter depends on whether the lesion sampled is homogeneous, as well as the volume and proportion of tissue acquired at biopsy. Based on these considerations and individual patient risk factors, excision is chosen as the recommended treatment option for a proportion of B3 lesions, while for those with lower risk, follow-up is usually recommended. B3 lesions may occur as pure or mixed lesions, and for any decisions concerning patient management the pathologic entity with the highest risk needs to be considered as the most important risk factor.

Percutaneous biopsy may significantly understate malignant change with regard to these lesions. According to an overview of literature data by Houssami, approximately 30% of those B3 lesions selected for subsequent excision eventually contained higher-grade lesions (DCIS or invasive carcinoma) (Houssami et al. 2007a). In another large series, two-thirds of such upgrades were from B3 to DCIS, while one-third were upgrades to invasive breast cancer (Houssami et al. 2007b). No significant difference in the rate of upgrade was reported for lesions presenting with microcalcifications versus lesions presenting as mass or architectural distortion. However, the rate of underestimation increased with lesion size (18% of 210 lesions < 20 mm were upgraded vs. 48% of 69 lesions > 20 mm). The rate of upgrades was approximately 50% higher with CNB than with VABB, which may be explained by the larger volume of tissue removed by VABB. Finally, underestimates were significantly more frequent among B3 lesions with atypical ductal or lobular hyperplasia than without (44% vs. 18%). Some authors have suggested subdividing B3 lesions into those at higher risk (ADH and LCIS) and those at low risk (papillary lesions, RSLs, FEAs, and fibroepithelial tumors) (Houssami et al. 2007b, Londero et al. 2008).

Atypical Intraductal Epithelial Proliferations

Atypical Ductal Hyperplasia

Definition

Atypical (intra)ductal hyperplasia (ADH) (Lakhani et al. 2012): ADH (like other B3 lesions) is a rare condition, and is seen in only 4% of symptomatic benign biopsies, but is far more frequent among biopsies with microcalcifications (van de Vijver 2005).

Histologically, ADH is a borderline breast lesion that demonstrates cellular changes identical to those of low-grade DCIS. It is a precursor of malignancy with an increased risk of developing to invasive breast cancer, which is 4–5 times the risk of the normal population, up to 6 times the risk if diagnosed premenopausally, and 10 times the risk if there is a first-degree relative with breast cancer (van de Vijver 2005).

Histopathology

ADH is currently considered a minute low-grade DCIS, measuring no more than 2 mm or incompletely occupying a terminal ductal lobular unit (TDLU) (Tavassoli and Norris 1990, NHSBSP 2001, Ellis et al. 2004).

Growth patterns and cytology are identical to low-grade DCIS, most often micropapillary and cribriform. ADH can be associated with microcalcifications, often of nonspecific lamellar type, and it can be clinically occult and an incidental histopathologic finding. ADH can be found in association with various lesions, notably UDH (usual ductal hyperplasia), FEA, LN, papilloma, radial scar, fibroadenoma, and also in proximity to fully developed DCIS of any grade, together with invasive carcinoma of any type.

Mammography

On mammography ADH is mostly detected by assessment of microcalcifications, which are often granular in nature. The microcalcifications may be clustered or exhibit ductal distribution and often demonstrate at least some degree of polymorphism. They are usually classified radiologically as BI-RADS (Breast Imaging Reporting and Data System) 4 (**Fig. 14.1**). ADH may also be found in papillomas, in radial scars, in fibroadenomas, and in association with other benign changes (with or without microcalcifications) at biopsy. There is no specific mammographic sign that could indicate presence or absence of ADH within the above entities. So, in many cases, ADH may be—strictly speaking—an incidental finding detected by the assessment of different underlying lesions.

Magnetic Resonance Imaging

There is little published literature on the use of MRI in ADH. One retrospective study examined the use of MRI for follow-up of 135 patients with ADH and 47 patients with lobular carcinoma in situ (LCIS) (Port et al. 2007). The authors reported a very high rate of false positive biopsies (25% of the patients) and an extraordinary rate of 6-month follow-up recommendations (48%) with a low overall yield of malignancy (six breast cancers in five patients detected by MRI, two interval cancers). Their conclusion was that MRI is not generally recommended in these patients. ADH may be detected as an incidental finding at MRI by detection of a suspicious area of enhancement. However, there are no specific features on MRI to point to or exclude the diagnosis of ADH (**Fig. 14.2**).

Management

Surgical excision biopsy is essential for correct classification and assessment of surrounding tissue when ADH is diagnosed at percutaneous breast biopsy. It is therefore generally recommended after this diagnosis. Exceptions may be made according to individual risk considerations.

The upgrade rate for ADH to DCIS is quoted as up to 50%, with a smaller percentage upgraded to invasive carcinoma (Jackman et al. 2002, Houssami et al. 2007b, Yu et al. 2010). The upgrade rate is lower for VABB devices (up to 24% reported) due to the larger volumes of tissue removed at VABB (Jackman et al. 2002, Pandelidis et al. 2003, Plantade et al. 2005, Kettritz 2004, Sohn et al. 2007, Eby et al. 2009, Jackman et al. 2009, Heywang-Köbrunner et al. 2010a,b, Kohr et al. 2010).

Follow-Up

There is a lack of evidence in the literature regarding frequency and length of surveillance, but annual mammography is a pragmatic approach given the increased risk of malignancy.

Flat Epithelial Atypia and Columnar Cell Lesions with Atypia

Definition

This group of lesions includes FEA—a term defined by the World Health Organization (WHO) classification of tumors which covers columnar cell change (CCC) with atypia, and columnar cell hyperplasia (CCH) with atypia (Tavassoli et al. 2003). They are usually identified in biopsies performed for microcalcifications. CCC and CCH with no cellular atypia are considered benign lesions and are classified as B2 lesions (Schnitt and Vincent-Salomon 2003, Amendoeira et al. 2006).

However, FEA is a B3 lesion and is often associated with other B3 lesions such as LN (50–86%) (Brandt et al. 2008, Leibl et al. 2007) and ADH (13%) (Leibl et al. 2007). These combinations are frequent. Infrequently, FEA may be associated with higher-grade lesions such as DCIS or invasive carcinoma—Pure FEA appears to have a low association with malignancy in most series: in a recent overview on small published series of FEA (patients, n = 8–63) by Sinn et al. (2010) the median upgrade rate was 10.2% (0–25%) with the highest number (25%) in the smallest series (David et al. 2006, Kunju and Kleer 2007, Senetta et al. 2009, Moinfar 2010). Thus FEA is also considered to be a precursor to low-grade DCIS and invasive carcinoma (Schnitt 2003, Tavassoli et al. 2003, Simpson et al. 2005, Nährig 2008).

However, these data should be interpreted with caution, since they are based on small numbers and differing definitions exist for FEA and, for part of the data, sampling error (with more significant lesions) cannot be excluded without exact radiologic–histopathologic correlation.

Histology

FEA is a low-grade atypical proliferation of TDLUs, often multifocal (61–75%) (Leibl et al. 2007, Martel et al. 2007) and bilateral. FEA describes lesions characterized by enlarged TDLUs in which the native epithelial cells are replaced by one to several layers of cuboidal or columnar cells that show mild cytologic atypia (Schnitt and Vincent-Salomon 2003, O'Malley et al. 2006). These proliferations are consistently found in cases with associated,

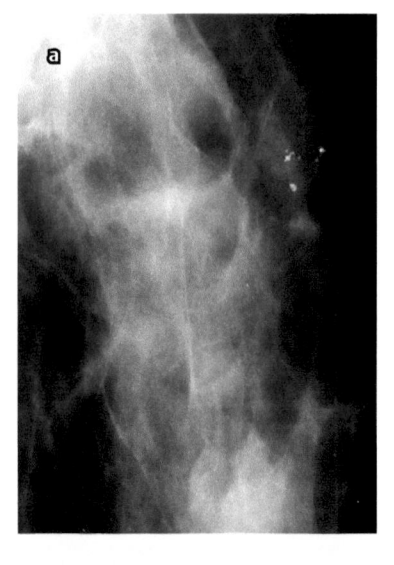

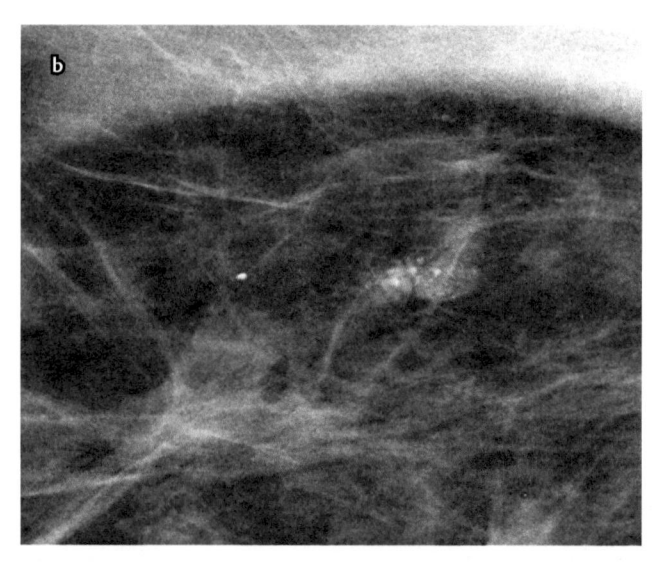

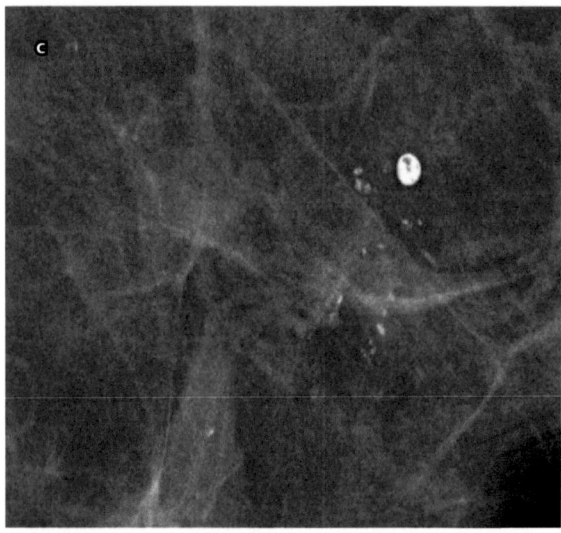

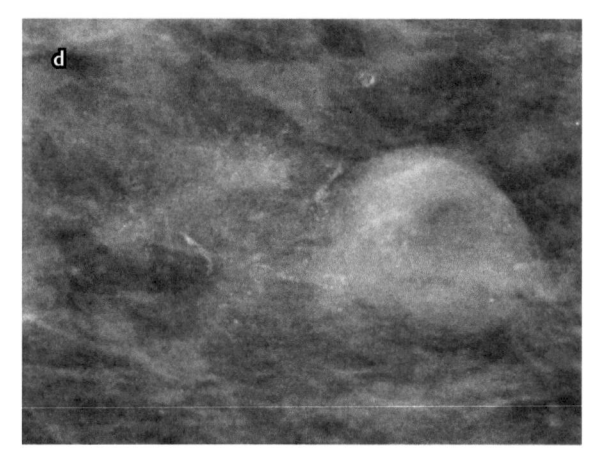

14 Lesions of Uncertain Malignant Potential (B3 Lesions)

Fig. 14.1a–e Varying radiographic presentations of atypical ductal hyperplasia (ADH). In the following cases (except **Fig. 14.1e**) malignancy was suspected or could not be excluded. Final diagnosis after vacuum-assisted breast biopsy (VABB) and excision was ADH, but there was no histologic proof of malignancy.

a Patient with a diagnosis of ADH at VABB. There is a small cluster of pleomorphic microcalcifications. Final histology yielded benign changes.
b Small indeterminate group of microcalcifications. VABB revealed ADH. Excision after VABB showed benign changes.
c Focal area of microcalcifications. The configuration of the calcifications is suggestive of a ductal pattern. VABB yielded ADH. Excision revealed benign changes.
d In this patient very fine microcalcifications were detected mammographically. Owing to their ductal distribution VABB was indicated and yielded ADH. Excision after VABB confirmed further atypias and benign changes.
e Patient with a diagnosis of ADH at VABB. The microcalcifications were partly removed. Final diagnosis yielded ductal carcinoma in situ grade 2.

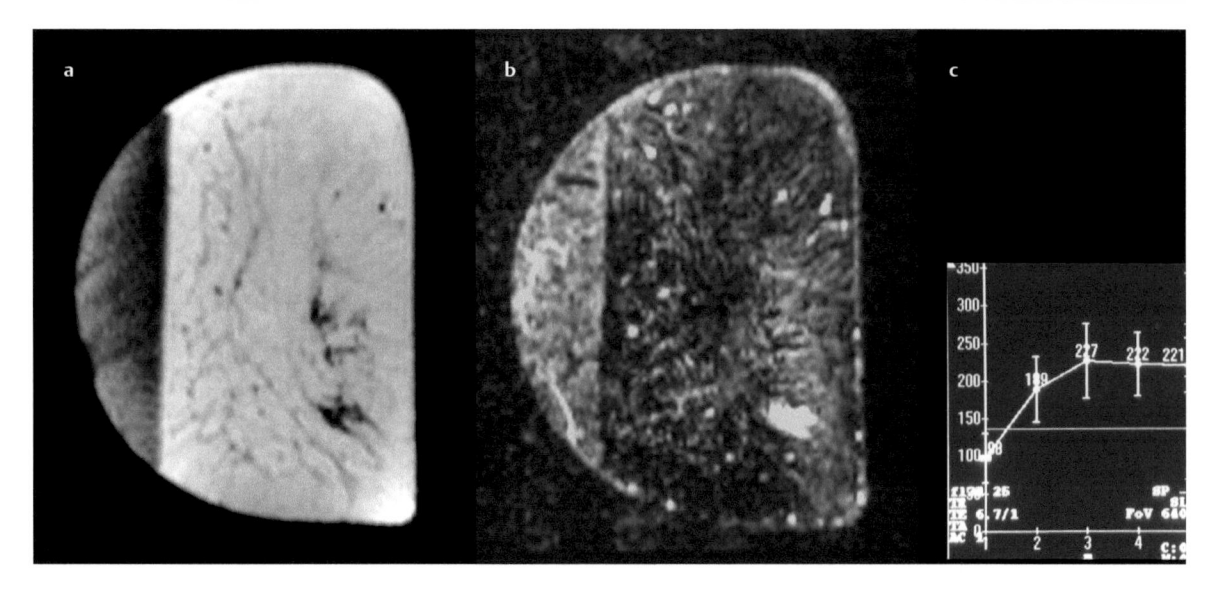

Fig. 14.2a–c Atypical ductal hyperplasia (ADH) detected by magnetic resonance imaging (MRI) within an area of asymmetric breast tissue. The enhancement was considered suspicious of malignancy. MR-guided vacuum-assisted breast biopsy yielded ADH. The diagnosis was confirmed after excision.

a Precontrast image.
b Subtraction image.
c Enhancement curve. (Reproduced with kind permission of Karger AG from Heywang-Köbrunner et al. 2010b.)

already fully developed DCIS and/or invasive carcinoma, most often of tubular type, a finding that, together with overlapping chromosomal abnormalities, indicates a possible role as direct precursor lesions or indicator lesions of increased risk of breast cancer.

Mammography

FEA is usually detected following biopsy for mammographic microcalcifications (up to 74%) or it can be an incidental finding in a biopsy for another lesion (Fraser et al. 1998, Martel et al. 2007). Lamellar microcalcifications are nonspecific and may be slightly pleomorphic, resembling microcalcifications in adenosis. However, sometimes also linear shapes or amorphous or fine pleomorphic microcalcifications are seen in a clustered or ductal distribution (Pandey et al. 2007). Rarely, FEA or CCM/CCH has also been described associated with a mass on mammography or ultrasound. It is, however, not yet clear whether this last appearance may just represent an incidental finding (**Fig. 14.3**).

Management

To date, there is no clear recommendation concerning the management of FEA.

Some authors generally recommend open surgical biopsy because of the inherent problems of sampling and possible associated malignancy (Schnitt and Vincent-Salomon 2003, Pinder et al. 2007).

Others give no general recommendation (de Mascarel et al. 2007), but recommend individual decision after interdisciplinary discussion. Excision is recommended for those cases with associated other risk lesions (LN or ADH) (Tavassoli 2008), or with remaining uncertainties concerning representative sampling and presence of further lesions after radiologic–histopathologic correlation (Martel et al. 2007). For the other cases of pure representatively sampled FEA without open questions, follow-up may be adequate.

The rate of upgrades after a VABB diagnosis of pure FEA ranges from 0–20% (Kunju and Kleer 2007, Senetta et al. 2009). Based on 40 cases diagnosed as FEA by VABB, David reported that if the size was below 10 mm and if the lesion was completely removed there was no upgrade to malignancy (David et al. 2006). Provided these results can be confirmed by further large-scale studies, benign surgical excisions could be reduced in these cases.

Follow-Up

There are no published long-term studies, but for FEA subsequent risk of invasion seems to be low following complete excision. One large study reviewed over 9,000 breast biopsies initially considered benign, with an average follow-up period of 19.2 years. Of 25 cases of so-called "clinging carcinoma" of monomorphic type (now classified as FEA), one patient (4%) developed recurrence of a histologically identical lesion, which was thought to be persistence rather than true recurrence. None of the 25 patients developed invasive breast carcinoma within

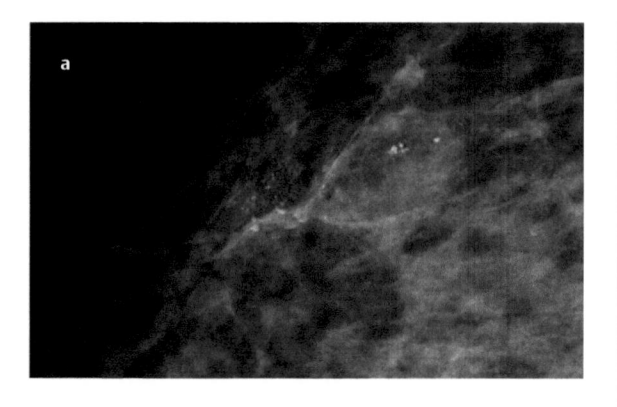

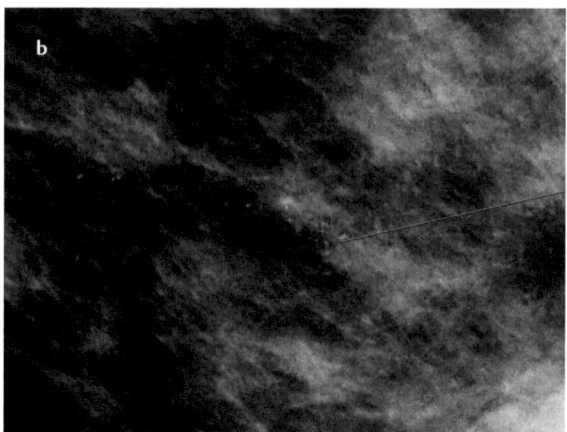

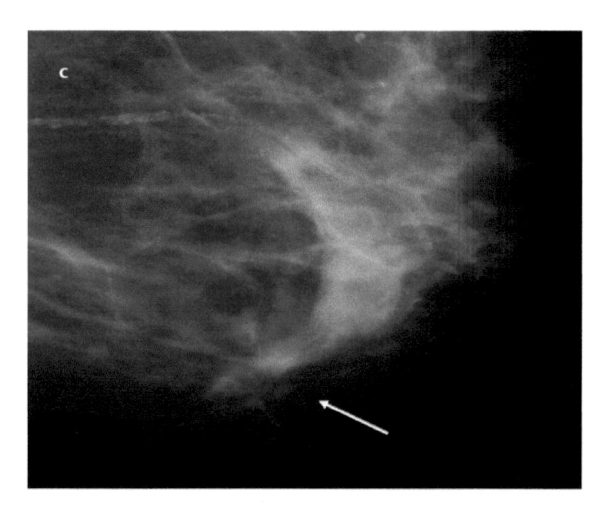

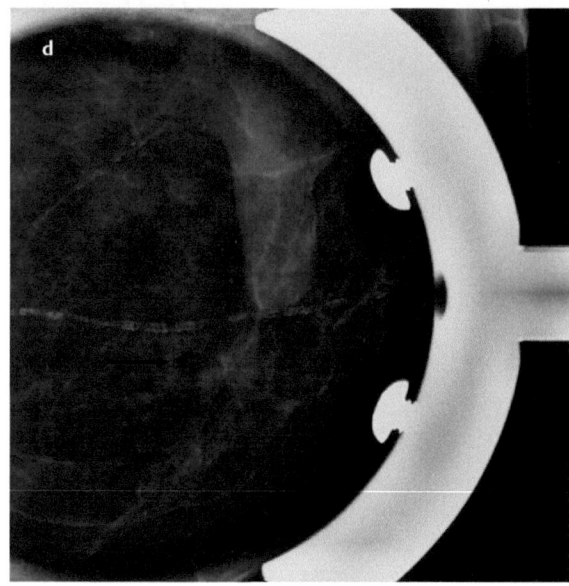

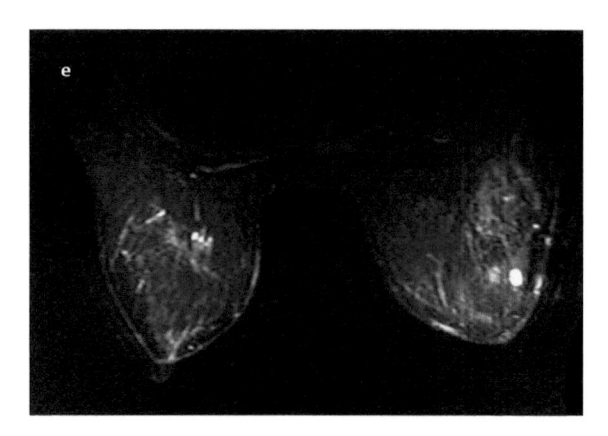

14 Lesions of Uncertain Malignant Potential (B3 Lesions)

Fig. 14.3a–e

a Classic LCIS and flat epithelial atypia (FEA) diagnosed at vacuum-assisted breast biopsy (VABB) and confirmed by excision. Prognostically the leading lesion is LCIS, the microcalcifications, however, were associated with FEA.

b These very fine microcalcifications were arranged suggesting a possible small segment. VABB and excision verified FEA.

c Magnified section of the mediolateral oblique view shows a subtle architectural distortion caudally.

d Spot compression confirms this subtle architectural distortion medially in the patient's left breast. *Histology*: Radial scar and FEA.

e Patient with histologically proven lobular neoplasia grade 2. The multiple areas of enhancement have not changed for more than 5 years. (Reproduced with kind permission of Karger AG from Heywang-Köbrunner et al. 2010b.)

the follow-up period (Eusebi et al. 1994). Evidence for or against long-term increased surveillance is lacking. For CCC and CCH with no cellular atypia there is no indication for increased follow-up (Schnitt 2003). In our opinion these lesions would be considered a normal finding and a variant of physiologic changes.

Atypical Lobular Hyperplasia, Lobular Carcinoma in Situ (and Pleomorphic-Type LCIS)

Definition

The term LN includes all forms of lobular proliferations with loss of E-cadherin mutations. LN comprises a spectrum of lesions including atypical lobular hyperplasia (ALH) and lobular carcinoma in situ including classic LCIS and pleomorphic-type LCIS (see also Chapter 15). ALH and LCIS share morphological features and the transition is gradual. They account for the great majority (approximately 90%) of all LNs. ALH and classic LCIS are incidental microscopic findings in breast biopsies targeting other lesions. Only occasionally are they associated with microcalcifications, for example in association with adenosis and rarely with the peculiar lesion collagenous spherulosis. LN is typically a process of premenopausal women with multifocal (60–85%) and bilateral (30–67%) distribution and is found in about 3% of all biopsies. Patients diagnosed with LCIS will develop invasive breast carcinoma in about 20–30% of cases in the ensuing 1 to 3 decades after biopsy diagnosis (Haagensen et al. 1978, Page et al. 1985, Contreras and Sattar 2009).

Whereas LN was initially thought to be simply a risk indicator for carcinoma (Haagensen et al. 1978), it is now thought that LN is also a nonobligate precursor of malignancy (mainly of invasive lobular carcinoma). Evidence for either role is both epidemiological and morphological (Tavassoli et al. 2003, Chuba et al. 2005, Contreras and Sattar 2009). While the risk of developing malignancy is increased in both breasts, it is over three times greater in the ipsilateral breast, with invasive lobular carcinomas over-represented (Page et al. 2003, Chuba et al. 2005).

Pleomorphic LCIS diagnosed from percutaneous breast biopsy is categorized as a B5 lesion, and will be discussed in detail in Chapter 15.

Histology

LCIS is invisible to the naked eye and can be recognized in histopathologic specimens only after excellent fixation, processing and staining, which, of course, should apply to all pathological specimens (optimal fixation time: 6–48 h; buffered formalin: 3.8% abs. conc.).

The neoplastic cells are specifically located in the acini which can be distended; the cells may also extend beyond the acini along adjacent ducts, and characteristically these cells spread as single cells between intact overlying epithelium and underlying basement membrane (so-called "Pagetoid spread"). Only rarely are ductal lumina distended by LCIS (characteristic of the very rare pleomorphic necrotic type). Tumor cells of invasive lobular carcinoma are morphologically identical to their noninvasive counterpart, which explains their designation. Both the in-situ lesions LCIS/ALH and invasive lobular carcinoma carry the same characteristic E-cadherin mutations or functional loss that is usually not found in other types of breast cancer.

Mammography

Many LN lesions (except pleomorphic LCIS; see Chapter 15) have no characteristic imaging features and are not visible on mammography. The majority (> 80%) are detected incidentally in or adjacent to areas with microcalcifications (**Fig. 14.3a**). However, histopathologically, ALH or classic LCIS is usually not associated with microcalcifications. The remaining LN lesions are found in breast biopsies performed for various further indications. Some LN lesions occur adjacent to radial scars, or coexist with other B3 lesions such as papilloma, ADH, or FEA; they may occur in fibroadenomas or are contained in benign changes.

Ultrasound and Magnetic Resonance Imaging

On ultrasound there are no specific sonographic features. There may be unspecific architectural changes, or a poorly defined area of decreased echogenicity. On MRI small enhancing masses or nonspecific regional areas of patchy enhancement may be detected. Enhancement curves are also uncharacteristic.

Since LCIS is associated with an increased risk (usually an intermediate risk) of invasive (more often lobular invasive) carcinoma, the value of additional MRI for screening such patients is of interest. So far, few retrospective studies have been published. The first study (Port et al. 2007) on 47 patients with preceding LCIS did not show significant advantages for MRI. More recent larger studies on screening MRI (Friedlander et al. 2011, Sung et al. 2011) demonstrated a significantly improved sensitivity by the additional use of MRI, while both MRI and mammography proved to be complementary. Even with a good positive predictive value of MRI of around 20%, the overall risk of a false positive recommendation for biopsy is significant. Prospective and multicenter studies will, however, be needed before general recommendations can be made. As again shown in this study, the availability of MR-guided minimally invasive interventions is another increasingly important prerequisite that needs to precede any general recommendation (see **Fig. 15.1a**).

Management

Overall the reported rates of upstaging after ALH or LCIS that has been diagnosed at percutaneous biopsy vary between 19% and 58% (Elsheikh and Silverman 2005, Mahoney et al. 2006, Houssami et al. 2007a, Londero et al. 2008) with a median upgrade rate in a recent review of 14.9% (Sinn et al. 2010). Many of these series, however, do not distinguish between ALH, classic LCIS or pleomorphic LCIS. Furthermore, information concerning associated clinical and imaging findings, including the initial indication for biopsy, is often not given. This is important, since areas of LN may constitute part of an invasive lobular carcinoma.

If needle biopsy yielded ALH or classic LCIS, close correlation with clinical findings and imaging is crucial to countercheck whether: the result is representative; the initial question is solved; and, based on clinical findings, imaging and histopathology, the presence of an adjacent lobular invasive carcinoma can be excluded with reasonable reliability. If this is not clear, open surgical biopsy has to be recommended. For pleomorphic LCIS, excision is indicated.

We advocate individual case discussion, which is supported by others (Menon et al. 2008, Albert et al. 2009), while some authors generally recommend excision (Pinder et al. 2007).

These issues are further complicated by a debate on optimum clinical management, which varies between systematic surgical excision and follow-up strategies with regular mammography. The desire for complete surgical excision is complicated by the fact that LN is frequently multifocal/-centric and bilateral. The authors of the latest version of the WHO classification point out that all data (including those concerning pleomorphic LCIS) are limited and that the evidence of improved outcome with excision to complete margins or mastectomy is lacking. However, the evidence for increased surveillance is lacking, too. So far the recommendation for annual mammography (usually including clinical examination and ultrasound, where indicated) for patients with a previous diagnosis of ALH or LCIS is adopted by most. There is no evidence to support MRI surveillance.

Radial Scars

Definition

Radial scar (lesion) (RSL) also known as complex sclerosing lesion (CSL) is another tumoral breast lesion (Tavassoli et al. 2003). Radial scar in a pure form is completely benign and the term refers to a lesion that macroscopically and mammographically simulates the patterns of low-grade invasive carcinoma, that is, invasive tubular carcinoma, invasive ductal carcinoma, and less often invasive lobular carcinoma.

RSL is characteristically associated with epithelial proliferations (92%). Some authors found a slightly elevated risk for subsequent breast cancer (Sanders et al. 2006), while others attributed the increased risk to associated epithelial proliferations (Tavassoli et al. 2003, Tavassoli and Eusebi 2009, Eusebi and Millis 2010). Associated benign proliferations include ductal papilloma, intraductal epithelial hyperplasia of usual type (UDH) and adenosis, but CSL can be associated with atypical proliferations such as ADH, FEA, and less often ALH or LCIS or invasive carcinoma, characteristically low-grade (G1) tubular or invasive ductal carcinoma. Therefore RSLs are included in the group of lesions of uncertain malignant potential (Amendoeira et al. 2006). A special task in the histopathologic evaluation of RSL is the diagnosis of specimens obtained by needle biopsies because the distribution and extent of any component of an individual lesion is often heterogeneous. In recent large series of CNB a rate of 9–17% underestimates (mostly low-grade DCIS or invasive tubular carcinoma G1) have been reported (Houssami et al. 2007a, El-Sayed et al. 2008, Linda et al. 2010). *Most important*: The risk of upgrade mainly concerns RSL associated with atypical epithelial proliferations. The published risk of RSL diagnosed at CNB was reported to be around 24–37% for RSL with atypical epithelial proliferations, whereas only 4–9% upgrades have been reported for CSL without atypia (Farshid 2004, Doyle et al. 2007, Tennant et al. 2008).

Radial scars mostly present as architectural distortion on mammography without a definite mass. They are rarely palpable clinically, and are therefore commonly detected by screening mammography. On the one hand radial sclerosing lesions thus represent a low-risk B3 lesion, on the other hand they may pose a diagnostic problem concerning differentiation from other stellate lesions like invasive carcinoma, DCIS, scarring, or superimposition.

Histology

RSLs are characteristically stellate and rarely nodular with a zone of central hypocellular dense center rich in fibroelastic stroma and strands of fibrous tissue radiating from the center resulting in parenchymal deformity. The periphery rather than the center of the lesion contains glandular components, that is, ducts and acini, entrapped within the sclerohyaline stroma This zoning phenomenon is characteristic of RSL. The histogenesis of RSL/CSL is still not resolved, but it is probably the result of an involutionary process (Jacobs et al. 1999). CSL overlaps with other sclerotic breast changes observed in involution and senescence—that is, obliterative mastitis, sclerosing papilloma, and sclerosing adenosis (Page and Anderson 1987, Eusebi and Millis 2010).

Radial Scars

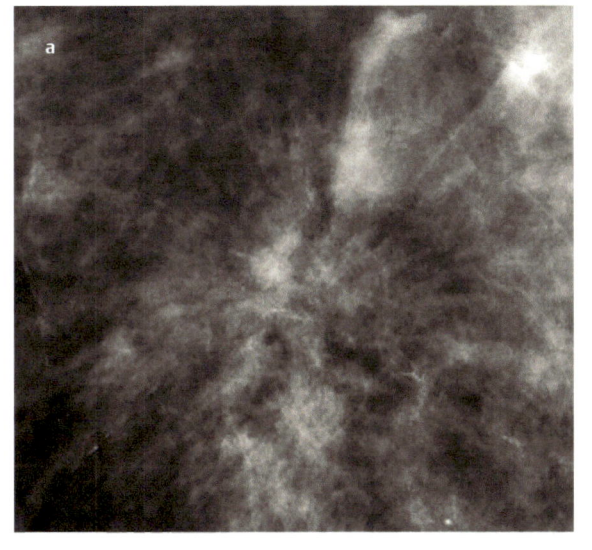

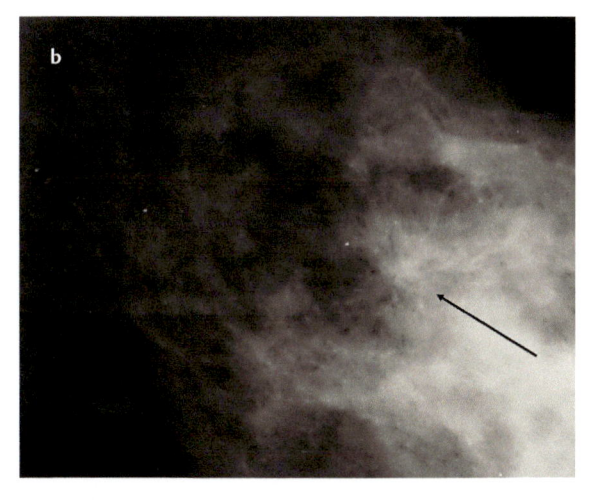

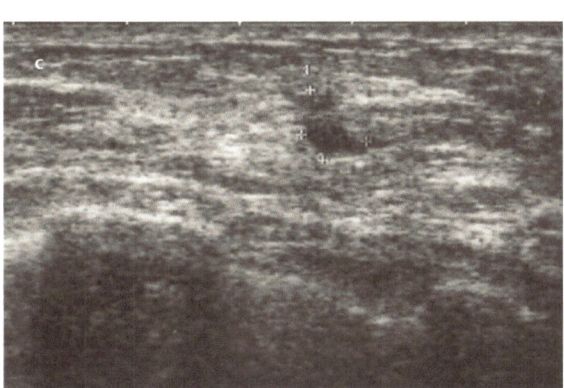

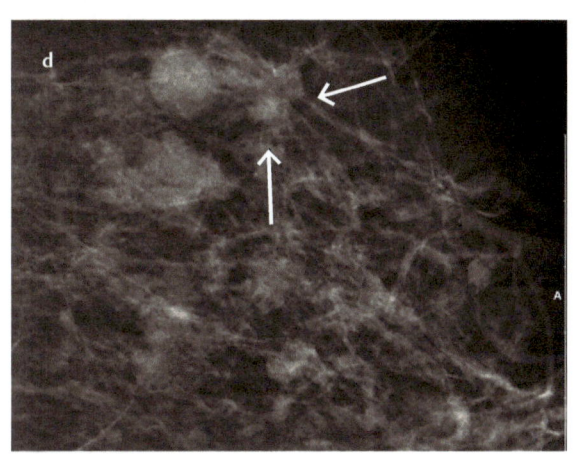

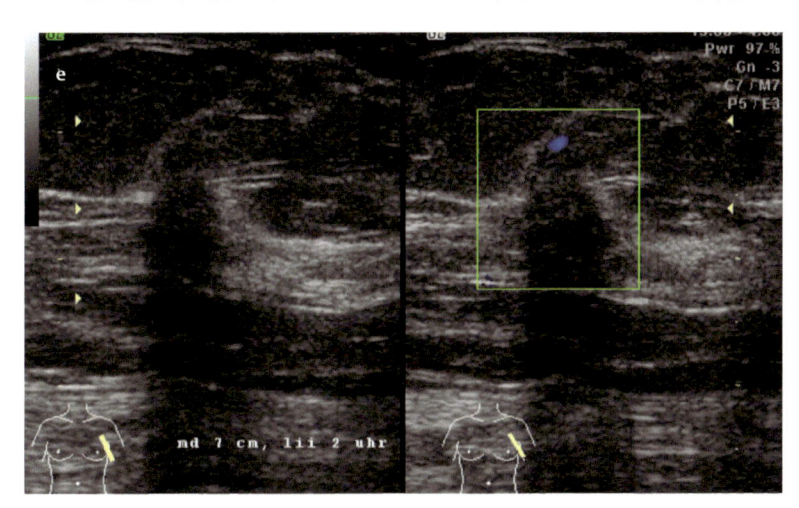

Fig. 14.4a–f

a Radial scar lesion (RSL), detected by screening mammography. *Histology* proved a typical radial scar without atypia.

b RSL with atypias, diagnosed at vacuum-assisted breast biopsy (VABB) and confirmed at surgery.

c On ultrasound a hypoechoic nodule is seen in the center of the lesion. *Final diagnosis*: RSL without atypia.

d,e Another small architectural distortion detected by screening mammography (**d**). Sonographically a small hypoechoic nodule interrupting the normal tissue with posterior sound attenuation and peripheral vascularization was detected (**e**). *Histology* revealed a tubular carcinoma.

Fig. 14.4f ▷

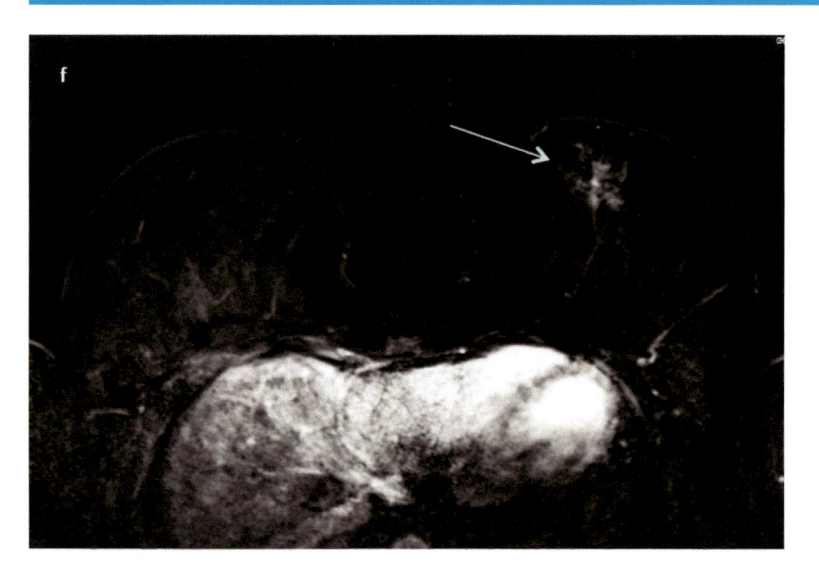

f In this patient (status after breast conservation right breast) this enhancing area was detected by magnetic resonance imaging (MRI) incidentally in the left breast. (Mammography and ultrasound exhibited dense and difficult to assess breast tissue—no abnormality.) MRI showed plateau-type enhancement dynamics. *Histology* (MRI-guided VABB, followed by excision) yielded an RSL.

In case of diagnostic doubts immune staining may be useful. Histologically it is important to exclude associated DCIS, invasive tubular, lobular or ductal carcinoma.

Mammography

As initially described by L. Tabar and P. B. Dean (1977), radial sclerosing lesions are usually seen as a parenchymal stellate distortion and may either have a small dense center (the so-called "white star" appearance) or a radiolucent center (the so-called "black star"). When an invasive carcinoma has a significant fibrotic stromal component, similar radiologic appearances are seen. Histologically, up to half of such mammographic abnormalities are invasive carcinoma.

Even though the risk of malignancy is higher with the "white star" imaging features, the "black star" may also be associated with malignancy (invasive or DCIS) in up to 20% of the cases. Mammographically indeterminate calcification may also be associated with radial sclerosing lesions. Unless an architectural distortion definitively corresponds to surgical or traumatic scarring or is proven as superimposition after additional mammographic views, no reliable mammographic sign exists that allows exclusion of malignancy (Alleva et al. 1999, Bouté et al. 2006, Lee et al. 2007, Linda et al. 2010) (**Figs. 14.3c** and **14.4**).

Ultrasound

Ultrasound should be performed routinely after further mammographic views. Although up to one-third of radial lesions show no abnormality on ultrasound, some benign radial scars will exhibit sufficient parenchymal distortion to be sonographically visible, usually as a hypoechoic mass with architectural distortion and sometimes with posterior acoustic attenuation. Even though ultrasound may be slightly more specific than mammography, no sonographic sign exists that can exclude malignancy in case of an architectural distortion and wherever possible ultrasound-guided core biopsy should be undertaken for diagnosis (Lee et al. 2007, Egyed et al. 2008) (**Fig. 14.4c–e**).

Magnetic Resonance Imaging

With MRI, radial scars mostly exhibit low or delayed enhancement. However, exceptions to this rule exist and there is overlap with the MR features of early malignancy (tubular carcinoma and DCIS). Overall published sensitivity and specificity is in the region of 85%, which does not allow the reliable exclusion of malignancy (Baum et al. 2000, Pediconi et al. 2005).

Management

If the diagnosis of RSL is obtained with a 14-gauge CNB, there is a 9–17% risk of associated DCIS or invasive breast cancer (Houssami et al. 2007a, El-Sayed et al. 2008, Linda et al. 2010) and therefore further surgical excision will be required. With VABB the rate of underestimation decreases, with various studies reporting that 11-gauge or larger VABB may eliminate the need for further surgical excision in benign RSLs where there is no cellular atypia, and all the radiologic abnormality has been excised (Tennant et al. 2008, Resetkova et al. 2011).

Following excision there is no evidence for increased follow-up.

Papillary Lesions

Definition

Papillary lesions of the breast can be divided into benign, atypical, and malignant variants. In this chapter benign and atypical papillary lesions will be discussed, which are included in the B3 category.

Histology

Papillary lesions can affect any part of the ductal tree. According to their location, papillomas can be further subdivided into central (solitary) papilloma, located in the collecting ducts of the subareolar region, and peripheral papilloma, which is often multiple and located within the peripheral ducts and TDLUs. Papillary lesions are characterized by intraductal macropapillary fronds containing stroma covered by glandular epithelium. The intraductal papillary configuration can be seen on macroscopic and microscopic examination. Papillomas can measure from a few millimeters to more than 4 cm, and the involved ducts can be cystically dilated. Superimposed changes are common that can obscure a papillary nature, that is, chronic erosion and inflammation which may cause partial or complete obliteration of the involved duct, periductal fibrosis, and inflammation. Infarction can occur either spontaneously or following biopsy, sometimes resulting in extensive squamous metaplasia of the ductal epithelia. Microcalcifications are regularly found in papilloma and most often associated within sclerosed papillary stroma (pleomorphic and coarse) or associated with epithelial proliferation (monomorphic or slightly pleomorphic and fine).

Any type of intraepithelial proliferation can occur in a papilloma: UDH, ADH and DCIS; these can develop primarily within the papilloma or secondarily involve a papilloma through surrounding ducts. These proliferations are more frequently found in peripheral papilloma than in central papilloma (Lakhani et al. 2012). Prognosis and risk of breast cancer in patients with papilloma is as yet not completely resolved. The risk is probably primarily related to associated lesions (UDH, ADH, DCIS). Also, it is probably lower for central papilloma than for peripheral papilloma without atypia. The risk of central papilloma without atypias appears to be similar to that of UDH (Lakhani et al. 2012). Most of the papillomas diagnosed by CNB (including both papillomas with and without epithelilal atypical proliferations) belong to the B3 category.

Accurate histopathologic diagnosis of papillary lesions remains challenging due to possible sampling error. The conversion rate of benign papillomas without atypia in biopsy to malignant lesions (more often DCIS) varies over a wide range from 0% (Agoff and Lawton 2004, Ivan et al. 2004, Renshaw et al. 2004) to 4–25% (Liberman et al. 2006, El-Sayed et al. 2008, Skandarajah et al. 2008). Except for two studies, which showed upgrades in 4% and 19%, respectively (El Sayed et al. 2008 and Skandarajah et al. 2008), the number of cases involved is low. Surgical proof was available in 20–70% of the patients in most studies, while only one study reported an excision rate of 100% (Skandarajah et al. 2008). The studies are heterogeneous concerning biopsy techniques, and a detailed analysis of imaging findings, lesion size, etc. is not given in most studies.

Papillary adenoma of the nipple/Nipple adenoma is a glandular ductal proliferation around segmental ducts of the subareolar region; however, it is not an intraductal proliferation like the ductal papillomas. Variant histopathologic growth pattern of this benign tumor occurs. It is frequently eroded and occurs unilaterally and bilaterally. Rare association with carcinoma has been described (Lakhani et al. 2012).

Clinical Findings

Papillomas usually show evidence of secretory activity (watery to yellowish discharge). They are very friable and bleed easily (brownish or bloody discharge). Papillomas also have the tendency to infarct. Old papillomas can become completely fibrosed and can contain calcifications.

Because of their intraductal location and high vulnerability, they can:
- Lead to watery or bloody discharge
- Distend ducts
- Distend cysts, and
- Be surrounded by a blood-containing cavity

Papillary lesions (most often central papillomas) are the most common cause of spontaneous discharge from the nipple, which may be serous or serosanguinous. Pathologic nipple discharge (PND) is a relatively common symptom accounting for approximately 5% of all symptomatic women attending breast clinics (Paterok et al. 1993). Papilloma is the commonest pathologic finding in women with PND accounting for 40–70% of cases.

Papillomas may also be palpable or are detected at screening mammography.

Discharge can be found in 80% of the papillomas and can be watery, yellowish, brownish, or bloody, whereby a bloody discharge strongly suggests a papilloma. Carcinomas can also cause a bloody discharge (in up to 25% of cases) and rarely a watery discharge, occurring in only 2–3% of carcinomas with discharge. A thorough diagnostic evaluation of women with PND is therefore indicated. Not infrequently, the localization of one or multiple papillomas can be suspected clinically if nipple discharge can be elicited by pressure on the so-called trigger points.

Only a few papillomas are primarily detected by palpation. These papillomas are usually large or superficial or have caused a retention cyst or "hemorrhagic cyst" through ductal obstruction.

Cytology of Nipple Discharge

The cytologic evaluation of nipple discharge can be easily performed and does not put any demand on the patient. A positive finding (cords of papillary cells, suspected cells, blood) should be an indication for further evaluation.

Cytology of the nipple discharge, which is based on the necrotic changes of the shed cells found in the discharge, is only of moderate sensitivity and specificity, mostly below 50% (Carvalho et al. 2009). A negative finding does not exclude a carcinoma. Furthermore, a reliable differentiation between carcinoma and papilloma cannot be expected from the cytologic assessment of the nipple discharge.

Diagnostic Strategy and Goals Assessing Patients with Nipple Discharge

Since most papillomas are detected by their secretory activity, the diagnostic questions to be answered are:
- *Confirmation of a papillary lesion*. In addition to papillary tumors, there are other causes of nipple discharge (as to the differential diagnosis of pathologic nipple discharge, see Chapter 24).
- *Localization* (search for the point of origin of the secretion).
- *Extent* (one papilloma or multiple papillomas).

Initially, noninvasive methods such as mammography, sonography, and a careful clinical examination are utilized.

Clinical examination (trigger point) as well as *mammography* (for large papillomas in a fatty breast) can point to the correct localization in some cases. The full extent is rarely appreciated mammographically or clinically.

Mammography serves to detect suspicious microcalcifications or masses with or without microcalcifications, which may be presentations of papillary benign or malignant lesions.

In some cases papillary lesions may be detected by ultrasound, mostly as hypoechoic solid or complex mass with or without a surrounding cyst filled with bloody material. Sometimes dilated hypoechoic ducts may correlate to papillary lesions.

In many instances, localization and extent cannot be adequately evaluated with noninvasive methods. In these cases, galactography may be helpful as a supplemental examination. By showing filling defects or, less frequently, truncated ducts, it can detect papillomas and allows an assessment of their extent. Absence of any filling defects or truncated ducts—together with cytologic absence of suspected cells or cords of papillary cells—makes an intraductal lesion unlikely.

Thus the imaging methods can suggest or exclude a papillary lesion in the majority of cases.

In cases where galactography is not possible or malignancy is unlikely, MRI may aid detecting or excluding an enhancing area that might correlate with a papillary lesion.

The important differentiation between papilloma and carcinoma is radiologically not possible. Consequently, *imaging is not adequate for determining the histology of suspected papillary lesions*, and should primarily support the planning of the inevitable diagnostic excision.

Whenever a focal lesion is identified it can be biopsied using imaging guidance. If this is not possible, surgical excision after filling of the ducts with methylene blue or after galactographic marking may be necessary to solve the diagnostic problem and treat the symptom.

Some authors have suggested the use of ductoscopy and ductoscopic biopsy. According to our experience, these methods may be useful for pathology that is close to the nipple. When using it, keep in mind that ductoscopic biopsy yields less tissue than percutaneous breast biopsy. The failure rate of ductoscopy, which usually requires general anesthesia, is higher than that of galactography. Also, it is mostly only possible to reach the proximal 3–5 cm of the retroareolar ducts.

Whenever preoperative marking is required, it should be remembered that methylene blue or contrast agent that was applied into the ductal system through the nipple may (in case of obliterated ducts) only mark the anterior part of the segment to be resected. Excision of diffuse papillary changes should therefore always include the complete segment in question. Thorough histopathologic examination of the margins is essential.

Mammography

(See **Fig. 14.5a–d.**)

Mammography (Cardenosa and Eklund 1991, Woods et al. 1992, Lam et al. 2006, Brookes and Bourke 2008, Muttarak et al. 2008) often does not reveal small papillomas surrounded by dense tissue. Sometimes high-resolution ultrasound can show an intraductal abnormality. If the cause of secretion or the exact extent of the pathologic intraductal changes cannot be determined with certainty, galactography can be performed.

If papillomas are surrounded by fatty tissue—as is often the case in older patients—they appear as nodular, round, or oval masses, ranging from a few millimeters to (though rarely) 2–3 cm in size. Owing to recurrent bleeding they are often not as sharply outlined as fibroadenomas, and are then not reliably distinguishable from a carcinoma.

Papillomas that cause cystic dilation of a ductal segment or a hemorrhagic cyst might be seen as a smoothly outlined, well-circumscribed mass, with or without halo. The smooth contour corresponds to the wall of the cyst.

If papillomas appear as a round or oval mass in the subareolar area, the correct diagnosis may be presumed on the basis of their location.

Only some of the papillomas develop sclerotic changes and can subsequently calcify. Typical calcifications appear intraductally, following a duct that may be dilated. They can be—resembling fibroadenoma-type calcifications—coarse or shell-like, but also punctate and densely aggregated in a round group (see **Fig. 24.44a**). Only this typical manifestation allows the mammographic assumption of a papillary tumor. Papillary lesions may also present as

Papillary Lesions

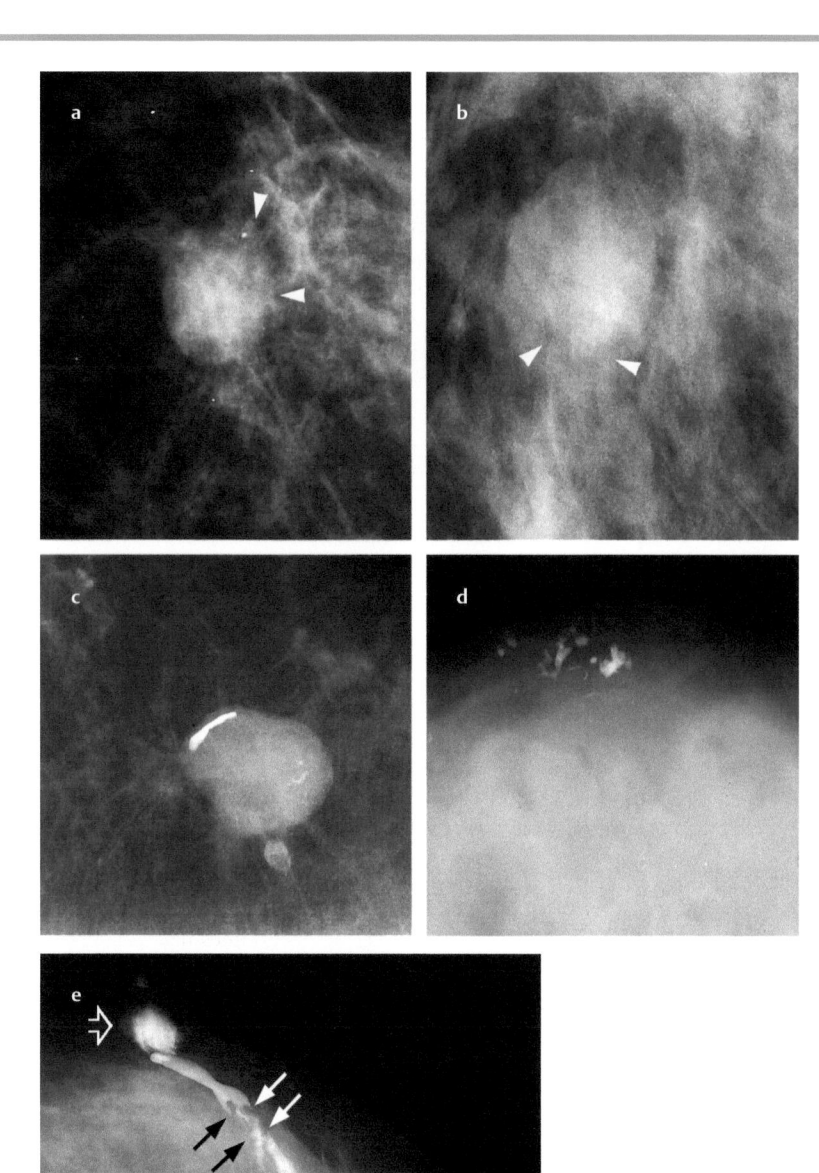

Fig. 14.5a–e Papilloma: Mammography (**a–d**) and galactography (**e**).

a As in this case, the papilloma is often visualized as a mass that frequently is incompletely outlined or even shows irregularities of contour (arrowheads). A papilloma can occasionally be suspected on the basis of the lesion's location in the region of the retromamillary ducts.

b Intracystic papillomas are often visualized—caused by the smooth wall of the surrounding cyst—as smoothly outlined lesions. In this case, the distal aspect of the cyst (arrowheads) is superimposed by dense surrounding tissue (for sonogram of this lesion, see **Fig. 14.6a**). The cyst surrounding the papilloma can be a true cyst or a hemorrhagic cavity around the papilloma.

c Nodular lesion with a shell-like calcification. A few uncharacteristic and V-shaped microcalcifications are visible. Although malignancy is possible because of the indistinct posterior border as well as the V-shaped microcalcifications, the shell-like calcification is consistent with a calcified wall of the cyst, as observed in a hemorrhagic cyst. By itself, such a marginal calcification could also be typical for a fibroadenoma. *Histology*: Benign intracystic papilloma with occasional calcifications and partially calcified hemorrhagic cyst.

d Some papillomas may contain characteristic calcifications. In this case, typical coarse calcifications as well as occasional elongated, delicate, suspicious calcifications in the retroareolar ducts are shown. Because of the latter calcifications, an excisional biopsy was obtained. *Histology*: Benign largely calcified retroareolar papilloma.

e Papilloma imaged by galactography. The galactographic delineation of a slightly dilated retroareolar duct reveals several small filling defects (arrows) caused by a benign papilloma growing along the duct (small retroareolar extravasation [open arrowhead]).

microcalcifications, which may be polymorphic, clustered, or linear in distribution and/or a mass lesion. Papillary lesions may also be contained in an RSW (**Fig. 14.5**).

Ultrasound

(See **Figs. 14.6 and 14.7**.)

Sonographically (Ganesan et al. 2006, Lam et al. 2006, Brookes and Bourke 2008, Muttarak et al. 2008) some intraductal papillomas can be identified in the subareolar ducts. Because of the unreliable detection of smaller and peripherally located papillomas, sonography cannot always replace galactography.

Usually ultrasound can detect intracystic or intraductal papillomas. They are recognized as hypoechoic lesions surrounded by echo-free cystic fluid or as hypoechoic lesions located within a dilated duct.

In contrast to intracystic sediment, their appearance remains constant with positional changes. If the papilloma occupies a cyst entirely or almost entirely, or if the

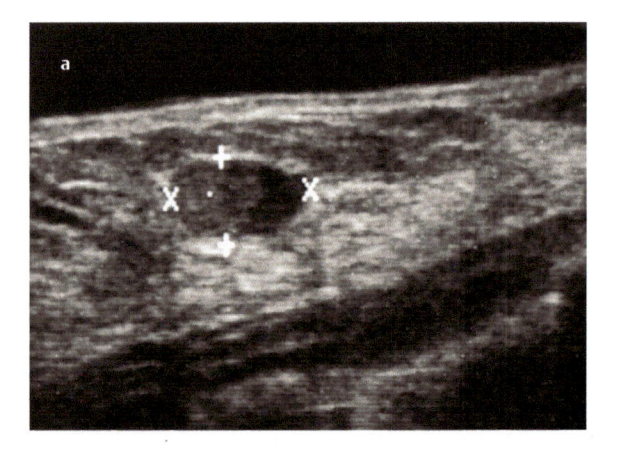

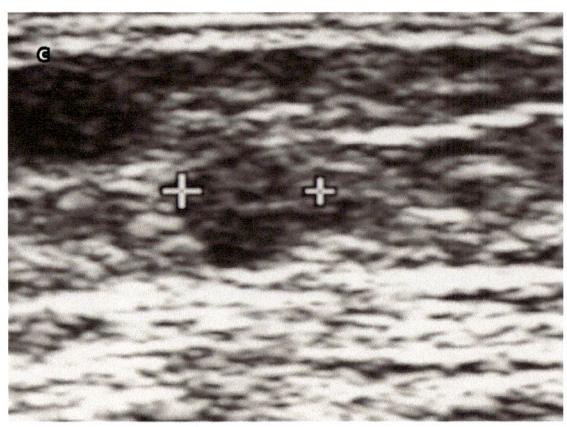

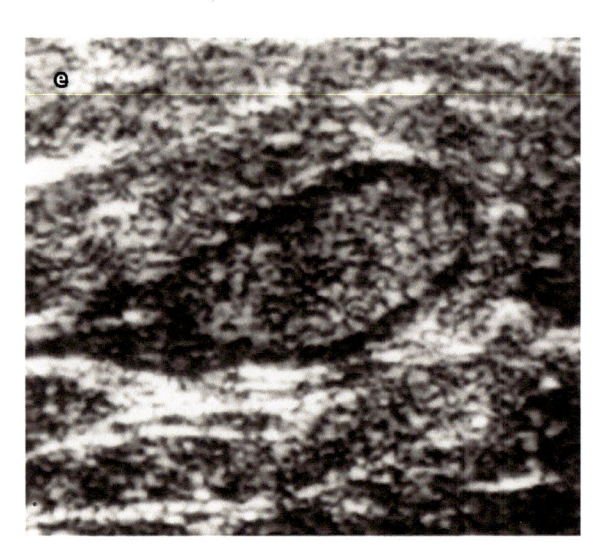

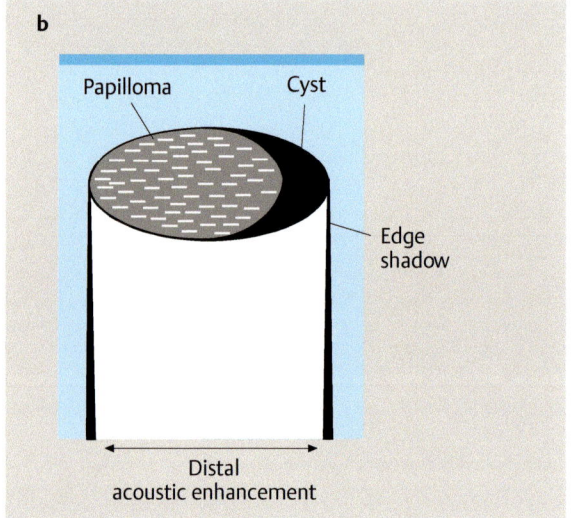

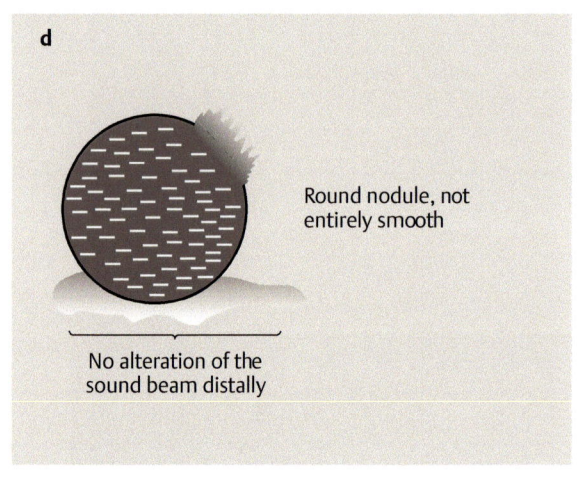

14 Lesions of Uncertain Malignant Potential (B3 Lesions)

Fig. 14.6a–e Papilloma: Sonography.

a The intracystic papilloma is characteristically seen as a hypoechoic to hyperechoic (as observed here) lesion within a mostly hypoechoic, smoothly outlined hemorrhagic "cyst."
b Diagram.
c A hypoechoic, not quite smoothly outlined lesion is found if the content of the cyst becomes thickened. In this case, a distinction of the papilloma itself and the surrounding echogenic fluid is no longer possible, and the complete complex lesion is only visible as a hypoechoic mass.
d Diagram.
e This oval solid mass distends the surrounding duct. Biopsy demonstrated it to be a papilloma.

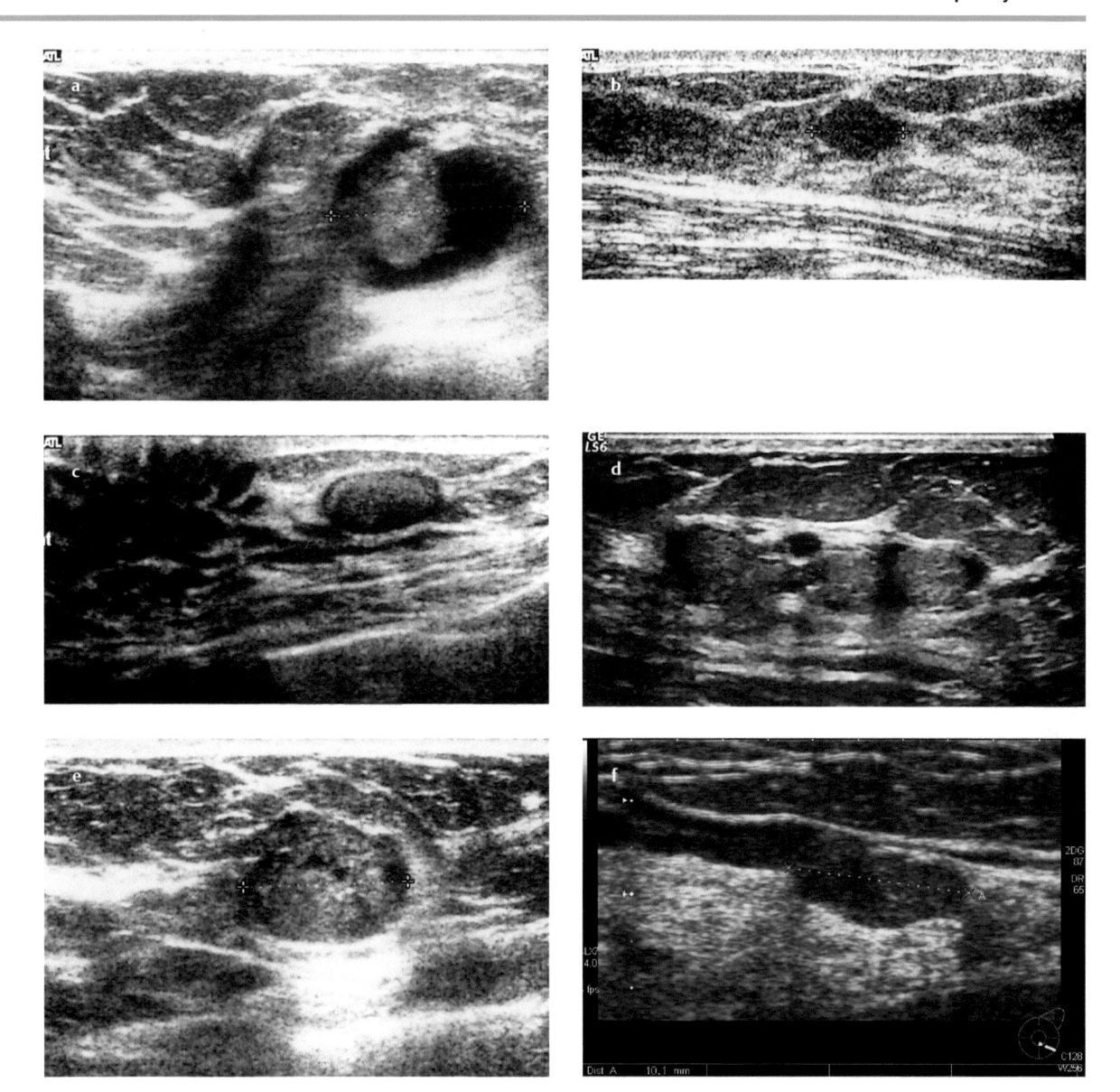

Fig. 14.7a–f Sonographic appearance of papillomas.

a   Intracystic irregular solid mass. Surgery yielded a papilloma without atypia.
b   Ill-defined hypoechoic lesion, detected because of nipple discharge. On core biopsy it turned out to be a papilloma.
c   Centrally located oval solid intraductal mass, yielding papilloma on core biopsy.
d   A dilated duct containing three roundish solid lesions: Multiple papillomas.
e   The same patient (**Fig. 14.7a**) showed another papilloma, which filled another cyst almost completely.
f   Papilloma detected on ultrsaound for nipple discharge. Note the surrounding dilated duct.

cystic fluid has become echogenic as a result of clotted hemorrhage, the hypoechoic-to-hyperechoic lesion may not be differentiated from other solid lesions.

Furthermore, benign papillomas may be imaged as a solid, smooth, well-defined nodule, compatible with a benign tumor. Sometimes contours may not be well-circumscribed. Irregularities of the contour may be caused by recurrent hemorrhage and resulting fibrosis. If calcifications are present in the papilloma, shadowing may be seen.

Therefore, papillary lesions may be visible as a hypoechoic mass, as a complex cystic lesion or as a hypoechoic lesion within a dilated duct. Even though homogenous echogenicity and a well-circumscribed margin (Kim et al. 2008, Shin et al. 2008) are indicative of a benign lesion, neither mammographic nor sonographic features allow a reliable distinction between benign and atypical papillary lesions. Ultrasound-guided biopsy is indicated if a mass or complex cystic lesion is demonstrated.

Galactography

(See **Fig. 14.5e**.)

Galactographically, papillomas appear as filling defects or truncated ducts. While small blood clots or debris can cause similar defects, multiple irregular filling defects and obstructed ducts strongly suggest the presence of intraductal papillary tumors. Uncertain findings can be differentiated from blood clots, debris, or even small air bubbles by emptying the ductal system, followed by a repeat instillation of contrast medium. Only true intraductal lesions reappear at the same site.

According to a recent series the sensitivity of galactography for malignancy has been reported to be around 80%, specificity around 27% (Carvalho et al. 2009). Thus galactography can confirm the presence of an intraductal lesion and is mostly able to determine its location in the ductal system. However, a negative galactogram cannot exclude malignancy. Also galactography may not demonstrate all of the extent. Since the contrast agent may only fill up to a stop, galactography may only demonstrate the ducts anterior to the stop. Differentiation of a benign lesion from an intraductal carcinoma is galactographically not possible, and excision of the suspicious ductal segment is always necessary.

When planning excision one should be aware that a galactographic stop may demonstrate only the proximal end of a segmental lesion.

Magnetic Resonance Imaging

(See **Fig. 14.8**.)

The role of MRI in the management of papillomas is currently limited (Sardanelli et al. 2010, Kurz et al. 2011, Lorenzon et al. 2011, Tominaga et al. 2011). Papillomas present with a variable appearance on contrast-enhanced MRI. Sclerosing papillomas do not or only minimally enhance, and nonsclerosing papillomas, even if small, demonstrate marked enhancement. Enhancing papillary lesions range from occult to "small luminal mass" papillomas to irregular rapidly enhancing lesions, which sometimes may even exhibit washout and cannot be reliably distinguished from invasive malignancy. Sometimes a papillary lesion may be suspected in complex lesions with blood-containing ducts or cysts and a solid component. MRI may help exclude malignancy in cases of nipple discharge with no mammographic or sonographic findings. While enhancing benign and malignant papillary lesions may exhibit overlapping morphological and dynamic MR features, absent enhancement may help exclude malignancy with a high negative predictive value.

Management

Percutaneous breast biopsy is indicated whenever a suspected papillary lesion becomes apparent as a mass with or without microcalcifications or as indeterminate microcalcifications. If a focal lesion or a definite area of ductal changes is detected by galactography, percutaneous biopsy (and/or clip marking for subsequent surgery) is possible under galactographic guidance. For lesions visualized by MRI only MR-guided VABB or preoperative marking is necessary.

Accurate histopathologic diagnosis of papillary lesions at CNB remains challenging. Based on a literature review, Ueng recommends surgical excision for all papillomas that have not been completely removed at CNB (Ueng et al. 2009). This is confirmed by the published negative predictive value of CNB diagnosis of a benign papilloma of 78–100%. Whenever atypical features are diagnosed at CNB, excision should be undertaken as subsequent malignancy is present in 22–75% of cases (Jackman et al. 2002, El-Sayed et al. 2008, Sakr et al. 2008, Skandarajah et al. 2008, Bernik et al. 2009, Hayes et al. 2009, Bennett et al. 2010, Jung et al. 2010).

There is increasing evidence for complete removal of small papillomas with no cellular atypia by VABB. For these lesions the reported rate of understaging is in the region of 0–5% (Carder et al. 2008, Tennant et al. 2008, Zografos et al. 2008) and follow-up instead of excision may be justified after close scrutiny of radiologic–histopathologic correlation.

There is no evidence for increased follow-up of patients with solitary benign papillomas.

A complete excision had been recommended for every papilloma by the WHO authors "regardless of the findings in a previous core biopsy" in 2003 (Tavassoli et al. 2003). The latest edition of the WHO classification does not contain this general recommendation (Lakhani et al. 2012).

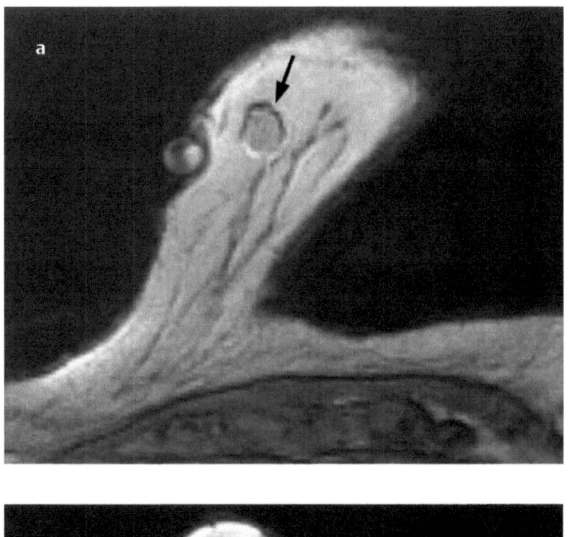

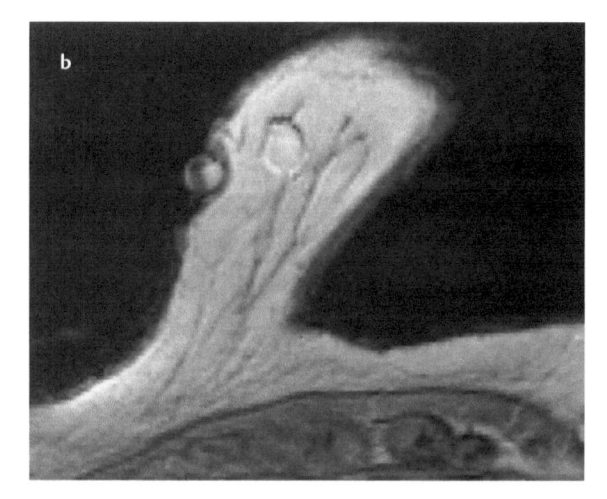

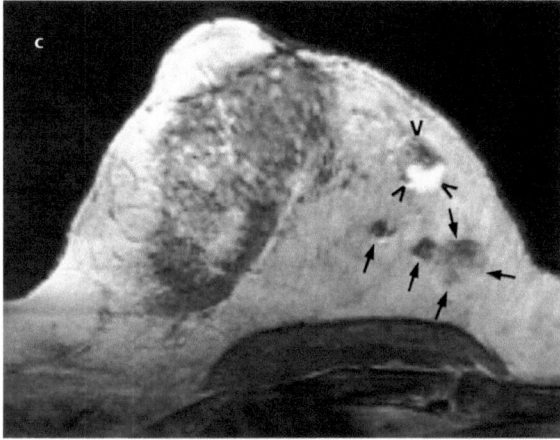

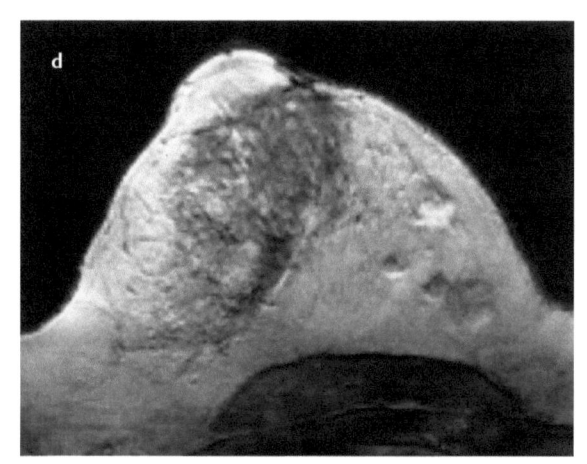

Fig. 14.8a–d Papilloma: Magnetic resonance imaging (MRI).

a,b Contrast-enhanced MRI of a nonsclerosing large papilloma. The papilloma (arrow), which was palpable, shows contrast enhancement and consequently is not distinguishable from an enhancing fibroadenoma or a smoothly outlined malignancy.

c,d In this patient with multiple, not quite smoothly outlined lesions, the T1-weighted image shows a moderately decreased signal intensity in three of the lesions (arrows) that is compatible with solid tumors. The fourth nodule (arrowheads) is seen as a complex lesion. The very high signal intensity, already seen in the unenhanced image (**c**), is characteristic of a hemorrhagic cyst. The anterior wall, which exhibits a low signal, is thickened and nodular. This finding of MRI already suggests a cystic papilloma before Gd-DTPA application.

All papillomas show only slight and delayed enhancement. Since papillary DCIS and rarely invasive carcinomas may show the same enhancement pattern, an excisional biopsy was advised. *Histology*: Fibrosed, nodular growing, and partially intracystic papillomas.

We advocate an individual approach for patients with papilloma: incidental (micro)papillomas without atypia (B2 category) do not warrant excision if diagnosed at VABB; on the other hand every papilloma with atypia (B3 category) is strongly recommended for excision independent of biopsy technique used. If papilloma without atypia (B3) is diagnosed at CNB (probably insufficient sampling), we generally recommend re-excision. Papilloma without atypia diagnosed at VABB according to recommendations (sample size, number of biopsies) is more challenging but a conservative approach can be considered appropriate if (1) the patient is not at increased risk of breast cancer, (2) clinical examination and imaging (mammograms, sonograms) are not suspicious, (3) complete or near-complete removal through biopsy is expected, (4) good compliance of the patient is anticipated, and (5) conservative strategy is accepted by the patient.

Fibroepithelial Lesions of Uncertain Malignant Potential

Definition

Fibroepithelial B3 lesions include phyllodes tumors and comparable cellular fibroepithelial lesions that have histopathologic similarities to phylloid tumors. Phyllodes tumors are rare fibroepithelial neoplasms that account for less than 1% of all breast neoplasms. They usually present in the 4th to 5th decade, but may develop in all age groups.

Phyllodes tumors mostly present as well-circumscribed oval or lobulated lesions similar to a fibroadenoma. Phyllodes tumors are characterized by rapid growth. Their histologic spectrum includes benign tumors, of which up to 30% recur, and malignant tumors, which can metastasize. In total, only about 5–10% of phyllodes tumors may metastasize (Ben Hassouna et al. 2006).

Benign and borderline phyllodes tumors are considered benign lesions of uncertain malignant potential. Malignant phyllodes tumors belong to the group of rare malignant tumors.

A needle biopsy diagnosis of a cellular fibroepithelial lesion that cannot for certain be distinguished from phyllodes tumor and the diagnosis of a (probably) benign phyllodes tumor are categorized as B3 lesions. Final histopathologic classification usually requires excision, since phyllodes tumors may be inhomogeneous.

In view of its biologic property (fast growth, tendency to recur, and low risk of dealing with a higher grade lesion), timely detection and complete excision with an adequate safety margin is generally recommended.

Histology

The phyllodes tumors are rare biphasic fibroepithelial neoplasms exhibiting the pattern analogous to fibroadenomas. They usually occur in middle-aged women (40–50 years). Most phyllodes tumors follow a benign course and local recurrences are the major problem. Prediction of the clinical course is difficult in the individual, but based on morphological features—that is, stromal cellularity, pleomorphism, mitoses, margins, stromal pattern, and heterologous stromal differentiation—subgroups have been defined; however, there is no clear delineation of benign, borderline, and malignant categories of phylloid tumors (Barth 1999, de Roos et al. 1999, Tavassoli et al. 2003) (see Chapter 18).

Most phyllodes tumors arise de novo, but development from fibroadenomas may occur. Macroscopically phyllodes tumors are well circumscribed; the smaller tumors in screening populations, usually 2–3 cm in size, may be indistinguishable from fibroadenomas, whereas larger lesions display their characteristic leaflike (phylloid) pattern. Larger tumors often show a cystic component and especially malignant tumors may develop necrosis. In contrast to benign phyllodes tumors, malignant tumors show invasive margins and the stromal component is malignant, usually with a high grade sarcoma component of variable and mixed differentiation (fibrosarcoma or heterologous differentiation like liposarcoma, osteosarcoma, chondrosarcoma, rhabdomyosarcoma, and others). The epithelial component is usually absent or very scarce in such tumors and only very rarely involved in malignant transformation (Lakhani et al. 2012).

Clinical Findings

Larger phyllodes tumors are mostly palpable:
- As a smoothly marginated, round, or lobulated mass, which is more or less elastic.
- Small tumors are generally moveable, but this characteristic is often lost with larger tumors.
- *Rapid growth* is suggestive of a phyllodes tumor. It can arise from a known fibroadenoma which was stable for a long time and then noted by its increasing growth. It can also be found as a mass that increases in size.

At the time of diagnosis, the majority of these neoplasms have reached a size of 3–5 cm, but occasionally small phyllodes tumors are also discovered. Due to the tension of the overlying skin, very large phyllodes tumors can cause erythematous or bluish discoloration of the skin, or even ulcerations.

Diagnostic Strategy and Goals

It is the major diagnostic goal to *differentiate* the phyllodes tumor from other nodular masses and mainly from the far more common solid nodular lesions that are *benign*. Only some phyllodes tumors have criteria that distinguish them from smoothly outlined benign lesions.

It is therefore important that a phyllodes tumor should be considered whenever a smoothly outlined mass increases in size. If suspected by CNB, excision is indicated. If a lesion that was diagnosed as fibroadenoma or fibroepithelial lesion exhibits rapid growth, a phyllodes tumor should be suspected and re-biopsy or -excision should be considered.

Mammography

(See **Fig. 14.9**.)

Mammographically (Liberman et al. 1996, Jorge Blanco et al. 1999, Muttarak and Chaiwun 2004), the phyllodes tumor often resembles a fibroadenoma. This means, it often presents as:
- An oval, round, or lobulated mass.
- Some phyllodes tumors are sharply outlined with or without a halo.

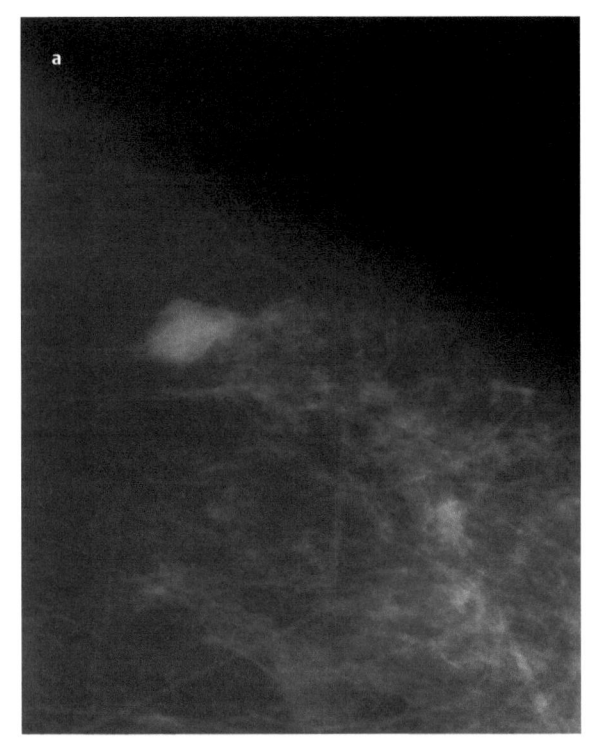

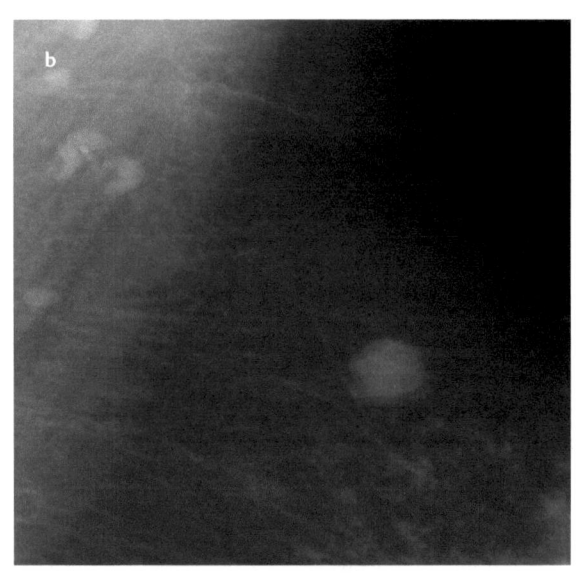

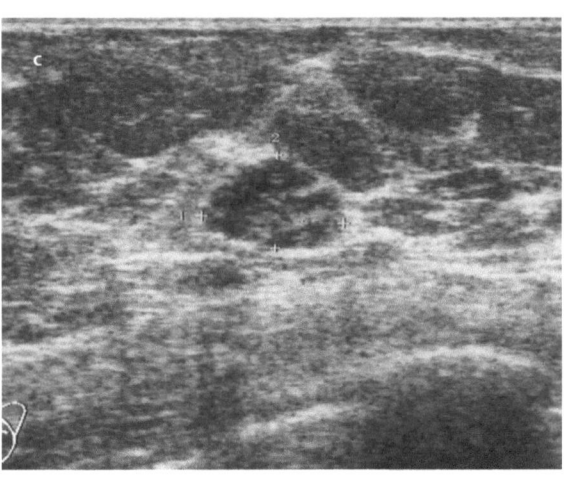

Fig. 14.9a–h

a–c Nonpalpable, oval, well-defined mass in the outer upper quadrant of the breast, sonographocally oval and well-defined as well. *Histology*: Benign phyllodes tumor.

d–f Mammogram of a patient with a large benign phyllodes tumor. (**d,e**) Note lobulated borders and cystic areas within the solid mass.

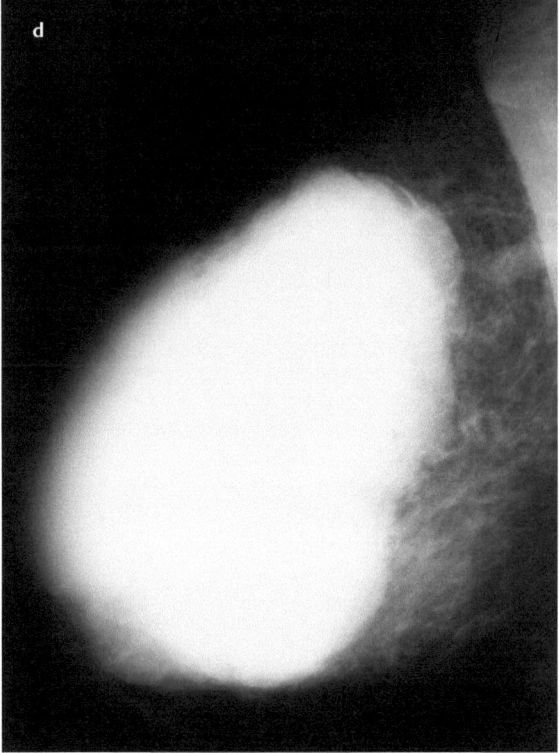

Fig. 14.9e–h ▷

14 Lesions of Uncertain Malignant Potential (B3 Lesions)

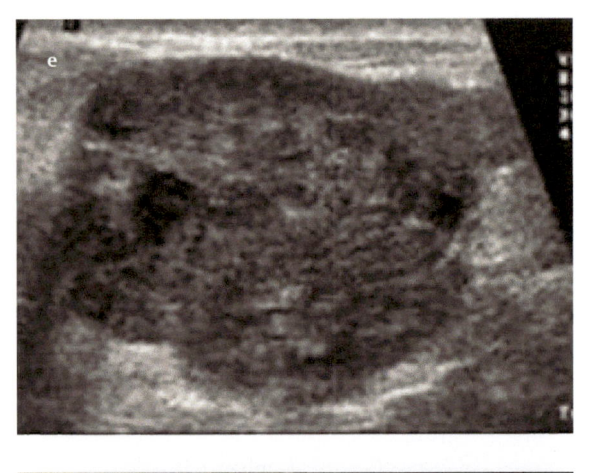

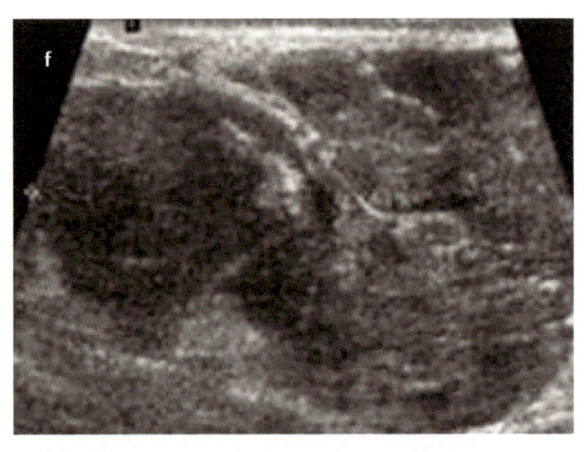

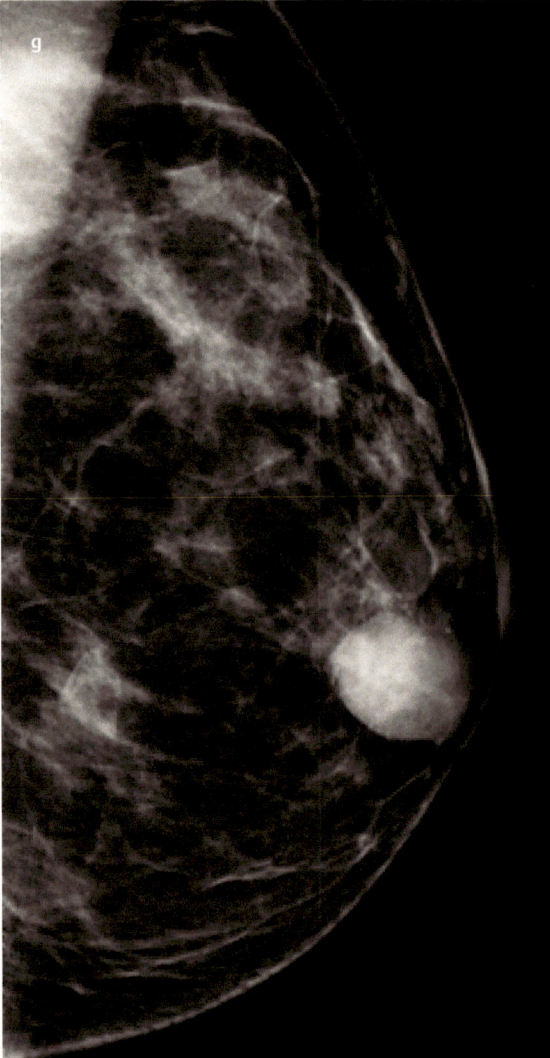

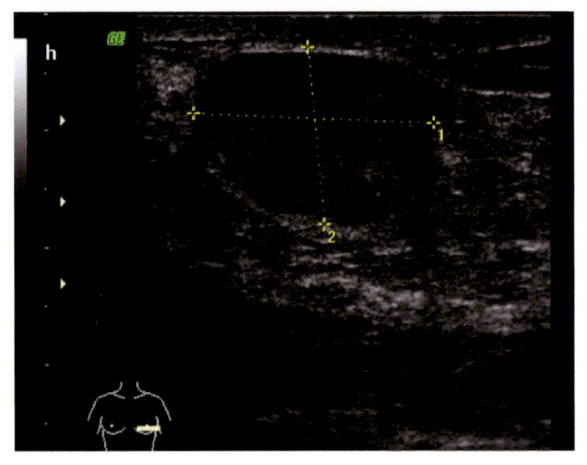

◁ continued

g,h Young woman presenting with a newly developed soft tumor behind the areola. Mammographically round, well-defined mass and sonographically (**h**) an oval circumscribed hypoechoic nodule with rather homogeneous texture. *Histology*: Benign phyllodes tumor.

- Depending on the surrounding tissue, the margin can be partially or completely obscured. In this situation, the phyllodes tumor is seen as a semicircular density or can be undetectable in dense parenchyma.
- Some irregularities in the contour are frequently, but not always, present. This can be caused by superimposition, vascular invasion, or infiltrating growth, and if present, indicates etiologies other than a fibroadenoma.
- Rarely, bizarre or coarse calcifications (as seen in fibroadenomas) can be found in portions of phyllodes tumors.

The indistinct outline of some phyllodes tumors can serve as evidence against the presence of a fibroadenoma. If an indistinct outline is absent or only minimal, there are, aside from a rapid increase in size and the often large extension, *no reliable mammographic differentiating criteria* between the phyllodes tumors and other smoothly or relatively smoothly outlined (usually benign) lesions.

Ultrasound

(See **Fig. 14.9a,c,d,f.**)

Sonographically (Liberman et al. 1996, Jorge Blanco et al. 1999, Muttarak and Chaiwun 2004, Gatta et al. 2011) the phyllodes tumor can resemble other smoothly or relatively smoothly outlined tumors. This means it often presents:
- As an oval, round, or lobulated mass
- With good acoustic enhancement
- With usually good compressibility and moveability
- Its contour is generally smooth

Though occasionally also exhibited by fibroadenomas, the *following findings* suggest the correct diagnosis:
- Indistinct outline (found in some phyllodes tumors), heterogeneity of the internal echo structure (in some phyllodes tumors, but often also in fibroadenomas, hamartomas, and malignancies).
- Cystic spaces within the solid tumor (corresponding to the gelatinous, cystic, or necrotic areas) are sonographically characteristic of the phyllodes tumor and should suggest its diagnosis. According to our experience they are rarely seen in small tumors.

Magnetic Resonance Imaging

(See **Fig. 14.10a–c.**)

Experience with contrast-enhanced MRI is limited (Heywang-Köbrunner and Beck 1996, Wurdinger et al. 2005, Yabuuchi et al. 2006, Yoo et al. 2010, Chung et al. 2011, Tan et al. 2012). As far as we know, phyllodes tumors enhance rapidly and intensely. About 33% of phyllodes tumors (compared with 22% of fibroadenomas) may exhibit a suspicious enhancement pattern. In general, however, the enhancement pattern does not permit a reliable differentiation from hypercellular fibroadenomas or from smoothly outlined malignancies. Heterogeneities or cystic spaces may be disclosed by MRI, as also seen on ultrasound. If present, they strongly suggest the diagnosis of phyllodes tumor. Also some phyllodes tumors may cause increased signal intensity of surrounding tissues on T2-weighted images.

All things considered, contrast-enhanced MRI offers no significant advantage over mammography or sonography in the differential diagnosis. The excellent visualization of the entire extent, in particular the relation of

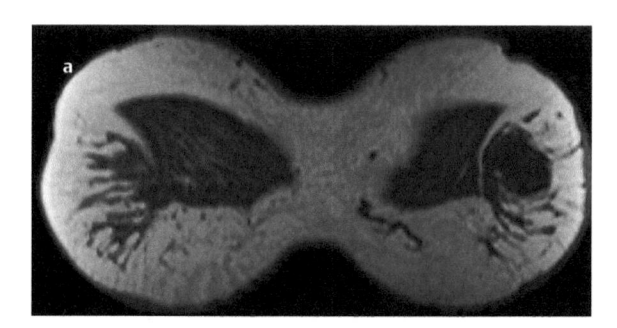

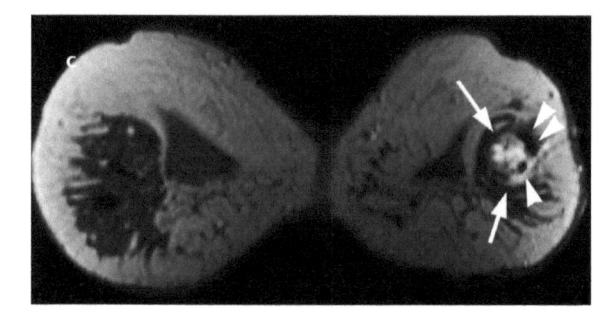

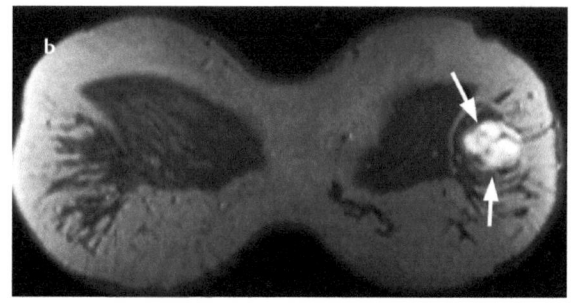

Fig. 14.10a–c Phyllodes tumor: Magnetic resonance imaging (MRI) (different patient).

a MRI (coronal plane) delineates a lesion of homogeneously low signal intensity and smooth outline before administration of contrast medium.

b,c After intravenous administration of contrast medium, the lesion (arrows) shows a lobulated internal structure (intense enhancement within the lobules, slight enhancement in the septa), with some nonenhancing clefts (arrowheads) seen in adjacent sections (c). *Histology*: Benign phyllodes tumor.

very large tumors to the thoracic wall, can be of interest to the surgeon. According to one publication low signal intensity on T2-weighted images and low apparent diffusion coefficient may correlate with higher grading of phyllodes tumors (Yabuuchi et al. 2006).

Percutaneous Biopsy

Percutaneous breast biopsy is generally the next step when assessing a well-circumscribed lesion that increases in size. In most cases a diagnosis of a fibroepithelial lesion or phyllodes tumor is possible from CNB; however, the diagnosis is not always possible and the distinction between benign phyllodes tumor and (juvenile) fibroadenoma may be challenging. Diagnosis of malignant phyllodes tumor is usually straightforward and should not be confused with rare primary sarcoma of the breast. (VABB is usually not needed, since most lesions are easily recognized and targeted by ultrasound guidance.)

Because of the multifarious changes of the stroma, which are decisive for establishing the diagnosis of phyllodes tumor, percutaneous biopsy may in some cases miss the diagnosis of phyllodes tumor or comparable fibroepithelial lesion. In some cases an unequivocal diagnosis of the tumor cannot be made, and the exact classification may not be possible from the limited volume of tissue available from percutaneous breast biopsy (Foxcroft et al. 2007, Resetkova et al. 2010, Gatta et al. 2011).

If a phyllodes tumor is suspected, owing to the rapid growth of a smoothly outlined mass, or if a lesion that was diagnosed as fibroadenoma or fibroepithelial lesion by percutaneous breast biopsy exhibits fast growth, excisional biopsy should be considered to establish the diagnosis.

Management

Although malignancy is infrequent, no radiologic features exist to differentiate benign from malignant lesions, and unless completely excised they tend to recur, with a recurrence rate of about 15% (Houssami et al. 2007a, El-Sayed et al. 2008). Therefore all phyllodes tumors as well as rare other fibroepithelial lesions that are classified as B3 (fibroadenomas or myxoid lesions that exhibit histopathologic changes suspicious of phyllodes tumors) require complete excision. Because of the risk of recurrence locally, annual follow-up with mammography is generally recommended.

Other B3 Lesions

Other rare lesions may be classified as B3 lesions at minimally invasive biopsy. These include mucocele-like lesions, mucinous or spindle cell lesions. The data on these lesions is very limited and therefore to date complete excision is recommended.

Summary

Lesions of uncertain malignant potential are a heterogeneous variety of histopathologic entities, which are considered benign but of unknown malignant potential. These entities are grouped together, since they have a comparable risk of malignancy, which is higher than that of benign changes. As supported by the results of genetic profiling, some of these lesions may indeed represent the link between early malignancy and benign changes. Even though they are known to have an unknown biological potential, they are still classified as benign changes, since, as yet, their malignant potential in the individual case is unclear, and they are classified as benign conditions.

These entities are challenging from the diagnostic and management perspectives.

Their imaging features may overlap with those of benign or early malignant change. Many of these lesions have no distinct imaging features, and constitute incidental findings.

Their histopathologic diagnosis and distinction from other entities is difficult, requiring a high level of expertise. Since many of these lesions may be inhomogeneous, the exact diagnosis and prediction of individual prognostic impact is more difficult still and even impossible from the small tissue volume gained at percutaneous breast biopsy. Lesions of uncertain potential are classified as B3 lesions when diagnosed at percutaneous breast biopsy.

Some of these lesions may indicate a generally increased bilateral risk of breast cancer or they may act as nonobligatory precursors of malignancy that might develop into malignancy.

They may also occur adjacent to higher-grade lesions (DCIS or invasive cancer). Thus, the diagnosis of a B3 lesion may be the only indicator of an adjacent breast cancer, which due to sampling error was not diagnosed at percutaneous breast biopsy.

International guidelines recommend that these cases be discussed in the multidisciplinary team and appropriate management decided for each individual patient, based on imaging, pathology, reliability of follow-up, and other risk factors such as family history.

Follow-up strategies for precursor lesions seem reasonable on current evidence:

- Annual mammography after complete excision is recommended for ADH, phyllodes tumor, and for LIN
- No increased follow-up for CCL, RSLs, and papillary lesions where there is no atypia
- There is no evidence to support MRI surveillance

While our knowledge of B3 lesions is still growing, it is important to collect and evaluate information on lesions of uncertain malignant potential. This will allow a better understanding of radiologic appearances, of histo-morphological appearances, and of potential future risk. This might eventually allow better management by limiting surgery to those women at risk and avoiding overtreatment in women at low risk.

References and Recommended Reading

Agoff SN, Lawton TJ. Papillary lesions of the breast with and without atypical ductal hyperplasia: can we accurately predict benign behavior from core needle biopsy? Am J Clin Pathol 2004;122(3):440–443

Albert US, Altland H, Duda V, et al. 2008 update of the guideline: early detection of breast cancer in Germany. J Cancer Res Clin Oncol 2009;135(3):339–354

Alleva DQ, Smetherman DH, Farr GH Jr, Cederbom GJ. Radial scar of the breast: radiologic-pathologic correlation in 22 cases. Radiographics 1999;19(Spec No):S27–S35; discussion S36–S37

Amendoeira I, Apostolikas N, Bellocq JP, et al. Quality assurance guidelines for pathology: cytological and histological non-operative procedures. In: Perry N, Broeders M, de Wolf C, Toernberg S, Holland R, von Karsa L (eds). European Guidelines for Quality Assurance in Breast Screening and Diagnosis. Luxembourg: Office for Official Publications of the European Communities; 2006:221–256

Azzopardi JG. Underdiagnosis of malignancy. In: Bennington JL (ed.). Problems in Breast Pathology, Vol. 11: Major Problems in Pathology. Philadelphia: WB Saunders; 1979: 192–233

Barth RJ Jr. Histologic features predict local recurrence after breast conserving therapy of phyllodes tumors. Breast Cancer Res Treat 1999;57(3):291–295

Bässler R, Zahner J. Recurrences and metastases of cystosarcoma phylloides (phylloid tumor, WHO). On the 150th birthday of a controversial diagnostic concept. [Article in German] Geburtshilfe Frauenheilkd 1989;49(1):1–10

Bässler R. Pathologie der Brustdrüse. In: Doerr W, Seifert G, Uehlinger E (eds). Spezielle Pathologische Anatomie. Berlin, Heidelberg, New York: Springer; 1995

Baum F, Fischer U, Füzesi L, Obenauer S, Vosshenrich R, Grabbe E. The radial scar in contrast media-enhanced MR mammography. [Article in German] Rofo 2000;172(10):817–823

Ben Hassouna J, Damak T, Gamoudi A, et al. Phyllodes tumors of the breast: a case series of 106 patients. Am J Surg 2006; 192(2):141–147

Bennett LE, Ghate SV, Bentley R, Baker JA. Is surgical excision of core biopsy proven benign papillomas of the breast necessary? Acad Radiol 2010;17(5):553–557

Bernik SF, Troob S, Ying BL, et al. Papillary lesions of the breast diagnosed by core needle biopsy: 71 cases with surgical follow-up. Am J Surg 2009;197(4):473–478

Bouté V, Goyat I, Denoux Y, Lacroix J, Marie B, Michels JJ. Are the criteria of Tabar and Dean still relevant to radial scar? Eur J Radiol 2006;60(2):243–249

Brandt SM, Young GQ, Hoda SA. The "Rosen Triad": tubular carcinoma, lobular carcinoma in situ, and columnar cell lesions. Adv Anat Pathol 2008;15(3):140–146

Brookes MJ, Bourke AG. Radiological appearances of papillary breast lesions. Clin Radiol 2008;63(11):1265–1273

Cardenosa G, Eklund GW. Benign papillary neoplasms of the breast: mammographic findings. Radiology 1991;181(3): 751–755

Carder PJ, Khan T, Burrows P, Sharma N. Large volume "mammotome" biopsy may reduce the need for diagnostic surgery in papillary lesions of the breast. J Clin Pathol 2008; 61(8):928–933

Carvalho MJ, Dias M, Gonçalo M, Fernandes G, Rodrigues V, de Oliveira CF. What is the diagnostic value of nipple discharge cytology and galactography in detecting duct pathology? Eur J Gynaecol Oncol 2009;30(5):543–546

Chivukula M, Haynik DM, Brufsky A, Carter G, Dabbs DJ. Pleomorphic lobular carcinoma in situ (PLCIS) on breast core needle biopsies: clinical significance and immunoprofile. Am J Surg Pathol 2008;32(11):1721–1726

Chuba PJ, Hamre MR, Yap J, et al. Bilateral risk for subsequent breast cancer after lobular carcinoma-in-situ: analysis of surveillance, epidemiology, and end results data. J Clin Oncol 2005;23(24):5534–5541

Chung J, Son EJ, Kim JA, Kim EK, Kwak JY, Jeong J. Giant phyllodes tumors of the breast: imaging findings with clinicopathological correlation in 14 cases. Clin Imaging 2011;35(2):102–107

Cohn-Cedermark G, Rutqvist LE, Rosendahl I, Silfverswärd C. Prognostic factors in cystosarcoma phyllodes. A clinicopathologic study of 77 patients. Cancer 1991;68(9): 2017–2022

Contreras A, Sattar H. Lobular neoplasia of the breast: an update. Arch Pathol Lab Med 2009;133(7):1116–1120

David N, Labbe-Devilliers C, Moreau D, Loussouarn D, Campion L. Diagnosis of flat epithelial atypia (FEA) after stereotactic vacuum-assisted biopsy (VAB) of the breast: What is the best management: systematic surgery for all or follow-up? [Article in French] J Radiol 2006;87(11 Pt 1):1671–1677

de Mascarel I, MacGrogan G, Mathoulin-Pélissier S, et al. Epithelial atypia in biopsies performed for microcalcifications. Practical considerations about 2,833 serially sectioned surgical biopsies with a long follow-up. Virchows Arch 2007;451(1):1–10

de Roos WK, Kaye P, Dent DM. Factors leading to local recurrence or death after surgical resection of phyllodes tumours of the breast. Br J Surg 1999;86(3):396–399

Dillon MF, McDermott EW, Hill AD, O'Doherty A, O'Higgins N, Quinn CM. Predictive value of breast lesions of "uncertain malignant potential" and "suspicious for malignancy" determined by needle core biopsy. Ann Surg Oncol 2007; 14(2):704–711

Doyle EM, Banville N, Quinn CM, et al. Radial scars/complex sclerosing lesions and malignancy in a screening programme: incidence and histological features revisited. Histopathology 2007;50(5):607–614

Eby PR, Ochsner JE, DeMartini WB, Allison KH, Peacock S, Lehman CD. Frequency and upgrade rates of atypical ductal hyperplasia diagnosed at stereotactic vacuum-assisted breast biopsy: 9-versus 11-gauge. AJR Am J Roentgenol 2009;192(1):229–234

Egyed Z, Péntek Z, Járay B, et al. Radial scar-significant diagnostic challenge. Pathol Oncol Res 2008;14(2):123–129

El-Sayed ME, Rakha EA, Reed J, Lee AH, Evans AJ, Ellis IO. Predictive value of needle core biopsy diagnoses of lesions of uncertain malignant potential (B3) in abnormalities detected by mammographic screening. Histopathology 2008;53(6):650–657

Ellis IO, Humphreys S, Michell M, Pinder SE, Wells CA, Zakhour HD; UK National Coordinating Commmittee for Breast Screening Pathology; European Commission Working Group on Breast Screening Pathology. Best Practice No 179. Guidelines for breast needle core biopsy handling and reporting in breast screening assessment. J Clin Pathol 2004;57(9):897–902

Elsheikh TM, Silverman JF. Follow-up surgical excision is indicated when breast core needle biopsies show atypical lobular hyperplasia or lobular carcinoma in situ: a correlative study of 33 patients with review of the literature. Am J Surg Pathol 2005;29(4):534–543

Eusebi V, Millis RR. Epitheliosis, infiltrating epitheliosis, and radial scar. Semin Diagn Pathol 2010;27(1):5–12

Eusebi V, Feudale E, Foschini MP, et al. Long-term follow-up of in situ carcinoma of the breast. Semin Diagn Pathol 1994; 11(3):223–235

Fadare O, Dadmanesh F, Alvarado-Cabrero I, et al. Lobular intraepithelial neoplasia [lobular carcinoma in situ] with comedo-type necrosis: a clinicopathologic study of 18 cases. Am J Surg Pathol 2006;30(11):1445–1453

Fahrbach K, Sledge I, Cella C, Linz H, Ross SD. A comparison of the accuracy of two minimally invasive breast biopsy methods: a systematic literature review and meta-analysis. Arch Gynecol Obstet 2006;274(2):63–73

Farshid G, Rush G. Assessment of 142 stellate lesions with imaging features suggestive of radial scar discovered during population-based screening for breast cancer. Am J Surg Pathol 2004;28(12):1626–1631

Fischer U, Schwethelm L, Baum FT, Luftner-Nagel S, Teubner J. Effort, accuracy and histology of MR-guided vacuum biopsy of suspicious breast lesions—retrospective evaluation after 389 interventions. [Article in German] Rofo 2009;181(8):774–781

Foxcroft LM, Evans EB, Porter AJ. Difficulties in the pre-operative diagnosis of phyllodes tumours of the breast: a study of 84 cases. Breast 2007;16(1):27–37

Fraser JL, Raza S, Chorny K, Connolly JL, Schnitt SJ. Columnar alteration with prominent apical snouts and secretions: a spectrum of changes frequently present in breast biopsies performed for microcalcifications. Am J Surg Pathol 1998;22(12):1521–1527

Friedlander LC, Roth SO, Gavenonis SC. Results of MR imaging screening for breast cancer in high-risk patients with lobular carcinoma in situ. Radiology 2011;261(2):421–427

Ganesan S, Karthik G, Joshi M, Damodaran V. Ultrasound spectrum in intraductal papillary neoplasms of breast. Br J Radiol 2006;79(946):843–849

Gatta G, Iaselli F, Parlato V, Di Grezia G, Grassi R, Rotondo A. Differential diagnosis between fibroadenoma, giant fibroadenoma and phyllodes tumour: sonographic features and core needle biopsy. Radiol Med (Torino) 2011;116(6): 905–918

Geisler DP, Boyle MJ, Malnar KF, et al. Phyllodes tumors of the breast: a review of 32 cases. Am Surg 2000;66(4):360–366

Grunwald S, Heyer H, Kühl A, et al. Radial scar/complex sclerosing lesion of the breast—value of ultrasound. Ultraschall Med 2007;28(2):206–211

Haagensen CD, Lane N, Lattes R, Bodian C. Lobular neoplasia (so-called lobular carcinoma in situ) of the breast. Cancer 1978;42(2):737–769

Han BK, Schnall MD, Orel SG, Rosen M. Outcome of MRI-guided breast biopsy. AJR Am J Roentgenol 2008; 191(6):1798–1804

Hayes BD, O'Doherty A, Quinn CM. Correlation of needle core biopsy with excision histology in screen-detected B3 lesions: the Merrion Breast Screening Unit experience. J Clin Pathol 2009;62(12):1136–1140

Heywang-Köbrunner SH, Beck R. Contrast-enhanced MRI of the breast. Heidelberg, New York: Springer; 1996

Heywang-Köbrunner SH, Nährig J, Hacker A, Hertlein M, Sedlacek S, Höfler H. Evaluation of B3-lesions diagnosed at percutaneous biopsy and surgical results after excision. Eur J Cancer Suppl. 2010a;8(3):175

Heywang-Köbrunner SH, Schreer I, Decker T, Böcker W. Interdisciplinary consensus on the use and technique of vacuum-assisted stereotactic breast biopsy. Eur J Radiol 2003;47(3):232–236

Heywang-Köbrunner SH, Sinnatamby R, Lebeau A, Lebrecht A, Britton PD, Schreer I; Consensus Group. Interdisciplinary consensus on the uses and technique of MR-guided vacuum-assisted breast biopsy (VAB): results of a European consensus meeting. Eur J Radiol 2009;72(2):289–294

Heywang-Köbrunner SH, Nährig J, Hacker A, Sedlacek S, Höfler H. B3 lesions: radiological assessment and multi-disciplinary Aspects. Breast Care (Basel) 2010b;5(4):209–217

Houssami N, Ciatto S, Bilous M, Vezzosi V, Bianchi S. Borderline breast core needle histology: predictive values for malignancy in lesions of uncertain malignant potential (B3). Br J Cancer 2007a;96(8):1253–1257

Houssami N, Ciatto S, Ellis I, Ambrogetti D. Underestimation of malignancy of breast core-needle biopsy: concepts and precise overall and category-specific estimates. Cancer 2007b;109(3):487–495

International Breast Cancer Consensus Conference. Image-detected breast cancer: state of the art diagnosis and treatment. J Am Coll Surg 2001;193(3):297–302

Ivan D, Selinko V, Sahin AA, Sneige N, Middleton LP. Accuracy of core needle biopsy diagnosis in assessing papillary breast lesions: histologic predictors of malignancy. Mod Pathol 2004;17(2):165–171

Jackman RJ, Birdwell RL, Ikeda DM. Atypical ductal hyperplasia: can some lesions be defined as probably benign after stereotactic 11-gauge vacuum-assisted biopsy, eliminating the recommendation for surgical excision? Radiology 2002;224(2):548–554

Jackman RJ, Marzoni FA Jr, Rosenberg J. False-negative diagnoses at stereotactic vacuum-assisted needle breast biopsy: long-term follow-up of 1,280 lesions and review of the literature. AJR Am J Roentgenol 2009;192(2):341–351

Jacobs TW, Byrne C, Colditz G, Connolly JL, Schnitt SJ. Radial scars in benign breast-biopsy specimens and the risk of breast cancer. N Engl J Med 1999;340(6):430–436

Johnson NB, Collins LC. Update on percutaneous needle biopsy of nonmalignant breast lesions. Adv Anat Pathol 2009;16(4):183–195

Jorge Blanco A, Vargas Serrano B, Rodríguez Romero R, Martínez Cendejas E. Phyllodes tumors of the breast. Eur Radiol 1999;9(2):356–360

Jung SY, Kang HS, Kwon Y, et al. Risk factors for malignancy in benign papillomas of the breast on core needle biopsy. World J Surg 2010;34(2):261–265

Kettritz U, Rotter K, Schreer I, et al. Stereotactic vacuum-assisted breast biopsy in 2874 patients: a multicenter study. Cancer 2004;100(2):245–251

Kim TH, Kang DK, Kim SY, Lee EJ, Jung YS, Yim H. Sonographic differentiation of benign and malignant papillary lesions of the breast. J Ultrasound Med 2008;27(1):75–82

Kohr JR, Eby PR, Allison KH, et al. Risk of upgrade of atypical ductal hyperplasia after stereotactic breast biopsy: effects of number of foci and complete removal of calcifications. Radiology 2010;255(3):723–730

Kunju LP, Kleer CG. Significance of flat epithelial atypia on mammotome core needle biopsy: Should it be excised? Hum Pathol 2007;38(1):35–41

Kurz KD, Roy S, Saleh A, Diallo-Danebrock R, Skaane P. MRI features of intraductal papilloma of the breast: sheep in wolf's clothing? Acta Radiol 2011;52(3):264–272

Lakhani SR, Elis IO, Schnitt SJ, et al. (eds) WHO classification of tumours of the breast. Lyon: IARC; 2012

Lam WW, Chu WC, Tang AP, Tse G, Ma TK. Role of radiologic features in the management of papillary lesions of the breast. AJR Am J Roentgenol 2006;186(5):1322–1327

Lee AH, Denley HE, Pinder SE, et al; Nottingham Breast Team. Excision biopsy findings of patients with breast needle core biopsies reported as suspicious of malignancy (B4) or lesion of uncertain malignant potential (B3). Histopathology 2003;42(4):331–336

Lee E, Wylie E, Metcalf C. Ultrasound imaging features of radial scars of the breast. Australas Radiol 2007;51(3):240–245

Leibl S, Regitnig P, Moinfar F. Flat epithelial atypia (DIN 1a, atypical columnar change): an underdiagnosed entity very frequently coexisting with lobular neoplasia. Histopathology 2007;50(7):859–865

Liberman L. Percutaneous image-guided core breast biopsy. Radiol Clin North Am 2002;40(3):483–500, vi

Liberman L, Bonaccio E, Hamele-Bena D, Abramson AF, Cohen MA, Dershaw DD. Benign and malignant phyllodes tumors: mammographic and sonographic findings. Radiology 1996;198(1):121–124

Liberman L, Bracero N, Morris E, Thornton C, Dershaw DD. MRI-guided 9-gauge vacuum-assisted breast biopsy: initial clinical experience. AJR Am J Roentgenol 2005; 185(1):183–193

Liberman L, Tornos C, Huzjan R, Bartella L, Morris EA, Dershaw DD. Is surgical excision warranted after benign, concordant diagnosis of papilloma at percutaneous breast biopsy? AJR Am J Roentgenol 2006;186(5):1328–1334

Linda A, Zuiani C, Bazzocchi M, Furlan A, Londero V. Borderline breast lesions diagnosed at core needle biopsy: can magnetic resonance mammography rule out associated malignancy? Preliminary results based on 79 surgically excised lesions. Breast 2008;17(2):125–131

Linda A, Zuiani C, Furlan A, et al. Radial scars without atypia diagnosed at imaging-guided needle biopsy: how often is associated malignancy found at subsequent surgical excision, and do mammography and sonography predict which lesions are malignant? AJR Am J Roentgenol 2010; 194(4):1146–1151

Londero V, Zuiani C, Linda A, Vianello E, Furlan A, Bazzocchi M. Lobular neoplasia: core needle breast biopsy underestimation of malignancy in relation to radiologic and pathologic features. Breast 2008;17(6):623–630

Lorenzon M, Zuiani C, Linda A, Londero V, Girometti R, Bazzocchi M. Magnetic resonance imaging in patients with nipple discharge: should we recommend it? Eur Radiol 2011;21(5):899–907

Mahoney MC, Robinson-Smith TM, Shaughnessy EA. Lobular neoplasia at 11-gauge vacuum-assisted stereotactic biopsy: correlation with surgical excisional biopsy and mammographic follow-up. AJR Am J Roentgenol 2006;187(4): 949–954

Malhaire C, El Khoury C, Thibault F, et al. Vacuum-assisted biopsies under MR guidance: results of 72 procedures. Eur Radiol 2010;20(7):1554–1562

Martel M, Barron-Rodriguez P, Tolgay Ocal I, Dotto J, Tavassoli FA. Flat DIN 1 (flat epithelial atypia) on core needle biopsy: 63 cases identified retrospectively among 1,751 core biopsies performed over an 8-year period (1992-1999). Virchows Arch 2007;451(5):883–891

Menon S, Porter GJ, Evans AJ, et al. The significance of lobular neoplasia on needle core biopsy of the breast. Virchows Arch 2008;452(5):473–479

Moinfar F. Flat ductal intraepithelial neoplasia of the breast: evolution of Azzopardi's "clinging" concept. Semin Diagn Pathol 2010;27(1):37–48

Murad TM, Contesso G, Mouriesse H. Papillary tumors of large lactiferous ducts. Cancer 1981;48(1):122–133

Muttarak M, Chaiwun B. Imaging of giant breast masses with pathological correlation. Singapore Med J 2004; 45(3):132–139

Muttarak M, Lerttumnongtum P, Chaiwun B, Peh WC. Spectrum of papillary lesions of the breast: clinical, imaging, and pathological correlation. AJR Am J Roentgenol 2008;191(3):700–707

Nährig J. Practical problems in breast screening. Columnar cell lesions including flat epithelial atypia and lobular neoplasia. [Article in German] Pathologe 2008;29(Suppl 2):172–177

NHSBSP. Publication No. 50: Guidelines for non-operative diagnostic procedures. Sheffield, UK: NHS Cancer Screening Programmes; 2001

Ohuchi N, Abe R, Kasai M. Possible cancerous change of intraductal papillomas of the breast. A 3-D reconstruction study of 25 cases. Cancer 1984;54(4):605–611

O'Malley FP, Mohsin SK, Badve S, et al. Interobserver reproducibility in the diagnosis of flat epithelial atypia of the breast. Mod Pathol 2006;19(2):172–179

Page DL, Anderson TJ. Diagnostic histopathology of the breast. Edinburgh: Churchill Livingstone; 1987

Page DL, Dupont WD, Rogers LW, Rados MS. Atypical hyperplastic lesions of the female breast. A long-term follow-up study. Cancer 1985;55(11):2698–2708

Page DL, Schuyler PA, Dupont WD, Jensen RA, Plummer WD Jr, Simpson JF. Atypical lobular hyperplasia as a unilateral predictor of breast cancer risk: a retrospective cohort study. Lancet 2003;361(9352):125–129. Erratum in: Lancet 2003;361(9373):1994

Pandelidis S, Heiland D, Jones D, Stough K, Trapeni J, Suliman Y. Accuracy of 11-gauge vacuum-assisted core biopsy of mammographic breast lesions. Ann Surg Oncol 2003; 10(1):43–47

Pandey S, Kornstein MJ, Shank W, de Paredes ES. Columnar cell lesions of the breast: mammographic findings with histopathologic correlation. Radiographics 2007;27(Suppl 1):S79–S89

Paterok EM, Rosenthal H, Säbel M. Nipple discharge and abnormal galactogram. Results of a long-term study (1964-1990). Eur J Obstet Gynecol Reprod Biol 1993;50(3):227–234

Pediconi F, Occhiato R, Venditti F, et al. Radial scars of the breast: contrast-enhanced magnetic resonance mammography appearance. Breast J 2005;11(1):23–28

Perlet C, Heywang-Köbrunner SH, Heinig A, et al. Magnetic resonance-guided, vacuum-assisted breast biopsy: results from a European multicenter study of 538 lesions. Cancer 2006;106(5):982–990

Pinder SE, Provenzano E, Reis-Filho JS. Lobular in situ neoplasia and columnar cell lesions: diagnosis in breast core biopsies and implications for management. Pathology 2007; 39(2):208–216

Plantade R, Hammou JC, Gerard F, et al. Ultrasound-guided vacuum-assisted biopsy: review of 382 cases. [Article in French] J Radiol 2005;86(9 Pt 1):1003–1015

Port ER, Park A, Borgen PI, Morris E, Montgomery LL. Results of MRI screening for breast cancer in high-risk patients with LCIS and atypical hyperplasia. Ann Surg Oncol 2007;14(3):1051–1057

Renshaw AA, Derhagopian RP, Tizol-Blanco DM, Gould EW. Papillomas and atypical papillomas in breast core needle biopsy specimens: risk of carcinoma in subsequent excision. Am J Clin Pathol 2004;122(2):217–221

Resetkova E, Khazai L, Albarracin CT, Arribas E. Clinical and radiologic data and core needle biopsy findings should dictate management of cellular fibroepithelial tumors of the breast. Breast J 2010;16(6):573–580

Resetkova E, Edelweiss M, Albarracin CT, Yang WT. Management of radial sclerosing lesions of the breast diagnosed using percutaneous vacuum-assisted core needle biopsy: recommendations for excision based on seven years of experience at a single institution. Breast Cancer Res Treat 2011;127(2):335–343

Rosen PP, Caicco JA. Florid papillomatosis of the nipple. A study of 51 patients, including nine with mammary carcinoma. Am J Surg Pathol 1986;10(2):87–101

Rosen PP, Holmes G, Lesser ML, Kinne DW, Beattie EJ. Juvenile papillomatosis and breast carcinoma. Cancer 1985;55(6):1345–1352

Sakr R, Rouzier R, Salem C, et al. Risk of breast cancer associated with papilloma. Eur J Surg Oncol 2008;34(12):1304–1308

Sanders ME, Page DL, Simpson JF, Schuyler PA, Dale Plummer W, Dupont WD. Interdependence of radial scar and proliferative disease with respect to invasive breast carcinoma risk in patients with benign breast biopsies. Cancer 2006;106(7):1453–1461

Sardanelli F, Boetes C, Borisch B, et al. Magnetic resonance imaging of the breast: recommendations from the EUSOMA working group. Eur J Cancer 2010;46(8):1296–1316

Schnitt SJ. The diagnosis and management of pre-invasive breast disease: flat epithelial atypia—classification, pathologic features and clinical significance. Breast Cancer Res 2003;5(5):263–268

Schnitt SJ, Vincent-Salomon A. Columnar cell lesions of the breast. Adv Anat Pathol 2003;10(3):113–124

Senetta R, Campanino PP, Mariscotti G, et al. Columnar cell lesions associated with breast calcifications on vacuum-assisted core biopsies: clinical, radiographic, and histological correlations. Mod Pathol 2009;22(6):762–769

Shin HJ, Kim HH, Kim SM, et al. Papillary lesions of the breast diagnosed at percutaneous sonographically guided biopsy: comparison of sonographic features and biopsy methods. AJR Am J Roentgenol 2008;190(3):630–636

Silverstein MJ. The University of Southern California/Van Nuys prognostic index for ductal carcinoma in situ of the breast. Am J Surg 2003;186(4):337–343

Simpson PT, Gale T, Fulford LG, Reis-Filho JS, Lakhani SR. The diagnosis and management of pre-invasive breast disease: pathology of atypical lobular hyperplasia and lobular carcinoma in situ. Breast Cancer Res 2003;5(5):258–262

Simpson PT, Gale T, Reis-Filho JS, et al. Columnar cell lesions of the breast: the missing link in breast cancer progression? A morphological and molecular analysis. Am J Surg Pathol 2005;29(6):734–746

Sinn HP, Elsawaf Z, Helmchen B, Aulmann S. Early breast cancer precursor lesions: lessions learned from molecular and clinical studies. Breast Care (Basel) 2010;5(4):218–226

Skandarajah AR, Field L, Yuen Larn Mou A, et al. Benign papilloma on core biopsy requires surgical excision. Ann Surg Oncol 2008;15(8):2272–2277

Sneige N, Wang J, Baker BA, Krishnamurthy S, Middleton LP. Clinical, histopathologic, and biologic features of pleomorphic lobular (ductal-lobular) carcinoma in situ of the breast: a report of 24 cases. Mod Pathol 2002;15(10):1044–1050

Sohn V, Arthurs Z, Herbert G, et al. Atypical ductal hyperplasia: improved accuracy with the 11-gauge vacuum-assisted versus the 14-gauge core biopsy needle. Ann Surg Oncol 2007;14(9):2497–2501

Sung JS, Malak SF, Bajaj P, Alis R, Dershaw DD, Morris EA. Screening breast MR imaging in women with a history of lobular carcinoma in situ. Radiology 2011;261(2):414–420

Tabar L, Dean PD. Atlas of mammography. Stuttgart: Thieme; 1977

Tan H, Zhang S, Liu H, et al. Imaging findings in phyllodes tumors of the breast. Eur J Radiol 2012;81(1):e62–e69

Tavassoli FA. Lobular and ductal intraepithelial neoplasia. Pathologe 2008;29(Suppl 2):107–111

Tavassoli FA, Norris HJ. A comparison of the results of long-term follow-up for atypical intraductal hyperplasia and intraductal hyperplasia of the breast. Cancer 1990;65(3):518–529

Tavassoli FA, Eusebi V. AFIP Atlas of tumor pathology: tumors of the mammary gland. Fascicle 10. Washington, DC: American Registry of Pathology; 2009

Tavassoli FA, Hoefler H, Rosai J, et al. Intraductal proliferative lesions. In: Tavassoli FA, Devilee P (eds). World Health Organization Classification of Tumours. Pathology and genetics of tumours of the breast and female genital organs. Lyon, France: IARC Press; 2003:63–73

Tennant SL, Evans A, Hamilton LJ, et al. Vacuum-assisted excision of breast lesions of uncertain malignant potential (B3)—an alternative to surgery in selected cases. Breast 2008;17(6):546–549

Tominaga J, Hama H, Kimura N, Takahashi S. Magnetic resonance imaging of intraductal papillomas of the breast. J Comput Assist Tomogr 2011;35(1):153–157

Ueng SH, Mezzetti T, Tavassoli FA. Papillary neoplasms of the breast: a review. Arch Pathol Lab Med 2009;133(6): 893–907

van de Vijver MJ. Biological variables and prognosis of DCIS. Breast 2005;14(6):509–519

Wellings SR, Alpers CE. Subgross pathologic features and incidence of radial scars in the breast. Hum Pathol 1984; 15(5):475–479

Werner M, Chott A, Fabiano A, Battifora H. Effect of formalin tissue fixation and processing on immunohistochemistry. Am J Surg Pathol 2000;24(7):1016–1019

Woods ER, Helvie MA, Ikeda DM, Mandell SH, Chapel KL, Adler DD. Solitary breast papilloma: comparison of mammographic, galactographic, and pathologic findings. AJR Am J Roentgenol 1992;159(3):487–491

Wurdinger S, Herzog AB, Fischer DR, et al. Differentiation of phyllodes breast tumors from fibroadenomas on MRI. AJR Am J Roentgenol 2005;185(5):1317–1321

Yabuuchi H, Soeda H, Matsuo Y, et al. Phyllodes tumor of the breast: correlation between MR findings and histologic grade. Radiology 2006;241(3):702–709

Yoo JL, Woo OH, Kim YK, et al. Can MR Imaging contribute in characterizing well-circumscribed breast carcinomas? Radiographics 2010;30(6):1689–1702

Yu YH, Liang C, Yuan XZ. Diagnostic value of vacuum-assisted breast biopsy for breast carcinoma: a meta-analysis and systematic review. Breast Cancer Res Treat 2010;120(2):469–479

Zografos GC, Zagouri F, Sergentanis TN, et al. Diagnosing papillary lesions using vacuum-assisted breast biopsy: should conservative or surgical management follow? Onkologie 2008;31(12):653–656

15 Carcinoma in Situ

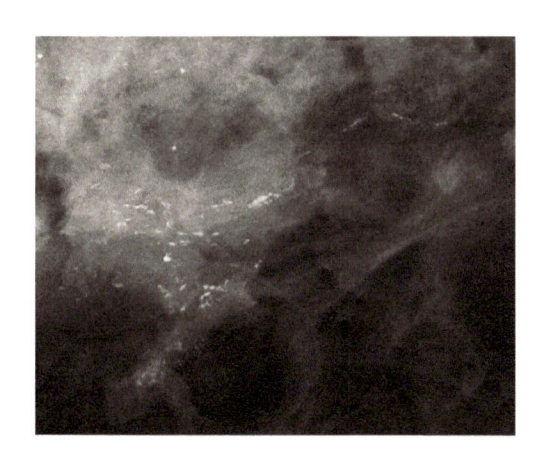

Definition, Terminology, and Biological Context → 366

Lobular Carcinoma in Situ, Pleomorphic Subtypes (Pleomorphic LCIS) → 366
Incidence → 366
Importance → 367
Histology → 368
Clinical Presentation and History → 368
Diagnostic Strategy → 368

Ductal Carcinoma in Situ (DCIS) → 370
Definition → 370
Incidence → 370
Histopathology → 370
Importance and Natural History → 371
Therapeutic Decisions → 372
Clinical Findings and History → 372
Diagnostic Methods: Value and Goals → 372

References and Recommended Reading → 386

15 Carcinoma in Situ

S. H. Heywang-Koebrunner, I. Schreer, J. Naehrig, S. Barter

Definition, Terminology, and Biological Context

Carcinomas in situ are lesions with cells which histologically have the same morphology and genetics as cells of invasive breast cancers. However, there is no extension across the basement membrane. Carcinomas in situ can therefore not metastasize. However, they are associated with a significant risk of developing into invasive malignancy and are therefore considered malignant nonobligatory precursors of invasive breast cancer.

Overall, it is assumed that there is a continuous progression from lobular neoplasia and from intraductal proliferative lesions to atypical hyperplasia, to in situ carcinoma to invasive carcinoma. It is also assumed that all invasive carcinomas develop from atypias through in situ carcinoma to invasive. However, for many invasive carcinomas (70–80%) this transition may be very fast and the interim stages will not be noted at all. All precursor lesions are considered nonobligatory precursors. This means that the precursor may persist, but it may also continue to develop into an invasive and thus potentially life-threatening disease.

Table 15.1 demonstrates the changes from intraductal proliferative lesions and from lobular neoplasias to invasive carcinoma.

Overall the risk appears to increase from flat epithelial atypia (FEA) to atypical ductal hyperplasia (ADH) to ductal carcinoma in situ (DCIS) grade 1 to grade 2 to grade 3 and potentially from atypical lobular hyperplasia (ALH)/classic lobular carcinoma in situ (LCIS) to pleomorphic LCIS (see below).

The various proliferations summarized under the designations ductal intraepithelial neoplasia (DIN) and lobular intraepithelial neoplasia (LIN or LN) are genetically and morphologically heterogeneous lesions. They are considered nonobligatory precursors and/or risk indicators of malignancy (invasive carcinoma): "precursors" means that an increased risk exists that the area in question develops into invasive malignancy, whereas the risk factor means that the risk of either breast increases. This implies that the precursors may persist, but may well continue to develop into an invasive carcinoma and thus potentially life-threatening disease (Collins et al. 2005).

Intraductal epithelial hyperplasia of usual type (UDH) is considered a benign change of only slightly increased risk. ADH, FEA, ALH, and ALH/classic LCIS belong to the group of lesions summarized under the terminological category of "benign change of uncertain malignant potential" or B3 lesion (see Chapter 14). Women with FEA have a very low risk for subsequent breast cancer (relative risk 1.6–1.9). However, data on the relative risk of ADH vary over a broad range of 2.4–13 (average probably 4–5) compared with a calculated relative risk of 8–11, which increases from DCIS grade 1 to 3 (Lakhani et al. 2012). *(The surprisingly large variations can best be explained by interobserver variability in classification of the lesions and definitions [Sloane et al. 1999, Verkooijen et al. 2003, Collins et al. 2004, Ellis et al. 2006, Ghofrani et al. 2006.])*

For intraductal changes the risk increases from ADH to DCIS and with the grade of DCIS. The relative risk of LN for subsequent development of an invasive carcinoma according to the literature ranges from approximately 4 to 12 (Lakhani 2012). It appears to increase from ALH to LCIS and to special types of LCIS which are summarized as pleomorphic LCIS (macroacinar, necrotic, pleomorphic, signet ring cell LCIS). Based on their morphological pattern and on part of the literature it is assumed that the latter are associated with a higher risk of invasive malignancy. According to EU guidelines the pleomorphic types of LCIS are thus classified as B5 lesions and discussed in this chapter. The World Health Organization emphasizes that data on pleomorphic LCIS are still limited and classify pleomorphic LCIS (that should be verified by excision) together with classic LCIS and ALH as lesion of uncertain malignant potential (Lakhani et al. 2012).

For lobular neoplasias both roles (as precursor lesion and as risk indicator) are important. For ADH and DCIS the role as precursor lesion appears more important.

Mixed lesions (ALH, LCIS, ADH, other B3 lesions, DCIS, invasive carcinoma) may occur. The lesion with the highest grade will determine the patient's risk of invasive breast cancer.

Lobular Carcinoma in Situ, Pleomorphic Subtypes (Pleomorphic LCIS)

Incidence

The overall incidence of lobular neoplasia including ALH and classic and pleomorphic LCIS was reported to be 1–3.8%, with most cases occurring in premenopausal women. LN is frequently a multicentric (60–85%) and bilateral (30–67%) finding (Lakhani et al. 2012). ALH and classic LCIS, which account for about 88% of LN and which belong to lesions of uncertain malignant potential, are mostly clinically and mammographically occult and often

Table 15.1 Terminology of the proliferations ranging from benign to malignant precursor lesions

Terminology	Lesion class (according to European guidelines*)	Discussed in Chapter
Intraductal proliferations		
UDH	Benign (B2)	10
CCC, CCH	Benign (B2)	10
FEA	Uncertain malignant potential (B3)	14
ADH	Uncertain malignant potential (B3)	14
DCIS grade 1 (low grade)	Malignant (B5)	15
DCIS grade 2 (intermediate grade)	Malignant (B5)	15
DCIS grade 3 (high grade)	Malignant (B5)	15
Lobular neoplasia		
ALH	Uncertain malignant potential (B3)	14
Classic LCIS	Uncertain malignant potential (B3)	14
Pleomorphic LCIS (including macroacinar, necrotic, pleomorphic, signet ring cell subtypes)	Malignant precursor/risk indicator (B5)	15

ADH, atypical ductal hyperplasia; ALH, atypical lobular hyperplasia; CCC, columnar cell change; CCH, columnar cell hyperplasia; DCIS, ductal carcinoma in situ; FEA, flat epithelial atypia; LCIS, lobular carcinoma in situ; UDH, usual ductal hyperplasia.

detected as an incidental histologic finding observed in a biopsy performed for microcalcifications or other reasons (Sgroi and Koerner 1995, Karabakhtsian et al. 2007, Lee et al. 2007). Histologically the microcalcifications are (except for some rare cases of classic LCIS with comedo necrosis) usually not associated with ALH or classic LCIS but with adjacent concomitant benign changes, most often adenosis and rarely with a peculiar lesion such as collagenous spherulosis. Pleomorphic LCIS makes up about 12% of all LN cases and thus is a rare lesion (Bratthauer and Tavassoli 2002). Pleomorphic LCIS is frequently (50%) associated with pleomorphic and casting microcalcifications and thus is typically detected through mammography.

Importance

For LN (without exact distinction of subtypes) an average risk of associated simultaneous invasive carcinoma in the ipsilateral breast of 4.2% and in the contralateral breast of 3.5% has been reported (Ansquer et al. 2010). The risk of developing invasive breast cancer within 25-year follow-up has been reported to be from 17% (Haagensen et al. 1978) to 35% within 35 years (McDivitt et al. 1967, Bodian et al. 1996, Tavassoli et al. 2003). The Nottingham data showed a risk of invasive breast cancer of 19% after an average follow-up of 15 years and a low rate of breast-cancer specific mortality (10% of women with invasive breast cancer after lobular neoplasia [LN] or 1% of all LN cases, respectively) (McLaren et al. 2006).

The relative risk of developing an invasive carcinoma within the first 15 years after a biopsy is thus increased by a factor of 3–5. The risk is slightly decreased if the diagnosis is made above the age of 45 years and is increased in women with a family history of breast cancer (factor of 5–10). Subsequent invasive cancers can be either lobular or ductal. Lobular invasive carcinoma appears to be about three times more frequent than invasive ductal carcinoma in patients with a previous diagnosis of LN. According to several reports pleomorphic LCIS appears to be associated with synchronous or metachronous invasive breast cancer in a much higher percentage (25–67%) than classic LCIS or ALH (Sneige et al. 2002, Fadare et al. 2006, Chivukula et al. 2008). In addition, invasive lobular carcinoma appears to be much more frequent than invasive ductal carcinoma in patients with pleomorphic LCIS (Bratthauer and Tavassoli 2002). However, the authors of the latest WHO classification (Lakhani et al. 2012) point out that there are significant variations among the studies, many of the studies are only anecdotal. Only a very low number have been completely documented and followed up and there is frequent confusion of pleomorphic LCIS with DCIS. Therefore, the exact biological potential of this entity remains uncertain. When diagnosed by percutaneous breast biopsy pleomorphic LCIS is, according to the EU guidelines (Perry et al. 2006), classified as a B5 lesion. Excision should be recommended after percutaneous breast biopsy of pleomorphic LCIS and classic LCIS with comedo necrosis. The authors of the latest WHO classification (Lakhani et al. 2012) point out that the importance of clear margins and thus the benefit of aggressive management strategies (complete excision to clear margins or mastectomy) remains uncertain. The same is, however, true for any other strategy, as well.

Histology

LNs by definition comprise all forms of lobular proliferations with functional loss of E-cadherin mutations (Lakhani et al. 2012). All LNs share some morphological features and the transition is gradual.

Pleomorphic LCIS is the rarest form and accounts for approximately 12% of all LNs. Pleomorphic LCIS presents either with extreme acinar distention (macroacinar type) or comedonecrosis (necrotic type) or high-grade nuclear features (pleomorphic cells) or signet ring cells type. The necrotic type is a specific variant characterized by a predominant ductal extension, which can be so extensive as to involve an entire segment and, rarely, an entire breast, simulating DCIS of intermediate or high grade. Morphology and immunohistochemistry distinguishes most LNs and DCIS; however, a minority of cases remains ambiguous: they are designated carcinoma in situ with mixed ductal and lobular features (Lakhani et al. 2012). Not infrequently LNs are associated with DCIS, ADH, or FEA (Leibl et al. 2007, Abdel 2008, Brandt et al. 2008). Among the lobular neoplasias, ALH and classic LCIS are still considered benign entities of uncertain malignant potential, but are risk indicators and partly also potential precursors of malignancy (Page et al. 1985, Contreras and Sattar 2009, O'Malley 2010).

Clinical Presentation and History

Clinically, there is no characteristic finding.

Diagnostic Strategy

Mammography

(See **Fig. 15.1**.)

Most lobular neoplasias have no characteristic mammographic findings. This implies that LN generally cannot be distinguished from benign changes or normal breast parenchyma or other concomitant borderline or malignant lesions. Rarely is an asymmetry found mammographically. Microcalcifications—which are generally uncharacteristic in morphology and distribution—are only found in a few cases of LN1 or LN2.

Pleomorphic LCIS is mostly associated with casting or pleomorphic microcalcifications. These microcalcifications are associated with histopathologic intraluminal necrosis and mimic high-grade DCIS.

Sonography

No specific finding characteristic of LN is known on ultrasound. The sonographic findings can usually be assigned to other concomitant benign, B3, or malignant lesions. Most of the LNs (including LN3) are sonographically occult.

Magnetic Resonance Imaging

On MRI, too, no specific findings are known for LIN. To date pleomorphic LCIS has not been treated separately. Variable presentations similar to those of DCIS (see below) may be expected. ALH and LCIS have been described as being associated with areas of patchy or milky enhancement or with an area of focal enhancement (as noted by us in some biopsy-proven cases with concomitant benign changes). Enhancement curves are usually uncharacteristic (mostly delayed, sometimes plateau-type enhancement).

Percutaneous Biopsy

The percutaneous biopsy diagnosis of a LN is usually an incidental finding, which was obtained during percutaneous biopsy of another abnormality (mass, microcalcifications). Correlation of the histopathologic and imaging findings must be checked to ensure that a definitive diagnosis of the lesion undergoing biopsy can be made with the material obtained (e.g., complete removal of the imaging finding of concern on vacuum-assisted breast biopsy (VABB) and absence of higher-grade lesions). If this is the case, the percutaneous biopsy diagnosis of incidental ALH or classic LCIS does not warrant a wider surgical excision (see Chapter 14). In case of discordance between pathologic changes present on biopsy and imaging or clinical findings, or if there are doubts about representative removal (e.g., additional palpable or imaging findings or small volume of tissue based on core needle biopsy [CNB] only, histopathologically suspected presence of higher-grade lesions), excisional biopsy should be recommended.

To date, excision should be recommended if percutaneous biopsy yields pleomorphic LCIS. However, as pre-

Fig. 15.1a–d

a Screening patient with a group of pleomorphic microcalcifications: *Histology*: Pleomorphic LCIS, diagnosed at vacuum-assisted breast biopsy (VABB) and confirmed at excision. Based on the histopathologic features and the known risk, excision was indicated, which confirmed the diagnosis. (Reproduced with kind permission of Karger AG from Heywang-Köbrunner et al. Breast Care 2010;5:209–217.)

b–d Asymptomatic patient. On the screening mammogram (**c**) a delicate architectural distortion is seen in the patient's right breast caudally and medially. Adjacent to the architectural distortion, which is more clearly seen on the magnification view (**d**), a group of punctate microcalcifications is shown. Both changes were verified by VABB. *Histology*: 3-mm invasive lobular carcinoma (which correlates well with the architectural distortion and pleomorphic LCIS, which correlates with the microcalcifications).

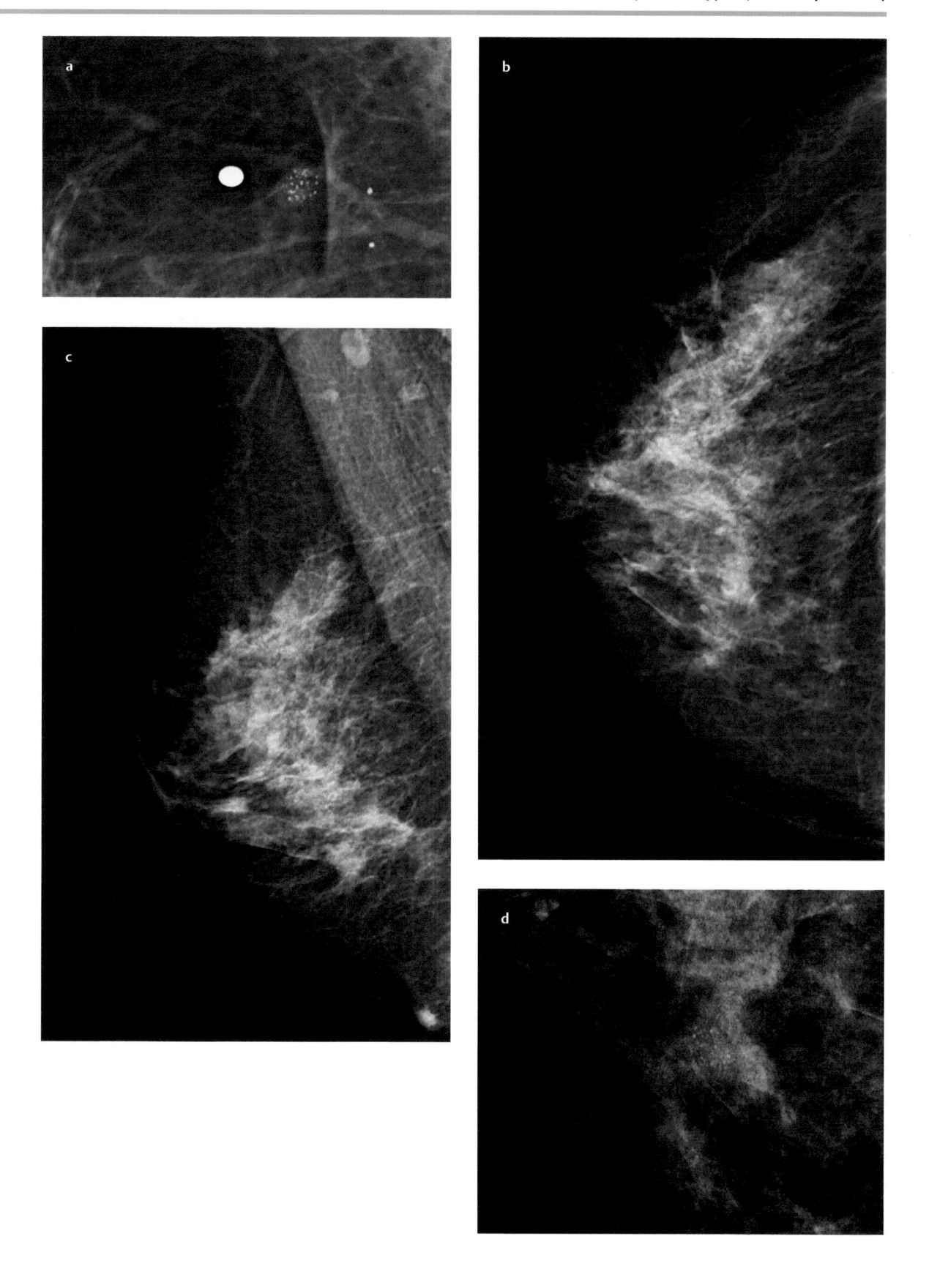

Lobular Carcinoma in Situ, Pleomorphic Subtypes (Pleomorphic LCIS)

viously mentioned, evidence for the benefits of excision for clearing margins (which may be impossible) or mastectomy is lacking (Lakhani et al. 2012); it is, however, lacking for other treatment strategies as well.

Following a histopathologic diagnosis of LN and adequate therapy, yearly follow-up by clinical examination and mammography is generally recommended. Since LN has no characteristic imaging findings, the follow-up does not serve the detection of residual or recurring LN, but early detection of (DCIS or) invasive carcinoma.

Ductal Carcinoma in Situ (DCIS)

Definition

Histopathologically, as well as clinically and prognostically, DCIS comprises a heterogeneous group of carcinomas. As a result of mammography and screening, the incidence of DCIS detected in biopsies has increased from 2–4% to 10–20%.

According to the pathologic definition of these tumors, malignant cells are exclusively found within the lactiferous ductal system—that is, intraductal, without destruction of the basement membrane.

They extend contiguously or noncontiguously through the ductal system, explaining the frequent multifocal tumor manifestations found on average in 30% of all DCIS and in over 60% of large-volume DCIS.

Incidence

The incidence of DCIS starts rising significantly after age 40 years. Since most cases of DCIS detectable by imaging contain microcalcifications, the detection rate has markedly increased with the expanding use of mammography. While the proportion of DCIS of all discovered carcinomas in patients with clinical findings amounts to only a few percent, it has now reached 20% in the screening group and values beyond 20% with digital mammography screening.

Noncalcified DCIS may be detected by MRI, in some cases by mammography, and rarely by ultrasound. It may be detected based on clinical symptoms (bloody discharge, rarely some unspecific palpable finding) or it may be incidentally discovered histologically in biopsies performed for other reasons.

Histopathology

Intraepithelial neoplasias are confined to basal membrane-bounded spaces of the lobular and ductal system and encompass a spectrum of epithelial proliferations with a broad range of cytologic grades and architectural patterns and a considerable number of combinations thereof. The spectrum of intraductal changes ranges from normal-appearing cells (UDH) to minimal deviations considered as mildly atypical (FEA or ADH) to highly atypical or anaplastic (DCIS grade 3).

DCIS grades 1–3 can be distinguished by cytonuclear features among others. ADH and DCIS grade 1 are separated by criteria of size (< or > 2 mm size) which finally suggests that ADH may be viewed as minute low-grade DCIS. According to the WHO classification (Lakhani et al. 2012), in every DCIS the documentation of histomorphologic parameter grading, presence or absence of comedonecrosis, and growth pattern/architecture are generally recommended. DCIS of all grades more or less show the same spectrum of patterns with some quite characteristic constellations—for example, the micropapillary pattern in DCIS grade 1 and the solid pattern with comedonecrosis in DCIS grade 3—thus histopathologic patterns may add valuable information to pathologic–radiologic correlation, at least to some cases (see below). DCIS are associated with radiologically and histopathologically detected microcalcifications in over 70% of cases but these can be distributed heterogeneously within an individual lesion.

While microcalcifications in DCIS grade 3 and in DCIS grade 2 with comedonecrosis correspond to mammographically casting, pleomorphic, and coarse granular microcalcifications (ranging around 50–500 μm), the microcalcifications of DCIS of lower grade (micropapillary or cribriform pattern) correspond to fine microcalcifications that arise within tiny lumina of the DCIS structure of the micropapillary or cribriform DCIS or within nondilated ducts. They are thus fine and powdery and are usually only mildly pleomorphic. The size of these very fine microcalcifications often ranges around 10 μm up to sometimes 200 μm.

With mammography the very fine microcalcifications of low-grade DCIS are often only recognized because the microcalcifications within the DCIS superimposed and thus add up to visible "dots." Unfortunately there is significant overlap of this type of microcalcifications seen in low-grade DCIS and microcalcifications seen in benign and in B3 changes. Owing to the higher resolution of digital mammography, these very fine microcalcifications are to date increasingly detected.

In addition about 15% of DCIS lesions are associated with increased density most often in the area of microcalcifications. This increased density surrounding pure DCIS may be explained by reactive stromal changes (desmoplasia, neoangiogenesis, and inflammation) around involved ducts. Some DCIS lesions (with or without microcalcifications) may have a nodular growth pattern (e.g., papillary DCIS).

Almost all (98%) DCIS are unicentric lesions; however, they frequently (50%) spread discontinuously and multifocally within the same segment/quadrant. Discontinuous means that 60% of DCIS show gaps of less than 5 mm distance and over 80% show gaps within 10 mm distance (Holland et al. 1990). Thus 90% of local recurrences after breast-conserving therapy occur in the same quadrant.

Mammography underestimates the extent of DCIS in more than 20–30% of cases (Thomas et al. 2010). Both overestimates and underestimates have been reported for MRI (see page 156). Due to higher vascularity and vascular permeability around the duct involved, DCIS of higher grade may be more easily detectable than some of the low-grade DCIS lesions. In some publications a reliable detection of high-grade DCIS has been stressed and it has been concluded that "MRI detects the biologically important lesions." According to our experience this can be confirmed to a certain degree. However, we have seen wide variations, and according to our experience MRI and mammography prove to be complementary for detecting both high- and low- grade DCIS. Both methods detect only part of the DCIS, both methods have false positives, and both methods also detect part of the biologically less important low-grade DCIS.

Considering that the extent of DCIS may sometimes be difficult to assess by histopathology alone (due to discontiguous growth, preceding intervention or the need for multiple excisions), the real extent of any DCIS should be determined only by interdisciplinary correlation between the pathology and radiology and surgery in each and every individual case!

After breast-conserving therapy there is an increased risk of recurrence in DCIS without microcalcifications due to residual DCIS; this accounts especially for DCIS of low and intermediate grades (grades 1 and 2) and specifically for the micropapillary type. This lesion is not infrequently underestimated and may involve an entire quadrant or even the entire ductal system of a breast without any radiologic sign. Even though the lesion is often still a pure noninvasive low-grade DCIS, this unfortunate constellation may require mastectomy if the lesion is too extensive.

Frequently (30–50%) mixed grades and growth patterns of DCIS can be seen within an individual lesion, and a combination of grades 1 and 2 or grades 2 and 3 is more common than that of all three grades. Increasing size of DCIS is correlated with increasing risk of invasion, whereby a significant increase in risk is expected in DCIS > 2.5 cm. A close correlation exists between nuclear grade of DCIS, extent of DCIS, positive margins after surgery, recurrence rate, and risk for progression to invasive cancer. Positive lymph nodes may be rarely seen in DCIS with occult invasion (1–4.5%) and very rarely this may be an initial clinical manifestation in patients with occult breast cancer (syndrome). Among patients with DCIS, 10–15% will suffer from bilateral disease—synchronous or metachronous. (This frequency is lower than for LN.)

Importance and Natural History

DCIS is an inhomogeneous entity. Indirect information on the natural history of DCIS is derived from a few reported cases that had been proven by needle biopsy or incisional biopsy and that had not undergone further treatment. Further knowledge is based on studies in which patients underwent excision only, and from randomized trials comparing groups of patients treated with or without radiation therapy and from trials comparing patients with or without antiestrogen treatment.

The risk of progression depends on the grade of lesion and increases from DCIS grade 1 (low risk) to DCIS grade 3 (high risk) (Lakhani et al. 2012, Tavassoli and Eusebi 2009).

Progression of DCIS grades 1–3 to invasive carcinoma has been reported in around 13–75% of patients without treatment (Leonard and Swain 2004, Collins et al. 2005, Sanders et al. 2005) and as much as 20–30% of local recurrences after lumpectomy alone have been reported from randomized trials, whereas approximately half the number is seen after lumpectomy plus irradiation. (Unfortunately none of the trials had a standardized protocol concerning the verification of complete excision—i.e., specimen radiography, standardized histopathology assessment, marking and orientation, histopathology–imaging correlation, postoperative imaging, and standardized assessment of size or margins) (Fisher et al. 2001, Fisher et al. 2002, Houghton et al. 2003, Emdin et al. 2006, Bijker and van Tienhoven 2010, Cuzick et al. 2011, Wapnir et al. 2011). It is assumed that there are different lines of progression that distinguish low-grade breast cancer types from high-grade breast cancer types (Abdel-Fatah et al. 2008), but a continuous progression from ADH and DCIS grades 1–3 or from LN to invasive carcinoma can be seen as well (Bijker et al. 2001, Tavassoli and Eusebi 2009). However, in actual fact a risk prediction in an individual patient with proven ADH, DCIS or LN is never possible. Most women develop invasive carcinoma within 10 years (Ernster et al. 2000); women with untreated DCIS develop invasive carcinoma in 30–50% of cases.

Not considering lesion size and margin status, the 10-year mortality caused by invasive breast cancer recurrence after DCIS is estimated to be around 2–3%. The recurrence rate of DCIS grade 3 compared with DCIS grade 1 is increased by a factor of 2–3 (Kerlikowske et al. 2003, Bijker and van Tienhoven 2010). Thus, DCIS is a potentially life-threatening entity. However, prognosis is very good for greater than 97% of the patients with DCIS who undergo state-of-the art treatment.

The following risk factors have been associated with more aggressive biological behavior:
- High nuclear grade and /or comedonecrosis
- Hormone-receptor negativity, erbB2 overexpression, p53 overexpression
- Abnormal DNA ploidy, high S-phase fraction
- Large tumor size (> 10 mm; Kerlikowske et al. 2003)

- Inadequate margins (Solin et al. 2005, Bijker and van Tienhoven 2010)
- Young patient age (Mokbel and Cutuli 2006, Bijker and van Tienhoven 2010)

A concordance rate concerning nuclear grade of the DCIS and the grading of the recurrence in around 70% of cases has been described (Idvall et al. 2005).

Considering the fact that DCIS is a nonobligatory precursor lesion, which in a certain percentage of cases may never develop into invasive (and thus potentially life-threatening) breast cancer, on the one hand, overdiagnosis and overtreatment is an important potential side effect of DCIS detection that should be considered, particularly in elderly women with low-grade DCIS. On the other hand, the low mortality rates reported for DCIS concern only treated DCIS.

Untreated DCIS is a proven precursor that may develop into invasive cancer (and thus is a potentially life-threatening disease). Such progression is described for 20–30% of low-grade DCIS (mostly within the following 15 years) and for about 50% of the high-grade DCIS (mostly within the following 5–10 years) (Millis and Thynne 1975, Lagios et al. 1982, 1989, Page et al. 1982, Holland et al. 1994, Eusebi et al. 1989, Fisher et al. 1995, Silverstein et al. 1996). Due to the delayed and highly variable onset of invasive disease the epidemiological proof of an effect of DCIS detection on mortality reduction is by principle, and predictably very difficult. In many individual cases, however, this onset of early invasion can be observed on histopathology in small or large areas of DCIS. In cases with extended DCIS the probability of invasion increases significantly and extended DCIS may lead to the sudden appearance of a large or diffusely involved area of invasive carcinoma with a poor prognosis.

According to our own experience and considering the patient's overall risk, DCIS should be taken most seriously with younger patient age, high grading, and increasing size. In contrast the risk of overdiagnosis and overtreatment will increase with high patient age (> age 70 years), low grade of the DCIS, and small size. Therefore future research may have to concentrate on further optimizing treatment considerations with respect to both the characteristics of the malignancy and individual patient factors.

Therapeutic Decisions

Standard treatment today for nonpalpable DCIS less than 40 mm in size is segmentectomy followed by irradiation. It is based on the results of four randomized clinical trials (Fisher et al. 2001, 2002, Houghton et al. 2003, Emdin et al. 2006, Bijker and van Tienhoven 2010, Cuzick et al. 2011, Wapnir et al. 2011), which demonstrated unanimously the benefit of 50 Gy whole-breast irradiation in breast-conserving therapy. The risk of both DCIS and invasive local recurrence is reduced by around 50% independent of histologic subtype. With up to 20 mm lesion size, breast conservation can be achieved in most women. If the DCIS reaches 40 mm, wide negative margins may be difficult to achieve. Evaluation of the above studies and data from Silverstein prove the importance of free margins (Silverstein and Buchanan 2003). New data suggest that a tumor-free margin of 2 mm should be achieved (Dunne et al. 2009). If mastectomy has to be performed, it is associated with a cure rate approaching 100%. Tamoxifen may decrease the rate of local recurrence and of contralateral disease by about 30%. But there is no proven influence of tamoxifen on the rate of invasive recurrences or on mortality. Thus the indication for adjuvant tamoxifen treatment has to be decided upon in multidisciplinary conferences.

Sentinel node biopsy is not recommended except for large DCIS (> 40 mm) because of the correlation of lesion extent and the probability of early invasion.

Clinical Findings and History

In population screening, only few percent of DCIS lesions are clinically apparent. The clinical findings mostly present as a pathologic secretion or Paget disease of the nipple. Rarely, it may be detected by an associated palpable abnormality. DCIS very rarely becomes symptomatic through localized pain, which is unilateral and usually not related to the menstrual cycle.

Diagnostic Methods: Value and Goals

Mammography alone detects a significant percentage of DCIS lesions. Most of this capability is based on the excellent detection of microcalcifications on mammography. This is associated with diagnostic challenges. Mammographically, DCIS may present with microcalcifications, with a mass or an architectural distortion. On the basis of current knowledge, good sensitivity and acceptable specificity may be achieved only by careful attention to the following:

- Thorough analysis of the mammographic calcifications (supported by magnification views and mediolateral projections). In some cases ultrasound may demonstrate a hypoechoic mass within an area of microcalcifications. Such a hypoechoic mass may correspond to a (sometimes small) invasive component. In such cases biopsy should target the hypoechoic mass.
- Full mammographic assessment and analysis of the microcalcifications will allow classification of the change as typically benign, indeterminate, or suspicious. In the two last cases percutaneous breast biopsy should be used for further assessment. Unless a focal sonographic finding exists, stereotactic VABB is the method of choice (Perry et al. 2006, Albert et al. 2008) for this task.

- Extent of microcalcifications should be assessed by additional magnification views where needed and—whenever decisive for the therapeutic approach—by additional percutaneous breast biopsy.

In the case of architectural distortions or masses, further evaluation may be made by ultrasound. Whenever the lesion can be targeted by ultrasound, subsequent percutaneous breast biopsy should be performed using ultrasound guidance. If this is not the case, stereotactic guidance is needed.

Owing to imperfect sensitivity and a specificity which is too low for microcalcifications, MRI should not be used for differentiation of mammographically indeterminate or suspicious lesions. However, MRI is able to detect DCIS lesions which are occult with mammography. Unless a sonographic correlate exists (which in the case of MR-detected DCIS is rare), MR-guidance is required for further histopathologic assessment.

Mammography

Microcalcifications are the cardinal finding of DCIS, but microcalcifications can be absent. DCIS can appear mammographically as a density or an asymmetry, can be clinically symptomatic, or can be incidentally diagnosed histologically (in excisional biopsies performed for an unrelated reason).

Image Presentation

Mammographically, DCIS can become visible:
- Through microcalcifications: they are the only finding in about 85–90% of DCIS lesions detected by mammography, rarely surrounded by soft tissue density. (The surrounding soft tissue density, encountered in some of the DCIS without invasion, can be explained as reactive periductal fibrosis.)
- As a spiculated mass often without central density (< 5% of DCIS lesions)
- As an irregularly outlined mass or asymmetry (< 5% of DCIS lesions)
- As a well-circumscribed nodular mass (~5% of DCIS lesions)
- As a filling defect or amputated duct visualized by galactography in patients who present with pathologic nipple discharge

Importance of Microcalcifications

Mammographic microcalcifications are the most important mammographic feature of DCIS, but their presence should by no means be equated with the presence of DCIS.

Around 70–80% of histopathologically assessed microcalcifications are ultimately found to be due to benign causes. Therefore, systematic analysis and the best possible differentiation of microcalcifications indicating benign versus malignant changes represent an important diagnostic challenge for the responsible interpretation of mammography.

Image Presentation of Microcalcifications

The following calcifications can be found in DCIS:
1. *Casting microcalcifications* occur in those DCIS lesions of intermediate or high grade, in which the central layers of the cells within the involved ducts undergo necrosis and calcify.

   These necrotic cylinders can be extruded under pressure from the macroscopic specimen—like common cutaneous comedos, as implied in the name given in analogy with this condition. Since this necrotic cellular material is always within the lactiferous ductal system, the following features may be seen:
   - Typical segmental arrangement following the ductal system (**Fig. 15.2a–c**). Such segments may be large or small depending on the involved part of the ductal tree. Often triangular arrangements result with the base of the triangle located distant from the nipple. When seen *en face*, the segmental distribution may not be obvious, but will mostly present differently from other areas within the breast and asymmetrically to the contralateral breast. Sometimes only one or few ducts and only a small part of a duct may be involved leading to a ductal or suggested ductal distribution. Segmental or ductal distribution, if present, is an important indicator of malignancy irrespective of the shape of the individual microcalcifications.
   - In small DCIS lesions only a small group of microcalcifications may be noted. Grouping of microcalcifications is only considered real if it is documented in at least two planes. (Otherwise grouping might be imitated in one projection by superimposition of microcalcifications from different areas.) Grouping is far less characteristic of malignancy than is the ductal or segmental arrangement. Even though grouping of microcalcifications may also be seen in benign changes, single groups of more than five microcalcifications require diligent analysis and often histopathologic assessment. For groups of fewer than five microcalcifications the probability of malignancy is decreased. Therefore histopathologic assessment is only recommended for such groups if the individual shapes are sufficiently suspicious, or if the microcalcifications have developed since previous mammograms (Müller-Schimpfle et al. 2010).
   - Microcalcifications arising in small papillomas or fibroadenomas may also be distributed in a rounded or oval area (corresponding to the shape of the underlying lesion, while the surrounding mass may or may not be visible).

15 Carcinoma in Situ

Fig. 15.2a–e

a Typical segmental arrangement of microcalcifications, extending from the prepectoral region to the nipple: ductal carcinoma in situ (DCIS), comedo type.
b This specimen radiograph (magnification) shows elongated casts of the individual calcifications and their branching pattern.
c Characteristic triangular group formation, with the apex of the triangle pointing toward the nipple. *Histology*: comedo DCIS.
d Pleomorphic linear and branching calcifications extending from the prepectoral tissue into the nipple: high grade DCIS.
e Typical branching group of calcifications with mostly linear, casting calcifications due to involved ducts filled with necrotic cells: high grade DCIS.

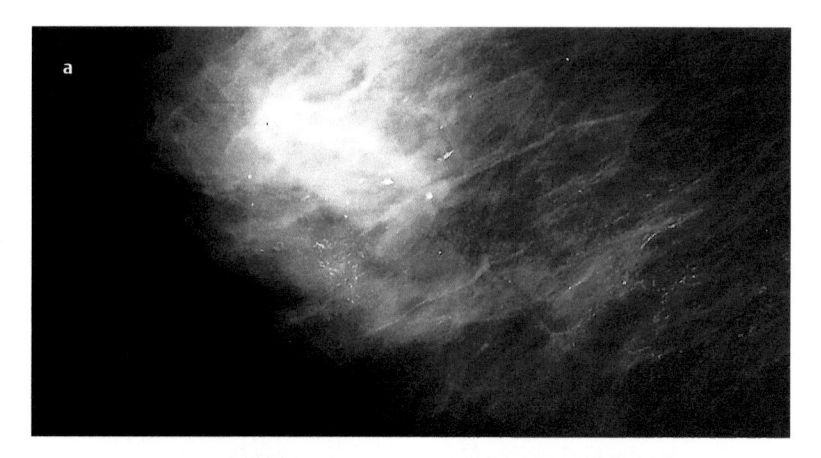

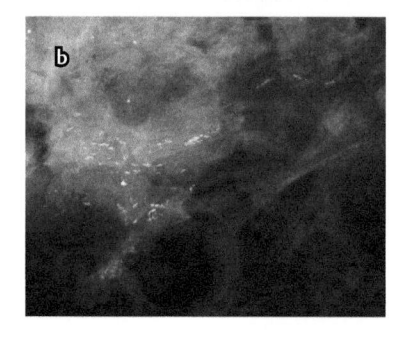

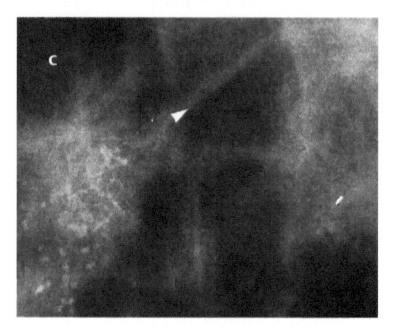

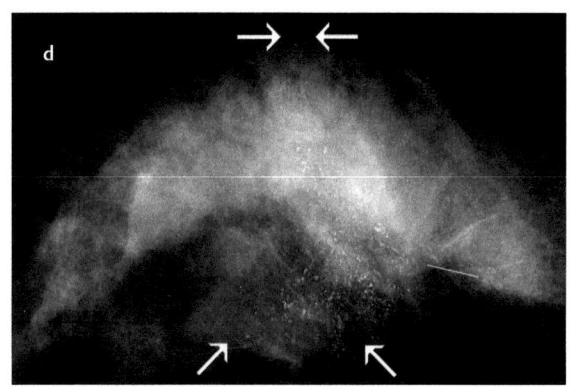

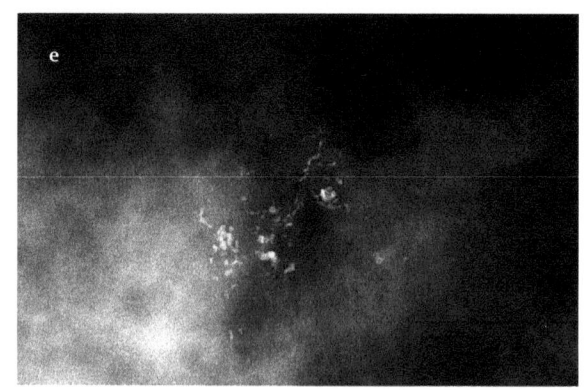

- The individual microcalcifications will also develop shapes which follow (in a more or less obvious arrangement) the ductal system. Shapes of such casting microcalcifications include elongated (sometimes fragmented) microcalcifications, which may be coarse or fine and sometimes very delicate.
- Typical shapes seen in comedo-type DCIS grade 2 and 3 lesions include Y-shaped, V-shaped, linear and/or comma-shaped calcifications (**Figs. 15.2d,e** and **15.3**).
- Furthermore, markedly pleomorphic, granular microcalcifications up to 2 mm in diameter (**Figs. 15.4 and 15.5l–n**) frequently, but not invariably, indicate the presence of DCIS, usually the comedo type, with a high degree of specificity (in ~80% of the cases).

It should be pointed out that DCIS does not always calcify and that about 20–25% of the cases of calcified comedo-type DCIS lesions fail to exhibit this characteristic pattern.

2. *In non–comedo-type DCIS which usually grows in a cribriform or micropapillary pattern*, mostly DCIS grades 1 or 2 that do not exhibit central intraductal necrosis (**Fig. 15.5b–k**), the very tiny, often round cavities that are part of the typical histomorphologic architecture of these DCISs fill with secretion and calcify. Therefore, calcific manifestation of the non-comedo DCIS is:
- Frequently very delicate
- Occasionally fine granular
- Sometimes irregular to bizarre, but
- Sometimes also fine granular, relatively monomorphic

This means that the rodlike casts characteristic of comedo-type DCIS lesions are less common.

The arrangement of the microcalcifications may often be ductal or segmental. For some DCIS, a ductal or segmental distribution may sometimes not be recognized.

Small DCIS may become apparent by grouped microcalcifications. Grouping of microcalcifications may also occur in papillary lesions and in papillary DCIS.

The fine microcalcifications of non–comedo-type DCIS are mostly less characteristic than those of comedo-type DCIS, and in those cases in which a ductal or segmental arrangement is not definitely recognizable, such microcalcifications are indicative of a malignancy in only 5–20% of the lesions. Thus detection of all calcified non-comedo DCIS lesions will not be possible unless unacceptably high rates of benign biopsies are performed. Since only a proportion of all DCIS is detectable by imaging and low-grade DCIS may progress to invasive carcinoma only after many years, a sensible and responsible threshold for initiation of histopathologic assessment versus follow-up should be sought, accepting that no perfect detection rate is possible.

In addition to these uncharacteristic calcifications, less frequently non-comedo DCIS may develop comedo-type calcifications, facilitating early detection and differentiation from benign changes.

Altogether, exact mammographic assignment to a certain histologic subtype only succeeds in some cases. The list presented above should be seen as a basis for a better understanding of the microcalcific formations, but by no means as a substitute for histology. Moreover, a subtype rarely manifests itself alone. More often, the various subtypes are mixed and occur together.

In addition, since the basement membrane cannot be seen mammographically, and because in some cases of pure DCIS a mass can be present (corresponding to the DCIS itself or to a reactive component adjacent to it), DCIS cannot be differentiated from invasive cancer based on

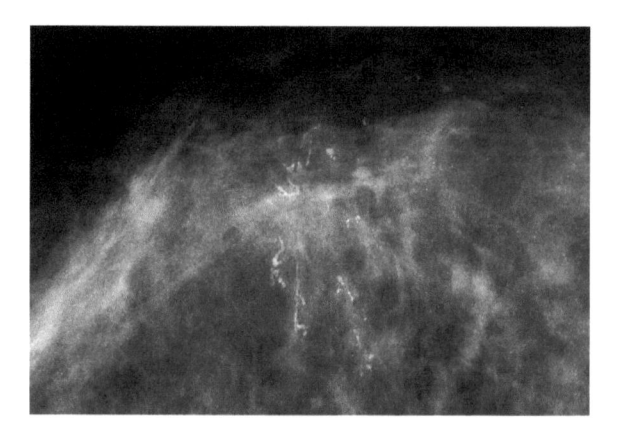

Fig. 15.3 Magnification mammography with typical irregular, linear calcifications and branching pattern: Comedo ductal carcinoma in situ.

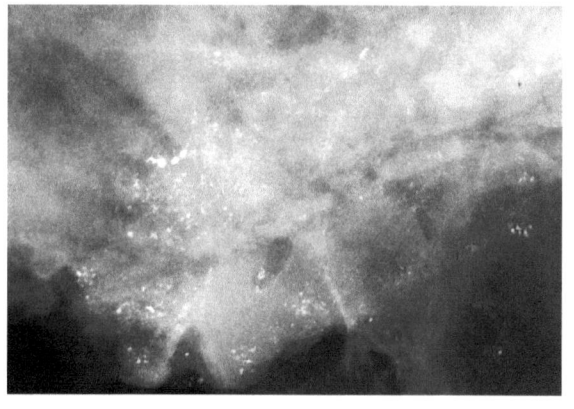

Fig. 15.4 Predominantly larger granular, pleomorphic microcalcifications next to a few elongated casts. *Specimen radiography*: Peripheral location of the calcifications.

15 Carcinoma in Situ

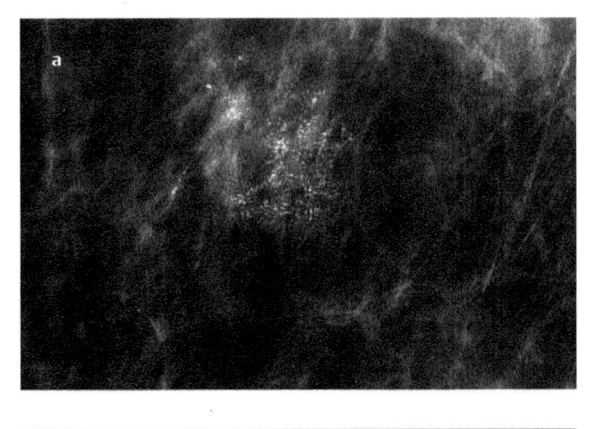

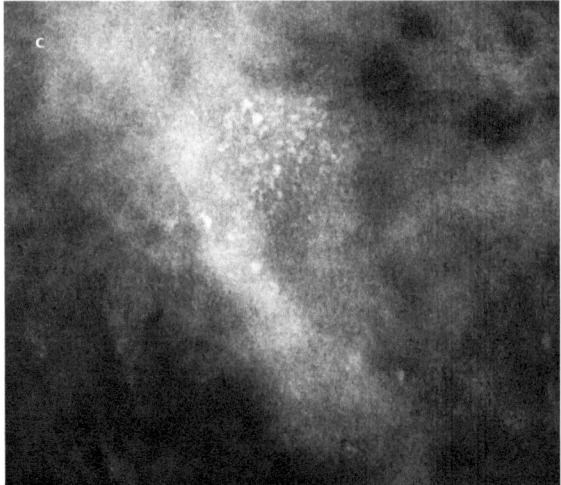

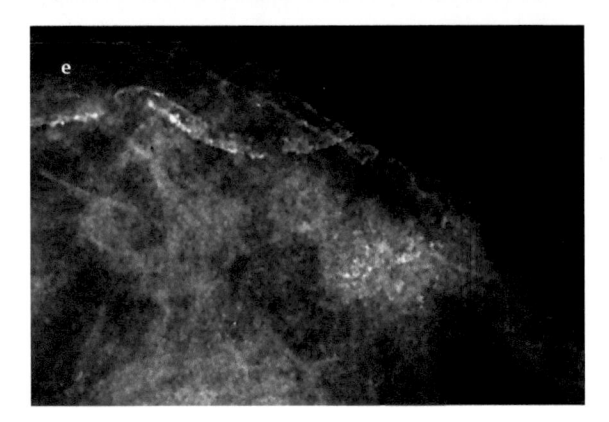

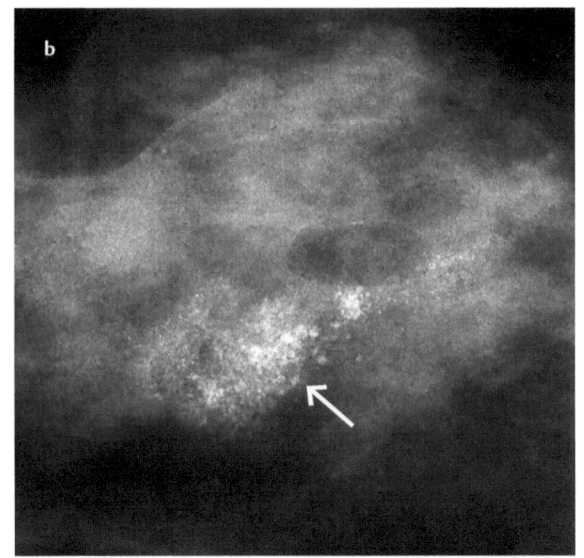

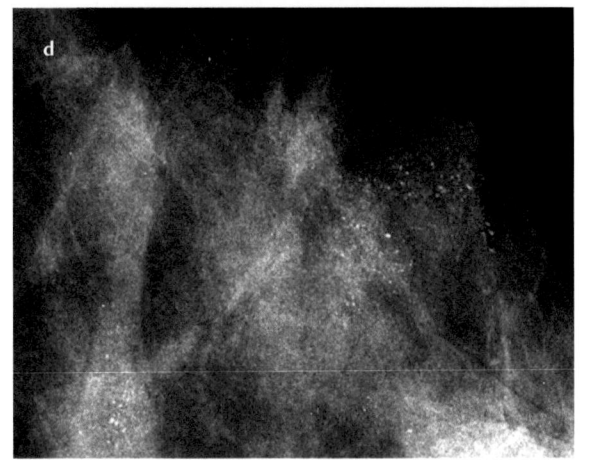

Fig. 15.5a–n

a Magnification mammography shows very fine granular but also casting-type calcifications: High-grade ductal carcinoma in situ (DCIS).
b A specimen radiograph clearly depicts the fine granular configuration as well as the ductal distribution. *Histology*: Micropapillary cribriform DCIS.
c Fine granular pleomorphic microcalcifications, in clusters, which contains casting shapes as well: Cribriform DCIS.
d Two groups of fine granular calcifications: DCIS grade 2.
e A small group of granular as well as pleomorphic calcifications next to a calcified vessel: DCIS grade 2.

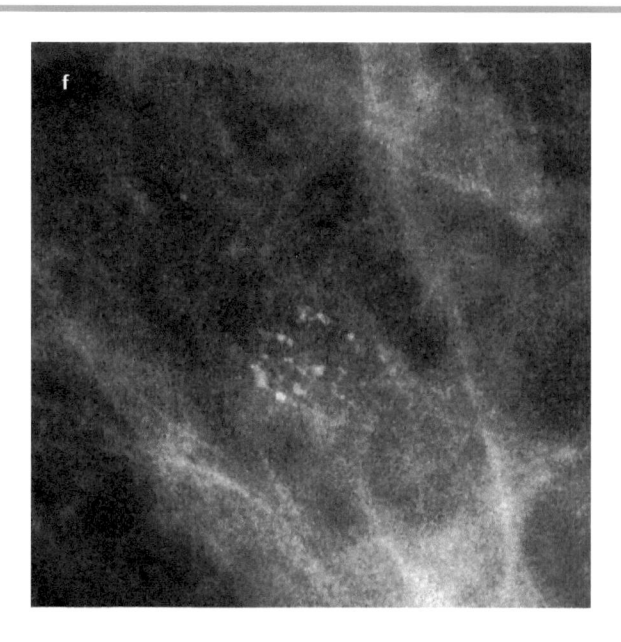

Ductal Carcinoma in Situ (DCIS)

f Small cluster of fine granular microcalcifications: DCIS, papillary type.
g Magnification specimen radiograph (excision after vacuum biopsy) shows very small, partially punctate, partially elongated fine granular microcalcifications in two areas arranged in a branching, ductal distribution: DCIS with micropapillary and solid subtypes.
h,i Small group of granular calcifications, yielding DCIS grade 2 on vacuum biopsy.
j Small group of predominantly fine granular microcalcifications within a focal mass with delicate spiculation: Small-cell DCIS, 5 mm in size, with desmoplastic reaction.

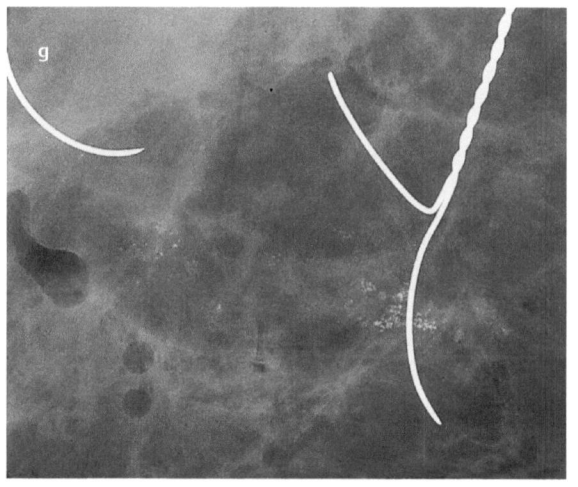

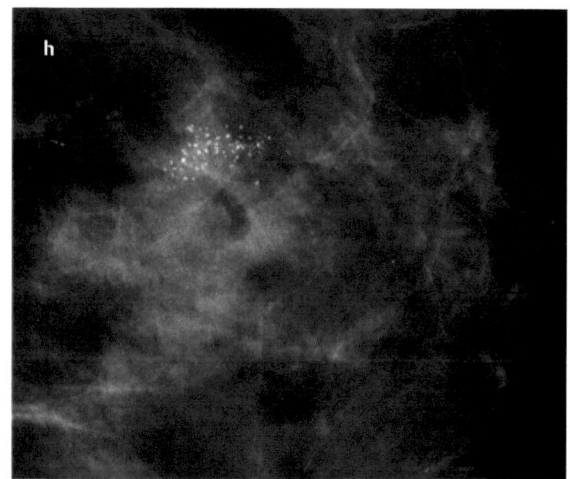

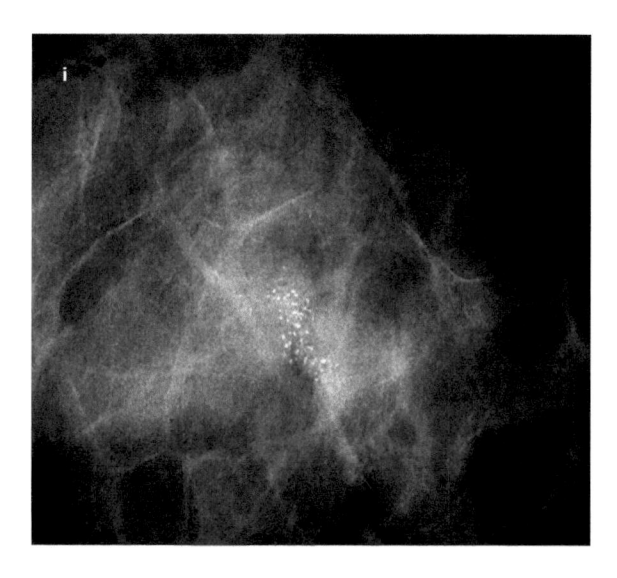

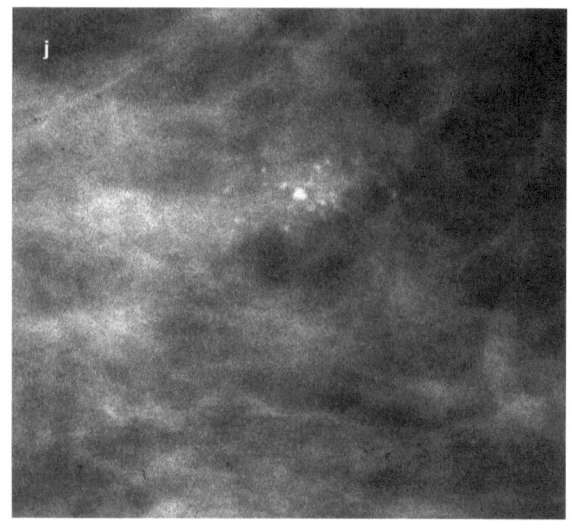

Fig. 15.5k–n ▷

15 Carcinoma in Situ

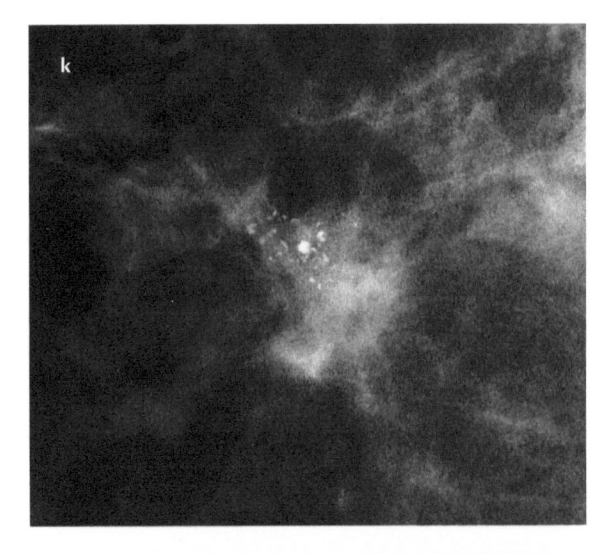

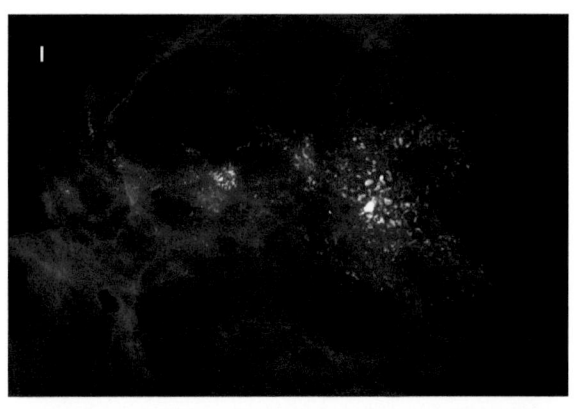

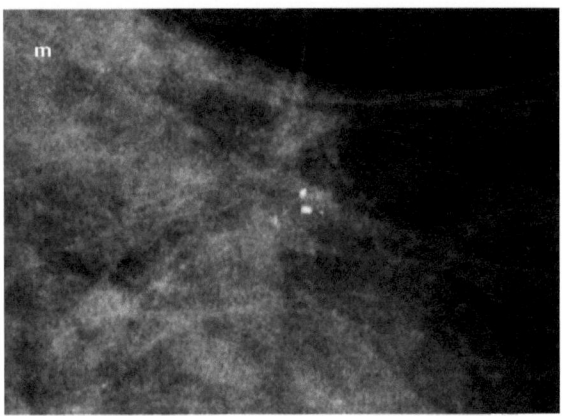

◁ continued

- **k** Magnification specimen radiography.
- **l** Specimen radiography showing microcalcifications of very variable sizes. Centrally in the group "crushed stone" calcifications are shown among the many elongated casting and very pleomorphic calcifications.
- **m–n** Tiny group of "crushed stone" calcifications, which indicated a DCIS grade 3.

imaging. Therefore, the radiologist should not attempt to predict the histology of DCIS on the basis of the mammographic pattern of calcifications or predict invasion based on the presence of a mass or density.

Methodical Prerequisites for the Analysis of Microcalcifications

The comprehensive evaluation of microcalcifications requires mammography in at least two projections. High image quality concerning optimized contrast, correct exposure of the area in question, and acceptable noise level are absolute prerequisites.

For demonstrating the "teacup" appearance of benign microcalcifications, an additional view in a 90° lateral projection.

Magnification mammography is of utmost importance for improving the analysis of the morphology of indeterminate microcalcifications and for assessment of the extent before surgery.

Other Mammographic Presentations

(See **Figs. 15.6 and 15.7**.)

Other presentations of DCIS include a spiculated lesion with or without a central density or a mass with smooth or irregular contours (usually without microcalcifications). Some DCIS lesions present neither as a mass nor as an architectural distortion nor with microcalcifications. These may be detected incidentally by histology (obtained for other reasons). In some cases a DCIS may present with nipple discharge, and can be detected by galactography (unless otherwise apparent by mammography) (**Fig. 15.6g**). Very rarely may a DCIS be apparent on the mammogram as a thickened duct only.

Accuracy of Mammography for Detection and Differential Diagnosis

Mammography has made it possible to detect DCIS on a large scale. It is therefore the most important method for detecting and diagnosing DCIS. Since DCIS not visible mammographically is generally clinically asymptomatic and since (except for highly selected indications) asymptomatic women usually do not undergo further investigations, the true sensitivity is unknown.

Some DCIS lesions which are mammographically occult may be detected by pathologic nipple discharge. Most of these will be visible by galactographic abnormalities or on MRI. Rarely DCIS presents as asymmetric palpable findings or is recognized as a mass (e.g., a papillary DCIS with mass-like growth pattern or intracystic papillary DCIS) or a diffusely altered area on ultrasound examination.

A significant proportion of mammographically occult DCIS can be detected by MRI. However, neither mammography nor MRI is able to detect all DCIS. They are, however, complementary.

Some DCIS lesions are detected only by MRI (if performed) or histopathology, either as an incidental finding during biopsy of other lesions or, quite commonly, they constitute part of a larger area of DCIS. While some parts of a DCIS are calcified, and therefore detectable by mammography, others may not be calcified (so-called "iceberg phenomenon") (**Fig. 15.8**).

DCIS presenting as "characteristic calcifications" or as a spiculated density is mammographically detectable with a very high sensitivity and good specificity. DCIS with less characteristic calcifications that are aggregated in groups too small for analysis, as well as DCIS presenting as an uncharacteristic or a smoothly outlined density, may not always be diagnosable by imaging. Since these changes are uncharacteristic, they cannot all be pursued by immediate biopsy in order to maintain an acceptable specificity.

It is well known that some DCIS lesions may not be visible mammographically and may only be discovered as an incidental histologic finding. The prevalence and significance of mammographically invisible DCIS cannot be assessed at the present time.

Additional Roles of Mammography for DCIS

In addition to detecting DCIS (usually on the basis of microcalcifications), mammography is used to define the extent of the mammographically visible portion of the DCIS. This is necessary since complete removal of DCIS is of therapeutic significance and also because DCIS generally is neither palpable nor macroscopically demarcated.

The mammographic assessment of size, however, is only a crude estimate, since noncalcified components of the DCIS are usually mammographically not apparent. This means that the extent of intraductal carcinomas is often mammographically underestimated (**Fig. 15.8**). To assess the extent as optimally as possible:

- *Preoperative mammography* should be performed using optimal technique (magnification). The area of suspicious microcalcifications should be optimally marked for the surgeon. Less characteristic microcalcifications or microcalcifications located in other quadrants should be assessed using percutaneous breast biopsy to avoid significant overestimates that might lead to mutilating surgery or even unnecessary mastectomy.
- *Specimen radiography* should be used routinely and with optimal technique, that is, as standard and magnification views. Specimens should be adequately marked and the specimen radiography should be provided to the pathologist to allow improved orientation.
- *Postoperative mammography* of the surgical site should be performed if complete removal of the area

15 Carcinoma in Situ

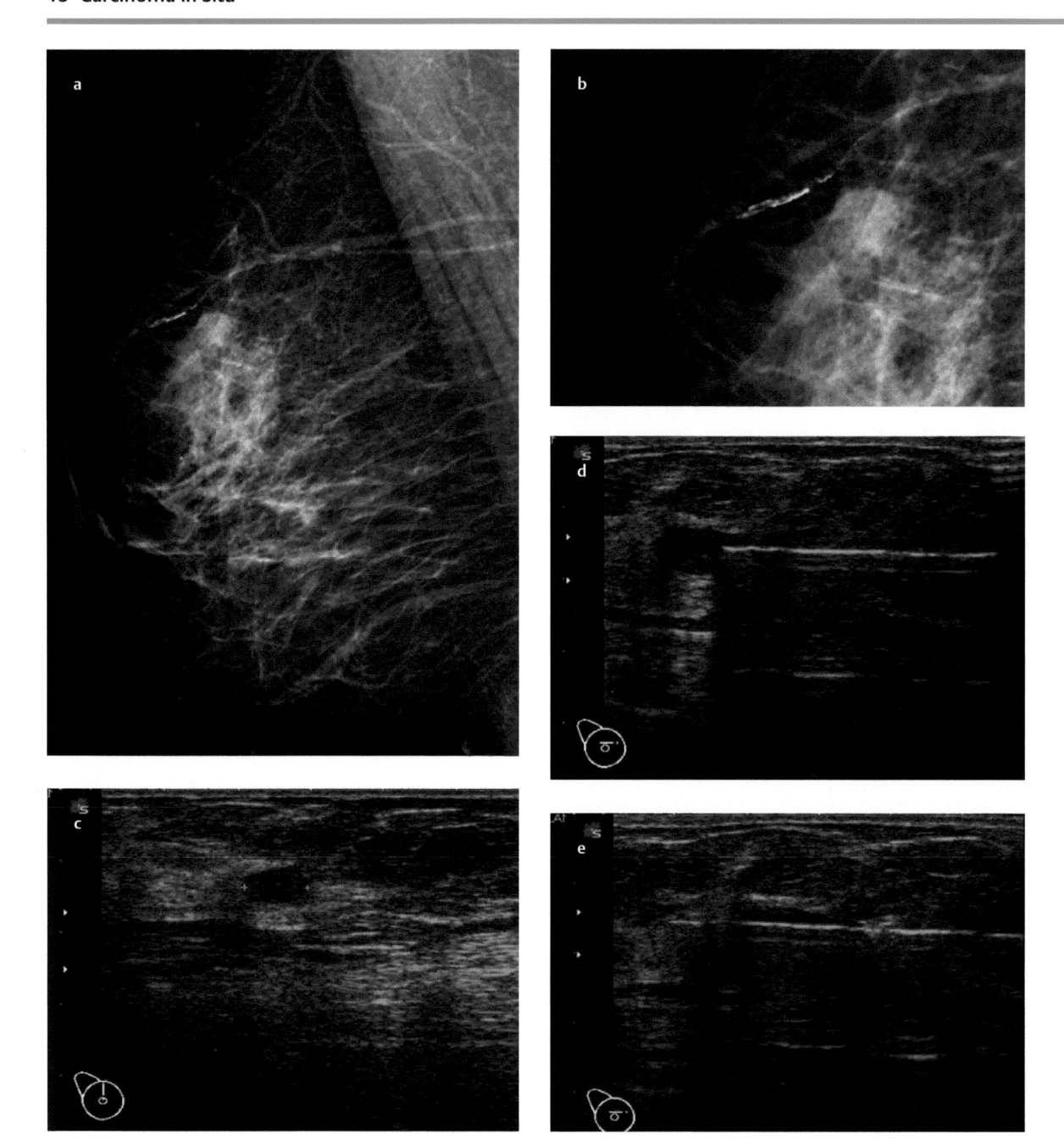

Fig. 15.6a–g Other presentations of ductal carcinoma in situ (DCIS).
a–e Rarely a DCIS may present as a mass.
a,b A round, partly obscured nodule was newly detected on the screening mammogram of this asymptomatic woman (craniocaudal view and spot; see **Fig. 3.25a,b**).

c Ultrasound confirmed a well-circumscribed very hypoechoic nodule with good posterior through-transmission, which might be confused with a cyst.
d,e The lesion was considered solid and, since it had newly appeared, core needle biopsy was performed. *Histology*: Highly differentiated papillary DCIS.

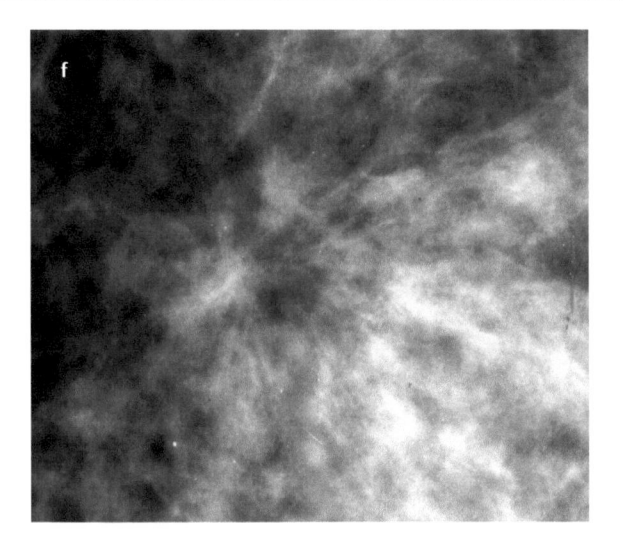

f Some ductal carcinomas in situ arise in radial scars. This radial scar has a dense center ("white scar") and contains some microcalcifications, two features which make it even more suspicious. *Histology*: Low-grade DCIS within a radial scar.

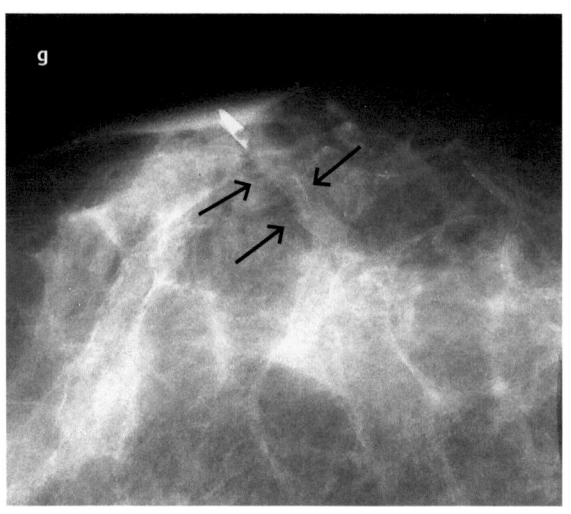

g Some ductal carcinomas in situ become apparent by nipple discharge. Galactography is indicated. In this patient there is a truncation of the duct directly behind the nipple. However, a dilated duct is visible for another 2 cm behind the truncation (arrows).

of suspicion is uncertain. This is possible from about 1 week after surgery and is important to detect any remaining calcifications that might necessitate a second resection before radiation therapy or mastectomy.

Sonography

(See **Figs. 15.6c–e** and **15.7**.)

Image Presentation

Most carcinomas in situ have no characteristic sonographic presentation, that is, they cannot be distinguished sonographically from normal parenchyma prospectively.

In retrospect, knowing the mammographic features, some sonographic correlation may be present in around 60% of cases.

Sometimes microcalcifications may be visualized or suspected by relatively strong echoes. However, owing to the high frequency of microcalcifications in benign changes and the inherent inability of ultrasound in analyzing and further characterizing these microcalcifications, detection of DCIS based on sonographic detection of microcalcifications is highly uncertain.

Sometimes dilated hypoechoic ductal structures may be seen in DCIS. However, there are numerous other causes of dilated ducts.

The most frequent sonographic finding concerns DCIS presenting as a mass, which includes papillary DCIS. However, a sonographically visible mass may also represent a small area of microinvasion (Lee et al. 2008, Izumori et al. 2010, Park et al. 2010, Gwak et al. 2011).

Accuracy

Considering all the evidence, sonography does not play a significant role in the prospective diagnosis of DCIS (Berg et al. 2004, 2008, Warner et al. 2011), even though some DCIS lesions may be detected by ultrasound (Izumori et al. 2010, Park et al. 2010).

Importance

Although sonography plays only a minor role in the prospective detection, exclusion, or differential diagnosis of DCIS, ultrasound may be useful to search for a mass within a suspicious area. The presence of a mass within such an area may be indicative of an invasive component and biopsy should be directed to the mass. (Proof of an invasive component is important, since surgical therapy should then include at least sentinel node biopsy.)

Magnetic Resonance Imaging

Image Presentation

Contrary to initial expectations, many DCISs (70–90%) enhance with contrast agents on MRI. However, the enhancement pattern of a proportion of DCIS (up to 40% of the lesions) differs from the patterns seen in most

15 Carcinoma in Situ

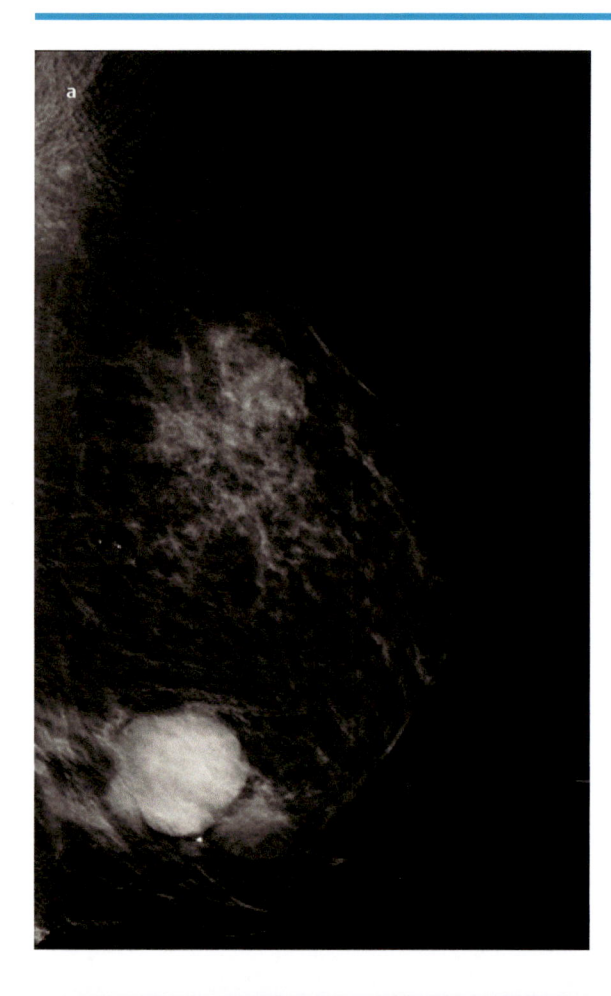

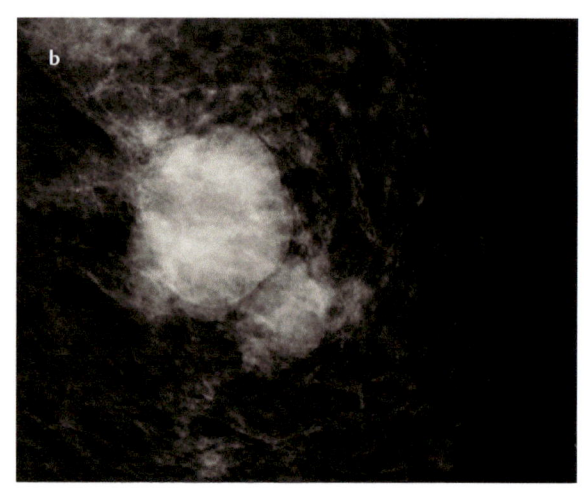

Fig.15.7a–c

a,b This 80-year-old patient presented with several palpable nodules and a skin retraction in the 6 o'clock region. Three years before a 15-mm mass had undergone core needle biopsy (CNB) in another institution and was diagnosed as benign papilloma based on the CNB only.
Mediolateral oblique view (**a**) and section of the craniocaudal view (**b**) demonstrate several large masses occupying the lower part of her breast, surrounded by asymmetrical increased density, which extends from the chest wall anteriorly at the 5 to 6 o'clock position. Furthermore skin retraction is visible on the mediolateral oblique view.

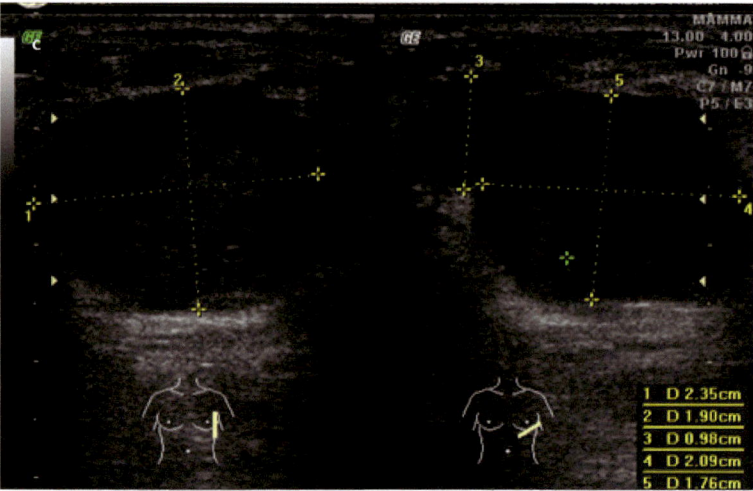

c Ultrasound images show lobulated complex masses. CNB yielded papillary ductal carcinoma in situ (DCIS).
The surgical diagnosis confirmed extensive DCIS and reactive changes. In spite of the skin retraction no invasion was noted on histopathology.
This case demonstrates that a diagnosis based on CNB is unreliable in papillary lesions.

Ductal Carcinoma in Situ (DCIS)

invasive carcinomas and shows an increased overlap with presentations seen in benign changes.

The following features, which occur in DCIS, have to be considered suspicious for malignancy and can thus lead to the correct diagnosis of DCIS based on MRI (**Figs. 5.4** and **15.8**:
- Mass with irregular or ill-circumscribed contours (positive predictive value [PPV] for malignancy, intermediate)
- Spiculated mass (mostly seen with invasive breast cancer) or spiculated architectural distortion (PPV high)
- Early enhancing mass with or without washout (PPV high or intermediate, respectively)
- Uncharacteristic mass with progressive or plateau-type enhancement (PPV low to intermediate)
- Focal enhancement with progressive or plateau-type enhancement (PPV low)
- Ductal or branching enhancement (irrespective of enhancement dynamics) (PPV low to intermediate)
- Segmental enhancement (irrespective of enhancement dynamics) (PPV intermediate to high)
- Regional enhancement (irrespective of enhancement dynamics) (PPV low to intermediate)
- Pattern of nonmass enhancement: confluent patchy, reticular or dendritic (PPV intermediate to high)
- Pattern of nonmass enhancement: milky or stippled (PPV low)

The above enhancement patterns of DCIS have been described by several authors as differing from those of many invasive carcinomas. Compared with invasive carcinoma, nonmass enhancement and progressive and

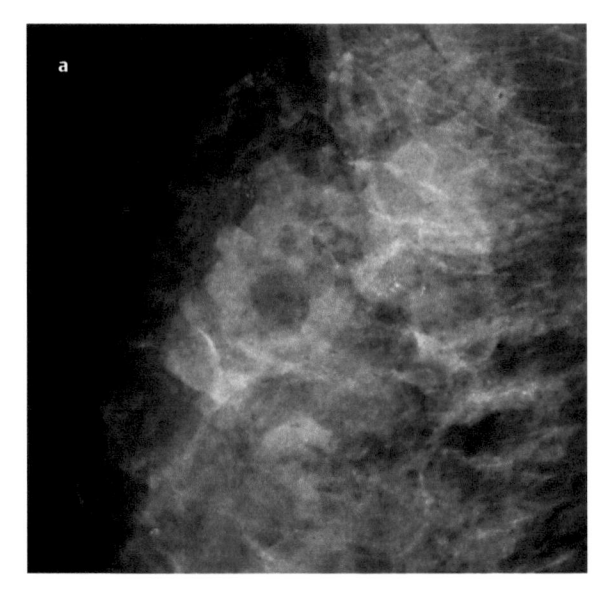

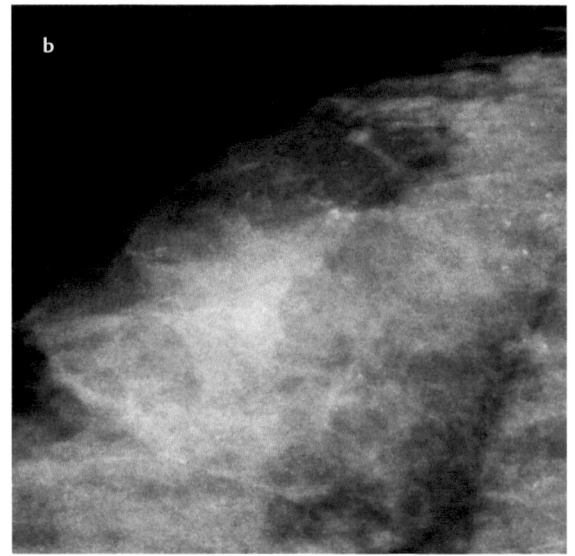

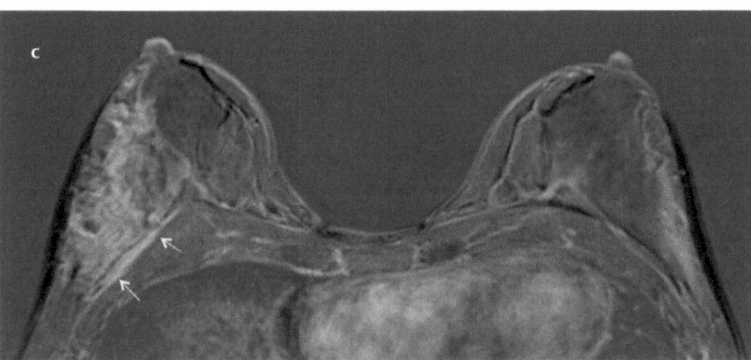

Fig. 15.8a–d This 30-year-old patient presented with an uncharacteristic palpable fullness of the upper outer quadrant of her right breast.

a,b Sections of the right mediolateral oblique and craniocaudal (CC) views. Mammography shows indeterminate, partly grouped microcalcifications in some areas of the upper outer quadrant. (Ultrasound showed no abnormality.)

c Magnetic resonance imaging (MRI) exhibits moderate and progressive segmental enhancement of more than the right upper outer quadrant. Owing to the segmental ditribution, the enhancement has to be considered suspicious. *Histology* proved an extended ductal carcinoma in situ (DCIS) grade 2.

Fig. 15.8d ▷

◁ continued

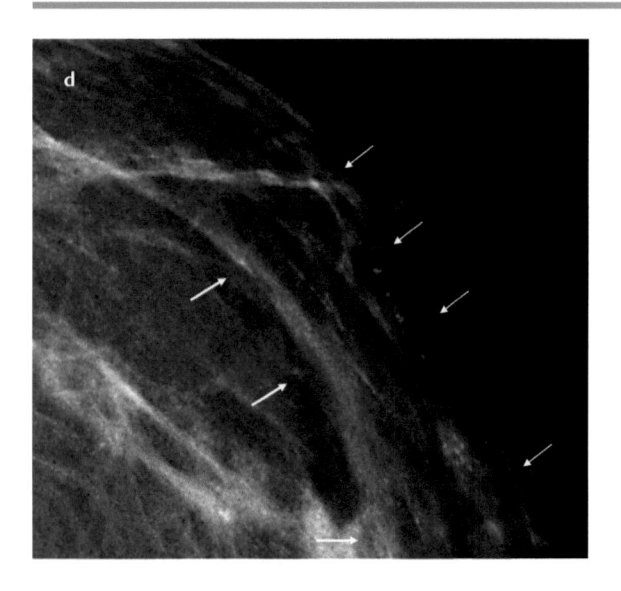

d This shows another case of unexpected extensive disease: The faint ductal microcalcifications were detected on screening mammography and extended in a thin segment of 2 cm width in a length of 5 cm. Vacuum-assisted breast biopsy confirmed high-grade DCIS. At surgery only a small part of the DCIS was calcified. Due to its very large extent (11 cm throughout the complete breast) the patient underwent mastectomy.

low to moderate enhancement are more frequent. The features with the highest PPV for DCIS include segmental enhancement, dendritic and reticular patterns of non-mass enhancement, any enhancement with washout, and masses with irregular or ill-defined contours. We recommend considering biopsy at least in those cases with the latter features. In other cases the combination of features and risk factors may have to be considered.

When analyzing the literature, a learning curve is evident, particularly among authors who strictly adhered to interpretation of dynamic enhancement criteria. Overall, with increasing awareness of the above-summarized variable features of DCIS, detection of DCIS lesions that are visible by MRI only has increased. However, this increased detection is associated with some loss of specificity owing to the overlap of some of the features of DCIS with enhancement patterns seen in benign changes (Lehman 2010, Warner et al. 2011).

As with mammography, MRI is able to detect only some DCIS lesions, since some will not enhance. Overall, as with mammography, detection of DCIS will depend on the chosen diagnostic threshold.

Depending on the thresholds used, the reported sensitivity of MRI for detection of DCIS has ranged between 63% and 92% (Heywang-Köbrunner et al. 2001, Neubauer et al. 2003, Shiraishi et al. 2003, Berg et al. 2004, Bluemke et al. 2004, Groves et al. 2005, Van Goethem et al. 2005, Kim et al. 2007, Kuhl et al. 2007, Rosen et al. 2007).

A multicenter study by Sardanelli, in which the results of a centralized prospective comparison of MR and mammography, verified by complete histopathologic assessment of the mastectomy specimens, yielded a sensitivity of 40% for MRI and of 37% for mammography.

In this study many small foci of DCIS that were detectable by histopathology only were included. The exact significance of small foci of DCIS is not known. However,

the study showed that both MRI and mammography are complementary but imperfect for the detection of DCIS (Sardanelli et al. 2004).

The large variations between the studies may probably be attributed to patient selection, differences in lesion size, mode of verification and different algorithms of interpretation, and to a learning curve.

Overall, for MRI detection of DCIS a sensible threshold has to be sought that allows a responsible balance between sensitivity and specificity, as with detection of DCIS by mammography.

Several authors evaluated enhancement patterns of high- versus low-grade and of comedo-type versus non–comedo-type DCIS (Viehweg et al. 2000, Heywang-Köbrunner et al. 2001, Neubauer et al. 2003, Oshida et al. 2005, Kim et al. 2007, Jansen et al. 2007, Kuhl et al. 2007). There may be some tendency toward earlier enhancement with comedo and high-grade DCIS compared with low-grade and non-comedo DCIS. Thus the former may be detected more reliably. However, the reported range is wide.

Considering that imaging presentation of DCIS exhibits more overlap with benign changes than invasive breast cancer, interpretation criteria that emphasize high sensitivity will detect more DCIS at the cost of specificity and vice versa.

Accuracy

Depending on patient preselection and interpretation rules, sensitivities ranging from 50% to 90% have been reported by different authors. Even though the sensitivity of MRI is lower for the detection of DCIS than for invasive breast cancer, MRI is able to prospectively detect a significant number of DCIS including mammographically occult DCIS and thus proves complimentary to mammography.

In general, diagnostic criteria that yield a higher sensitivity are usually associated with lower specificity, and vice versa. It should, however, be understood that some ductal carcinomas in situ (10–20%) do not enhance.

Considering that DCIS is a non-obligatory precursor of malignancy, detection and adequate therapy is considered important particularly for DCIS of higher grade (intermediate or high grade) and for extended areas of DCIS, since in these patients the risk of progression to invasive disease is increased. This applies in particular to those groups of women for whom MRI is recommended due to an increased risk (owing to personal or family history).

Considering the complimentary information obtained from mammography and MRI, their combined use will yield the best results for these women.

Even though the extent of DCIS is depicted more correctly by MRI alone than by mammography alone (Hwang et al. 2003, Hata et al. 2004, Menell et al. 2005, Chung et al. 2005, Van Goethem et al. 2007, Kim et al. 2007, Schouten van der Velden et al. 2006, Santamaría et al. 2008, Hollingsworth et al. 2008), there is over- and underestimation even with the combined use of both methods, which ranges around 15–25%. Considering the as yet uncertain role of MRI in preoperative staging before breast conservation with radiation therapy there is no general recommendation for a preoperative MRI in patients with proven DCIS.

In selected cases with extended disease, where the best possible surgical planning may be needed, MRI may be helpful for preoperative marking or for an optimum assessment of the volume that should be removed. In the latter case MRI may need to be combined with percutaneous breast biopsy.

Significance

To avoid false negative diagnoses on otherwise suspicious lesions, MRI is not recommended for differentiation of mammographically suspected DCIS. If suspicious microcalcifications or other signs compatible with the potential presence of ductal carcinoma in situ (radial scar) are present on conventional imaging, biopsy is necessary irrespective of the MRI findings.

However, MRI is capable of detecting DCIS not visualized by other methods.

Whether MRI should be recommended for preoperative local staging to assess the extent or multicentricity of ductal carcinoma in situ is controversial.

Percutaneous Biopsy

The accuracy of CNB is lower for DCIS than for invasive carcinoma. The reason may be that many DCISs exhibit discontinuous growth and that microcalcifications indicative of DCIS may be remote from the malignant cells. Thus sampling error may occur. Entities, for which there is an increased risk of sampling error, include lesions that present with microcalcifications only and radial scars.

Since vacuum biopsy allows acquisition of a much higher volume of tissue, an improved accuracy can be achieved with VABB compared with CNB, particularly concerning the detection of DCIS. According to the literature and our own experience missed diagnoses are rare with VABB, provided it is performed according to strict standards (see Chapter 7).

DCIS may be suspected based on atypia at histology. In these circumstances the DCIS is not missed since surgery will be correctly recommended based on the diagnosis of atypias. However, the diagnosis will be considered an underestimate. Such underestimates can be reduced from approximately 40% with CNB to approximately 20% with VABB. On the other hand, percutaneous breast biopsy may yield a DCIS. Depending on the volume sample and the extent of the DCIS, an invasive focus or area within this lesion may be missed. This type of underestimate is considered an underestimate of DCIS. It can be reduced from around 20–25% at CNB to around 10–15% with VABB (Fahrbach et al. 2006, Yu et al. 2010).

Overall today with modern imaging and intervention including VABB, the vast majority of diagnostic surgical biopsies that were performed some 5–10 years ago can be avoided. The increasing capabilities of minimal invasive procedures also allow the achievement of even better sensitivity with a lower rate of surgical procedures (Perry et al. 2006, Albert et al. 2009, Utzon-Frank et al. 2011).

Advantages of vacuum biopsy over conventional biopsy have been confirmed for microcalcifications; the role of vacuum biopsy in radial scars, however, which may be associated with DCIS in their periphery, is under evaluation. DCIS, which presents as a mass, may be worked-up by conventional percutaneous biopsy or vacuum biopsy under stereotactic or sonographic guidance.

Whenever malignancy or DCIS is a differential diagnosis and biopsy does not confirm the suspicion, correlation of imaging and histopathology is required to check representative removal. A diagnosis of pleomorphic LCIS, ADH, DCIS or invasive carcinoma (at CNB or VABB) should lead to appropriate surgical treatment (excision with or without irradiation or—in the case of extended involvement—mastectomy). If the DCIS is associated with an invasive component, sentinel lymph node biopsy is required.

Whereas fine needle aspiration cannot distinguish between invasive and in situ carcinoma, with CNB this is possible in some patients. VABB is able to correctly diagnose associated invasion in an even higher percentage of the patients, which is advantageous for treatment planning.

Summary

LN cannot be diagnosed clinically or mammographically. It is often discovered incidentally through excisional or percutaneous biopsies performed because of questionable abnormal palpation or indeterminate mammographic findings. Whereas ALH and classic LCIS (corresponding to atypical lobular hyperplasia) are considered B3 lesions or lesions of uncertain biological potential (see Chapter 14), pleomorphic LCIS diagnosed at percutaneous breast biopsy is considered a non-obligatory precursor of malignancy and categorized (like DCIS) as a B5 lesion. Whereas ALH/classic LCIS is rarely associated with microcalcifications and mostly an incidental finding, pleomorphic LCIS is often associated with microcalcifications representing intraluminal calcified necrosis. Pleomorphic LCIS diagnosed at percutaneous biopsy should be followed by excisional biopsy to remove the lesion completely. Evidence for the exact biological potential of pleomorphic LCIS remains limited, as is evidence for the optimum treatment strategy. Strict imaging–histopathologic correlation is mandatory. Also imaging should exclude the presence of an associated invasive carcinoma in another quadrant of the breast.

The term DCIS encompasses a group of histologically and prognostically heterogeneous non invasive carcinomas. Its discovery has risen with the increasing use of mammography. Microcalcifications are the cardinal mammographic finding in DCIS. Mammography is the primary imaging method since it permits the detection and analysis of microcalcifications.

While the comedo subtypes of high- and intermediate-grade DCIS often produce a mammographically characteristic (ductal) pattern of individual forms and distribution, the non-comedo subtypes are more difficult to differentiate from the numerous microcalcifications that are associated with benign breast conditions. The use of magnification mammography adds to increased accuracy.

Other presentations of DCIS are less frequent. They include masses or architectural distortions. Some DCIS may present with uncharacteristic clinical symptoms, others with bloody nipple discharge. Some DCIS are detected only by histopathology. This includes many small foci of non-calcified DCIS.

Sonography plays no significant role in the detection, exclusion, or differential diagnosis of DCIS.

MRI is able to detect mammographically occult DCIS, which appears important in women at high risk. Overall MRI presentations of DCIS are less specific than those of most invasive breast cancers.

Features with a relatively high predictive value include segmental enhancement, dendritic and reticular patterns of non-mass enhancement, which all may exhibit very variable features concerning enhancement dynamics. Furthermore DCIS may present with features imitating either invasive malignancy (focal enhancement, washout) or benign changes (uncharacteristic mass-like enhancement, non-mass enhancement, etc.).

MRI and mammography are complementary concerning the detection of DCIS. Due to limited specificity MRI does not contribute to the differential diagnosis of microcalcifications.

To date, VABB is considered the method of choice for histopathologic assessment of microcalcifications. Ultrasound-guided CNB may be useful to target areas suspected of invasion that may be contained in larger areas of microcalcifications.

References and Recommended Reading

Abdel-Fatah TM, Powe DG, Hodi Z, Lee AH, Reis-Filho JS, Ellis IO. High frequency of coexistence of columnar cell lesions, lobular neoplasia, and low grade ductal carcinoma in situ with invasive tubular carcinoma and invasive lobular carcinoma. Am J Surg Pathol 2007;31(3):417–426

Abdel-Fatah TM, Powe DG, Hodi Z, Reis-Filho JS, Lee AH, Ellis IO. Morphologic and molecular evolutionary pathways of low nuclear grade invasive breast cancers and their putative precursor lesions: further evidence to support the concept of low nuclear grade breast neoplasia family. Am J Surg Pathol 2008;32(4):513–523

Albert US, Altland H, Duda V, et al. 2008 update of the guideline: early detection of breast cancer in Germany. J Cancer Res Clin Oncol 2009;135(3):339–354

Anderson BO, Calhoun KE, Rosen EL. Evolving concepts in the management of lobular neoplasia. J Natl Compr Canc Netw 2006;4(5):511–522

Ansquer Y, Santulli P, Colas C, et al. Lobular intra-epithelial neoplasia: atypical lobular hyperplasia and lobular carcinoma in situ. [Article in French] J Gynecol Obstet Biol Reprod (Paris) 2010;39(2):91–101

Ballesio L, Maggi C, Savelli S, et al. Role of breast magnetic resonance imaging (MRI) in patients with unilateral nipple discharge: preliminary study. Radiol Med (Torino) 2008;113(2):249–264

Berg WA, Gutierrez L, NessAiver MS, et al. Diagnostic accuracy of mammography, clinical examination, US, and MR imaging in preoperative assessment of breast cancer. Radiology 2004;233(3):830–849

Berg WA, Blume JD, Cormack JB, et al; ACRIN 6666 Investigators. Combined screening with ultrasound and mammography vs mammography alone in women at elevated risk of breast cancer. JAMA 2008;299(18):2151–2163

Bijker N, Peterse JL, Duchateau L, et al. Risk factors for recurrence and metastasis after breast-conserving therapy for ductal carcinoma-in-situ: analysis of European Organization for Research and Treatment of Cancer Trial 10853. J Clin Oncol 2001;19(8):2263–2271

Bijker N, van Tienhoven G. Local and systemic outcomes in DCIS based on tumor and patient characteristics: the radiation oncologist's perspective. J Natl Cancer Inst Monogr 2010;2010(41):178–180

Bluemke DA, Gatsonis CA, Chen MH, et al. Magnetic resonance imaging of the breast prior to biopsy. JAMA 2004;292(22):2735–2742

Bodian CA, Perzin KH, Lattes R. Lobular neoplasia. Long term risk of breast cancer and relation to other factors. Cancer 1996;78(5):1024–1034

Brandt SM, Young GQ, Hoda SA. The "Rosen Triad": tubular carcinoma, lobular carcinoma in situ, and columnar cell lesions. Adv Anat Pathol 2008;15(3):140–146

Bratthauer GL, Tavassoli FA. Lobular intraepithelial neoplasia: previously unexplored aspects assessed in 775 cases and their clinical implications. Virchows Arch 2002;440(2):134–138

Carder PJ, Khan T, Burrows P, Sharma N. Large volume "mammotome" biopsy may reduce the need for diagnostic surgery in papillary lesions of the breast. J Clin Pathol 2008;61(8):928–933

Chivukula M, Haynik DM, Brufsky A, Carter G, Dabbs DJ. Pleomorphic lobular carcinoma in situ (PLCIS) on breast core needle biopsies: clinical significance and immunoprofile. Am J Surg Pathol 2008;32(11):1721–1726

Chuba PJ, Hamre MR, Yap J, et al. Bilateral risk for subsequent breast cancer after lobular carcinoma-in-situ: analysis of surveillance, epidemiology, and end results data. J Clin Oncol 2005;23(24):5534–5541

Chung A, Saouaf R, Scharre K, Phillips E. The impact of MRI on the treatment of DCIS. Am Surg 2005;71(9):705–710

Collins LC, Connolly JL, Page DL, et al. Diagnostic agreement in the evaluation of image-guided breast core needle biopsies: results from a randomized clinical trial. Am J Surg Pathol 2004;28(1):126–131

Collins LC, Tamimi RM, Baer HJ, Connolly JL, Colditz GA, Schnitt SJ. Outcome of patients with ductal carcinoma in situ untreated after diagnostic biopsy: results from the Nurses' Health Study. Cancer 2005;103(9):1778–1784

Contreras A, Sattar H. Lobular neoplasia of the breast: an update. Arch Pathol Lab Med 2009;133(7):1116–1120

Correa C, McGale P, Taylor C, et al; Early Breast Cancer Trialists' Collaborative Group (EBCTCG). Overview of the randomized trials of radiotherapy in ductal carcinoma in situ of the breast. J Natl Cancer Inst Monogr 2010;2010(41):162–177

Cuzick J, Sestak I, Pinder SE, et al. Effect of tamoxifen and radiotherapy in women with locally excised ductal carcinoma in situ: long-term results from the UK/ANZ DCIS trial. Lancet Oncol 2011;12(1):21–29

de Roos MA, de Bock GH, de Vries J, van der Vegt B, Wesseling J. p53 overexpression is a predictor of local recurrence after treatment for both in situ and invasive ductal carcinoma of the breast. J Surg Res 2007;140(1):109–114

Di Saverio S, Catena F, Santini D, et al. 259 Patients with DCIS of the breast applying USC/Van Nuys prognostic index: a retrospective review with long term follow up. Breast Cancer Res Treat 2008;109(3):405–416

Dunne C, Burke JP, Morrow M, Kell MR. Effect of margin status on local recurrence after breast conservation and radiation therapy for ductal carcinoma in situ. J Clin Oncol 2009;27(10):1615–1620

Ellis IO, Humphreys S, Michell M, Pinder SE, Wells CA, Zakhour HD; UK National Coordinating Commmittee for Breast Screening Pathology; European Commission Working Group on Breast Screening Pathology. Best Practice No 179. Guidelines for breast needle core biopsy handling and reporting in breast screening assessment. J Clin Pathol 2004;57(9):897–902

Ellis IO, Coleman D, Wells C, et al. Impact of a national external quality assessment scheme for breast pathology in the UK. J Clin Pathol 2006;59(2):138–145

Emdin SO, Granstrand B, Ringberg A, et al; Swedish Breast Cancer Group. SweDCIS: Radiotherapy after sector resection for ductal carcinoma in situ of the breast. Results of a randomised trial in a population offered mammography screening. Acta Oncol 2006;45(5):536–543

Erbas B, Provenzano E, Armes J, Gertig D. The natural history of ductal carcinoma in situ of the breast: a review. Breast Cancer Res Treat 2006;97(2):135–144

Ernster VL, Barclay J, Kerlikowske K, Wilkie H, Ballard-Barbash R. Mortality among women with ductal carcinoma in situ of the breast in the population-based surveillance, epidemiology and end results program. Arch Intern Med 2000;160(7):953–958

Eusebi V, Foschini MP, Cook MG, Berrino F, Azzopardi JG. Long-term follow-up of in situ carcinoma of the breast with special emphasis on clinging carcinoma. Semin Diagn Pathol 1989;6(2):165–173

Evans AJ, Wilson AR, Burrell HC, Ellis IO, Pinder SE. Mammographic features of ductal carcinoma in situ (DCIS) present on previous mammography. Clin Radiol 1999;54(10):644–646

Facius M, Renz DM, Neubauer H, et al. Characteristics of ductal carcinoma in situ in magnetic resonance imaging. Clin Imaging 2007;31(6):394–400

Fadare O, Dadmanesh F, Alvarado-Cabrero I, et al. Lobular intraepithelial neoplasia [lobular carcinoma in situ] with comedo-type necrosis: a clinicopathologic study of 18 cases. Am J Surg Pathol 2006;30(11):1445–1453

Fahrbach K, Sledge I, Cella G, Linz H, Ross SD. A comparison of the accuracy of two minimally invasive breast biopsy methods: a systematic literature review and meta-analysis. Arch Gynecol Obstet 2006;274(2):63–73

Fischer U, Schwethelm L, Baum FT, Luftner-Nagel S, Teubner J. Effort, accuracy and histology of MR-guided vacuum biopsy of suspicious breast lesions—retrospective evaluation after 389 interventions. [Article in German] Rofo 2009;181(8):774–781

Fisher B, Land S, Mamounas E, Dignam J, Fisher ER, Wolmark N. Prevention of invasive breast cancer in women with ductal carcinoma in situ: an update of the National Surgical Adjuvant Breast and Bowel Project experience. Semin Oncol 2001;28(4):400–418

Fisher B, Land S, Mamounas E, et al. Preventation of invasive breast cancer in woman with ductal carcinoma in situ: an update of the National Surgical Adjuvant Breast and Bowel Project Experience. In: Silverstein MJ, Recht A, Lagios M (eds). Ductal carcinoma in situ of the breast. 2nd ed. Philadelphia: Lippincott Williams and Wilkins; 2002: 432–446

Fisher ER, Costantino J, Fisher B, Palekar AS, Redmond C, Mamounas E; The National Surgical Adjuvant Breast and Bowel Project Collaborating Investigators. Pathologic findings from the National Surgical Adjuvant Breast Project (NSABP) Protocol B-17. Intraductal carcinoma (ductal carcinoma in situ). Cancer 1995;75(6):1310–1319

Ghofrani M, Tapia B, Tavassoli FA. Discrepancies in the diagnosis of intraductal proliferative lesions of the breast and its management implications: results of a multinational survey. Virchows Arch 2006;449(6):609–616

Gilles R, Zafrani B, Guinebretière JM, et al. Ductal carcinoma in situ: MR imaging-histopathologic correlation. Radiology 1995;196(2):415–419

Groves AM, Warren RM, Godward S, Rajan PS. Characterization of pure high-grade DCIS on magnetic resonance imaging using the evolving breast MR lexicon terminology: can it be differentiated from pure invasive disease? Magn Reson Imaging 2005;23(6):733–738

Gwak YJ, Kim HJ, Kwak JY, et al. Ultrasonographic detection and characterization of asymptomatic ductal carcinoma in situ with histopathologic correlation. Acta Radiol 2011;52(4):364–371

Haagensen CD, Lane N, Lattes R, Bodian C. Lobular neoplasia (so-called lobular carcinoma in situ) of the breast. Cancer 1978;42(2):737–769

Hata T, Takahashi H, Watanabe K, et al. Magnetic resonance imaging for preoperative evaluation of breast cancer: a comparative study with mammography and ultrasonography. J Am Coll Surg 2004;198(2):190–197

Hermann G, Keller RJ, Drossman S, et al. Mammographic pattern of microcalcifications in the preoperative diagnosis of comedo ductal carcinoma in situ: histopathologic correlation. Can Assoc Radiol J 1999;50(4):235–240

Heywang-Köbrunner SH, Bick U, Bradley WG Jr, et al. International investigation of breast MRI: results of a multicentre study (11 sites) concerning diagnostic parameters for contrast-enhanced MRI based on 519 histopathologically correlated lesions. Eur Radiol 2001;11(4):531–546

Hieken TJ, Cheregi J, Farolan M, Kim J, Velasco JM. Predicting relapse in ductal carcinoma in situ patients: an analysis of biologic markers with long-term follow-up. Am J Surg 2007;194(4):504–506

Holland R, Hendriks JHCL. Microcalcifications associated with ductal carcinoma in situ: mammographic-pathologic correlation. Semin Diagn Pathol 1994;11(3):181–192

Holland R, Hendriks JHCL, Vebeek AL, Mravunac M, Schuurmans Stekhoven JH. Extent, distribution, and mammographic/histological correlations of breast ductal carcinoma in situ. Lancet 1990;335(8688):519–522

Holland R, Peterse JL, Millis RR, et al. Ductal carcinoma in situ: a proposal for a new classification. Semin Diagn Pathol 1994;11(3):167–180

Hollingsworth AB, Stough RG, O'Dell CA, Brekke CE. Breast magnetic resonance imaging for preoperative locoregional staging. Am J Surg 2008;196(3):389–397

Houghton J, George WD, Cuzick J, Duggan C, Fentiman IS, Spittle M; UK Coordinating Committee on Cancer Research; Ductal Carcinoma in situ Working Party; DCIS trialists in the UK, Australia, and New Zealand. Radiotherapy and tamoxifen in women with completely excised ductal carcinoma in situ of the breast in the UK, Australia, and New Zealand: randomised controlled trial. Lancet 2003;362(9378):95–102

Hwang ES, Kinkel K, Esserman LJ, Lu Y, Weidner N, Hylton NM. Magnetic resonance imaging in patients diagnosed with ductal carcinoma-in-situ: value in the diagnosis of residual disease, occult invasion, and multicentricity. Ann Surg Oncol 2003;10(4):381–388

Idvall I, Ringberg A, Anderson H, Akerman M, Fernö M. Histopathological and cell biological characteristics of ductal carcinoma in situ (DCIS) of the breast—a comparison between the primary DCIS and subsequent ipsilateral and contralateral tumours. Breast 2005;14(4):290–297

Izumori A, Takebe K, Sato A. Ultrasound findings and histological features of ductal carcinoma in situ detected by ultrasound examination alone. Breast Cancer 2010;17(2):136–141

Jansen SA, Newstead GM, Abe H, Shimauchi A, Schmidt RA, Karczmar GS. Pure ductal carcinoma in situ: kinetic and morphologic MR characteristics compared with mammographic appearance and nuclear grade. Radiology 2007;245(3):684–691

Karabakhtsian RG, Johnson R, Sumkin J, Dabbs DJ. The clinical significance of lobular neoplasia on breast core biopsy. Am J Surg Pathol 2007;31(5):717–723

Kerlikowske K, Molinaro A, Cha I, et al. Characteristics associated with recurrence among women with ductal carcinoma in situ treated by lumpectomy. J Natl Cancer Inst 2003;95(22):1692–1702

Kettritz U, Rotter K, Schreer I, et al. Stereotactic vacuum-assisted breast biopsy in 2874 patients: a multicenter study. Cancer 2004;100(2):245–251

Kim Y, Moon WK, Cho N, et al. MRI of the breast for the detection and assessment of the size of ductal carcinoma in situ. Korean J Radiol 2007;8(1):32–39

Kuhl CK, Schrading S, Bieling HB, et al. MRI for diagnosis of pure ductal carcinoma in situ: a prospective observational study. Lancet 2007;370(9586):485–492

Lagios MD, Silverstein MJ. Ductal carcinoma in situ. The success of breast conservation therapy: a shared experience of two single institutional nonrandomized prospective studies. Surg Oncol Clin N Am 1997;6(2):385–392

Lagios MD, Westdahl PR, Margolin FR, Rose MR. Duct carcinoma in situ. Relationship of extent of noninvasive disease to the frequency of occult invasion, multicentricity, lymph node metastases, and short-term treatment failures. Cancer 1982;50(7):1309–1314

Lagios MD, Margolin FR, Westdahl PR, Rose MR. Mammographically detected duct carcinoma in situ. Frequency of local recurrence following tylectomy and prognostic effect of nuclear grade on local recurrence. Cancer 1989;63(4):618–624

Lakhani SR, Ellis IO, Schnitt SJ, Tan PH, van de Vijver MJ (eds). WHO classification of tumours of the breast. Lyon: IARC; 2012

Lee JM, Kaplan JB, Murray MP, et al. Underestimation of DCIS at MRI-guided vacuum-assisted breast biopsy. AJR Am J Roentgenol 2007;189(2):468–474

Lee JW, Han W, Ko E, et al. Sonographic lesion size of ductal carcinoma in situ as a preoperative predictor for the presence of an invasive focus. J Surg Oncol 2008;98(1):15–20

Lehman CD, Isaacs C, Schnall MD, et al. Cancer yield of mammography, MR, and US in high-risk women: prospective multi-institution breast cancer screening study. Radiology 2007;244(2):381–388

Lehman CD. Magnetic resonance imaging in the evaluation of ductal carcinoma in situ. J Natl Cancer Inst Monogr 2010;2010(41):150–151

Leibl S, Regitnig P, Moinfar F. Flat epithelial atypia (DIN 1a, atypical columnar change): an underdiagnosed entity very frequently coexisting with lobular neoplasia. Histopathology 2007;50(7):859–865

Leonard GD, Swain SM. Ductal carcinoma in situ, complexities and challenges. J Natl Cancer Inst 2004;96(12):906–920

McDivitt RW, Hutter RV, Foote FW Jr, Stewart FW. In situ lobular carcinoma. A prospective follow-up study indicating cumulative patient risks. JAMA 1967;201(2):82–86

McLaren BK, Schuyler PA, Sanders ME, et al. Excellent survival, cancer type, and Nottingham grade after atypical lobular hyperplasia on initial breast biopsy. Cancer 2006;107(6):1227–1233

Menell JH, Morris EA, Dershaw DD, Abramson AF, Brogi E, Liberman L. Determination of the presence and extent of pure ductal carcinoma in situ by mammography and magnetic resonance imaging. Breast J 2005;11(6):382–390

Millis RR, Thynne GSJ. In situ intraduct carcinoma of the breast: a long term follow-up study. Br J Surg 1975;62(12):957–962

Mokbel K, Cutuli B. Heterogeneity of ductal carcinoma in situ and its effects on management. Lancet Oncol 2006;7(9):756–765

Morrogh M, Morris EA, Liberman L, Van Zee K, Cody HS III, King TA. MRI identifies otherwise occult disease in select patients with Paget disease of the nipple. J Am Coll Surg 2008;206(2):316–321

Müller-Schimpfle MP, Heindel W, Kettritz U, Schulz-Wendtland R, Bick U. Consensus Meeting of Course Directors in Breast Imaging, 9 May 2009, in Frankfurt am Main—Topic: Masses. [Article in German] Rofo 2010;182(8):671–675

Nakahara H, Namba K, Watanabe R, et al. A comparison of MR imaging, galactography and ultrasonography in patients with nipple discharge. Breast Cancer 2003;10(4):320–329

Neubauer H, Li M, Kuehne-Heid R, Schneider A, Kaiser WA. High grade and non-high grade ductal carcinoma in situ on dynamic MR mammography: characteristic findings

References and Recommended Reading

for signal increase and morphological pattern of enhancement. Br J Radiol 2003;76(901):3–12

Nofech-Mozes S, Spayne J, Rakovitch E, Hanna W. Prognostic and predictive molecular markers in DCIS: a review. Adv Anat Pathol 2005;12(5):256–264

O'Malley FP. Lobular neoplasia: morphology, biological potential and management in core biopsies. Mod Pathol 2010;23(Suppl 2):S14–S25

Orel SG, Mendonca MH, Reynolds C, Schnall MD, Solin LJ, Sullivan DC. MR imaging of ductal carcinoma in situ. Radiology 1997;202(2):413–420

Oshida K, Nagashima T, Ueda T, et al. Pharmacokinetic analysis of ductal carcinoma in situ of the breast using dynamic MR mammography. Eur Radiol 2005;15(7):1353–1360

Page DL, Dupont WD, Rogers LW, Landenberger M. Intraductal carcinoma of the breast: follow-up after biopsy only. Cancer 1982;49(4):751–758

Page DL, Dupont WD, Rogers LW, Rados MS. Atypical hyperplastic lesions of the female breast. A long-term follow-up study. Cancer 1985;55(11):2698–2708

Park JS, Park YM, Kim EK, et al. Sonographic findings of high-grade and non-high-grade ductal carcinoma in situ of the breast. J Ultrasound Med 2010;29(12):1687–1697

Perlet C, Heywang-Kobrunner SH, Heinig A, et al. Magnetic resonance-guided, vacuum-assisted breast biopsy: results from a European multicenter study of 538 lesions. Cancer 2006;106(5):982–990

Perry N, Broeders M, de Wolf C, Toernberg S, Holland R, von Karsa L, Eds. European Guidelines for quality assurance in breast screening and diagnosis. Luxembourg: Office for Official Publications of the European Communities; 2006: 221–256

Port ER, Park A, Borgen PI, Morris E, Montgomery LL. Results of MRI screening for breast cancer in high-risk patients with LCIS and atypical hyperplasia. Ann Surg Oncol 2007;14(3):1051–1057

Provenzano E, Hopper JL, Giles GG, Marr G, Venter DJ, Armes JE. Biological markers that predict clinical recurrence in ductal carcinoma in situ of the breast. Eur J Cancer 2003;39(5):622–630

Rosen EL, Smith-Foley SA, DeMartini WB, Eby PR, Peacock S, Lehman CD. BI-RADS MRI enhancement characteristics of ductal carcinoma in situ. Breast J 2007;13(6):545–550

Sanders ME, Schuyler PA, Dupont WD, Page DL. The natural history of low-grade ductal carcinoma in situ of the breast in women treated by biopsy only revealed over 30 years of long-term follow-up. Cancer 2005;103(12):2481–2484

Santamaría G, Velasco M, Farrús B, Zanón G, Fernández PL. Preoperative MRI of pure intraductal breast carcinoma—a valuable adjunct to mammography in assessing cancer extent. Breast 2008;17(2):186–194

Sardanelli F, Giuseppetti GM, Panizza P, et al; Italian Trial for Breast MR in Multifocal/Multicentric Cancer. Sensitivity of MRI versus mammography for detecting foci of multifocal, multicentric breast cancer in fatty and dense breasts using the whole-breast pathologic examination as a gold standard. AJR Am J Roentgenol 2004;183(4):1149–1157

Sardanelli F, Boetes C, Borisch B, et al. Magnetic resonance imaging of the breast: recommendations from the EUSOMA working group. Eur J Cancer 2010;46(8):1296–1316

Schnall MD, Blume J, Bluemke DA, et al. Diagnostic architectural and dynamic features at breast MR imaging: multicenter study. Radiology 2006;238(1):42–53

Schnitt SJ, Silen W, Sadowsky NL, Connolly JL, Harris JR. Ductal carcinoma in situ (intraductal carcinoma) of the breast. N Engl J Med 1988;318(14):898–903

Schouten van der Velden AP, Boetes C, Bult P, Wobbes T. The value of magnetic resonance imaging in diagnosis and size assessment of in situ and small invasive breast carcinoma. Am J Surg 2006;192(2):172–178

Sgroi D, Koerner FC. Involvement of collagenous spherulosis by lobular carcinoma in situ. Potential confusion with cribriform ductal carcinoma in situ. Am J Surg Pathol 1995;19(12):1366–1370

Shiraishi A, Kurosaki Y, Maehara T, Suzuki M, Kurosumi M. Extension of ductal carcinoma in situ: histopathological association with MR imaging and mammography. Magn Reson Med Sci 2003;2(4):159–163

Silverstein MJ, Lagios MD, Craig PH, et al. A prognostic index for ductal carcinoma in situ of the breast. Cancer 1996;77(11):2267–2274

Silverstein MJ, Lagios MD. Use of predictors of recurrence to plan therapy for DCIS of the breast. Oncology (Williston Park) 1997;11(3):393–406, 409–410; discussion 413–415

Silverstein MJ, Buchanan C. Ductal carcinoma in situ: USC/Van Nuys Prognostic Index and the impact of margin status. Breast 2003;12(6):457–471

Sloane JP, Amendoeira I, Apostolikas N, et al; European Commission Working Group on Breast Screening Pathology. Consistency achieved by 23 European pathologists from 12 countries in diagnosing breast disease and reporting prognostic features of carcinomas. Virchows Arch 1999;434(1):3–10

Sneige N, Wang J, Baker BA, Krishnamurthy S, Middleton LP. Clinical, histopathologic, and biologic features of pleomorphic lobular (ductal-lobular) carcinoma in situ of the breast: a report of 24 cases. Mod Pathol 2002;15(10):1044–1050

Solin LJ, Fourquet A, Vicini FA, et al. Long-term outcome after breast-conservation treatment with radiation for mammographically detected ductal carcinoma in situ of the breast. Cancer 2005;103(6):1137–1146

Stomper PC, Connolly JL. Ductal carcinoma in situ of the breast: correlation between mammographic calcification and tumor subtype. AJR Am J Roentgenol 1992;159(3):483–485

Tavassoli FA, Eusebi V. AFIP Atlas of Tumor Pathology, Tumors of the Mammary Gland, Fourth Series, Fascicle 10. Washington, DC: American Registry of Pathology; 2009.

Thomas J, Evans A, Macartney J, et al; Sloane Project Steering Group. Radiological and pathological size estimations of pure ductal carcinoma in situ of the breast, specimen handling and the influence on the success of breast conservation surgery: a review of 2564 cases from the Sloane Project. Br J Cancer 2010;102(2):285–293

Uematsu T, Yuen S, Kasami M, Uchida Y. Dynamic contrast-enhanced MR imaging in screening detected microcalcification lesions of the breast: is there any value? Breast Cancer Res Treat 2007;103(3):269–281

Ueng SH, Mezzetti T, Tavassoli FA. Papillary neoplasms of the breast: a review. Arch Pathol Lab Med 2009;133(6): 893–907

Utzon-Frank N, Vejborg I, von Euler-Chelpin M, Lynge E. Balancing sensitivity and specificity: sixteen years of experience from the mammography screening programme in Copenhagen, Denmark. Cancer Epidemiol 2011;35(5):393–398

Van Goethem M, Schelfout K, Kersschot E, et al. Comparison of MRI features of different grades of DCIS and invasive carcinoma of the breast. JBR-BTR 2005;88(5):225–232

Van Goethem M, Schelfout K, Kersschot E, et al. MR mammography is useful in the preoperative locoregional staging of breast carcinomas with extensive intraductal component. Eur J Radiol 2007;62(2):273–282

Verkooijen HM, Peterse JL, Schipper ME, et al; COBRA Study Group. Interobserver variability between general and expert pathologists during the histopathological assessment of large-core needle and open biopsies of non-palpable breast lesions. Eur J Cancer 2003;39(15):2187–2191

Viehweg P, Lampe D, Buchmann J, Heywang-Köbrunner SH. In situ and minimally invasive breast cancer: morphologic and kinetic features on contrast-enhanced MR imaging. MAGMA 2000;11(3):129–137

Wapnir IL, Dignam JJ, Fisher B, et al. Long-term outcomes of invasive ipsilateral breast tumor recurrences after lumpectomy in NSABP B-17 and B-24 randomized clinical trials for DCIS. J Natl Cancer Inst 2011;103(6):478–488

Warner E, Causer PA, Wong JW, et al. Improvement in DCIS detection rates by MRI over time in a high-risk breast screening study. Breast J 2011;17(1):9–17

Yu YH, Liang C, Yuan XZ. Diagnostic value of vacuum-assisted breast biopsy for breast carcinoma: a meta-analysis and systematic review. Breast Cancer Res Treat 2010;120(2):469–479

16 Invasive Carcinoma

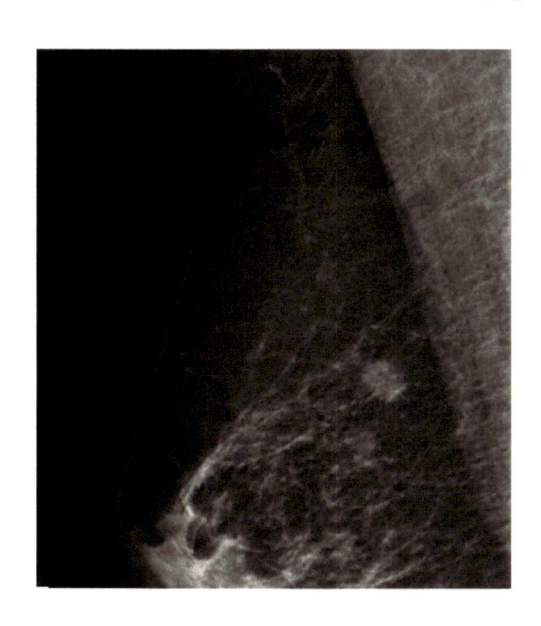

Epidemiology and Etiology → *392*
Definition and Problems Posed → *392*
Spectrum and Detectability → *393*
Diagnostic Strategy and Goals → *394*
Histology → *400*
Breast Cancer and Prognosis → *402*
Clinical Examination → *403*

Mammography → *405*
Radiographic Density of Breast Carcinomas → *405*
Direct Signs of Focally Invasive Breast Carcinoma → *407*
Indirect Signs (Secondary Criteria of Malignancy) of Focally Growing Invasive Carcinomas → *417*
Signs of Diffusely Growing Carcinomas → *420*
Value of Follow-up and Prior Studies → *420*
The Influence of Histology on Mammographic Presentation → *428*
Sensitivity and Specificity of Mammography → *431*
Differential Diagnostic Considerations → *431*

Sonography → *432*
Diagnostic Role → *432*
Indications → *432*
Image Presentation of Breast Carcinoma → *433*
Correlation between Sonographic Image Presentation and Histology → *440*
Accuracy and Differential Diagnosis → *440*

Magnetic Resonance Imaging → *441*
Diagnostic Role → *441*
Imaging Presentation of Carcinomas → *441*
Indications → *445*

Percutaneous Biopsy Methods → *448*
Diagnostic Role → *448*
Indications → *450*
Disposition after Percutaneous Biopsy → *450*

References and Recommended Reading → *450*

16 Invasive Carcinoma

I. Schreer, S. H. Heywang-Koebrunner, S. Barter, J. Naehrig

Epidemiology and Etiology

Invasive breast carcinoma is the most frequent malignancy among women and the most frequent cause of death due to malignancy in women. Currently, it can be expected that 1 in every 8 to 10 women will develop a breast carcinoma in her lifetime. The incidence of breast cancer is low below age 40 years, with less than 2% of breast cancers occurring before age 40. At age 40–45 the yearly incidence is around 1/1,000 and after age 50 around 2–3/1,000. Thus about 10% of breast cancers occur at age 40–50, whereas about 50% of breast cancers occur at age 50–69. Since the absolute number of women aged 70 and above is lower than that in younger age groups, the absolute number of breast cancers does not continue to increase with age at the same pace as for the younger age groups. However, the incidence of breast cancer within each age group continues to rise with age throughout all age groups. Altogether 38% of breast cancers occur beyond age 70. The maximum number of breast cancers occurs around age 60. After age 70, other causes of death increase considerably.

The causes of breast cancer are not exactly known. Only 5–10% of breast cancers are monogenic hereditary breast cancers. For "true" hereditary breast cancers an association with one certain (monogenic) gene aberration is assumed, which explains their occurrence in families and their high prevalence in these families. For about two-thirds of hereditary breast cancers gene mutations or familial syndromes are known. The most important gene mutations concern the *BRCA1* mutation (which is located on chromosome 17q21) and *BRCA2* mutation (located on chromosome 13q12-13). Together these make up about 50% of the hereditary breast cancers. Other rare hereditary syndromes include ataxia telangiectasia, Li–Fraumeni syndrome, Fanconi anemia, Cowden syndrome, Peutz–Jeghers syndrome, and hereditary diffuse gastric cancer syndrome. The above genes have a high penetrance. The risk of being affected by breast cancer ranges up to 80% for female *BRCA1* or *BRCA2* carriers. Their risk for ovarian cancer ranges up to 40%. The other above-mentioned syndromes are associated with lifetime risks for breast cancer of 30–80%. Recently another gene associated with familial breast cancer, *RAD51C/BRCA3*, has been described. It is not yet included in systematic testing, since mutations appear to be rare and its penetrance is not yet known. Other genes are not yet identified and the subject of further research.

Multiple further genes are known to increase the overall risk of breast cancer. However, manifestation of breast cancer appears to depend on other genes, as well, and probably on further as yet unknown factors (Walsh et al. 2010, Meindl et al. 2011).

About 90% of the breast cancers are sporadic and are suspected to be associated with a multifactorial genesis. There are certain risk factors which are known to increase the risk of breast cancer. These include family history, certain gene variants, individual history of breast cancer, precursor lesions, and possibly even proliferative benign changes (status after benign biopsies). Furthermore, breast density, endogenous and exogenous hormone intake and irradiation of the breast appear to play a role (Chapters 1 and 9).

Assessing the patient's approximate risk helps identify and counsel women at high or intermediate risk. In the future risk-adapted surveillance may gain increasing importance.

Definition and Problems Posed

With the development of invasion—recognizable by the extension of tumor cells through the basement membrane—there is the possibility of metastases, and therefore death. According to cancer registry data an almost linear correlation exists between tumor size at detection and lymph node involvement and tumor size at detection and mortality. For invasive tumors, lethality increases by approximately 1.3% per additional millimeter in diameter.

Furthermore, grading of the malignant cell changes allows assessment of the aggressiveness of a tumor and estimation of the risk of progression or death. Cancer registry data also show that grading increases with increasing size at detection. This change in grading and aggressiveness with time is supported by fundamental knowledge on tumor growth and DNA changes.

Based on a large amount data, the most important prognostic features include tumor size at detection, grading, receptor status (estrogen receptor, progesterone receptor, Her2 neu status), lymph node involvement, vascular and lymphatic invasion, and completeness of excision (Blamey et al. 2007, 2010).

There is some correlation between these factors (e.g., correlation of size at detection and grading or lymph node involvement). However, the named factors also act independently.

Based on our present knowledge, prognosis can be influenced by early detection, by complete surgical elimination of tumor tissue, and by (neo)adjuvant antihormonal or chemotherapy.

It is thus desirable to detect the invasive carcinoma when it is as small as possible. Based on evaluation of Swedish screening data Tábar suggested that detection at a tumor size below 15 mm should be an important goal of screening (Tabár et al. 1992). Furthermore, imaging and interventions should attempt to optimally support and guide the surgeon when planning therapy with the goal of removing as little tissue as possible but as much as necessary to achieve free margins.

Spectrum and Detectability

While detecting the carcinoma that is already large and exhibits characteristic findings usually does not represent a problem, the timely detection of tumors in their early stage or with atypical manifestations remains a diagnostic challenge. Both breast carcinomas and various benign breast conditions exhibit a considerable range of variability, and the signs of an early carcinoma frequently overlap with those of benign conditions, making detection and diagnosis more difficult. With all modalities, the detectability of the breast carcinoma depends on size, histology (e.g., difficult recognition of lobular carcinoma), growth pattern (difficult recognition of diffusely growing carcinoma), and surrounding tissue (difficult recognition of carcinomas within dense tissue).

It should be kept in mind that so far no available clinical or diagnostic method can detect all invasive carcinomas. Even though the chances for early and timely detection increase with screening and could probably increase further with the use of multiple modalities and shorter time intervals, no guarantee is possible in the individual case. When intensifying surveillance or screening, other potential side effects also need to be taken into account. Overall, false negative findings can be encountered with all methods and concepts.

Diffusely growing cancers are generally difficult to detect. These and some lobular cancers pose a diagnostic problem to all imaging methods, including magnetic resonance imaging (MRI).

It is important to understand that microcalcifications can be detected in almost any type of breast tissue (irrespective of tissue density). Most of the very small and early breast cancers are detected by microcalcifications, associated with a DCIS component of the invasive carcinoma. Polymorphic microcalcifications are often the only indicator for grade 3 ductal carcinoma in situ (DCIS), which may contain microinvasion. Detection of such changes is prognostically relevant. While mammography is thus able to detect many invasive cancers that present with microcalcifications at very early stages irrespective of the density of surrounding tissue, the sensitivity of mammography for masses, asymmetries, and also for some architectural distortions decreases according to the density of the surrounding tissue.

If surrounded by dense tissue, even large breast cancers may be obscured or may just cause unspecific asymmetry that is often indistinguishable from the many other benign asymmetries.

The sensitivity of sonography for larger and palpable carcinomas is mostly excellent. However, sensitivity of sonography is low in fatty breast tissue or fatty areas of the breast and decreases in those breasts with inhomogeneous echogenicity and/or shadowing. The sensitivity of sonography decreases with lesion size.

Contrast-enhanced MRI is the most sensitive method for the detection of breast cancer. However, a small percentage of invasive breast cancers do not enhance and about 10% of the invasive breast cancers exhibit moderate progressive enhancement and may thus be mistaken for a benign lesion unless they show clearly suspicious morphology. Sensitivity of MRI decreases with increasing enhancement of the surrounding tissue, which may pose some problem in up to 15% of patients. Patient motion may severely impair diagnostic accuracy. Also, hormonal factors may disturb image interpretation and therefore should always be considered when scheduling MRI (see Chapter 5).

Sensitivity will usually increase when combining several diagnostic methods. Since specificity usually decreases with additional methods and since costs thus increase, the optimum combination of methods depends on the diagnostic question, on the existing risk, on patient age, and on individual features.

The sensitivity that can be reached in a prospective screening situation, where small malignant changes without any clinical sign are to be detected among many benign changes and variations, is very different from the sensitivity of a targeted examination performed for the assessment of a known abnormality. And this problem exists in a similar way for each imaging method and for combinations of different methods.

The specificity indicates the percentage of benign lesions that can correctly be diagnosed as benign. Considering that any screening examination is a repeated procedure that is applied to large parts of the population, a high specificity is a must for any test that is considered as screening test. Side effects of false positives include psychological stress and the need for additional examinations, additional minimally invasive methods, or even surgery. For a screening test mostly specificities above 95–97% are expected. The positive predictive value of biopsy indications should usually range around 25–50%.

In the diagnostic situation (assessing a known abnormality), in contrast, a specificity of 70–80% may be excellent. The reason is that in the diagnostic situation (where a symptom exists) the main goal is reliable exclusion of malignancy. If reliable exclusion of malignancy is possible without requiring surgery, this is usually of advantage. (In the screening situation, however, detecting benign abnormalities is of no advantage to the patient. It is a side effect that has to be accepted in the quest for detection of malignancy at an early stage.)

Specificity and positive predictive value depend on patient selection, on the age distribution, on the methods used, on the individual threshold of the examiner, and on litigation issues.

All things considered, there is an inverse proportional relationship between sensitivity and specificity. However, the additional gain in sensitivity decreases with decreasing specificity.

Selecting a very low threshold for a positive diagnosis (recommending a biopsy even for findings with a low likelihood of being malignant) increases the number of malignancies detected by a few percent. The positive predictive value, however, decreases markedly because more benign changes have to be removed. Selecting a very high threshold for a positive diagnosis increases the positive predictive value, but several carcinomas that would have been detected with a lower threshold remain undetected.

Considering the possibilities and limitations of imaging methods, it remains important to combine imaging with palpation, inspection, and patient history for symptomatic patients.

Overall, it must be accepted that no modality is capable of detecting all breast cancers with the limit of acceptable side effects for the patient. Usually mammography and sonography provide the necessary complementary information. In patients at high risk or for selected indications, MRI may be very valuable.

Summarizing, for the interpretation of imaging methods in asymptomatic patients, a compromise has to be made between a detection rate that is as high as possible and the number of additional examinations and biopsies that can be justified medically and economically.

The evaluation of symptomatic patients with an uncertain finding requires the utilization of supplemental methods to avoid unnecessary biopsies combined with the greatest safety for the patient.

Diagnostic Strategy and Goals

It should be understood that screening of asymptomatic women has to be distinguished from assessment of clinical or imaging abnormalities, from regional staging, from monitoring of therapy response, and eventually from surveillance after breast cancer.

Screening

In asymptomatic patients, diagnostic methods are used as screening for early detection of breast carcinoma. The only method currently appropriate for screening of asymptomatic women at low to moderate risk is mammography. The effectiveness of mammographic screening to reduce mortality through improved early detection has been established in numerous studies (see Chapter 23). Limitations of mammography screening concern limitations of mammography (e.g., decreased sensitivity in dense breast tissue) and limitations caused by the interval (too long intervals may act as a filter for preferable detection of lower-grade tumors). Side effects of any screening (caused by false positive call or overdiagnosis) should be known. Side effects of screening examinations are important, since they may affect asymptomatic women.

Currently, for screening of women at high risk yearly mammography, yearly MRI, and clinical examination are internationally recommended to be performed in special surveillance programs.

- Yearly mammography is presently recommended to start at age 30 years; MRI is recommended to start at age 25 until (at least) age 55 in most countries. The definition of high risk may vary from country to country. An exact assessment of the risk is possible using special calculation models.
- In Germany and Great Britain intensified surveillance is recommended for a lifetime risk greater than 30%; in the United States a recommendation for a lifetime risk greater than 20% exists (see Chapter 5) (National Institute for Health and Clinical Excellence [NICE guideline] 2006, Albert et al. 2009; Sardanelli et al. 2010).

To date there is no uniform recommendation for women at intermediate risk. In most Western countries yearly mammography is recommended for these women. The additional use of ultrasound is indicated in cases with abnormal findings where sonography may contribute (usually assessment of all abnormalities except microcalcifications only) and in difficult-to-assess breasts with dense tissue.

Assessment

In clinically symptomatic patients and in patients with abnormal screening examinations, further evaluation is indicated to avoid unnecessary biopsies and to reveal or exclude possible additional findings. For this diagnostic evaluation, special supplemental mammographic techniques (magnification views, additional projections, galactography), sonography, and percutaneous biopsy techniques are regularly used. With systematic use of state-of-the-art diagnostic mammography, sonography, and percutaneous breast biopsy, the use of MRI will rarely be needed for the assessment of indeterminate findings.

Preceding any additional evaluation of a potentially malignant finding, a technically adequate mammogram consisting of two views should be available. Taking a complete history and performing a clinical examination is considered standard.

- *Mammographically*, additional views should be obtained for palpable findings that are not included on the standard views because of atypical location, also for mammographically suspicious densities possibly caused by superimposition, and for microcalcifications. For the evaluation of microcalcifications, mammography (lateral view and magnification view) is the crucial imaging method. Since ultrasound may sometimes be able to identify an invasive component within larger areas of DCIS, it may be applied as an additional check to guide biopsy to the most suspicious area. (Preoperative diagnosis of the invasive component is of importance, since proof of invasive disease will support the decision for a sentinel node biopsy, for example.) However, sonography usually does not contribute to differentiation of microcalcifications.

- *Sonography* is the supplemental modality for palpable changes in mammographically dense tissue and for all changes that might be attributable to simple cysts. Sonography is also valuable for assessing the margins of a mass, especially when it lies in dense tissue. It should always be remembered that a negative sonographic finding may not exclude a suspected malignancy, since carcinomas that are small and preinvasive can be unapparent sonographically.
- *Percutaneous biopsy* is appropriate for further evaluation of findings that are indeterminate by palpation or imaging. Its use is contingent on high-quality technique, procurement of adequate tissue, and review of the accuracy of one's own patient material. A positive finding can confirm malignancy. A negative finding must be critically checked as to the accuracy of the localization procedure and the possibility of sampling error. If the histologic result and the imaging findings are non-concordant, a repeat percutaneous or open biopsy is necessary.
- *Contrast-enhanced MRI* presently is the most sensitive method for detecting breast cancer. However, the sensitivity and negative predictive value of MRI is lower than the sensitivity of quality-assured percutaneous breast biopsy. Because of this and the relatively high false positive rate (which may also concern further areas of the breast), contrast-enhanced MRI is currently not recommended for workup of indeterminate lesions. However, in selected cases MRI may be very helpful. Indications concern detection or exclusion of malignancy in women with severe scarring, in women with diagnostic problems after breast conservation or silicone implants, and in patients with positive axillary lymph nodes and cancer of unknown primary origin. It may also be helpful in patients with increasing nipple retraction, in patients with nipple discharge if galactography is impossible, or rarely if a lesion can only be visualized on one mammographic view but not on ultrasound. Even though absent enhancement is associated with a high probability of benignity (~95%), neither MRI nor percutaneous biopsy alone can dismiss a highly suspicious lesion the assessment of which is negative with these techniques.
- *Galactography* should follow mammography as the method of choice for further evaluation of the breast with pathologic discharge, if ultrasound does not show an abnormality.

Legal aspects

Because of the increasing number of lawsuits claiming that carcinomas have been discovered too late, it is important to document one's own accuracy. This applies not only to screening but also to diagnostic examinations performed for further evaluation. This is particularly important considering that a high percentage of interval carcinomas and up to 50% of all carcinomas detected by screening can, in retrospect, be seen as discrete abnormality in the preceding examination (Bird et al. 1992, Ikeda et al. 1992, van Dijck et al. 1993, Harvey et al. 1993, Duncan et al. 1998, Saarenmaa et al. 1999). The dividing line is blurred between findings that unquestionably need further evaluation and findings that cannot be differentiated, even by an experienced mammographer, from benign lesions. Having one's own accuracy well documented is particularly advantageous for cases subject to litigation.

Staging

In the presence of a suspicious finding, the available imaging methods are used for preoperative staging. This involves assessing the extent of the known tumor, detecting or excluding multifocality or multicentricity, assessment for a possible tumor in the contralateral breast, and a check of the regional lymph nodes (see Chapter 17, pp. 460–462). Findings that might change the surgical approach or therapeutic strategy (e.g., extension of findings over a wide area or the presence of a second focus) should be verified histologically. Histologic verification should be performed using percutaneous biopsy whenever possible or—only if this is not possible—excision after localization. Therapy should only be changed after adequate confirmation of the diagnosis.

Preoperative marking of significant findings (e.g., marking of lesion extent) guides the surgeon and supports his or her attempt to achieve free margins with the best possible cosmetic result.

Therapeutic planning must consider:
- The extent of the cancer in the breast
- Exclusion/detection of additional foci in the ipsilateral or contralateral breast, and
- Nodal involvement

Even though no generally agreed consensus exists concerning the exact measurement of free margins needed for invasive breast cancer and DCIS, the extent of free margins has proven to be an independent prognostic factor concerning both survival and avoidance of local recurrence.

Even though 20-year follow-up of the initial studies has shown that survival after breast conservation (quadrantectomy followed by radiation therapy for tumors < 3 cm) is equal to survival after mastectomy, recurrence rates vary significantly between the studies and range from 8.8% (initial studies with quadrantectomy) up to 25% for subsequent studies (Blichert-Toft et al. 1992, Arriagada et al. 1996, van Dongen et al. 2000, Fisher et al. 2002, Poggi et al. 2003). Approximately 50% of the recurrences are invasive, and it is known that local recurrence is associated with a worse prognosis (Ghossein et al. 1992, Silverstein et al. 1996). Furthermore, it is a psychologically disturbing and threatening event for the patient that affects quality of life and should be avoided. Therefore complete excision of the malignant change should always be attempted.

Comparing the available imaging methods, in most cases an acceptable accuracy may be achieved by combining mammography and sonography. Direct comparison of MRI, mammography and sonography, however, shows that MRI is the most sensitive method. As shown in large studies, MRI has proven capable of detecting both additional foci of invasive carcinoma and additional DCIS (Fischer et al. 1999, Heywang-Köbrunner et al. 2001, Hwang et al. 2003, Berg et al. 2004, Bluemke et al. 2004, Hata et al. 2004, Sardanelli et al. 2004, Van Goethem et al. 2004, 2007, Schnall et al. 2005, Schouten van der Velden et al. 2006, Gutierrez et al. 2011).

These capabilities of MRI allow improvement of the assessment of lesion extent, detection of additional foci remote from the primary tumor (multicentricity that otherwise might go undetected even histologically since these areas would not be excised), and detection of occult synchronous or metachronous malignancy of the contralateral breast. Detection of additional contralateral malignancy by MRI alone has been reported to occur in around 3–4% of women after breast conservation and usual staging (Lehman et al. 2007, Brennan et al. 2009, Bernard et al. 2010). However, the rate of biopsy recommendations in women undergoing MR screening of the contralateral breast ranges around 13–17% and histopathologic assessment requires special training, specialized personnel, and significant additional costs.

According to two recent meta-analyses (Houssami et al. 2008, Plana et al. 2012), one large and one small randomized study (Turnbull et al. 2010, Peters et al. 2011), MRI leads to incremental detection of some (benign or malignant) abnormality in 16–20% of the patients. Unexpected abnormalities of the contralateral breast have been reported in 3–5.5% of the patients. The positive predictive value of a biopsy recommendation in the ipslateral breast (~67%) appears to be higher than in the contralateral breast (37%).

Overall, this resulted in an increased rate of more radical surgery in about 19% of patients, which was caused by a false positive finding in about 12.8% of patients, and by a true positive finding in 6.3% of the examined patients. More radical surgery mostly concerned wider excision, but partly also an increased rate of mastectomies (Houssami et al. 2008).

In spite of the incremental detection of malignancy (and thus the more accurate detection of malignancy) so far no proof exists for a better patient outcome with MRI. Contrary to expectations the randomized studies could not demonstrate the expected decrease of re-excisions (needed by the surgeon to obtain clear margins). An initial evaluation of a large British randomized study (Turnbull et al. 2010) did not show a significant difference in recurrence rates or rates of contralateral breast cancer, which confirms a previous retrospective observation study (Solin et al. 2008).

In fact the lack of proof of any improved outcome together with the known effect of causing more aggressive surgery does not support a general recommendation for preoperative MRI.

These results are astonishing and contradict our present knowledge concerning the prognostic impact of clear margins and their impact on recurrence rates. There are two major possible explanations for this phenomenon. Possibly MRI detects additional disease, but due to insufficient guidance (by preoperative marking) excisions are on average not more accurate. The other (more probable) explanation is that MRI preferentially detects very small additional foci, which otherwise are eliminated by radiation therapy and adjuvant chemotherapy or hormone therapy. As to contralateral disease (which occurs in 3–4% of the patients), adjuvant therapy will also have some effect. Also prognosis may mainly be determined by the primary tumor, whereas state-of-the art conventional imaging might allow detection of significant contralateral disease at an early stage.

Thus, based on the present data, a general recommendation for preoperative MRI (Schwartz et al. 2006, Albert et al. 2009, Sardanelli et al. 2010) does not appear justified in spite of the high sensitivity of MRI. Since subgroups may not be adequately evaluated by meta-analyses or randomized studies yet and since different biology or prerequisites may exist for certain subgroups, the European recommendations (Sardanelli et al. 2010) explicitly exclude certain subgroups from the above recommendation against general use of preoperative MRI.

Exceptions where, based on expert consensus, MRI may be of benefit include (Schwartz et al. 2006, Sardanelli et al. 2010):

- Lobular cancers: Detection of lobular cancer by conventional imaging is known to be more difficult (with a higher probability of missing cancers of significant size) and MRI has proven to be by far superior for this special entity (Trecate et al. 2001, Kneeshaw et al. 2003, Schelfout et al. 2004).
- Women at high risk: Possibly on account of the younger age groups involved, the increased breast density at a young age, and the special histopathologic subtypes, sensitivity of mammography and sonography is low, whereas MRI has proven to be the most sensitive method for this entity.
- Based on one study, better assessment of extent or multicentricity has been reported in particular for

tumors which on mammography display a significantly different size compared with sonography.
- Owing to its better assessment of lesion extent, MRI may be helpful for planning the surgical approach to larger tumors which may be close to critical structures such as the chest wall or the nipple.

Extent of Tumor

The following findings have to be observed since their presence precludes a breast-conserving therapy or requires at least more demanding oncoplastic surgery:
- Tumor size too large to permit resection with good cosmetic results, or evidence of widely separated multifocal or multicentric carcinoma
- Invasion of the nipple or subareolar ducts, or a narrow space between the tumor and these structures, does not preclude breast conservation but requires sacrificing the nipple
- Invasion of the skin

To assess the extension in fatty or normal breasts, examination by standard methods is generally sufficient. In mammographically dense, small, and normal-sized breasts, supplemental sonography has been used. High-resolution ultrasound is capable of detecting additional foci or demonstrating larger extension than shown on mammography (Skaane 1999, Berg and Gilbreath 2000). Being the most sensitive method, MRI may be useful for appropriate indications (see above). Since both MRI and sonography have a high rate of false positive calls, however, any finding suggestive of in situ or invasive carcinoma that would change treatment needs verification.

Percutaneous breast biopsy should be used to determine the histology of suspicious or indeterminate mammographic (microcalcifications), sonographic, or MR findings. For MR-detected abnormalities, second look ultrasound should be used to countercheck whether the lesion is in retrospect detectable by ultrasound and can thus be accessed under ultrasound guidance.

The volume of tissue including nonpalpable areas of verified or suspected malignancy should be marked preoperatively to allow adequate excision.

Excision of nonpalpable mammographic abnormalities should be counterchecked by specimen radiography. Care should be taken to correctly orient the specimen (Chapter 8). In case of incomplete excision correct orientation of the specimen and marking on both the specimen and the specimen radiograph will help in excising residual tissue.

Care should be taken to excise all suspicious areas and to mark them in the specimen so that they can be found and evaluated by the pathologist to determine the extent of the tumor. Otherwise, small foci can remain undetected by the surgeon as well as by the pathologist (Kollias et al. 1998). We also recommend sending a copy of the specimen radiograph to the pathologist to allow direct correlation of pathology and imaging findings. Conversely, the pathologist might find malignancy that is occult to imaging.

If specimen radiography reveals marginal or possibly incompletely excised areas of microcalcifications, a wider resection at the time of the lumpectomy should be considered by the surgeon. Abnormalities visible only by ultrasound can be imaged by specimen ultrasound.

While specimen radiography or ultrasound may be attempted to countercheck for MR-detected lesions, a direct correlation between MR enhancement and specimen imaging is usually impossible due to the interrupted blood supply, which is a prerequisite for demonstrating enhancement.

In suspected incomplete excision or unsuccessful excision following a wider resection, a postoperative mammogram should be obtained if the original tumor contained calcifications. A postoperative mammogram for assessment of residual microcalcifications is usually possible starting 8–10 days after surgery. Residual uncalcified tumor, which often cannot be adequately assessed by postoperative mammography or ultrasound, can be evaluated by MRI up to the 10th postoperative day (before too much granulation tissue develops). While neither method can exclude residual microscopic foci, they can disclose most remaining foci.

Exclusion and Detection of Additional Foci

Additional foci may be detected close to the primary lesion (multifocal disease). In this case wider excision is indicated. It may be detected remote to the primary lesion (multicentric disease*) or even in the contralateral breast.

Preoperative evaluation to find or exclude additional foci* is important for two reasons:
- Any additional malignancy (or indeterminate finding that cannot be assessed by percutaneous breast biopsy) should, if possible, be removed during the same surgical procedure.
- If multicentric growth is confirmed, breast-conserving therapy is often no longer appropriate because of the expected high recurrence rate and the deformity of the breast resulting from removal of tumors at multiple sites.

---

* The definition of multicentricity is variable. Some define multicentricity as presence of foci in other quadrants than the primary carcinomas, others as presence of foci that are > 4 cm distant from the primary carcinoma. Overall, multicentricity suggests foci in more than one duct system, whereas multifocality suggests foci just in one duct system.

For these reasons, a thorough diagnostic evaluation of both breasts is indicated before any scheduled breast surgery. Surgery on the basis of palpable findings alone without further diagnostic evaluation is no longer considered standard care. The preoperative exclusion or detection of additional foci begins with the standard diagnostic evaluation. Microcalcifications as suggestive evidence for additional invasive or in situ foci (associated with a DCIS component) can be detected by additional magnification views. Ultrasound may complement mammography in dense breasts and may detect additional foci not seen by mammography. Contrast-enhanced MRI is the most sensitive method. Its additional use may be appropriate for the above-mentioned indications or in case a problem cannot be solved by percutaneous breast biopsy and state-of-the-art conventional breast imaging.

A suspected secondary focus (in the ipsi- or contralateral breast) should be confirmed, as described above, before altering the therapy.

Diagnostic Evaluation of the Lymph Nodes

Lymph node involvement is still the most important prognostic factor. Therefore knowledge of lymph node involvement is important for many therapeutic decisions. Adequate treatment of involved axillary lymph nodes is important to avoid painful suffering of extensive axillary disease and involvement of the plexus. Imaging of other lymph node regions (parasternal lymph nodes, supraclavicular lymph nodes, etc.) is not usually indicated, but may be performed in case of symptoms. To date this knowledge is obtained from sentinel node biopsy (SNB) or from axillary dissection.

For SNB a radioactive tracer or methylene blue (or both) is injected around the tumor or underneath the nipple. The tracer and/or dye travels with the lymphatic fluid and thus allows identification of the first lymph nodes; this first filter station is called the sentinel node or nodes and is likely to harbor the first metastases. These one to five lymph nodes can be directly identified by the surgeon tracking the blue dye or using a gamma counter and can thus be excised with a small incision and examined histopathologically.

SNB requires adequate expertise and logistics. However, it allows avoidance of unnecessary axillary dissection, which is often associated with side effects, which are sometimes severe.

To date SNB is performed for evaluation of clinically unsuspicious axilla, mostly for tumor sizes below 3 cm (since the probability of lymph node involvement is lower for tumors < 3 cm).

In cases of macroscopically enlarged axillary lymph nodes (due to malignancy or other lymph node disease) SNB may be inaccurate since the usual drainage is disturbed. Therefore SNB is not indicated in these cases. In cases of positive sentinel lymph nodes axillary dissection is standard today.

Ultrasound imaging of the axillary lymph nodes is performed:
- To evaluate clinically abnormal findings or to evaluate axillary changes detected by mammography or MRI
- To screen for (macroscopically detectable) lymph node involvement during locoregional staging
- To screen the axilla during surveillance after breast cancer
- To guide biopsy to axillary findings, which are suspicious clinically or by imaging

Since after percutaneous breast biopsy reactive lymph node enlargement may rarely occur, ultrasound imaging of the axilla is recommended whenever a suspicious lesion is detected in the breast.

With a published sensitivity of 60–85% (depending on the selection patients with palpable vs. nonpalpable lymph nodes), ultrasound is moderately sensitive for detecting lymph node involvement (Alvarez et al. 2006, Sidibé et al. 2007, Mainiero et al. 2010, Mills et al. 2010). This complies with expectations, since—like all other modalities—ultrasound cannot detect microscopic involvement. However, depending on the histology, sometimes even large lymph nodes may be isoechoic to fat and may be missed (Neal et al. 2010).

Various causes of axillary abnormalities and lymph node abnormalities exist. (The most frequent benign causes of lymph node changes include acute and chronic inflammatory changes; see also Chapter 17). Therefore, if lymph node involvement is suspected histopathologic or cytologic assessment is indicated. For the assessment of lymph node involvement both methods appear to be equivalent provided there is sufficient local experience.

The reported specificity of combined sonography and ultrasound (US)-guided biopsy ranges greater than 97% (Sidibé et al. 2007).

Based on the given accuracy, sonography and US-guided biopsy are quite valuable in those cases where lymph node involvement can be proven. In such cases unnecessary SNB can be avoided. If sonography and/or US-guided biopsy are negative, exclusion of involvement remains uncertain and SNB remains necessary.

Mammography may show evidence of involvement if rarely suspicious microcalcifications are visualized within a lymph node, if its margins assume an irregular shape, or if the lymph node increases in density and loses its central fat. In most of these cases ultrasound may help to detect the lymph node in question and can be used to guide percutaneous breast biopsy.

Based on the existing literature, MRI and positron emission tomography are not superior to sonography plus US-guided biopsy. Thus the latter proves a cost-effective combination for avoiding unnecessary surgery.

Recurrent disease (above all, axillary, supraclavicular, or infraclavicular recurrence) can be best evaluated by sonography. Contrast-enhanced CT and contrast-enhanced MRI (using a technique different from that used for breast imaging) may be helpful as well.

Monitoring of Response to Therapy

Neoadjuvant chemotherapy is used to downstage large breast cancers to make surgical therapy possible (inflammatory breast cancer or T4 breast cancer with involvement of muscle or chest wall) or to allow breast conservation.

Imaging is used to support monitoring of the response. The tasks of imaging include:
- Confirming a suspicion of insufficient response. Early detection of insufficient response may support the decision to perform a salvage mastectomy and to switch the therapeutic regimen. Even though imaging has a better accuracy than clinical examination, over- and underestimates occur (see below). Therefore, histopathologic confirmation of insufficient response is generally needed, before changing the therapeutic approach. Imaging, however, may be very valuable when guiding percutaneous breast biopsy, since it helps avoid areas of necrosis. MRI may even guide biopsy to areas of increased perfusion, which mostly correspond to areas of metabolically active tissue.
- Preoperative assessment to guide surgical therapy. Imaging can help define areas of residual disease. Optimally such areas should undergo image-guided percutaneous breast biopsy to define the volume of tissue that has to be removed and support the decision for or against mastectomy.

When assessing response it should be understood that complete response is defined as complete disappearance of invasive tumor. This definition of complete response correlates with prognosis. It should be understood that only complete response correlates with a good prognosis as to survival. Residual DCIS is acceptable for a histopathologic classification of complete response, even though residual DCIS should be completely removed at surgery. Thus, strictly speaking, information on the extent of DCIS is important for therapy planning but not for assessment of response.

While imaging cannot detect microscopic disease, it may be able to guide biopsy to areas of increased perfusion and metabolism. Imaging can only visualize part of the DCIS and it cannot distinguish between DCIS and invasive tumor reliably. Thus some false positive calls (as to assessment of response) may concern correctly identified areas of DCIS. Other false positive calls of imaging may be due to areas of residual granulation tissue or fibrosis or residual calcifications. The imaging modalities achieve different accuracy. By and large assessment by imaging is more accurate than clinical assessment. However, there are limitations and the role of imaging for assessing response is not yet exactly defined and further research is necessary.
- Guide clip marking of residual tumor or (in cases with excellent response) of the tumor bed. In cases with suspected excellent response imaging should be used over time to guide clip marking of the tumor bed over time (as long as the tumor bed or residual tissue can still be defined. Preoperative marking of the areas to be excised is performed like preoperative marking of small tumors. Areas that, if involved, might change the therapeutic approach should optimally be assessed by percutaneous breast biopsy before planning the access. (Biopsied areas can easily be marked by a clip.) Since the volume of tissue to be removed by the surgeon may be quite large, and since optimum removal may be decisive for breast conservation, positioning of several markers may be indicated.

Monitoring of Neoadjuvant Chemotherapy

The exact role of imaging is not yet defined.

Ultrasound has been used as a supplement to clinical examination. In most cases with concentric shrinkage, correct assessment and improved information compared with clinical examination may be expected. Overestimates of residual tumor may occur, since residual granulation tissue and fibrosis may mimic malignant tissue. Underestimates may concern diffuse or fragmented shrinkage and assessment within areas of necrosis. Elastography may increase the objectivity of clinical imaging and quantitative measurement of elasticity (as this is possible with shear wave elastography) and may be promising in monitoring neoadjuvant chemotherapy.

Mammography allows assessment and measurement of masses in fatty breast tissue and large breasts. In breasts with diffuse changes and response, overall density will regress. Mammography like sonography may overestimate residual viable tissue and cannot identify small areas of residual malignant tissue in dense areas. However it may yield complementary information in cases with confusing ultrasound imaging.

Mostly, regression of microcalcifications will correspond to response. However, due to changed pH milieu in the tumor or residual tissue, microcalcifications may newly appear within previously uncalcified areas of tumor or DCIS, which may not indicate lack of response. Also disappearing microcalcifications may not necessarily indicate response. Thus for interpreting significant change in microcalcifications, histopathologic assessment is needed.

On MRI complete regression of enhancement usually corresponds well with response. So does change of enhancement dynamics from early rising to progressive enhancement. Concentric shrinkage of enhancing tumor indicates good response.

However, fragmented patterns of enhancement and residual multicentric or dendritic enhancement usually indicate insufficient response.

Interpretation of diffuse enhancement is difficult, as it may be caused by residual nests of tumor cells, DCIS, or just granulation tissue (see also Chapter 5 and **Figs. 5.17, 5.18, 5.19**).

Incorrect assessment is known to occur in women with diffusely growing malignancy (which often will not respond well). Also, in women treated with taxanes and with antiangiogenetic agents residual tumor may be underestimated (Nakamura et al. 2002, Denis et al. 2004, Bahri et al. 2009, Chen et al. 2009a).

Overall, using contrast-enhanced MRI, response may best be assessed after (one or) two cycles of chemotherapy. Measurement of residual tumor should follow RECIST or WHO criteria (see **Table 5.5**).

The accuracy of imaging to date ranges around 60% for conventional imaging using mammography and sonography and around 70% for MRI (Sardanelli et al. 2010). However, the available data are still limited.

Possibly diffusion weighted imaging or proton spectroscopy (see **Fig. 5.20**) may improve the achieved accuracy of assessing response (Meisamy et al. 2004, Manton et al. 2006, Pickles et al. 2006, Baek et al. 2009, Sharma et al. 2009). The latter method measures the choline peak and may indicate response in tumors that produce phosphocholines. An ACRIN study investigating the value of contrast-enhanced MRI, diffusion weighted imaging, and proton spectroscopy is ongoing.

Histology

Major reasons for the difficulty encountered in recognizing and differentiating breast carcinomas through breast imaging are (1) the multitude of macroscopic and (microscopic) growth patterns that may be attributed to the various histopathologic types observed, (2) the multitude of benign mimics of breast cancer, and (3) the "background noise" of normal breast parenchyma and concurrent benign breast lesions that can obscure especially small tumors and innocent-looking tumor types. Therefore knowledge of tumor types and their histopathologic growth patterns is of particular importance for diagnosing breast carcinoma.

To pathologists the histopathologic spectrum of breast cancer and benign breast disease is extremely heterogeneous and it may be quite confusing for nonpathologists. Some basic considerations can clarify the considerable confusion of terminology and classification.

Invasive and/or in situ carcinomas can be detected owing to soft tissue density and/or microcalcifications and by the detection of changes in focal lesions and/or changes in adjacent structures over time (Azzopardi, 1979). Increased density results from the degree and composition of (1) cellular and (2) noncellular stromal components (in contrast to fat). The cellular components include in particular tumor cells, fibroblasts, and inflammatory cells, whereas the stromal components include extracellular matrix proteins (fibrosis) and in some tumors specific extracellular tumor cell products, for example mucin. An increase in the extracellular matrix of tumors results in fibrosis of breast parenchyma within a tumor, which can be dense, sclerotic, and paucicellular or desmoplastic, that is, rich in fibroblasts and mucosubstances. The histologic components can vary to a great extent between tumor types and even among tumors of the same type. However, some degree of fibrosis is present in almost all invasive breast carcinomas and even about 15% of noninvasive carcinomas can develop periductal desmoplasia. Tumors with fibrosis usually show a stellate distortion while cellular tumors often display less desmoplasia and can be perfectly rounded and well circumscribed. Thus, specific tumor types and their variants often show characteristic patterns in histopathology and in radiology but exceptions to the general rules are not uncommon.

The growth patterns are generally characterized as:
- Spiculated as well as lobulated growing carcinomas with irregular margins
- Nodular and lobulated carcinomas
- Round as well as smoothly demarcated carcinomas
- Diffusely growing carcinomas

Frequent Types of Invasive Carcinomas

(Lakhani et al. 2012 WHO classification)

The most frequent type of carcinoma is the invasive ductal carcinoma, of no special type (NST) (up to 75% of carcinomas), followed by the invasive lobular carcinomas (~5–15%) with several different architectural patterns and other types, including tubular carcinoma (~2–8%), medullary carcinoma (3–4%), mucinous carcinoma (~3%), and micropapillary carcinoma (~2%). There are several other rather rare types of carcinoma.

In the most common invasive carcinoma, the ductal invasive carcinoma of NST, more than 90% of the individual tumor is composed of a nonspecific histopathologic pattern. Wide variations in the morphology of these tumors are found. In gross morphology the IDC, NST most often presents as a stellate tumor with an irregular contour, but it can have a circumscribed rounded, oval, or discoid contour, and another well known pattern is that of a multinodular tumor as well as combined patterns. At higher magnification tumor borders are always blurred. However, IDC, NST grade 3 can have a round shape with a relatively smooth contour simulating fibroadenoma. A marked fibrotic central component can be found in the majority of tumors. An in situ component is found in up to 75% of IDCs, NST to varying extent, most often of intraductal type (DCIS). Infrequently, extensive areas of DCIS are present within or in the periphery of the invasive component. About 40% of IDCs, NST contain microcalcifications, predominantly in the DCIS component and less frequently in the invasive component. These calcifications can—as in DCIS—characteristically appear as rodlike casts along the ductal system, but calcifications exhibiting less characteristic manifestations can occur. Central necrotic areas in invasive tumors can harbor coarse calcifications. Diffuse infiltrative patterns are less frequent, but may occur in a few percent of the IDCs.

Invasive lobular carcinoma (ILC) is the second most frequent type and may present with several architectural patterns and variants. Characteristically, this type exhibits a diffuse infiltrative growth pattern with isolated tumor cells extending diffusely through the parenchyma and adipose tissue; it may or may not be associated with moderate to signficant fibrosis, desmoplastic stroma, or a localized mass. ILCs can even be invisible to the pathologist by macroscopy in up to 30% of cases, and in these cases only palpation may help identify induration in the tumor's area, often of a multinodular pattern. Most striking, even extensive ILC involving the entire breast may be invisible mammographically or sonographically. ILC presenting with a diffuse growth pattern is thus often discovered late. Rarely, ILC contains microcalcifications (e.g., within DCIS or within rare variants of LCIS that may be associated with ILC). Most diffusely growing ILC may, however, become visible only after accompanying fibrosis leads to retraction within the breast tissue, retraction or infiltration of the skin, or even reduced size of the entire breast. Some may only be detected through secondary signs, for example, lymph node enlargement. ILC can produce an architectural distortion but also lobulated or spiculated masses or, rarely, even a fairly well-circumscribed mass (solid variant). Lobular carcinoma is more often multicentric or bilateral than the other types (~20%, which is twice the likelihood of bilateral tumors observed in IDC, NST). In breast cancer screening a significant number of interval carcinomas are of the invasive lobular type (Porter et al. 1999) As with most other types of breast cancer prognosis of lobular carcinoma depends on the stage and histopathologic grading (frequently G2) at detection, and stage-by-stage prognosis is similar to that of invasive ductal carcinoma (Moran et al. 2009).

Tubular carcinoma (TC) presents with spicules and a stellate contour producing the mammographic features of an architectural distortion with or without a mass, sometimes with long spiculations, which are suggestive of this type of carcinoma. Even small TCs present with a stellate contour and central core of fibrotic or desmoplastic stroma. Microcalcifications can be present in TC, typically fine lamellar microcalcifications, which are often found in an associated intraductal component (i.e., low-grade DCIS and flat epithelial atypia (FEA); for nomenclature and notation see Chapter 14, pp. 340–342 and **Table 15.1**). TC is a low-grade carcinoma with a very favorable prognosis. Radial scar (complex sclerosing lesion) is a well recognized differential diagnosis for both radiologists and pathologists. Even though radial scars may be associated with DCIS or TC, a pure radial scar is a benign lesion (see Chapter 10, p. 257).

Carcinoma with medullary features (consisting of medullary carcinoma, atypical medullary carcinoma and invasive carcinoma NST with medullary features) is another special type of invasive duct carcinoma. A typical medullary carcinoma is a highly cellular tumor consisting of anaplastic tumor cells and a dense infiltration of lymphocytes. Characteristically, the tumor is smoothly outlined, but it can be lobulated. Indistinct image presentation of a characteristic medullary carcinoma can occur because of superimposed surrounding tissue or through the characteristic extensive lymphoid infiltrates. Not infrequently, large medullary carcinomas develop central necroses that can calcify. Medullary carcinoma occurs in all age groups and an increased incidence has been described among women affected by familial breast cancer, especially in *BRCA1* germline mutations (Honrado et al. 2006). However, the presence of medullary carcinoma per se is not yet an indicator of familial breast cancer (Iau et al. 2004). The prognosis of medullary carcinoma is better than that of IDC, NST grade 3, which contrasts with the high-grade histopathologial features. For this reason grading of pure medullary carcinoma is not recommended.

Mucinous (colloid) carcinoma is characterized by extensive mucin deposits "injected" by the tumor cells into stroma of the surrounding breast tissue. The characteristic mucinous carcinoma is smoothly marginated, sometimes lobulated, placing it among the mimics of fibroadenoma and other benign rounded lesions. Calcifications can develop in up to 30% of mucinous carcinomas, frequently within DCIS components. There are different types of mucinous carcinoma; type A produces a high content of mucin and has an excellent prognosis in its pure form. Type B is rich in cells and partly solid. The typical mucinous carcinoma appears primarily in older age.

Other rare types of invasive breast carcinoma which may exhibit a predominantly nodular growth with well-defined contours are metaplastic carcinomas (a diverse group of tumours from low- to high-grade carcinomas with epithelial or mixed epithelial/mesenchymal variants), invasive ductal carcinoma with osteoclastic giant cells, and carcinoma with neuroendocrine features.

Further very rare invasive carcinomas include the cribriform carcinoma, adenoid cystic carcinoma, carcinomas with neuroendocrine features, apocrine carcinoma, and myoepithelial carcinomas.

A note of caution: There are specific variants of intraductal carcinoma that can also present as a tumoral mass:

papillary intracystic carcinoma and solid papillary in situ carcinoma. Their nodular manifestation is an exception to the mostly nontumoral longitudinal intraductal growth fashion of usual DCIS, which, however, may still be adjacent. The surrounding cyst wall can give the tumor an entirely smooth outline. Only after penetration of the cyst wall does it become an invasive carcinoma. Penetration beyond the cyst wall can be seen mammographically as irregularity of the margin if visualized tangentially or sonographically. However, small areas of invasion may not be detectable by imaging. The cyst itself frequently contains blood in cases where the invasion has a smooth contour ("blunt invasion"), and even evaluation by a pathologist may be difficult.

Finally, an extensive high-grade DCIS with accompanying periductal desmoplasia may also manifest as a mass or density on mammography.

Specific Clinical Manifestations of Breast Carcinomas

Paget disease of the nipple and inflammatory carcinoma are specific clinical manifestations of breast carcinomas.

Paget carcinoma/Paget disease is an intraepidermal adenocarcinoma in situ of the nipple and areola with or without invasive component. Most cases of Paget carcinoma have an underlying true DCIS of high grade with involvement of retroareolar sinuses and large ducts. An invasive component is found in more than half of patients. Clinically, the epidermal tumor infiltrate induces an inflammatory reaction with erythema, moisture, and ulceration. Cancer (DCIS or invasive) can also be found elsewhere within the breast. In these cases Paget disease is caused by intraductal (mostly noncontiguous) tumor spread through the ductal system. Paget carcinoma of the nipple is diagnosed by cytologic smear of the weeping nipple eczema, punch biopsy, or excisional biopsy of the suspicious lesion. This diagnosis must lead to a thorough search for a carcinoma in the parenchyma away from the nipple.

Inflammatory carcinoma indicates a breast cancer with a very poor prognosis. The underlying carcinoma is usually NST grade 3 with extensive vascular invasion. The diagnosis is made by excisional biopsy, by a punch biopsy of the skin, or by core needle biopsy showing emboli of tumor cells in lymphatic vessels of the dermis, which are responsible for the clinical presentation of edema, erythema, and hyperthermia. Not infrequently punch biopsies or core needle biopsies show only dilated lymphatics without tumors cells, requiring repeated biopsies to confirm the clinical diagnosis and for determining tumor biology (i.e., receptor status and HER2 status) before therapy. Inflammatory carcinoma is treated with neoadjuvant (primary) chemotherapy.

Breast Cancer and Prognosis

As mentioned above, prognosis of breast cancer correlates very well with tumor size, lymph node involvement, and grading (Elston and Ellis 1991, Ellis et al. 1992). There are certain carcinoma types with low-grade malignancy and/or a better prognosis: invasive tubular carcinoma, mixed tubulo-lobular carcinoma, invasive cribriform carcinoma, adenoid cystic carcinoma, endocrine carcinoma (not all variants), medullary carcinoma, and other very rare types.

Further indicators of a good prognosis include positivity for estrogen and progesterone receptors.

Due to the good response to trastuzumab (an antibody to HER2), HER2 positivity meanwhile has become a good prognostic parameter, even though it genuinely is an indicator of less favorable prognosis.

A poor prognosis is usually associated with so-called triple negative carcinomas (testing negative for estrogen receptor, for progesterone receptor, and for HER2).

Based on the excellent reproducibility of the above features, they are considered the main and classic indicators for predicting prognosis (Gusterson 2009, Blamey et al. 2010, Kreipe 2011). Further features which aid prediction of recurrence or metastases include the presence of vascular and lymphatic invasion of the tumor. The prognostic value has also been proven for the presence of isolated tumor cells in the blood or bone marrow. However, the added value so far has not justified their use for routine staging.

To better distinguish prognostically between more versus less favorable tumors additional tests have been developed and propagated. These include testing for PAI and UPA1 (only possible on fresh material or frozen sections) or gene expression tests which include multiple features and Ki67 (e.g., MammaPrint and OncotypeDX) (Stuart-Harris et al. 2008, Kreipe 2011). While the testing for PAI and UPA1 has been recommended, testing of gene profiling with OncotypeDX and MammaPrint is still under discussion.

Based on molecular biology and mRNA expression, profiling a new classification of breast cancers has been proposed. It is hoped that in the future it may allow improved prediction of prognosis and stratification for therapy. However, to date it is not regularly used, since the methods for testing are not yet reliably reproducible and thresholds are still under discussion (Goldhirsch et al. 2011, Kreipe 2011).

With the new classification the distinction of following four types is proposed: Luminal A, Luminal B, Her2 neu positive, and Basal type (Sørlie et al. 2001). When this typing is attempted with the available immunohistological methods (currently not standardized, which would be essential for routine use), the following approximate typing results:

- Luminal A (ER+; Ki67 low—threshold not yet agreed)
- Luminal B (ER+, Ki67 high—threshold not yet agreed)
- HER2-positive
- Basal type (mostly overlapping with triple negative tumors)

Antiestrogen therapy is recommended for Luminal A and B type cancers; HER2 for all HER2-positive tumors, and chemotherapy for all types except Luminal A (Goldhirsch et al. 2011).

Since reproducibility is not yet established, the use of the existing nomenclature is still recommended (e.g., triple negative vs. estrogen/progesterone receptor [ER/PR]-positive, etc.) (Badve et al. 2011).

Clinical Examination

Corresponding to the multifarious histologic presentation, the clinical presentation also varies considerably.

Since mammography, the only screening method, and other imaging methods are not able to detect all breast carcinomas, clinical breast examination remains an important tool for the detection of breast carcinoma. Even though the impact of both self-examination and clinical breast examination on mortality reduction is small compared with imaging, it should be remembered that for certain age groups there is no recommendation for imaging, that interval cancers are mostly detected by self- or clinical breast examination, and that in individual cases even small breast cancers and some DCIS lesions may be detectable as palpable or otherwise apparent clinical findings.

History

In addition to assessing risk factors, attention should be paid to all changes reported by the patient (palpable abnormality, newly developed pain, discharge, nipple changes).

While pain related to the menstrual cycle is common in benign changes, unilaterally localized pain, not related to the menstrual cycle, should be taken seriously, since it may rarely be the only sign of malignancy. Therefore unilateral pain, which may also be caused by benign changes, should always be subject to thorough evaluation.

Taking a detailed history is important, since the risk of malignancy of a lesion partly depends on the lesion characteristics; however, it is also influenced by overall risk factors. Knowledge about preceding surgery or interventions may help avoid misinterpretation of scarring and unnecessary re-interventions. In addition certain information (e.g., bloody nipple discharge) may give hints to questions that require further assessment.

The following recommendations exist for surveillance of asymptomatic women:

- Usual screening is recommended for women at low risk.
- At intermediate risk shorter intervals (usually yearly) and the use of additional methods (mainly ultrasound) may be considered.
- For women at high risk special surveillance and counseling are recommended in some countries.

Women are considered to belong to the high-risk group if lifetime risk exceeds 25–30% or if the woman can be identified as a carrier of a known gene mutation or a known syndrome (see Chapter 1). Furthermore, women are considered to belong to the high-risk group, if radiation treatment was been applied to the chest wall more than 10 years before.

All of these women are presently recommended to obtain genetic counseling and intensified surveillance (see Chapter 5).

The presence of a known mutation or a genetic syndrome is usually assessed by geneticists, who can calculate the probability of being affected or even perform specific blood tests.

Knowledge of the presence of the above-mentioned mutations is important for the carriers and their family members (being potential carriers) for several reasons:

- The monogenic hereditary breast cancers occur at earlier ages than sporadic breast cancers (on average 20 years earlier than sporadic breast cancers), sometimes in very young women and less frequently in older women (> age 55). For *BRCA1* or *BRCA2* carriers affected by breast cancer there is a significant risk of contralateral breast cancer (up to 50%).
- Overall breast cancers associated with the *BRCA1* mutation (and to a lesser degree the *BRCA2* mutation) may be particularly difficult to detect by mammography and ultrasound. Due to this fact and the faster growth rates of many genetic types of breast cancer, different schemes of surveillance are recommended (see Chapter 5).
- Since breast cancers of *BRCA1* carriers tend to be very aggressive, other prophylactic measures may need to be considered: For bilateral prophylactic mastectomy a mortality reduction of 90% has been proven. Bilateral salpingo-oophorectomy allows a 50% reduction in breast cancer incidence and 90% reduction in ovarian cancers. Intensified surveillance may also be discussed with the individual affected woman. However, its mortality reduction is not proven and will not approach that of bilateral mastectomy.

Hereditary breast cancer is often associated with hereditary ovarian cancer and sometimes with other malignancies such as lymphoma, gastrointestinal tumors, pancreatic, lung, bladder, and kidney cancer, prostate cancer in men, and melanoma. The lifetime risk of breast cancer

16 Invasive Carcinoma

among gene carriers ranges around 50–90% and for ovarian cancer around 10–40%. Owing to the high incidence of malignancy with these syndromes and the special features of the associated malignancies, genetic and interdisciplinary counseling and special surveillance is recommended for women that might belong to the high-risk group (National Breast Cancer Care Centre 2006; National Institute for Health and Clinical Excellence, National Collaborating Centre for Primary Care 2006, Schmutzler et al. 2008; Albert et al. 2009). (For identification of risks, see Chapter 1.)

Genetic counseling and testing is important for three reasons:

- If in a high-risk family a certain mutation is proven (e.g., *BRCA1* positivity) and this mutation cannot be detected in the woman, the probability of being a gene carrier and that of being affected by breast cancer drops significantly. (If, however, in a family affected by breast cancer no mutation can be detected, the family might be affected by a yet unknown mutation and the risk of breast cancer for the woman in question cannot be downgraded.)
- Carriers of gene mutations should consider prophylactic measures or increased surveillance for breast cancer and other malignancies.
- There is some evidence emerging that these breast cancers may also require different therapy (including cisplatin, Her2neu or PARP inhibitors) compared with sporadic breast cancers.

To detect women who might be at risk of having a hereditary breast cancer, an adequate history should be taken in every woman. If—based on the family history—hereditary breast cancer might be suspected (see Chapter 1, **Table 1.2**), genetic counseling and testing should be considered.

Inspection and Palpation

While inspecting the patient, *skin retraction* should be looked for. It can be caused by reactive fibrosis that can even be induced by a small carcinoma.

It is noteworthy that retraction can precede a definite palpatory finding.

During the clinical examination, retraction can be elicited by asking the patient to raise her arms and thereafter to lean on them. (By contracting the pectoral muscle, discrete retraction can be accentuated). Finally, the breast must be systematically evaluated for the Jackson phenomenon (see pp. 17 and 78). Any skin retraction must be considered suggestive until proven otherwise and should lead to a thorough evaluation.

Any possible *deviation, decreased erectility of the nipple*, or a definite *retraction of the nipple* should be thoroughly looked for. In particular, unilateral nipple changes must be considered suspicious unless unequivocally explained by scar formation or mastitis. (Bilateral nipple retraction can be associated with the so-called plasma cell mastitis.)

In the presence of moist eczematous changes of the *nipple* or *areola*, Paget disease of the nipple must be excluded at least by cytologic smear, by mammography, including a magnification view of the retroareolar region, and by ultrasound. Unless a definite diagnosis is possible based on these findings, a small biopsy of the involved skin and underlying tissue should be taken.

If malignant cells are detected without suspicious mammographic or sonographic findings, MRI may be considered as a supplement to exclude another malignant focus in the breast. Such a focus may cause Paget disease by seeding of single cells while it is still occult by mammography or ultrasound.

Localized skin changes (edema, erythema, induration, peau d'orange) overlying a palpatory finding can be evidence of tumor infiltration.

Diffuse skin changes, such as thickening, edema, and erythema, as well as peau d'orange and induration of the breast, warrant the exclusion of an inflammatory carcinoma unless it can be definitely explained by an underlying benign condition (mastitis), which should resolve completely after adequate antibiotic therapy. Inflammatory changes that do not resolve with antibiotics must be considered suspicious until proven otherwise.

Palpation (technique, see Chapter 2) must pay attention to any area different from its surroundings or from the corresponding area of the contralateral breast. It should be remembered that breast carcinomas do not always present as discrete nodules. Often only a diffuse, viscous (rubberlike) consistency and impaired moveability of the soft tissue is found. Some medullary and mucinous carcinomas, as well as the phyllodes tumor when it is still small, can be relatively soft to palpation. Some of these malignancies are also moveable.

Each palpatory abnormality must be correlated with the image presentation. Vice versa, it may be helpful to review mammographically and sonographically abnormal areas in context with the palpatory finding.

A palpatory finding larger than the corresponding mammographic finding increases the suspicion of a carcinoma since many scirrhous carcinomas elicit a palpable reaction in the surrounding area. However, a mammographically large density immediately under the skin without a corresponding palpatory finding reduces the likelihood of a malignancy.

Any spontaneous abnormal nipple discharge that is hemorrhagic or clear, cytologically suspicious, or unilateral, or attributable to a single duct needs further evaluation. On the contrary, discharge that occurs only after strong compression or manipulation is not considered suspicious and does not require further evaluation. Manipulation, which may be done by some patients regularly in the misunderstanding that ducts should be "emptied," provokes secretion and should be stopped.

It is worthwhile obtaining a *cytologic smear* in the evaluation of every spontaneous unilateral nonmilky discharge despite the unreliability of a negative cytologic finding and the cytologic evaluation of nipple discharge in general. The smear cytology can be repeated at any time and occasionally discovers nonmalignant causes underlying a persistent galactorrhea.

Regardless of the cytologic findings, the source of the pathologic discharge must be further assessed by imaging (usually ultrasound, mammography, and if needed galactography). Rarely (if galactography is impossible) MRI may be necessary.

Mammography

Mammographically, invasive carcinoma—corresponding to its various histologic patterns—has many features.

Since mammography is the only primary imaging modality for breast screening, it is particularly important to know the various presentations of breast carcinomas.

While spiculated and nodular breast carcinomas are diagnosed without difficulty in fatty breasts, it is a challenge even for the experienced mammographer (1) to detect invasive carcinoma in its early stage when its features are often still indeterminate, (2) to find carcinoma without microcalcifications within dense tissue, and, in particular, (3) to diagnose the diffusely spreading carcinoma.

Table 16.1 summarizes the direct and indirect findings for detecting focally growing invasive breast carcinomas.

The listed findings can be present alone or in combination (**Fig. 16.1**).

Before explaining and illustrating these findings further, the principles that govern the radiographic density of breast carcinomas will be briefly discussed.

Radiographic Density of Breast Carcinomas

(See **Fig. 16.2**.)

All breast carcinomas visible as density have a higher mass attenuation coefficient than fat. The mass attenuation coefficient can also be higher than that of parenchyma, though this only applies, unfortunately, to some carcinomas. Indeed, only about half of carcinomas have

Table 16.1 Mammographic signs of breast carcinoma

Direct signs of a focally growing invasive carcinoma
1. Focal lesion of increased density in comparison with the parenchyma
2. Focal lesion equal in density in comparison with the parenchyma
   The outline of the density can be:
   - Spiculated or irregular
   - Similar to parenchyma, lobulated, geographically ill defined (= indeterminate mass)
   - Round or rarely entirely smooth
3. Microcalcifications (with or without surrounding soft-tissue density)
4. Distorted architecture
5. Asymmetry in comparison with the contralateral side
(6. Single dilated duct)

Indirect signs of a focally growing invasive carcinoma (secondary signs of malignancy)
1. Nipple retraction (sometimes only mammographically apparent)
2. Local retraction of the skin or the parenchyma overlying the lesion
3. Thickening of Cooper ligaments in the vicinity of the lesion (subcutaneous or prepectoral)
4. Local thickening of skin overlying the lesion
5. Trabecular thickening in the subcutaneous space or in the prepectoral adipose tissue
6. Retraction or fixation on the pectoral muscle
7. Enlarged, multiple, homogeneously dense, smoothly or unsharply outlined lymph nodes in the axillary extension

Signs of a diffusely growing carcinoma
1. Diffuse microcalcifications
2. Diffuse density, hyperdense in comparison with the contralateral parenchyma
3. Diffuse density, isodense in comparison with the parenchyma, but asymmetric in location compared with the contralateral side
4. Contour deformity
5. Thickened Cooper ligaments
6. Distorted architecture
7. Indistinctness of the structures of the mammary tissue
8. Trabecular–reticular marking in the subcutaneous and prepectoral fatty tissue
9. Skin thickening (generally in inflammatory carcinoma)

16 Invasive Carcinoma

a Spiculated mass or architectural distortion

Spiculated mass with center (frequent)

Indistinctly outlined mass (frequent)

Spiculated mass or architectural distortion without central mass

b Lobulated mass

Visualized in two views

Visualized because of atypical location

Visualized as asymmetry

Visualized through changes on serial examinations

As neodensity

By increase in size

By decrease in size and retraction

c Nodular mass

Not entirely smoothly outlined, sometimes with microlobulation

Smoothly outlined with indistinct areas

Smoothly outlined (< 2 % of all malignancies)

d Suspicious morphology of microcalcifications

Pleomorphism of the individual calcification (linear or granular)

Casting rod-like, V-, or Y-shaped individual calcifications (multiple or in one group) with irregular shape

Any uncharacteristic area of microcalcifications with significant change

e Suggestive distribution of microcalcifications

Ductal distribution

Segmental distribution

Regional distribution

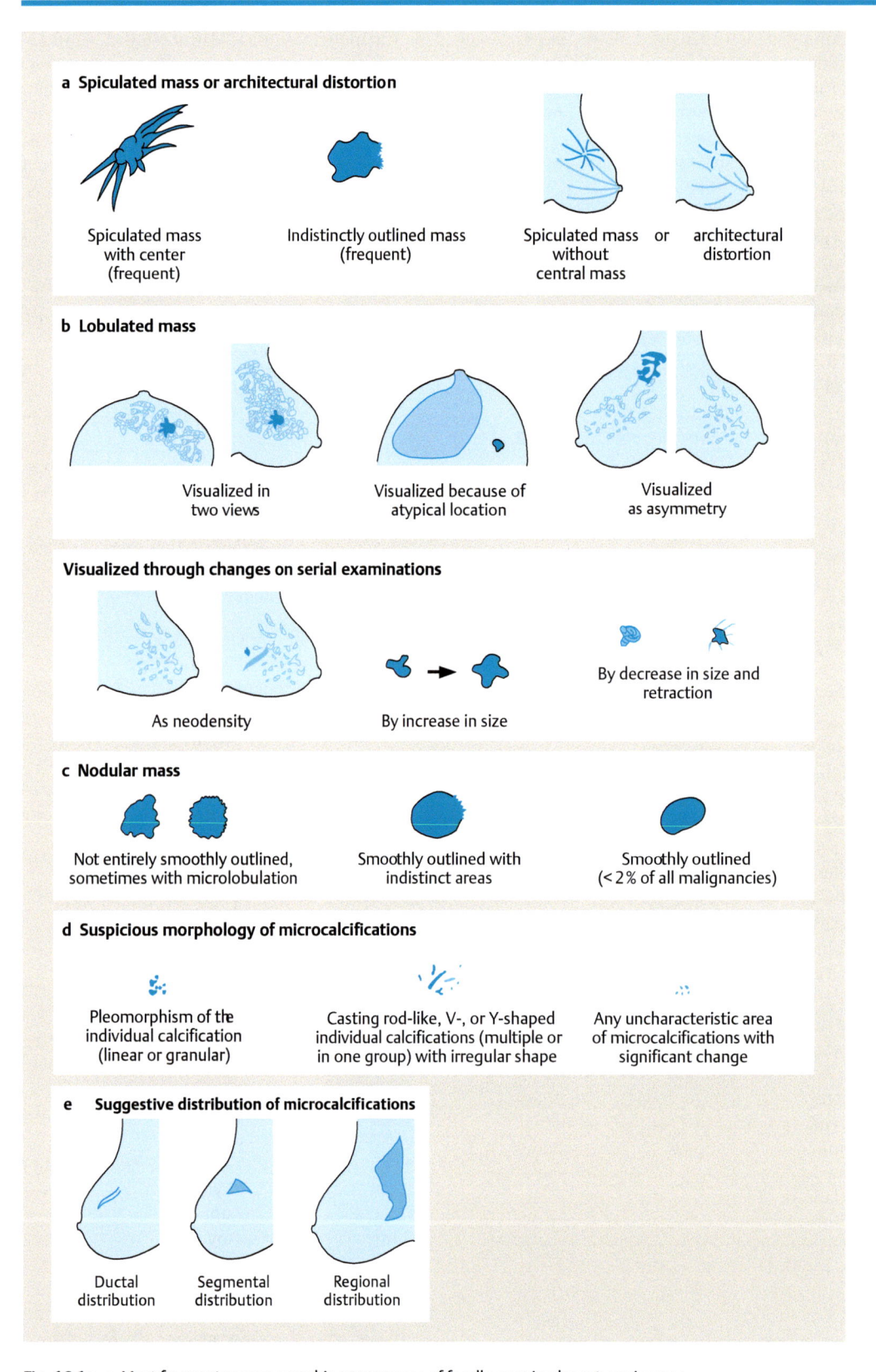

Fig. 16.1a–e Most frequent mammographic appearances of focally growing breast carcinomas.
- **a** Spiculated and/or indistinctly outlined mass.
- **b** Lobulated mass.
- **c** Nodular mass.
- **d** Malignant microcalcifications.
- **e** Suggestive distribution of microcalcifications.

a higher attenuation than parenchyma, while the parenchyma may well show considerable variation in its attenuation. The remaining carcinomas have equal or even less mass attenuation in comparison with parenchyma or dense tissue (**Fig. 16.2h,i,l,m**) (Jackson et al. 1991).

In particular, early carcinomas frequently have the same density as parenchyma. In those cases, other morphological criteria are important (configuration, architectural distortion, asymmetry, secondary signs of malignancy, etc.).

Furthermore, mammographically increased density can be technical in nature. In the majority of cases, areas with increased density found in the normal mammogram are caused by the summation of several parenchymal lobules or lobules of dense tissue.

Foci with truly increased radiodensity must be identifiable in several planes. Otherwise, the increased radiodensity only represents superimposition.

Direct Signs of Focally Invasive Breast Carcinoma

(See **Fig. 16.2a–m.**)

A schematic summary of the most frequent features of the focal breast carcinoma is presented in **Fig. 16.1**.

The *focal, irregularly outlined, and spiculated mass* is a very important and frequent sign of breast carcinoma. If surrounded by adipose tissue or tissue of less density, such a change can be perceived very early (**Fig. 16.2a**).

In mammographically dense tissue, these carcinomas are often detected by their spiculated extensions, that is, their characteristic morphology (**Fig. 16.2b,c**). Some of them may present with increased density in comparison with the surrounding parenchyma. As already stated, this increased density is neither necessary nor confirmatory.

Some carcinomas show a *lobulated parenchyma-like growth pattern*. Some of these carcinomas are recognized by increased density, while others are recognized only by a disturbance of the normal distribution pattern of the parenchyma, by architectural distortion, by asymmetry, or by atypical location (**Fig. 16.2d,e,h,i,l,m**).

Depending on the severity of the changes, size of the lesion, and density of the surrounding tissue, these indistinct masses may or may not be readily identifiable. Magnification mammography, palpatory findings, sonography, MRI, and percutaneous biopsy help in their detection and differentiation.

Again, depending on the density of surrounding tissues, *nodular, round or oval shaped carcinomas may or may not be readily visible*.

Medullary, mucinous, papillary in situ, including intracystic papillary carcinomas are characteristically nodular or smoothly outlined carcinomas. Because of its high prevalence, however, ductal carcinoma NST is the most frequent oval carcinoma. Whereas medullary and mucinous, and, of course, papillary in situ and intracystic carcinomas are usually associated with a better prognosis, ductal carcinomas with nodular or rounded contours tend to be of higher grade (often grade 3) than carcinomas which exhibit spiculations. (Invasive papillary and micropapillary carcinomas are rare and do not usually present as well-circumscribed nodules. Other non-carcinomatous malignancies that can present as round masses include malignant lymphomas, phyllodes tumors, malignant lymph nodes, and rare sarcomas of the breast, as well as metastases.)

Because of the frequent benign round lesions (mastopathic nodules, fibroadenomas), the differentiation of these round carcinomas from the many benign findings with similar presentation can be difficult, compromising their detection (**Fig. 16.2n–s**).

In the approximately 5–10% of the carcinomas that show a round growth pattern, some indistinctness of the contour is often observed and, until proven otherwise, should be considered a sign of malignancy. It is rare that carcinomas exhibit an entirely smooth outline or are surrounded by a halo (**Fig. 16.2s**; see also **Fig. 16.9**).

Actually, less than 2% of the lesions that are entirely smooth in outline are malignant (Sickles 1994). This implies that all nodular or round lesions with a contour that is not entirely distinct need further evaluation. If considered suspicious (e.g., increase in size), even lesions with entirely smooth outlines need further workup.

As a general rule, multiple lesions mostly indicate benign changes. In the case of single smooth lesions further workup should be considered in cases with increased density, new growth, or an increase in size as compared with prior studies. Follow-up examinations at intervals of 6, 12 and 24 months are sufficient for those focal lesions that are smoothly outlined.

Depending on the radiodensity and composition of the surrounding tissue and of the carcinoma itself, not all focal carcinomas are visible as focal densities. They can be obscured by or be equal to—and indistinguishable from—dense surrounding tissue.

Therefore, it is important to look for other signs, such as distorted architecture, and asymmetry, as well as for any possible secondary signs of malignancy (see **Table 16.1**). Very rarely a single dilated duct may be the only hint of a carcinoma.

Finding architectural distortion and asymmetry means looking for distortion of normal structures:
- Looking for masses (which can resemble parenchyma) outside the normal parenchymal distribution. Most parenchymal tissue is in the upper outer quadrant and extends toward the nipple. Any parenchyma-like density in atypical location (asymmetry in comparison with the contralateral side, increased density anterior, medial, and especially, deep to the parenchyma) needs special attention. Thorough evaluation, including comparison with prior studies, additional projections, spot compression views and ultrasound imaging should be considered (**Fig. 16.2k–m**).
- Looking for any distortion in the usual course of the

16 Invasive Carcinoma

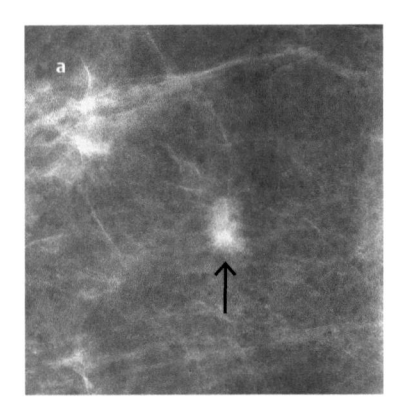

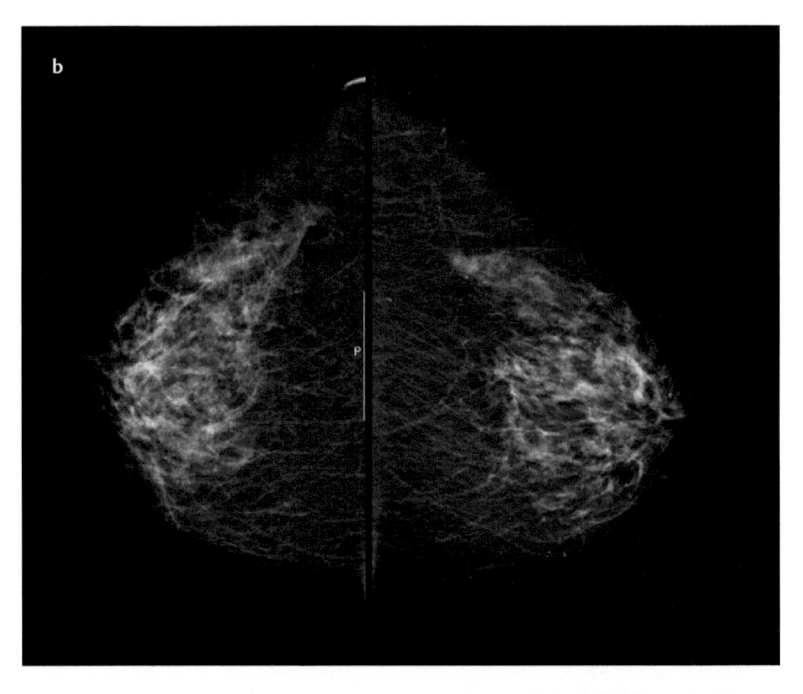

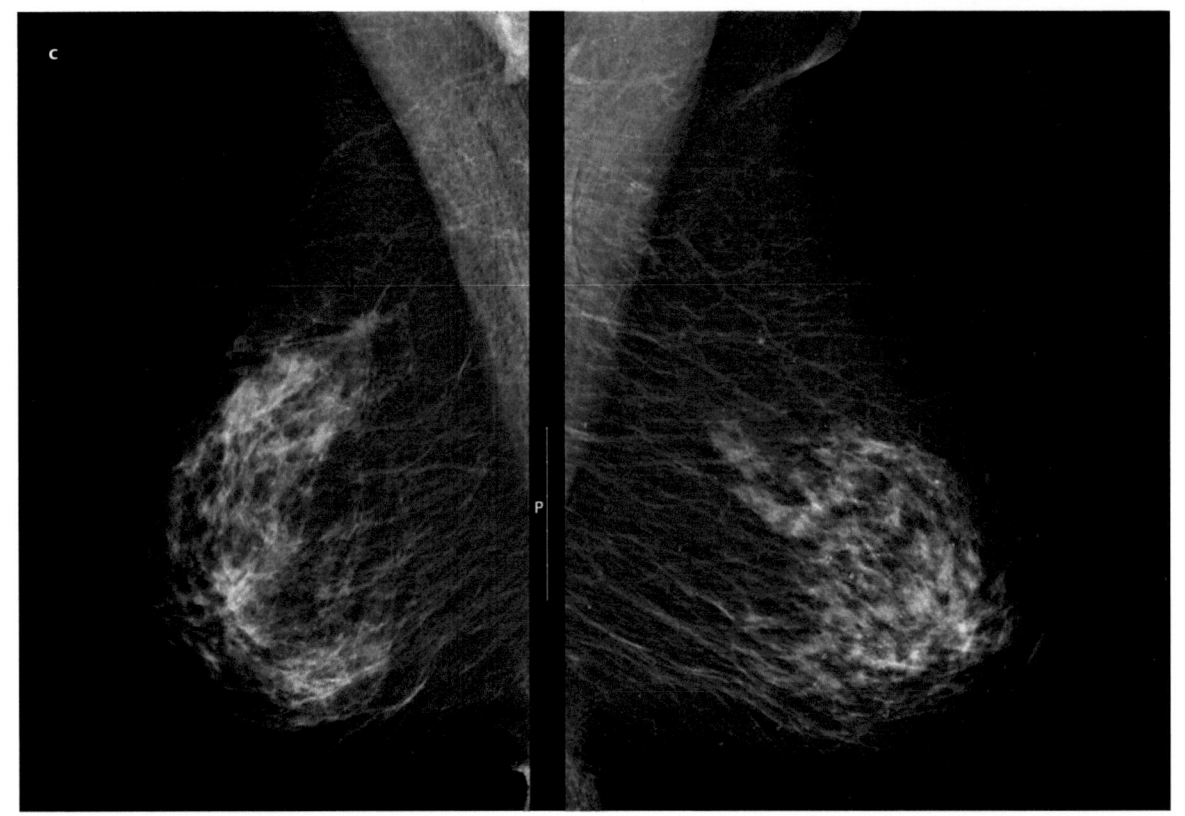

Fig. 16.2a–w Focally growing carcinomas.

a   Spiculated small mass, typical of malignancy. *Histology*: Small ductal carcinoma with tubular differentiation.

b,c   Oblique and craniocaudal views of a spiculated *ductal scirrhous carcinoma* at the posterolateral margin of the breast parenchyma of the patient's right breast (arrow). The carcinoma is easily discernible by its spiculation and its location (atypical site for normal tissue) at the periphery of the parenchyma on the mediolateral oblique and craniocaudal views. (The slightly increased density at the posterolateral edge of the breast tissue on the left craniocaudal view resolves completely on the left mediolateral oblique view and is thus explained as superimposition.)

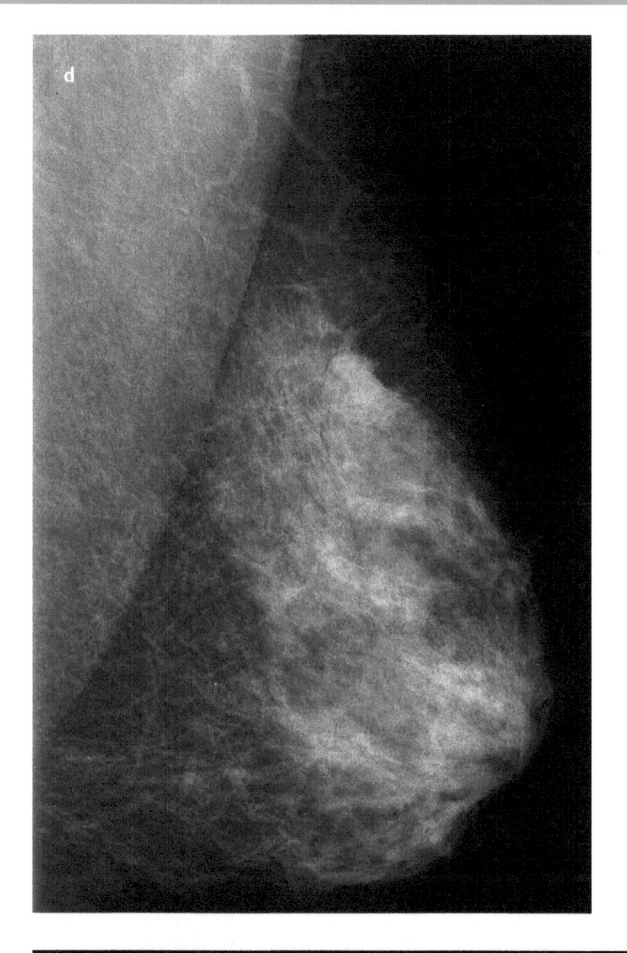

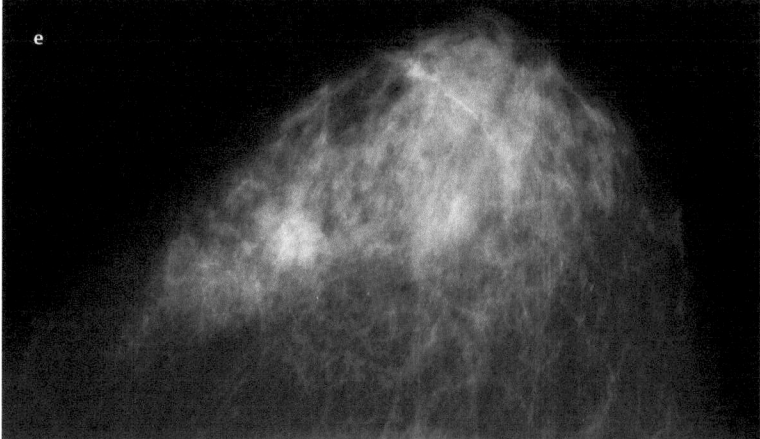

d,e Oblique and craniocaudal views of a ductal carcinoma that mimics the lobular architecture. On the mediolateral oblique view the mass is apparent by its increased density. Very faint spiculations may be perceived. Note the slight retraction of the glandular tissue over the carcinoma. On the craniocaudal view, the ducts appear to converge toward the mass, disturbing their usual orientation toward the nipple.

Fig. 16.2f–w ▷

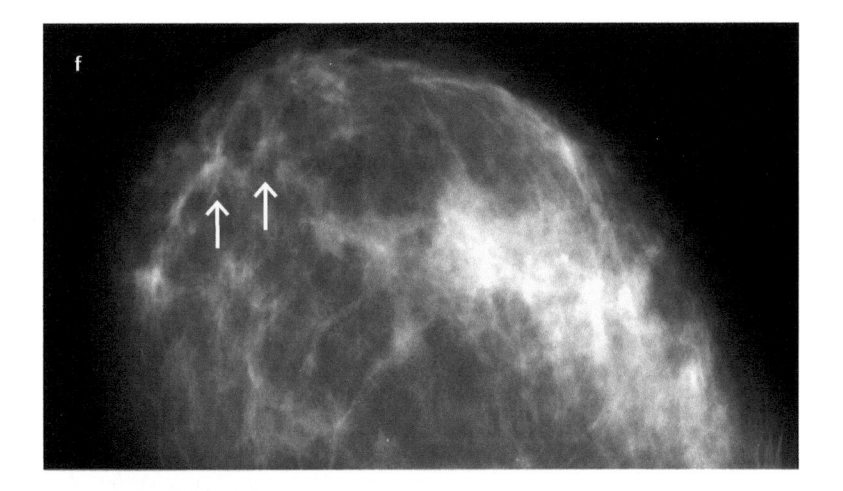

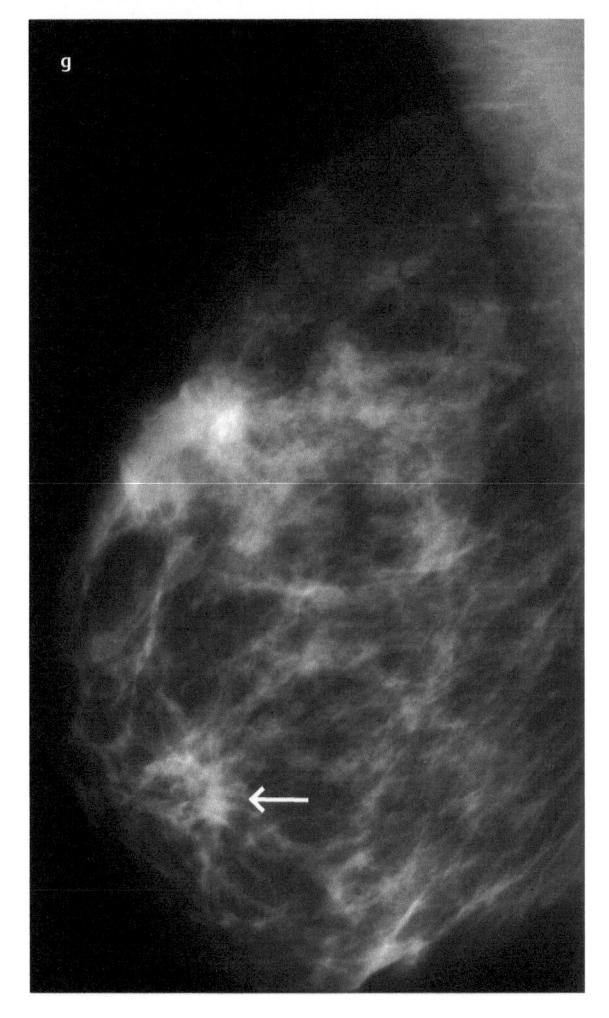

f,g This patient presented with a palpable thickening medial to the nipple. Even though the tissue in the upper outer quadrant is denser than in the area of the palpable abnormality, the latter is suspicious: while the tissue density is not increased on the craniocaudal view the ducts appear to converge toward two centers located ~3 cm behind the nipple (arrows). The ducts are thus disturbed during their course toward the nipple. On the mediolateral view this area appears dense, partly due to superimposition of the two centers shown in the craniocaudal view. Except for the architectural distortion, this lobular carcinoma imitates breast tissue very well.

Mammography

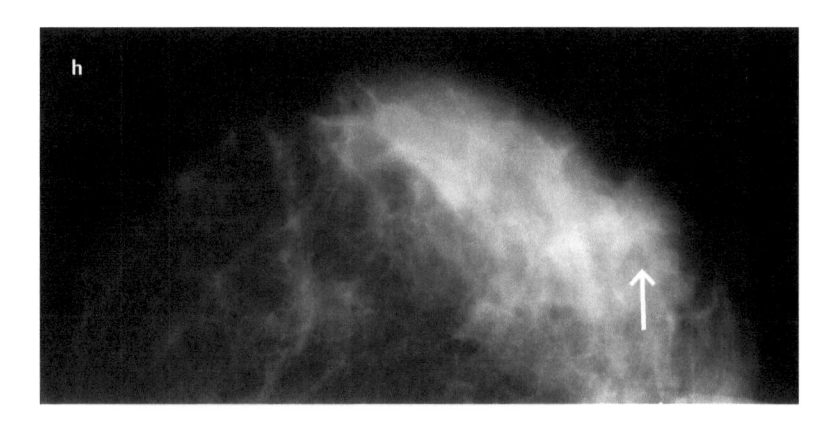

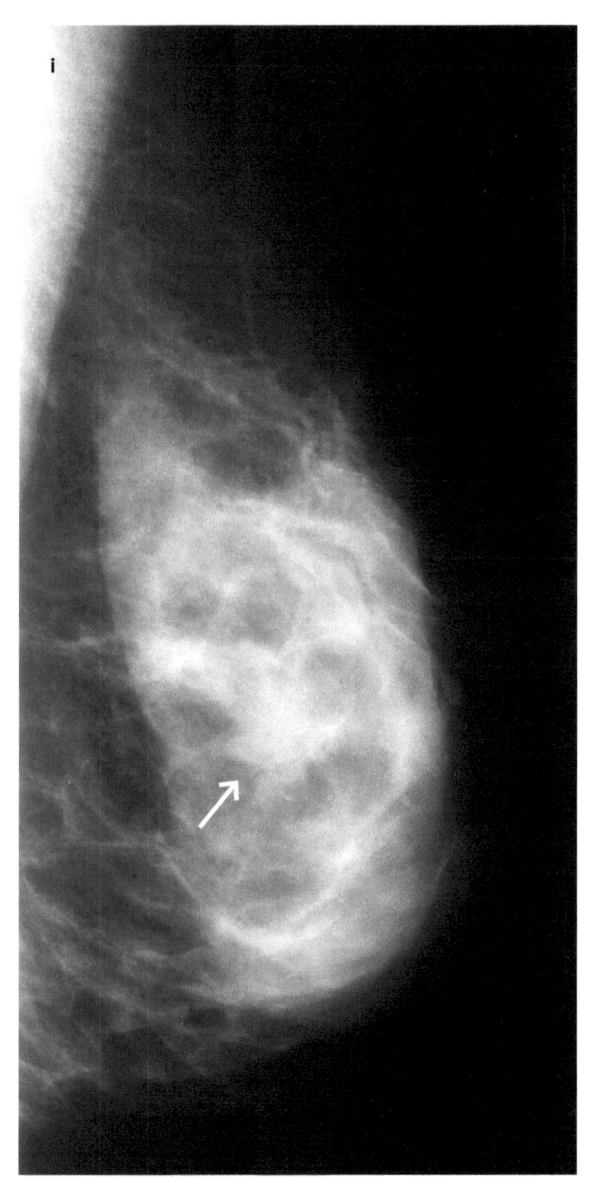

h,i In dense breast tissue carcinomas may be completely obscured. In this case the carcinoma is visible (arrows) in both views as an irregular mass. It is only difficult to perceive since it has identical density to the breast tissue. It does not show retraction, but the usual architecture of ducts converging toward the nipple is disturbed. *Histology*: Ductal breast cancer (NST).

Fig. 16.2l–w ▷

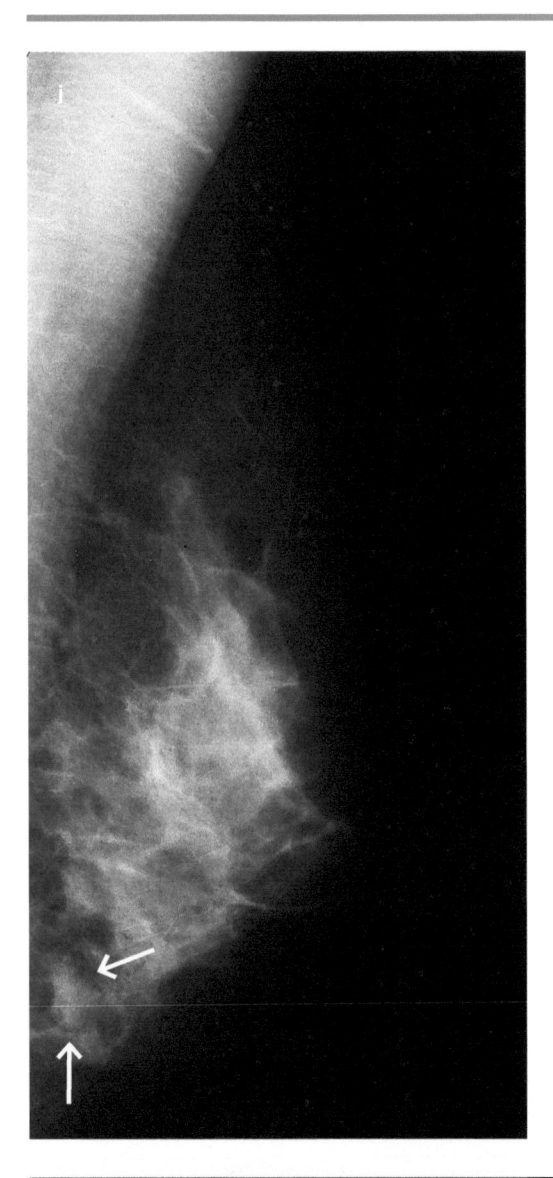

◁ continued

j *Invasive ductal carcinoma* NST G3, isodense with the glandular tissue. The nodular carcinoma (arrows) is not reliably distinguishable from other nodules in breast tissue.

k Same carcinoma as shown in **Fig. 16.2i**. In the craniocaudal view (medially exaggerated), it is conspicuously delineated by its location deep to the parenchyma. Asymmetric densities in the retromammary fat are to be considered suspect until proven otherwise.

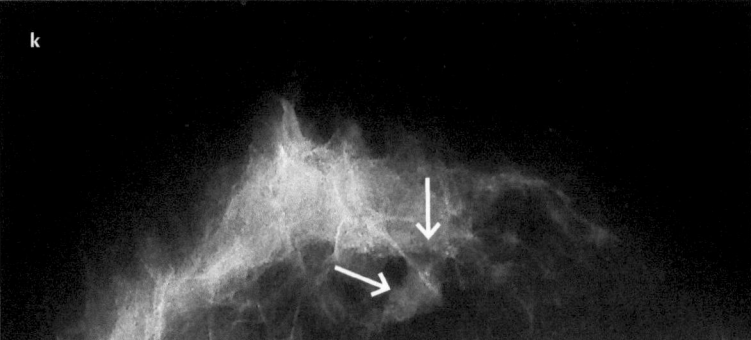

Mammography

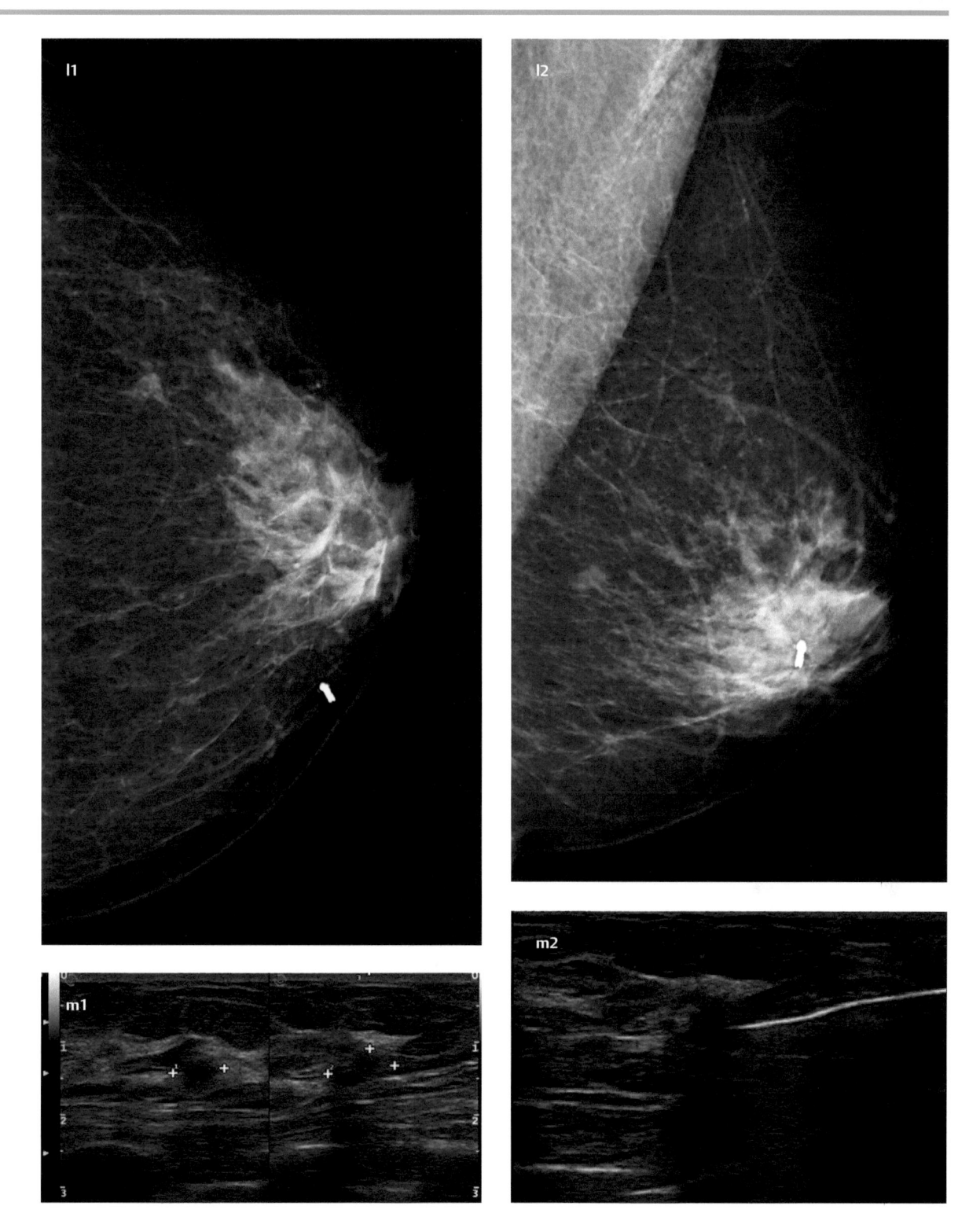

l   Screening mammogram of an asymptomatic patient with a subtle uncharacteristic finding in the "no man's land" (the area anterior to the pectoral muscle, which should contain fatty tissue), craniocaudal and mediolateral oblique views.

m   The finding in **Fig 16.2l** is very subtle on ultrasound, as well. Ultrasound-guided core biopsy proved an invasive ductal carcinoma.

Fig. 16.2n–w ▷

16 Invasive Carcinoma

◁ continued

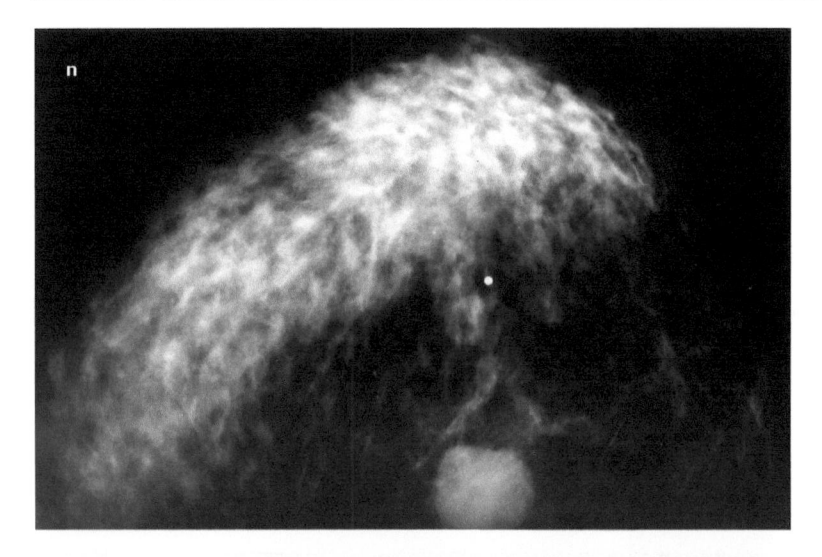

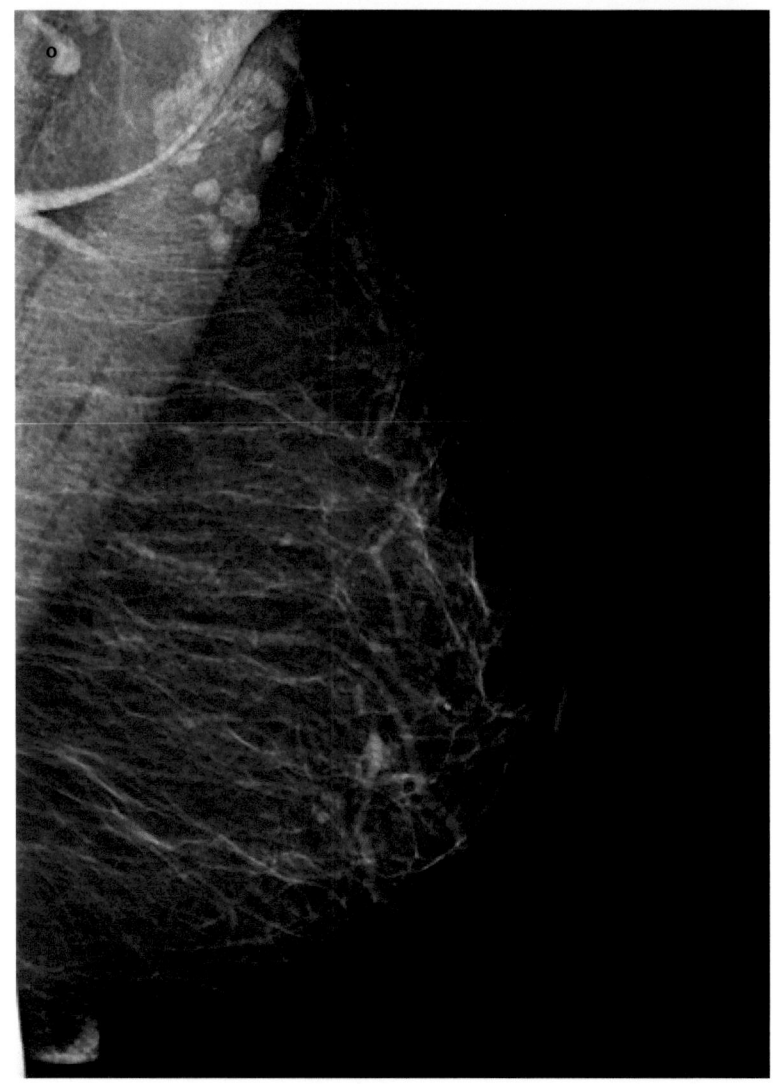

n A round fairly well-circumscribed mass is seen. Biopsy is warranted since it was newly developed. *Histology*: Invasive ductal carcinoma (NST G3). Ductal carcinomas (mostly NST G3, often triple negative, and often carcinomas with medullary features) are the most frequent histology encountered among well-circumscribed carcinomas.

o–q Screening patient with a small round and only partly well-defined mass at 9 o'clock position (**o,p**). On ultrasound (**q**) it is hypoechoic and fairly well defined. The lesion itself is not vascularized. However, numerous vessels are seen in the surroundings. *Histology* verified a mucinous carcinoma.

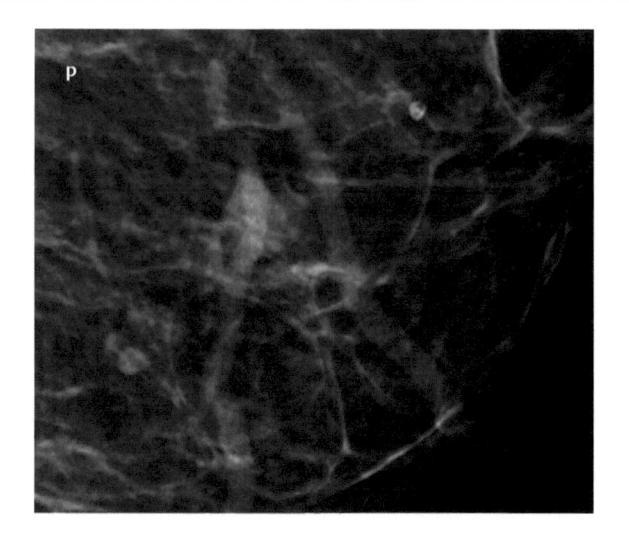

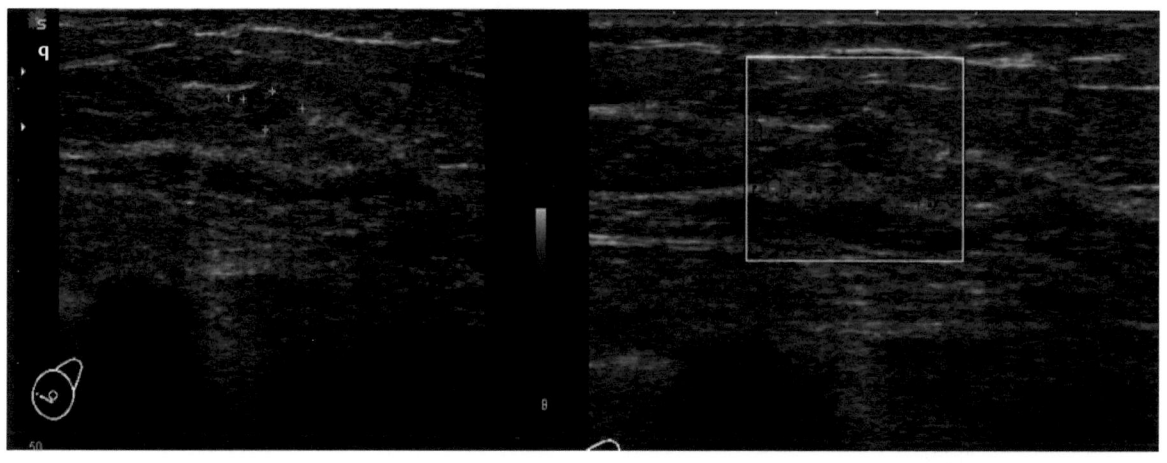

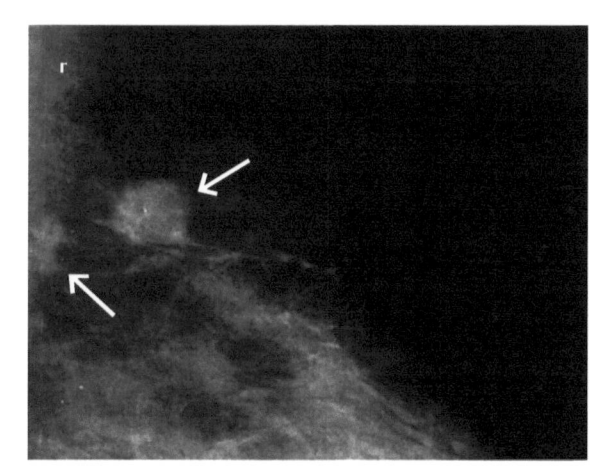

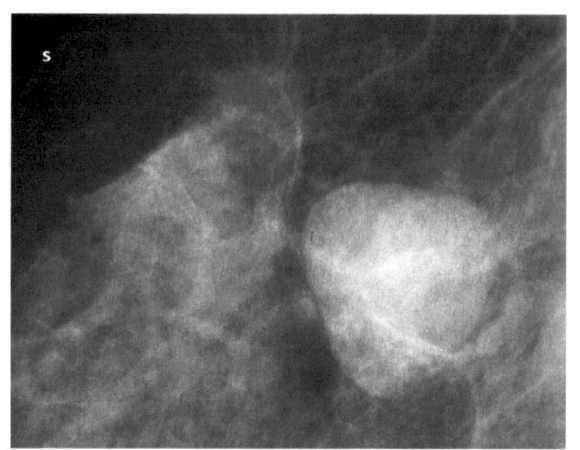

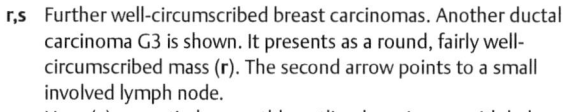

Mammography

r,s Further well-circumscribed breast carcinomas. Another ductal carcinoma G3 is shown. It presents as a round, fairly well-circumscribed mass (**r**). The second arrow points to a small involved lymph node.
Here (**s**), an entirely smoothly outlined carcinoma with halo is shown. Despite the smooth outline and a relatively soft moveable lesion on palpation, it is not a benign lesion but a *mucinous carcinoma*. The lesion was newly discovered in this 63-year-old patient.

Fig. 16.2t–w ▷

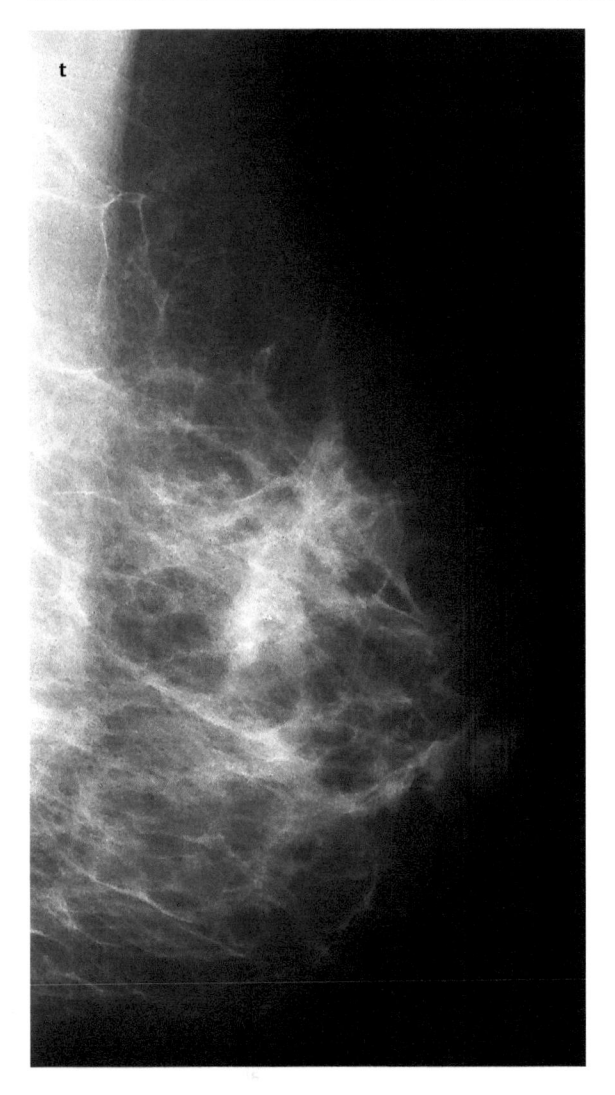

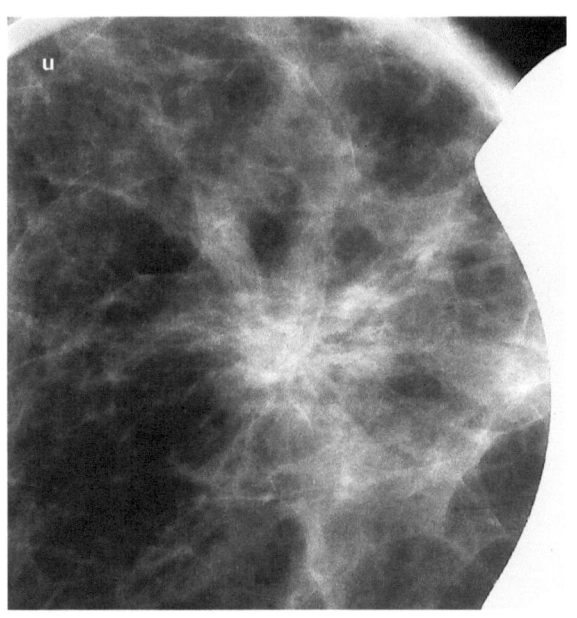

t,u Invasive ductal carcinoma with distorted architecture. The oblique view shows an increased density. The course of the ductal structures toward the nipple is altered, and these structures appear to converge toward this area. This impression is confirmed by the magnification view (**u**), which better demonstrates this spiculated mass.

parenchyma toward the nipple. Such distortions are suspicious, regardless of whether a real center can be recognized or not (**Fig. 16.2t–w**).
- Looking for any retractive changes in the parenchyma (**Fig. 16.2d**).
- Looking for secondary signs of malignancy in the skin and subcutaneous tissue (**Table 16.1**; see also **Fig. 16.4a,b**).

The likelihood of malignancy based on these signs depends primarily on their severity. If any of these signs is present and cannot be explained (e.g., a scar), they must be further evaluated (mammographic compression views, additional projections, repeat and targeted palpation, sonography, MRI, and—if indicated—histopathologic assessment).

A very rare sign of malignancy is the appearance of a single dilated duct. Multiple dilated ducts, in contrast, are usually caused by benign changes (such as duct ectasia or papillomas). The likelihood of malignancy increases with additional suggestive findings (microcalcifications, ductal discharge, progressing nodularity, or retraction (**Fig. 16.3**).

Detection of microcalcifications, which are usually associated with the DCIS component within or around invasive carcinomas, may be of great importance for the detection of invasive carcinomas. Depending on patient selection, microcalcifications are associated with 30–40% of invasive carcinomas.

This means that microcalcifications are important evidence for diagnosing a carcinoma, but they are by no means mandatory for such a diagnosis.

The malignant criteria for microcalcifications found in invasive carcinomas correspond to those found in carcinomas in situ and are, therefore, only briefly repeated here (**Table 16.1** and **Fig. 16.3**).

Linear, V-shaped, and Y-shaped calcifications as intraductal casts are very suggestive of malignancy.

Clustered, larger granular, pleomorphic calcifications, usually ranging between 0.3 mm and 2 mm, are strongly

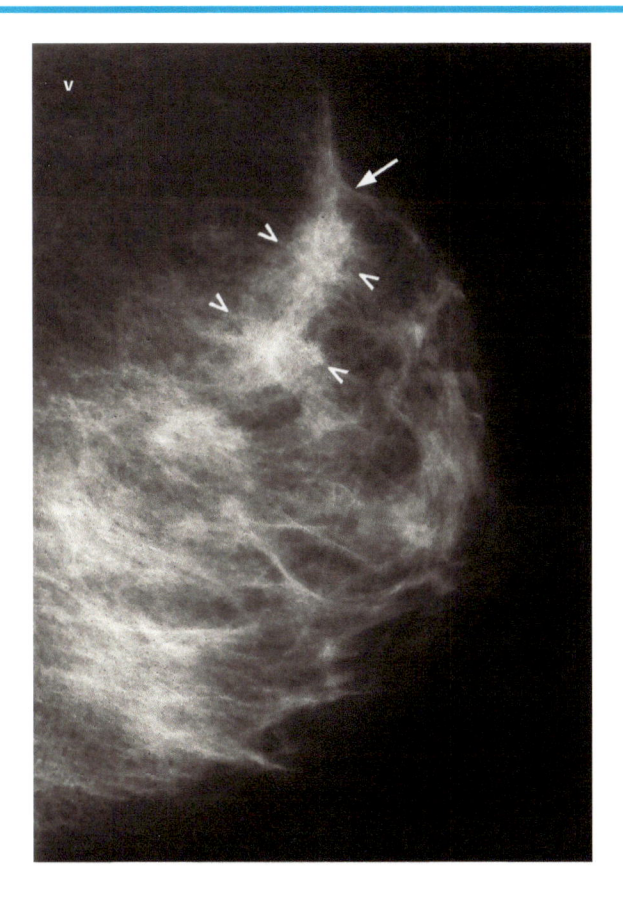

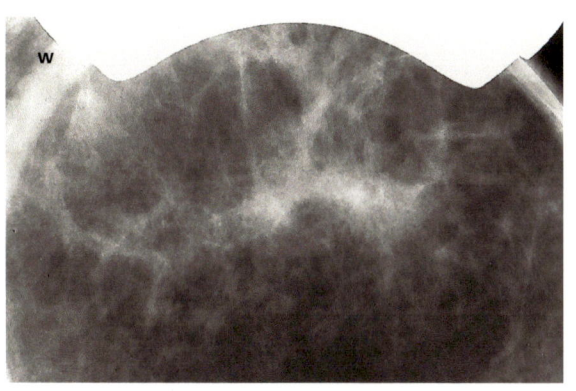

v,w Only the mediolateral view disclosed a suspicious dense area (arrowheads). In addition to the density, the subcutaneous fascia is displaced by a focal retraction. The magnification craniocaudal view confirms the presence of an area of slightly increased density, which persists despite spot compression. The excisional biopsy revealed an intraductal carcinoma with early invasion.

suspicious for malignancy. Furthermore, fine granular calcifications ≤0.3 mm that follow a segmental distribution may be indicative of malignancy, in particular, if they are new. Any distribution pattern (segmental or ductal) that suggests a ductal origin of the microcalcifications must be considered suspicious for malignancy.

Indeterminate microcalcifications are more worrisome if they are clearly localized and asymmetric to the contralateral side. Microcalcifications which increase or appear newly in comparison with the previous examination require special attention (see **Fig. 16.8g,h**), even if there are only a few calcifications.

Calcifications that are clearly benign (e.g., coarse calcifications), however, do not need to undergo biopsy.

An associated soft-tissue density (if it is distinguishable from dense tissue) may be an additional sign of malignancy, in particular, if it is irregularly outlined or if it follows the ductal structures (see **Fig. 16.3**).

Whenever the mass or the microcalcifications or both appear suspicious, further evaluation is indicated.

Surrounding soft-tissue density does not indicate that a carcinoma is invasive. Though such a soft-tissue density may be caused by invasion, it can also represent reactive fibrosis induced by DCIS without invasion. Absent soft-tissue density does not exclude an invasive growth.

Indirect Signs (Secondary Criteria of Malignancy) of Focally Growing Invasive Carcinomas

Secondary signs of malignancy (**Table 16.1**) often *accompany advanced breast carcinomas*. Together with a focal finding, they increase the likelihood of malignancy (**Figs. 16.4, 16.5, 16.6**) and *often suggest a widespread extension*:
- Nipple retraction with extension into the subareolar space or even nipple
- Reticular subcutaneous thickening, thickening of Cooper ligaments with extension into the subcutaneous space or into the prepectoral adipose tissue
- Skin thickening or retraction with extension into the skin
- Retraction or fixation on the musculature with extension into the musculature
- Axillary adenopathy

These signs, however, do not prove direct infiltration. They can be caused by *reactive changes* (retraction or edema) *in the vicinity of a carcinoma*, for example:
- Dimpling and retraction of the skin caused by reactive fibrosis affecting the tissues surrounding the tumor
- Parenchymal retraction along the subcutaneous or retromammary fascia caused by reactive fibrotic strands

16 Invasive Carcinoma

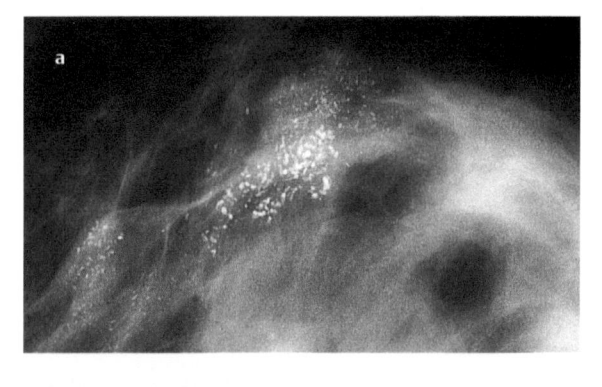

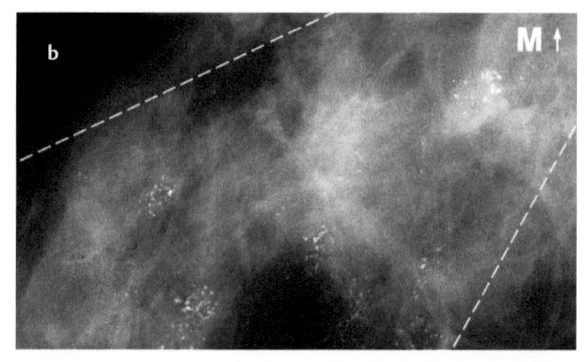

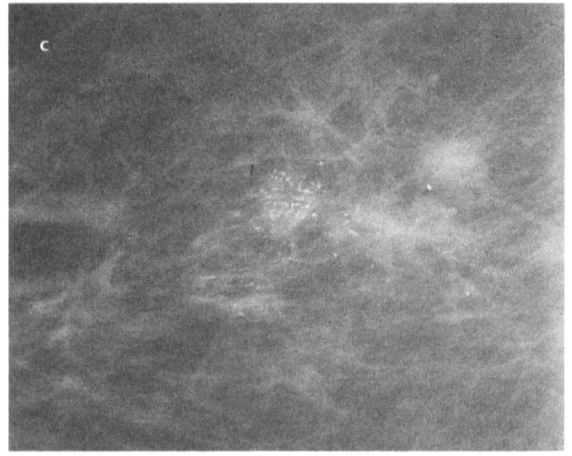

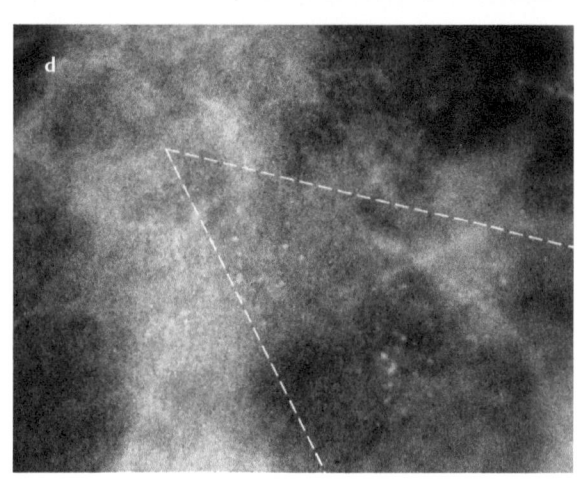

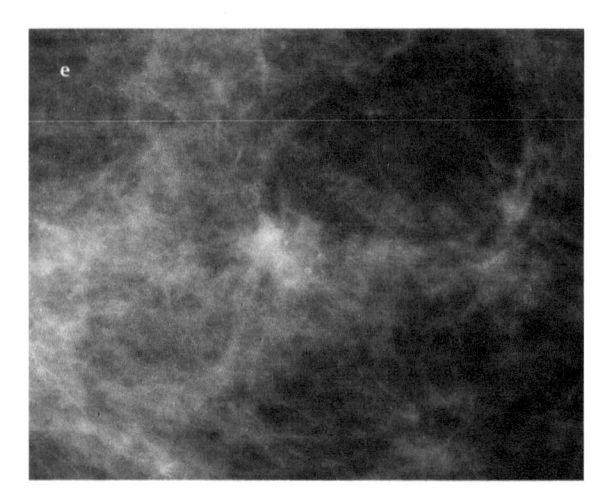

Fig. 16.3a–g Malignant microcalcifications as evidence of a carcinoma.

a Extensive pleomorphic granular microcalcifications measuring up to 2 mm in diameter. These microcalcifications are characteristic of a carcinoma. Rarely do early calcifying fibroadenomas exhibit similar individual forms. The typical distribution along the ducts (segmental) is consistent with malignancy: *Histologically*, invasive ductal carcinoma with extensive in situ comedo component. Concomitant soft-tissue changes—if present—are indistinguishable from the dense surrounding tissue.

b Very pleomorphic microcalcifications. Despite the almost round configuration of individual clusters, the overall pattern is clearly suspicious for malignancy: Extensive pleomorphism, several elongated, in part very fine calcifications (casts), and a segmental arrangement (triangular configuration) with the apex pointing toward the nipple (M). Extensive carcinoma in situ with microcalcifications.

c Fine microcalcifications with typical elongated casts. Also in this case, the calcifications are oriented along the ductal system toward the nipple (not visualized). There may be some minimal associated architectural distortion and soft-tissue density. *Histology*: Comedo ductal carcinoma in situ.

d Extremely fine, granular microcalcifications, barely discernible (twice the magnification of that shown in (**c**), with minimal pleomorphism. They are less typical of a carcinoma than those shown in (**a–c**) and similar calcifications are also found in the various benign changes. *Histology*: Ductal carcinoma with extensive intraductal component.

e An irregularly outlined mass with microcalcifications is suggestive of a carcinoma, even if it contains only a few or uncharacteristic calcifications. *Histology*: Ductal carcinoma, 6 mm.

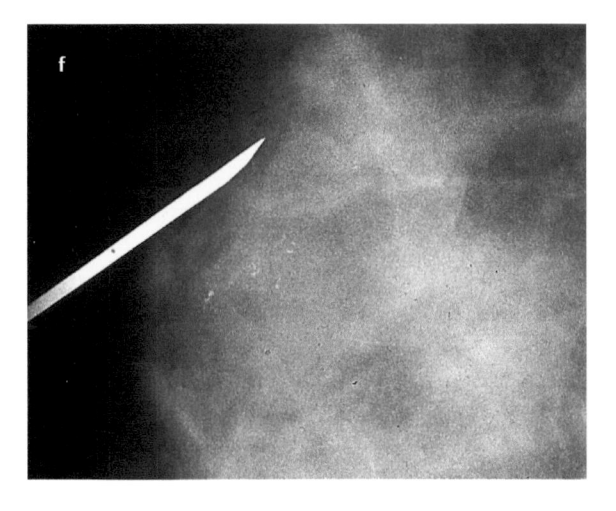

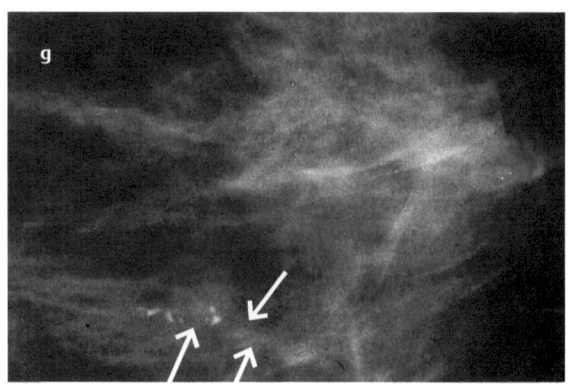

f,g Less characteristic groups of microcalcifications as evidence of malignancy. In particular, the analysis is limited with only very few tiny microcalcifications. Because of their pleomorphism and clustering, they were biopsied. **f** Intraductal non-comedo carcinoma with microinvasion (the trace of a segmental distribution as well as individual casting elongated forms should be noted). **g** Subtle ductal thickening and typical arrangement of very few pleomorphic calcifications with a ductal distribution. Small ductal breast carcinoma.

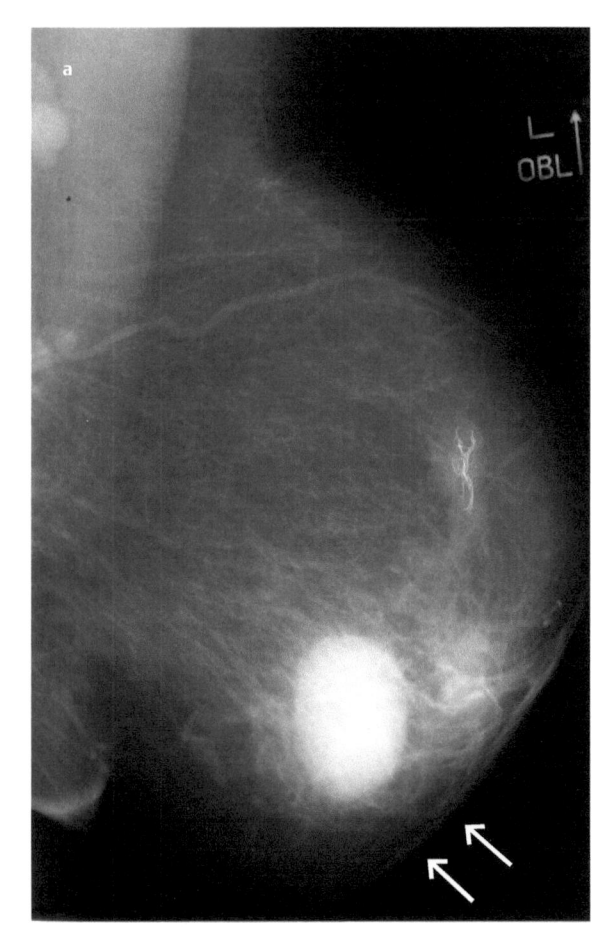

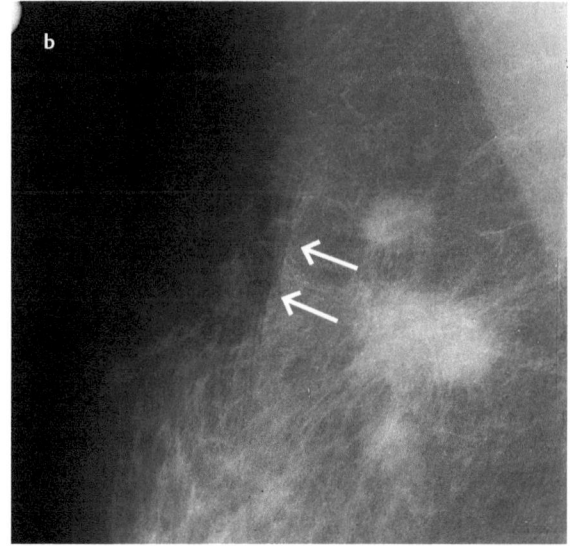

Fig. 16.4a,b Secondary signs of malignancy.

a   A large oval mass is shown in the lower aspect of this breast (arrows). The lesion has spiculations. Furthermore, there is increased interstitial density around the lesion compatible with lymphangiosis. The lower aspect of the breast is flattened; the overlying skin and also the Cooper ligaments are thickened. Note the dense axillary lymph nodes. The faint density and the bizarre dystrophic calcifications in the upper breast are due to previous trauma.
b   A large, spiculated carcinoma has retracted adjacent breast tissue and the overlying skin (arrows).

- Nipple retraction caused by reactive fibrotic strands (**Fig. 16.5**)
- Thickening confined to Cooper ligaments caused by reactive fibrosis and peri-tumoral edema
- Reticular linear thickening in the subcutaneous or prepectoral fatty tissue caused by lymphedema

Finally, such changes can also be observed in nonmalignant findings, such as scars, inflammatory changes, or fat necrosis.

In the presence of a carcinoma, whether these signs represent reactive changes or direct tumor invasion can only be determined histologically.

If the reactive changes are induced by small tumors, they may be the only evidence of a small malignancy within dense mammary tissue. Accentuated by good mammographic compression, they can become visible on the mammogram before they are clinically apparent (**Fig. 16.5**, compare also with **Fig. 16.2v,w**). Therefore, searching for secondary malignant criteria, such as retraction affecting skin, subcutaneous tissue, prepectoral space, or nipple, is also important.

Signs of Diffusely Growing Carcinomas

(See **Fig. 16.7**.)

The detection of diffusely growing carcinomas may be quite difficult, especially if these carcinomas do not contain microcalcifications.

If *microcalcifications* are present, the same differentiating criteria are valid as applied to the evaluation of microcalcifications in general. Especially V-shaped and Y-shaped casts and larger granular or pleomorphic microcalcifications are suggestive for malignancy, as is the ductal distribution pattern. Fine granular or monomorphic calcifications may, on occasion, require further evaluation as well:
- If they follow a ductal distribution pattern
- If they are new
- If additional soft tissue changes are present
- If associated with a clinically suspicious finding

The problem of early mammographic detection of diffusely growing, noncalcifying carcinoma is the divergent spread of these carcinomas without inducing any mammographically visible increase in density. Increased density or retractive changes, or both, often become visible only after a clinically apparent finding has developed. Therefore, clinical correlation is very important for the detection of diffusely growing carcinomas.

To detect *diffusely growing carcinomas* without microcalcifications, the following has to be looked for (**Fig. 16.6**):
- *Asymmetry* in comparison to the contralateral side (close correlation with palpation, and possibly with sonography and MRI)
- Already present or newly developed *increased density*
- Increased *blurring* of the ligamentous structures in the parenchyma (caused by cellular infiltrates or edema)
- *Densities in the subcutaneous region* and in the *retromammary fatty tissue* (usually caused by accompanying inflammation or direct infiltration)
- Any *retractive changes* of the breast tissue or nipple
- *Thickening of Cooper ligaments*, whereby this thickening usually begins deep in the ligament near the parenchyma rather than more superficially (**Fig. 16.6a**)

The signs of an *inflammatory carcinoma*, which is generally clinically apparent, are:
- Skin thickening
- Trabecular thickening in the subcutaneous space and prepectoral space
- Blurring of structures caused by edema (**Fig. 16.6g**)

All of these signs are typically present in an inflammatory carcinoma. While these signs can also be found in inflammation, the presence of additional malignant-type calcifications strongly suggests the diagnosis of an inflammatory carcinoma.

Value of Follow-up and Prior Studies

As shown by several studies, diagnostic accuracy increases with prior mammograms. While sensitivity appears to remain quite stable, significant improvement has been reported for specificity in particular. Therefore, if available, prior mammograms should be *compared with the current mammogram* (Thurfjell et al. 2000, Sumkin et al. 2003, Varela et al. 2005, Roelofs et al. 2007).

A mammographic finding that has increased in size or is *new* suggests a malignancy (**Fig. 16.8a–f**). Recognizing such changes will increase sensitivity.

While increasing or new masses, microcalcifications, or densities may be an indicator of early malignancy, some lesions may show unexpected behavior:
- Some early malignancies may stay stable for years before they suddenly start growing. Rarely, microcalcifications may even regress when a DCIS turns into an invasive malignancy; this change may be due to a changed pH milieu. And, decreasing size combined with increasing density can be evidence of malignant retraction caused by invasion with accompanying fibrosis. Knowledge of these pitfalls is important, since for stable or decreasing findings biopsy might still be indicated, if the finding is sufficiently suspicious (**Fig. 16.8e,f**).

Therefore, a *change in a finding*, mainly an increase, a new appearance, and rarely a decrease, might indicate the possibility of a carcinoma.

This implies that a stable appearance makes malignancy less likely but can exclude it only after long-term follow-up examinations over an extended period (**Fig. 16.8g,h**). In particular, this must be considered in the

Mammography

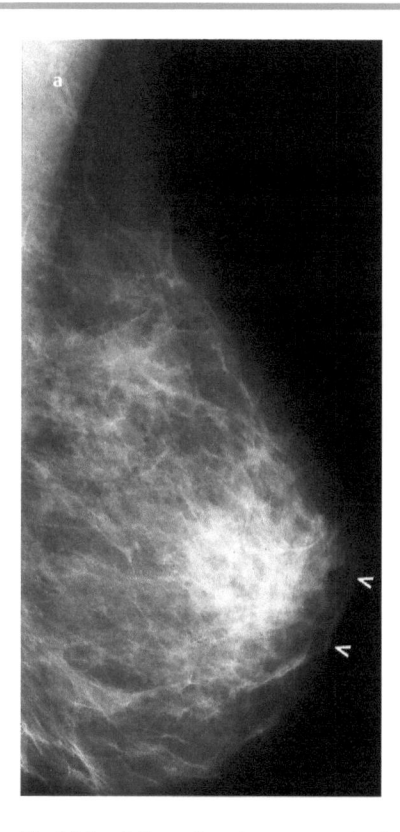

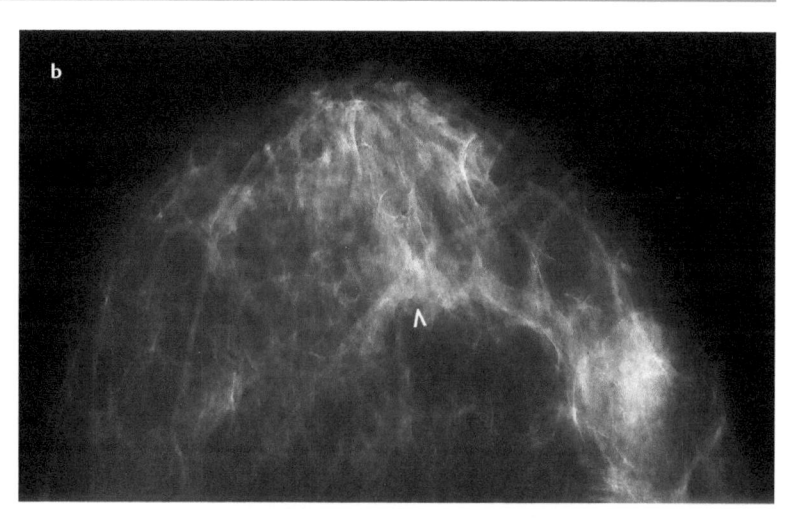

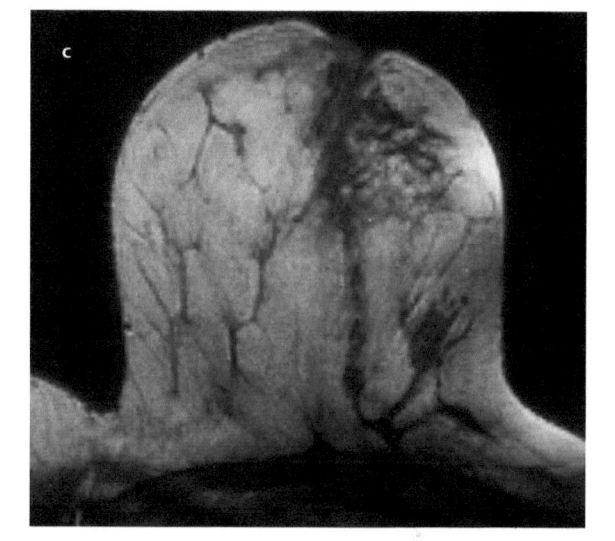

Fig. 16.5a–d Secondary signs may rarely also be the first hint of a small carcinoma. This series shows a 40-year-old patient who noticed impaired erectility of the nipple.

a Only the mediolateral view—provoked by good compression—reveals flattening of the areola (arrowheads). The central parenchyma appears slightly thickened but without definite evidence of malignancy.

b This craniocaudal view, as well as the corresponding oblique view, was interpreted as negative by an experienced radiologist. Retrospectively, focal mass and architectural distortion (arrowhead) can be discerned deep in the breast but without corresponding findings in the mediolateral view.

c Transverse magnetic resonance image at the level of the nipple before administration of contrast medium.

d The same image shown in (**c**) but after injection of contrast medium. There is strong, rapid focal enhancement in the breast tissue, strongly suggestive of malignancy (arrow). The small satellite foci should be noted (arrowheads). The laterally situated parenchyma shows moderate enhancement in this patient. Without mammographic–clinical suspicion, this is suggestive of an enhancing mastopathy (e.g., proliferative mastopathy).

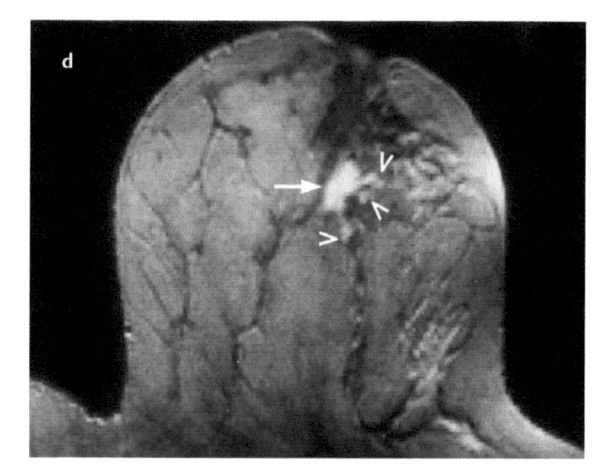

16 Invasive Carcinoma

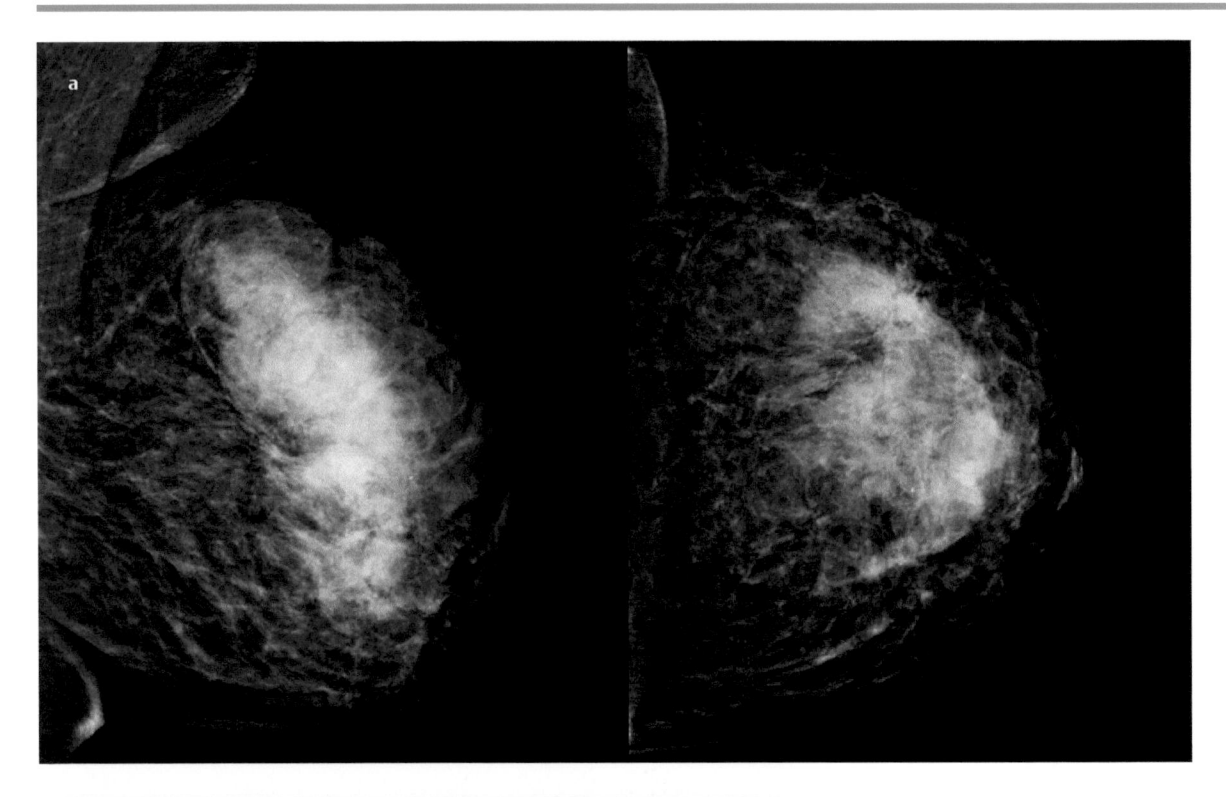

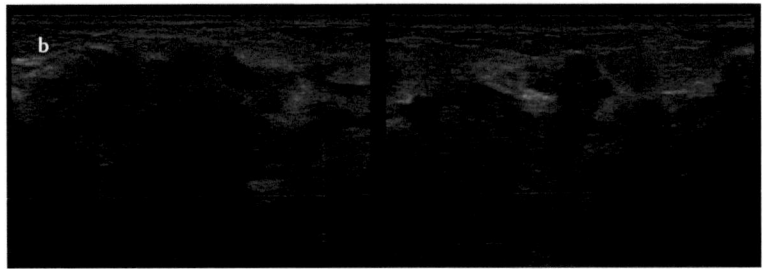

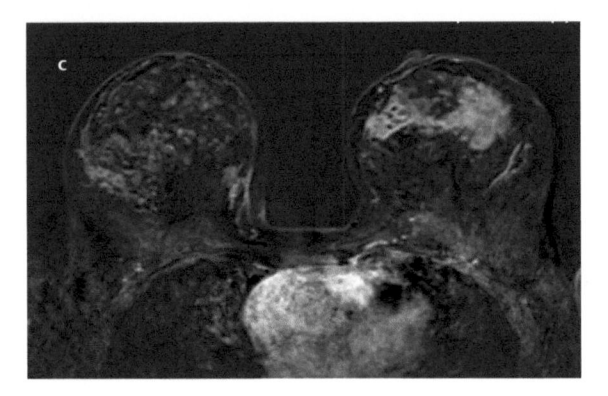

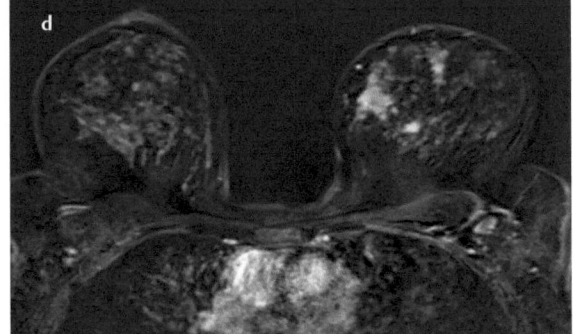

Fig. 16.6a–g

a–d The patient presented with a diffuse thickening of the breast tissue.

a The tissue is very dense, but retraction of the central tissue of the gland is seen. At 6 o' clock position the skin is retracted (arrow) and a double contour of the skin is shown.

b Ultrasound demonstrates dilated ductal structures, some architectural distortion and diffuse shadowing. However, the three-dimensional extent is difficult to visualize.

c Magnetic resonance imaging shows diffuse moderate plateau-type enhancement. It demonstrates that the diffuse extent obviously corresponds well with the mammographically perceivable area of increased density.

d In other quadrants (cranially) multicentric involvement is seen.

The patient underwent mastectomy, which confirmed extensive ductal breast cancer (G2).

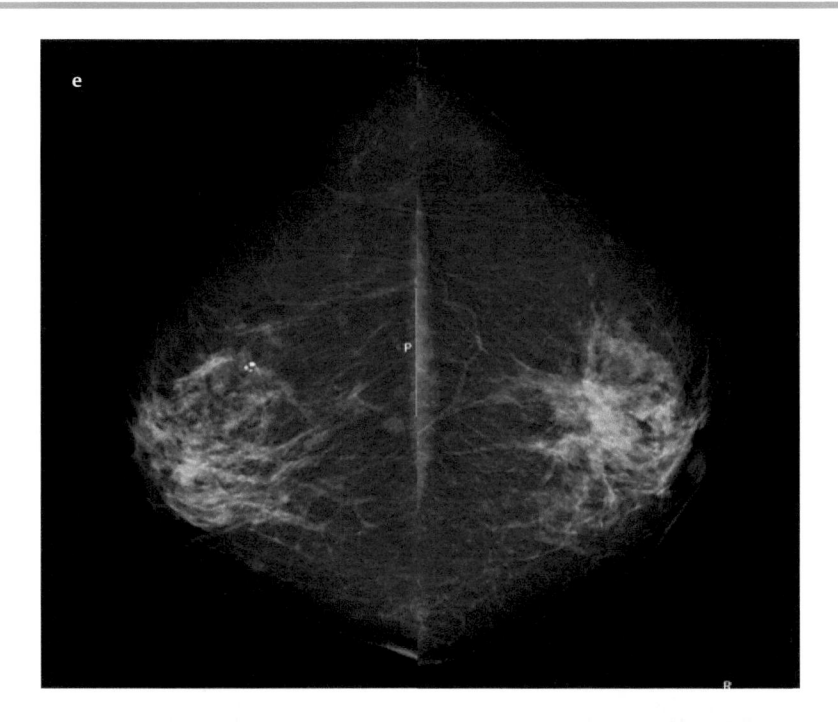

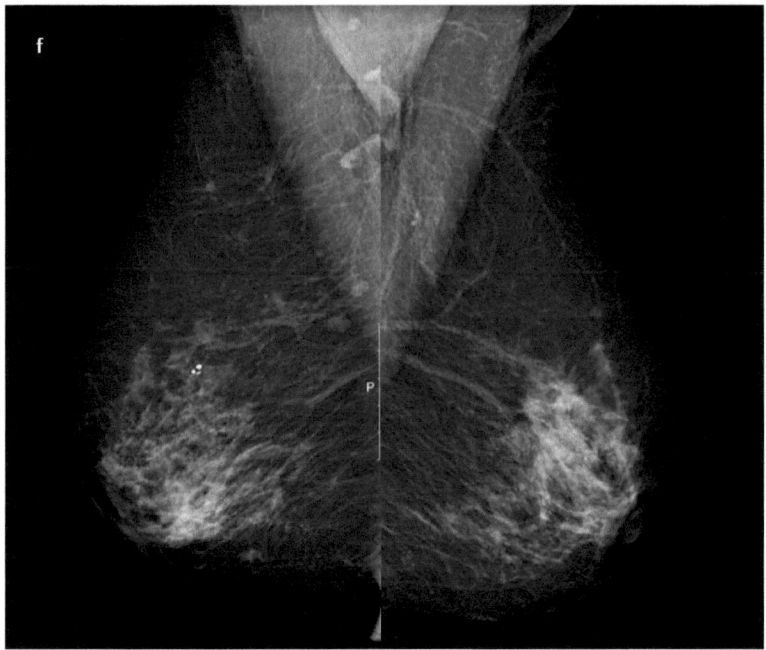

e,f Another patient with a diffusely growing breast cancer: Craniocaudal and mediolateral oblique images show a diffusely increased density of the breast tissue centrally in the left breast and some architectural distortion and nipple retraction, which did not allow imaging of the nipple in profile. *Histology* demonstrated an extensive lobular carcinoma on the left (pT2 G2).

Fig. 16.6g ▷

16 Invasive Carcinoma

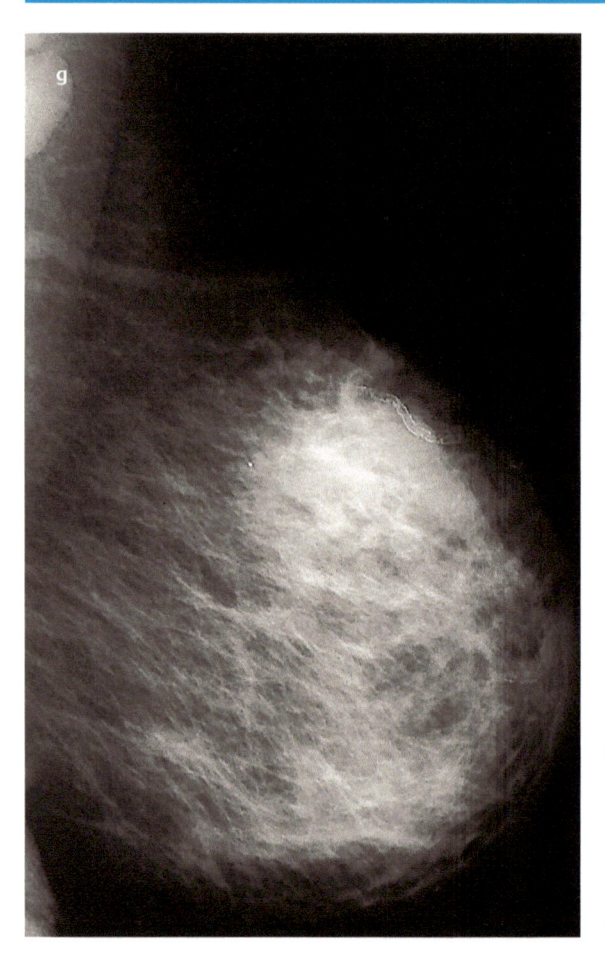

◁ continued

g Patient with an inflammatory breast cancer: There is diffuse thickening of the entire parenchyma as well as definite skin thickening that is most pronounced in the central periareolar region. The reticular densities in the subcutaneous and retromammary fat can be explained as edematous thickening. In the axilla, a large and a small, very dense lymph node are partially visualized.

a Diffuse spiculation

b Diffuse reticular densities (with or without skin thickening)

c Asymmetry

d Extensive microcalcifications

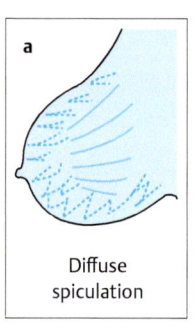

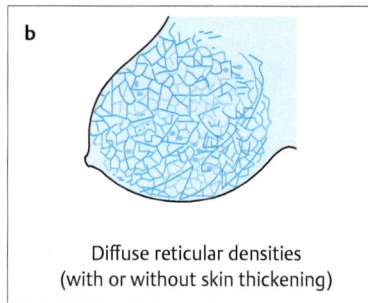

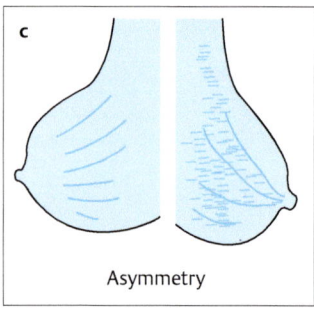

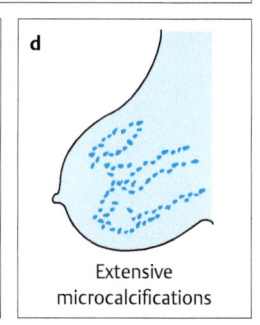

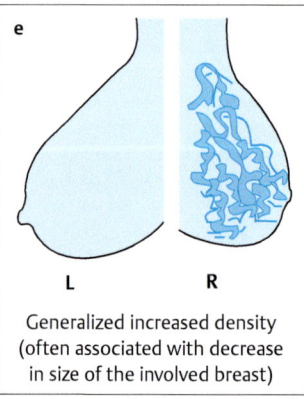

e Generalized increased density (often associated with decrease in size of the involved breast)

Fig. 16.7a–e Diffusely growing carcinoma (diagram), mammographic appearance.

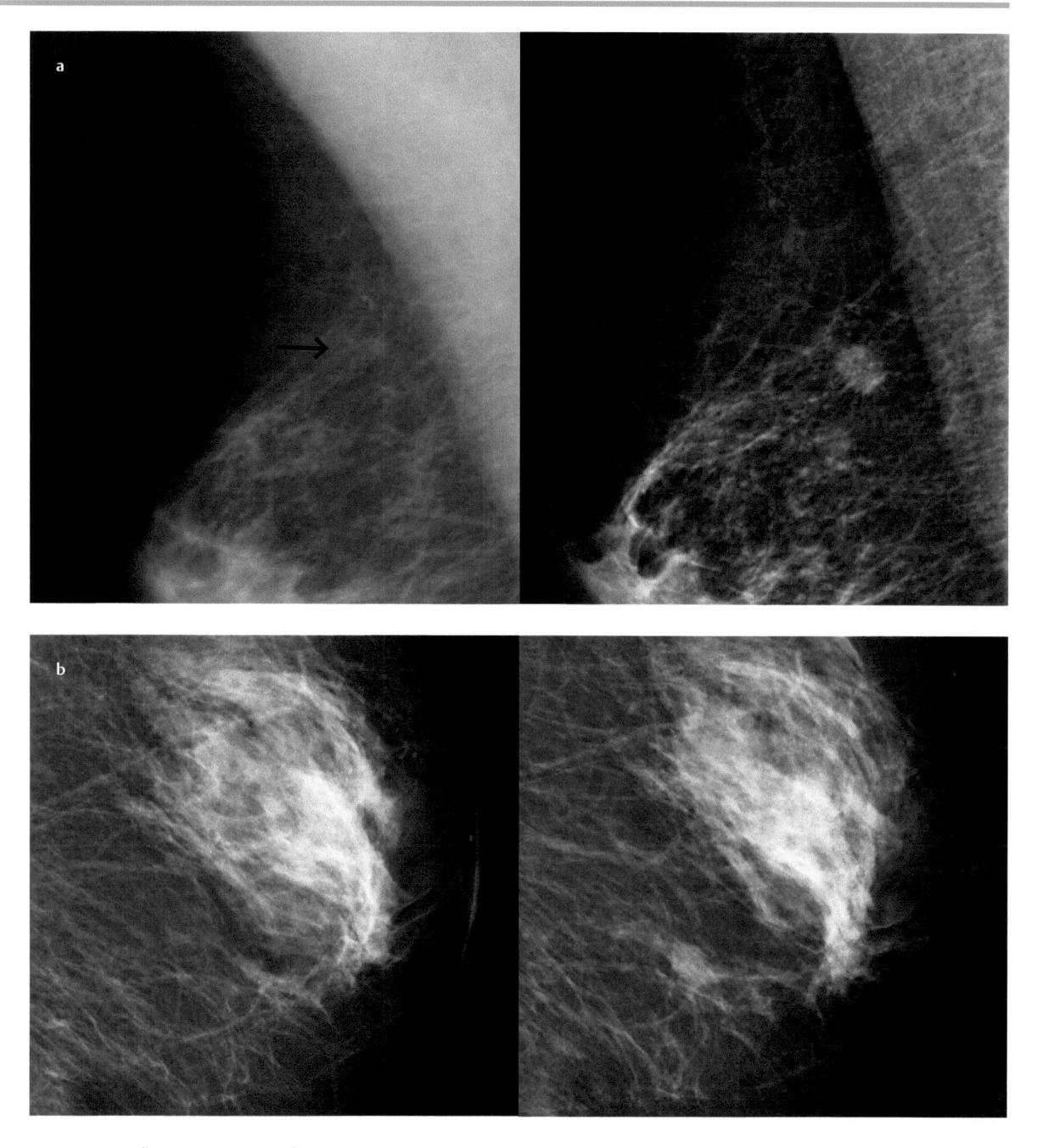

Fig. 16.8a–i Follow-up mammography

a   Current oblique view (on the right) and previous view obtained 2 years earlier (on the left). In comparison with the previous view, the current screening mammography shows that a spiculated density has developed. In retrospect, a faint nodular density is seen in this area, which, however, could not have been expected to be diagnosed at the time of the original mammography. The faint nodular change that imitates the usual nodularity of breast tissue would be classified as no or minimal sign. *Core needle biopsy* confirmed an invasive ductal carcinoma.

b   Another example of a newly developed, small, ill-defined density. The patient had obtained this mammogram (on the right) 9 months after her previous mammogram (on the left, for another reason). *Core needle biopsy* proved an invasive ductal carcinoma.

Fig. 16.8c–i ▷

16 Invasive Carcinoma

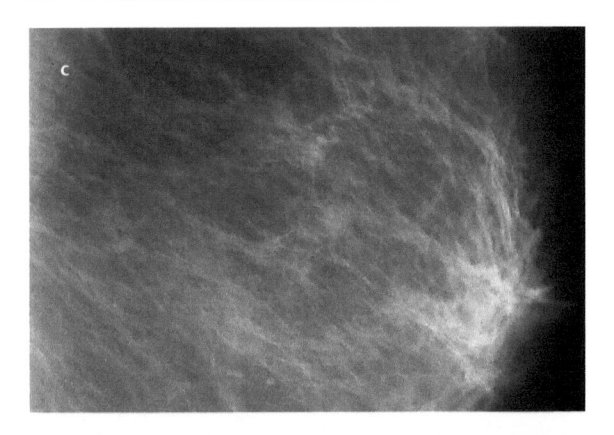

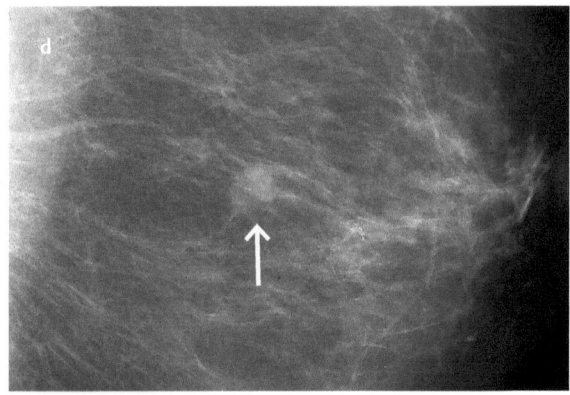

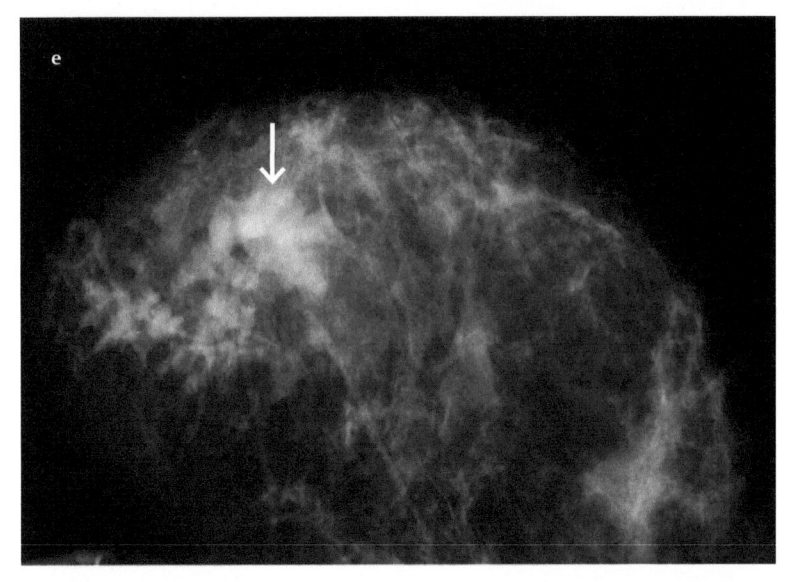

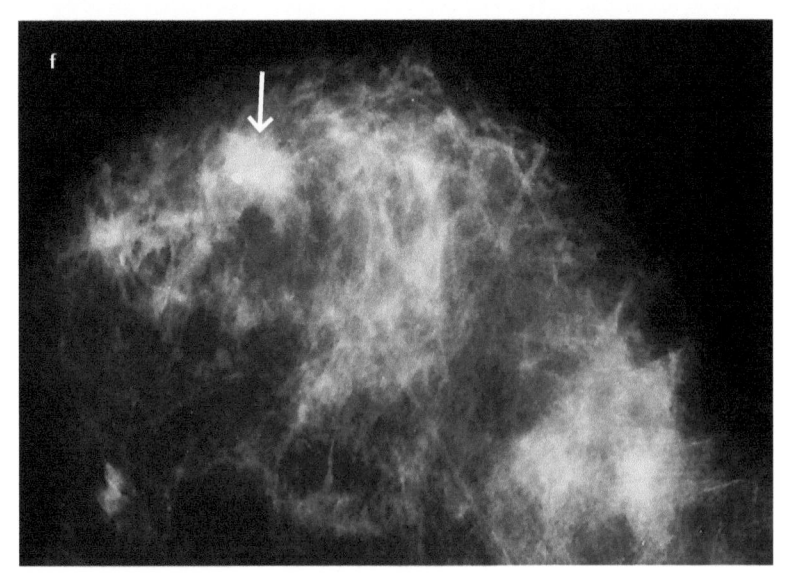

◁ continued

c,d A round structure measuring a few millimeters is shown here. It could represent a small cyst, a very small fibroadenoma, or a papilloma in the parenchyma. The next follow-up examination revealed an increase in size, rendering this structure (arrow)—which does not correspond to a cyst sonographically—very suspicious for malignancy (close-up of an oblique view). *Histology*: Intraductal carcinoma with minimal invasion (pT1a).

e,f The previous mammogram of a 46-year-old patient reveals asymmetric densities with distorted architecture and slightly increased density medially, which were not mentioned as suspicious by the interpreting radiologist (**e**). Three years later, the density of the mass has increased, and its margins are now spiculated (**f**). (The density of the entire parenchyma appears increased since a high-contrast film was used.) A decrease in size is certainly not a sign of benignity and can be explained by retraction due to fibrosis. Another small mass has appeared adjacent to the thoracic wall. Additional examinations and follow-up after breast conservation therapy showed no further malignant changes. *Histology*: Unifocal well-differentiated tubular carcinoma.

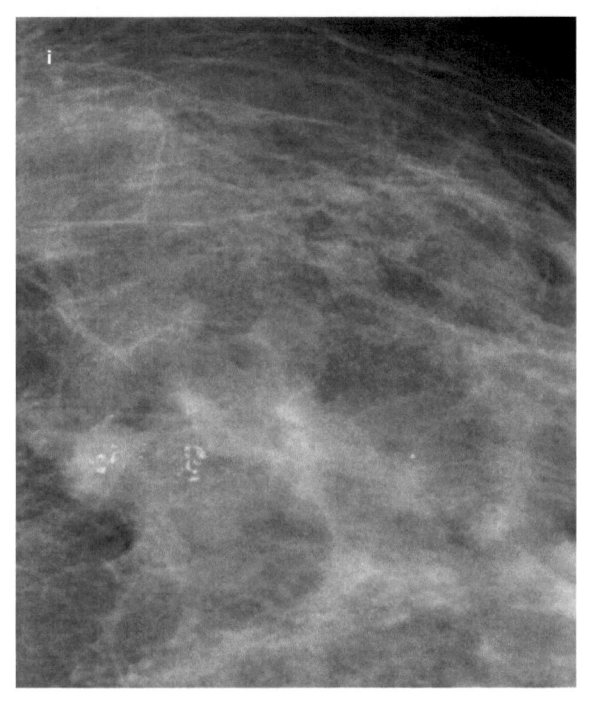

g,h Mammography with unequivocally suspicious calcifications (elongated individual forms), confined to the upper inner quadrant, which were not categorized as suspicious initially by the interpreting radiologist (**g**). Six years later, the microcalcifications are essentially unchanged. The surrounding soft tissues have even decreased in density owing to postmenopausal involution (**h**). Because of the suspicious appearance of the individual calcifications and despite the lack of any interval change, excisional biopsy was recommended. *Histology*: Extensive ductal carcinoma in situ with microinvasion.
This finding confirms that any progression seen on follow-up examination mandates prompt definitive evaluation, but that stability—as illustrated in this case—cannot be taken as assurance of benignity of an otherwise suspicious finding.

i Mammographically two groups of polymorphic microcalcifications (at a distance of 1 cm from one another) had newly developed within dense nodular breast tissue. They indicated a T2 ductal breast cancer of 2.5 cm size, which may in retrospect be suspected within the dense tissue. The example also demonstrates the difficulty of delineating the exact extent of masses or other noncalcified malignant tissue, which are partly obscured by dense tissue.

evaluation of microcalcifications, since these (when representing a DCIS) may stay stable for years while development of the invasive carcinoma may start suddenly.

Suspicious changes—even if unchanged in comparison with the previous examination—have to be further evaluated by biopsy.

To follow changes judged to be benign, the generally accepted approach is:
- The follow-up intervals should—because of the usual slow doubling time of breast carcinomas—generally not be shorter than (4–) 6 months for masses and may range around 6–12 months for microcalcifications. Follow-up examinations must be continued for a sufficient time span (in general, at least 2 years).
- If possible, the current mammogram should be compared with previous and older mammograms.
- In patients undergoing hormone replacement therapy, false positive calls are often increased. However, it has been reported that the false positive rate may be decreased when comparing mammograms during hormone replacement therapy with older (premenopausal) mammograms.
- If the intervals are too short, discrete and slowly developing changes are not sufficiently appreciated or cannot be distinguished from usual fluctuations of technique (different projection, compression, and distance to the film).
- Finally it should be remembered that short-term follow-up may be associated with long-term distress, since the patient will not have a definite diagnosis. As is known from psychological studies, long-term uncertainty is far less well tolerated than short-term stress (e.g., caused by a diligently performed percutaneous breast biopsy).
- Therefore organized screening programs recommend limiting the number of short-term follow-up examinations. Also any recommendation for short-term follow-up should be carefully explained to the patient. It should also be remembered that—in the case of finding malignancy—the delay will have to be explained to the patient.

The Influence of Histology on Mammographic Presentation

As already mentioned, histologic type and growth pattern of the carcinoma affect the mammographic presentation. Knowing the histologic features and the different manifestations of the various types of carcinomas is important for detecting breast carcinomas. Though the histopathologic classification cannot be deduced, it can sometimes be suspected from the particular presentation of the carcinoma.

In this context, the relationships between histology and mammographic features are recapitulated.

Invasive ductal carcinoma can have diverse manifestations, and any of the signs of malignancy listed in **Table 16.1** can be present, alone or with others (e.g., irregularly outlined mass, circumscribed mass, diffuse growth pattern, focal microcalcifications, diffusely distributed microcalcifications, or no microcalcifications).

Invasive lobular carcinoma frequently grows along established tissue planes without forming a mass and sometimes without inciting fibrosis. Therefore, it is often difficult to recognize. In some lobular carcinomas a spiculated mass or other focal lesion (not infrequently similar to the density of the normal parenchyma) is observed. Very rarely even a round mass can be present. Because of their diffuse growth, lobular carcinomas have the highest percentage of mammographically and sonographically occult carcinomas. Lobular carcinoma does not form microcalcifications. If present, microcalcifications are within associated DCIS or pleomorphic LCIS MRI has the by far highest detection rate of primary lobular carcinomas or of foci of lobular carcinoma. However, some diffusely growing and/or extensively fibrosed lobular carcinomas may exhibit low and progressive or even no enhancement. Such—sometimes even extensive—malignancies may be extremely difficult to detect or are undetectable by MRI. About 10% of the lobular carcinomas will show such growth patterns.

Tubular carcinoma frequently presents as a spiculated mass with long, reactive, fibrotic strands. It can contain microcalcifications. Regardless of the individual shapes of these microcalcifications, the spiculated mass is an indication for biopsy. Microcalcifications are often the manifestation of DCIS accompanying a tubular carcinoma and can assume characteristic configuration or arrangement. Tubular carcinomas may also exhibit quite moderate and sometimes low progressive enhancement on MRI.

Carcinomas with medullary features and mucinous carcinomas belong to the invasive carcinoma that present as round lesions. However, the most frequent round, well-defined carcinoma histologically is the invasive ductal carcinoma, NST G3 (**Fig. 16.2n**). Round carcinomas frequently show areas of indistinctness or subtle undulation (microlobulation) that suggest that they are not benign (**Fig. 16.9a**). Some of these carcinomas, however, can be smoothly outlined throughout and might even be surrounded by a halo. *Intracystic "papillary carcinoma"* may also present as a well-circumscribed nodule. The well-circumscribed border is caused by the surrounding cyst. Thus, this is really an in situ carcinoma. Any macroscopic infiltration is detected only if the affected portion of the cyst wall is seen tangentially (**Fig. 16.9c**). Sometimes extension beyond the wall of the surrounding cyst, which is very rare, may be noted sonographically. Carcinomas with a completely smooth outline (some with a halo sign) constitute around 2% of the smoothly outlined solid lesions. Completely smooth outlines may also occur in papillary DCIS (mostly papillary DCIS with

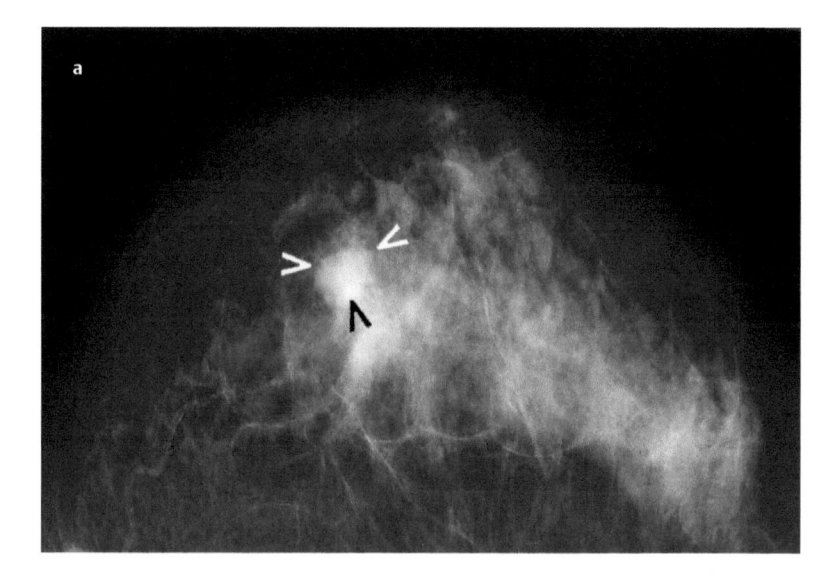

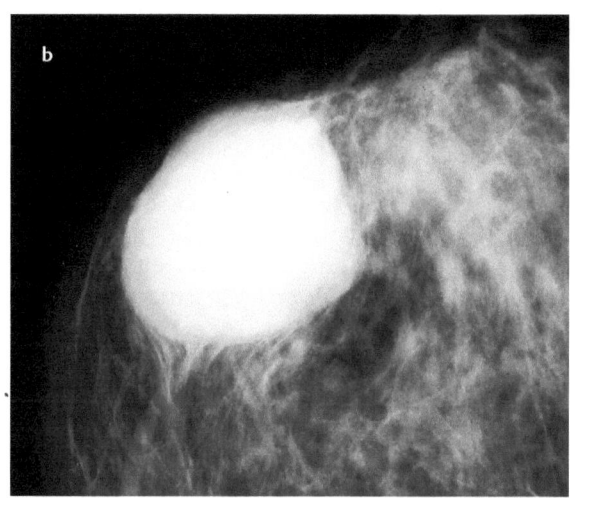

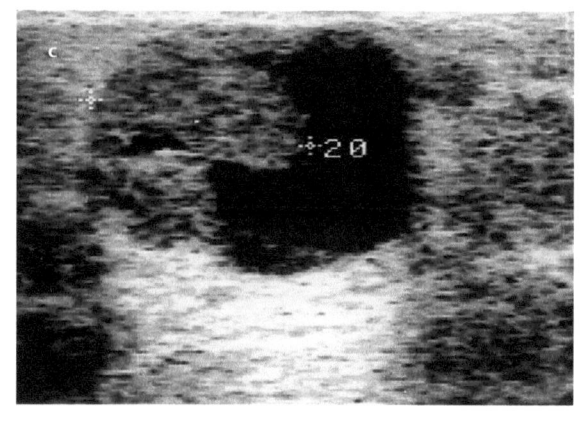

Fig. 16.9a–c Additional specific manifestations

a Medullary carcinoma, 1 cm in size. In this case, the outline of the round carcinoma is relatively sharp, but microlobulation (arrowheads) raises the possibility of a malignancy.

b,c Mammographically smoothly outlined lesion in a different patient. Some areas of indistinctness might be explained by superimposed tissue, but the pattern should raise concern about possible spiculation (**b**). Sonography shows that the smoothly outlined lesion with good sound transmission consists of a solid and a liquid component (**c**). *Histology*: Papillary DCIS with surrounding cyst and small area of invasive carcinoma.

Remark: Invasion outside the wall of the cyst is only detectable if this segment of the wall (not illustrated here) is tangentially projected on the mammographic view. Sonographically, macroscopic invasion can be noted as an irregular interface with the adjacent tissue.

surrounding cyst). While medullary and mucinous carcinomas only rarely show microcalcifications (usually single atypical ones), papillary DCIS, can have microcalcifications. On MRI papillary DCIS, which may present as a well-circumscribed nodule, may exhibit very variable enhancement, ranging from low progressive to strong enhancement with washout. Most papillary and micropapillary invasive carcinomas exhibit growth patterns similar to those of usual invasive ductal carcinomas (NST) and do not present as well-circumscribed masses. However, large variations in enhancement, ranging from no enhancement to very strong enhancement, have been described for mucinous carcinomas. Medullary carcinomas may sometimes be recognized by increased peripheral (rim) enhancement on MRI. However, they may also mimic fibroadenomas. Some may be recognized by washout, but absence of washout cannot exclude a medullary carcinoma.

Paget disease of the nipple becomes clinically apparent through eczema of the nipple or areola. The eczema is induced by seeding of malignant cells into the nipple or areola or both. It can arise from any invasive carcinoma or DCIS within the ductal system of the breast. A direct retroareolar site of origin in the major ducts is also possible. Eczema suggestive of Paget disease of the nipple always demands a thorough evaluation of the breast to the level of the thoracic wall (mammography, magnification mammography, supplemental methods). In many cases, Paget disease of the nipple has no mammographic findings. Occasionally focal changes in the nipple–areolar complex are seen. Mammograms should always be obtained, since suspicious microcalcifications might indicate an underlying tumor within the breast tissue.

Sonography should complement mammography in such cases. Unless the tumor is detected by mammography or ultrasound, MRI should be applied to detect or exclude further areas requiring histopathologic assessment.

Inflammatory carcinoma (**Fig. 16.6g**) is characterized by diffuse thickening of the skin as well as by increased trabecular markings in the subcutaneous tissue and parenchyma, caused by carcinomatous lymphangiosis. Focal masses as well as malignant-type microcalcifications may be present. The former may be detectable by mammography, sonography, or MRI, the latter by MRI. If focal pathology is visualized, percutaneous biopsy should target that area. If no focal changes are visible, percutaneous biopsy with a fanned distribution of passes may be attempted. Due to the diffuse growth pattern and sometimes dispersed cells of inflammatory breast cancer, however, a negative percutaneous biopsy may not be reliable. Therefore, if inflammatory cancer is suspected (e.g., after unsuccessful antibiotic treatment) surgical biopsy including skin biopsy should be considered.

Breast carcinoma associated with nipple discharge: Pathologic discharge is always an indication for mammography; supplemental cytologic examination may be helpful. Positive cytology confirms an underlying malignancy, but negative cytology does not exclude it. The majority of discharge-inducing breast carcinomas are mammographically detectable. Rarely can such breast carcinomas be hidden in mammographically dense tissue. To localize these carcinomas, first ultrasound imaging (and in case of positive findings US-guided biopsy) should be applied. If ultrasound cannot determine the origin of discharge, *galactography* is indicated.

Filling defects in the ductal system and truncated ducts indicate a carcinoma (**Fig. 16.10**). A definite differentiation between papillomatosis, papilloma, or malignancy cannot be achieved by galactography. This means that galactographically suggestive changes must be clarified histologically. The rare cases of negative galactography despite a definite positive cytology should be considered for MRI.

When analyzing the growth pattern of *invasive carcinomas*, spiculated and irregular shapes appear to indicate a somewhat better prognosis. Microcalcifications may be present in both fast- and slow-growing carcinomas and are not predictive of a good or bad prognosis. High-grade and fast-growing carcinomas are unfortunately more often rounded or oval and may thus even be mistaken for benign lesions with almost all modalities. On MRI at least part of these carcinomas may be recognized correctly due to washout of contrast agent.

Diffusely growing carcinomas are usually quite difficult to detect irrespective of the imaging modality.

In younger women diagnosis may be quite difficult, partly because of the very dense breast tissue, which on mammography may obscure noncalcified breast cancers and which on MRI may exhibit disturbing enhancement and benign enhancing lesions. Well-circumscribed, round or oval carcinomas may be confused with the much more frequent fibroadenomas.

Breast cancers, which occur in *hereditary breast cancer* and predominantly in *BRCA1* carriers may pose special diagnostic problems:
- Microcalcifications (which are an important sign of sporadic breast cancer) are rarely seen in *BRCA1*-positive women. Rounded and well-circumscribed cancers (medullary cancers or ductal G3 and often triple negative cancers) are more frequent in these women. Due to the younger average age of onset, confusion with benign changes is frequent.
- The cancers detected in *BRCA2* carriers appear to have features similar to sporadic breast cancers and may be associated with microcalcifications. However, for *BRCA2* mutation carriers an increased risk of radiation has been discussed (see Chapter 3).

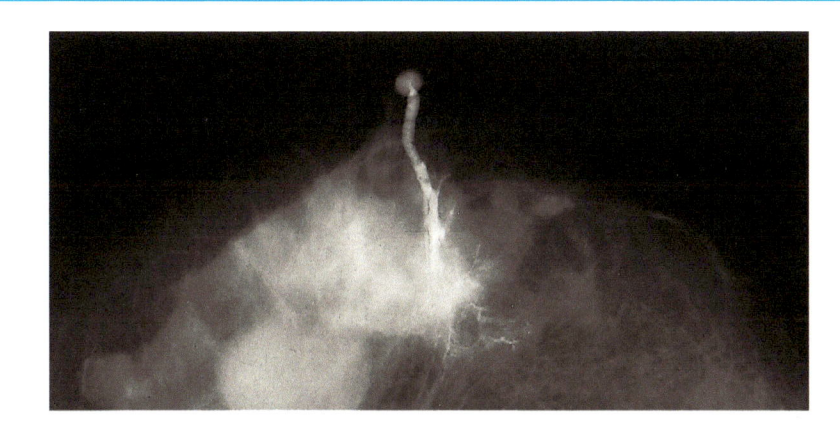

Fig. 16.10 Galactography (craniocaudal view) of a patient with pathologic nipple discharge and suspicious cytologic smear. Mammography, sonography, and palpation were unremarkable. There are small persistent filling defects, best explained as remnants of debris and an appreciable change in caliber and ductal cutoff, 2–3 cm behind the nipple. This region must be considered suspicous. *Histology*: Extensive, partially intraductal, partially invasive, poorly differentiated ductal carcinoma.

Sensitivity and Specificity of Mammography

State-of-the-art mammography approaches a sensitivity of 85–90%. The sensitivity of detecting lesions in fatty tissue is close to 100%. With increasing density of tissue, the accuracy of mammography decreases because small carcinomas without microcalcifications or diffusely growing malignancies can be hidden in isodense tissue (van Gils et al. 1998). In a screening situation, when mammography is performed in asymptomatic women only (and for which interval carcinomas during the subsequent two years are counted as false negative) sensitivity ranges around 70–80% (Duncan et al. 1998, van Gils et al. 1998, Saarenmaa et al. 1999). Depending on their histology and growth pattern, large carcinomas are in most cases obvious. However, diffusely growing carcinomas may sometimes be difficult to detect and may thus only be detected late. Depending on the growth pattern of the carcinoma and on the surrounding tissue, sometimes even palpable carcinomas may not be detectable by mammography. Therefore assessment of symptomatic patients and of patients with any indeterminate imaging abnormality should always include a thorough clinical examination.

The specificity of mammography depends on the finding itself. In general, the appearance of an early carcinoma may be less characteristic than that of an advanced palpable carcinoma. To detect as many early carcinomas as possible, biopsies for benign changes cannot be avoided. Adequate evaluation, regular review of one's own accuracy, and selecting an acceptable threshold for detecting carcinomas are required to keep both sensitivity and specificity in an acceptable range.

Differential Diagnostic Considerations

Any mammographic pattern, even if most suspicious for carcinoma, can be caused by benign entities.

Spiculated masses have a high likelihood of malignancy, unless they correspond to a surgical scar. The appearance can be mimicked by the superimposition of breast tissue, which can be excluded further by a compression view or views in additional projections. Other causes of a spiculated mass include radial scar, fat necrosis, hematoma, abscess, or rare causes such as extra-abdominal desmoid or myoblastoma.

A lobulated mass has a moderate probability of malignancy. The differential diagnosis should include asymmetrically developed parenchyma, mastopathic changes, superimpositions, hormone-induced changes, fat necrosis, and scar formation.

Round and smoothly outlined changes can be a manifestation of malignancy. The probability of malignancy, however, is low. It is less than 2% for lesions exhibiting an outline that is entirely smooth. After sonographic exclusion of a cyst, the main differential diagnosis of benign entities with this presentation includes fibroadenomas, papillomas, or masses caused by fibrocystic alteration (see also Chapter 24).

Microcalcifications are found in about 30% of invasive carcinomas and can be a sign of malignancy, with or without surrounding soft tissue density. Depending on their features, various benign conditions are to be considered as well, primarily microcalcifications in benign changes with or without atypia, in fibroadenomas, "plasma cell mastitis," or scarring (see also Chapter 24).

Diffuse changes, such as *asymmetry, increased density, thickening, and indistinctness of structures*, are particularly suspicious if associated with an abnormal palpatory finding. If the palpation is normal, the likelihood of malignancy is low, but further evaluation (supplemental image studies, percutaneous biopsy) may still be indicated, depending on the severity of the abnormality. The differential diagnosis should include developmental asymmetries, benign fibrocystic changes, hormone-induced changes, and postsurgical or postradiation changes (see also Chapter 24).

Diffuse architectural distortion and retraction are suggestive of malignancy, particularly if found unilaterally. They are often—if caused by a malignancy—associated with diffusely increased consistency to palpation. The differential diagnosis should primarily consider chronic mastitis, in addition to postsurgical scarring and radial scar. Thorough evaluation (MRI, core biopsy, and surgical biopsy) is necessary.

Diffuse skin thickening, if associated with peau d'orange, hyperthermia, and erythema, should first raise the possibility of an inflammatory carcinoma rather than a nonpuerperal mastitis, in particular in patients who are not pregnant, nursing, or postpartum. Furthermore, other rare causes of skin thickening should be mentioned, such as lymphoma, metastatic involvement, and venous or lymphatic stasis.

In cases with signs of *inflammation* a tentative antibiotic therapy using one or two different combinations should be attempted. If unsuccessful and in cases with diffuse changes without inflammation, biopsy of the representative skin should be the next diagnostic procedure unless further imaging studies have already revealed a suspicious focus. In case of such a finding, these methods will also be applied to guide biopsy.

Sonography

Diagnostic Role

Sonography is the most important method supplementing mammography and is primarily used for *further diagnostic evaluation*. It can provide the following important information complementing mammography.

Sonography is indicated for all localized findings that might represent a cyst.

Since many palpable carcinomas are sonographically hypoechoic compared with normal breast tissue, sonography can directly visualize a carcinoma that is hidden in dense tissue on mammography. Therefore, sonography can contribute to immediate further evaluation of an abnormal palpatory finding in mammographically dense breasts.

Sonography may also allow assessment of the borders of lesions which are partially hidden behind dense breast tissue. Therefore sonography may be a valuable tool for complementary evaluation of indeterminate mammographic findings.

Since the sensitivity of sonography is limited, great care is necessary when excluding malignancy in cases with a palpable or mammographically indeterminate findings. In general ultrasound examination cannot exclude malignancy in cases of small mammographic masses, architectural distortions or suspicious microcalcifications. This takes into account the limited sensitivity of sonography for small nonpalpable or preinvasive carcinomas. Therefore, sonography should not be used to exclude malignancy in mammographically detected suspicious lesions that do not prove to be cysts.

In the case of a mass that fulfils all mammographic and sonographic criteria of benignity (see Chapter 4) short-term follow-up may be considered instead of biopsy in women at low risk (Graf et al. 2004, Mainiero et al. 2005). In women at high risk the frequency of well-circumscribed cancers is, however, higher than in other populations. Therefore, in these women percutaneous biopsy is recommended for all solid lesions.

In cases of asymmetric tissue without mammographic signs of malignancy and without palpable findings, the sonographic exclusion of malignancy is quite reliable in cases with homogeneously hyperechoic tissue or hyperechoic tissue with some interspersed fat lobules if the tissue proves elastic and mobile (Stavros et al. 1995, Dennis et al. 2001). If surrounded by hypoechoic fatty tissue, hypoechoic carcinomas exhibit minimal contrast, particularly if no characteristic echogenic rim or acoustic shadowing is present. Furthermore, when surrounded by mixed fatty and glandular tissue, small hypoechoic carcinomas can be mistaken for hypoechoic fat lobules imbedded in the parenchyma.

In the case of a palpable thickening or a suspiciously palpable mass (increased consistency, decreased elasticity, or decreased mobility) percutaneous breast biopsy should always be considered. This takes into account the limited sensitivity of all methods for diffusely growing carcinomas and the rare possibility of a hyperechoic malignancy (see also **Fig. 16.12i,j**).

Indications

For the diagnostic evaluation of breast carcinoma, sonography has the following *indications*:

- Exclusion of a simple cyst as cause of a mammographically or clinically indeterminate focal finding (avoidance of unnecessary biopsies).
- Detection of malignancy in the presence of uncharacteristic and questionable palpatory findings in mammographically dense tissue. Sonographic exclusion of a malignancy, however, apart from the diagnosis of a simple cyst, is unreliable.
- Complementary assessment of focal lesions and asymmetries.
- Sonographically guided puncture (for percutaneous biopsy or preoperative localization of focal findings) is often done faster than mammographically guided stereotactic puncture. In addition, it allows direct documentation of the correct position of the needle (in contrast to the stereotactic localization that only shows the correct projection of the needle during the procedure; see also Chapter 7).

Image Presentation of Breast Carcinoma

In general, breast carcinoma expresses a wide sonographic spectrum (**Figs. 16.11, 16.12, 16.13**).

Sonographically, breast carcinoma is characteristically seen as:

- A hypoechoic mass, often with varying echogenicity. Hyperechoic carcinomas are rare.
- A mass with irregular margin (spiculation, angulation, microlobulation, or indistinct contours is typical). Infrequently carcinomas may present as a well-circumscribed mass.
- A mass with or without hyperechoic rim ("echogenic halo"). If present, a hyperechoic rim is quite specific.

In addition:

- The shape of the mass is mostly irregular, sometimes round and rarely oval (except high risk).
- The orientation of the mass is mostly vertical or indeterminate, infrequently horizontal.
- Acoustic shadowing may be present posterior to malignant masses and may be an important hint for detection. It is, however, not specific, and—if absent—malignancy cannot be excluded. Some malignancies even exhibit posterior enhancement. Other malignancies (mostly very early or diffusely growing malignancy) may exhibit shadowing without a definite mass.
- Distorted architecture (often associated with shadowing) may be a subtle sign of malignancy, but may also be due to other causes (scarring, radial lesions) or even benign structures (e.g., Cooper ligaments).
- Most cancers are poorly to moderately compressible or moveable.
- A significant number of small breast cancers which are surrounded by fatty tissue or diffusely growing breast cancers may not be visible at all by ultrasound. Therefore absence of a sonographic finding cannot be used to rule out a suspicious mammographic or MR finding. In the case of clinical findings sonography may aid excluding malignancy, if it allows explaining the findings as a benign change (which may be possible together with other imaging or interventional methods).

1. Echogenicity

- Characteristically, a *hypoechoic mass* is found. In general, it is easily recognized if surrounded by more hyperechoic parenchyma (**Fig. 16.12a–f**). The differentiation from interposed hypoechoic fat lobules as well as its demarcation within fat can be difficult, primarily in the absence of an echogenic rim or acoustic shadow.
- Some carcinomas are isoechoic with surrounding fat (**Fig. 16.12h**) (primarily early carcinomas and carcinomas in situ). In general, they are indistinguishable from fatty tissue and may thus be easily missed by ultrasound imaging.

2. Demarcation (Margins) and Shape

- *Irregular* margins are a characteristic feature of most carcinomas (**Fig. 16.12c,f**). Evaluating the lateral margin of a mass may be more difficult sonographically than mammographically, but the superficial margins can be more accurately assessed with sonography than with mammography.
- If a thick *hyperechoic* rim is encountered, a malignancy should be considered first, even if the mass is relatively smooth in outline.
- A hyperechoic thick rim (as opposed to the thin hyperechoic capsule seen in fibroadenoma) (**Fig. 16.12b,c**) is a strong indication for malignancy but is by no means found in all carcinomas (**Fig. 16.12d–f**). It could correspond to the zone of carcinomatous infiltration into the surrounding tissue, representing the numerous lamellated interfaces induced by this infiltration.
- A smooth outline (compare **Fig. 18.5b,c** and **Fig. 16.11f,g**), which is usually combined with a round or oval shape (but not vice versa) can be found in nodular growing malignancies (mostly ductal and ductal grade 3, medullary, mucinous, sometimes DCIS, and rarely lobular carcinoma, as well as other rare malignancies or metastases). Its incidence is comparable to that found in mammography. Well-circumscribed cancers are, however, more common among high-risk women.

3. Orientation

A lesion with a sonographic *height exceeding its width* is strongly suspicious for a malignancy. This finding is only seen in some malignancies (**Fig. 16.12b,d**). An oval lesion oriented parallel to the transducer (its width exceeding its height) favors a fibroadenoma if it is smoothly outlined, but this does not exclude a malignancy. Such a horizontal orientation in fact strongly favors a benign lesion (e.g., fibroadenoma) if the horizontal axis exceeds the vertical axis by more than a factor of 1.5. Carcinomas with this presentation are rare except among women at high risk.

4. Attenuation

- A *central or eccentric acoustic shadow* seen behind one or more areas within the lesion and not characteristic of a delicate edge shadow is strongly *suspicious for malignancy* if a (partly) calcified fibroadenoma is excluded mammographically. Extensively fibrosed noncalcified fibroadenomas can have this feature as well. They can often be distinguished from malig-

16 Invasive Carcinoma

a Irregularly outlined hypoechoic lesion with echogenic rim (frequent and typical)

b Irregularly outlined hypoechoic lesion (frequent)

c Hyperechoic lesion (rare! difficult to discern!)

d Hypoechoic lesion (see above) with acoustic shadowing

e Acoustic shadowing (lesion itself not discernible)

f Lesion with partial acoustic shadowing

g Lesion with broad edge shadow

h Lesion without altered sound transmission

i Lesion with acoustic enhancement (hypercellular or edematous carcinoma)

Nodular lesion

j Height exceeds width (typical of carcinoma)

k Round (malignant or benign)

l Oval, width exceeds height (rare!)

Echogenicity

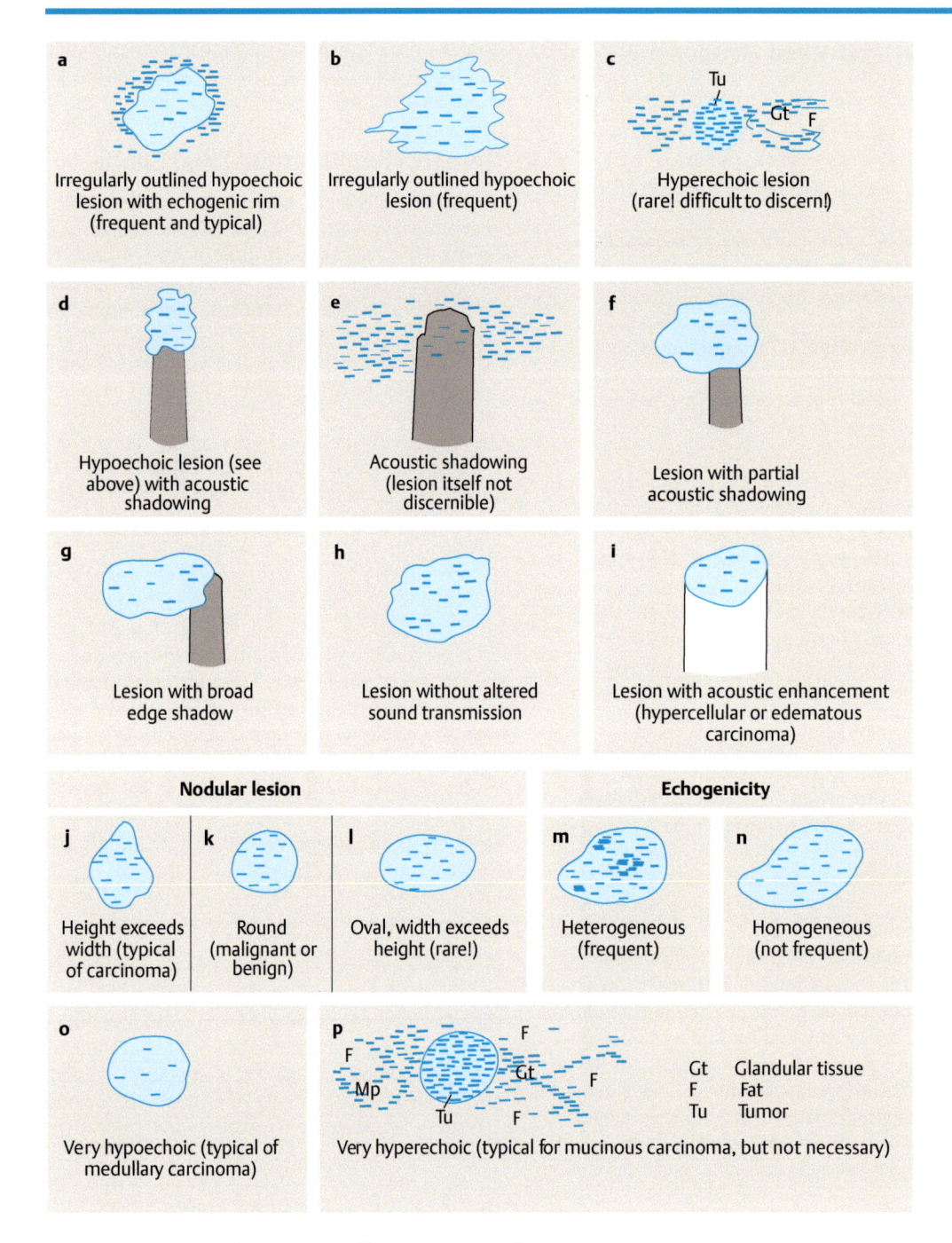

m Heterogeneous (frequent)

n Homogeneous (not frequent)

o Very hypoechoic (typical of medullary carcinoma)

p Very hyperechoic (typical for mucinous carcinoma, but not necessary)

Gt Glandular tissue
F   Fat
Tu Tumor

Fig. 16.11a–p Sonographic appearance of breast carcinomas: diagram.

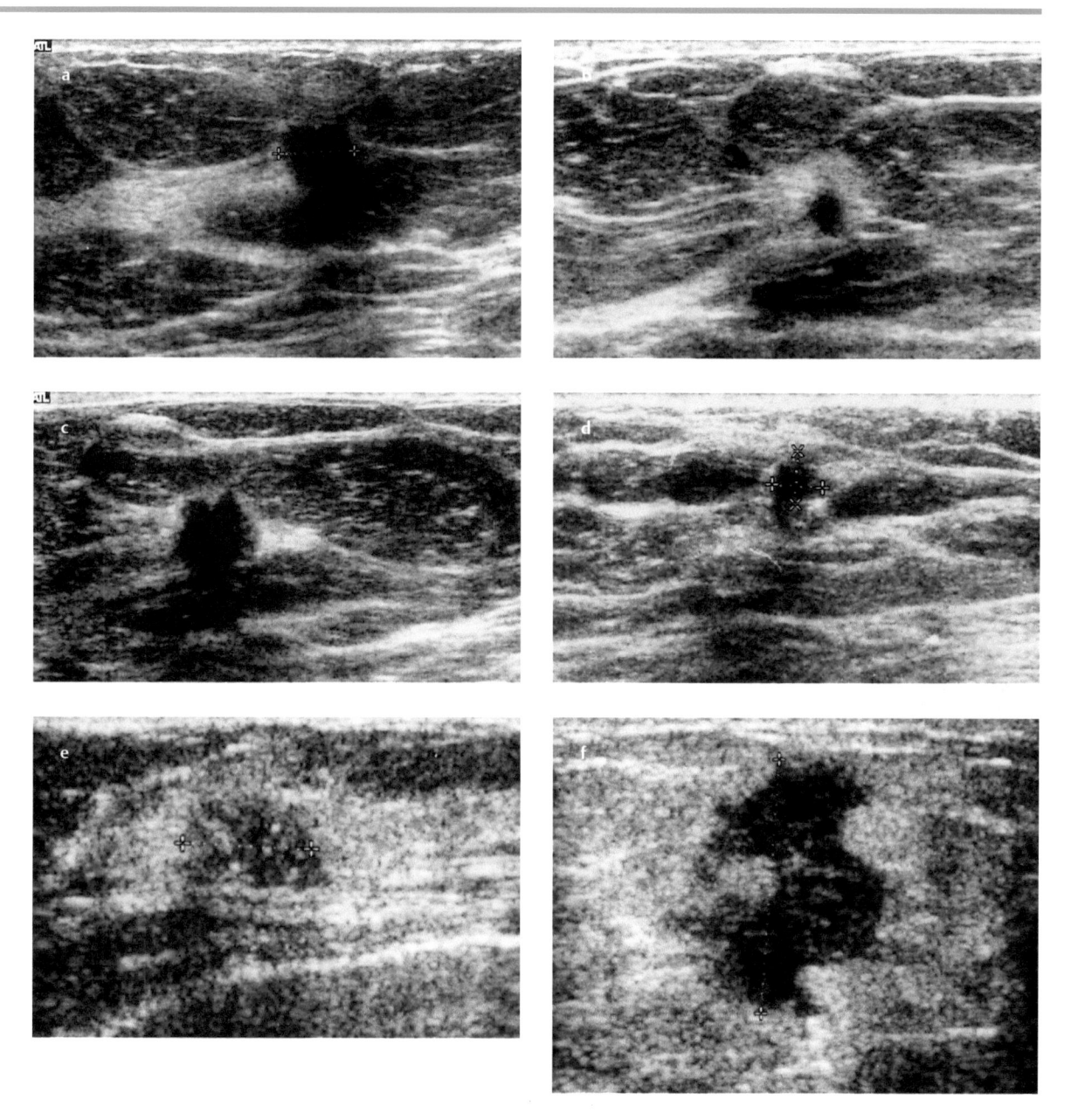

Fig. 16.12a–o

a Typical hypoechoic breast carcinoma with abrupt interface. The Cooper ligaments are interrupted and on the left border of the lesion microlobulation can be recognized. *Histology*: Invasive ductal NST carcinoma.

b Tiny very hypoechoic lesion taller than wide surrounded by a broad echogenic rim. The broad, hyperechoic rim suggests a malignancy. It corresponds to the histologically identifiable infiltration zone. Another sign of malignancy is the observation that the lesion's height exceeds its width. *Histology*: Invasive ductal carcinoma G1.

c Typical hypoechoic carcinoma with a spiculated, partly angular contour. The carcinoma, however, causes neither appreciable sound attenuation nor appreciable acoustic enhancement. This carcinoma also is surrounded by a subtle hyperechoic rim. Histologically, both the rim, corresponding to the infiltrative zone, and the hypoechoic central region are part of the carcinoma. A thickened Cooper ligament is incidentally visualized (arrowheads). *Histology*: Invasive ductal carcinoma.

d Tiny hypoechoic invasive ductal carcinoma, which does not cause appreciable sound attenuation or enhancement. It is perceivable only by the architectural distortion.

e This patient presented with a newly developed group of microcalcifications. Sonography shows that a corresponding small ill-defined and hypoechoic mass contains calcifications. *Histologically* it proved to be infiltrating ductal carcinoma.

f Typical angular margins of this palpable cancer.

Fig. 16.12g–o ▷

16 Invasive Carcinoma

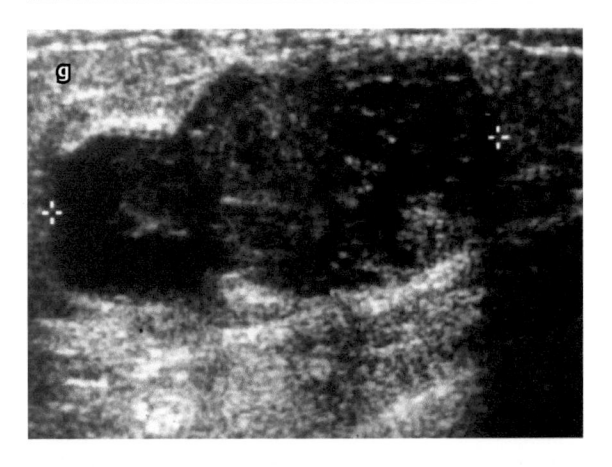

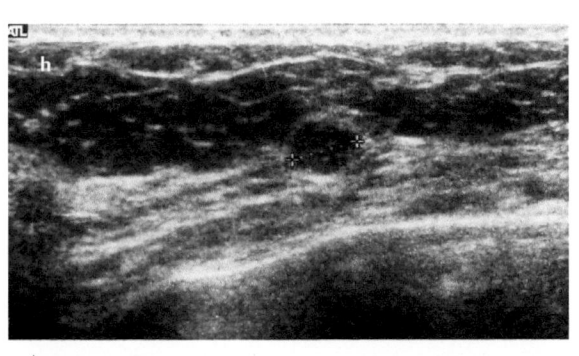

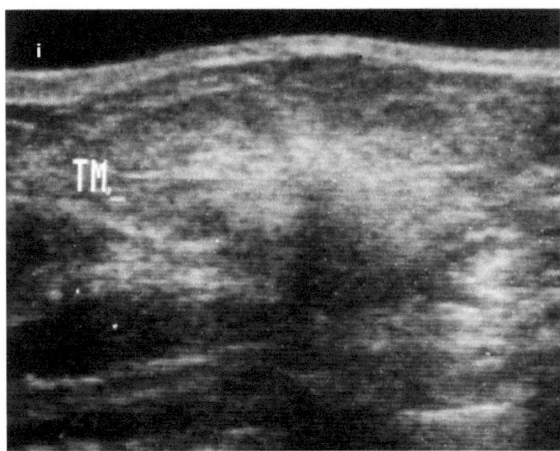

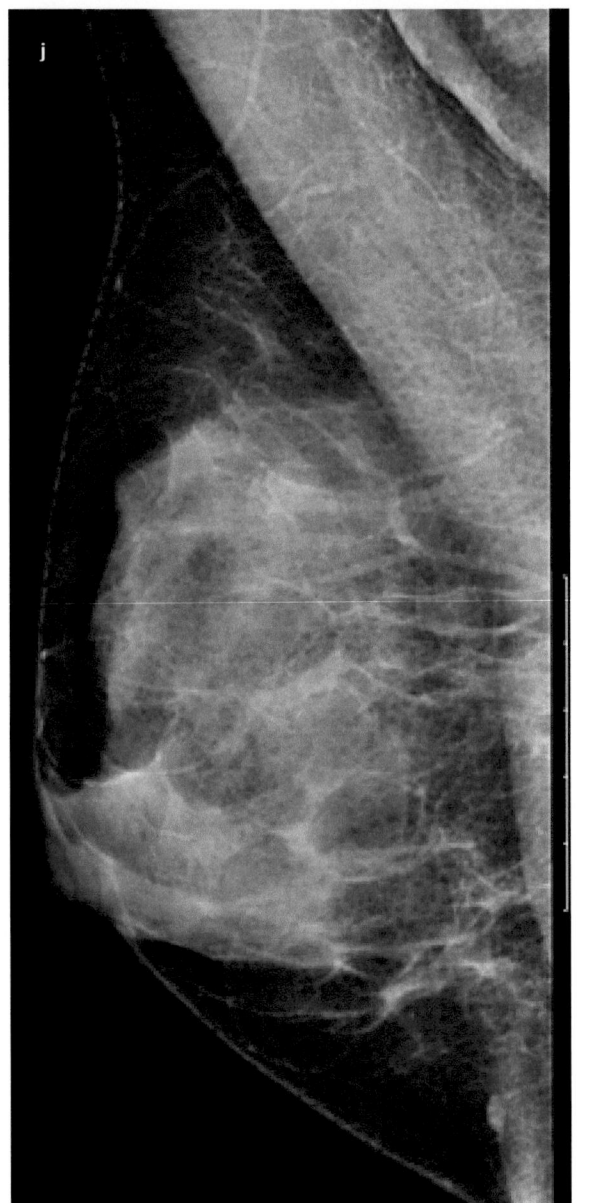

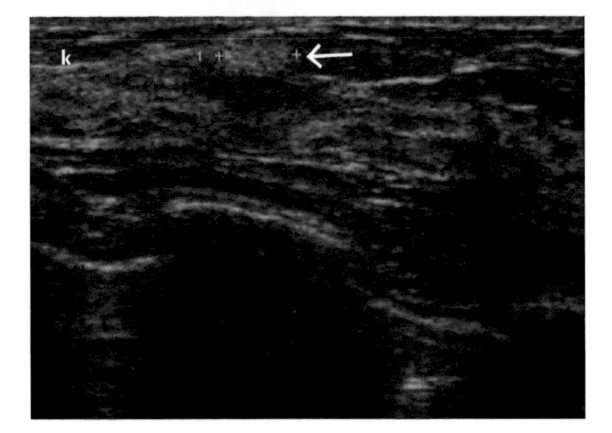

◁ continued

g This oval, wider than tall, inhomogeneous but largely hypoechoic mass shows some lobulation of its margins and distal enhancement of the sound beam. *Histologic analysis* showed this to be a mucinous carcinoma.

h A round mass, hypoechoic without sound attenuation, but with a small echogenic rim and discrete acoustic enhancement: *Histology* proved it to be a medullary cancer.

i Predominantly hyperechoic carcinoma with distal acoustic shadowing. *Histology*: NST carcinoma.

Sonography

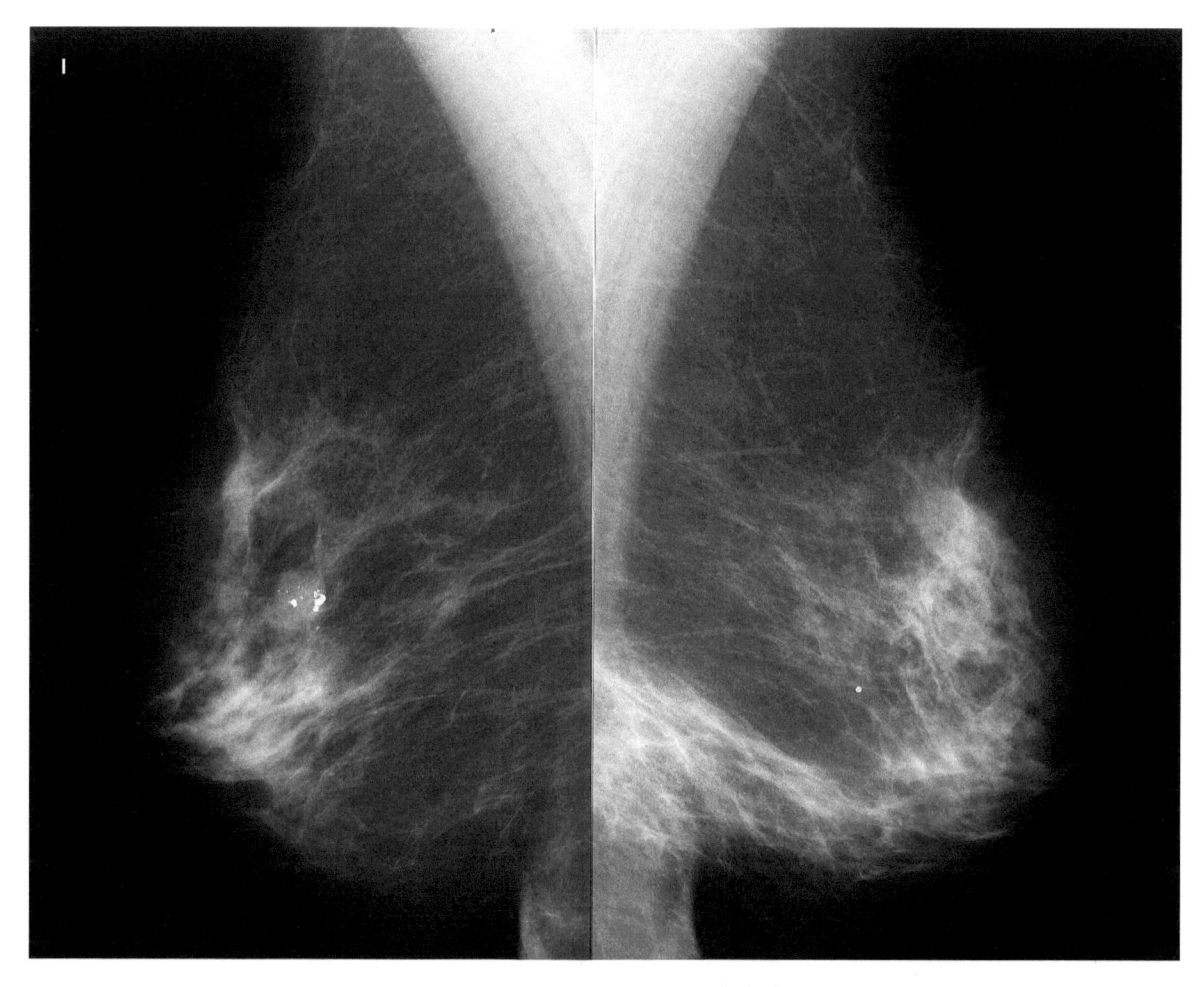

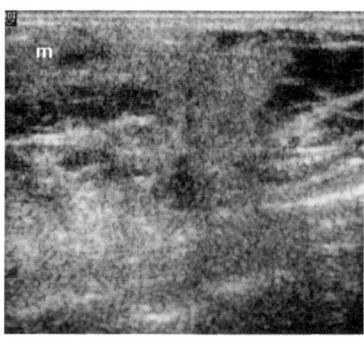

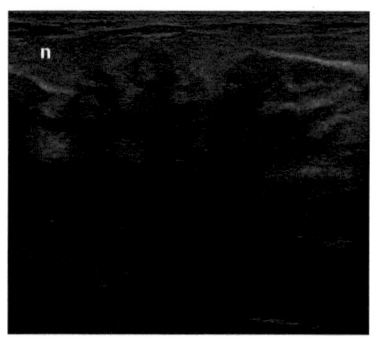

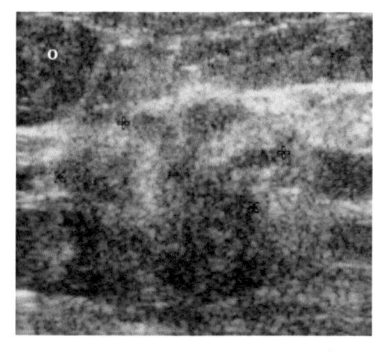

j,k Another hyperechoic carcinoma is shown: This 49-year-old patient presented with a 9-mm palpable nodule (arrow) subcutaneously in the upper outer quadrant. Mammographically the nodule cannot be identified in this ACR 4 breast. On ultrasound the nodule was completely hyperechoic. US-guided biopsy was performed and verified an invasive breast cancer with mixed ductal and lobular features. *Histologically* cells growing in strands with interleaved fat and connective tissue explain this very unusual ultrasound image of the mixed ductulo-lobular invasive breast cancer.

l,m A palpable thickening of the left breast, mammographically visible as a diffuse area with increased homogeneous density (l) corresponded to an irregular and diffusely expanding hyperechoic region reaching into the subcutaneous fat and the prepectoral, fascia. *Histology* revealed an invasive ductal carcinoma.

n A different patient with a G3 ductal diffusely growing breast cancer, which was occult on mammography (ACR 4). The carcinoma is only visible by the diffuse shadowing, by some ductlike hypoechoic structures that mimic mastopathic changes, and by some architectural distortion on sonography.

o Another patient with a diffusely growing cancer. The patient presented with a large, diffusely thickened area. On ultrasound no definite mass is visible. Within an irregular and diffusely increased echogenicity a coarse architectural distortion is visible. *Histology*: Extensive, diffusely growing lobular carcinoma.

16 Invasive Carcinoma

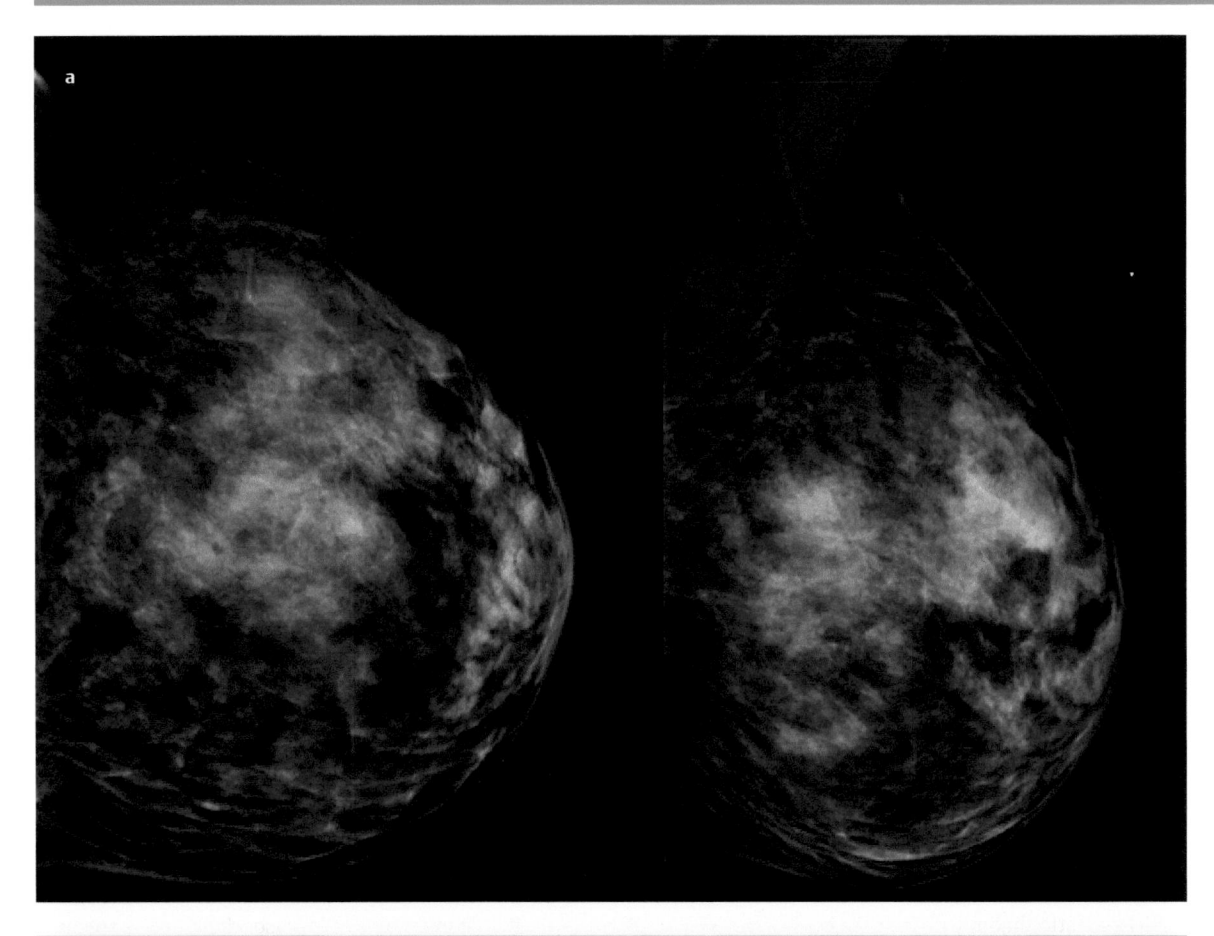

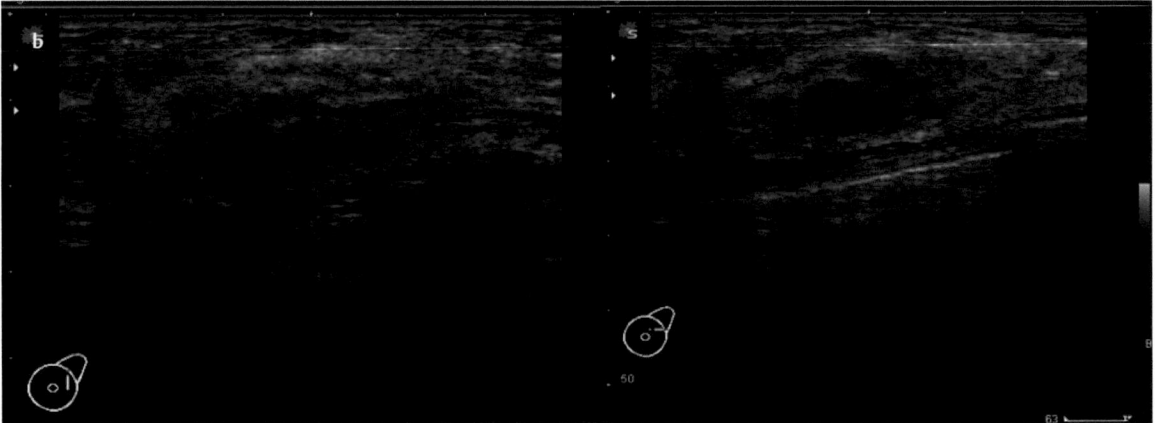

Fig.16.13a–e Advantages and limitations of sonography.

a The 69-year-old patient presented without any clinical findings. The routine examination was performed because of a moderate family history (postmenopausal breast cancer of her mother) and uncharacteristic pain. Mammography showed very dense, nodular tissue.

b On ultrasound an uncharacteristic hypoechoic area was noted within the posterior breast tissue. Owing to the uncharacteristic findings magnetic resonance imaging (MRI) was performed.

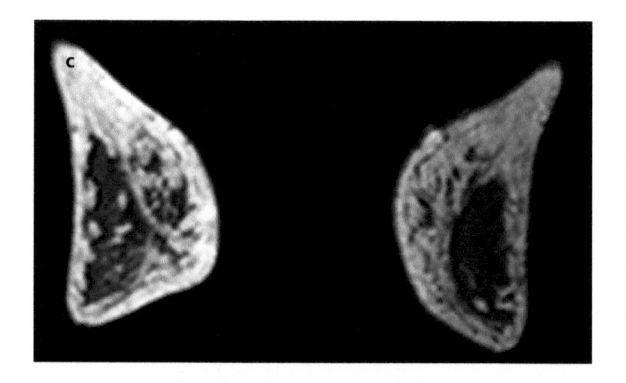

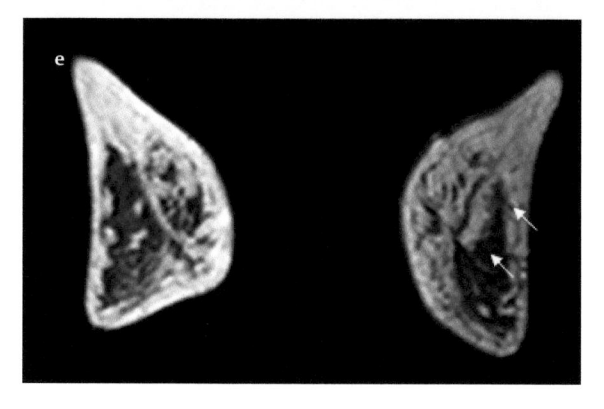

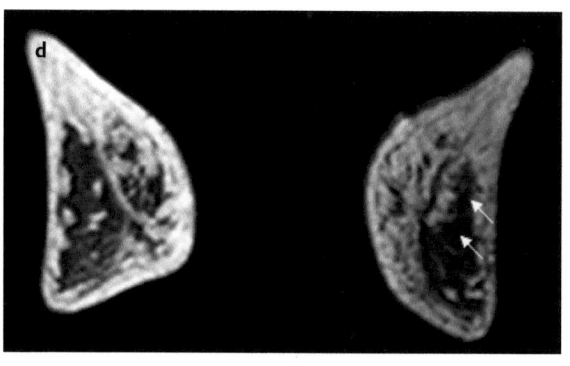

c–e Contrast-enhanced MRI: precontrast, representative early (2 min) and late (5 min) postcontrast images demonstrate a flat area of regional progressive enhancement at the posterior border of the breast tissue.
Histology revealed a lobular invasive breast cancer.

nancy by MRI. The acoustic shadow can be explained by sound absorption in fibrotic tissue. The posterior border of the lesion is not always distinguishable from the acoustic shadow (**Fig. 16.12a,c**).
- Presence of a *thickened edge shadow* also suggests that a lesion is not benign (compare also **Fig. 16.11g**).
- Some carcinomas show *no significant attenuation difference* in comparison with the surrounding structures (**Fig. 16.12b, e,f**) or may even exhibit (relative) *posterior enhancement* as compared with surrounding tissue (**Fig. 16.11i, 16.12g**). Such carcinomas contain very few reflective surfaces. They are usually homogeneously cellular or consist of a homogeneously gelatinous matrix. Such malignancies include some ductal, medullary and mucinous carcinomas, some lymphomas, and some metastases (**Fig. 18.5b,d**).
- *Acoustic shadows without focal findings* in the tissue itself—but not originating from Cooper ligaments—can be evidence of a diffusely growing carcinoma, but such acoustic shadows are nonspecific since they can frequently be seen in fibrotic benign changes (fibrocystic alterations) (**Fig. 16.12n**).

5. Distorted Architecture

- Sonographically, *architectural distortion* (**Fig. 16.12l,m**) can be identified and suggests a malignancy. It corresponds to an interruption of parenchymal and stromal surfaces, which in the supine position orient parallel to the transducer.

- Usually these normal structures are interrupted by the cancer or by edematous or fibrous reaction in the vicinity of a cancer. Thus the cancer may become detectable even though it is isoechoic or hyperechoic to fat. Architectural distortion is, however, often difficult to recognize sonographically because of the variable echo pattern of the normal breast.

6. Elasticity

Corresponding to their palpable findings, many carcinomas also exhibit sonographically detectable diminished elasticity (for evaluation of the elasticity, see Chapter 4). This can assist in the differentiation of less elastic carcinomas from fat lobules and in the very difficult detection of isoechoic carcinomas. However, good compressibility may be found with approximately 10% of the carcinomas. Few carcinomas present as quite soft (Wojcinski et al. 2010).

7. Mobility

Restricted mobility—that is, less displacement by the palpating finger—is also a property of most carcinomas. Some carcinomas with a nodular growth pattern may, however, be quite mobile. The vast majority of these carcinomas, however, are recognizable by increased consistency compared with benign tissues. Thus, overall, carcinomas that are very mobile and soft are extremely rare.

8. Internal Structure

Some carcinomas show heterogeneous internal echoes (**Fig. 16.12f,g**; for exception see **Fig. 16.12h**). This feature is, however, unreliable.

The following secondary signs of a malignancy can be sonographically observed:
- Thickening and possibly shortening of Cooper ligaments (which may be responsible for the vertical orientation of malignant lesions)
- Skin infiltration recognizable as interruption of the interface between the hyperechoic skin and hypoechoic subcutaneous tissues and as thickening of the skin
- Skin thickening which can occur locally or, in the case of the inflammatory carcinoma, diffusely

Correlation between Sonographic Image Presentation and Histology

The sonographic detectability of carcinomas, like their mammographic detectability, is affected by their size, type, growth pattern, and surrounding tissue.

As in mammography, understanding the different manifestations of breast carcinomas in relation to their histology is an important prerequisite for the correct interpretation of sonography and sensitive detection of carcinomas. Likewise it is only rarely possible to deduce the exact histology from the sonographic presentation.

- Corresponding to its diverse composition and growth pattern, *ductal carcinoma* also has a variable sonographic presentation.
  The usual invasive carcinoma with a significant fibrous component has a discrete acoustic shadow, a hyperechoic rim, and decreased elasticity. Hypercellular types can also be round, occasionally even oval, and smoothly outlined with delicate lateral acoustic shadows. Because of its homogeneous structure, the hypercellular carcinoma often shows distal acoustic enhancement, similar to that seen with the hypercellular fibroadenoma. Some ductal carcinomas may exhibit extended (mainly intraductal) growth along the ducts, just distending them. Unless microcalcifications exist within the EIC, such carcinomas may go undetected on mammography or cause only nonspecific diffuse changes such as increased density. Sonographically no specific change may be seen or somewhat prominent ductal structures. Occasional hypoechoic foci are found in areas with nodular growth. Diffuse shadowing and diminished elasticity can also be occasionally detected. Finally, small carcinomas are often sonographically isoechoic and consequently difficult to identify.
- *Lobular carcinoma* can grow focally or diffusely (**Figs. 16.12o and 16.13b**). In the latter case, it presents in a similar way to a ductal carcinoma whereby diffuse malignant growth is difficult to recognize.
- In addition to the nodular manifestation of some ductal carcinomas (**Fig. 16.12g**), *medullary* (**Fig. 16.12h**), and *mucinous* (**Fig. 16.2q,s**) carcinomas present a characteristically nodular or round appearance. These types of carcinomas are not always easily differentiated from fibroadenomas because they can also exhibit regular internal echoes and deep acoustic enhancement. If a sharply outlined focus shows only moderate compressibility, moderate mobility, or even vertical orientation (e.g., its height exceeds its width), a carcinoma must be seriously considered. If these findings are not present, a carcinoma cannot be excluded with certainty. An increase in size always requires further evaluation.
- It should be mentioned as a peculiarity that the *mucinous carcinoma* can be hypoechoic, but is often isoechoic and in these cases shows little difference relative to surrounding tissue. Papillary in situ carcinoma can, in addition to showing a nodular growth or a growth along the ducts, also be intracystic and is then sonographically easily recognizable as a hypoechoic intracystic structure. A differentiation between intracystic papilloma and papillary DCIS is generally not possible (Kim et al. 2008). Papillary invasive carcinoma is mostly indistinguishable from IDC NST.
- *Inflammatory carcinoma* presents sonographically with marked skin thickening, thickened Cooper ligaments, and edematous changes in the subcutaneous space. Additional foci of tumor nodules might be detectable within the parenchyma. Detecting such foci can be helpful in mammographically dense tissue to select areas for biopsy.

Accuracy and Differential Diagnosis

It is generally felt that the accuracy of sonography is not adequate without mammography in the patient above 40 years of age (Albert et al. 2009). Below age 40 the assessment of symptomatic patients should start with clinical examination and sonography. Unless malignancy can be excluded based on sonography (e.g., in patients who present with a simple cyst or with homogeneous hyperechoic breast tissue and benign appearing clinical findings), mammography should be supplemented in all indeterminate cases to exclude a malignancy that could easily be detected mammographically (e.g., by microcalcifications). In the very young patient (below age 30) without increased risk who presents with a palpable abnormality which is compatible with a benign fibroadenoma, US-guided percutaneous breast biopsy may be considered before a mammogram. However, if percutaneous breast biopsy does not confirm the expected diagnosis, mammography should be re-considered. This recommendation takes into account the high probability of a fibroadenoma, the low probability of malignancy at that age, and issues of radiation protection.

Because of limited accuracy, time commitment (physician time), and operator dependence, sonography is not suitable as a stand-alone method for screening (Berg et al. 2006, Lazarus et al. 2006).

When used as a supplementary tool for selected groups of patients and by selected institutions sonography has proven capable of detecting small cancers which were occult to mammography (Berg et al. 2008, Nothacker et al. 2009).

If sonography is used selectively as a supplemental method to solve problems, it can increase accuracy.

- If palpation reveals a questionable finding, sonography can contribute to the correct diagnosis in mammographically dense tissue and in this way contributes in the timely detection of carcinomas (= avoidance of false negative findings). It may help evaluate margins of a lesion that is partially obscured by mammography.
- In clinical and mammographic findings that can be sonographically explained as one or several simple cysts, sonography can markedly eliminate unnecessary biopsies (= avoidance of false positive diagnoses).
- The sensitivity of sonography is limited for the detection of small and pre-invasive carcinomas. Therefore, negative sonography with a noncystic finding does not refute a mammographic or clinical suspicion.
- Because of the wide range of variations found with benign as well as malignant tumors (smooth or irregular outline, acoustic shadowing to acoustic enhancement, and different compressibility of benign and malignant findings), great care is necessary when averting biopsy in cases with probably benign findings. Such a decision should usually be based on a combined evaluation of clinical findings, mammography, and sonography.

In all sonographically detected findings:
- Fat lobules and tumors must be carefully distinguished (accuracy depends on the examiner and his/her experience and the size and depth of the lesion).
- The differential diagnosis of hypoechoic findings includes (in addition to malignant tumors) complex cysts, fibroadenomas, and papillomas, as well as hypoechoic areas that can be multiple in the presence of pronounced fibrocystic changes or adenosis. Depending on the degree of suspicion, follow-up examinations in 6 months, sonographically guided percutaneous needle biopsy, or excisional biopsy is indicated.

All things considered, the sonographic accuracy of detecting tumors in sonographically homogeneous, echogenic tissue (mastopathy, dense parenchyma) is better than in heterogeneous tissue (fibrocystic changes with hypoechoic areas and acoustic shadowing, or glandular tissue with multiple interspersed fat lobules). In adipose tissue, mammography is the method of choice.

Magnetic Resonance Imaging

Diagnostic Role

Contrast-enhanced MRI is the most sensitive method for the detection of invasive carcinomas. About 90–95% of the invasive carcinomas show moderate to marked enhancement following injection of Gd-DTPA (Heywang-Köbrunner et al. 2001, Schnall et al. 2006, Peters et al. 2008), so that contrast-enhanced MRI, as a method complementary to mammography, can provide valuable additional information. This information is most valuable for selected diagnostic questions that cannot be solved otherwise (see below and Chapter 5).

There is no international recommendation that would support MRI as a screening method except for women at high risk (National Institute for Health and Clinical Excellence, National Collaborating Centre for Primary Care 2006, National Breast Care Centre 2006, Sardanelli et al. 2010). Its use for screening is not recommended since the specificity of MRI is too low (Heywang-Köbrunner et al. 2001, 2008, Peters et al. 2008), and because of the expensive and time-consuming assessment of lesions detected by MRI only.

Imaging Presentation of Carcinomas

Invasive carcinomas can be visualized as follows (**Fig. 16.14a–i**, see also Chapter 5).
- Focal, moderate to marked enhancement is the cardinal finding for detecting 85–90% of the carcinomas. The focal enhancement is:
  - Mostly irregularly outlined or indistinct (**Fig. 16.14a,b**)
  - Occasionally linear or segmental by following ductal structures (this corresponds histologically to a partial intraductal growth (**Fig. 16.14c–e**)
  - Occasionally nodular (**Fig. 16.14f,g**)
  - Rarely smoothly outlined (see also **Fig. 16.14a,b**)
  - More intense or earlier enhancement along the periphery is characteristic of a carcinoma. The peripheral areas of early and intense enhancement generally correspond to the hypercellular growth zone of the carcinoma, whereas the central zone of progressive and moderate enhancement is explained by central fibrosis or necrosis (**Fig. 16.14g**)
- Regional or diffuse enhancement (= milky or patchy-confluent enhancement, without distinct border, covering large areas of the parenchyma) is seen in approximately 10–15% of carcinomas. About half of these cases with diffuse enhancement correspond to diffusely growing carcinomas (**Fig. 16.14h,i**). In the remaining cases, a histologically focal tumor is surrounded by diffusely enhancing, mostly proliferative fibrocystic changes, rarely by inflammatory tissue.

16 Invasive Carcinoma

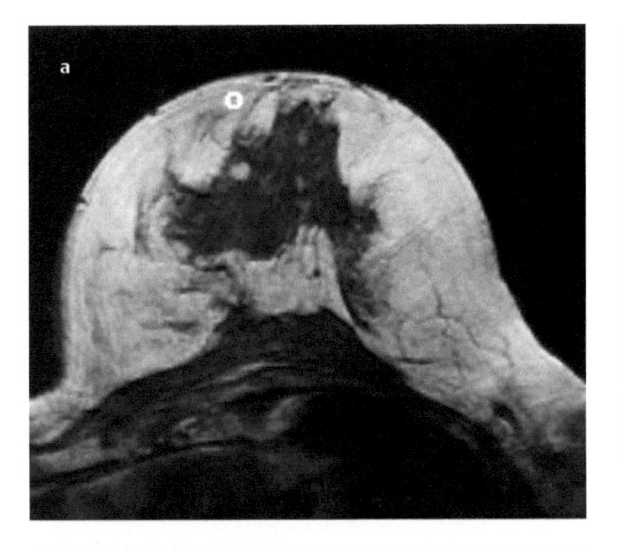

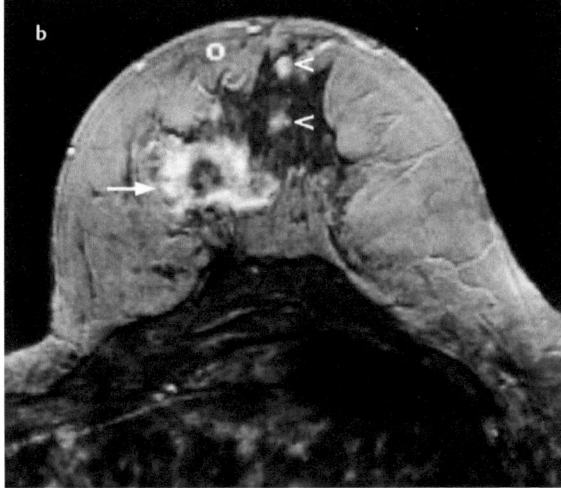

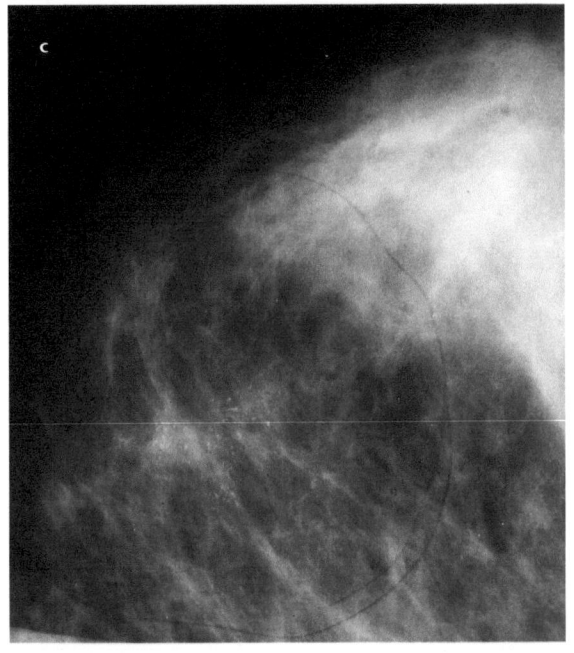

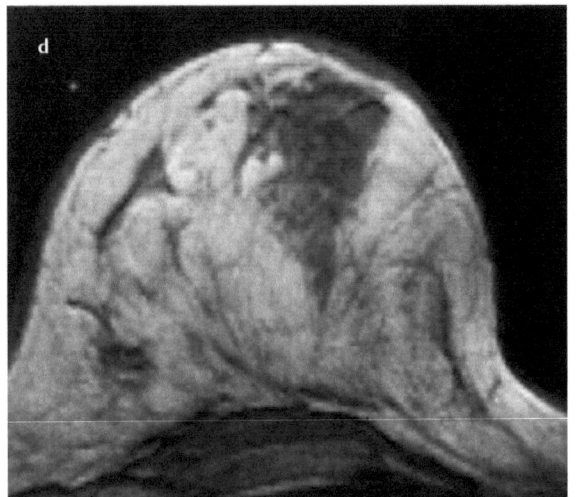

Fig. 16.14a–i Magnetic resonace imaging (MRI) appearance of carcinomas.

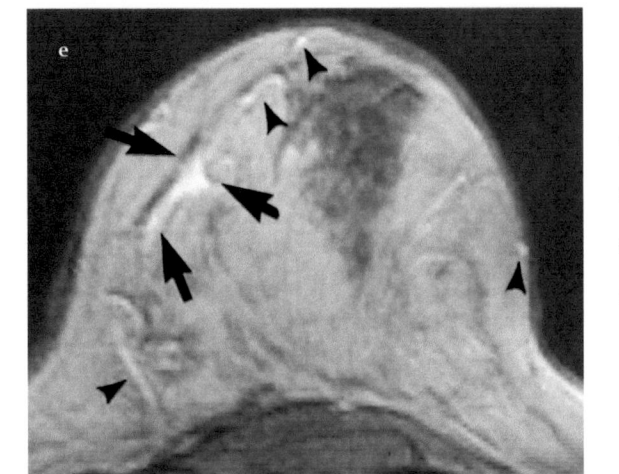

a,b Preoperative MRI before (**a**) and after (**b**) intravenous injection of the paramagnetic contrast agent Gd-DTPA. In addition to the large, medially located focus (large arrow) corresponding to a mammographic and sonographic finding, there are several additional foci (arrowheads) that are visible only by magnetic resonance imaging. The central zone without enhancement corresponds to central necrosis. *Histology*: Multifocal ductal carcinoma.

c–e Preoperative MRI in a patient with suspicious microcalcifications.

c Mammographically pleomorphic microcalcifications with a suggested ductal arrangement.

d Transverse image at the level of the suspicious microcalcifications.

e Intense rapid enhancement of the involved ductal system (arrows) after administration of the contrast agent. In contrast to the enhancing ductal segments, the transected vessels (arrowheads) appear punctate or linear and follow a curved course in the subcutaneous space but do not converge toward the nipple. *Histology*: Intraductal carcinoma with microinvasion. (Reproduced with kind permission of Springer Science+Business Media from Heywang-Köbrunner and Beck 1996.)

f Contrast-enhanced MRI (from left upper corner to right lower corner), unenhanced and 1, 3, and 5 minutes after intravenous injection of Gd-DTPA, shows a slowly enhancing nodule corresponding to an uncertain palpable finding. Even delayed enhancement (maximum at 3 min or later after injection) is an indication for biopsy of a lesion found to be suspicious by other imaging modalities or clinically. *Histology*: Papillary carcinoma with microinvasion (5 mm). (Reproduced with kind permission of Springer Science+Business Media from Heywang-Köbrunner and Beck 1996.)

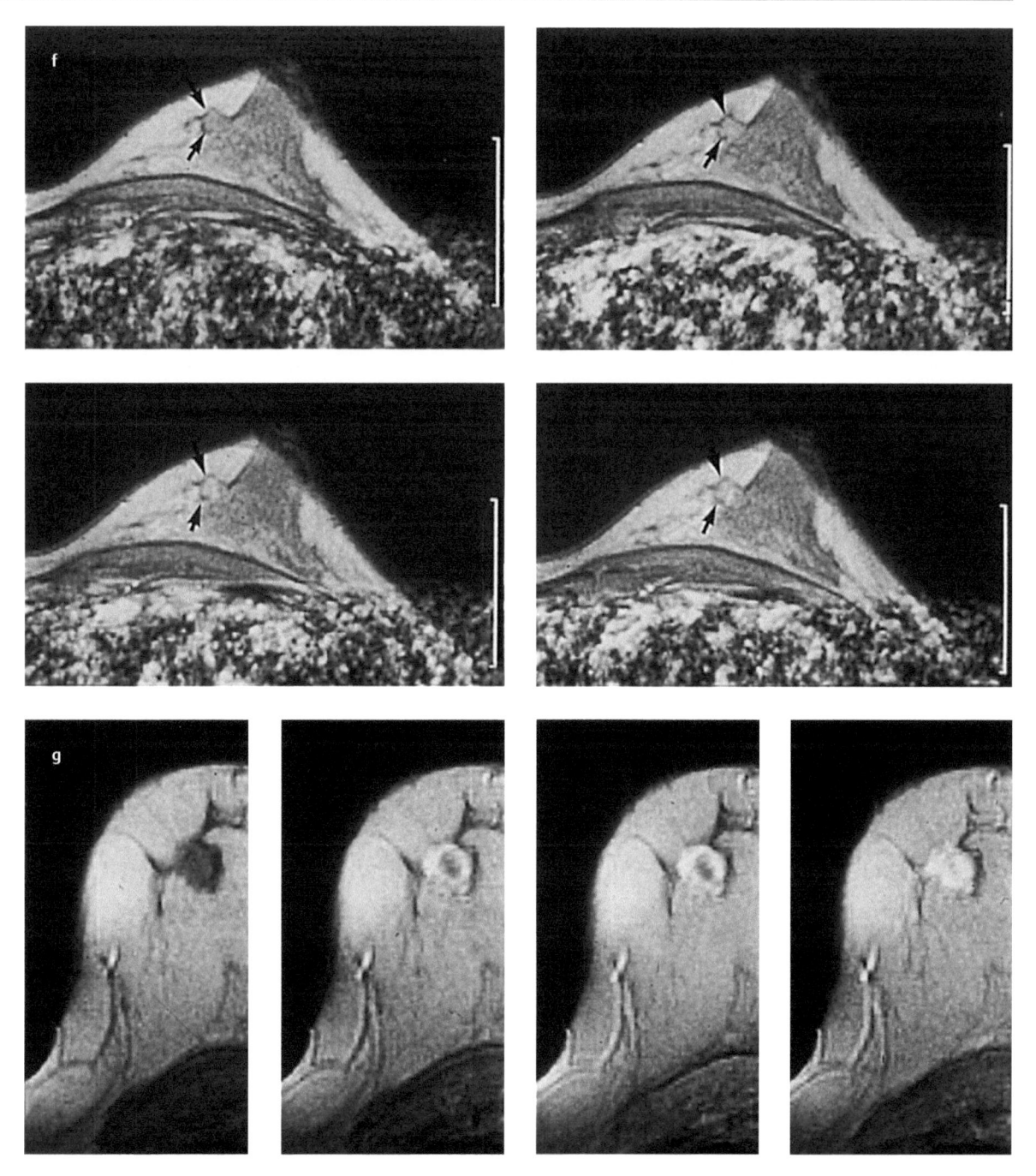

g Ringlike enhancement in a focal finding. The contrast-enhanced MRI (from left upper corner to right lower corner), unenhanced and 1, 3, and 5 minutes after intravenous application of Gd-DTPA shows a ringlike enhancement. This pattern of enhancement must be considered as highly suggestive of a malignancy. *Histology*: Invasive ductal NST carcinoma.

◁ continued

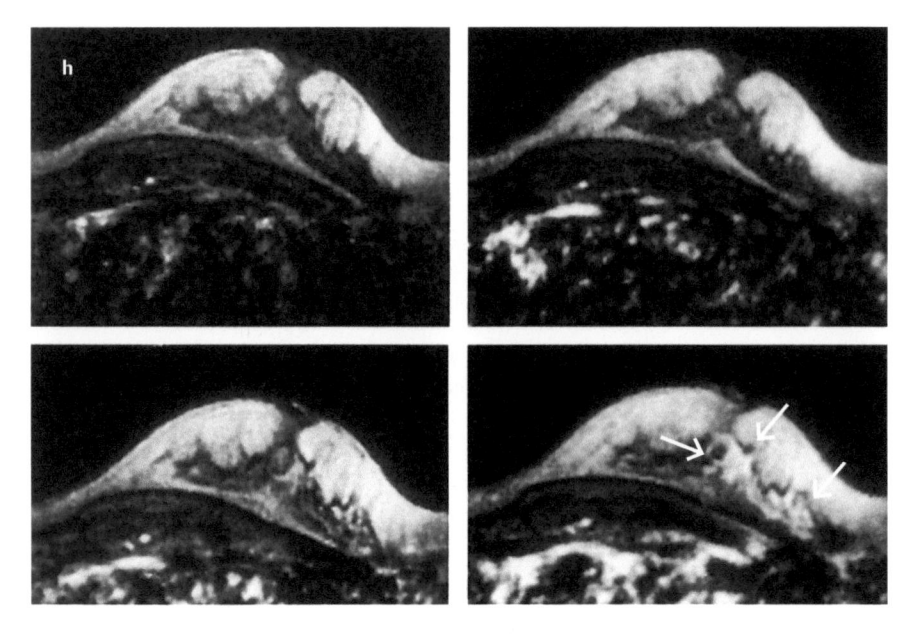

h Diffuse and delayed enhancement in a carcinoma permeating the upper outer quadrant. MRI before scheduled biopsy (from left upper corner to right lower corner), unenhanced and 1, 3, and 5 minutes after intravenous application of Gd-DTPA, shows a delayed enhancement in the entire upper outer quadrant (arrows).
As explained in conjunction with the case illustrated in **Fig. 16.15f**, the excision of an area found to be suspicious by other imaging modalities is always indicated—even if the enhancement is diffuse or slow. *Histology*: Lobular scirrhous carcinoma. (Reproduced with kind permission of Springer Science+Business Media from Heywang-Köbrunner and Beck 1996.)

In these cases of enhancing surrounding tissue, the tumor cannot reliably be delineated and can usually not be detected by MRI alone.
- Most carcinomas show rapidly increasing enhancement, that is, the maximum enhancement is achieved 1–3 minutes after injection of the contrast medium. About half of these carcinomas show a subsequent decrease in signal intensity, beginning 3–5 minutes after the injection and corresponding to a washout effect. Washout is associated with a high probability of malignancy. However, as mentioned above, only about half of the cancers exhibit washout. The other rapidly enhancing malignancies do not show significantly changed enhancement after the first rapid increase. This enhancement is called plateau-type enhancement. Such enhancement is frequently also seen in benign lesions or changes (such as benign changes, adenosis, fibroadenomas, papillomas).
- Continuously increasing enhancement (progressive enhancement) was observed in our patients in 12% of the carcinomas. In view of these progressively enhancing carcinomas, progressive enhancement that is otherwise characteristic of many benign changes cannot be used to exclude malignancy in cases with mammographic, clinical, or sonographic suspicion.
- Absent enhancement is rare with invasive malignancy (< 5%). However, it is seen in up to 40% of the in situ malignancies (Heywang-Köbrunner et al. 2001, Sardanelli et al. 2004, Schnall et al. 2006).

Correlation between MRI and Tumor Extension

To date ample literature confirms that MRI is the most sensitive method for demonstrating invasive tumor, second foci, and extensive intraductal component (EIC). Concerning visualization of DCIS or EIC all methods are only moderately sensitive and specific, but MRI and mammography prove complementary (Berg et al. 2004, Sardanelli et al. 2004, Schelfout et al. 2004). Concerning lesion extent, for the EIC in particular, overestimates and underestimates exist with both mammography and MRI. However, the combined information from MRI and mammography is superior to mammography alone or mammography plus sonography, and currently allows the best assessment with respect to histopathology (Schouten van der Velden et al. 2006, Kim et al. 2007b, Van Goethem et al. 2007). As proven by a large randomized study and by meta-analyses on the performance of preoperative MRI, the additional use of MRI allows detection of malignant extent or foci more accurately than conventional imaging (Houssami et al. 2008, Turnbull et al. 2010, Plana et al. 2012). Since, however, existing data so far cannot prove a benefit (improved outcome, fewer re-excisions, or fewer recurrences) for patients undergoing breast conservation, the general use of MRI for preoperative staging is not recommended. This lack of proof of benefit may probably be explained by the effect of radiation therapy and adjuvant therapy administered with standard breast conservation.

It may be assumed that the small lesions detected by MRI alone mostly concern foci, which—due to their small size—respond excellently to these therapies and therefore would not require to be detected.

While an overall improved outcome could not be proven, this may not concern subgroups or women who undergo different types of treatment.

According to present consensus papers and recommendations, preoperative MRI may be considered in preoperative patients with proven lobular breast cancer, in patients at high risk, and in patients who present with significantly different lesion size on mammography compared with sonography (Albert et al. 2009, Sardanelli et al. 2010). Schwartz points out that contrast-enhanced MRI may be useful when planning therapy and deciding for or against breast conservation in T2-stage breast cancers (Schwartz et al. 2006).

Also, preoperative MRI may be of value in women who are not planned to undergo standard breast conservation, but rather partial breast irradiation or oncoplastic partial breast surgery without radiation.

When performing MRI preoperatively, the following may be encountered:
- In focally growing invasive carcinomas, the area enhancing on MRI mostly corresponds very well to the histologically determined size of the invasive carcinoma.
- If an area with a poorly differentiated carcinoma in situ is histologically found next to an invasive carcinoma, the contrast enhancement of the carcinoma in situ may be similar to that of the invasive carcinoma and consequently cannot be distinguished from it. In these cases, the enhancing area seen on MRI often corresponds to the site of the invasive carcinoma plus the site of the carcinoma in situ.
- Some DCIS lesions enhance less and more slowly than the invasive carcinoma. These may be demarcated from the invasive carcinoma, with the focally strong enhancement corresponding to the invasive carcinoma itself. In other cases, the DCIS component may be indistinguishable from benign proliferative changes. In cases with strong underlying enhancement or additional foci detected in other parts of the breast great care is necessary not to overdiagnose and overtreat. Thus findings that might lead to more extensive surgery should be verified first by percutaneous breast biopsy.
- In other cases DCIS may not enhance and may thus only be detectable by mammography (by presence of microcalcifications) or by histopathology.

So overall, MRI may add valuable information. However, it is not able to replace percutaneous breast biopsy. Whenever additional extent is detected, percutaneous breast biopsy should be considered. Preoperative MRI should not be performed unless the possibility of MR-guided percutaneous breast biopsy and MR-guided marking exists.

Fig. 16.15 demonstrates advantages and limitations of contrast-enhanced MRI used for local staging.

Variations and Pitfalls

The following situations should be dealt with cautiously:
- Carcinomas with a pronounced fibrous component, mainly the lobular carcinoma, can have moderate, diffuse, or delayed enhancement (**Fig. 16.14h,i**). Such enhancement should not lead to the exclusion of a carcinoma, even if it is most often associated with benign changes.
- While most invasive carcinomas demonstrate strong enhancement, individual cases with very low or even absent enhancement have been observed. Histologically and according to our own experience, this may concern any type of breast cancer. Also, according to our experience, nonenhancing breast cancer may be lethal like other breast cancers. Absent or low and progressive enhancement occurs more frequently among lobular breast cancers, among diffusely growing fibrosed breast cancers, and among very early and small breast cancers.
- For the differential diagnosis of microcalcifications, mammography rather than MRI is still the method of choice.

Indications

Current indications for MRI include questions for which MRI can provide relevant information in addition to conventional methods, and cases where a significant prevalence of breast cancer can be expected.

MRI is not recommended in the following situations:
- Systematic MR screening beyond high-risk groups (e.g., women with dense breasts or young women). In women with low risk there is a significant risk of false positive calls caused by benign tumors, adenosis, or hormonally induced changes. There is also a significant risk of unnecessary biopsy, and when a lesion is visible only by MRI, MR-guided percutaneous breast biopsy may be needed, which is not widely available and associated with significant costs and unnecessary stress to the patient.
- Indications that can be solved by percutaneous biopsy. Since the negative predictive value of MRI is lower than that of percutaneous breast biopsy, MRI should not generally be used as a tool to exclude malignancy. Exceptions should be well founded. False positive calls may concern the lesion in question and additional areas in the same or contralateral breast and may require unnecessary assessment. And the probability of false positive calls rises in patients in whom the primary lesion proves to be benign.

16 Invasive Carcinoma

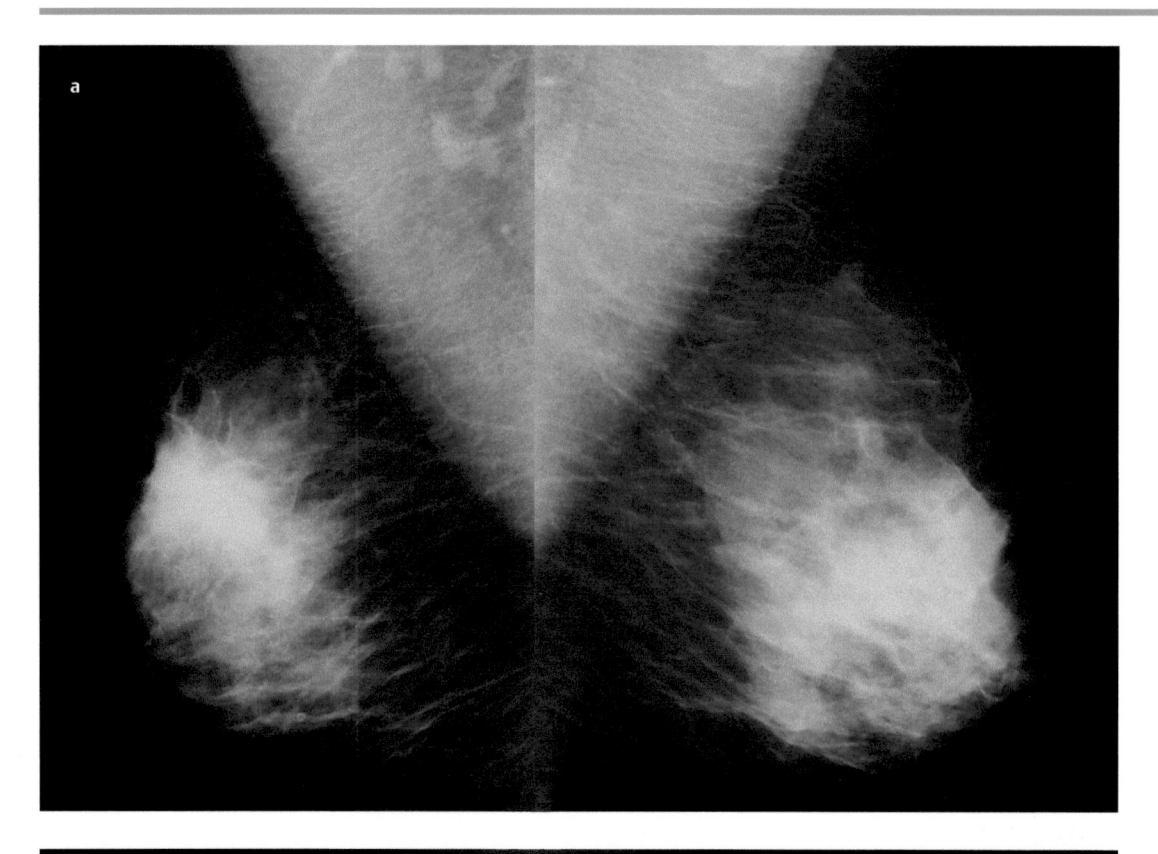

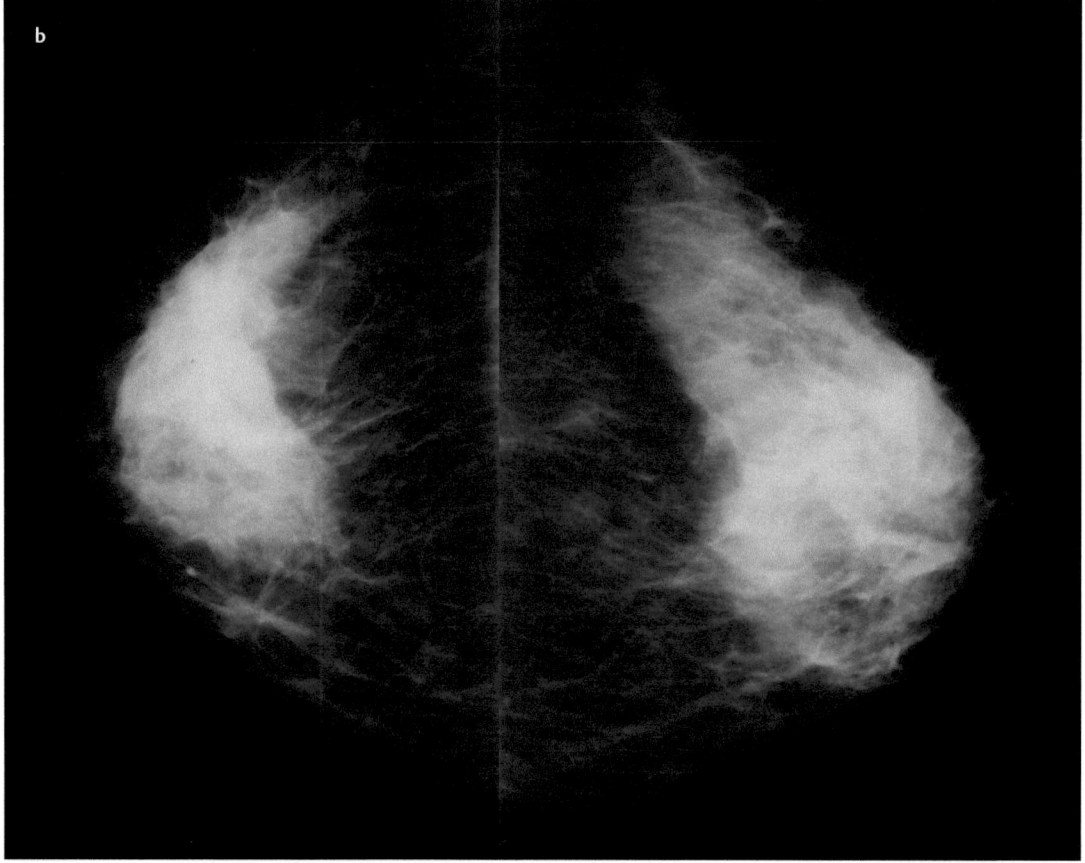

446

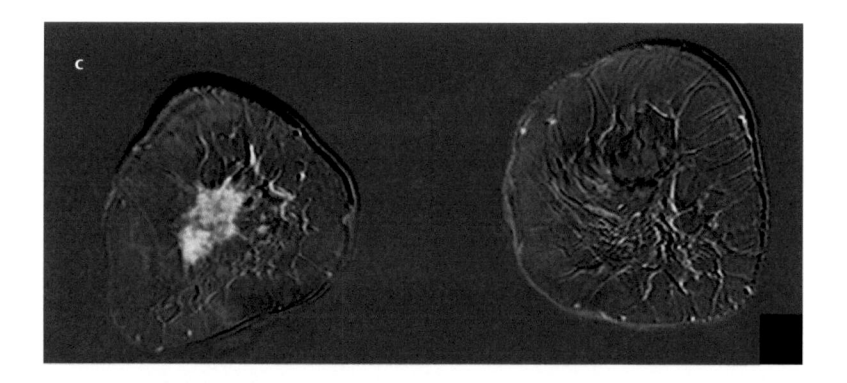

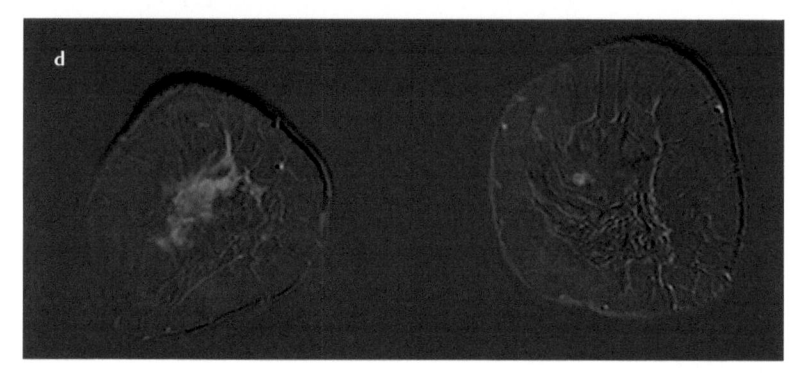

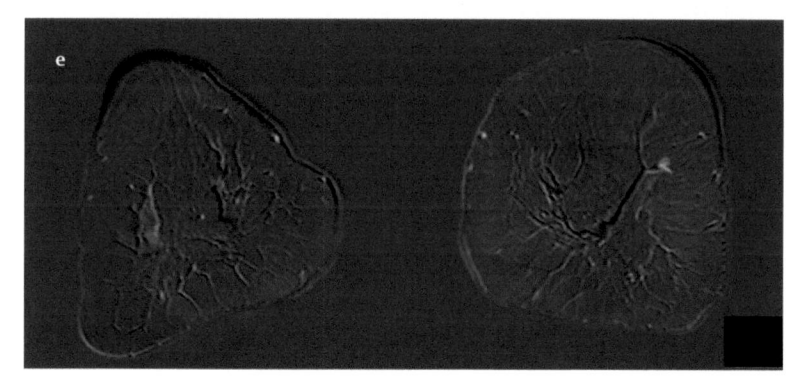

Fig. 16.15a–e This postmenopausal patient presented with a palpable thickening of the right breast.

- **a,b** Mammographically (and clinically) some shrinkage of the right breast compared with the left breast is seen; there is also slight nipple retraction of the right. The density on the right is diffusely increased. Overall the findings are highly suspicious. On the left, mammographically no abnormality is noted.
- **c** Magnetic resonance imaging (MRI) (subtraction image) confirms strong plateau-type enhancement and some shrinkage of the breast tissue on the right–overall highly suspicious findings.
- **d** On MRI two small enhancing foci were detected on the left side. This subtraction image shows the enhancing focus (> 5 mm) in the left inner upper quadrant (plateau-type, round, fairly well-circumscribed enhancement, which is more pronounced peripherally. Due to this peripheral enhancement malignancy was suspected. *Histology* yielded a papilloma. (The central area probably corresponded to some central bleeding.)
- **e** Another focus (well circumscribed, plateau-type enhancement) was excised during the same surgery after MR-guided marking and turned out to correspond to a well-circumscribed small additional focus of invasive lobular carcinoma.

Thus MRI proves capable of detecting additional malignant foci. Its specificity is limited. Considering the extensive disease on the right the prognostic value of detecting the second focus is questionable.

Indications where MRI may add valuable information include:
- Screening for women at high risk. (The scheme should follow the general guidelines for this particular indication (see Chapter 5, pp. 152–156) and patients should be adequately informed about potential prophylactic measures, their reliability and side effects.
- Search for primary tumor in cases with positive axillary lymph nodes and no findings on conventional imaging (**Fig. 16.16**).
- Detection or exclusion of malignancy in breasts with diagnostic problems after conservative therapy for breast carcinoma with or without radiation, and after silicone implants (see also **Figs. 19.16** and **19.17**, as well as **Fig. 24.16**).
- Detection or exclusion of multicentricity or bilateral involvement before planning conservative therapy in the above-mentioned restricted indications.
- Monitoring of neoadjuvant chemotherapy. While MRI (like any other imaging modality) cannot exclude microscopic residual tissue, it may allow recognition of poor response and depiction of macroscopic residual tissue preoperatively. This indication is, however, still under investigation (see Chapter 5, pp. 162–166).
- Complementary use for questions that could not be adequately answered with conventional methods and are not suitable for percutaneous biopsy (nipple retraction of unclear origin, nipple discharge and unsuccessful galactogram, evaluation of multiple unclear findings, and findings that are problematic to puncture, such as densities only visible on one mammographic view) (see **Fig. 16.7**).

It is mandatory that all nonpalpable findings seen only by MRI and considered suspicious are further evaluated by MR-guided percutaneous biopsy or by excision after MR-guided localization, which is necessary for the surgeon and pathologist.

All things considered, MRI can add important and decisive information to the diagnostic evaluation of carcinomas. As a general rule, it should be reserved as a complementary method for specific indications.

Percutaneous Biopsy Methods

Diagnostic Role

For further evaluation of clinically, mammographically, and sonographically abnormal findings, or even abnormal findings by MRI, percutaneous needle biopsy is currently the method of choice.

If compatible benign findings are present, unnecessary surgical biopsy can be avoided. A malignancy percutaneous breast biopsy allows improved therapy planning, by supporting preoperative planning to minimize the volume of tissue to be removed, while decreasing the number of excisions needed to obtain free margins and increasing the number of cases with free margins. Based on this proven effect the use of percutaneous breast biopsy is recommended to confirm the diagnosis before surgery for breast malignancy. The European guidelines recommend that in certified breast centers at least 70%, optimally 90%, of the malignancies should be verified by percutaneous breast biopsy before surgery (Perry et al. 2006).

Histologic results of percutaneous biopsy must be critically assessed to determine whether the procured material is representative and, consequently, the result definitive. In case of incompatible findings or remaining uncertainty repeat percutaneous or surgical biopsy must be considered.

Cognizance of the achievable *accuracy* of the particular percutaneous biopsy method is crucial for the *appropriate application* and *correct assessment* of the cytologic or histologic results in the diagnostic workup. The accuracy can be estimated from data in the literature but should also be continuously validated for the respective diagnostic team and the given technical conditions (correlation of percutaneous biopsy with the results of surgery or subsequent follow-up).

The accuracy achieved for diagnosing or excluding breast carcinoma indeed depends on several factors (see Chapter 7):
- Experience of the diagnostic team
- Methodical factors (accuracy of targeting, volume of tissue removed compared with the area in question, duration of the procedure, standards of procedure used, systematic countercheck with all imaging material and histopathology)
- Biological factors (special care is necessary with diffuse changes and lesions which may exhibit discontinuous growth or inhomogeneous composition such as suspected lobular breast cancer or DCIS; for large areas it must be diligently checked whether the sampled tissue can be representative for the whole area)

Sensitivity of core needle biopsy (before interdisciplinary correlation and consensus) ranges around 92–98% and specificity approximates 100%. The accuracy in the diagnosis of masses exceeds that of microcalcifications or architectural distortion.

Improved diagnostic accuracy may be expected for assessment of microcalcifications and other very small findings with vacuum-assisted breast biopsy (95–99%). Also a decreased rate of upgrades among B3 lesions is possible with this technique. For image-guided cytology, sensitivities of 53–98% and specificities of 89–100% have been reported (see Chapter 7). Therefore cytology should only be used by highly experienced diagnostic and multidisciplinary teams.

Percutaneous Biopsy Methods

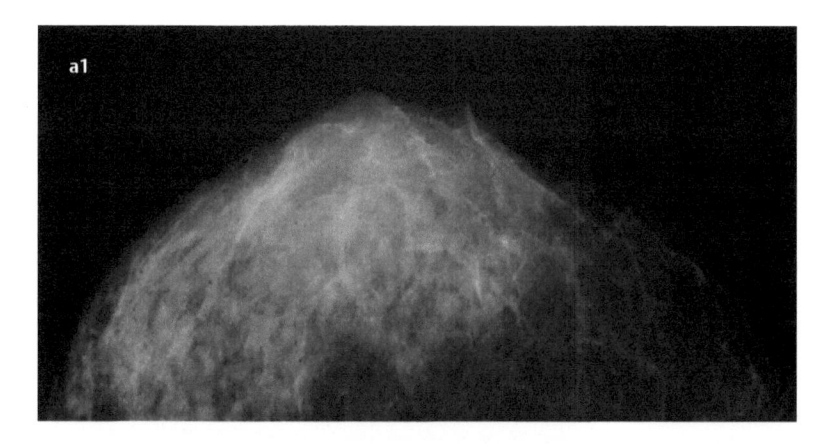

Fig. 16.16a,b A 57-year-old patient, symptomatic with a lymph node in the left axilla positive for breast cancer.
a Mammography and ultrasound did not show an abnormality.
b On MRI (repesentative pre- and postcontrast slices are shown) the enhancing lymph node is clearly visible (thin arrow). Furthermore a suspicious focal plateau-type enhancement (thick arrow) is seen in the left upper outer quadrant. *Histology*: Invasive ductal NST carcinoma.

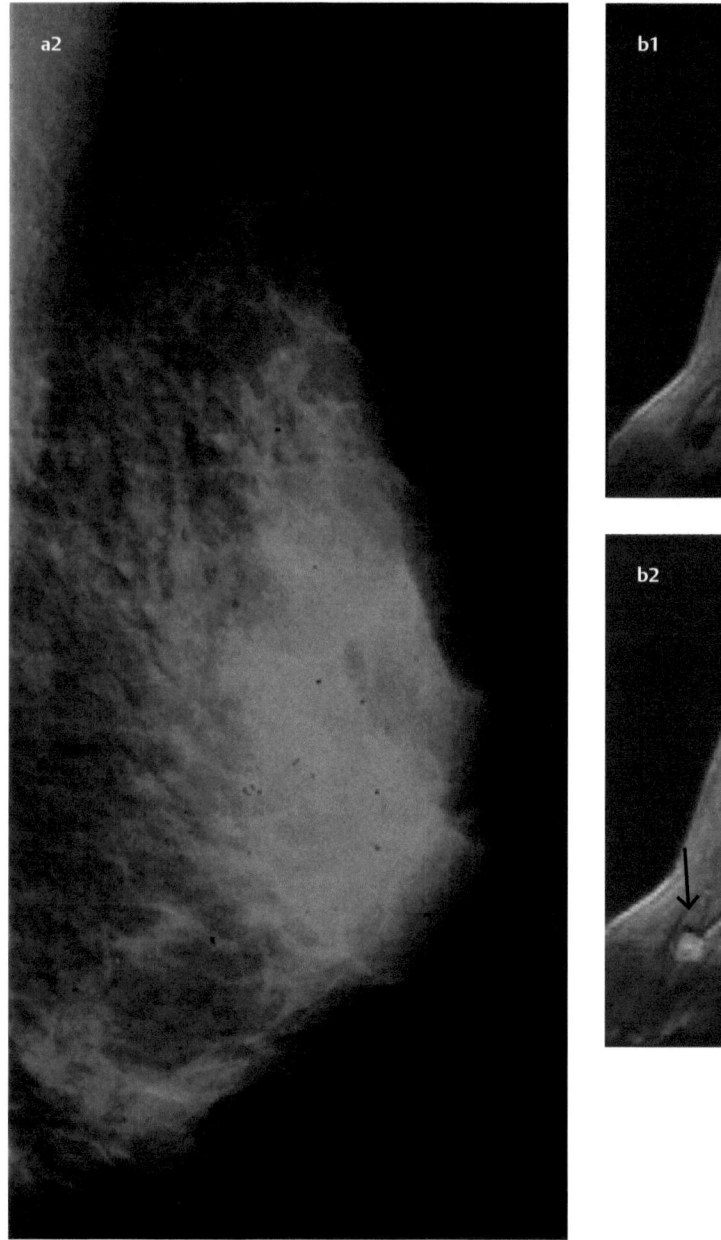

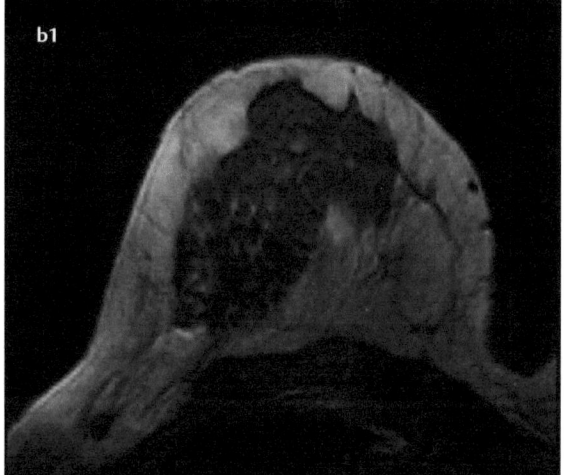

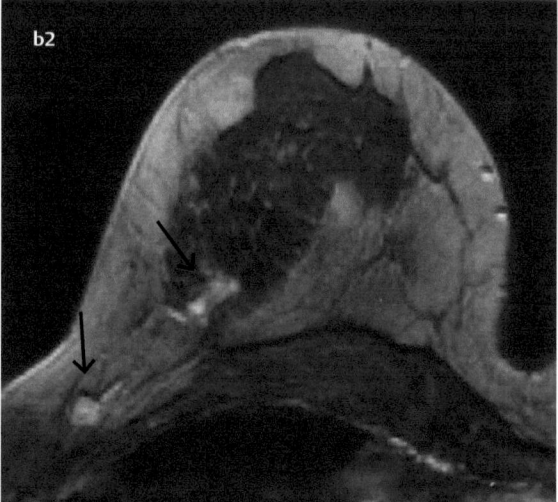

Indications

- Based on the experience so far, percutaneous biopsy is indicated as the method of choice for the assessment of indeterminate lesions, for suspected second foci, and for assessing the extent of changes that may require excision.
- With a suspicious finding, histology from percutaneous biopsy can confirm the diagnosis before surgery and chemotherapy or radiation, or both. In most European countries and in the United States cytology is generally not considered sufficiently reliable to initiate primary treatment of a cancer (mastectomy, chemotherapy).
- A suspicious clinical or imaging finding is to be dismissed judiciously on the basis of the results of percutaneous biopsy. Both accuracy of the localization and possibility of sampling error must be critically considered in view of both imaging and histologic findings.

Disposition after Percutaneous Biopsy

After percutaneous biopsy, it is the task of the examining physician to *correlate the histologic or cytologic findings with the available information* obtained through imaging and clinical examination. All lesions with uncertain correlation, all B3 lesions and all histologies leading to a therapeutic change should be discussed in an interdisciplinary conference. Only then should the recommendation of the further approach be issued.

Summary

Because of the histologic variability and multiple patterns of growth, invasive breast carcinoma can have diverse presentations. Knowing these variations is important for early detection.

Except for women at high risk, mammography with or without clinical correlation is the only recognized screening method. Mammography and clinical examination are complementary. The accuracy of mammography depends on the type of tumor, growth pattern, and surrounding tissue. While the sensitivity of mammography in adipose tissue approaches 100%, it markedly decreases in mammographically dense tissue. In this situation, a negative mammogram cannot be taken to dismiss a clinical suspicion of malignancy. Since most nonpalpable carcinomas are first diagnosed or suspected on the basis of the mammographic finding, optimal technique, continued education, and review of one's own accuracy are important prerequisites for good results.

While mammography and clinical examination as screening methods aim to detect suggestive findings as early as possible, supplemental methods serve to evaluate these findings further.

By delineating cysts and in selected cases with mammographically and sonographically benign findings, sonography may help prevent unnecessary biopsies of uncertain palpable findings or mammographic masses. In mammographically dense tissue, sonography used as a complementary method can improve the detection of carcinomas. Exclusion of a malignancy in cases of mammographically suspicious noncystic findings is usually not possible by sonography alone. MRI is the most sensitive method for detecting malignancy. However, it is only indicated for use as a screening tool in high-risk women. Even though it is the most sensitive method for demonstrating extent of invasive breast cancer, DCIS, and second foci, its recommended preoperative use is restricted to selected indications, where an effect of outcome appears possible.

Being very sensitive MRI is particularly suitable for detecting or excluding malignancy in scarred tissue. The use of MRI for monitoring neoadjuvant therapy is still under investigation. Apart from these indications, use of MRI should be limited to findings that could not be resolved by conventional methods and percutaneous biopsy.

Percutaneous biopsy is the method of choice for assessing indeterminate primary lesions, suspected second foci, or therapeutically decisive lesion extent. The accuracy of state-of-the-art percutaneous breast biopsy followed by an interdisciplinary conference is comparable to open surgery but associated with fewer side effects. State-of-the art standards of procedures and discussion of the results in a multidisciplinary conference are crucial for good results. Also the limitations of percutaneous breast biopsy (depending on the biopsy method, the individual patient and the expected histology) must be known.

References and Recommended Reading

Abdullah N, Mesurolle B, El-Khoury M, Kao E. Breast imaging reporting and data system lexicon for US: interobserver agreement for assessment of breast masses. Radiology 2009;252(3):665–672

Albert US, Altland H, Duda V, et al. 2008 update of the guideline: early detection of breast cancer in Germany. J Cancer Res Clin Oncol 2009;135(3):339–354

Alvarez S, Añorbe E, Alcorta P, López F, Alonso I, Cortés J. Role of sonography in the diagnosis of axillary lymph node metastases in breast cancer: a systematic review. AJR Am J Roentgenol 2006;186(5):1342–1348

American College of Radiology. ACR breast imaging reporting and data system (BIRADS): breast imaging atlas. Reston, VA: American College of Radiology; 2003

Arpino G, Bardou VJ, Clark GM, Elledge RM. Infiltrating lobular carcinoma of the breast: tumor characteristics and clinical outcome. Breast Cancer Res 2004;6(3):R149–R156

References and Recommended Reading

Arriagada R, Lê MG, Rochard F, Contesso G; Institut Gustave-Roussy Breast Cancer Group. Conservative treatment versus mastectomy in early breast cancer: patterns of failure with 15 years of follow-up data. J Clin Oncol 1996;14(5):1558–1564

Azzopardi JG. Problems in breast pathology. London: WB Saunders; 1979

Badve S, Dabbs DJ, Schnitt SJ, et al. Basal-like and triple-negative breast cancers: a critical review with an emphasis on the implications for pathologists and oncologists. Mod Pathol 2011;24(2):157–167

Baek HM, Chen JH, Nie K, et al. Predicting pathologic response to neoadjuvant chemotherapy in breast cancer by using MR imaging and quantitative 1H MR spectroscopy. Radiology 2009;251(3):653–662

Bahri S, Chen JH, Mehta RS, et al. Residual breast cancer diagnosed by MRI in patients receiving neoadjuvant chemotherapy with and without bevacizumab. Ann Surg Oncol 2009;16(6):1619–1628

Ballesio L, Maggi C, Savelli S, et al. Role of breast magnetic resonance imaging (MRI) in patients with unilateral nipple discharge: preliminary study. Radiol Med (Torino) 2008;113(2):249–264

Baum F, Fischer U, Vosshenrich R, Grabbe E. Classification of hypervascularized lesions in CE MR imaging of the breast. Eur Radiol 2002;12(5):1087–1092

Beresford M, Padhani AR, Goh V, Makris A. Imaging breast cancer response during neoadjuvant systemic therapy. Expert Rev Anticancer Ther 2005;5(5):893–905

Berg WA, Gilbreath PL. Multicentric and multifocal cancer: whole-breast US in preoperative evaluation. Radiology 2000;214(1):59–66

Berg WA, Gutierrez L, NessAiver MS, et al. Diagnostic accuracy of mammography, clinical examination, US, and MR imaging in preoperative assessment of breast cancer. Radiology 2004;233(3):830–849

Berg WA, Blume JD, Cormack JB, Mendelson EB. Operator dependence of physician-performed whole breast US: lesion detection and characterization. Radiology 2006;241(2):355–365

Berg WA, Blume JD, Cormack JB, et al; ACRIN 6666 Investigators. Combined screening with ultrasound and mammography vs mammography alone in women at elevated risk of breast cancer. JAMA 2008;299(18):2151–2163

Bernard JR Jr, Vallow LA, DePeri ER, et al. In newly diagnosed breast cancer, screening MRI of the contralateral breast detects mammographically occult cancer, even in elderly women: the Mayo Clinic in Florida experience. Breast J 2010;16(2):118–126

Bhattacharyya M, Ryan D, Carpenter R, Vinnicombe S, Gallagher CJ. Using MRI to plan breast-conserving surgery following neoadjuvant chemotherapy for early breast cancer. Br J Cancer 2008;98(2):289–293

Bird RE, Wallace TW, Yankaskas BC. Analysis of cancers missed at screening mammography. Radiology 1992;184(3):613–617

Blamey RW, Pinder SE, Ball GR, et al. Reading the prognosis of the individual with breast cancer. Eur J Cancer 2007;43(10):1545–1547

Blamey RW, Hornmark-Stenstam B, Ball G, et al. ONCOPOOL—a European database for 16,944 cases of breast cancer. Eur J Cancer 2010;46(1):56–71

Blichert-Toft M, Rose C, Andersen JA, et al; Danish Breast Cancer Cooperative Group. Danish randomized trial comparing breast conservation therapy with mastectomy: six years of life-table analysis. J Natl Cancer Inst Monogr 1992;11(11):19–25

Bluemke DA, Gatsonis CA, Chen MH, et al. Magnetic resonance imaging of the breast prior to biopsy. JAMA 2004;292(22):2735–2742

Boetes C, Strijk SP, Holland R, Barentsz JO, Van Der Sluis RF, Ruijs JH. False-negative MR imaging of malignant breast tumors. Eur Radiol 1997;7(8):1231–1234

Brennan ME, Houssami N, Lord S, et al. Magnetic resonance imaging screening of the contralateral breast in women with newly diagnosed breast cancer: systematic review and meta-analysis of incremental cancer detection and impact on surgical management. J Clin Oncol 2009;27(33):5640–5649

Buchanan CL, Morris EA, Dorn PL, Borgen PI, Van Zee KJ. Utility of breast magnetic resonance imaging in patients with occult primary breast cancer. Ann Surg Oncol 2005;12(12):1045–1053

Chen JH, Feig BA, Hsiang DJ, et al. Impact of MRI-evaluated neoadjuvant chemotherapy response on change of surgical recommendation in breast cancer. Ann Surg 2009a;249(3):448–454

Chen LL, Nolan ME, Silverstein MJ, et al. The impact of primary tumor size, lymph node status, and other prognostic factors on the risk of cancer death. Cancer 2009b;115(21):5071–5083

Ciatto S, Rosselli del Turco M, Catarzi S, Morrone D, Bonardi R. The diagnostic role of breast echography. [Article in Italian] Radiol Med (Torino) 1994;88(3):221–224

de Roos MA, de Bock GH, de Vries J, van der Vegt B, Wesseling J. p53 overexpression is a predictor of local recurrence after treatment for both in situ and invasive ductal carcinoma of the breast. J Surg Res 2007;140(1):109–114

DeMartini W, Lehman C, Partridge S. Breast MRI for cancer detection and characterization: a review of evidence-based clinical applications. Acad Radiol 2008;15(4):408–416

Denis F, Desbiez-Bourcier AV, Chapiron C, Arbion F, Body G, Brunereau L. Contrast enhanced magnetic resonance imaging underestimates residual disease following neoadjuvant docetaxel based chemotherapy for breast cancer. Eur J Surg Oncol 2004;30(10):1069–1076

Dennis MA, Parker SH, Klaus AJ, Stavros AT, Kaske TI, Clark SB. Breast biopsy avoidance: the value of normal mammograms and normal sonograms in the setting of a palpable lump. Radiology 2001;219(1):186–191

Duncan KA, Needham G, Gilbert FJ, Deans HE. Incident round cancers: what lessons can we learn? Clin Radiol 1998;53(1):29–32

Eby PR, Demartini WB, Peacock S, Rosen EL, Lauro B, Lehman CD. Cancer yield of probably benign breast MR examinations. J Magn Reson Imaging 2007;26(4):950–955

Ellis IO, Galea M, Broughton N, Locker A, Blamey RW, Elston CW. Pathological prognostic factors in breast cancer. II. Histological type. Relationship with survival in a large study with long-term follow-up. Histopathology 1992;20(6):479–489

Elston CW, Ellis IO. Pathological prognostic factors in breast cancer. I. The value of histological grade in breast cancer: experience from a large study with long-term follow-up. Histopathology 1991;19(5):403–410

Evaluation of Genomic Applications in Practice and Prevention (EGAPP) Working Group. Recommendations from the EGAPP Working Group: can tumor gene expression profiling improve outcomes in patients with breast cancer? Genet Med 2009;11(1):66–73

Fischer U, Kopka L, Grabbe E. Breast carcinoma: effect of preoperative contrast-enhanced MR imaging on the therapeutic approach. Radiology 1999;213(3):881–888

Fischer U, Schwethelm L, Baum FT, Luftner-Nagel S, Teubner J. Effort, accuracy and histology of MR-guided vacuum biopsy of suspicious breast lesions—retrospective evaluation after 389 interventions. [Article in German] Rofo 2009;181(8):774–781

Fisher B, Anderson S, Bryant J, et al. Twenty-year follow-up of a randomized trial comparing total mastectomy, lumpectomy, and lumpectomy plus irradiation for the treatment of invasive breast cancer. N Engl J Med 2002;347(16):1233–1241

Ghossein NA, Alpert S, Barba J, et al. Breast cancer. Importance of adequate surgical excision prior to radiotherapy in the local control of breast cancer in patients treated conservatively. Arch Surg 1992;127(4):411–415

Godinez J, Gombos EC, Chikarmane SA, Griffin GK, Birdwell RL. Breast MRI in the evaluation of eligibility for accelerated partial breast irradiation. AJR Am J Roentgenol 2008;191(1):272–277

Goldhirsch A, Wood WC, Coates AS, Gelber RD, Thürlimann B, Senn HJ; Panel members. Strategies for subtypes—dealing with the diversity of breast cancer: highlights of the St. Gallen International Expert Consensus on the Primary Therapy of Early Breast Cancer 2011. Ann Oncol 2011;22(8):1736–1747

Gordon PB. Ultrasound for breast cancer screening and staging. Radiol Clin North Am 2002;40(3):431–441

Graf O, Helbich TH, Fuchsjaeger MH, et al. Follow-up of palpable circumscribed noncalcified solid breast masses at mammography and US: can biopsy be averted? Radiology 2004;233(3):850–856

Gusterson B. Do 'basal-like' breast cancers really exist? Nat Rev Cancer 2009;9(2):128–134

Gutierrez RL, DeMartini WB, Eby PR, Kurland BF, Peacock S, Lehman CD. BI-RADS lesion characteristics predict likelihood of malignancy in breast MRI for masses but not for nonmasslike enhancement. AJR Am J Roentgenol 2009;193(4):994–1000

Gutierrez RL, DeMartini WB, Silbergeld JJ, et al. High cancer yield and positive predictive value: outcomes at a center routinely using preoperative breast MRI for staging. AJR Am J Roentgenol 2011;196(1):W93-9

Harvey JA, Fajardo LL, Innis CA. Previous mammograms in patients with impalpable breast carcinoma: retrospective vs blinded interpretation. 1993 ARRS President's Award. AJR Am J Roentgenol 1993; 161(6):1167–1172

Hata T, Takahashi H, Watanabe K, et al. Magnetic resonance imaging for preoperative evaluation of breast cancer: a comparative study with mammography and ultrasonography. J Am Coll Surg 2004;198(2):190–197

Hattangadi J, Park C, Rembert J, et al. Breast stromal enhancement on MRI is associated with response to neoadjuvant chemotherapy. AJR Am J Roentgenol 2008;190(6):1630–1636

Heywang-Köbrunner SH, Beck R. Contrast-Enhanced MRI of the Breast. Berlin; Heidelberg: Springer; 1996

Heywang-Köbrunner SH, Bick U, Bradley WG Jr, et al. International investigation of breast MRI: results of a multicentre study (11 sites) concerning diagnostic parameters for contrast-enhanced MRI based on 519 histopathologically correlated lesions. Eur Radiol 2001;11(4):531–546

Heywang-Köbrunner SH, Möhrling D, Nährig J. The role of MRI before breast conservation. Semin Breast Dis 2007;10(4):137–144

Heywang-Köbrunner SH, Schreer I, Heindel W, Katalinic A. Imaging studies for the early detection of breast cancer. Dtsch Arztebl Int 2008;105(31-32):541–547

Hlawatsch A, Teifke A, Schmidt M, Thelen M. Preoperative assessment of breast cancer: sonography versus MR imaging. AJR Am J Roentgenol 2002;179(6):1493–1501

Holland DW, Boucher LD, Mortimer JE. Tubular breast cancer experience at Washington University: a review of the literature. Clin Breast Cancer 2001;2(3):210–214

Hong AS, Rosen EL, Soo MS, Baker JA. BI-RADS for sonography: positive and negative predictive values of sonographic features. AJR Am J Roentgenol 2005;184(4):1260–1265

Honrado E, Benítez J, Palacios J. Histopathology of BRCA1- and BRCA2-associated breast cancer. Crit Rev Oncol Hematol 2006;59(1):27–39

Houssami N, Ciatto S, Macaskill P, et al. Accuracy and surgical impact of magnetic resonance imaging in breast cancer staging: systematic review and meta-analysis in detection of multifocal and multicentric cancer. J Clin Oncol 2008;26(19):3248–3258

Hrung JM, Sonnad SS, Schwartz JS, Langlotz CP. Accuracy of MR imaging in the work-up of suspicious breast lesions: a diagnostic meta-analysis. Acad Radiol 1999;6(7):387–397

Hwang ES, Kinkel K, Esserman LJ, Lu Y, Weidner N, Hylton NM. Magnetic resonance imaging in patients diagnosed with ductal carcinoma-in-situ: value in the diagnosis of residual disease, occult invasion, and multicentricity. Ann Surg Oncol 2003;10(4):381–388

Iau PT, Marafie M, Ali A, et al. Are medullary breast cancers an indication for BRCA1 mutation screening? A mutation analysis of 42 cases of medullary breast cancer. Breast Cancer Res Treat 2004;85(1):81–88

Ikeda DM, Andersson I, Wattsgård C, Janzon L, Linell F. Interval carcinomas in the Malmö Mammographic Screening Trial: radiographic appearance and prognostic considerations. AJR Am J Roentgenol 1992;159(2):287–294

Ikeda DM, Hylton NM, Kinkel K, et al. Development, standardization, and testing of a lexicon for reporting contrast-enhanced breast magnetic resonance imaging studies. J Magn Reson Imaging 2001;13(6):889–895

Institute for Clinical Systems Improvement. Health care guideline: Diagnosis of breast disease. Institute for Clinical Systems Improvement (www.icsi.org); 2012

Jackson VP, Dines KA, Bassett LW, Gold RH, Reynolds HE. Diagnostic importance of the radiographic density of noncalcified breast masses: analysis of 91 lesions. AJR Am J Roentgenol 1991;157(1):25–28

Kaplan SS. Clinical utility of bilateral whole-breast US in the evaluation of women with dense breast tissue. Radiology 2001;221(3):641–649

Kettritz U, Rotter K, Schreer I, et al. Stereotactic vacuum-assisted breast biopsy in 2874 patients: a multicenter study. Cancer 2004;100(2):245–251

Kim HJ, Im YH, Han BK, et al. Accuracy of MRI for estimating residual tumor size after neoadjuvant chemotherapy in locally advanced breast cancer: relation to response patterns on MRI. Acta Oncol 2007a;46(7):996–1003

Kim Y, Moon WK, Cho N, et al. MRI of the breast for the detection and assessment of the size of ductal carcinoma in situ. Korean J Radiol 2007b;8(1):32–39

Kim TH, Kang DK, Kim SY, Lee EJ, Jung YS, Yim H. Sonographic differentiation of benign and malignant papillary lesions of the breast. J Ultrasound Med 2008;27(1):75–82

Kneeshaw PJ, Turnbull LW, Smith A, Drew PJ. Dynamic contrast enhanced magnetic resonance imaging aids the surgical management of invasive lobular breast cancer. Eur J Surg Oncol. 2003;29(1):32–37

Kolb TM, Lichy J, Newhouse JH. Occult cancer in women with dense breasts: detection with screening US—diagnostic yield and tumor characteristics. Radiology 1998;207(1):191–199

Kolb TM, Lichy J, Newhouse JH. Comparison of the performance of screening mammography, physical examination, and breast US and evaluation of factors that influence them: an analysis of 27,825 patient evaluations. Radiology 2002;225(1):165–175

Kollias J, Gill PG, Beamond B, Rossi H, Langlois S, Vernon-Roberts E. Clinical and radiological predictors of complete excision in breast-conserving surgery for primary breast cancer. Aust N Z J Surg 1998;68(10):702–706

Kreipe HH. Histopathologie—Immunhistochemie—Intrinsic Typing. In: Untch M, Thomssen C, Costa SD, Eds. Munich Aegileum: Colloquium Senologie; 2011:36–51

Kriege M, Brekelmans CT, Boetes C, et al; Magnetic Resonance Imaging Screening Study Group. Efficacy of MRI and mammography for breast-cancer screening in women with a familial or genetic predisposition. N Engl J Med 2004;351(5):427–437

Kuhl CK, Schrading S, Leutner CC, et al. Mammography, breast ultrasound, and magnetic resonance imaging for surveillance of women at high familial risk for breast cancer. J Clin Oncol 2005;23(33):8469–8476

Lakhani SR, Ellis IO, Schnitt SJ, Tan PH, van de Vijver MJ (eds). WHO classification of tumours of the breast. Lyon: IARC; 2012

Lazarus E, Mainiero MB, Schepps B, Koelliker SL, Livingston LS. BI-RADS lexicon for US and mammography: interobserver variability and positive predictive value. Radiology 2006;239(2):385–391

Leach MO, Boggis CR, Dixon AK, et al; MARIBS study group. Screening with magnetic resonance imaging and mammography of a UK population at high familial risk of breast cancer: a prospective multicentre cohort study (MARIBS). Lancet 2005;365(9473):1769–1778

Lee CH, Dershaw DD, Kopans D, et al. Breast cancer screening with imaging: recommendations from the Society of Breast Imaging and the ACR on the use of mammography, breast MRI, breast ultrasound, and other technologies for the detection of clinically occult breast cancer. J Am Coll Radiol 2010;7(1):18–27

Lehman CD, Isaacs C, Schnall MD, et al. Cancer yield of mammography, MR, and US in high-risk women: prospective multi-institution breast cancer screening study. Radiology 2007;244(2):381–388

Liberman L, Mason G, Morris EA, Dershaw DD. Does size matter? Positive predictive value of MRI-detected breast lesions as a function of lesion size. AJR Am J Roentgenol 2006;186(2):426–430

Lieberman S, Sella T, Maly B, Sosna J, Uziely B, Sklair-Levy M. Breast magnetic resonance imaging characteristics in women with occult primary breast carcinoma. Isr Med Assoc J 2008;10(6):448–452

Lord SJ, Lei W, Craft P, et al. A systematic review of the effectiveness of magnetic resonance imaging (MRI) as an addition to mammography and ultrasound in screening young women at high risk of breast cancer. Eur J Cancer 2007;43(13):1905–1917

Madjar H, Ohlinger R, Mundinger A, et al. BI-RADS-analogue DEGUM criteria for findings in breast ultrasound—consensus of the DEGUM Committee on Breast Ultrasound. [Article in German] Ultraschall Med 2006;27(4):374–379

Mainiero MB, Goldkamp A, Lazarus E, et al. Characterization of breast masses with sonography: can biopsy of some solid masses be deferred? J Ultrasound Med 2005;24(2):161–167

Mainiero MB, Cinelli CM, Koelliker SL, Graves TA, Chung MA. Axillary ultrasound and fine-needle aspiration in the preoperative evaluation of the breast cancer patient: an algorithm based on tumor size and lymph node appearance. AJR Am J Roentgenol 2010;195(5):1261–1267

Manton DJ, Chaturvedi A, Hubbard A, et al. Neoadjuvant chemotherapy in breast cancer: early response prediction with quantitative MR imaging and spectroscopy. Br J Cancer 2006;94(3):427–435

Meindl A, Ditsch N, Kast K, Rhiem K, Schmutzler RK. Hereditary breast and ovarian cancer: new genes, new treatments, new concepts. Dtsch Arztebl Int 2011;108(19):323–330

Meisamy S, Bolan PJ, Baker EH, et al. Neoadjuvant chemotherapy of locally advanced breast cancer: predicting response with in vivo (1)H MR spectroscopy—a pilot study at 4 T. Radiology 2004;233(2):424–431

Meissnitzer M, Dershaw DD, Lee CH, Morris EA. Targeted ultrasound of the breast in women with abnormal MRI findings for whom biopsy has been recommended. AJR Am J Roentgenol 2009;193(4):1025–1029

Mendelson EB. Problem-solving ultrasound. Radiol Clin North Am 2004;42(5):909–918, vii

Mills P, Sever A, Weeks J, Fish D, Jones S, Jones P. Axillary ultrasound assessment in primary breast cancer: an audit of 653 cases. Breast J 2010;16(5):460–463

Moran MS, Yang Q, Haffty BG. The Yale University experience of early-stage invasive lobular carcinoma (ILC) and invasive ductal carcinoma (IDC) treated with breast conservation treatment (BCT): analysis of clinical-pathologic features, long-term outcomes, and molecular expression of COX-2, Bcl-2, and p53 as a function of histology. Breast J 2009;15(6):571–578

Morrogh M, Morris EA, Liberman L, Van Zee K, Cody HS III, King TA. MRI identifies otherwise occult disease in select patients with Paget disease of the nipple. J Am Coll Surg 2008;206(2):316–321

Moy L, Elias K, Patel V, et al. Is breast MRI helpful in the evaluation of inconclusive mammographic findings? AJR Am J Roentgenol 2009;193(4): 986–993

Nakahara H, Namba K, Watanabe R, et al. A comparison of MR imaging, galactography and ultrasonography in patients with nipple discharge. Breast Cancer 2003;10(4):320–329

Nakamura S, Kenjo H, Nishio T, Kazama T, Doi O, Suzuki K. Efficacy of 3D-MR mammography for breast conserving surgery after neoadjuvant chemotherapy. Breast Cancer 2002;9(1):15–19

National Breast Cancer Centre. Magnetic resonance imaging for the early detection of breast cancer in women at high risk: a systematic review of the evidence. Camperdown, NSW: NBCC; 2006

National Comprehensive Cancer Network. Clinical Practice Guidelines in Oncology. Breast cancer screening and diagnosis guidelines V.I 2008. National Comprehensive Cancer Network (www.nccn.org); 2008

National Institute for Health and Clinical Excellence, National Collaborating Centre for Primary Care. Clinical Guideline 41. Familial breast cancer: the classification and care of women at risk of familial breast cancer in primary, secondary and tertiary care. London: National Institute for Health and Clinical Excellence (www.nice.org.uk); 2006

Neal CH, Daly CP, Nees AV, Helvie MA. Can preoperative axillary US help exclude N2 and N3 metastatic breast cancer? Radiology 2010;257(2):335–341

Nothacker M, Duda V, Hahn M, et al. Early detection of breast cancer: benefits and risks of supplemental breast ultrasound in asymptomatic women with mammographically dense breast tissue. A systematic review. BMC Cancer 2009;9:335–344

Padhani AR, Ollivier L. The RECIST (Response Evaluation Criteria in Solid Tumors): implications for diagnostic radiologists. Br J Radiol 2001;74(887):983–986

Pamilo M, Soiva M, Anttinen I, Roiha M, Suramo I. Ultrasonography of breast lesions detected in mammography screening. Acta Radiol 1991;32(3):220–225

Pengel KE, Loo CE, Teertstra HJ, et al. The impact of preoperative MRI on breast-conserving surgery of invasive cancer: a comparative cohort study. Breast Cancer Res Treat 2009;116(1):161–169

Perlet C, Heywang-Köbrunner SH, Heinig A et al. Magnetic resonance-guided, vacuum-assisted breast biopsy: results from a European multicenter study of 538 lesions. Cancer 2006;106(5):982–990

Perry N, Broeders M, de Wolf C, Toernberg S, Holland R, von Karsa L, eds. European guidelines for quality assurance in breast screening an diagnosis. Luxembourg: Office for Official Publications of the European Communities; 2006

Peters NH, Borel Rinkes IH, Zuithoff NP, Mali WP, Moons KG, Peeters PH. Meta-analysis of MR imaging in the diagnosis of breast lesions. Radiology 2008;246(1):116–124

Peters NH, van Esser S, van den Bosch MA, et al. Preoperative MRI and surgical management in patients with nonpalpable breast cancer: the MONET - randomised controlled trial. Eur J Cancer 2011;47(6):879–886

Pickles MD, Gibbs P, Lowry M, Turnbull LW. Diffusion changes precede size reduction in neoadjuvant treatment of breast cancer. Magn Reson Imaging 2006;24(7):843–847

Plana MN, Carreira C, Muriel A, et al. Magnetic resonance imaging in the preoperative assessment of patients with primary breast cancer: systematic review of diagnostic accuracy and meta-analysis. Eur Radiol 2012;22(1):26–38

Poggi MM, Danforth DN, Sciuto LC, et al. Eighteen-year results in the treatment of early breast carcinoma with mastectomy versus breast conservation therapy: the National Cancer Institute Randomized Trial. Cancer 2003;98(4):697–702

Porter PL, El-Bastawissi AY, Mandelson MT, et al. Breast tumor characteristics as predictors of mammographic detection: comparison of interval- and screen-detected cancers. J Natl Cancer Inst 1999;91(23):2020–2028

Potterton AJ, Peakman DJ, Young JR. Ultrasound demonstration of small breast cancers detected by mammographic screening. Clin Radiol 1994;49(11):808–813

Raza S, Goldkamp AL, Chikarmane SA, Birdwell RL. US of breast masses categorized as BI-RADS 3, 4, and 5: pictorial review of factors influencing clinical management. Radiographics 2010;30(5):1199–1213

Riedl CC, Ponhold L, Flöry D, et al. Magnetic resonance imaging of the breast improves detection of invasive cancer, preinvasive cancer, and premalignant lesions during surveillance of women at high risk for breast cancer. Clin Cancer Res 2007;13(20):6144–6152

Roelofs AA, Karssemeijer N, Wedekind N, et al. Importance of comparison of current and prior mammograms in breast cancer screening. Radiology 2007;242(1):70–77

Saarenmaa I, Salminen T, Geiger U, et al. The visibility of cancer on earlier mammograms in a population-based screening programme. Eur J Cancer 1999;35(7):1118–1122

Sardanelli F, Boetes C, Borisch B, et al. Magnetic resonance imaging of the breast: recommendations from the EUSOMA working group. Eur J Cancer 2010;46(8):1296–1316

Sardanelli F, Giuseppetti GM, Panizza P, et al; Italian Trial for Breast MR in Multifocal/Multicentric Cancer. Sensitivity of MRI versus mammography for detecting foci of multifocal, multicentric breast cancer in fatty and dense breasts using the whole-breast pathologic examination as a gold standard. AJR Am J Roentgenol 2004;183(4):1149–1157

Saslow D, Boetes C, Burke W, et al; American Cancer Society Breast Cancer Advisory Group. American Cancer Society guidelines for breast screening with MRI as an adjunct to mammography. CA Cancer J Clin 2007;57(2):75–89

Schelfout K, Van Goethem M, Kersschot E, et al. Preoperative breast MRI in patients with invasive lobular breast cancer. Eur Radiol 2004;14(7):1209–1216

Schmutzler R, Schlegelberger B, Meindl A, et al. Spezielle strategie – familiäre belastung. In: Schulz KD, Albert U, eds. Stufe 3 Leitlinie. Brustkrebsfrüherkennung in Deutschland. Munich: Zuckschwerdt Verlag; 2008

Schnall MD, Blume J, Bluemke DA, et al. MRI detection of distinct incidental cancer in women with primary breast cancer studied in IBMC 6883. J Surg Oncol 2005;92(1):32–38

Schnall MD, Blume J, Bluemke DA, et al. Diagnostic architectural and dynamic features at breast MR imaging: multicenter study. Radiology 2006;238(1):42–53

Schott AF, Roubidoux MA, Helvie MA, et al. Clinical and radiologic assessments to predict breast cancer pathologic complete response to neoadjuvant chemotherapy. Breast Cancer Res Treat 2005;92(3):231–238

Schouten van der Velden AP, Boetes C, Bult P, Wobbes T. The value of magnetic resonance imaging in diagnosis and size assessment of in situ and small invasive breast carcinoma. Am J Surg 2006;192(2):172–178

Schouten van der Velden AP, Boetes C, Bult P, Wobbes T. Magnetic resonance imaging in size assessment of invasive breast carcinoma with an extensive intraductal component. BMC Med Imaging 2009;9:5

Schwartz GF, Veronesi U, Clough KB, et al; Consensus Conference Committee. Proceedings of the Consensus Conference on Breast Conservation, April 28 to May 1, 2005, Milan, Italy. Cancer 2006;107(2):242–250

Schwartz GF, Hughes KS, Lynch HT, et al; Consensus Conference Committee. Proceedings of the International Consensus Conference on Breast Cancer Risk, Genetics, & Risk Management, April, 2007. Breast J 2009;15(1):4–16

Sharma U, Danishad KK, Seenu V, Jagannathan NR. Longitudinal study of the assessment by MRI and diffusion-weighted imaging of tumor response in patients with locally advanced breast cancer undergoing neoadjuvant chemotherapy. NMR Biomed 2009;22(1):104–113

Sickles EA. Quality assurance. How to audit your own mammography practice. Radiol Clin North Am 1992;30(1):265–275

Sickles EA. Nonpalpable, circumscribed, noncalcified solid breast masses: likelihood of malignancy based on lesion size and age of patient. Radiology 1994;192(2):439–442

Sidibé S, Coulibaly A, Traoré S, Touré M, Traoré I. Role of ultrasonography in the diagnosis of axillary lymph node metastases in breast cancer: a systematic review. [Article in French] Mali Med 2007;22(4):9–13

Silverstein MJ, Lagios MD, Craig PH, et al. A prognostic index for ductal carcinoma in situ of the breast. Cancer 1996;77(11):2267–2274

Skaane P. The additional value of US to mammography in the diagnosis of breast cancer. A prospective study. Acta Radiol 1999;40(5):486–490

Skaane P, Engedal K. Analysis of sonographic features in the differentiation of fibroadenoma and invasive ductal carcinoma. AJR Am J Roentgenol 1998;170(1):109–114

Solin LJ, Orel SG, Hwang WT, Harris EE, Schnall MD. Relationship of breast magnetic resonance imaging to outcome after breast-conservation treatment with radiation for women with early-stage invasive breast carcinoma or ductal carcinoma in situ. J Clin Oncol 2008;26(3):386–391

Soo MS, Rosen EL, Baker JA, Vo TT, Boyd BA. Negative predictive value of sonography with mammography in patients with palpable breast lesions. AJR Am J Roentgenol 2001;177(5):1167–1170

Sørlie T, Perou CM, Tibshirani R, et al. Gene expression patterns of breast carcinomas distinguish tumor subclasses with clinical implications. Proc Natl Acad Sci U S A 2001;98(19):10869–10874

Stavros AT. Breast ultrasound. Philadelphia: Lippincott Williams and Wilkins; 2003

Stavros AT, Thickman D, Rapp CL, Dennis MA, Parker SH, Sisney GA. Solid breast nodules: use of sonography to distinguish between benign and malignant lesions. Radiology 1995;196(1):123–134

Stuart-Harris R, Caldas C, Pinder SE, Pharoah P. Proliferation markers and survival in early breast cancer: a systematic review and meta-analysis of 85 studies in 32,825 patients. Breast 2008;17(4):323–334

Sumkin JH, Holbert BL, Herrmann JS, et al. Optimal reference mammography: a comparison of mammograms obtained 1 and 2 years before the present examination. AJR Am J Roentgenol 2003;180(2):343–346

Swayampakula AK, Dillis C, Abraham J. Role of MRI in screening, diagnosis and management of breast cancer. Expert Rev Anticancer Ther 2008;8(5):811–817

Tabár L, Fagerberg G, Day NE, Duffy SW, Kitchin RM. Breast cancer treatment and natural history: new insights from results of screening. Lancet 1992;339(8790):412–414

Tendulkar RD, Chellman-Jeffers M, Rybicki LA, et al. Preoperative breast magnetic resonance imaging in early breast cancer: implications for partial breast irradiation. Cancer 2009;115(8):1621–1630

Therasse P, Arbuck SG, Eisenhauer EA, et al. New guidelines to evaluate the response to treatment in solid tumors. J Natl Cancer Inst 2000;92(3):205–216

Thurfjell MG, Vitak B, Azavedo E, Svane G, Thurfjell E. Effect on sensitivity and specificity of mammography screening with or without comparison of old mammograms. Acta Radiol 2000;41(1):52–56

Trecate G, Tess JD, Vergnaghi D, et al. Lobular breast cancer: how useful is breast magnetic resonance imaging? Tumori 2001;87(4):232–238

Turnbull L, Brown S, Harvey I, et al. Comparative effectiveness of MRI in breast cancer (COMICE) trial: a randomised controlled trial. Lancet 2010;375(9714):563–571

Uematsu T, Yuen S, Kasami M, Uchida Y. Dynamic contrast-enhanced MR imaging in screening detected microcalcification lesions of the breast: is there any value? Breast Cancer Res Treat 2007;103(3):269–281

van Dijck JAAM, Verbeek ALM, Hendriks JH, Holland R. The current detectability of breast cancer in a mammographic screening program. A review of the previous mammograms of interval and screen-detected cancers. Cancer 1993;72(6):1933–1938

van Dongen JA, Voogd AC, Fentiman IS, et al. Long-term results of a randomized trial comparing breast-conserving therapy with mastectomy: European Organization for Research and Treatment of Cancer 10801 trial. J Natl Cancer Inst 2000;92(14):1143–1150

van Gils CH, Otten JD, Verbeek AL, Hendriks JH, Holland R. Effect of mammographic breast density on breast cancer screening performance: a study in Nijmegen, the Netherlands. J Epidemiol Community Health 1998;52(4):267–271

Van Goethem M, Schelfout K, Dijckmans L, et al. MR mammography in the pre-operative staging of breast cancer in patients with dense breast tissue: comparison with mammography and ultrasound. Eur Radiol 2004;14(5):809–816

Van Goethem M, Schelfout K, Kersschot E, et al. MR mammography is useful in the preoperative locoregional staging of breast carcinomas with extensive intraductal component. Eur J Radiol 2007;62(2):273–282

Varela C, Karssemeijer N, Hendriks JH, Holland R. Use of prior mammograms in the classification of benign and malignant masses. Eur J Radiol 2005;56(2):248–255

Veronesi U, Cascinelli N, Mariani L, et al. Twenty-year follow-up of a randomized study comparing breast-conserving surgery with radical mastectomy for early breast cancer. N Engl J Med 2002;347(16):1227–1232

Wagner TD, Wharton K, Donohue K, et al. Pure tubular breast carcinoma: a 34 year study of outcomes. Breast J 2008;14(5):512–513

Walsh T, Lee MK, Casadei S, et al. Detection of inherited mutations for breast and ovarian cancer using genomic capture and massively parallel sequencing. Proc Natl Acad Sci U S A 2010;107(28):12629–12633

Wang LC, DeMartini WB, Partridge SC, Peacock S, Lehman CD. MRI-detected suspicious breast lesions: predictive values of kinetic features measured by computer-aided evaluation. AJR Am J Roentgenol 2009;193(3):826–831

Warner E, Messersmith H, Causer P, Eisen A, Shumak R, Plewes D. Systematic review: using magnetic resonance imaging to screen women at high risk for breast cancer. Ann Intern Med 2008;148(9):671–679

Weinstein SP, Hanna LG, Gatsonis C, Schnall MD, Rosen MA, Lehman CD. Frequency of malignancy seen in probably benign lesions at contrast-enhanced breast MR imaging: findings from ACRIN 6667. Radiology 2010;255(3):731–737

Wojcinski S, Farrokh A, Weber S, et al. Multicenter study of ultrasound real-time tissue elastography in 779 cases for the assessment of breast lesions: improved diagnostic performance by combining the BI-RADS®-US classification system with sonoelastography. Ultraschall Med 2010;31(5):484–491

Yeh E, Slanetz P, Kopans DB, et al. Prospective comparison of mammography, sonography, and MRI in patients undergoing neoadjuvant chemotherapy for palpable breast cancer. AJR Am J Roentgenol 2005;184(3):868–877

17 Lymph Nodes

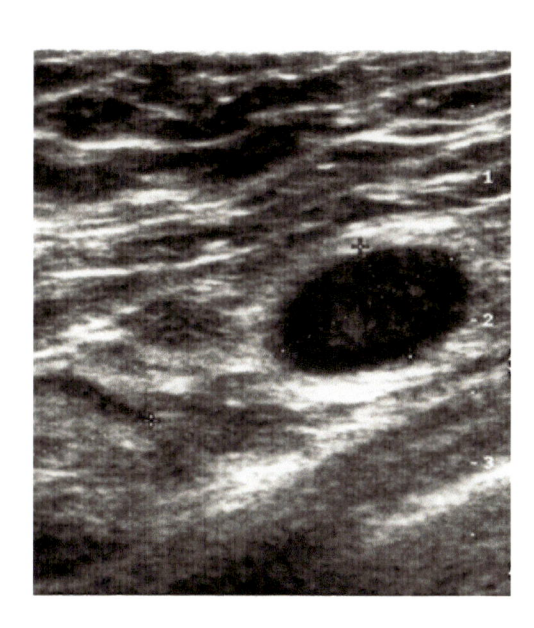

Sentinel Lymph Node Biopsy → 458
The Role of Imaging → 459
Anatomy → 459

Normal Lymph Nodes → 459

Pathologic Changes in Lymph Nodes → 464
Metastatic Adenopathy → 464
Other Causes of Adenopathy → 469
Nodal Calcifications → 469

Percutaneous Biopsy → 471

Further Techniques in Nodal Imaging: MRI and PET → 471

References and Recommended Reading → 473

17 Lymph Nodes

I. Schreer, S. H. Heywang-Koebrunner, S. Barter

Of all the prognostic factors in breast cancer, nodal involvement is the most important. Based on 30-year follow-up, Adair reported that breast cancer patients with negative nodes had a 75% survival. Women with level I involvement had only a 40% survival, and this deteriorated with higher levels involved (Adair et al. 1974). The number of lymph nodes involved is also important. Veronesi reported that on 60-month follow-up of women with breast cancer with 1–3, 4–10, and more than 10 nodes involved, disease-free survival was 80%, 62%, and 35%, respectively (Veronesi et al. 1993). He found that nodal involvement is usually progressive, with nodes closest to the breast (level I) involved before those at higher levels. However, in about 9% of cases, skipped metastases occur with higher levels involved without evidence of level I nodal disease. This means that in about 95% of women, the status of level I nodes truly indicates the presence or absence of nodal disease. Today, overall survival has significantly improved with the use of adjuvant therapy. However, even today mortality directly correlates with tumor size at detection and lymph node status (Blamey et al. 2007, 2010).

Some breast cancers drain into internal mammary nodes. As is also the case for axillary lymph nodes, dissection or irradiation of internal mammary nodes does not improve survival (Veronesi et al. 1999). However, involvement of these nodes appears to be an independent additional indicator for a worse prognosis.

Thus, knowledge about absence or presence of lymph node involvement has proven to be of prognostic importance and thus important for therapeutic decisions. This is the main rationale for the exact histopathologic assessment of axillary lymph nodes.

Axillary dissection has been considered the most accurate method for lymph node staging. However, it may be associated with long-term side effects such as lymphedema or radiation damage to the axillary plexus.

It had long been assumed that axillary dissection might have an impact on survival (e.g., by preventing distant metastases).

To date it is proven that for assessing the clinically uninvolved axilla, sentinel node biopsy (SNB) is equivalent to axillary dissection. The latest research even indicates that axillary dissection is unlikely to influence survival or distant metastases (Giuliano et al. 2011).

Considering the high morbidity resulting from axillary dissection, the high number of surgically treated uninvolved axillae and the predominant prognostic importance of lymph node staging, SNB has been developed to identify the node or nodes that are the first site of drainage of a carcinoma. If these are negative, there is a likelihood of over 90% that no metastatic disease is present within the axilla. This technique has increasingly replaced axillary dissection (Giuliano et al. 1994). Today SNB is considered state-of-the-art assessment in women with clinically negative axillary findings. A recent systematic review (Pepels et al. 2011) has confirmed the safety of omitting axillary lymph node dissection (ALND) in sentinel-negative patients. Replacing ALND in women with negative axillary findings contributes decisively to improvement in their quality of life.

Axillary dissection is indicated as local treatment of the clinically involved axilla. So far, it has also been considered indicated in all cases with clinically negative axillary findings and positive SNB. Lately, however, even the necessity and prognostic value of axillary lymph node dissection in women with clinically occult axillary involvement (women with clinically negative axillary findings but positive SNB) is being questioned (Giuliano et al. 2011).

Sentinel Lymph Node Biopsy

SNB implies that the sentinel node or nodes represent the first lymphatic filter of the breast and breast cancer. The sentinel lymph nodes are detected (and distinguished as the first filter station from the other axillary lymph nodes) by injection of technetium colloid or blue dye, or both. The agent is injected into the breast around the tumor or in the overlying skin several hours before surgery. If isotopes are used, the temporal sequence of the drainage can be monitored by scintigraphic imaging and the location of the first draining nodes can be identified and demonstrated to the surgeon before planning the surgery (**Fig. 17.1**). Scintigraphic imaging, however, cannot distinguish between involved and noninvolved lymph nodes.

Intraoperatively the group of lymph nodes is located by the surgeon using a hand-held scintillation detector and/or visually by blue staining.

Occasionally, sentinel nodes are located in the internal mammary chain or in the breast (intramammary nodes). Based on lack of evidence of any benefit, extensive surgery is usually avoided and these sentinel nodes are usually not excised.

SNB appears to be very reliable in patients with clinically negative axillary findings. In patients with a large burden of involved lymph nodes or in patients after axillary surgery the usual lymphatic drainage may be blocked or circumvented. Therefore, because of altered drainage routes, SNB may not be sufficiently reliable in this group of patients.

Normal Lymph Nodes

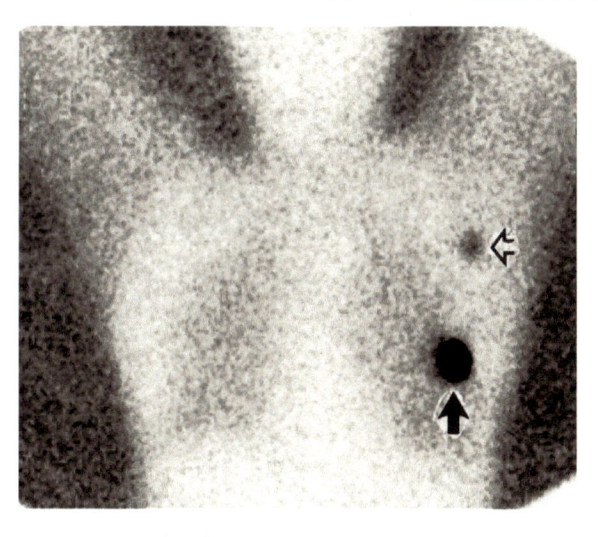

Fig. 17.1 Sentinel node imaging. The intense concentration of tracer is at the site of injection of $^{99}Tc^m$ over the tumor site (closed arrow). The fainter concentration of isotope (open arrow) is within the sentinel node, the initial site of drainage of the tumor.

The Role of Imaging

Traditionally, lymph node imaging has not played a significant role in staging of patients with breast cancer. The reasons for this included the inability of imaging to detect microscopic nodal metastases, the desire for exact staging (which up to the 1990s was only possible by ALND) and the belief that ALND was a prognostically important therapeutic measure needed for all breast cancer patients.

To date SNB is performed in women with clinically negative axillary findings and followed by ALND in the event of positive findings at SNB.

Based on the changed algorithms and the reduced reliability of SNB, imaging and image-guided biopsy may contribute to a correct staging and assessment of the axilla and to problem-solving.

Imaging, mostly by ultrasound (US) and where indicated by US-guided biopsy, can be used:
- For the workup of indeterminate clinical findings in the axilla
- For the workup of indeterminate findings at imaging of the breast (where axillary lymph nodes may be included)
- For complementary assessment of the axilla during primary staging. If a suspicious lymph node is detected by imaging and confirmed by US-guided needle biopsy, SNB is not indicated and is (according to the present algorithm) replaced by ALND.
- For complementary lymph node staging before neoadjuvant therapy and (in case of involved lymph nodes) for monitoring response
- For surveillance after breast cancer treatment

Since lymph nodes of the lower axilla are often imaged during assessment of the breast and for the above questions, it is important to know the typical imaging features of normal and diseased axillary lymph nodes.

Unfortunately, imaging techniques are often not able to differentiate inflammatory and neoplastic nodal disease. Imaging can never exclude microscopic involvement. Where there are abnormal clinical or imaging findings, the imaging is frequently unspecific. Unless the clinical history (preceding surgery or infection) or other clinical findings (known rheumatic or collagen disease) can explain the findings, imaging may need to be complemented by percutaneous lymph node biopsy.

Anatomy

The lymph nodes in the axilla are divided into three levels, defined by their relation to the pectoralis minor muscle. Those nodes which are inferior and lateral to this muscle are level I, those that are deep to the muscle are level II, and those that are superior and medial to the pectoralis minor are level III (see **Fig. 17.3b**). Nodes that are found between the pectoralis major and minor are called Rotter nodes.

As noted above, a small percentage of breast cancers drain medially into the internal mammary chain. These nodes are parasternal, deep to the intercostal muscles, and extrapleural. They follow the internal mammary vessels and are usually present in the first three intercostal spaces.

Normal Lymph Nodes

The normal mammographic pattern of lymph nodes is reniform or coffee bean shaped with a fatty hilum (**Fig. 17.2**).

On mammography this classic configuration is often obvious. However, depending on the projection of the individual node or on overlying structures (vessels, axillary breast tissue, pectoral muscle) this may not always be the case. If smooth margins, a coffee bean shape, and fatty hilum can be demonstrated, the mass can be definitely identified as lymph node. The size of normal nodes is variable, and the overall size of a lymph node is not of any clinical significance. Nodes with very large fatty hila and a small crescent of nodal tissue can measure up to 5 cm. If only the parenchyma (excluding the fatty hilum) of the short axis is determined, this measurement allows some correlation with the presence of malignant involvement (accuracy: 70–80%). However, an exact diagnosis is not possible because microscopic involvement does not lead to an increase in the lymph node size, and benign lymph nodes may have an increased parenchymal diameter due to postinflammatory changes. Nodes are seen

Fig. 17.2a–c Mammography of normal lymph nodes.

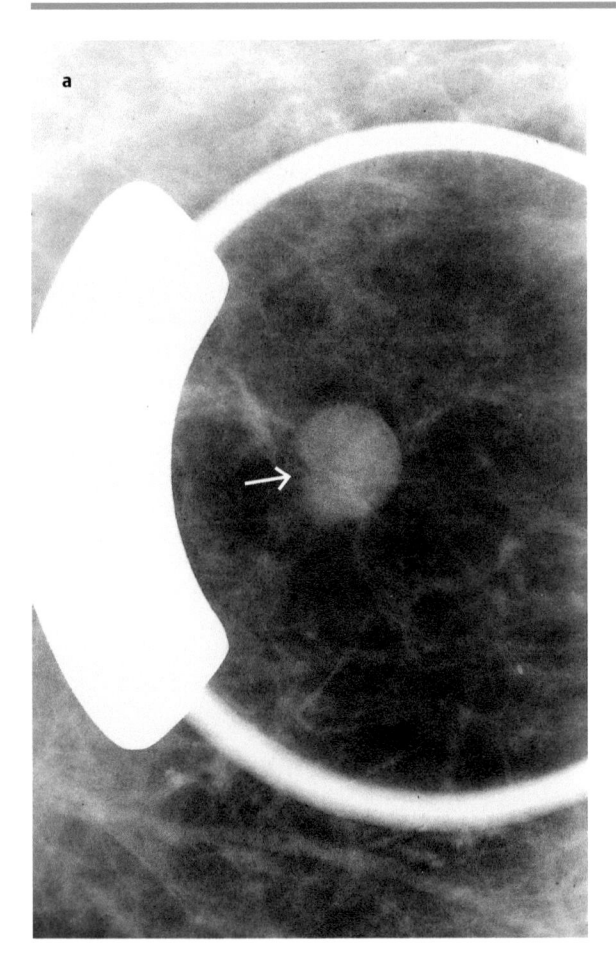

a This coned view of an intramammary lymph node shows the classic coffee bean-shaped pattern with the fatty notch of the nodal hilum (arrow). The node is well defined, and its density is equal to that of breast tissue.

b The fatty hilum of this node is more prominent, but the node is well defined, and its density is not greater than surrounding normal tissues.

c As fatty replacement of a node increases, it will progressively enlarge. This large, palpable axillary node is almost all fat with a thin rim of nodal tissue. Another, smaller node overlies the inferior portion of this large lymph node, suggesting a lobulated contour to the node.

in about one-third of axillae on mammography. The mammographic density of the node is usually equal to or less than that of normal breast tissue. Furthermore, some lymph nodes may occur within the breast. These are intramammary lymph nodes (**Fig. 12.12a**). Although they may occur in any location within the breast, they are most often situated on the posterior half of the upper outer quadrant. Mammographically these nodes become apparent if they are not obscured by dense breast tissue. They are recognized as such if they exhibit the typical morphology of a lymph node.

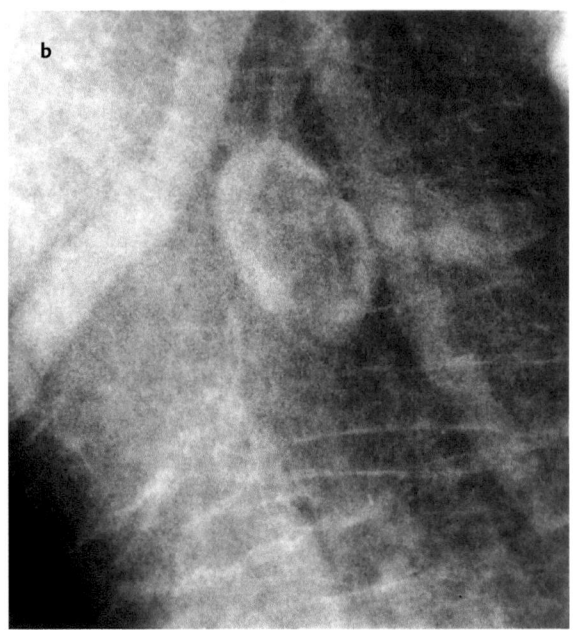

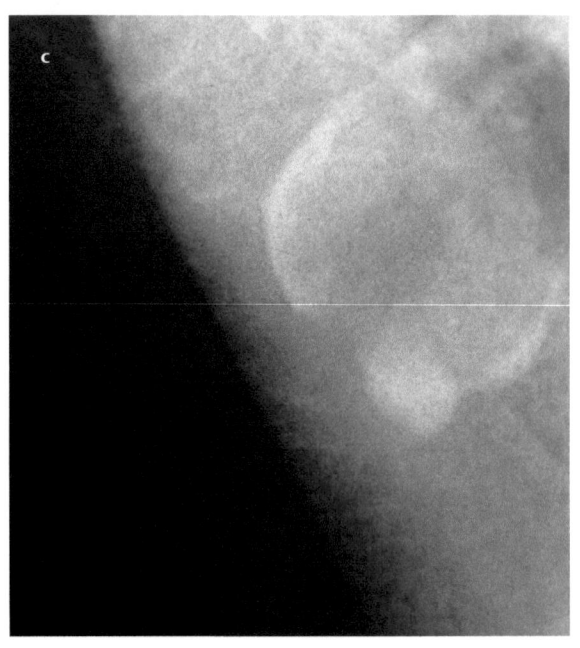

When mammographic imaging of the axilla is desired, this can be optimized using the axillary view. This view is performed using a small, rectangular compression paddle over the axilla and angling the view at 40°. Even with this optimized view, only about the lower half of level I can be imaged mammographically.

For lymph node assessment *sonography* is more accurate than clinical examination and mammography. Also, unlike mammography, sonography is capable of imaging the entire axilla.

Normal Lymph Nodes

However, accuracy depends on the equipment and the examination technique.

A standardized examination technique and knowledge of the anatomical landmarks for identifying lymph nodes of level I or II is very important (**Fig. 17.3**):

- The thoraco-acromial artery, which originates medially and cranially from the axillary artery, marks the medial border of level II, since it follows the medial margin of the minor pectoral muscle.

- The lateral thoracic artery originates caudally from the axillary artery and marks the lateral border of the minor pectoral muscle.
- Furthermore, the lateral subscapular artery, which originates laterally from the lateral thoracic artery, is another landmark for distinguishing lymph nodes of level I versus II (**Fig. 17.3**)

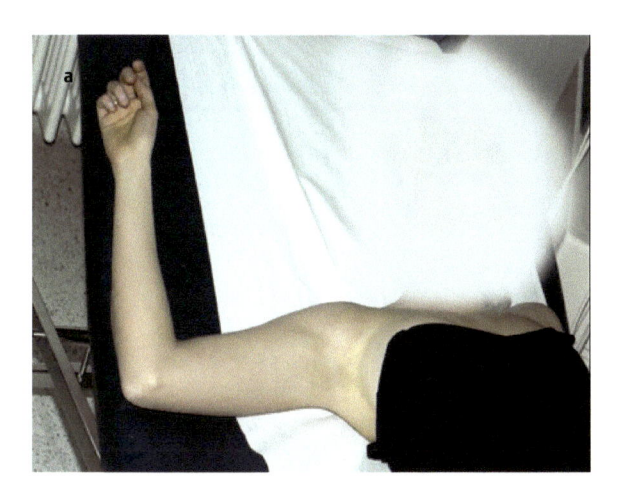

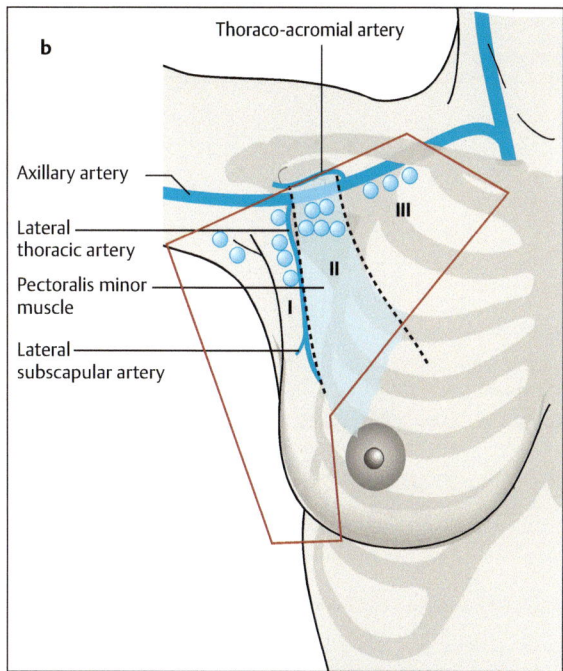

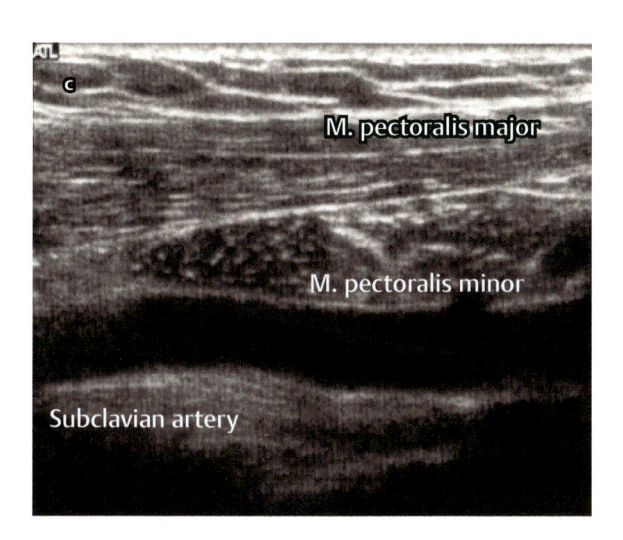

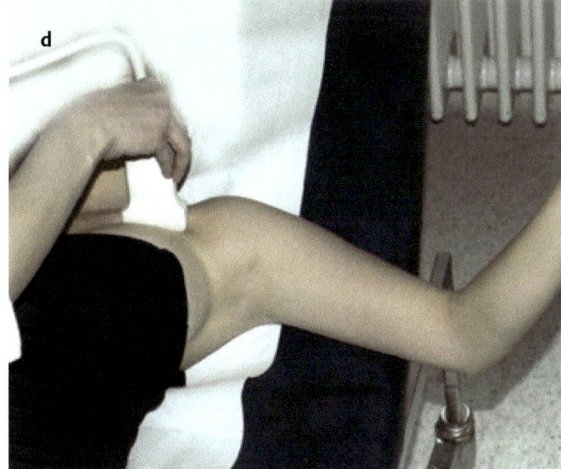

Fig. 17.3a–j Systematic axillary investigation.
a Positioning with 90-degree arm abduction.
b Anatomy. I, II, and III indicate lymph node levels 1, 2, and 3, respectively. The red lines indicate the area that should be covered when looking for involved lymph nodes.
c Sonographic anatomy.
d Transducer position to investigate level I / II border.

Fig. 17.3e–j ▷

17 Lymph Nodes

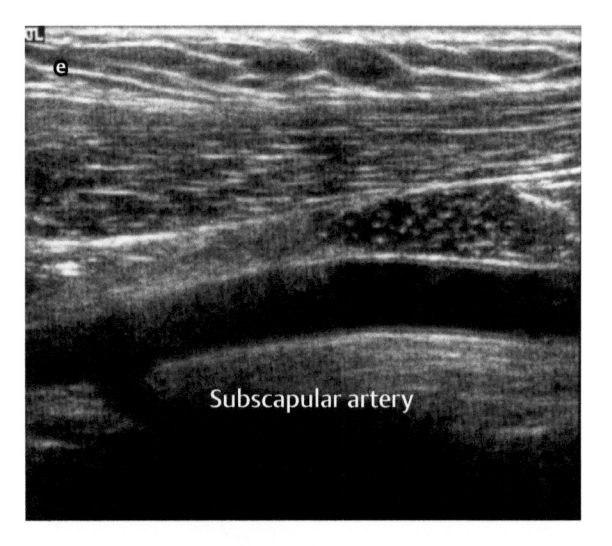

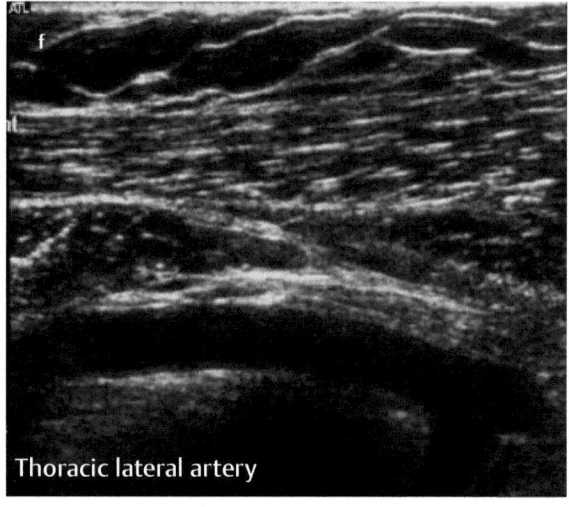

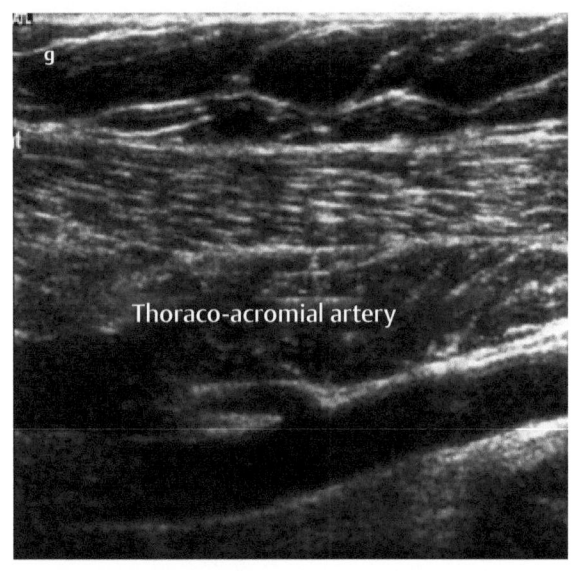

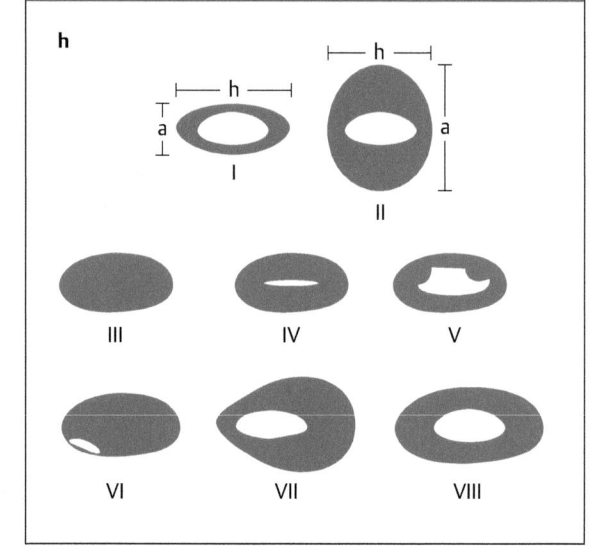

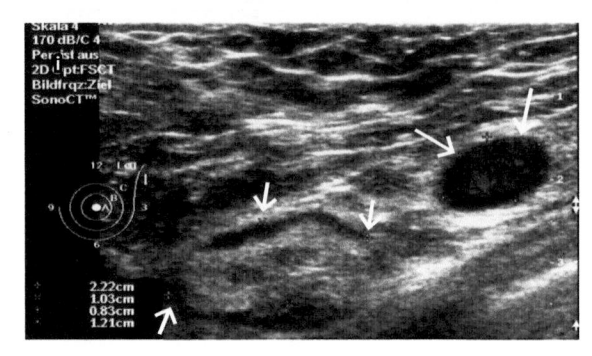

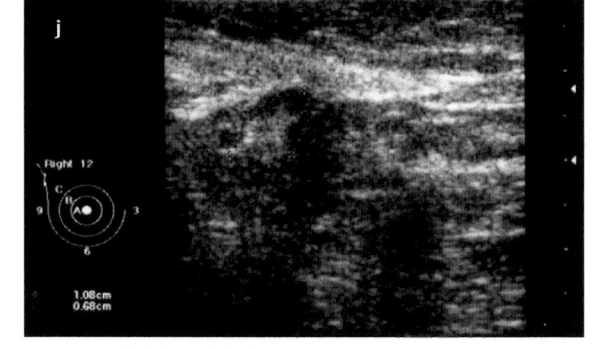

◁ continued

- **e** Sonogram of level I.
- **f** Sonogram of level I/IIA thoracica lateralis.
- **g** Sonogram of level II/IIIA thoracica acromialis.
- **h** Criteria of lymph node interpretation:
  Size
  Form (length/width)
  Hilum and cortex morphology:
  –Normal: oval, echorich hilum, small cortex (**I**)
  –Normal hilum but thickened cortex (>3mm); round shape (**II**)
  –Loss of echogenic hilum (**III**)
  –Narrowing of the central hilum reflex (**IV–VI**)
  –Eccentric enlargement of the cortex (**V, VI**)
  –Concentric enlargement of the cortex (**VII**)
  –Diameter of cortex more than 3mm? (**VIII**)
- **i** Normal lymph node morphology (scheme [**I**]) (short arrows) beside a suspicious lymph node with rather hypoechoic and enlarged cortex (long arrows).
- **j** Irregularly enlarged cortex (scheme [**V**]).

Normal Lymph Nodes

The complete region of levels I and II should be examined systematically. This includes an area, which reaches from the clavicle and humerus (upper border with patients examined with the laterally extended arm) down to the inframammary fold and from the posterior axillary line medially to the anterior serratus muscle (which area overlaps the area covered by breast sonography):

- It should be known that the sentinel node mostly is located in the lower axilla. Therefore the area down to the inframammary fold should be examined with special care.

Lymph nodes are assessed according to their shape and the morphology of hilum and cortex. The thickness of the cortex is more important than lymph node size. Lymph nodes with a fatty hilum may be very large but are unlikely to be involved if the cortex is very thin.

Sonographically, lymph nodes are also coffee bean shaped, smoothly marginated, with an echo-poor cortex and a central, echogenic fatty hilum (**Fig. 17.4**). Focal thickening should be absent. The cortex should generally not be thicker than 3 mm. On Doppler ultrasound, vessels should enter only through the hilum.

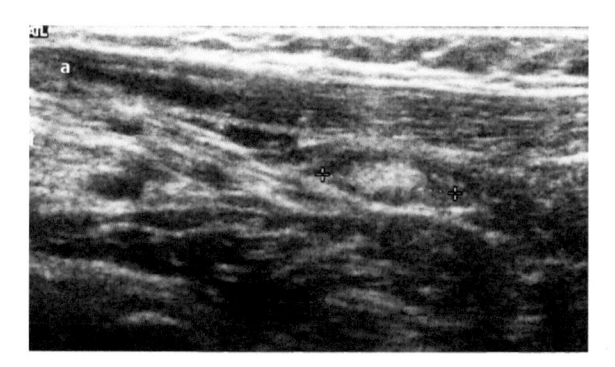

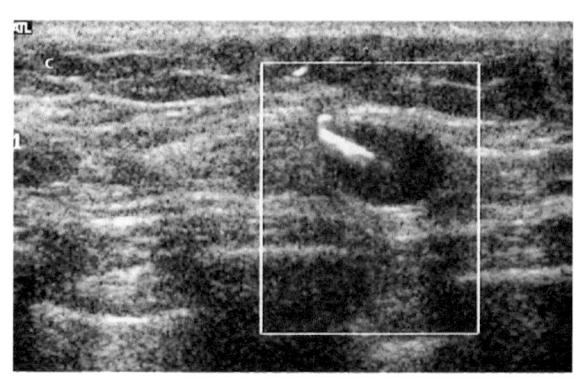

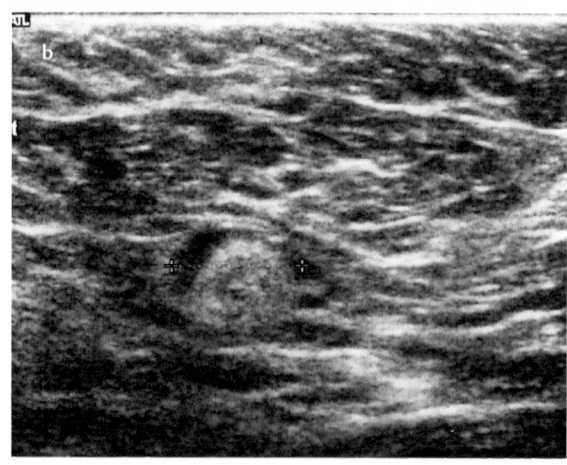

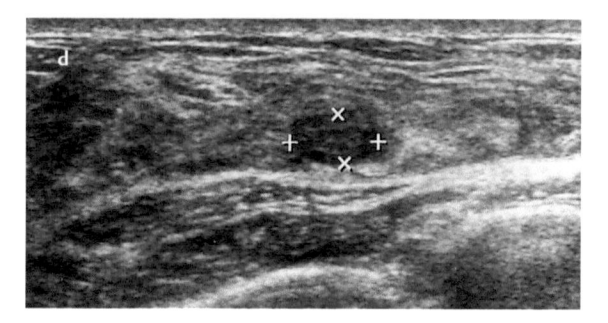

Fig. 17.4a–d Sonography of normal lymph nodes.

a This hypoechoic mass has a pattern similar to that seen in **Fig. 17.2a**. The coffee bean-shaped mass is well defined, and the echo pattern throughout the mass is uniform. The fatty hilum appears sonographically as an echogenic area indenting the mass.

b Another normal lymph node shown in two projections.

c Using color Doppler the central afferent vessels can be visualized.

d Normal intramammary lymph node.

Pathologic Changes in Lymph Nodes

Criteria indicating pathologic changes include:
- Absence of an echogenic hilum
- Disappearance or compression of the echogenic hilum
- Focal thickening of the cortex
- Diffuse thickening of the cortex > 3 mm
- Infrequently irregular contours (indicating invasion beyond the capsule) may be seen

Metastatic Adenopathy

Women with metastatic disease in the axilla from breast cancer usually have a known primary in the breast.

Rarely, enlarged lymph nodes are the first manifestation of a breast cancer, which is not apparent clinically, mammographically, or sonographically. In most of these cases, axillary lymph node involvement is detected clinically by palpation of suspicious nodes in the axilla. Infrequently axillary or intramammary lymph node involvement is discovered by imaging alone.

It should be remembered that nodes with metastatic involvement are often comingled with normal lymph nodes. It should also be remembered that, using any imaging modality, a lymph node with a normal appearance does not exclude the possibility of metastatic disease within the node.

If (by any imaging modality) enlargement of lymph node parenchyma or replacement of the fatty hilum is noted, it is often impossible without biopsy to differentiate metastatic disease in axillary nodes from reactive hyperplasia.

Mammographically metastatic nodes can have a density greater than that of normal breast tissue. Furthermore, lymph nodes containing metastases may show loss of the normal fatty hilum (**Fig. 17.5a**). Lymph nodes

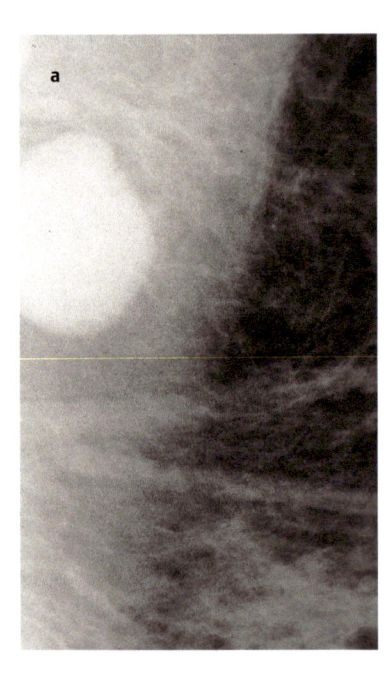

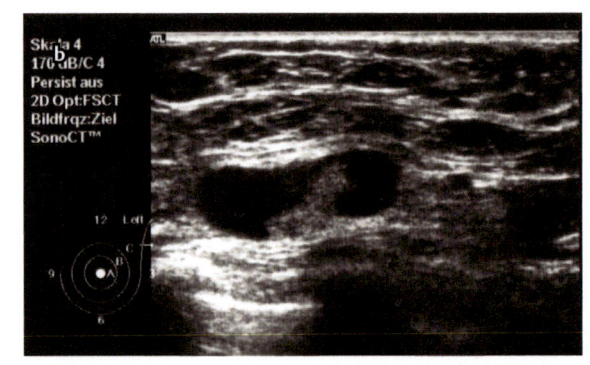

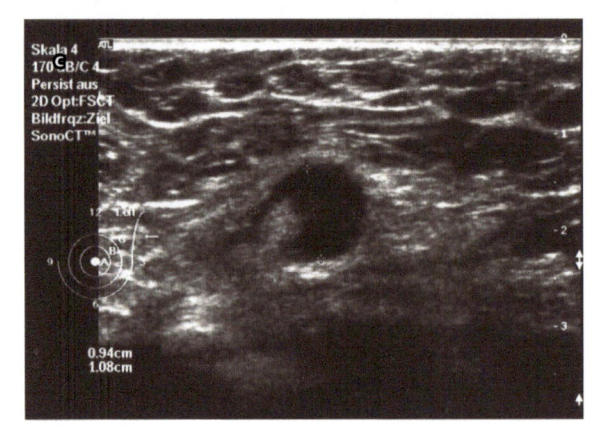

Fig. 17.5a–h Metastatic lymph nodes.

a This axillary node contains metastatic disease from breast carcinoma. It is dense, and the fatty hilum has been replaced. In the context of known breast carcinoma, the pattern is suggestive of a metastasis.

b This axillary node contains metastatic disease from breast carcinoma. It is very hypoechoic, and the fatty hilum has been partly replaced. In the context of known breast carcinoma, the pattern is suggestive of a metastasis.

c Sonographically, nodes containing metastases can develop a lobulated configuration. The focal bulging in the contour of this node was due to metastatic breast carcinoma.

Pathologic Changes in Lymph Nodes

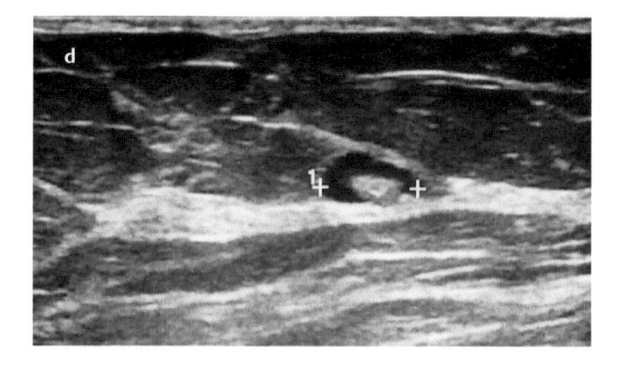

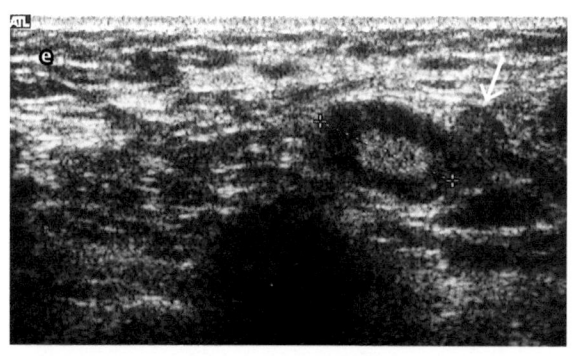

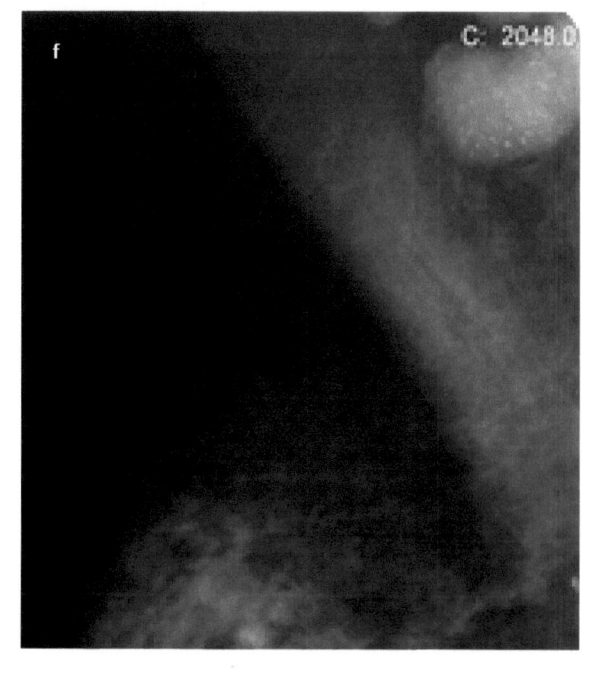

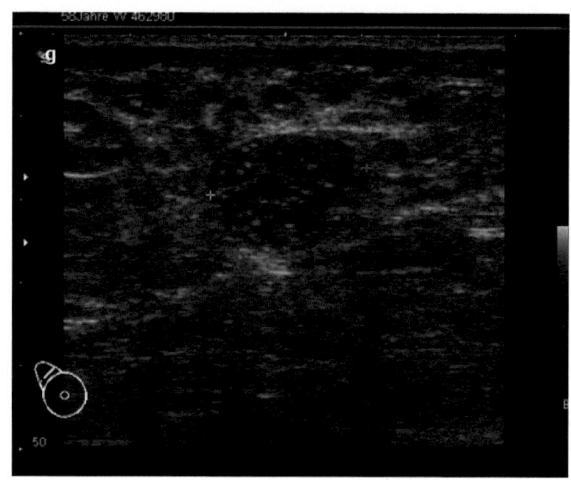

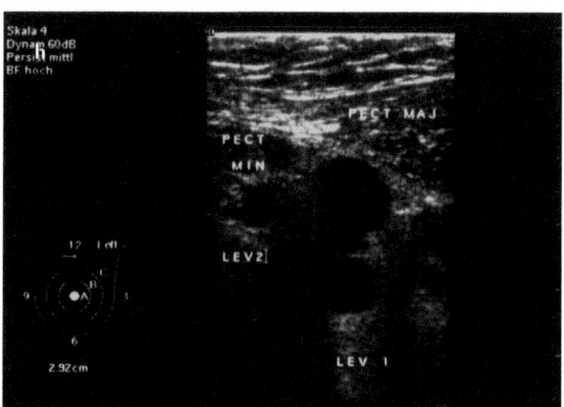

d Very low echogenicity of the cortex may be a sign of malignancy. The cortex is, however, homogeneous and smooth and does not exceed 3 mm. This lymph node proved to be normal.

e Another example of a lymph node with a hypoechoic cortex. Here the cortex is, however, eccentrically enlarged (arrow) and the hilum shows rather low echogenicity (involved lymph node).

f This involved lymph node is lobulated, the hilum irregular and the hypoechoic cortex is eccentrically enlarged.

g This involved lymph node is rounded, the cortex enlarged and very hypoechoic, and the hilum corresponds to a small linear and irregular reflex.

h Levels I and II involved with highly suspicious ill-defined nodes with loss of the hilum.

containing metastatic disease are usually smoothly marginated. Irregularity and gross spiculation of the node can occasionally occur (**Fig. 17.6a**). This pattern is due to extranodal extension of tumor into perinodal fat and indicates a biologically aggressive cancer.

Although calcifications are common in primary breast cancers, they are infrequently present within sites of metastatic disease, including axillary nodes. If a node contains pleomorphic microcalcifications, metastatic involvement should be suspected (**Fig. 17.7**).

Sonographically the following changes should raise the suspicion of lymph node involvement in women with known breast cancer or other malignancies: partial or complete replacement of the echogenic fatty hilum (**Fig. 17.5b,h,i**), focal or diffuse decrease of echogenicity within the nodal cortex (**Figs. 17.5b,d, Fig. 17.6b**), and focal bulges or marginal irregularity (**Fig. 17.5c**).

Further signs may include a round (vs. oval) shape (Yang et al. 2000) or demonstration of a peripheral versus central flow pattern with Doppler imaging.

Malignancies other than breast cancer can be responsible for metastatic axillary adenopathy. The most common of these are lymphoproliferative malignancies such as lymphomas and leukemias, especially chronic lymphocytic leukemia. Nodes in lymphoproliferative malignancies are usually grossly enlarged and dense. These nodes are usually well defined and often massive (**Fig. 17.8**). On palpation these lymph nodes are mostly softer than those of metastatic breast cancer.

Other common sites of metastatic disease to the axilla include contralateral breast, lung, melanoma, gastrointestinal, thyroid, and ovarian cancers. There are no characteristic patterns to these metastases.

Even though the published sensitivity and specificity of sonography (being the most appropriate imaging modality today) ranges only around 60–80% and 85–85%, respectively, and is even lower for nonpalpable lymph nodes (Alvarez et al. 2006, Sidibé et al. 2007, Mainiero et al. 2010, Mills et al. 2010), the combination of ultrasound and US-guided biopsy has proven quite reliable (accuracy > 95%) and may help to support therapeutic decisions (Sidibé et al. 2007).

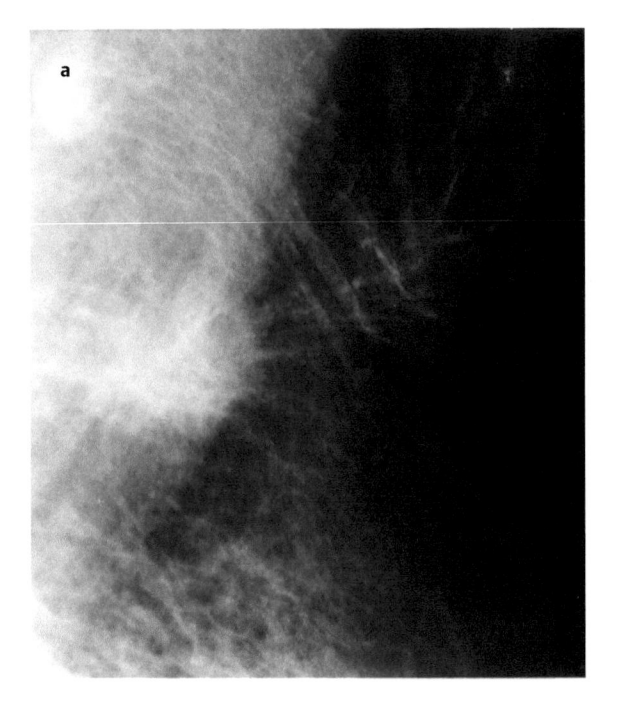

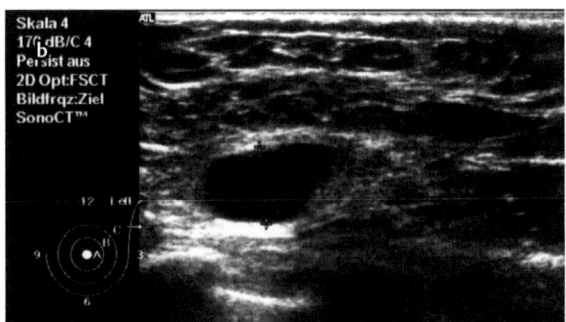

Fig. 17.6a,b Spiculated axillary adenopathy. In the context of known breast carcinoma, spiculated axillary nodes are due to extranodal extension of metastatic disease into perinodal fat.

a This axillary node has a spiculated contour owing to perinodal extension of metastatic disease from a primary carcinoma within this breast. The second smaller lymph node also exhibits a loss of hilum and increased density.
b The sonographic pattern of this lymph node shows a very hypoechoic mass without hilum.

Pathologic Changes in Lymph Nodes

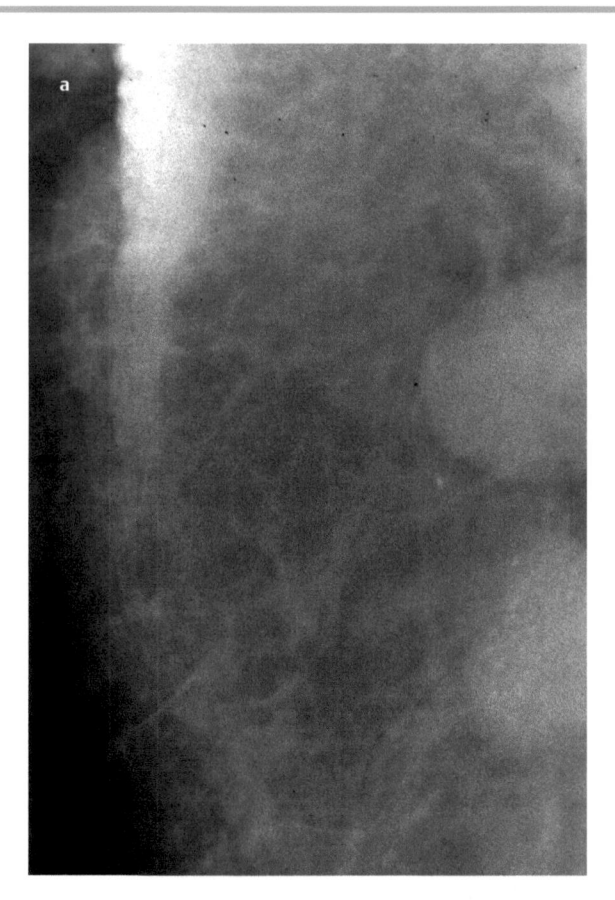

Fig. 17.7a–f

a Faint calcifications are present in the lower of these two enlarged, dense axillary nodes containing metastatic breast carcinoma.

b–d Patient with ovarian cancer, showing faint microcalcifications in an enlarged palpable axillary lymph node. Another smaller lymph node looks normal. Fine needle aspiration (FNA) proved metastasis from ovarian cancer in the calcified node and no malignant change in the smaller one.

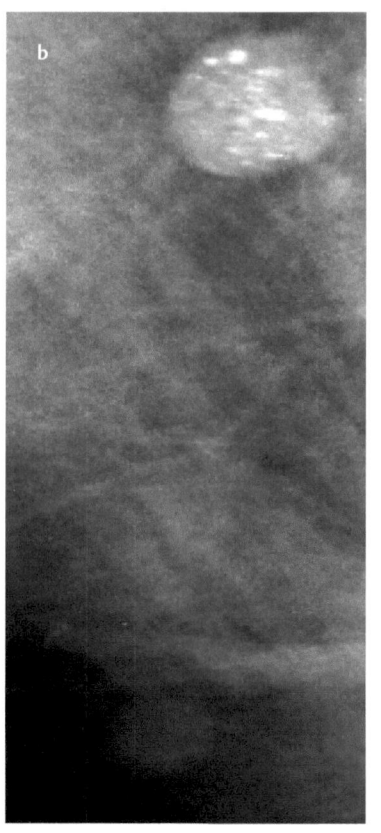

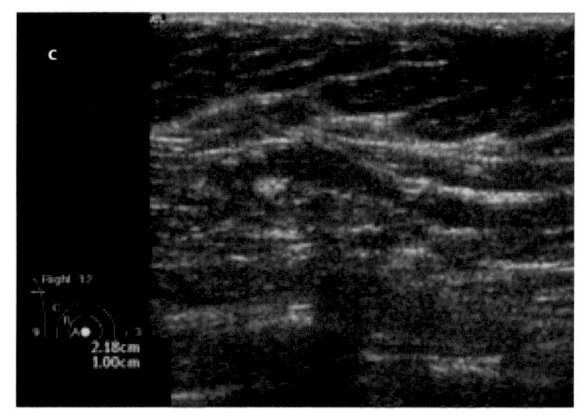

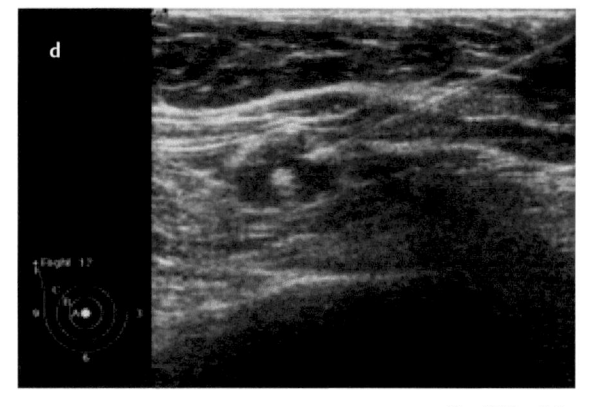

Fig. 17.7e–f ▷

17 Lymph Nodes

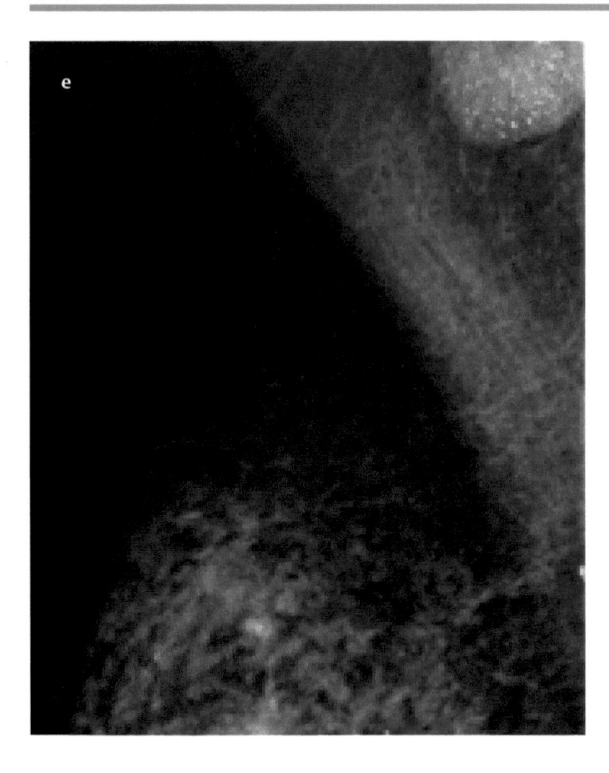

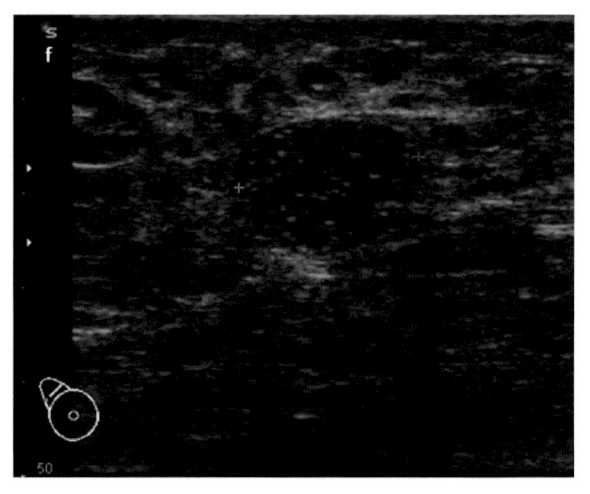

◁ continued

e,f Three years after breast-conserving therapy this woman presented with a newly visible rounded, hyperdense lymph node with microcalcifications in the axilla. Ultrasound examination showed an enlarged lymph node with loss of the hilum. The calcifications are visible on ultrasound too. FNA revealed metastatic lymph node involvement.

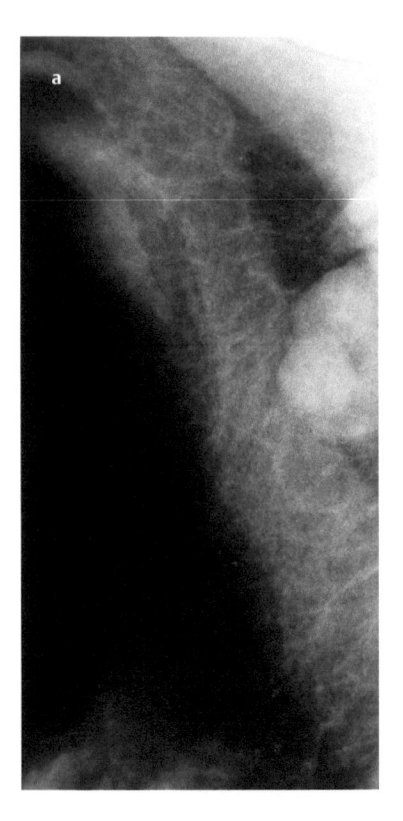

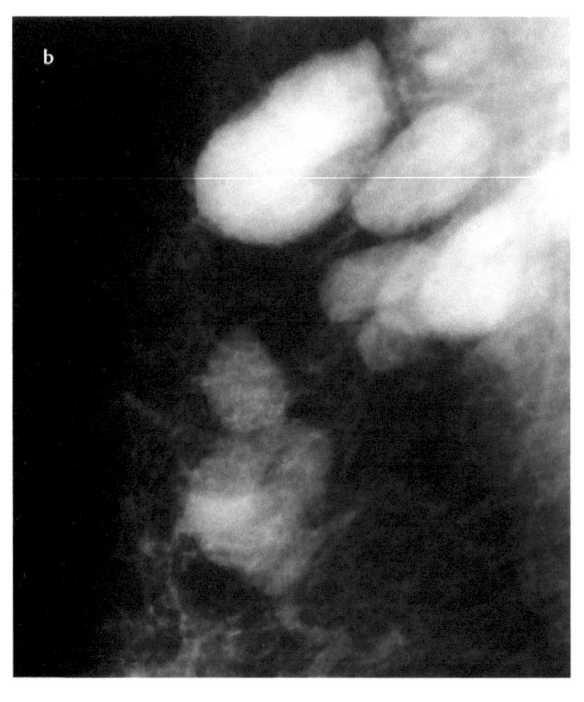

Fig. 17.8a–b Malignant axillary adenopathy not due to breast carcinoma.

a Multiple, enlarged, dense axillary nodes are present in this patient with metastatic thyroid carcinoma. A similar pattern was present in both of her axillae.

b Another woman with multiple, bulky lymph nodes. These are due to lymphoma. Lymphoproliferative diseases can produce some of the most impressive adenopathy seen in the axillae.

Pathologic Changes in Lymph Nodes

Other Causes of Adenopathy

Interval enlargement of lymph nodes on serial mammography can be a source of worry; but without a history of cancer, this is infrequently the first indicator of malignant disease.

According to Lee et al. (1997) who examined 24 women with lymph nodes enlarging by 20% to over 300% on serial mammograms, metastatic disease was found in only two. Both of them had a known history of cancer.

The most common cause of axillary nodal involvement is nonspecific benign adenopathy. A series by Walsh et al. (1997) reported this as the cause in 29% of cases, although this percentage would depend upon the population under study. Causes of this change can include skin and nail infections or inflammatory processes in the arm, breast infections, or inflammation.

A large number of nonmalignant diseases have been reported as causing axillary lymphadenopathy. These include any type of acute bacterial or viral infection, tuberculosis, HIV (human immunodeficiency virus), sarcoidosis, rheumatoid arthritis, psoriasis, and other collagen vascular diseases (Irshad et al. 2008, Cao et al. 2011) (**Fig. 17.9**).

In women who have recently had surgery for breast carcinoma, enlargement of axillary nodes may just be caused by the preceding therapy. In the vast majority of cases it will be benign and should thus not be a source of concern. We usually would recommend imaging follow-up.

Finally, benign nodal enlargement may even occur as a mere reactive change in patients with breast cancer (sometimes medullary carcinoma) without metastatic disease (Neuman and Homer 1996).

To avoid unnecessary interventions, patient history and short-term follow-up may be considered first. If the enlargement persists, the question can mostly be solved by percutaneous biopsy.

Nodal Calcifications

Occasionally, calcifications will be present in axillary nodes (Bruwer et al. 1987, Dunnington et al. 1995, Hooley et al. 1996, Feder et al. 1999). These can be due to benign or malignant causes (**Fig. 17.10**). Coarse calcifications due

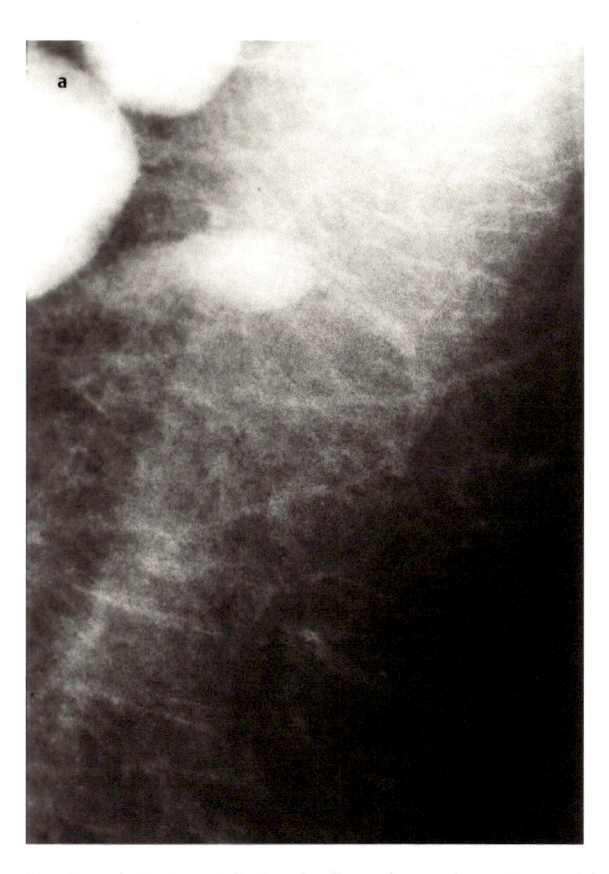

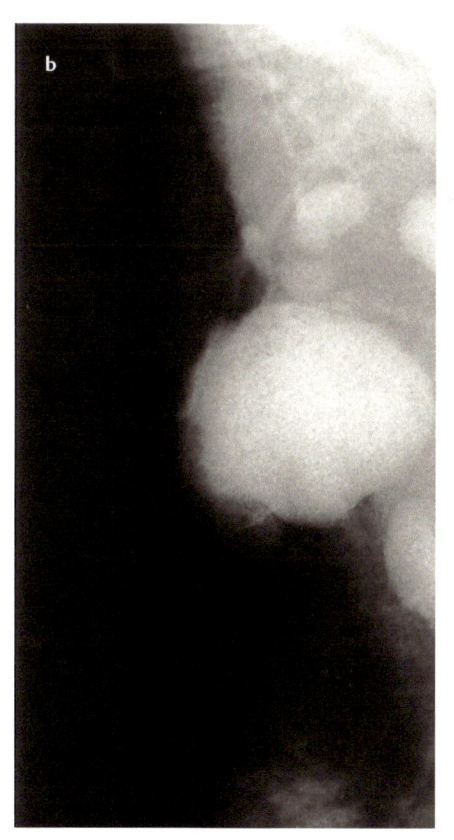

Fig. 17.9a,b Benign etiologies of axillary adenopathy. Axillary nodal enlargement due to benign causes can appear identical to malignant axillary nodal enlargement.

a Multiple, dense nodes without central fatty hila are seen in this woman with adenopathy due to HIV disease.

b Marked axillary adenopathy in this patient is caused by histiocytosis X.

17 Lymph Nodes

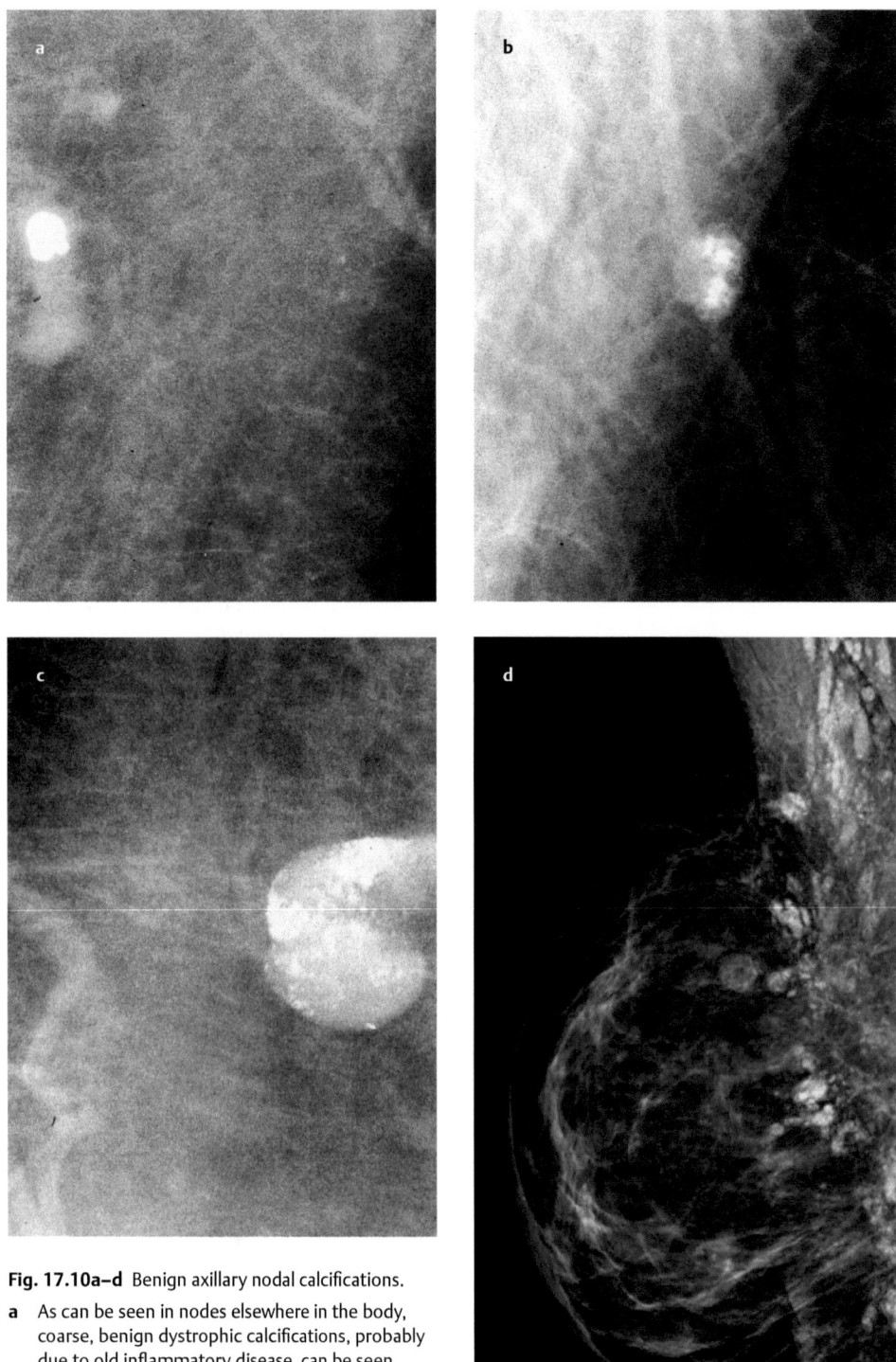

Fig. 17.10a–d Benign axillary nodal calcifications.
a As can be seen in nodes elsewhere in the body, coarse, benign dystrophic calcifications, probably due to old inflammatory disease, can be seen in axillary lymph nodes. The calcification in this node was unchanged over many years and is presumably due to old inflammation.
b Dystrophic calcification is also seen in this axillary node.
c Fine calcifications and increased nodal density in this patient were caused by gold treatment given for rheumatoid arthritis.
d Silicon-containing lymph nodes and silicon granulomas.

to old granulomatous disease or fat necrosis can be found. Punctate or fine elongated calcifications from gold given for treatment of rheumatoid arthritis can also be seen. Dense nodes, simulating those containing calcifications, can also be found in women with silicone injected into the breast or silicone leaks from breast augmentation prostheses (**Fig. 17.10d**). Silicone drains into the axilla and can be taken up by axillary nodes, causing them to appear extremely dense.

Although microcalcifications are present in around 50% of invasive breast cancers on mammography, microcalcifications are rarely present in involved lymph nodes. When metastatic adenopathy due to breast carcinoma contains calcifications, these calcifications are usually pleomorphic and often faint (**Fig. 17.7**). Similar calcifications within nodes can also be seen with metastatic ovarian and thyroid carcinomas. A case of papillary carcinoma of the breast has been reported as presenting as axillary nodal calcifications.

Percutaneous Biopsy

If further diagnostic workup in addition to imaging is required, needle biopsy can be performed.

Concerning verification of malignancy, the reported accuracy is around 95% (de Kanter et al. 1999, Sidibé et al. 2007, Britton et al. 2009a). Core needle biopsy may allow a more exact verification of the various benign causes. Although a negative diagnosis cannot definitely exclude malignant involvement, a positive diagnosis is quite reliable and can be used to influence treatment decisions.

The risk of side effects (bleeding close to the axillary plexus) may be lower with fine needle aspiration biopsy.

Further Techniques in Nodal Imaging: MRI and PET

Some studies have suggested that magnetic resonance imaging (MRI) using Gd-chelate as contrast agent has a high positive predictive value for axillary nodal metastases (Mumtaz et al. 1997, Mussurakis et al. 1997) (**Fig. 17.11a**).

In a study including 75 axillae in women with breast carcinoma, Mumtaz found a sensitivity of 90% and a specificity of 82% in detecting nodal metastases. His criteria were nodal size sensitivity greater than 5 mm, higher than soft tissue intensity on short inversion time inversion recovery images, and enhancement after the injection of Gd-dimeglumine. Mussurakis demonstrated that of 51 women studied with MRI after the administration of gadopentetate dimeglumine, uptake patterns in lymph nodes in about one-quarter of women made it possible to define groups with less than 5% or greater than 95% likelihood of nodal metastases. For Gd-chelate-enhanced MRI the most important criteria for nodal involvement used by Baltzer have been asymmetry of lymph nodes, inhomogeneous cortex (using T2-weighted images and dynamic contrast-enhanced MRI), and surrounding edema (Baltzer et al. 2011). Mortellaro et al. (2009) mentioned absence of a fatty hilum as an important criterion, but pointed out that lymph node size and kinetics

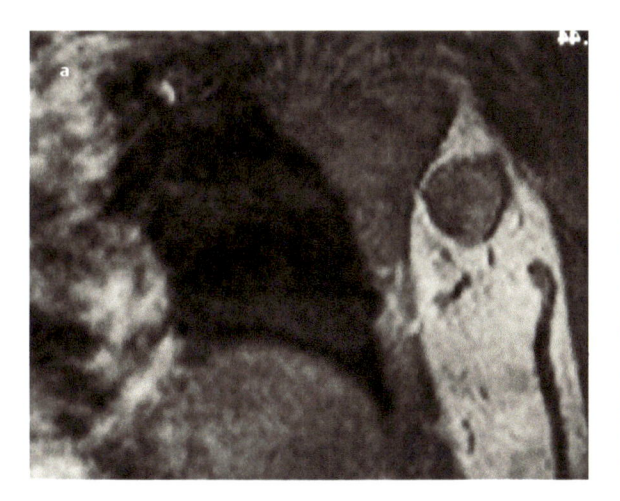

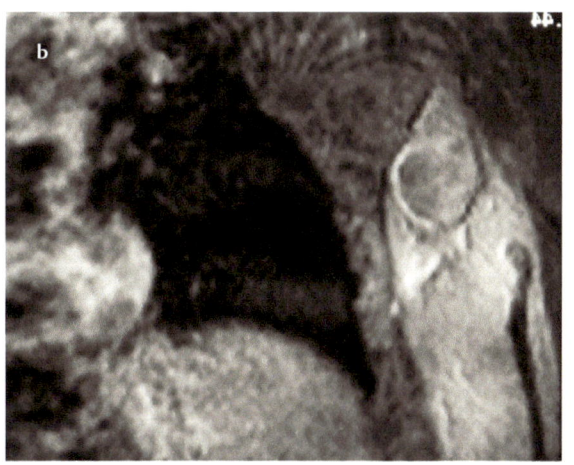

Fig. 17.11 Magnetic resonance imaging

a,b Images before and after intravenous administration of Gd-DTPA demonstrate a 2.4-cm inhomogeneously enhancing lymph node metastasis. There is another smaller indistinct mass, suspicious of a lymph node with perinodal infiltration, as proven by histology.

Fig. 17.11c,d ▷

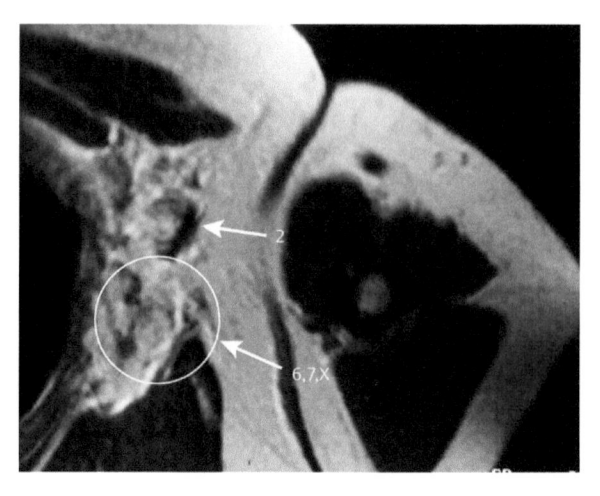

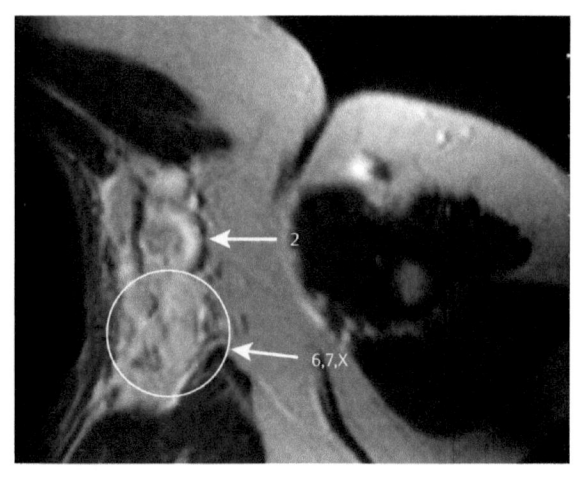

c,d T2-weighted images before and 24 hours after administration of ultrasmall super-paramagnetc iron oxide contrast agent (USPIO). The anterior normal lymph nodes decrease in signal intensity due to accumulation of USPIO. The posterior lymph nodes (circled), which are involved, do not accumulate USPIO and thus do not change their signal intensities.

of enhancement were unreliable, an observation that is supported by us.

Another possibility concerns the use of a more specific contrast agent: USPIO contrast medium (ultrasmall super-paramagnetic iron oxide) is administered intravenously 24–48 hours before the scheduled MRI study. It accumulates in the reticuloendothelial system of normal lymph node tissue and causes a decrease of signal intensity on T2-weighted images by its ferromagnetic properties. However, in metastatic tissue USPIO does not accumulate, and therefore signal intensity does not change (Stets et al. 2002).

Overall MR imaging of the axillary lymph nodes is not yet a generally used method. However, a first systematic review has shown a good future potential for both Gd-chelate-enhanced MRI and USPIO-enhanced MRI (Cooper et al. 2011) (**Fig. 17.11b,e**). In spite of existing variations between the studies and a limited number of examinations, MRI appears to be by far more sensitive and specific than positron emission tomography (PET) imaging and may be even cost-effective for low-risk groups when compared with SNB. According to these results the mean sensitivity and specificity of USPIO-enhanced MRI is greater than 95%. The mean sensitivity and specificity of Gd-chelate-enhanced MRI are reported as 88% and 73%, respectively.

In another set of women with nodal disease, MRI may be especially helpful, namely, in those women who present with axillary metastases and no known primary, MRI may be able to detect the primary tumors in a high percentage of cases (see Chapter 5).

PET using ^{18}F-fludeoxyglucose (FDG) has also been reported as useful in assessing axillary lymph nodes (Scheidhauer et al. 1996, Adler et al. 1997) (**Fig. 17.12**). A recent systematic review and meta-analysis (Cooper et al. 2011) regarding PET for assessment of axillary lymph node status in early breast cancer showed, for PET only,

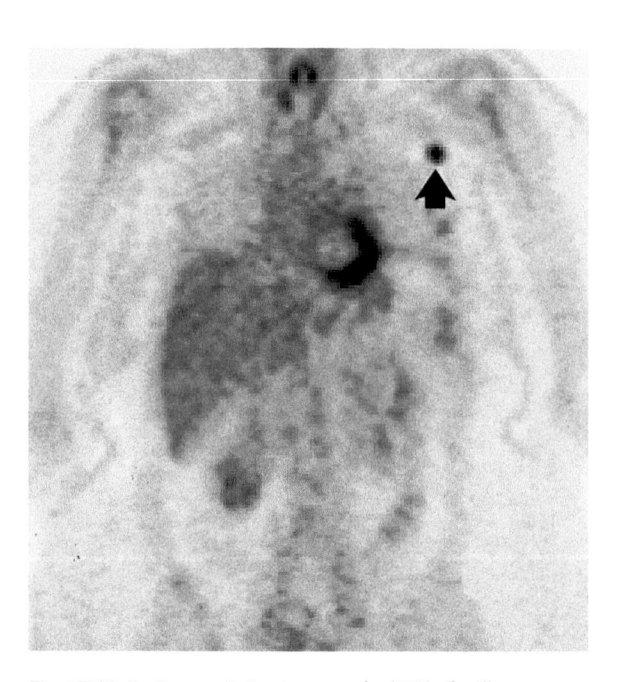

Fig. 17.12 Positron emission tomography (PET) of axillary adenopathy. FDG-PET imaging of a woman with known metastatic breast carcinoma shows an axillary node containing metastatic disease (arrow).

a mean sensitivity of 63% and a mean specificity of 94%. With PET/computed tomography (CT) the mean sensitivity was 56% and mean specificity 93%. The mean sensitivity was 11% for micrometastases and 57% for macrometastases (> 2 mm). The authors' conclusion was that the available evidence does not support the routine use of PET or PET/CT for the assessment of the clinically negative axilla.

Summary

At the time when axillary dissection was still considered state of the art for staging the axilla of every breast cancer patient, imaging of the axilla played a minor role. The reason was that imaging cannot detect microscopic axillary metastases.

To date ALND has been increasingly replaced by SNB. In cases with negative clinical findings and a negative SNB no further measures are needed. Since positive SNB is today considered to require subsequent ALND, imaging may be useful to check for positive lymph nodes. Even if the sensitivity of imaging is limited, detection of an involved lymph node by imaging and subsequent verification (e.g., by percutaneous biopsy) is helpful, since the surgeon can proceed straight to ALND, saving the patient marking of the sentinel node with sentinel node biopsy before ALND.

In this situation imaging may be helpful to support therapeutic decisions. Furthermore, imaging may be useful for the assessment of clinical findings and as a method of surveillance after breast cancer. A lymph node change may be noted on imaging studies of the breast.

Knowledge of the typical anatomy of the axilla and the location of different groups of lymph nodes, knowledge of the various benign and malignant changes, and the use of a standardized technique are essential.

Mammographically, a benign lymph node typically has a fatty hilum and smooth contour. Its parenchyma has a density comparable to breast parenchyma. Overall size is of no importance. Replacement of the hilum by dense tissue, irregular contours, and the rare presence of microcalcifications may be indicators of malignant involvement.

Sonographically smooth contours, homogeneous texture of the lymph node parenchyma, and presence of a hyperechoic hilum are usually seen in benign lymph nodes. Irregular contours, bulging of the parenchyma, loss of the hilum reflex, strong hypoechogenicity of the cortical rim, eccentric cortex enlargement, and a linear hilum reflex suggest malignant involvement.

If biopsy of indeterminate or suspicious imaging findings is required, this is usually done by US-guided percutaneous biopsy, usually fine needle aspiration biopsy or core needle biopsy.

MRI has so far shown promising results. But even in 2011 our experience is still limited. PET and PET/CT have so far not proven superior to sonography and are inferior to MRI.

Considering that so far no imaging modality is capable of reliably detecting or excluding microscopic lymph node involvement, imaging cannot replace histopathologic assessment. But when combined with appropriate histopathologic assessment (using percutaneous breast biopsy, SNB, or ALND), imaging may help to optimize the individual diagnosis and therapy.

References and Recommended Reading

Adair F, Berg J, Joubert L, Robbins GF. Long-term followup of breast cancer patients: the 30-year report. Cancer 1974;33(4):1145–1150

Adler LP, Faulhaber PF, Schnur KC, Al-Kasi NL, Shenk RR. Axillary lymph node metastases: screening with [F-18]2-deoxy-2-fluoro-D-glucose (FDG) PET. Radiology 1997;203(2):323–327

Alvarez S, Añorbe E, Alcorta P, López F, Alonso I, Cortés J. Role of sonography in the diagnosis of axillary lymph node metastases in breast cancer: a systematic review. AJR Am J Roentgenol 2006;186(5):1342–1348

Baltzer PA, Dietzel M, Burmeister HP, et al. Application of MR mammography beyond local staging: is there a potential to accurately assess axillary lymph nodes? Evaluation of an extended protocol in an initial prospective study. AJR Am J Roentgenol 2011;196(5):W641–647

Blamey RW, Pinder SE, Ball GR, et al. Reading the prognosis of the individual with breast cancer. Eur J Cancer 2007;43(10):1545–1547

Blamey RW, Hornmark-Stenstam B, Ball G, et al. ONCOPOOL—a European database for 16,944 cases of breast cancer. Eur J Cancer 2010;46(1):56–71

Britton PD, Goud A, Godward S, et al. Use of ultrasound-guided axillary node core biopsy in staging of early breast cancer. Eur Radiol 2009a;19(3):561–569

Britton PD, Provenzano E, Barter S, et al. Ultrasound guided percutaneous axillary lymph node core biopsy: how often is the sentinel lymph node being biopsied? Breast 2009b;18(1):13–16

Britton P, Moyle P, Benson JR, et al. Ultrasound of the axilla: where to look for the sentinel lymph node. Clin Radiol 2010;65(5):373–376

Bruwer A, Nelson GW, Spark RP. Punctate intranodal gold deposits simulating microcalcifications on mammograms. Radiology 1987;163(1):87–88

Cao MM, Hoyt AC, Bassett LW. Mammographic signs of systemic disease. Radiographics 2011;31(4):1085–1100

Cooper KL, Meng Y, Harnan S et al. Positron emission tomography (PET) and magnetic resonance imaging (MRI) for the assessment of axillary lymph node metastases in early breast cancer: systematic review and economic evaluation. Health Technol Assess 2011;15(4)

de Kanter AY, van Eijck CH, van Geel AN, et al. Multicentre study of ultrasonographically guided axillary node biopsy in patients with breast cancer. Br J Surg 1999;86(11):1459–1462

Dershaw DD, Selland DG, Tan LK, Morris EA, Abramson AF, Liberman L. Spiculated axillary adenopathy. Radiology 1996;201(2):439–442

Dunnington GL, Pearce J, Sherrod A, Cote R. Breast carcinoma presenting as mammographic microcalcifications in axillary lymph nodes. Breast Dis 1995;8:193–198

Feder JM, de Paredes ES, Hogge JP, Wilken JJ. Unusual breast lesions: radiologic-pathologic correlation. Radiographics 1999;19(Spec No):S11–S26, quiz S260

Giuliano AE, Kirgan DM, Guenther JM, Morton DL. Lymphatic mapping and sentinel lymphadenectomy for breast cancer. Ann Surg 1994;220(3):391–398, discussion 398–401

Giuliano AE, Hunt KK, Ballman KV, et al. Axillary dissection vs no axillary dissection in women with invasive breast cancer and sentinel node metastasis: a randomized clinical trial. JAMA 2011;305(6):569–575

Hooley R, Lee C, Tocino I, Horowitz N, Carter D. Calcifications in axillary lymph nodes caused by fat necrosis. AJR Am J Roentgenol 1996;167(3):627–628

Irshad A, Ackerman SJ, Pope TL, Moses CK, Rumboldt T, Panzegrau B. Rare breast lesions: correlation of imaging and histologic features with WHO classification. Radiographics 2008;28(5):1399–1414

Lee CH, Giurescu ME, Philpotts LE, Horvath LJ, Tocino I. Clinical importance of unilaterally enlarging lymph nodes on otherwise normal mammograms. Radiology 1997;203(2):329–334

Leibman AJ, Wong R. Findings on mammography in the axilla. AJR Am J Roentgenol 1997;169(5):1385–1390

Mainiero MB, Cinelli CM, Koelliker SL, Graves TA, Chung MA. Axillary ultrasound and fine-needle aspiration in the preoperative evaluation of the breast cancer patient: an algorithm based on tumor size and lymph node appearance. AJR Am J Roentgenol 2010;195(5):1261–1267

Mills P, Sever A, Weeks J, Fish D, Jones S, Jones P. Axillary ultrasound assessment in primary breast cancer: an audit of 653 cases. Breast J 2010;16(5):460–463

Moriggl B, Steinlechner M. Ultrasono-anatomy for evaluation of the local lymphatic groups of the mamma. Surg Radiol Anat 1994;16(1):77–85

Mortellaro VE, Marshall J, Singer L, et al. Magnetic resonance imaging for axillary staging in patients with breast cancer. J Magn Reson Imaging 2009;30(2):309–312

Motomura K, Ishitobi M, Komoike Y, et al. SPIO-enhanced magnetic resonance imaging for the detection of metastases in sentinel nodes localized by computed tomography lymphography in patients with breast cancer. Ann Surg Oncol 2011;18(12):3422–3429

Mumtaz H, Hall-Craggs MA, Davidson T, et al. Staging of symptomatic primary breast cancer with MR imaging. AJR Am J Roentgenol 1997;169(2):417–424

Mussurakis S, Buckley DL, Horsman A. Prediction of axillary lymph node status in invasive breast cancer with dynamic contrast-enhanced MR imaging. Radiology 1997;203(2):317–321

Neuman ML, Homer MJ. Association of medullary carcinoma with reactive axillary adenopathy. AJR Am J Roentgenol 1996;167(1):185–186

Pandharipande PV, Harisinghani MG, Ozanne EM, et al. Staging MR lymphangiography of the axilla for early breast cancer: cost-effectiveness analysis. AJR Am J Roentgenol 2008;191(5):1308–1319

Pepels MJ, Vestjens JH, de Boer M, et al. Safety of avoiding routine use of axillary dissection in early stage breast cancer: a systematic review. Breast Cancer Res Treat 2011;125(2):301–313

Scheidhauer K, Scharl A, Pietrzyk U, et al. Qualitative [18F]FDG positron emission tomography in primary breast cancer: clinical relevance and practicability. Eur J Nucl Med 1996;23(6):618–623

Sidibé S, Coulibaly A, Traoré S, Touré M, Traoré I. Role of ultrasonography in the diagnosis of axillary lymph node metastases in breast cancer: a systematic review. Mali Med 2007;22(4):9–13 [Article in French]

Stets C, Brandt S, Wallis F, Buchmann J, Gilbert FJ, Heywang-Köbrunner SH. Axillary lymph node metastases: a statistical analysis of various parameters in MRI with USPIO. J Magn Reson Imaging 2002;16(1):60–68

Sugg SL, Ferguson DJ, Posner MC, Heimann R. Should internal mammary nodes be sampled in the sentinel lymph node era? Ann Surg Oncol 2000;7(3):188–192

Veronesi U, Galimberti V, Zurrida S, Merson M, Greco M, Lini A. Prognostic significance of number and level of axillary node mestases in breast cancer. Breast 1993;2:224–228

Veronesi U, Marubini E, Mariani L, Valagussa P, Zucali R. The dissection of internal mammary nodes does not improve the survival of breast cancer patients. 30-year results of a randomised trial. Eur J Cancer 1999;35(9):1320–1325

Walsh R, Kornguth PJ, Soo MS, Bentley R, DeLong DM. Axillary lymph nodes: mammographic, pathologic, and clinical correlation. AJR Am J Roentgenol 1997;168(1):33–38

Yang WT, Chang J, Metreweli C. Patients with breast cancer: differences in color Doppler flow and gray-scale US features of benign and malignant axillary lymph nodes. Radiology 2000;215(2):568–573

18 Other Semi-Malignant and Malignant Tumors

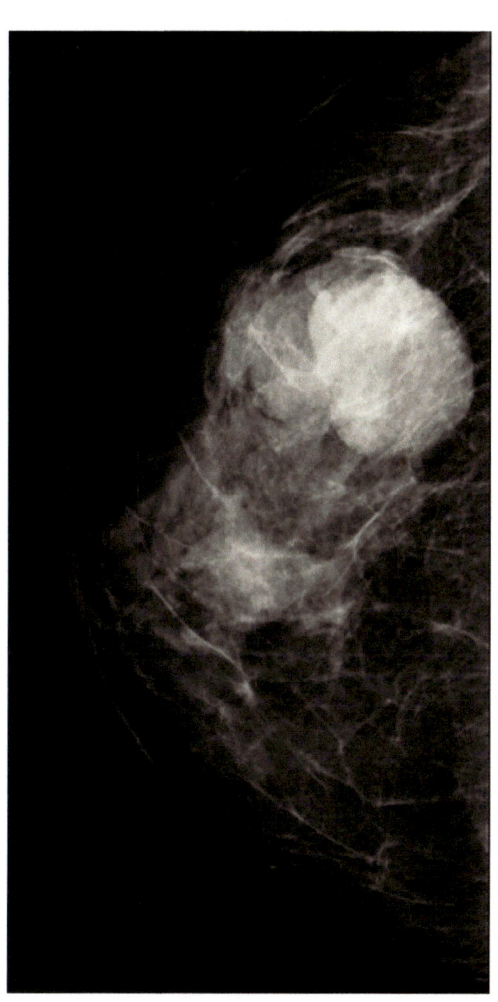

Phyllodes Tumor (Cystosarcoma Phyllodes) → 476
Histology → 476
Clinical Findings → 476
Diagnostic Strategy and Goals → 476

Fibromatosis (= Extra-Abdominal Desmoid) → 479

Hemangiopericytoma and Hemangioendothelioma → 479

Adenomyoepithelioma → 480

Sarcomas → 480
Histology → 480
Clinical Findings → 480
Diagnostic Strategy and Goals → 480

Malignancies of the Breast of Hematologic Origin → 484
Histopathology → 484
Clinical Findings → 484
Diagnostic Strategy and Goals → 485

Metastases → 487
Histology → 487
Clinical Findings → 487
Diagnostic Strategy and Goals → 487

References and Recommended Reading → 489

18 Other Semi-Malignant and Malignant Tumors

S. H. Heywang-Koebrunner, I. Schreer, S. Barter

Phyllodes Tumor (Cystosarcoma Phyllodes)

The phyllodes tumor is a rare tumor (~0.5% of all breast tumors). Its histologic spectrum includes benign tumors, of which up to 30% recur, semi-malignant, and malignant tumors. The latter can metastasize. In toto, only around 5–15% of phyllodes tumors may metastasize. In view of its biological properties, timely detection and complete excision with an adequate safety margin is critical for the malignant variant (Geisler et al. 2000, Ben Hassouna et al. 2006).

Larger tumors may require a mastectomy, since recurrence is best prevented by complete excision (with a small safety margin). Axillary dissection should not be performed because these tumors metastasize hematogenously, not lymphogenously.

Clinically and by imaging methods, the phyllodes tumor mostly presents as an oval or lobulated mass. Larger and malignant tumors may exhibit indistinct margins. It can develop in all age groups and generally shows rapid growth.

Benign and semi-malignant phyllodes tumors, when diagnosed at needle biopsy, are usually classified as B3 (or B4) lesions (see Chapter 14). Malignant phyllodes tumors (if recognized correctly at needle biopsy) will be classified as B5 lesions. Whenever a phyllodes tumor is diagnosed at needle biopsy, excision is indicated. It allows the final classification and is necessary to avoid recurrence, which is frequent in benign and malignant phyllodes tumors that are incompletely excised. Excision therefore is the standard treatment. Benign phyllodes tumors have been discussed in Chapter 14, malignant and semi-malignant phyllodes tumors are described in this chapter.

Histology

As mentioned in Chapter 14, phyllodes tumors belong to the group of fibroepithelial lesions. Typically phyllodes tumors present as a round, oval, or lobulated mass consisting of a hypercellular myxoid stroma with wide leaflike (phyllodes) interspaces covered with epithelium. The stroma contains fibroblasts, myofibroblasts and giant cells in varying distributions.

Phyllodes tumors are subclassified based on the degree of cellular proliferation and differentiation within the stroma (Tan et al. 2012):

- *Benign phyllodes tumor* (prevalence: 70%). Sharp demarcation, no atypical cells, no pleomorphic cells, low mitotic rate
- *Malignant phyllodes tumor* (prevalence: 5–15%). Infiltrative growth, atypical cells, pleomorphic cells, obliteration of the fibroepithelial configuration, high mitotic rate: > 5/10 HPF (high-power fields)
- *Borderline phyllodes tumor* (up to 20%). Usually sharply demarcated, minimal atypia of the pleomorphic cells, mitotic rate 5/10 HPF

Following incomplete excision, the phyllodes tumor has a high recurrence rate of 20–30%, whereby the proportion of multiple recurrences is relatively high if a wide margin of normal breast tissue is not included at the time of surgical excision.

Clinical Findings

- The phyllodes tumor is generally palpable as a smoothly marginated, round or lobulated mass, which is more or less elastic.
- Small tumors are generally moveable, but this characteristic is often lost with larger tumors.
- Rapid growth is suggestive of a phyllodes tumor. It can arise from a known fibroadenoma that was stable over a long period of time and is then noted by its increasing growth. It can also be found as a mass that increases in size.

At the time of the diagnosis, the majority of these neoplasms have reached a size of 3–5 cm, but occasionally small phyllodes tumors are also discovered (see also **Fig. 14.9a–h**). Owing to the tension of the overlying skin, very large phyllodes tumors can cause erythematous or bluish discoloration of the skin, or even ulcerations.

Diagnostic Strategy and Goals

Most phyllodes tumors present as a mass that rapidly increases in size. Today these masses usually undergo needle biopsy. The histology of a phyllodes tumor will be classified as B3, B4 (suspected of being malignant), or B5 at core biopsy. The therapeutic consequence for phyllodes tumors classified as B3, B4, or B5 will always be complete excision of the tumor with a tumor-free margin. For extremely large tumors simple mastectomy may be necessary. Since malignant phyllodes tumors metastasize hematogenously, axillary dissection is not indicated.

Mammography

(See **Fig. 18.1a,g**.)

Mammographically (Liberman et al. 1996, Jorge Blanco et al. 1999, Muttarak and Chaiwun 2004), the phyllodes tumor usually presents as a round, oval, or lobulated mass. Its presentations range from sharply outlined masses to masses with partially or completely obscured margins (depending on the density of the surrounding tissue) to masses with indistinct margins. Even though indistinct margins may represent a zone of infiltration or vascular invasion, malignant phyllodes tumors may also be completely well circumscribed. Some irregularities in the contour are frequently, but not always, present with larger phyllodes tumors. Rarely, bizarre or coarse calcifications (as seen in fibroadenomas) can be found in portions of phyllodes tumors.

There is no mammographic feature that reliably allows the distinction of other round, oval, or lobulated masses from phyllodes tumors or the distinction between malignant or benign phyllodes tumors.

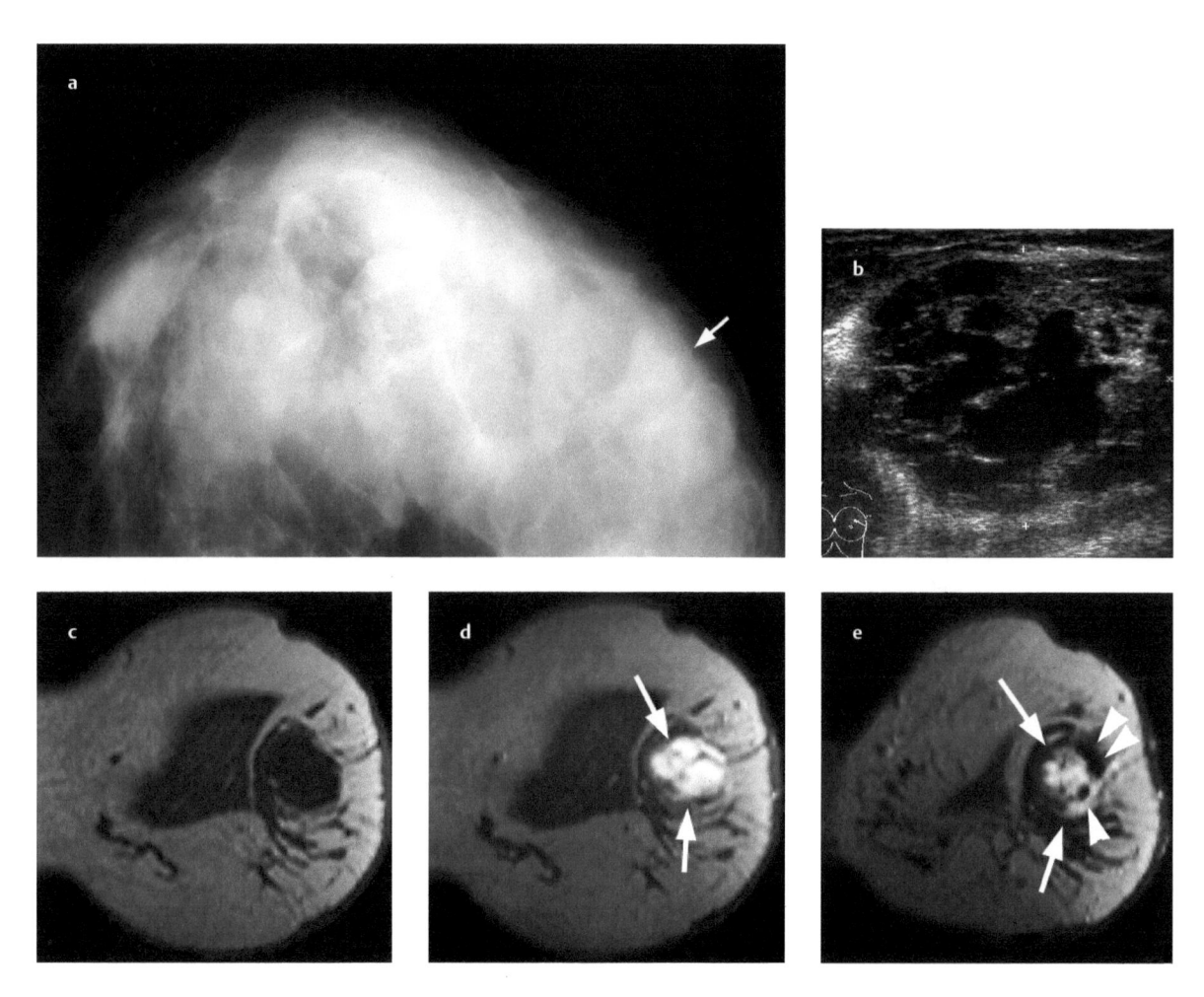

Fig. 18.1a–h Phyllodes tumor.

a The phyllodes tumor, being an oval, smoothly outlined lesion, cannot be discerned among the very dense parenchyma amid numerous sonographically documented cysts.
b Sonographically, the lesion is heterogeneous with intervening cystic spaces.
c Magnetic resonance imaging (coronal plane) delineates a lesion of homogeneously low signal intensity and smooth outline before administration of contrast medium.

d,e After intravenous administration of contrast medium, the lesion (arrows) shows a lobulated internal structure (intense enhancement within the lobules, slight enhancement in the septa), with some nonenhancing clefts (arrowheads) seen in adjacent sections (**e**). *Histology*: Benign phyllodes tumor.

Fig. 18.1f–h ▷

18 Other Semi-Malignant and Malignant Tumors

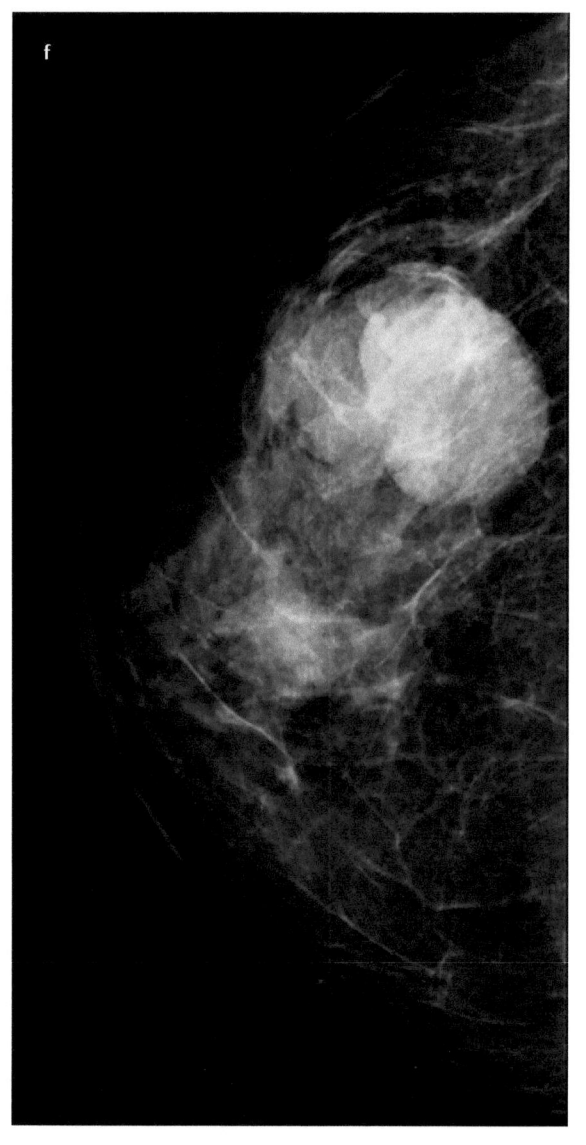

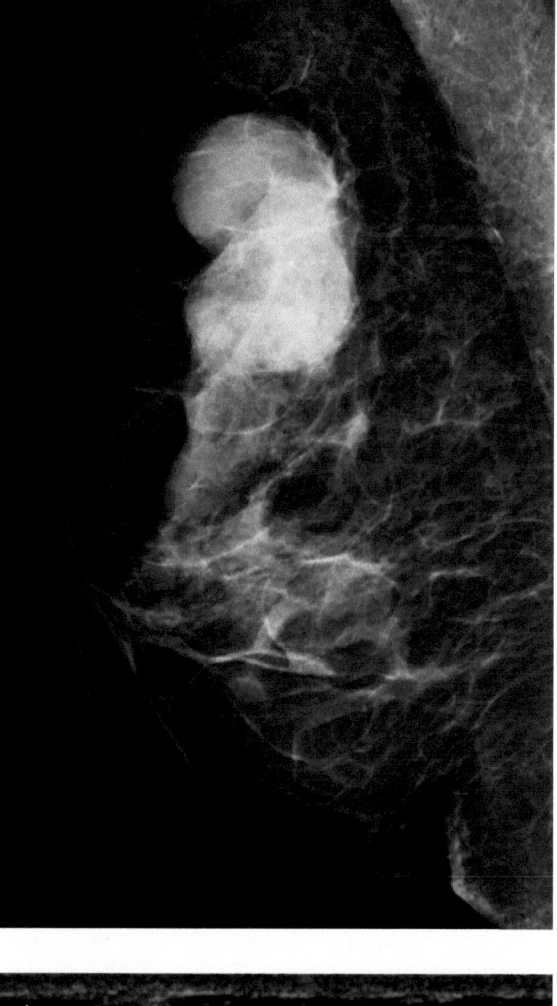

◁ continued

f–h Shows a 60-year-old woman who felt a lump in her breast. Mammograms show a lobulated, dense, well-defined mass (**f,g**). On sonography, a well-defined, solid mass with variable internal echogenicity can be seen. *Histology*: Malignant phyllodes tumor.

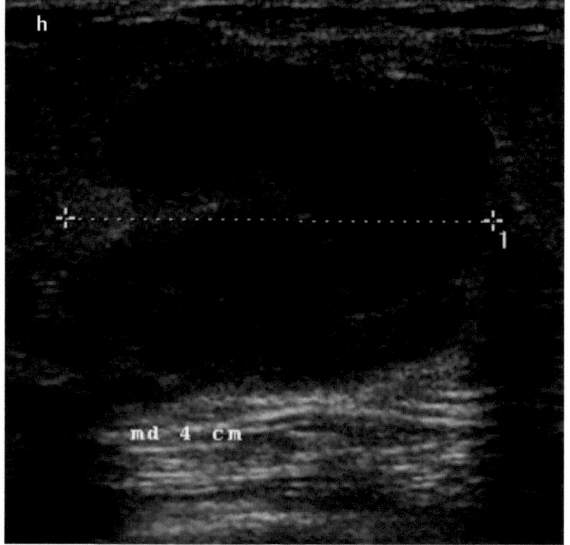

Sonography

(See **Fig. 18.1b,f.**)

Sonographically (Jorge Blanco et al. 1999, Muttarak and Chaiwun 2004, Gatta et al. 2011), the phyllodes tumor usually resembles other round or oval tumors, and often even smoothly outlined benign tumors.

Some phyllodes tumors may have indistinct margins or exhibit a heterogeneous internal echo pattern. Cystic spaces within the tumor are considered characteristic of phyllodes tumors. They correspond to the gelatinous, cystic, or necrotic areas, but are (according to our experience) predominantly seen in larger tumors. There is no sonographic feature that could allow reliable distinction of malignant and benign phyllodes tumors.

Magnetic Resonance Imaging

(See **Fig. 18.1c–e.**)

Contrast-enhanced magnetic resonance imaging (MRI) (Heywang-Köbrunner and Beck 1996, Wurdinger et al. 2005, Yabuuchi et al. 2006, Yoo et al. 2010, Chung et al. 2011, Tan et al. 2012) may be useful for planning surgery in very large tumors. According to the literature, phyllodes tumors enhance rapidly and intensely. Heterogeneities or cystic spaces may be visible on MRI, as well, mainly in larger tumors. If present they may be a hint that this is the diagnosis. However, the enhancement pattern generally does not permit a reliable distinction from other round, oval, or lobulated benign or malignant lesions. Nor does it permit a reliable distinction of benign from malignant phyllodes tumors. One author reported that in a series of 30 tumors including 5 malignant phyllodes tumors (Yabuuchi et al. 2006), a higher signal intensity on T1-weighted images, lower signal on T2-weighted images, and low apparent diffusion coeffcient values (indicating hypercellularity) were seen more frequently in malignant phyllodes tumors.

Percutaneous Biopsy

Phyllodes tumors can usually be diagnosed at core needle biopsy. Since phyllodes tumors are frequently inhomogeneous, a reliable distinction between malignant, semi-malignant, and benign phyllodes tumors requires excision, a measure that also represents the only therapeutic option (Foxcroft et al. 2007, Resetkova et al. 2010, Gatta et al. 2011).

> **Summary**
>
> Microscopically, clinically, and by imaging, the phyllodes tumor presents a as smooth or relatively smoothly outlined mass. *Reliable differentiation from other relatively smoothly outlined masses* and, in particular, from benign lesions is *often impossible*.
>
> In addition to the clinically noticed, usually rapid, increase in size, mammographic or sonographic irregularities of the outline as well as a sonographic heterogeneous internal echo structure suggest the presence of a fibroadenoma. Cystic spaces within the solid, smoothly outlined tumor disclosed by sonography or MRI are considered characteristic and should raise the suspicion of a phyllodes tumor.
>
> Because of the unreliable differentiation of smoothly outlined solid masses that increase in size, a phyllodes tumor must always be considered. The diagnosis of such a tumor should be established by excisional biopsy.

Fibromatosis (= Extra-Abdominal Desmoid)

Fibromatosis of the breast is a benign mass that may be locally invasive. It is more common in the abdominal wall and very rare in the breast. Local recurrence occurs frequently following incomplete excision. Therefore it is also considered a semi-malignant lesion. It does not metastasize.

It arises from the fascia and consequently is frequently fixed to the pectoral muscle. Histologically, it consists of proliferative fibroblasts and extensive fibrosis (Wargotz et al. 1987, Brogi 2004).

- Mammographically (Feder et al. 1999, Porter et al. 2006, Neuman et al. 2008) it is seen as an irregular mass or density with fibrous strands and retractions, and cannot be distinguished from the growth of a scirrhous carcinoma. Skin retraction is possible.
- Sonographically, extensive acoustic shadowing can be expected, as is found in scirrhous carcinoma.
- On MRI fibromatosis has been reported to enhance and present with a morphology that is indistinguishable from breast cancer.

Excision is recommended for diagnosis and therapy.

Hemangiopericytoma and Hemangioendothelioma

Both of these tumors are extremely rare in the breast. They arise from the pericytes and endothelium of blood vessels. Benign, semi-malignant, semi-malignant (recurring), and malignant variants are possible. The malignant variant has a similar appearance to angiosarcoma. The diagnosis is made histologically.

On imaging such lesions present as a rounded, oval mass with variable contours. The lesion may contain fat, which makes it one of the very rare fat-containing malignant lesions. Doppler ultrasound will usually show high perfusion (Buecker et al. 2008, Jesinger et al. 2011).

Adenomyoepithelioma

Adenomyoepithelioma is a myoepithelial breast tumor, of which benign and malignant variants exist. However, even benign adenomyoepitheliomas tend to recur. Thus, excision of these tumors is generally recommended.

Histologically these lesions can be diagnosed by immunostaining.

On mammography and sonography benign adenomyoepithelioma may present as a circumscribed mass with or without lobulations. On ultrasound imaging indifferent posterior enhancement or shadowing has been described (Tait et al. 2005, Irshad et al. 2008, Adejolu et al. 2011, Hayes 2011).

Sarcomas

Sarcomas are rare tumors of the breast, comprising less than 1% of all malignant neoplasms of this organ. About 15% of breast sarcomas are seen in men. Sarcomas can occur in any age group. Since the manifestation of most sarcomas—except for their rapid growth—is uncharacteristic, the *diagnosis must be made histologically*.

Histology

The sarcomas of the breast mainly include malignant fibrous histiocytoma, angiosarcoma, stromal sarcoma, liposarcoma, fibrosarcoma, leiomyosarcoma, rhabdomyosarcoma, osteochondrosarcoma, and chondrosarcoma.

Some sarcomas may occur late after radiotherapy (mostly > 10 years) and are considered to be radiation induced.

The prognosis of breast sarcoma depends on the tumor size and, partly, on grading.

Angiosarcomas are vessel-forming sarcomas with a poor prognosis, which can be further defined by the degree of malignancy. While the growth pattern of most soft tissue sarcomas is generally nodular (round, oval, with or without formation of a pseudocapsule, with a well-defined or irregular outline), angiosarcomas can be nodular or multinodular, but can also spread diffusely and infiltrate into the connective tissue. From the differential diagnostic and radiologic standpoints, it is relevant that the very rare liposarcoma, angiosarcomas, and the malignant hemangiopericytoma constitute the few very rare malignancies of the breast containing neoplastically transformed fatty tissue.

Clinical Findings

Corresponding to their growth pattern, most sarcomas present as round, oval, or lobulated lesions that—depending on the degree of infiltration—are smoothly or indistinctly outlined, moveable or fixed. While fibrous sarcomas and malignant fibrous histiocytomas present as palpable firm lesions, leiomyosarcomas as well as all liposarcomas are palpated as elastic to soft lesions. Some of the sarcomas might present clinically with pain. Angiosarcomas are palpated as soft and spongelike lesions, based on their vascular composition, and in 15–20% of the cases present with a bluish skin discoloration.

The *cardinal finding* of all sarcomas is their rapid growth.

Diagnostic Strategy and Goals

Because of their rapid growth, sarcomas are generally discovered clinically rather than by screening examinations. They lack any characteristic presentation. A rapidly growing lesion must, in addition to other considerations, raise the possibility of a sarcoma. Since rapidly growing lesions need surgical intervention, the diagnosis is generally made histologically.

Mammography

(See **Fig. 18.2a,d,e,f.**)

Mammographically (Ciatto et al. 1992, Yang et al. 2007a, Surov et al. 2011), soft tissue sarcomas generally present as nodular (round, oval, or lobulated) lesions. If seen without superimposition, their outline can be smooth, but also indistinct, or even show signs of infiltrating growth (compare **Fig. 18.2e**). If lobulated or diffusely growing sarcomas are completely or partly obscured by breast tissue, they may only present as unspecific asymmetry or may remain occult in spite of their sometimes large extent.

Coarse calcifications may develop in necrotic or vascular areas, and typical calcifications of osteoblastic or chondroblastic transformation have rarely been described in sarcomas of the breast.

Liposarcoma, angiosarcoma, and hemangiopericytoma constitute the rare malignancies which may contain fatty areas. Because of their very rare occurrence, they do not play a role in the differential diagnosis of fatty lesions but have to be considered if a fatty tumor shows rapid growth.

Angiosarcomas and lymphangiosarcomas usually cause indeterminate densities. If the growth is diffusely infiltrating—found in about one-third of cases—they cannot be disclosed mammographically within dense tissue or may present as unspecific asymmetry only. Less frequently, they present as solitary, smooth, or indistinctly outlined nodular lesions or even as multiple nodules. Very rarely (< 10%), bizarre calcifications have been described within angiosarcomas.

Sonography

(See **Fig. 18.2b,g.**)

Sonographically, soft tissue sarcomas (Yang et al. 2007a, Surov et al. 2011) present as hypoechoic nodular or lobulated lesions, with a smooth or indistinct contour. Such masses may be hyperechoic, hypoechoic, or exhibit mixed echogenicity. Central necrosis causing a complex cystic appearance is frequent. Some of the sarcomas (often angiosarcomas) exhibit infiltrative growth. Multinodular growth has also been described. Diffusely infiltrating sarcomas may be visualized by heterogeneous mixed hyper-/hypo-echogenicity with lobulated or indistinct contours with or without architectural distortion. Hyperechoic areas may represent hemorrhage.

Depending on the consistency of the underlying sarcomatous type (liposarcomas and angiosarcomas have a soft consistency, while fibrous histiocytomas and fibrosarcomas are very firm), very good to minimal compressibility can be encountered sonographically.

Magnetic Resonance Imaging

The current knowledge of the MRI properties of soft tissue sarcomas is still based on a limited number of cases (Yang et al. 2007a, Uematsu and Kasami 2009, Surov et al. 2011).

On MRI so far, sarcomas are described as strongly enhancing lesions with or without washout with a rounded well-circumscribed, lobular or nodular growth pattern. Most sarcomas exhibit heterogeneous enhancement. Tubular structures corresponding to vessels may be seen in angiosarcomas.

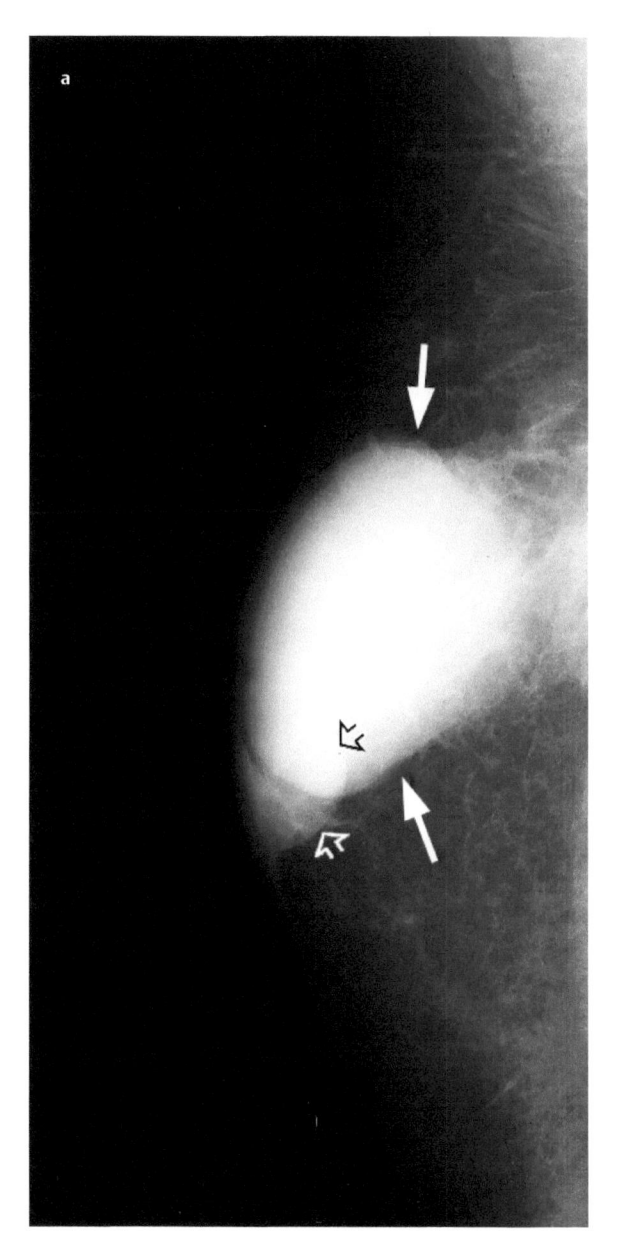

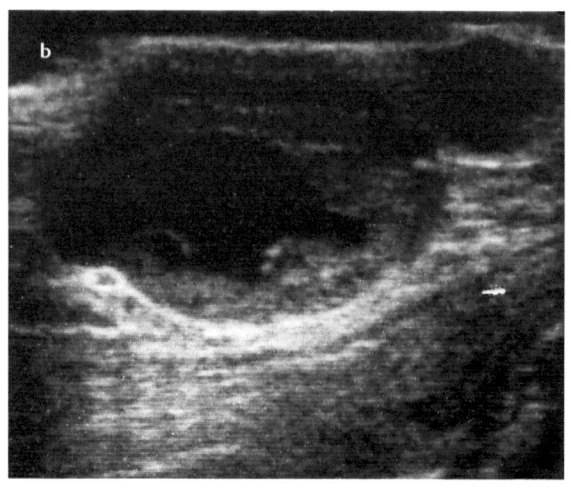

Fig. 18.2a–g Various types of sarcomas and differential diagnosis.

a,b Malignant fibrous histiocytoma in an 18-year-old man. **a** The mediolateral view, which was technically difficult because of infiltration of the thoracic wall, shows a large tumor (arrows), in part smooth (ventral), in part indistinct (dorsal) in outline. In addition (open arrows), directly behind the nipple is a second nodule. **b** Sonographically, the tumor appears smoothly outlined on the section shown. It is apparent that the small nodule and the large nodule are connected. Like many sarcomas, this malignant fibrous histiocytoma shows extensive necrosis, which is anechoic.

Fig. 18.2c–g ▷

18 Other Semi-Malignant and Malignant Tumors

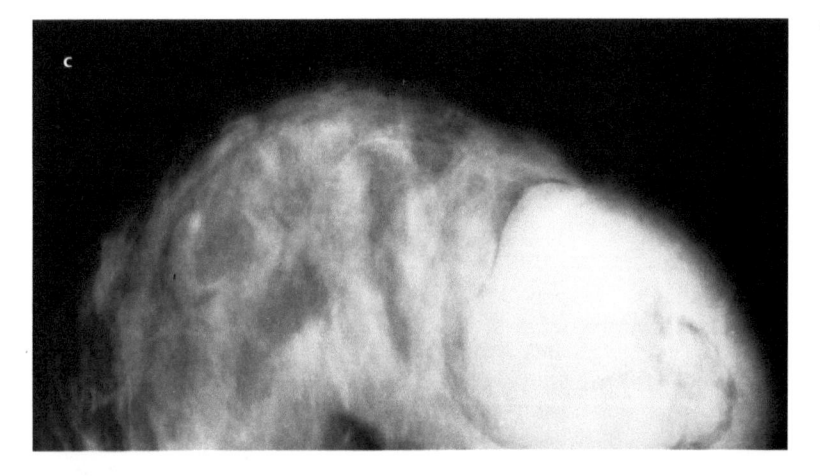

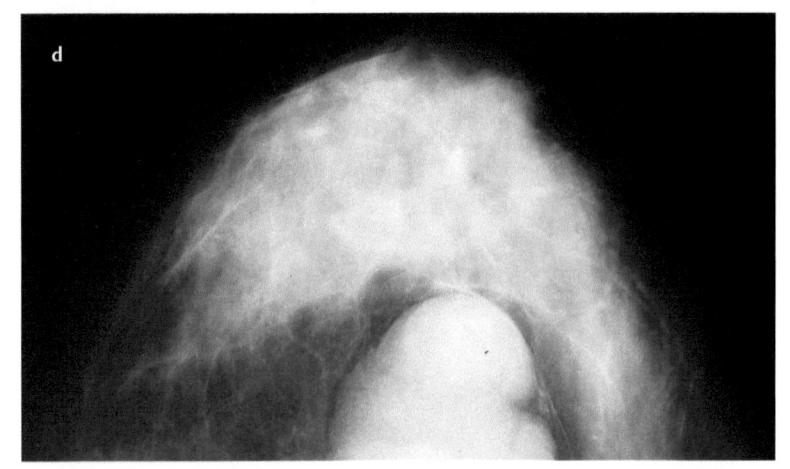

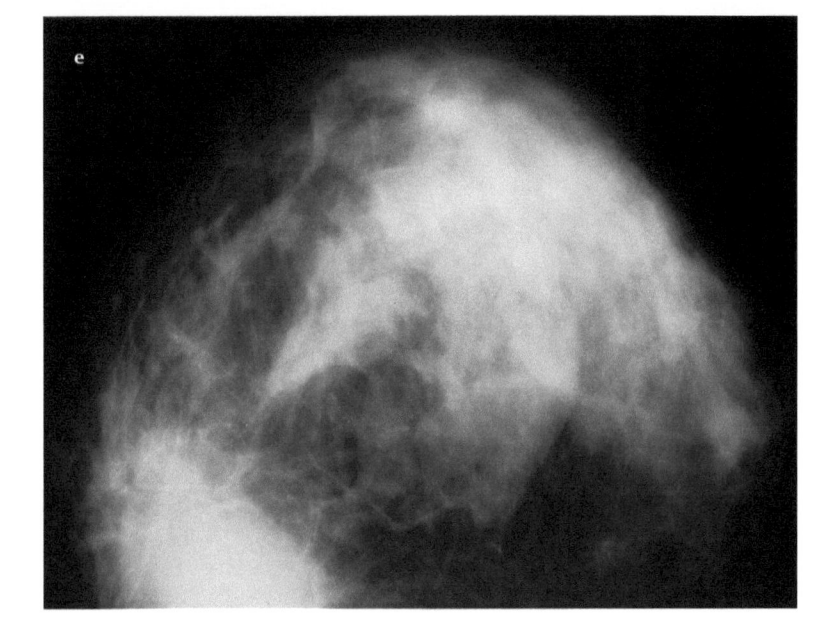

◁ continued

c This large mass containing fat underwent biopsy. *Histology*: In spite of its size and relatively fast growth the lesion proved to be a benign fibroadenoma (juvenile fibroadenoma).

d A similar-appearing mass in another patient was also readily palpable. *Histology*: Leiomyosarcoma. Even though this sarcoma contains areas of fat, the general policy of considering fat-containing masses as benign should not be changed unless rapid growth is noted. The reason is that sarcomas, and in particular fat-containing sarcomas, are very rare.

e A soft, ill-defined mass developed in the posterior aspect of this breast. *Histology*: Angiosarcoma.

Sarcomas

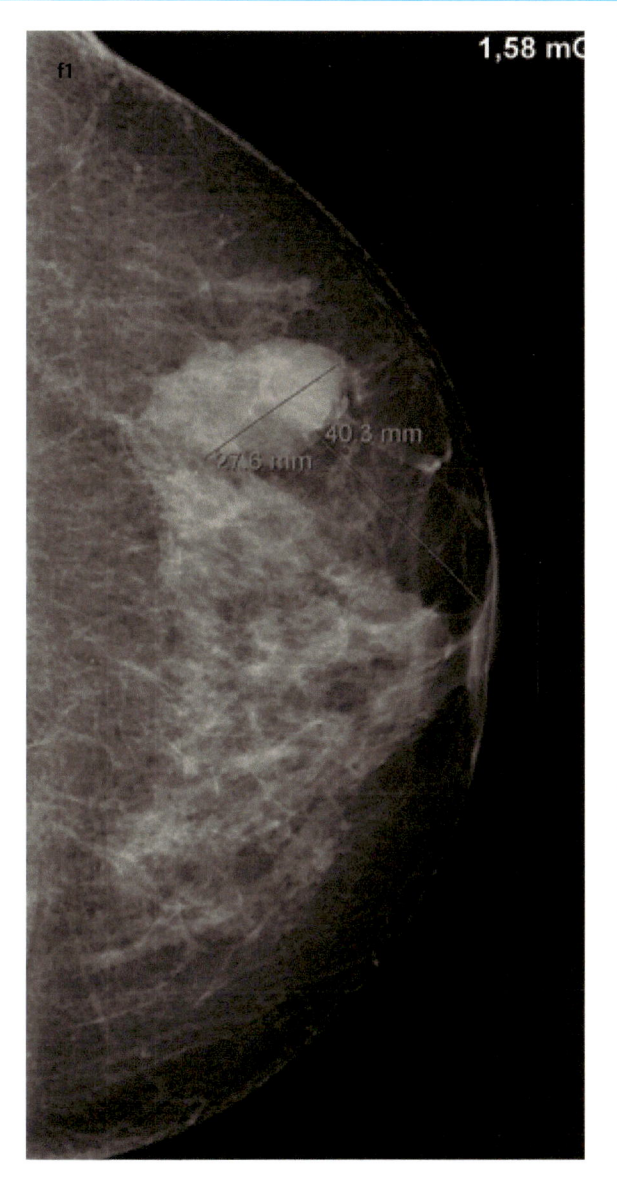

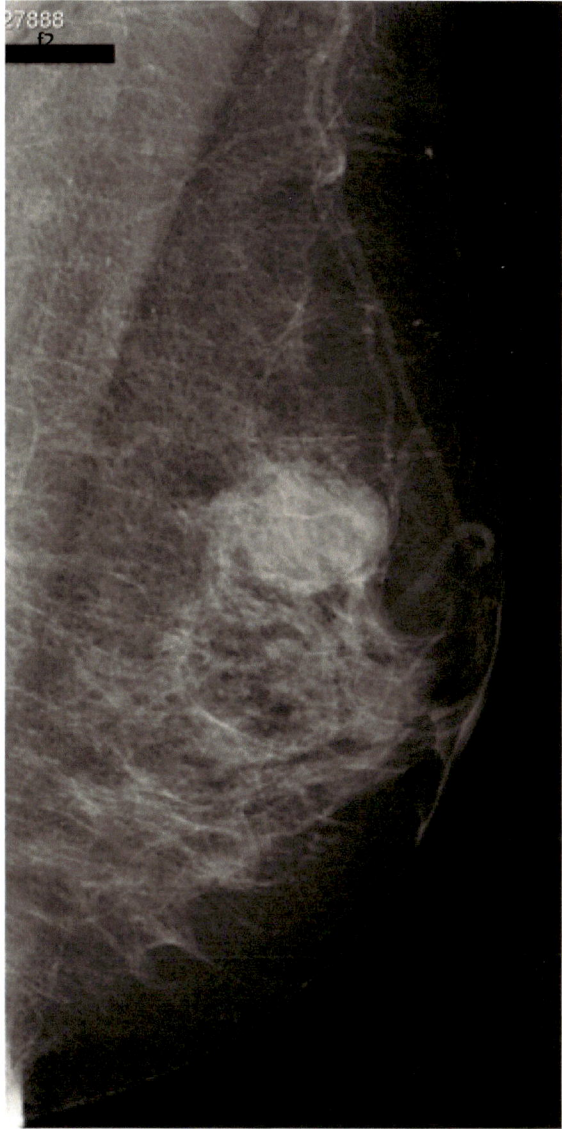

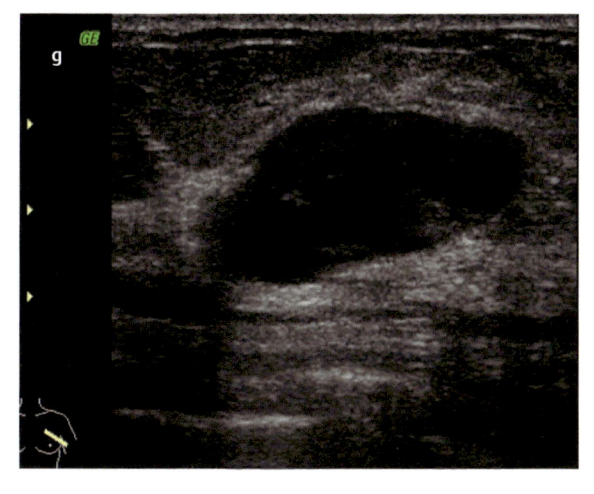

f,g Craniocaudal and mediolateral oblique mammograms and sonogram of a patient who presented with a palpable mass. **f** Mammographically the oval mass exhibits some large lobulations. The mass is partly obscured by overlying breast tissue. There is suggestion of a slight lack of sharpness. Also, the mass is fairly dense. **g** Ultrasound confirms a fairly well-circumscribed mass with a somewhat inhomogenous texture. On the left margin some sharpness may be suggested. Due to its fast growth excision was considered necessary. *Final histology*: Primary soft tissue sarcoma.

Percutaneous Biopsy

According to all present knowledge, seeding from breast cancer due to percutaneous breast biopsy is not a feature. For sarcomas this may be different. Since there is no specific imaging finding of breast sarcoma, however, the histopathologic result of a sarcoma may only become apparent after a needle biopsy has been performed. Therefore, in these cases only, excision of the needle tract (combined with wide excision of the lesion itself) should be considered.

> **Summary**
>
> Sarcomas are very rare tumors of the breasts. They usually present as a mass with a well-circumscribed to ill-defined contour, rarely with diffuse extension. Almost exclusively, they are detected as an abnormal palpatory finding. Mammographically and sonographically, there are no characteristic findings differentiating them from other nodular or diffusely growing processes.
>
> Mammography can reveal dystrophic calcifications. Very rarely, characteristic calcifications of chondrogenic or osteogenic transformation or fatty areas are found. Sonographically, central necrotic areas are characteristic but not pathognomonic. Some sarcomas (like angiosarcoma) present with a diffuse growth pattern and mainly become apparent by heterogeneous echogenicity or some architectural distortion.
>
> Some of the angiosarcomas present with a pattern of alternating hyperechoic and pronounced hypoechoic areas. Typically, angiosarcomas are very well perfused. On MRI sarcomas enhance strongly and often heterogeneously.
>
> If a nodular lesion shows rapid growth, a rapidly growing carcinoma, phyllodes tumor, or lymphoma must be considered, in addition to a sarcoma. The diagnosis must be made histologically.

Malignancies of the Breast of Hematologic Origin

Malignancies of the breast of hematologic origin include various forms of lymphoma as well as leukemia (Tavassoli and Devilee 2003, Irshad et al. 2008). Overall less than 1% of the breast malignancies are malignancies of hematologic origin. Lymphomatous involvement of the breast can be a manifestation of primary or secondary lymphoma. The latter is more frequent. Histologically, primary and secondary manifestations are indistinguishable.

Of course, hematologic malignancy may also present as axillary adenopathy and then has to be distinguished from other causes of lymphadenopathy (infection, granulomatous disease, sarcoidosis, nodal hyperplasia, immunodeficiency, connective tissue disease, metastatic disease).

The age distribution is wide—comparable to the hematologic malignancies involving other sites—and thus not helpful in the differential diagnosis. In the presence of an extra mammary manifestation, suspicious changes in the breast may raise the possibility of a concomitant mammary involvement. However, some hereditary syndromes may be associated with an increased risk of both breast cancer and lymphoma.

Histopathology

Hematologic malignancies of the breasts do not vary from corresponding malignancies at other sites within the body. Macroscopically, most hematologic malignancies present as a localized finding. These foci (singular or multiple) generally grow in a nodular fashion. They are oval to round or lobulated. They can be sharply demarcated (with a complete or partial halo). In general, they show some irregularities and indistinctness of the contour. A spiculated configuration, as seen with scirrhous carcinoma, is not found. Lymphoma may present as a singular mass with or without involved axillary nodes. Multifocal and bilateral involvement is possible. Diffuse infiltration of the breast is another possible presentation of hematologic malignancies.

Characteristic differences in the macroscopic growth pattern between the individual hematologic malignancies have not been recognized.

The non-Hodgkin lymphomas of the breast are exclusively B-cell lymphomas. The highly malignant lymphoblastic Burkitt lymphomas are primarily found in young women during pregnancy and lactation, and present as bilateral bluish macromastia.

Hodgkin lymphomas, plasmocytomas, and leukemic involvement are very rare. They, too, manifest as lesions of nodular or diffuse growth.

Histopathologically the differentiation from lobular carcinoma, from medullary carcinoma, or from inflammatory conditions may be difficult.

To establish the primary diagnosis and to determine the exact type, retrieving an adequate tissue sample is important. Special stains and immunohistology are mandatory today.

It should be mentioned that hematologic malignancies can occasionally be receptor positive and that estrogen receptor positivity by no means proves the presence of a breast carcinoma.

Clinical Findings

Corresponding to their growth pattern, hematologic malignancies can present as:
- A palpable nodule that is:
  - More or less moveable
  - Mostly elastic, relatively soft, and therefore difficult to distinguish from a fibroadenoma

Malignancies of the Breast of Hematologic Origin

- Diffuse skin thickening, increased consistency of the breast, enlargement of the breast, rarely erythema
- Palpable axillary adenopathy

Rapid growth is characteristic.

Diagnostic Strategy and Goals

In a patient with known systemic lymphoma, new changes in the breasts should raise the possibility of a lymphomatous involvement. If a malignancy of hematologic origin elsewhere in the body is not known, lymphomatous involvement of the breast is usually only suggested as one possibility in the differential diagnosis of nodular or diffusely growing lesions.

Histopathology, including immunohistology, is necessary for the primary diagnosis and exact classification.

Mammography

(See **Figs. 18.3a and 18.4**.)

Hematologic malignancies generally occur as (Sabaté et al. 2002, Lyou et al. 2007, Yang et al. 2007b, Irshad et al. 2008):

- A nodular mass (ovoid or lobulated, frequently with irregularities in its contour rather than a completely smooth contour)
- An irregularly outlined lesion (less frequently)
- Asymmetrically increased density (or completely obscured behind dense tissue)

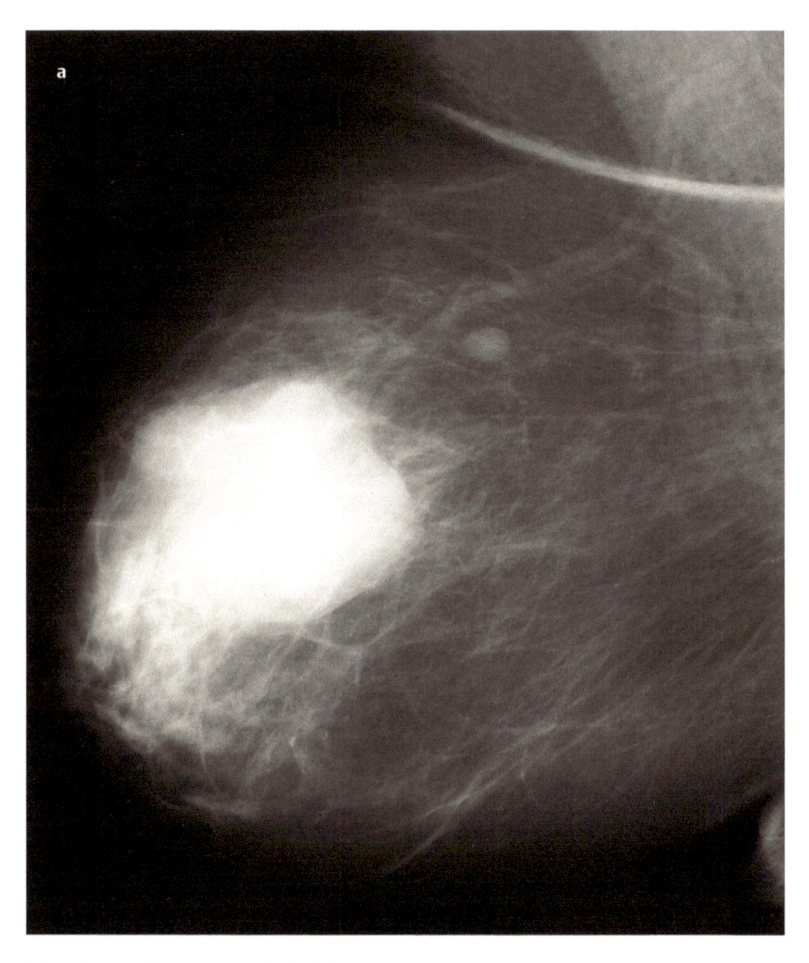

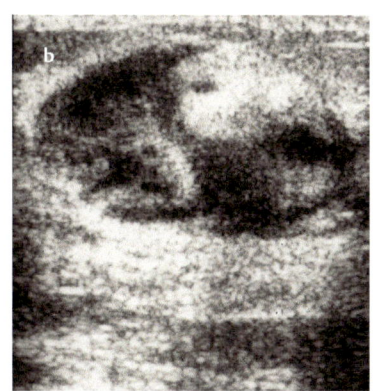

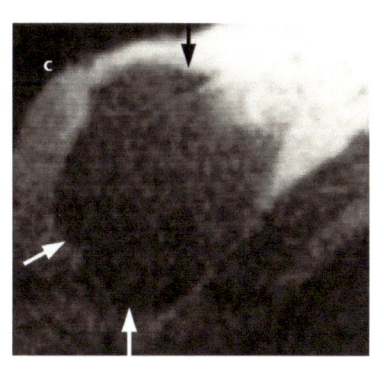

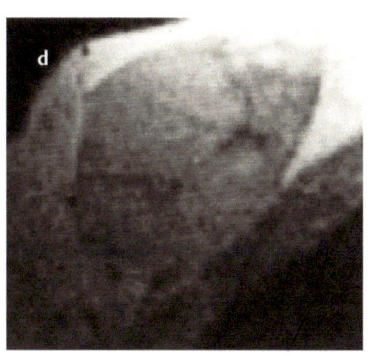

Fig. 18.3a–d Nodular non-Hodgkin lymphoma.
a A 76-year-old woman with a left breast mass that is largely well defined. *Histology*: Lymphoma.
b Sonographically, this lymphoma is seen as a lobulated, inhomogeneous hypoechoic lesion.
c It is low signal on the T1-weighted images (arrows).
d Lobulation is apparent on the T2-weighted images (contrast medium was not available at the time of this examination), whereby the areas of high signal intensity corresponded histologically to lymphomatous tissue and the low signal intensity linear bands were fibrous structures.

18 Other Semi-Malignant and Malignant Tumors

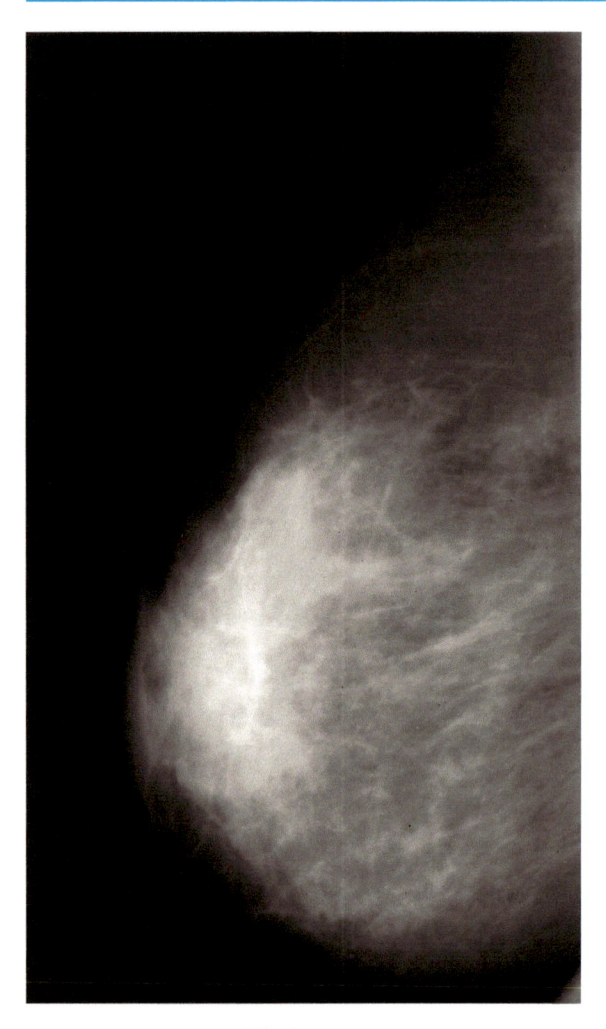

Fig. 18.4 Diffuse non-Hodgkin lymphoma.
In addition to predominantly periareolar skin thickening, this mediolateral mammogram shows diffuse interstitial thickening throughout the mammary tissue.

Extensive spiculations or microcalcifications are not part of the appearance found with a malignancy of hematologic origin. Rarely, an echogenic rim has been described.
Furthermore, hematologic malignancies may sometimes present as:
- Diffuse pattern with skin thickening, trabecular coarsening, and generalized increased density (like inflammatory breast cancer)
- Axillary adenopathy

Hematologic malignancies have no pathognomonic changes.

Diffuse involvement can only be distinguished histologically from diffuse lymphedema secondary to axillary nodal metastases, with therapeutic implications. A reliable differentiation is mammographically impossible.

Sonography

(See **Fig. 18.3b**.)
Sonographic presentations of hematologic malignancies include (Lyou et al. 2007, Yang et al. 2007b, Irshad et al. 2008):
- One (or several) ovoid or lobulated mass(es)
- Outlines are mostly somewhat indistinct, sometimes completely well-circumscribed or irregular
- The mass is mostly hypoechoic, sometimes very hypoechoic (and can be mistaken for a cyst!)
- Sometimes the mass can have mixed echogenicity, rarely it may be hyperechoic
- Often with very good distal acoustic enhancement, less frequently with heterogeneous or absent enhancement

Because of the generally good elasticity and partly because of the encountered moveability, the lesions may be mistaken for fibroadenomas or, if very hypoechoic, for cysts.

Diffuse involvement is characterized by:
- Skin thickening
- Diffusely decreased or increased echogenicity (uncharacteristic)
- Architectural distortion

Magnetic Resonance Imaging

On MRI lymphomas will mostly exhibit masslike (sometimes smoothly outlined, sometimes with irregularities) enhancement and sometimes diffuse contrast enhancement. Enhancement dynamics have been described as mostly plateau-type, and sometimes progressive, sometimes with washout. The pattern has been described as homogeneous or heterogeneous (Yang et al. 2007b, Irshad et al. 2008, Rizzo et al. 2009).

Percutaneous Biopsy

The diagnosis of a lymphoma can generally be made by fine needle or core biopsy. The immunohistochemical subclassification is generally based on the adequate material obtained from core needle biopsy and/or excisional biopsy.

> **Summary**
> Hematologic malignancies can present as a focal lesion or as an indistinct diffuse process. There are no morphologic criteria to distinguish the individual hematologic malignancies, nor are there reliable differentiating criteria toward benign tumors (for well-circumscribed masses), carcinomas (for irregularly outlined lesions), or inflammatory carcinoma, lymphedema, or inflammation (for diffuse involvement). The final diagnosis and exact classification rest on the histopathology.

Metastases

Metastases in the breasts are rare (~0.5–2% of the breast malignancies). They can arise from:
1. An extramammary malignancy of any origin (carcinoma, melanoma, sarcoma, or hematologic malignancy)
2. A contralateral breast carcinoma

Metastases should be considered in findings with multiple masses or diffuse increased breast density in patients with a history of known primary carcinoma or metastases, but for whom a specific manifestation is not known.

The therapeutic approach depends on the overall prognosis.

Histology

Metastases may arise from the opposite breast, or they may be caused by malignancies of hematologic origin or malignant melanomas, followed by bronchial carcinomas, ovarian carcinomas, sarcomas, and carcinoid. Moreover, metastases can arise from any carcinoma or sarcoma. In men, prostate cancer is the most common primary of metastases in the breast (Feder et al. 1999, Bartella et al. 2003, Lee et al. 2010, Cao et al. 2011). The metastases of most extramammary *malignancies* exhibit a *nodular* growth: round rather than oval, and sometimes lobulated.

Metastatic spread can produce *single or multiple* lesions. Metastases are usually distinct in outline and rarely somewhat indistinct. Spiculations are extremely rare.

Metastases are usually located in subcutaneous fat rather than in the core of the breast tissue.

Some extramammary malignancies also have metastases that show a *diffuse growth pattern*. This is most frequently observed in ovarian carcinomas, but has been occasionally described with other malignancies.

Metastases from a carcinoma of the contralateral breast can be hematogenous or lymphogenous via the lymphatics crossing the sternum.

Clinical Findings

If adequate in size and situated superficially, *focal metastases* may be palpated as:
- Smoothly outlined, round
- Usually moveable, rarely fixed—they generally do not tend to cause skin or nipple retraction (Feder et al. 1999).
- More often firm than soft lesions (depending on the property of the primary tumor)
- A finding the size of which approximates to the mammographic size
- Frequently located in subcutaneous fat

Reliable criteria differentiating these from fibroadenomas and cysts do not exist. History of rapid growth often suggests the diagnosis.

If the *involvement is diffuse*, skin thickening and diffuse swelling are observed. Pain is infrequent.

Metastases from a carcinoma of the contralateral breast usually occur via direct extension. They are detectable through skin thickening, palpable thickening, peau d'orange, nodules, or swelling.

Diagnostic Strategy and Goals

With the appropriate history (preceding primary tumor with or without known metastatic disease in other organs) metastases should be considered if single or multiple, new or growing lesions are found clinically or mammographically, or if diffuse changes of undetermined etiology are encountered.

If the histopathology of a breast lesion—without appropriate history—suggests a metastasis, the search for a primary tumor is warranted.

Appropriate special stains and immunohistology of the excised tissue may assist in determining the origin of the metastasis.

Mammography

(See **Fig. 18.5a,c**; see also **Fig. 24.4a,b**)

Focal metastases are generally visualized mammographically (Feder et al. 1999, Bartella et al. 2003, Lee et al. 2010, Cao et al. 2011, Glazebrook et al. 2011):
- As round, sharply outlined lesions, frequently without any significant marginal indistinctness. Particularly suggestive is the perfectly round shape. Some metastases are lobulated.
- Sometimes outlines may be indistinct. Irregular outlines are extremely rare.
- Metastases may be single or multiple.
- They can also be partially or totally hidden in dense tissue.
- Coarse calcifications may be seen in necrotic areas; microcalcifications are rare and may occur in breast or ovarian (or very rarely other) carcinomas. However, the vast majority of metastases (including those from primary breast cancers with microcalcifications) do not contain microcalcifications.
- Multiple round lesions containing subgroups of lesions that are about equal in size—reflecting intermittent dissemination—are characteristic and considered important evidence of the presence of metastases.

Reliable criteria that distinguish individual metastases from smoothly outlined benign lesions (fibroadenomas) do not exist.

Elongated, polymorphic or ductally oriented microcalcifications or spicules are rare for metastases. They have

18 Other Semi-Malignant and Malignant Tumors

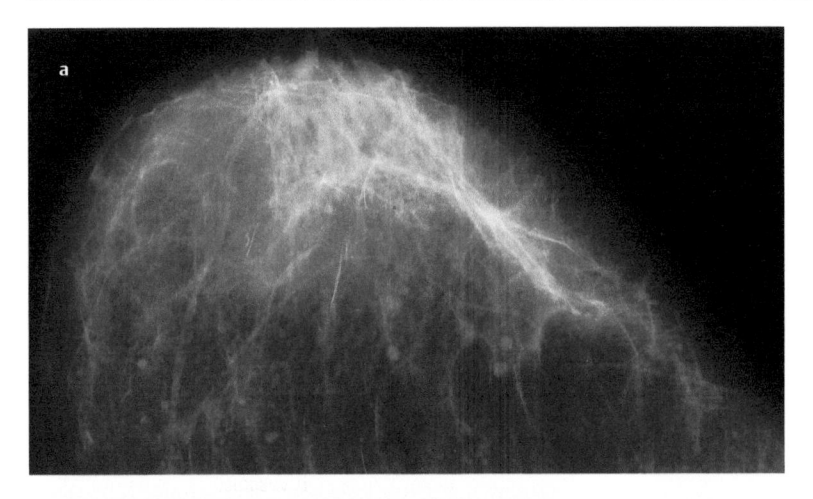

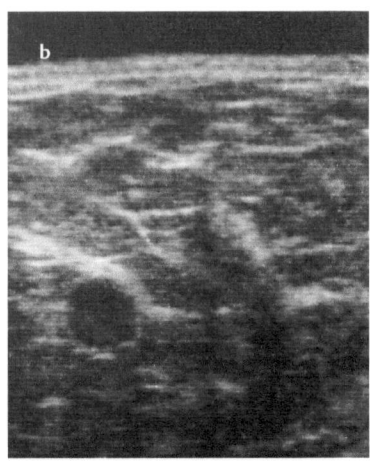

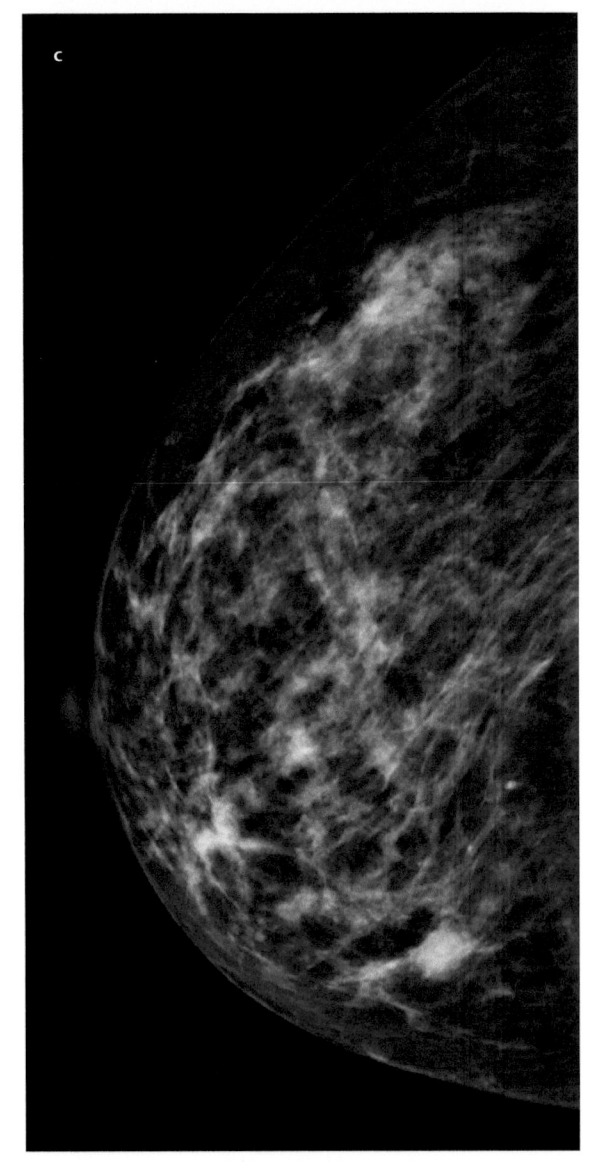

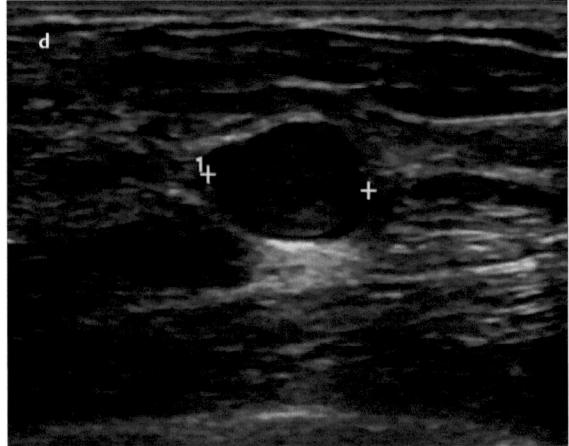

Fig. 18.5a–d

a,b Multiple small nodular metastases in a patient with known metastatic malignant melanoma. **a** Craniocaudal mammogram. The multitude of nodules with several nodules of equal size suggests (even without the clinical history) a metastatic process. Despite the smooth outline, the perfectly round configuration favors metastases over benign lesions.
b Sonography of a small metastasis also exhibiting a perfectly round configuration.
c Craniocaudal screening mammogram of a 54-year-old asymptomatic women presenting with a partly well-defined, partly obscured mass in the inner half of the breast.
d On ultrasound the nodule was heterogeneously hypoechoic, showing a lobulated form and completely circumscribed margins. Core biopsy yielded a metastasis of a bronchial carcinoma.

been described in a few cases of primary breast and ovarian carcinomas and very rarely for other carcinomas. Such changes usually indicate a primary breast cancer.

Diffuse metastases may present as:
- Skin thickening
- Thickened trabecular markings
- Diffuse, asymmetrically increased density of the parenchyma

A reliable distinction between diffuse metastatic spread and other causes of diffuse lymphedema is usually not possible by mammography.

Metastases from a carcinoma of the contralateral breast can involve the entire breast diffusely, or appear as cutaneous and subcutaneous thickening extending from the parasternal region laterally.

Sonography

(See **Fig. 18.5b**.)

Sonography is used to exclude a simple cyst and to verify the presence of palpable findings in mammographically dense tissue.

Sonographically localized metastases display the following features (Feder et al. 1999, Bartella et al. 2003, Lee et al. 2010, Cao et al. 2011):
- They mostly present as sharply outlined, round masses, with homogeneous internal structure, and with no or only minimal reactive changes in the surrounding tissue.
- Sometimes their margins may be instinct, and sometimes surrounding (echogenic) edema may be seen.
- Some metastases may be inhomogeneous (with central necrosis or bleeding). Rarely echogenic metastases are seen.
- Usually the lesions show distal acoustic enhancement; sometimes no enhancement or acoustic shadowing (in the presence of intense fibrosis) is seen.
- Metastases are mostly easily moveable, rarely fixed.
- The consistency of lesions varies from firm to soft elastic.

Consequently, *sonography does not allow a reliable differentiation* from benign lesions or from well-circumscribed other malignancies that are sharply outlined.

Diffuse metastatic spread is sonographically recognized by (Feder et al. 1999, Bartella et al. 2003, Lee et al. 2010, Cao et al. 2011):
- Diffuse skin thickening and obliteration of the echogenic interface with the subcutaneous layer
- Cooper ligaments may be thickened and appear hypoechoic, secondary to lymphatic stasis caused by tumor cells
- The changes of the parenchyma are often uncharacteristic; overall, the parenchyma appears somewhat hypoechoic, whereas the echogenicity of fat increases with the underlying edema

However, distinction of diffuse metastatic spread from edema of other origin is not possible by sonography.

Magnetic Resonance Imaging

Experience is based on only a few individual cases (Bartella et al. 2003, Lee et al. 2010, Glazebrook et al. 2011), which showed the metastases as being nodular, enhancing lesions (with the same morphological range of presentations as on mammography).

Internal signal intensity is mostly homogeneous. It may be heterogeneous due to central necrosis or bleeding.

Diffuse metastatic spread may present as skin thickening with dilated lymph vessels and sometimes with tubular intra- and subcutaneous enhancing structures, which correspond to involved lymph vessels.

Percutaneous Biopsy

Percutaneous biopsy is very well suited to confirm the presence of malignancy. If metastatic disease is suspected immunohistology may give important hints.

> **Summary**
>
> Metastatic spread can become manifest by forming single or several nodular lesions or (less frequently) as diffuse, ill-defined changes (skin thickening, increased consistency).
>
> Reliable criteria distinguishing metastases from other nodular, usually sharply outlined lesions or from other diffuse changes (mastitis, inflammatory carcinoma, lymphedema) do not exist. Several round lesions, including subgroups of equal size, suggest a metastasizing process.
>
> With the history of a known carcinoma, metastases should be considered if nodular or diffuse changes are found. Confirmation and analysis as to their site of origin rest on the histologic examination.

References and Recommended Reading

Adejolu M, Wu Y, Santiago L, Yang WT. Adenomyoepithelial tumors of the breast: imaging findings with histopathologic correlation. AJR Am J Roentgenol 2011;197(1):W184–W190

Bartella L, Kaye J, Perry NM, et al. Metastases to the breast revisited: radiological-histopathological correlation. Clin Radiol 2003;58(7):524–531

Barth RJ Jr. Histologic features predict local recurrence after breast conserving therapy of phyllodes tumors. Breast Cancer Res Treat 1999;57(3):291–295

Bässler R, Zahner J. Recurrences and metastases of cystosarcoma phylloides (phylloid tumor, WHO). On the 150th birthday of a controversial diagnostic concept. [Article in German] Geburtshilfe Frauenheilkd 1989;49(1):1–10

Ben Hassouna J, Damak T, Gamoudi A, et al. Phyllodes tumors of the breast: a case series of 106 patients. Am J Surg 2006;192(2):141–147

Brogi E. Benign and malignant spindle cell lesions of the breast. Semin Diagn Pathol 2004;21(1):57–64

Buecker B, Kapsimalakou S, Stoeckelhuber BM, Bos I, Wulf-Brodnjak S, Fischer D. Malignant hemangiopericytoma of the breast: a case report with a review of the literature. Arch Gynecol Obstet 2008;277(4):357–361

Cao MM, Hoyt AC, Bassett LW. Mammographic signs of systemic disease. Radiographics 2011;31(4):1085–1100

Chung J, Son EJ, Kim JA, Kim EK, Kwak JY, Jeong J. Giant phyllodes tumors of the breast: imaging findings with clinicopathological correlation in 14 cases. Clin Imaging 2011;35(2):102–107

Ciatto S, Bonardi R, Cataliotti L, Cardona G. Sarcomas of the breast: a multicenter series of 70 cases. Neoplasma 1992;39(6):375–379

Cohn-Cedermark G, Rutqvist LE, Rosendahl I, Silfverswärd C. Prognostic factors in cystosarcoma phyllodes. A clinicopathologic study of 77 patients. Cancer 1991;68(9): 2017–2022

de Roos WK, Kaye P, Dent DM. Factors leading to local recurrence or death after surgical resection of phyllodes tumours of the breast. Br J Surg 1999;86(3):396–399

Feder JM, de Paredes ES, Hogge JP, Wilken JJ. Unusual breast lesions: radiologic-pathologic correlation. Radiographics 1999;19(Spec No):S11–S26, quiz S260

Foxcroft LM, Evans EB, Porter AJ. Difficulties in the pre-operative diagnosis of phyllodes tumours of the breast: a study of 84 cases. Breast 2007;16(1):27–37

Gatta G, Iaselli F, Parlato V, Di Grezia G, Grassi R, Rotondo A. Differential diagnosis between fibroadenoma, giant fibroadenoma and phyllodes tumour: sonographic features and core needle biopsy. Radiol Med (Torino) 2011;116(6):905–918

Geisler DP, Boyle MJ, Malnar KF, et al. Phyllodes tumors of the breast: a review of 32 cases. Am Surg 2000;66(4):360–366

Glazebrook KN, Jones KN, Dilaveri CA, Perry K, Reynolds C. Imaging features of carcinoid tumors metastatic to the breast. Cancer Imaging 2011;11:109–115

Hayes MM. Adenomyoepithelioma of the breast: a review stressing its propensity for malignant transformation. J Clin Pathol 2011;64(6):477–484

Heywang-Köbrunner SH, Beck R. Contrast-Enhanced MRI of the Breast. Heidelberg, New York: Springer; 1996

Irshad A, Ackerman SJ, Pope TL, Moses CK, Rumboldt T, Panzegrau B. Rare breast lesions: correlation of imaging and histologic features with WHO classification. Radiographics 2008;28(5):1399–1414

Jesinger RA, Lattin GE Jr, Ballard EA, Zelasko SM, Glassman LM. Vascular abnormalities of the breast: arterial and venous disorders, vascular masses, and mimic lesions with radiologic-pathologic correlation. Radiographics 2011;31(7):E117–E136

Jorge Blanco A, Vargas Serrano B, Rodríguez Romero R, Martínez Cendejas E. Phyllodes tumors of the breast. Eur Radiol 1999;9(2):356–360

Lee SK, Kim WW, Kim SH, et al. Characteristics of metastasis in the breast from extramammary malignancies. J Surg Oncol 2010;101(2):137–140

Liberman L, Giess CS, Dershaw DD, Louie DC, Deutch BM. Non-Hodgkin lymphoma of the breast: imaging characteristics and correlation with histopathologic findings. Radiology 1994;192(1):157–160

Liberman L, Bonaccio E, Hamele-Bena D, Abramson AF, Cohen MA, Dershaw DD. Benign and malignant phyllodes tumors: mammographic and sonographic findings. Radiology 1996;198(1):121–124

Lyou CY, Yang SK, Choe DH, Lee BH, Kim KH. Mammographic and sonographic findings of primary breast lymphoma. Clin Imaging 2007;31(4):234–238

Magri K, Demoulin G, Millon G, Duvert B. Metastasis to the breast from non mammary metastasis. Clinical, radiological characteristics and diagnostic process. A report of two cases and a review of literature. [Article in French] J Gynecol Obstet Biol Reprod (Paris) 2007;36(6):602–606

Mussurakis S, Carleton PJ, Turnbull LW. MR imaging of primary non-Hodgkin's breast lymphoma. A case report. Acta Radiol 1997;38(1):104–107

Muttarak M, Chaiwun B. Imaging of giant breast masses with pathological correlation. Singapore Med J 2004;45(3):132–139

Neuman HB, Brogi E, Ebrahim A, Brennan MF, Van Zee KJ. Desmoid tumors (fibromatoses) of the breast: a 25-year experience. Ann Surg Oncol 2008;15(1):274–280

Ng CS, Taylor CB, O'Donnell PJ, Pozniak AL, Michell MJ. Case report: mammographic and ultrasound appearances of Kaposi's sarcoma of the breast. Clin Radiol 1996;51(10):735–736

Ormándi K, Lázár G, Tószegi A, Palkó A. Extra-abdominal desmoid tumor mimicking malignant male breast tumor. Eur Radiol 1999;9(6):1120–1122

Pameijer FA, Beijerinck D, Hoogenboom HH, Deurenberg JJ, Nortier JW. Non-Hodgkin's lymphoma of the breast causing miliary densities on mammography. AJR Am J Roentgenol 1995;164(3):609–610

Paulus DD. Lymphoma of the breast. Radiol Clin North Am 1990;28(4):833–840

Porter GJ, Evans AJ, Lee AH, Hamilton LJ, James JJ. Unusual benign breast lesions. Clin Radiol 2006;61(7):562–569

Resetkova E, Khazai L, Albarracin CT, Arribas E. Clinical and radiologic data and core needle biopsy findings should dictate management of cellular fibroepithelial tumors of the breast. Breast J 2010;16(6):573–580

Rizzo S, Preda L, Villa G, et al. Magnetic resonance imaging of primary breast lymphoma. Radiol Med (Torino) 2009;114(6):915–924

Sabaté JM, Gómez A, Torrubia S, et al. Lymphoma of the breast: clinical and radiologic features with pathologic correlation in 28 patients. Breast J 2002;8(5):294–304

Surov A, Holzhausen HJ, Ruschke K, Spielmann RP. Primary breast sarcoma: prevalence, clinical signs, and radiological features. Acta Radiol 2011;52(6):597–601

Tait R, Pinder SE, Ellis IO, Purushotham AD. Adenomyoepithelioma of the breast; a case report and literature review. J BUON 2005;10(3):393–395

Tan H, Zhang S, Liu H, et al. Imaging findings in phyllodes tumors of the breast. Eur J Radiol 2012;81(1):e62–e69

Tavassoli FA, Devilee P. World Health Organization classification of tumors. Tumors of the breast and female genital organs, 2nd edition. Lyon: IARC Press; 2003

Uematsu T, Kasami M. MR imaging findings of benign and malignant circumscribed breast masses: part 1. Solid circumscribed masses. Jpn J Radiol 2009;27(10):395–404

Vizcaíno I, Torregrosa A, Higueras V, et al. Metastasis to the breast from extramammary malignancies: a report of four cases and a review of literature. Eur Radiol 2001;11(9):1659–1665

Wargotz ES, Norris HJ, Austin RM, Enzinger FM. Fibromatosis of the breast. A clinical and pathological study of 28 cases. Am J Surg Pathol 1987;11(1):38–45

Wurdinger S, Herzog AB, Fischer DR, et al. Differentiation of phyllodes breast tumors from fibroadenomas on MRI. AJR Am J Roentgenol 2005;185(5):1317–1321

Yabuuchi H, Soeda H, Matsuo Y, et al. Phyllodes tumor of the breast: correlation between MR findings and histologic grade. Radiology 2006;241(3):702–709

Yang WT, Hennessy BT, Dryden MJ, Valero V, Hunt KK, Krishnamurthy S. Mammary angiosarcomas: imaging findings in 24 patients. Radiology 2007a;242(3):725–734

Yang WT, Lane DL, Le-Petross HT, Abruzzo LV, Macapinlac HA. Breast lymphoma: imaging findings of 32 tumors in 27 patients. Radiology 2007b;245(3):692–702

Yoo JL, Woo OH, Kim YK, et al. Can MR Imaging contribute in characterizing well-circumscribed breast carcinomas? Radiographics 2010;30(6):1689–1702

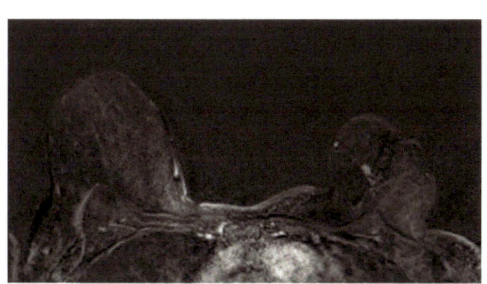

19 Post-Traumatic, Post-Surgical, and Post-Therapeutic Changes

Post-Traumatic and Post-Surgical Changes → 494
Histology → 494
Clinical History and Findings → 494
Diagnostic Strategy and Goals → 494

Reduction Mammoplasty → 507
Definition → 507
Surgical Procedures → 507
Diagnostic Strategy → 507

Changes Following Reconstruction → 509
Definition → 509
Surgical Procedures → 509
Diagnostic Strategy → 509

Changes Following Breast-Conserving Therapy without Irradiation → 512
Definition → 512
Clinical and Imaging Findings → 512
Differential Diagnosis and Diagnostic Strategy → 512

Changes Following Breast-Conserving Therapy with Irradiation → 512
Definition → 512
Clinical Findings → 513
Diagnostic Strategy and Goals → 513

References and Recommended Reading → 529

19 Post-Traumatic, Post-Surgical, and Post-Therapeutic Changes

I. Schreer, S. H. Heywang-Koebrunner, S. Barter

Post-Traumatic and Post-Surgical Changes

Following surgery or trauma, characteristic tissue changes can develop.

Acute changes can be separated from late changes:
1. *Acute changes*: Hematoma, seroma, edema, fat necrosis (acute)
2. *Late changes*: Scar formation, retraction, dystrophic calcifications, fat necrosis (chronic): oil cyst, lipophagic granuloma

Histology

Hematomas and seromas occupy either a surgical cavity or a traumatic tear, or spread into the surrounding parenchyma, connective tissue, and adipose tissue.

After the formation of these fluid collections, resorption takes place. Tissue necrosis is generally called "fat necrosis," even though it only partially involves fat cells. It is caused by traumatic injury of the cell membrane. The subsequent healing process is marked by the appearance of foam cells as well as leukocytic, round cell, and histiocytic infiltrates, permeating the affected area or causing resorption and repair along the border of the cavity. Beginning along the cavity border, granulation tissue, rich in fibroblasts, grows centripetally. Initially, this tissue is hypervascular and is later transformed into a poorly vascularized, densely packed scar fibrosis. Confluent foci of necrotic fat can liquefy centrally, producing oil cysts, which have a tendency to calcify.

Clinical History and Findings

Following surgery or major injury, the location and time of the trauma are well known. Both hematoma and fat necrosis can, however, also occur "spontaneously." The eliciting trauma is often not remembered. Instead, the patient notices a nodule, which may or may not be painful and is caused by a hematoma or fat necrosis. Sometimes an associated subcutaneous hematoma suggests the site of the trauma or hemorrhage.

Hematomas are generally completely resolved and transformed into scar tissue, while fat necroses present as tumorlike lipophagic granulomas or oil cysts. The lipophagic granuloma presents as a clinically suggestive palpable nodule, usually of medium to firm consistency and of poor demarcation. Despite their smooth mammographic demarcation, oil cysts are also generally palpated as indistinctly demarcated fixed nodules.

Diagnostic Strategy and Goals

Fresh hematomas and seromas are easily diagnosed by sonography in the context of preceding surgery and corresponding clinical findings. This is, however, rarely necessary. An oval, sometimes even ill-defined mass at the surgical site may normally be present up to a year after surgery. For objective exclusion of a malignancy, mammographic evaluation of the lesion is necessary in all cases where doubts exist whether the suspected hematoma, seroma, or fat necrosis can explain all of the changes. The patient's statement of a preceding trauma may not prove a traumatic etiology, and it should be verified that findings are consistent with trauma rather than malignancy. Complementary sonography may be helpful. It is also particularly useful to monitor regression.

With time, hematomas mostly resorb. Sometimes seromas, oil cysts, or scars may persist. Oil cysts mostly have a pathognomonic appearance on mammography, which allows their unequivocal diagnosis. Seromas are mostly recognized as anechoic cystic lesions, which—even when they contain septations—can mostly be correctly diagnosed.

Scarring can often be correctly diagnosed by mammography in context with the clinical findings and the patient's history. Since, however, carcinomas may develop in any area of the breast, carcinoma needs to be diligently excluded. Availability of prior imaging studies is often very helpful and therefore attempts should always be made to obtain them.

In difficult cases sometimes marking of the skin and/or additional views may be helpful. On occasion it may be difficult, however, to exclude a malignant lesion without further workup.

Sometimes palpable nodules or increased consistency on clinical examination can pose a problem as to the exclusion of residual or newly evolving malignancy, with mammographically increased density and architectural distortion, an atypical dense center of the scar, or suspicious calcifications. In cases with severe scarring magnetic resonance imaging (MRI) may be very helpful, since usually scar tissue older than 4–6 months does not enhance, whereas the vast majority of invasive malignancies will enhance. In the case of a focally suspicious finding or a finding that changes, or increases in size, percutaneous breast biopsy should be considered.

Dystrophic calcifications are usually clearly identified by mammography on the basis of their form, size, and location within or along scars. When these calcifications are first forming, differential diagnostic problems can be encountered. If early dystrophic calcifications are suspected, magnified views may demonstrate a confluent or shell-like pattern indicating the beginning of possible fat necrosis. Short-term follow-up may be considered to avoid unnecessary biopsy. In cases with indeterminate or suspicious microcalcifications histopathologic assessment may be necessary. The least invasive and sufficiently reliable method in these cases will usually be stereotactic vacuum-assisted breast biopsy (VABB).

Fat necroses are readily diagnosed by mammography if they present as calcifying liponecrosis or oil cysts. Fat necrosis presenting as lipophagic granuloma (fat necrosis consisting of granulation tissue without typical oily liquefaction), however, usually requires histopathologic verification, unless it can be diagnosed by its characteristic clinical course. On MRI a lipophagic granuloma usually enhances and generally cannot be distinguished from malignancy owing to its irregular contours and the focal enhancement.

Mammography

Acute Changes

Fresh hematomas/seromas are seen as an ill-defined mass (**Fig. 19.1a–f**), sometimes obscured by dense breast tissue. Hematomas, which occupy a surgical cavity, usually present as round to oval masses with some contour irregularity. Air–fluid levels can be found in the acute postoperative period (**Fig. 19.2a–c**). Fresh fat necrosis initially produces an ill-defined mass that can be more or less radiodense. With time its density may decrease and it may eventually progress to an oil cyst or it may persist as lipophagic granuloma. Often skin thickening and an increased indistinct density is visualized along the scar.

Late Changes

Scars in the skin are visualized as focal skin thickening if seen tangentially (**Fig. 19.2b,c**; see also **Fig. 19.13**), or as more or less round to elongated streaky densities if seen en face. Fibrous stranding into the subcutaneous fat may be present.

Scars within the breast usually are seen as elongated or spiculated and are usually associated with architectural distortion. In the majority of cases they can be correctly diagnosed as scars. In some cases (**Fig. 19.3a,b**), differential diagnostic problems occur when differentiating scars from carcinomas or other spiculated masses. Whereas scars usually do not have a central mass and present differently on different projections compatible with a flat extension, carcinomas tend to grow more concentrically.

The following options can be used to define a radial structural change as a scar-related change as accurately as possible:

1. Sometimes marking the location on the skin by placing a thin metal wire over the scar on the skin may be useful. In general, the surgeon will select the most direct approach so that the parenchymal scar can be expected underneath the cutaneous scar.
2. Additional projections can help to clarify the findings. Scars can often be seen better on one orthogonal view than on the other, and change their appearance in different projections (**Fig. 19.3a,b**). Cancers, however, mostly but not always have a similar pattern in different projections.
3. Spot compression views can often better demonstrate the absence of a focal central mass. Fat can frequently be present in the center of the scar. Neither absence of a focal density nor presence of fat, however, can exclude a carcinoma with absolute certainty—a few carcinomas only elicit spiculation without forming a hyperdense center—but detecting a newly developed central mass strongly suggests a neoplasm arising in the scar.
4. The interpretation of scar-related parenchymal structural changes is most definitive if serial postoperative mammographic studies can be reviewed. Changes caused by a scar are a definite possibility if the findings remain unchanged or decrease in density.
   Length or thickness of the spicules is not a criterion for the *differential diagnosis*: markedly fibrosed ductal carcinomas and tubular carcinomas can have very long thick or delicate radial extensions mammographically.
5. The lipophagic granuloma is a manifestation of granulomatous fat necrosis. It is visualized as an ill-defined mass (**Fig. 19.3c**). It cannot be distinguished from malignancy by imaging and consequently necessitates biopsy.

Dystrophic calcifications within a scar are caused by deposition of calcium salts in necrotic tissue.

The following calcifications occur:
- Calcifications of the stroma
- Calcifications within fat necroses
- Calcifications around suture material

Calcifications in the stroma have a characteristic coarse oblong form and are located within the scar (**Fig. 19.4a,b**). Furthermore, they can appear amorphous and plaquelike (**Fig. 19.4c**).

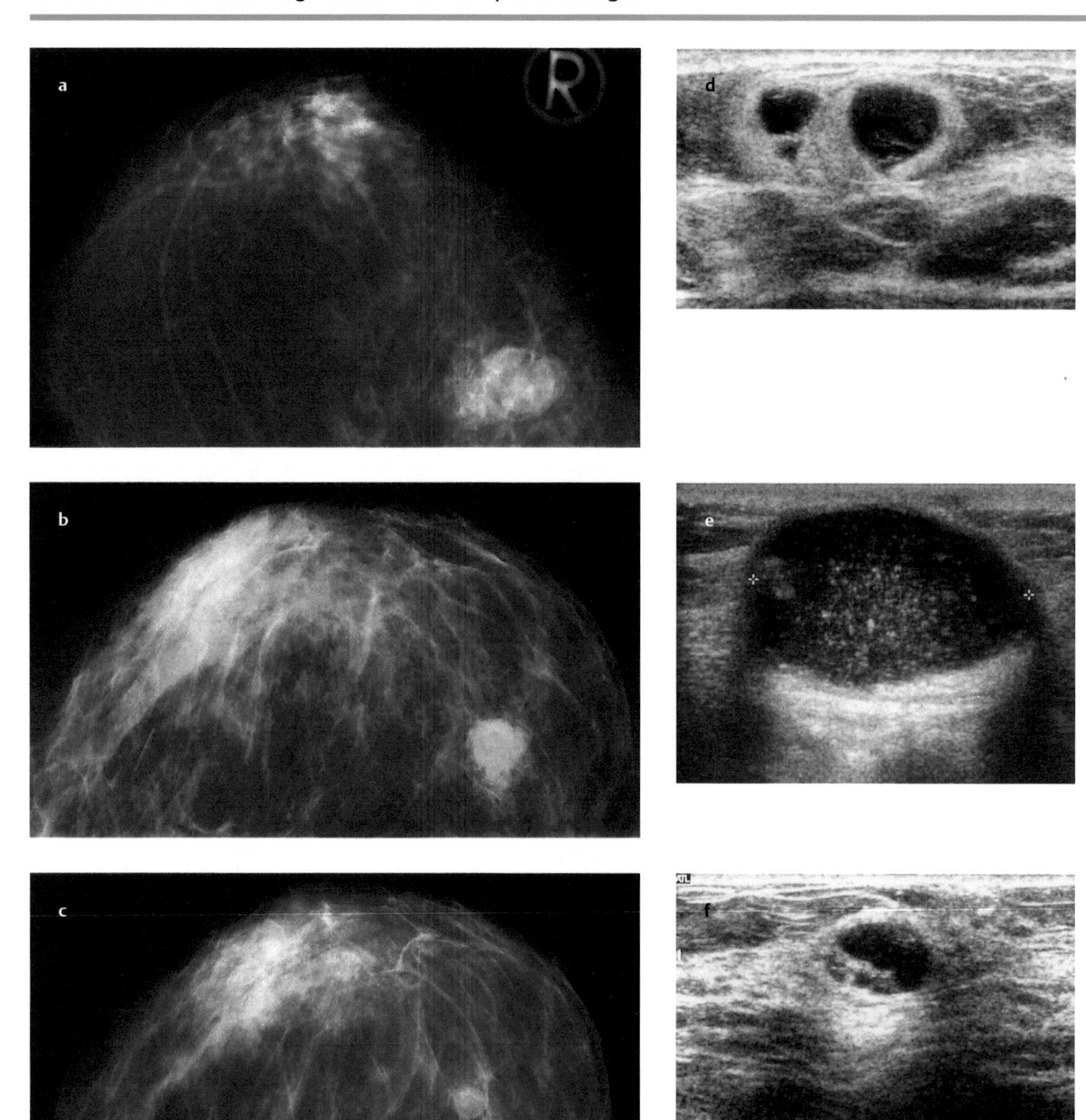

19 Post-Traumatic, Post-Surgical, and Post-Therapeutic Changes

Fig. 19.1a–f

a Patient after trauma. A soft, circumscribed mass is palpated beneath a cutaneous hematoma, corresponding mammographically to a lobulated, indistinctly outlined soft tissue density: Hematoma.

b,c Trauma while working in the garden. Irregularly outlined focal lesion in the medial half of the breast (**b**); 9 days later (**c**), markedly resolved.

d Sonography of hematomas. Two oval hypoechoic lesions surrounded by a broad echogenic rim: Fresh hematomas after trauma.

e Postoperative hematoma showing strong posterior enhancement and speckles in the center corresponding to blood clots.

f This complex lesion represented a partly organized hematoma after breast-conserving therapy.

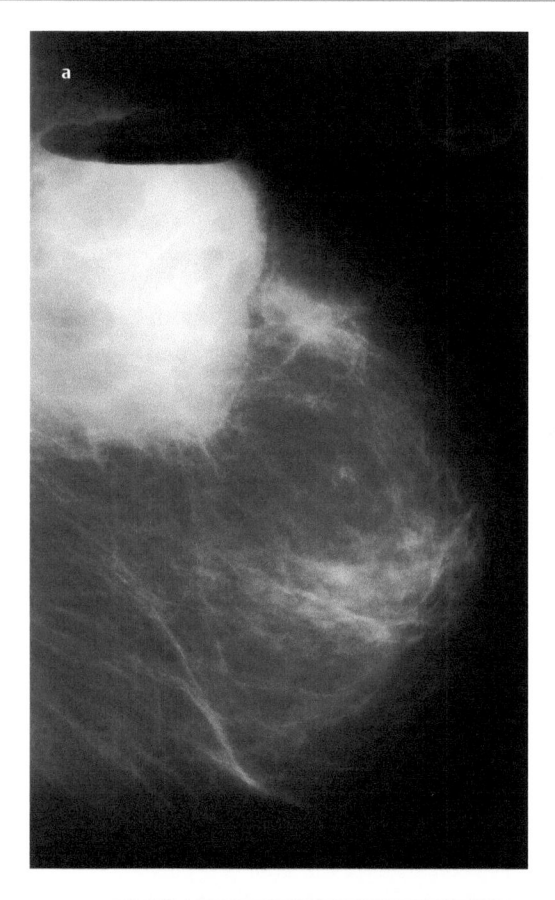

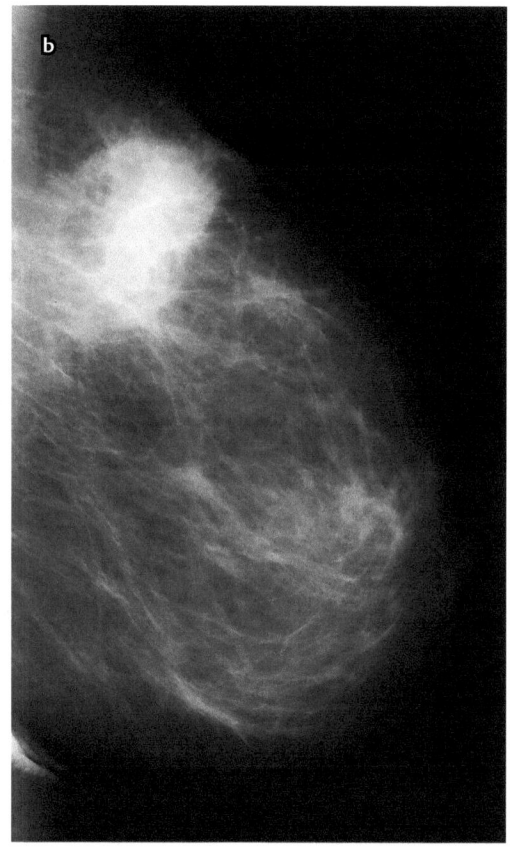

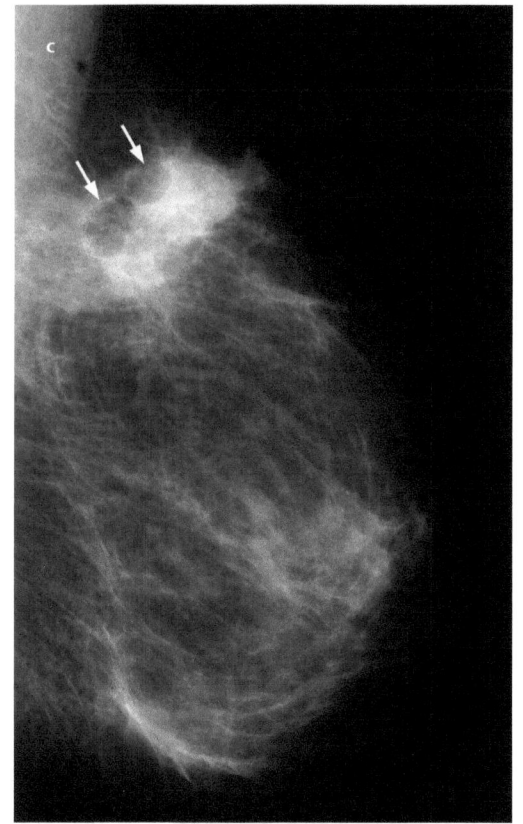

Fig. 19.2a–c Evolving scar formation (mediolateral views). Follow-up of large fluid collection with air–fluid level 5 days after surgery (**a**). Five weeks later, decrease in size of the mass, decreased radiodensity, and increasing spiculation as well as thickening and retraction of the skin (**b**). Three months later, scar formation with progressive retraction and demarcation of two oil cysts (arrows) (**c**).

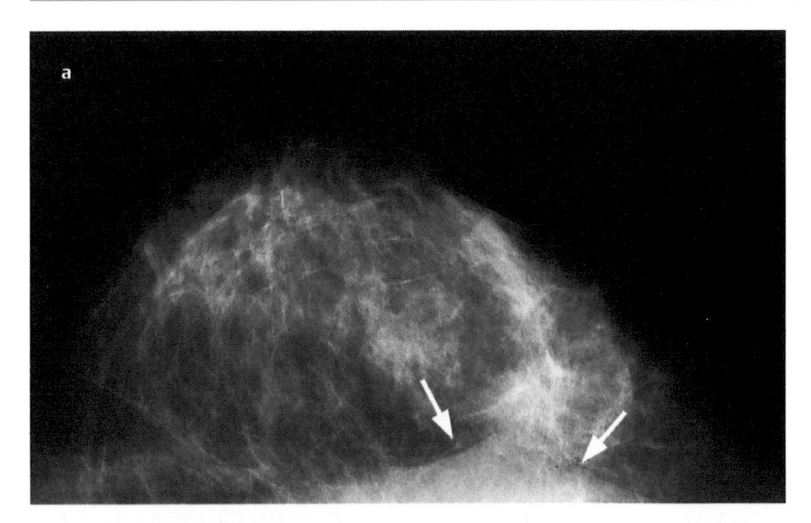

19 Post-Traumatic, Post-Surgical, and Post-Therapeutic Changes

Fig. 19.3a–c

a,b Scar formation in the upper outer quadrant with skin retraction and thickening and architectural distortion, as well as retraction of the pectoral muscle (arrows). The craniocaudal view reveals a localized mass with a central density, which is not visible in the mediolateral view (scar). Different appearance on different views is typical for scarring.

c Granuloma: In the upper half of the breast, a 7-mm focal finding with relatively thick spicules (mediolateral view).

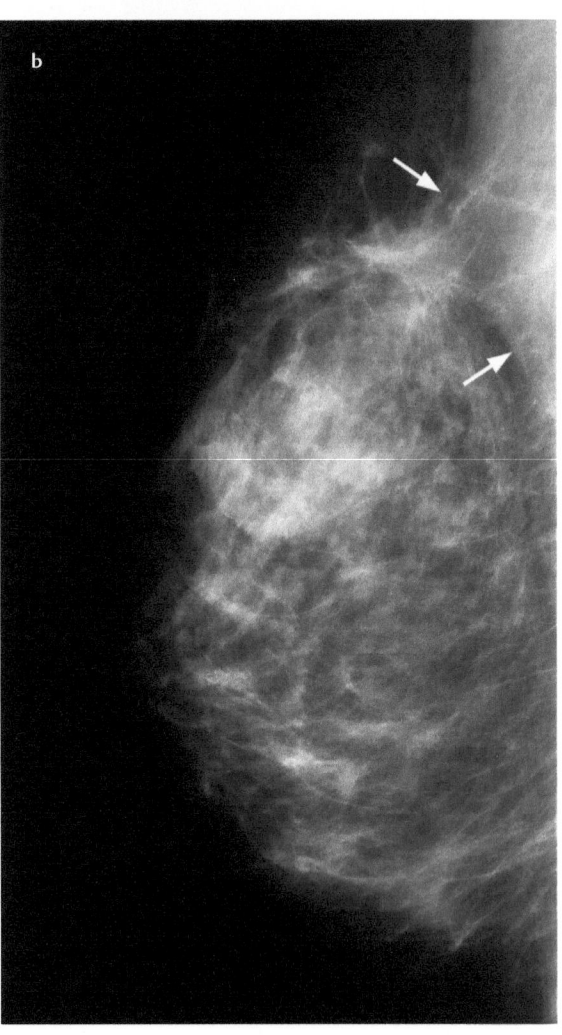

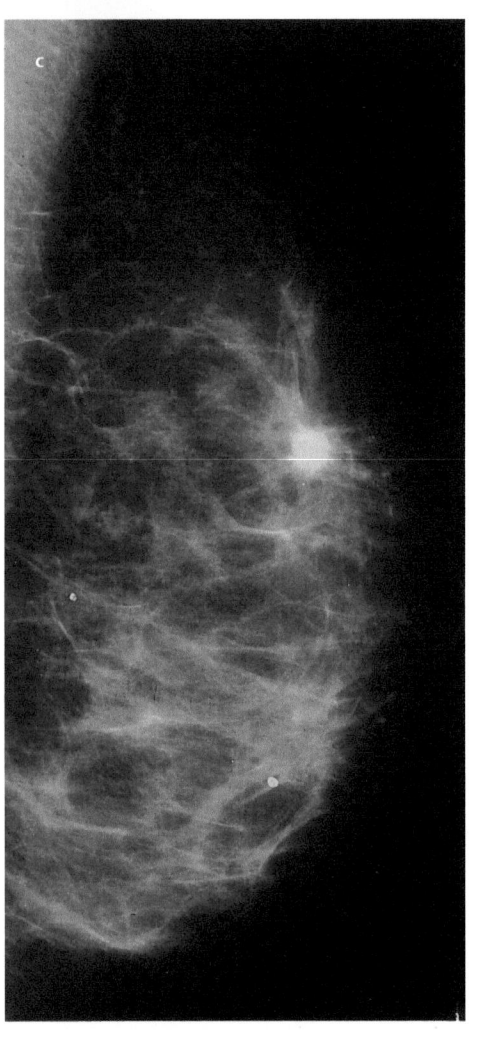

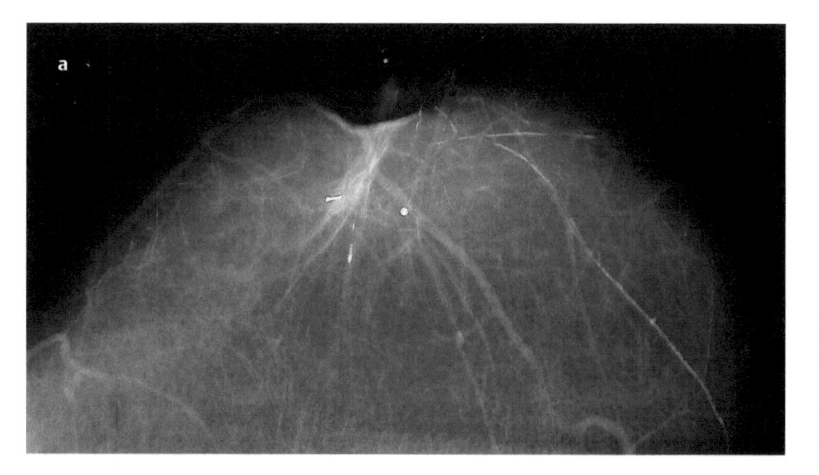

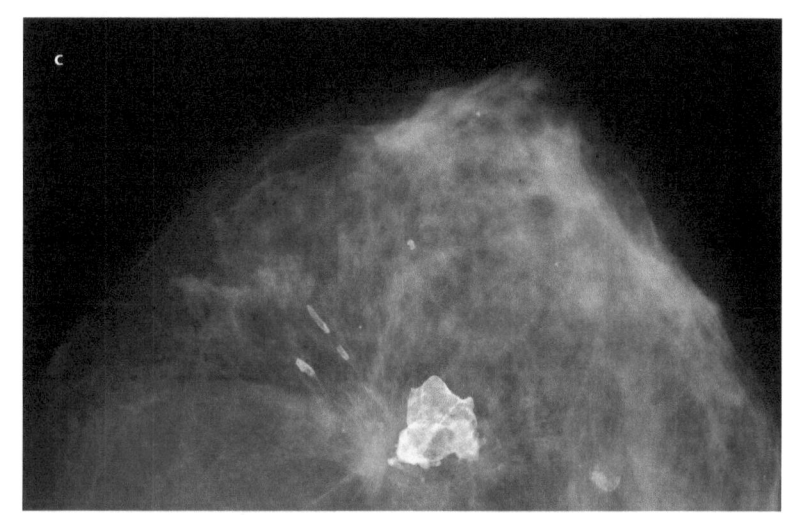

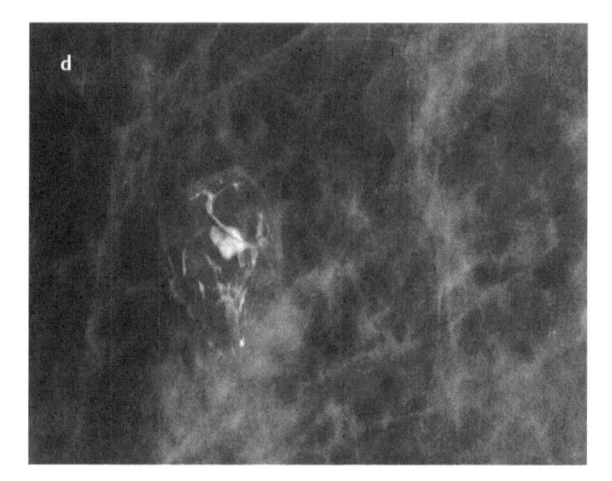

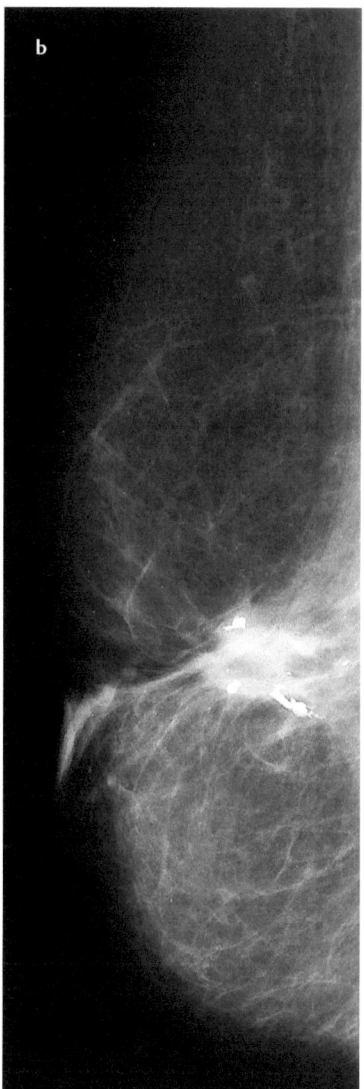

Post-Traumatic and Post-Surgical Changes

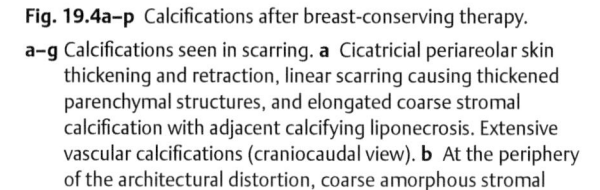

Fig. 19.4a–p Calcifications after breast-conserving therapy.

a–g Calcifications seen in scarring. **a** Cicatricial periareolar skin thickening and retraction, linear scarring causing thickened parenchymal structures, and elongated coarse stromal calcification with adjacent calcifying liponecrosis. Extensive vascular calcifications (craniocaudal view). **b** At the periphery of the architectural distortion, coarse amorphous stromal calcifications are seen. Areolar retraction (mediolateral view). **c** Coarse calcifications adjacent to a spiculated mass are due to fat necrosis following lumpectomy and breast conservation. **d** Magnification mammography shows oval radiolucency with delicate capsule and typical eggshell-like calcifications: Oil cyst.

Fig. 19.4e–p ▷

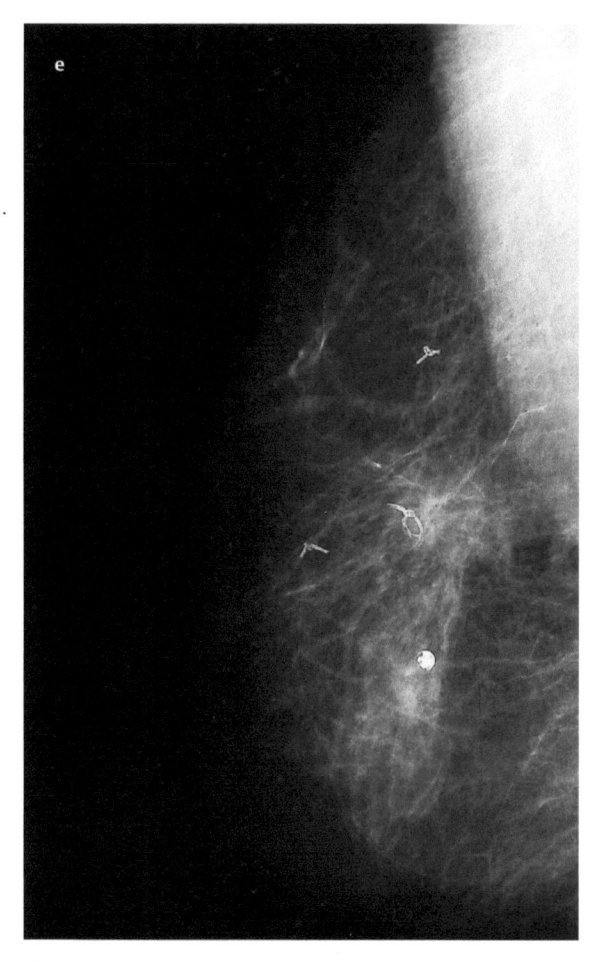

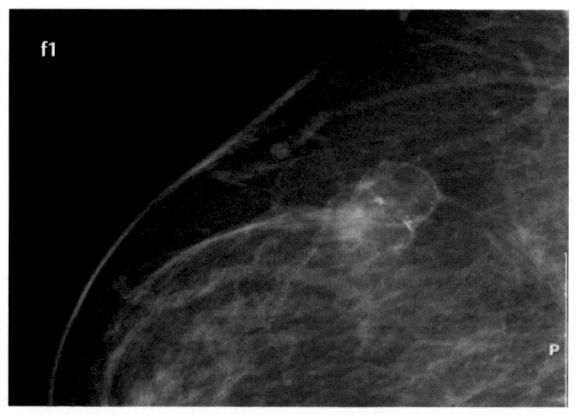

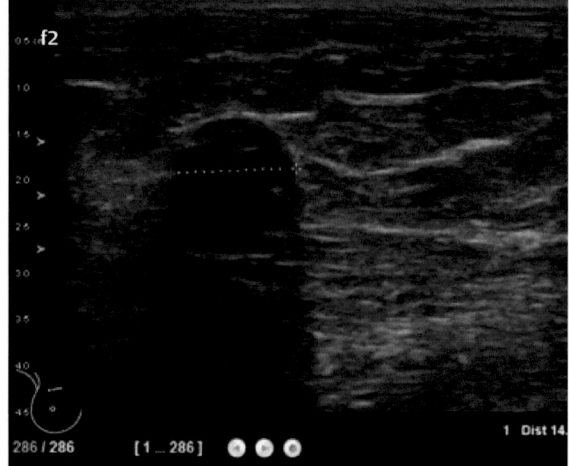

◁ continued

e Calcified suture material and calcifying liponecrosis.
f,g After breast-conserving therapy a typical oil cyst developed, mammographically (**f1**) representing an oval fat-equivalent mass surrounded by fibrous tissue. On ultrasound scan it correlated well with a partly well-defined hypoechoic mass with a few linear internal echoes and posterior shadowing (**f2**). On follow-up the scar became more pronounced and spiculated and showed microcalcifications (**g**). The microcalcifications, however, are compatible with dystrophic microcalcifications in the wall of the accompanying oil cyst, and thus do not require histopathologic assessment.

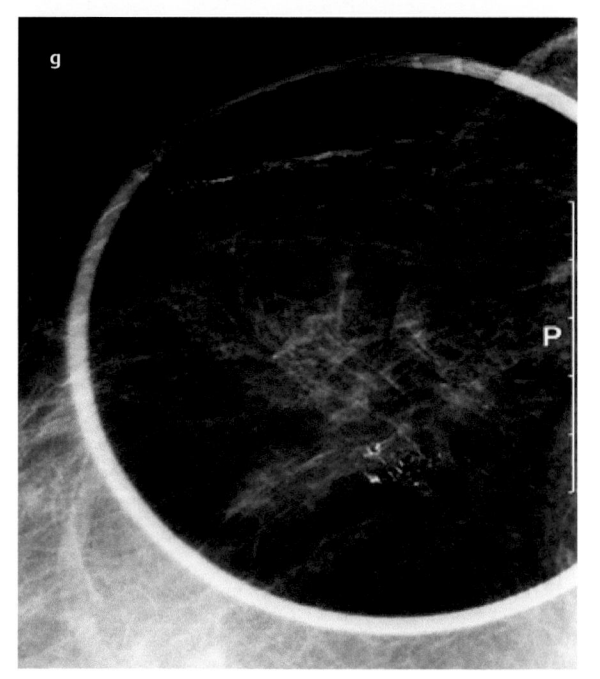

Post-Traumatic and Post-Surgical Changes

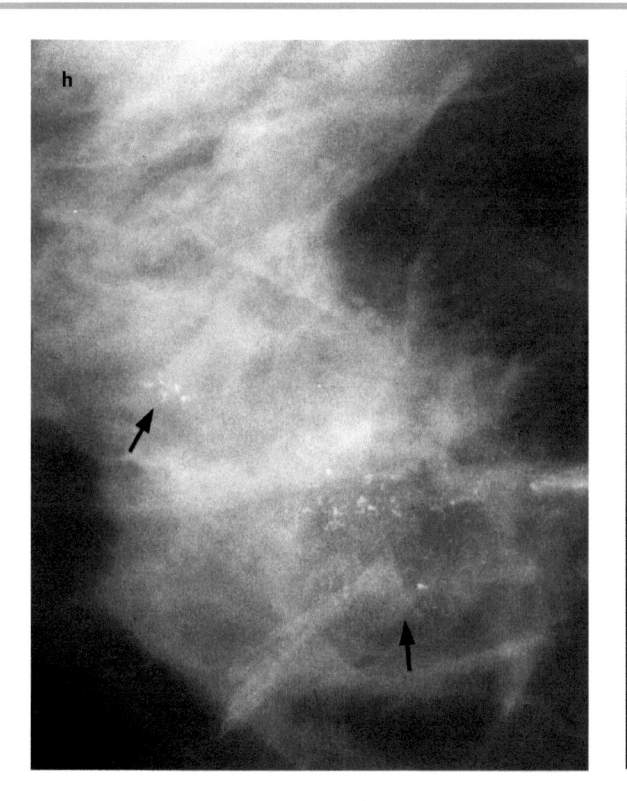

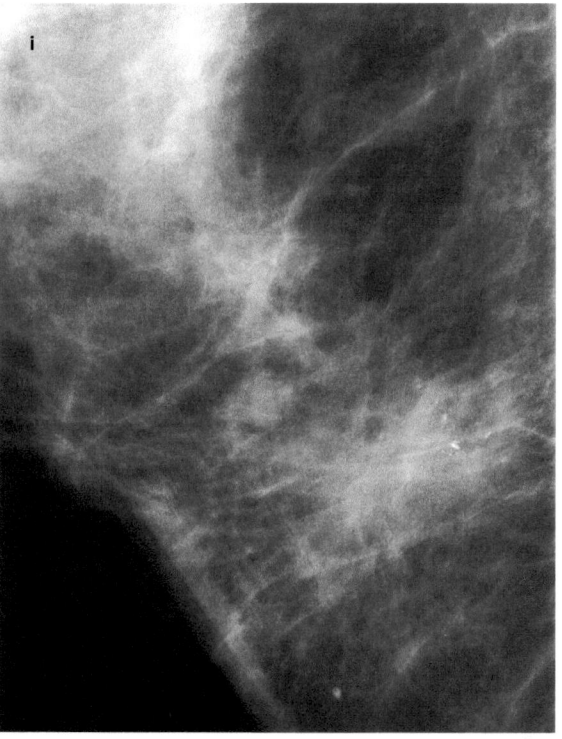

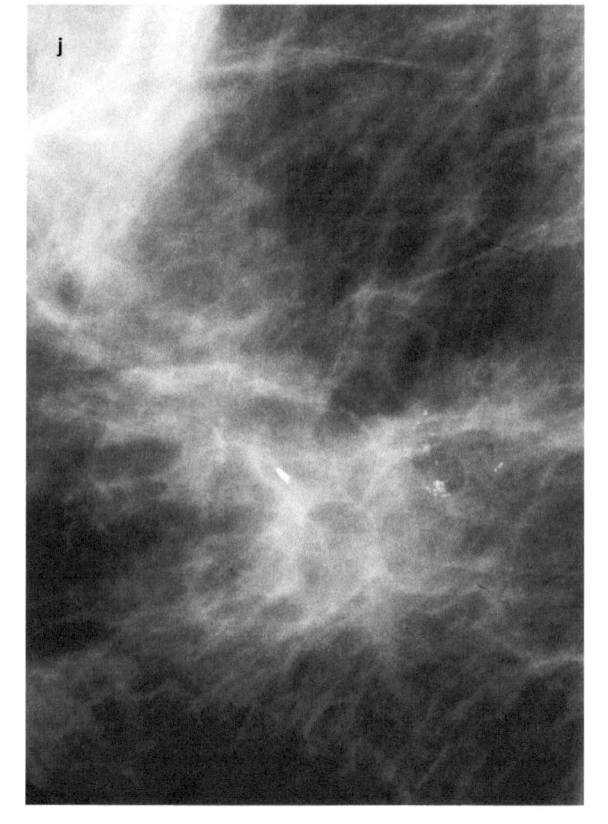

h–j Preoperative mammography of a primary tumor in the upper half of the breast. Two groups of granular microcalcifications are seen: Invasive ductal carcinoma, measuring 21 mm in diameter, as well as ductal carcinoma in situ (DCIS). Four years after therapy of the primary tumor, new pleomorphic microcalcifications are seen (**i**). On magnification mammography (**j**) they can be unequivocally assigned to two small oil cysts.

Fig. 19.4k–p ▷

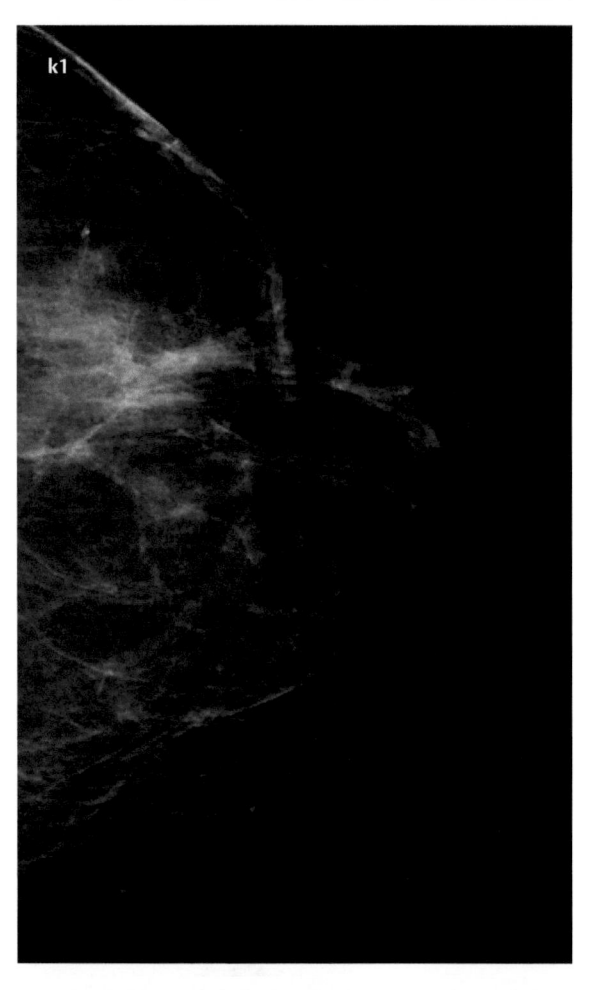

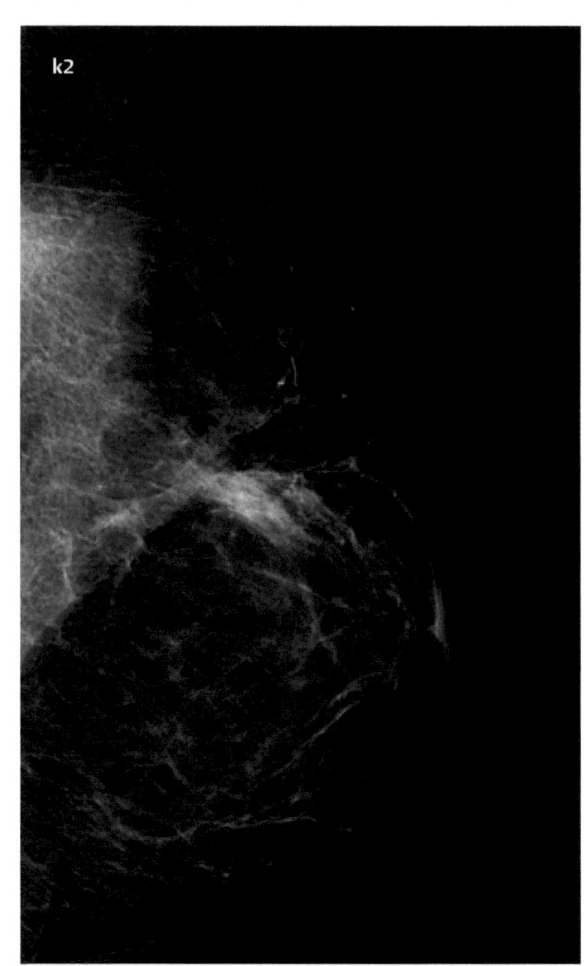

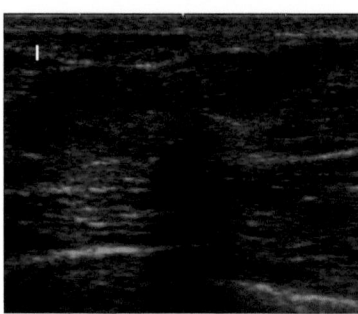

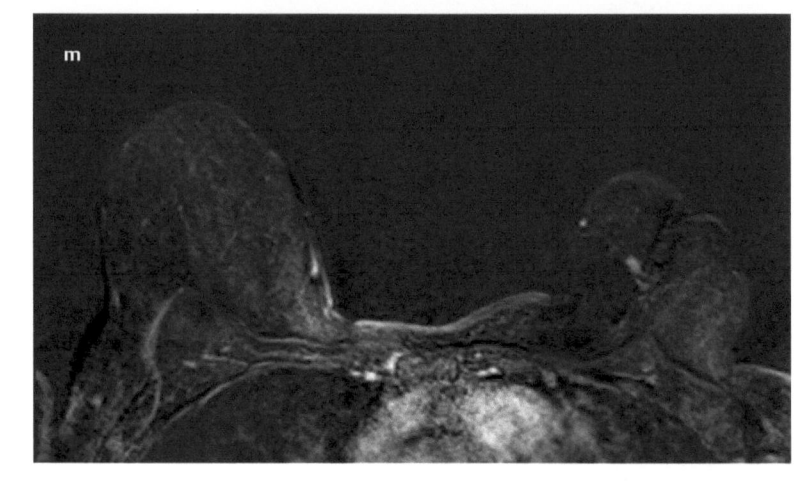

◁ continued

k This patient with a positive family history of breast cancer following breast-conserving therapy for a magnetic resonance imaging (MRI)-detected DCIS, initially resected with close margins. Mammography 4 years after breast-conserving treatment is shown. The scarring process produced both a skin and a pectoralis retraction.

l Ultrasound exhibits shadowing which appeared slightly more prominent than documented in the preceding examination.

m On MRI (subtraction image is shown early after contrast injection) a slightly indistinct 5-mm mass with plateau-type enhancement appeared. The lesion was completely removed by MR-guided vacuum-assisted breast biopsy (VABB) and yielded the diagnosis of fresh fat necrosis.

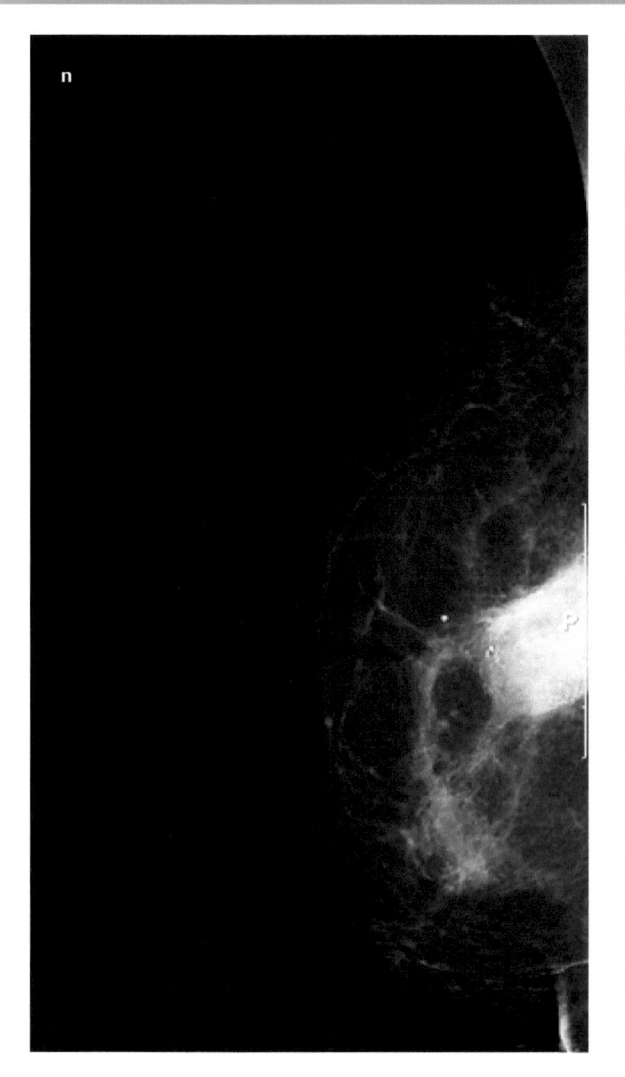

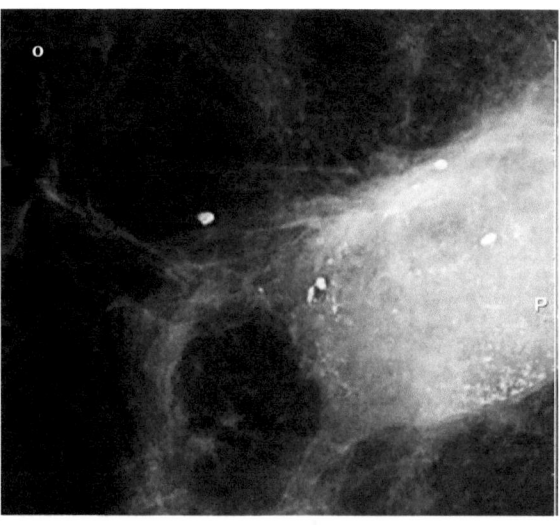

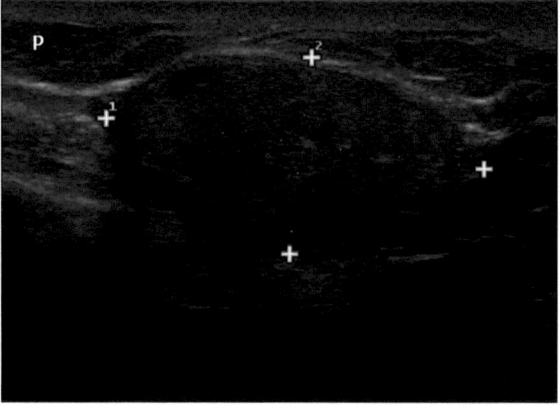

n–p In this patient (previous bilateral breast cancer which had presented with uncharacteristic microcalcifications and subsequent recurrence on the left), an oval mass had occurred after surgery which showed increasing microcalcifications (n,o) Even though morphology more likely indicates calcifications within scarring, VABB was performed to rule out recurrence on the right. Ultrasound shows a well-circumscribed hypoechoic mass (p). *Histology*: Calcified fibroma after surgery.

Calcifications in fat necrosis can present as:
- Calcifying liponecrosis: small fat droplets are formed and become calcified, producing coarse, round, or ringlike calcifications (**Fig. 19.4a,c**).
- Oil cysts: a large cystic mass containing oily necrotic material may evolve. It produces a round or oval radiolucency surrounded by a capsule. Furthermore, typical eggshell-like calcifications can develop in the capsule (**Fig. 19.4d,f**).
- Small, circumscribed, calcified cellular necrosis: in this case, pleomorphic, clustered microcalcifications can evolve that are not always distinguishable from ductal calcifications (**Fig. 19.4g,h**).

Calcifying liponecrosis and oil cysts are definitively diagnosed by mammography and do not require further evaluation. Evolving microcalcifications in fat necrosis, however, can appear rather pleomorphic as well as clustered (**Fig. 19.4f**). Magnification mammography can improve the morphological evaluation by better visualizing any evolving round and ringlike configurations as signs of benignity. Furthermore, demonstrating the relationship to a typically round or oval radiolucent area (**Fig. 19.4h,i**) can be helpful. If uncertainty remains, biopsy is indicated.

Calcified suture material is identified as elongated stringlike structures, sometimes with knots (**Fig. 19.4e**). Their double contour resembles periductal calcifications and chronic galactophoritis ("plasma cell mastitis").

Sonography

Acute Changes

Diffuse hemorrhage into the tissue can appear sonographically as an area of:
- Increased echogenicity compared with fat (usually indistinctly outlined) (**Fig. 19.5a**)
- Decreased or same echogenicity as glandular tissue
- Architectural distortion

In the acute stage, *hematomas* are visualized as an ill-defined hypoechoic area on sonography.

With increasing age of the hematoma, it becomes more sharply demarcated from surrounding tissues and tends to become more hypoechoic. The hematoma can contain hypoechoic fluid but also echogenic components (e.g., clots), which are distinguished from solid lesions by showing fluctuating echoes on palpation (**Fig. 19.1e**).

Seromas present like hematomas. Echogenic internal structures are generally absent. Oil cysts may exhibit very variable appearance on ultrasound. Usually they present as solid or complex masses with variable sound transmission. They are usually not moveable. Even though they mostly have smooth external contours, they usually have to be classified as indeterminate or suspicious based on the usual sonographic criteria. Sometimes their appearance may mimic an intracystic mass. Irrespective of the sonographic appearance, oil cysts do not require further workup if mammography is characteristic (see **Fig. 11.5a,b**).

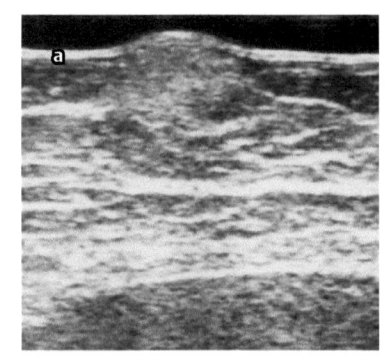

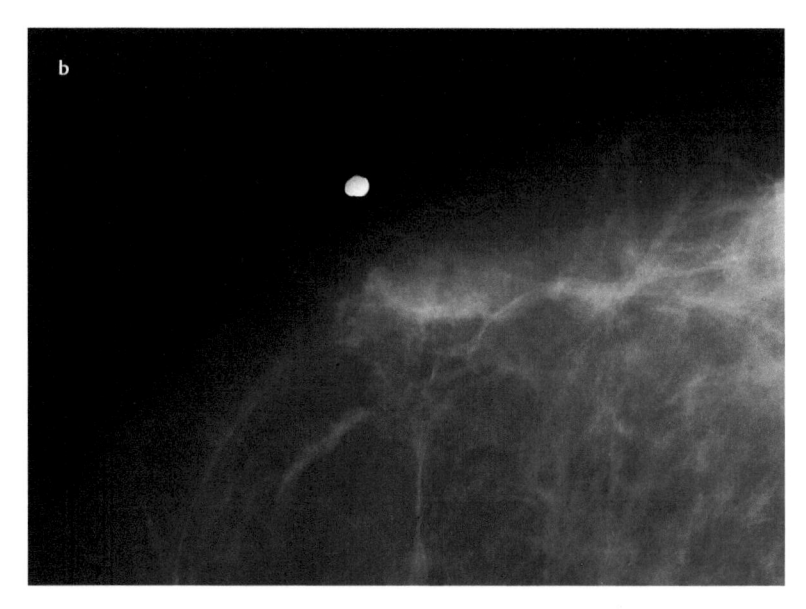

Fig. 19.5a,b Sonographic (**a**) and mammographic (**b**) visualization of hematomas.

a Oval, hyperechoic lesion in the subcutaneous space with bulging of the overlying skin: Hematoma following trauma (see also **Fig. 19.1d–f**).

b The same patient as in (**a**): magnification mammography with lead marker over the palpable finding shows an ill-defined subcutaneous soft tissue density corresponding to a hematoma.

The diagnosis is unequivocal if reviewed together with the mammogram.

Fresh *fat necroses* containing necrotic and granulation tissue generally are seen as ill-defined masses with or without distal acoustic shadowing. A differentiation between fat necrosis and malignancy is, therefore, not possible on the basis of sonographic criteria or by any other method.

Hypoechoic areas in a scar that increase in size require further workup to exclude a tumor. Such changes can also be caused by impaired wound healing. A differentiation between fat necrosis and tumor is sonographically impossible. Doppler is usually unreliable as a tool to distinguish between small malignancies and granulomas due to variations of perfusion in both.

Late Changes

Scar Formation

With progressive scar formation, the hypoechoic areas caused by fresh fat necrosis and granulation tissue decrease in size.

In the final stage, the following findings remain (**Fig. 19.6a–i**):
- A more or less pronounced skin thickening along the scar in the skin
- Discrete to marked architectural distortion with occasional hypoechoic structures in the subcutaneous space, acoustic shadowing, interruptions, or distortion of the parenchyma
- Occasionally one or more hypoechoic, indistinctly outlined areas with or without distal acoustic shadowing
- Areas with marked acoustic attenuation
- Often hypoechoic areas within scars present with triangular shapes—a connection to the skin is considered indicative of scar tissue

However, the sonographic exclusion or detection of a malignancy can be considerably impaired or even impossible in the presence of hypoechoic areas and marked acoustic shadowing. Well-documented serial sonographic studies, if available, can be helpful.

Magnetic Resonance Imaging

Acute Changes

Hemorrhage can—depending on its age—have variable signal intensity on precontrast T1-weighted images. Following injection of Gd-DTPA, minimal to moderate, mostly progressive enhancement can be observed. Early or intense enhancement or both may occur infrequently in fresh hematomas.

Hematomas and seromas are visualized as a cavity of low to high signal intensity, depending on their age and fluid composition. Following injection of contrast medium, the signal intensity of the nonenhancing content of the seroma or hematoma remains unchanged. The capsule—as far as it is developed—and the traumatized surrounding tissues usually show minimal to moderate enhancement, which generally is delayed.

Fresh granulation tissue within scarring usually shows moderate and delayed enhancement. However, in some cases fast enhancement may occur, which may cause false positive calls.

Utility

MRI is usually not necessary to image hemorrhage, seromas, or hematomas. Owing to the usual pattern of moderate and mostly progressive enhancement, assessment may be slightly impaired. In fresh scarring (usually up to 6 months after surgery), however, focally enhancing granulation tissue may cause diagnostic problems. (The few progressively enhancing malignancies such as some diffusely growing malignancies, some lobular carcinomas, and a proportion of ductal carcinomas in situ (DCISs) may not be recognized within such tissue. Therefore, it is recommended that a contrast-enhanced MRI is performed later than (4–) 6 months after surgery or major interventions (such as vacuum biopsy) whenever possible. If, however, residual or missed tumor (without microcalcifications) is suspected within mammographically dense tissue, contrast-enhanced MRI might provide valuable additional information.

In spite of the above-mentioned limitations, MRI is often capable of diagnosing residual or missed tumor if present, because most tumors enhance faster, exhibiting a typical washout or a typical morphology that allows distinction even from fresh scarring. Since the presence of residual or missed noncalcified tumor may be even more difficult to assess by mammography or sonography early after therapy, MRI should be considered if residual or missed tumor has to be excluded in equivocal cases (Orel et al. 1997, Soderstrom et al. 1997).

Late Changes

While fresh scar tissue generally shows some enhancement, old scar tissue after complete fibrosis no longer exhibits relevant enhancement.

This usually is the case after the sixth postoperative month, and thereafter MRI often allows a much better differentiation between scar tissue and malignancy. The rare exceptions of nonenhancing malignancies should always be considered. But overall assessment of severely scarred tissue is often excellent by MRI.

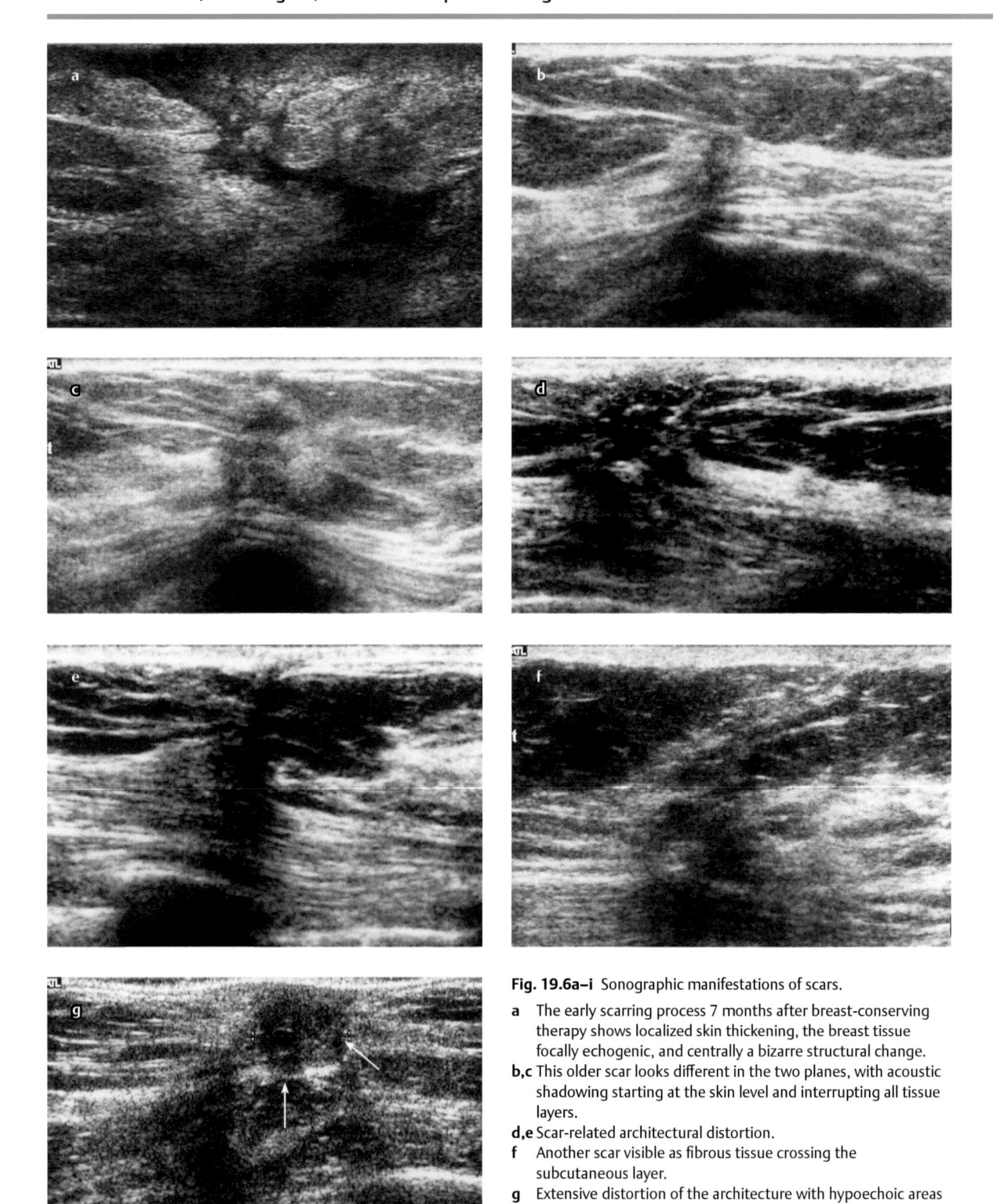

19 Post-Traumatic, Post-Surgical, and Post-Therapeutic Changes

Fig. 19.6a–i Sonographic manifestations of scars.
- **a** The early scarring process 7 months after breast-conserving therapy shows localized skin thickening, the breast tissue focally echogenic, and centrally a bizarre structural change.
- **b,c** This older scar looks different in the two planes, with acoustic shadowing starting at the skin level and interrupting all tissue layers.
- **d,e** Scar-related architectural distortion.
- **f** Another scar visible as fibrous tissue crossing the subcutaneous layer.
- **g** Extensive distortion of the architecture with hypoechoic areas (arrows).

Reduction Mammoplasty

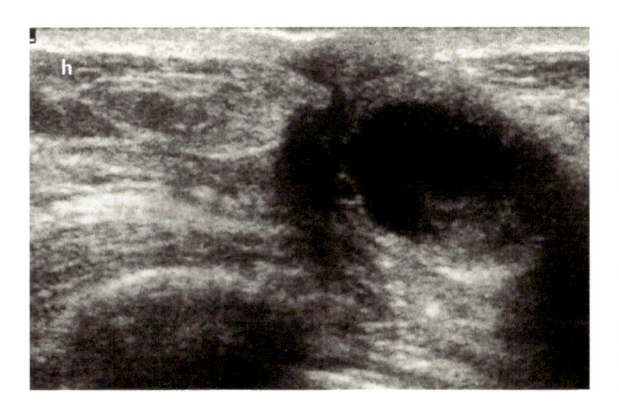

h Scar-related complex area that appears as an anechoic and hypoechoic mass. *Histology* showed oil cyst in the vicinity of a scar.

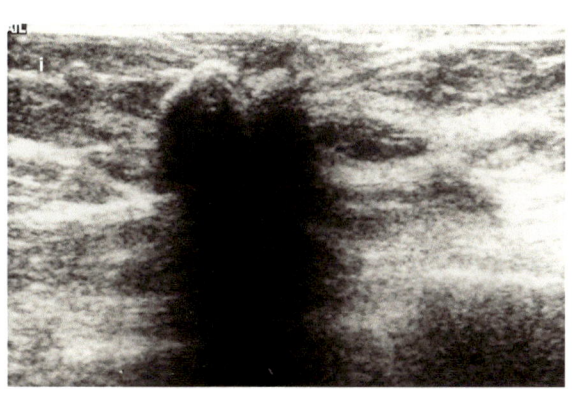

i Hypoechoic, irregularly outlined nodules with strong acoustic shadowing caused by two calcified oil cysts.

Utility

As a supplemental method, contrast-enhanced MRI offers new information relevant for the detection or exclusion of malignancy if evaluation by mammography and ultrasound is difficult or diagnostic uncertainty persists.

Mammography remains the method of choice for detection and assessment of microcalcifications.

Percutaneous Biopsy

Scar tissue can compromise percutaneous biopsy because of needle deviation and the difficulty of retrieving an adequate specimen from fibrotic tissue. This is most important to consider when interpreting biopsy results. Whenever a definite mass exists clinically, mammographically, sonographically, or on MRI, evaluation by core biopsy may be useful. For very small or uncharacteristic changes within scarred tissues VABB may improve reliability owing to the larger amount of acquired tissue.

Reduction Mammoplasty

Definition

Reduction refers to making the breast smaller to achieve symmetry following mastectomy and reconstruction or because of anisomastia. Furthermore, macromastia is a frequent indication for reduction mammoplasty, which is also performed in conjunction with breast lifting.

Surgical Procedures

To reduce the volume of the breasts, portions of the parenchyma and skin are removed, and the areola and nipple are repositioned. This is achieved by means of a characteristic "key-hole" incision technique (**Fig. 19.7a,b**), with a scar around the areola and along the inferior mammary fold, as well as a vertical scar in the 6-o'clock position connecting the periareolar scar to the inframammary scar.

Diagnostic Strategy

Palpable nodules that represent oil cysts or contain typical calcifications are easily diagnosed mammographically (**Fig. 19.7e**). It has proven helpful to have a baseline mammographic documentation, which should be performed to exclude unexpected malignancy before extensive surgery will change the anatomy. It is equally valuable for the correct evaluation of parenchymal asymmetries after reduction mammoplasty (**Fig. 19.7c,d**).

The differential diagnosis of calcifications, which can be related to scar formation, rests on the meticulous analysis of microcalcifications. Punctate or rounded microcalcifications following the scars are frequently seen after reduction mammoplasty.

In the presence of extensive scar formation and diagnostic problems, contrast-enhanced MRI can provide useful supplemental information, beginning about 6 months after surgery. However, it will rarely be needed.

Imaging and Percutaneous Biopsy

The image evaluation of scars following reduction and of any focal findings within these scars (oil cysts, lipophagic granulomas, and calcifications) is the same as the evaluation of scars of other origin.

Owing to the architectural distortion that results from this special surgical procedure, it is recommended that a baseline mammogram is obtained 3–6 months postoperatively.

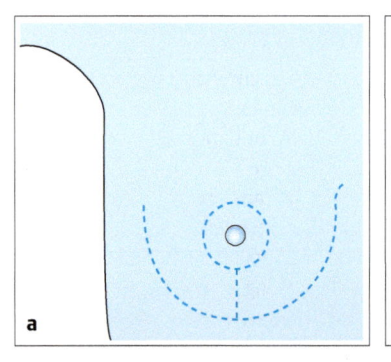

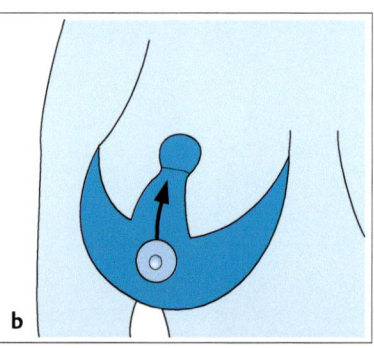

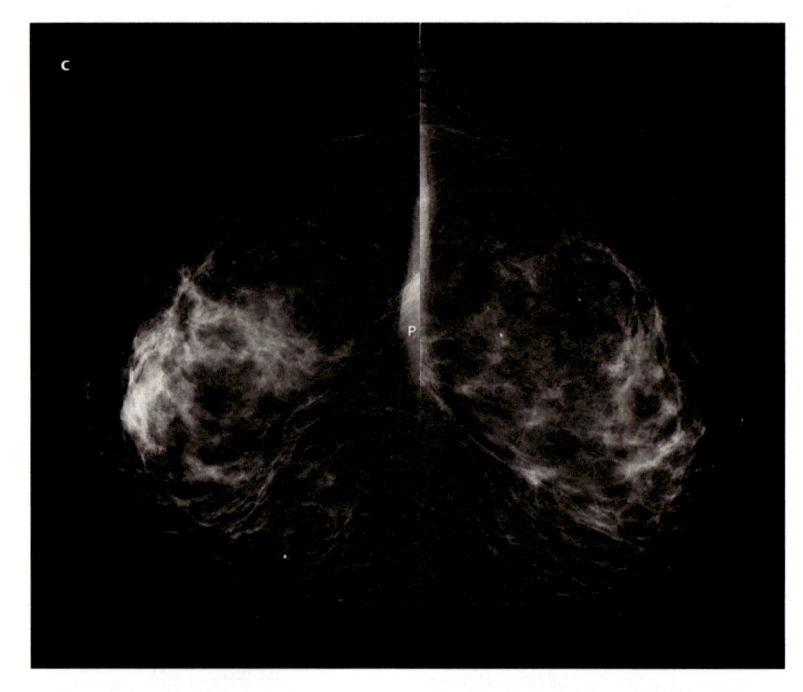

19 Post-Traumatic, Post-Surgical, and Post-Therapeutic Changes

Fig. 19.7a–e Scars after reduction mammoplasty.

a,b Incisions for reduction mammoplasty: Circumareolar incision connected by a vertical incision with the inframammary incision (**a**). At the end of the procedure, the nipple, which remains on a vascular pedicle, is pulled upward and reimplanted (**b**).

c,d Mammographic craniocaudal (**c**) and mediolateral oblique (**d**) views after reduction mammoplasty: In typical scarring, as in this case, increased density often extends centrally at the 6 o'clock position toward the chest wall. The nipple is positioned somewhat medially. However, the breast tissue appears to be well included. The central density extending toward the chest wall is compatible with the shifted tissue and the scarring. In mediolateral oblique views (**d**) the skin folds caudally are due to the scar at the 6 o'clock position. Owing to the scar it may be difficult to completely include the inframammary fold.

Changes Following Reconstruction

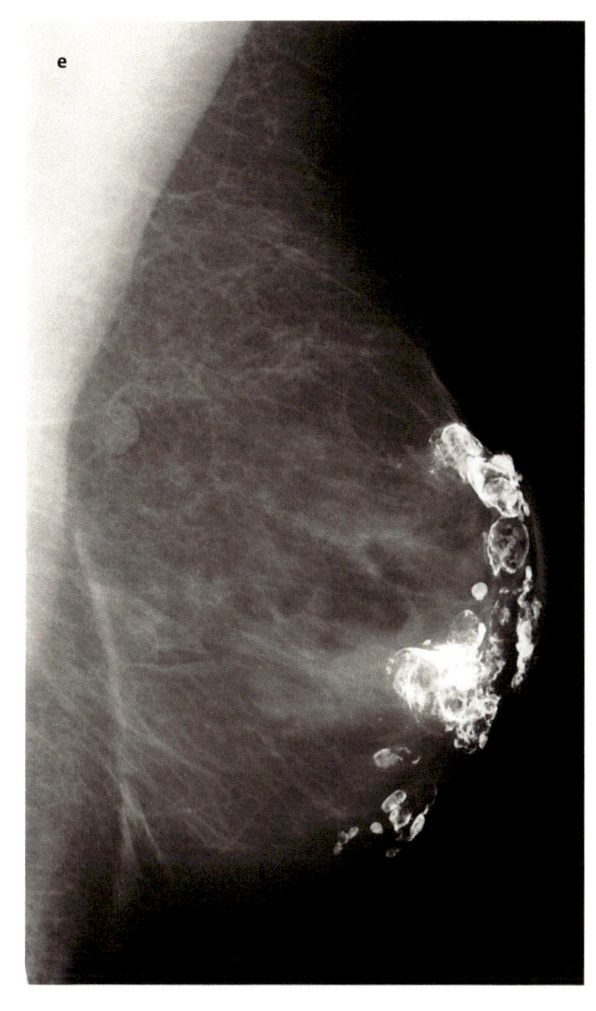

e Extensive calcification due to fat necrosis after reduction mammoplasty.

Changes Following Reconstruction

Definition

Reconstruction refers to surgical reconstitution after mastectomy.

Surgical Procedures

Breast reconstruction can be achieved by means of implants or myocutaneous flaps.

Imaging of implants is discussed in Chapter 20.

Reconstruction with autogenous tissue transfer is most frequently done with the help of pedunculated or free myocutaneous flaps. The flaps are most frequently taken from the latissimus dorsi and transverse rectus abdominis muscle (TRAM flap) or from perforator vessels ([deep inferior epigastric perforator] DIEP flap).

Diagnostic Strategy

Imaging is used to characterize clinically suspicious findings that may be due to malignancy, to benign changes within remaining breast tissue, or to postsurgical changes, and to detect a rupture of the prosthesis (see Chapter 20).

Since most myocutaneous flaps are quite transparent, mammography is indicated both for surveillance after breast cancer and for evaluation of symptoms. Sonography may be helpful for assessing seromas. However, the value of sonography within fatty tissue and its capabilities for the distinction of scarring and malignancy are limited.

Thus in the case of diagnostic problems, contrast-enhanced MRI may be useful for its excellent capability for distinguishing scarring from carcinoma and for assessing changes close to the chest wall. Indeterminate masses, which may, however, be caused by granulomatous fat necrosis, require histopathologic workup; this can usually be obtained by percutaneous biopsy.

Mammography

Myocutaneous Flap

(See **Fig. 19.8a–c.**)

Mammography is indicated and can be performed without problems for surveillance after breast cancer. It is also indicated for diagnostic evaluation of suspicious abnormalities. When performed after breast reconstruction with autogenous tissue transfer, the mammographic evaluation of areas with dense scars or muscle tissue may be impaired. Regressive dystrophic changes of the adipose and connective tissue, such as oil cysts, are frequently found, producing clinically conspicuous palpatory findings. They can be correctly diagnosed as benign by mammography. Microcalcifications or ill-circumscribed masses may indicate recurrence. However, dystrophic microcalifications, granulomatous fat necroses, and scarring may mimic malignancy.

Sonography

The accuracy of sonography is limited by the difficult differentiation of changes caused by scar formation. It is used for further evaluation of palpatory findings. Here, it may support the suspicion for a malignancy. It is also helpful for evaluating areas that (owing to scarring) cannot be included on the mammogram.

Granulomas cannot be distinguished mammographically or sonographically from small malignant foci.

Magnetic Resonance Imaging

Owing to its excellent distinction between fibrosed scarring or fibrosed granulomas and malignancy, and the excellent visualization of all the tissue as far back as the chest wall, MRI may be helpful in solving selected diagnostic problems.

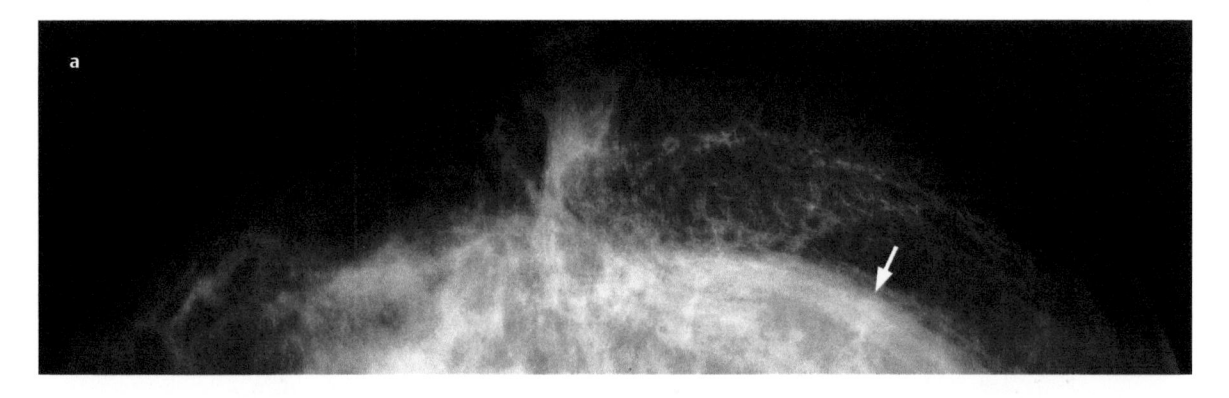

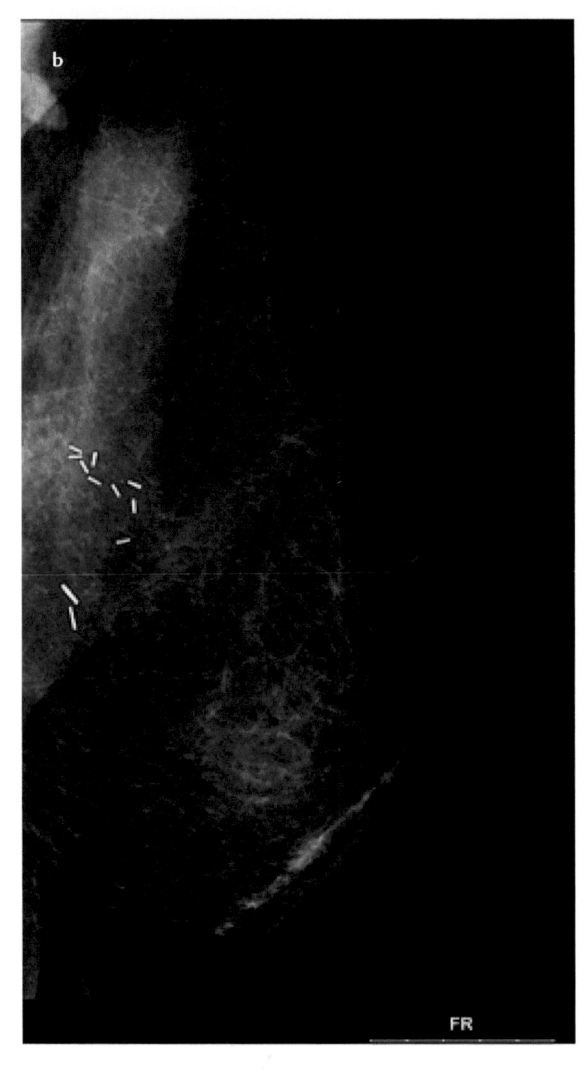

19 Post-Traumatic, Post-Surgical, and Post-Therapeutic Changes

Fig. 19.8a–f

a Myocutaneous flap. The craniocaudal view delineates the coarse fascicular structure of the implanted myocutaneous flap in the upper outer quadrant as well as the coarse subcutaneous reticular connective tissue structure, in comparison with the other side.

b–e Deep inferior epigastric perforator (DIEP) flap with swelling, lymphedema, and tissue necrosis. Mammography (**b,c**) and magnetic resonance imaging (**d,e**).

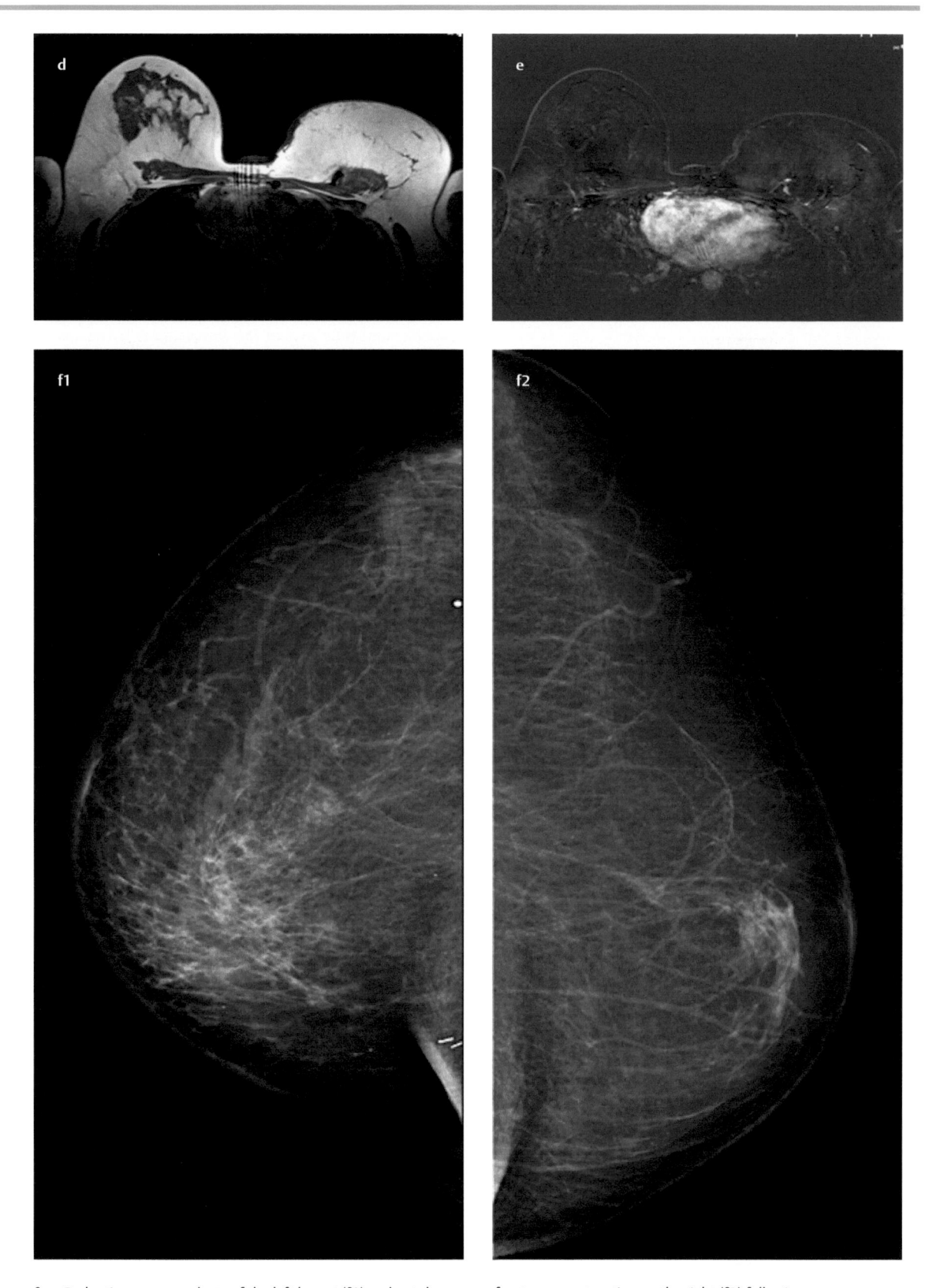

f Reduction mammoplasty of the left breast (**f1**) and autologous perforator reconstruction on the right (**f2**) following mastectomy.

Changes Following Breast-Conserving Therapy without Irradiation

Definition

Whereas breast-conserving treatment with radiation therapy is considered state-of-the-art treatment for women with invasive breast cancer and for most women with DCIS, breast-conserving treatment without irradiation may be considered for completely excised small, low-grade DCIS and selected early malignancy grade 1 (tubular carcinoma). Outside these indications breast conservation without irradiation is not considered state of the art and is associated with a significantly increased risk of recurrence (factor of 3–4).

Clinical and Imaging Findings

Both clinical and imaging findings are identical to the findings after surgery described above. The amount of scarring and deformity of the breast is usually related to the volume of tissue excised. In addition, edematous changes of the breast tissue corresponding to lymphedema after axillary resection can be superimposed.

Marked changes, however, require exclusion of a diffuse (or even inflammatory) recurrence.

Differential Diagnosis and Diagnostic Strategy

Differential diagnosis and diagnostic strategy are the same as explained for postoperative scarring in general. Unless a very small G1 tumor was treated, we recommend assessing these patients thoroughly, including MRI whenever doubts exist.

Changes Following Breast-Conserving Therapy with Irradiation

Definition

Breast-conserving treatment involves surgical removal of the breast cancer, often with axillary node dissection, and is usually followed by breast irradiation. In numerous studies, survival rates of women treated by breast-conserving surgery and radiation therapy have been comparable to those achieved with mastectomy (Veronesi et al. 2002, Fisher et al. 2002, Poggi et al. 2003).

Breast-conserving surgery implies surgical removal of the tumor, which should be performed with a tumor-free margin, followed by radiotherapy of the breast. The tumor-free margin should be larger if in situ carcinoma is present versus mere invasive carcinoma. The exact required margin is still disputed (Ghossein et al. 1992, Houssami et al. 2010).

It has become the standard therapy for breast carcinomas up to a size of 3 cm, with an increasing number of patients benefitting from this therapeutic approach today. Optimal interdisciplinary cooperation between surgeon, radiologist, radiotherapist, and pathologist is decisive for the success of this approach.

For larger tumors neoadjuvant therapy has evolved as a new option. It offers the possibility of monitoring response and thus may in the future allow better use of individualized therapy. It may be used in cases for which adjuvant therapy is recommended. According to the existing data there is no significant difference in outcome for patients undergoing adjuvant versus neoadjuvant therapy (Kaufmann et al. 2007, Wöckel and Kreienberg 2008, Untch et al. 2011). To date it is often used in patients with larger tumors. Furthermore it is indicated as the method of choice for all inoperable and inflammatory breast cancers. If sufficient shrinkage of the tumor and free margins can be achieved, breast conservation followed by radiation therapy may be possible.

For small and locally limited tumors, partial breast irradiation may be another option. Depending on the chosen method scarring of the biopsy site may be somewhat more pronounced and may exhibit dense fibrosis or oil cysts. However, the skin and breast tissue of the other quadrants of the affected breast may be softer. Currently this treatment is mostly performed in controlled studies.

The radiologic assessment of women treated with one of the above options of breast-conserving treatment is identical.

The role of radiology is:
- The best possible preoperative staging
- Preoperative localization of nonpalpable lesions
- Intraoperative specimen radiography to detect obvious areas of incomplete resection
- Postsurgical documentation of complete removal of calcifications, and
- Regular follow-up and further assessment of any changes that may occur

In addition to postsurgical changes (see above) of the breast, changes following axillary node dissection and radiotherapy can also occur. Recurrence always has to be excluded.

Overall the rate of malignancy in the ipsi- or contralateral breast is about 2 to 3-fold higher than in the normal population. Diagnostic accuracy of standard imaging may be impaired by post-therapeutic changes. However, early detection of recurrence or second malignancy is proven to be important for patient outcome (Montgomery et al. 2007, Houssami et al. 2009, 2011).

Owing to the 2 to 3-fold increased risk of malignancy and the known diagnostic problems after breast-conserving therapy, at least yearly imaging by mammography and—where indicated—by sonography is considered state-of-the-art surveillance. Malignancy may present as ipsilateral recurrence or (with almost the same frequency) as a newly developing breast cancer on the contralateral side. About 70–90% of recurrences are located in the scar, which means that thorough investigation of the scar is very important (Khatcheressian et al. 2006, Houssami et al. 2011, Kontos et al. 2011).

In contrast to the pattern discussed above for postsurgical scars, the changes induced by breast-conserving therapy with irradiation affect the entire breast and are superimposed on the changes at the surgical site. Furthermore, changes following breast-conserving therapy can be more severe than after excisional biopsy alone. Post-therapy changes can both mimic and obscure malignancy. To avoid diagnostic errors, knowledge of, and experience with, the expected changes are a prerequisite for the radiologist caring for these women. The interpretation of systematically performed follow-up examinations and the selection of supplemental methods is an important part of their treatment.

Clinical Findings

Depending on the extent of postoperative edema, the breast is regionally or diffusely dense and swollen in the early postoperative phase. This limits the value of palpation.

Axillary dissection and radiotherapy can lead to acute lymphedema of the breast with swelling and peau d'orange. Furthermore, a postoperative seroma in the axilla can cause lymphedema of the breast.

Radiotherapy induces hyperemia caused by vascular dilation and capillary damage as well as by disturbed microcirculation, increased transudation, inflammation, and development of microscopic and, less frequently, macroscopic areas of fat necrosis and granulation tissue. This leads to erythema, skin thickening, and swelling of the entire breast. A dry epitheliosis of the skin and an edema-induced induration may develop, as well as hyperpigmentation to a variable degree. In large breasts, sometimes a wet epitheliosis may be seen along the inferior mammary fold.

The entire radiated tissue and particularly the surgical bed show delayed resorption of exudates, and fluid might remain detectable for many months and sometimes years after completion of therapy.

In general, erythema, edema, and skin thickening largely resolve during the first 2 years, but considerable variations can be observed.

The resolution of edema is particularly slow around the areola and in the dependent regions of the breast, that is, in the lower half of the breast, especially in the lower inner quadrant.

During the first few years after radiotherapy, the acute radiation changes can diminish. Simultaneously, scars are formed and dystrophic calcifications can appear. In some patients mammary fibrosis can develop.

While the scar region is palpable as a flat plateau-like consistency, new nodular, rather firm areas can develop. They can be induced by the evolution of large dystrophic calcifications and oil cysts, as well as by emerging lipophagic granulomas. Clinically, these changes cannot usually be distinguished from recurrence.

Mammary fibrosis is palpable as diffusely increased consistency of the parenchyma in comparison with the contralateral breast. This fibrosis is often particularly pronounced in the lower half of the breast and around the scar. It may also be the cause of skin dimpling. Both pronounced fibrosis and skin dimpling can be the cause of diagnostic problems clinically or by conventional imaging.

A pronounced tissue defect can usually be palpated in the dissected axilla, in addition to various manifestations of cicatricial induration. In the case of supraclavicular radiation, a diffusely increased firmness can develop in this region as well.

Diagnostic Strategy and Goals

Important *goals* are:
- Early detection of recurrent disease.
- The lowest possible rate of diagnostic excisional biopsies on benign lesions—that is, a high positive predictive value. Avoiding diagnostic biopsies of early benign post-therapeutic changes is of particular importance because radiation changes can lead to impaired wound healing that can compromise the cosmetic result of breast conservation.

Approach

- Mammography, combined with clinical examination, is the most important diagnostic modality in the fatty breast. The highest accuracy can be achieved if both the preoperative mammogram and the postoperative studies are regularly available at the time a new mammogram is obtained. Many, but not all, recurrences exhibit a similar appearance to the primary tumor (presence of microcalcifications, visibility on mammography) (Günhan-Bilgen and Oktay 2007). Ultrasound is useful as an adjunct in mammographically dense tissue, for supplementary monitoring of the scar. It is most valuable for monitoring of the axilla and chest wall (Kim et al. 2011). It allows good assessment of early changes if needed. Sonographic assessment may, however, also be impaired by scarring. This causes shadowing and hypoechoic areas, which may lead to false negative or false positive results. Therefore, the value of ultrasound in the irradiated breast is assessed differently by various investigators (Bock et al. 1998, Viehweg et al. 1998).

- If evaluation by conventional methods is impaired by dense tissue or scarring or if the findings are equivocal, supplemental contrast-enhanced MRI can provide important information, allowing not only early detection of recurrences but also correct identification of scar-induced changes.
- Some authors have noted an increased false positive rate when MRI is performed during the first year after irradiation. Therefore its use more than 1 year after irradiation is preferred unless there are urgent diagnostic problems that need evaluation.

Mammography

Technical Difficulties

The following different conditions must be considered following breast-conserving therapy.

Complete mammographic evaluation of the parenchyma, particularly of the scar region, is often more difficult because of retraction of skin and muscle toward the tumor bed.

Indeterminate structural changes or newly developing fine microcalcifications are best assessed initially by additional views. Coned compression and magnification views should be applied to obtain the maximum possible information. Owing to the changing tissue, serial examinations should always be compared.

The same adequate exposure conditions for serial examinations (kVp, type of anode, position of the photocell, degree of compression) and optimum positioning should be attempted. Otherwise, discrete increases in size or density as early evidence of a recurrence can be overlooked amid the cicatricial changes.

Complete visualization of the entire scar and inclusion of all breast tissue and pectoral muscle, despite the known retractive changes, should be attempted, if necessary by using individually adapted additional views. In some cases with scars that are adherent to the chest wall this may, however, not be possible.

Post-Therapeutic Changes

The following changes are usually seen:
1. Diffuse changes including trabecular coarsening, skin thickening, and diffusely increased breast density secondary to irradiation and axillary dissection
2. Localized parenchymal changes of the skin and breast tissue due to the surgical scar
3. Localized parenchymal changes secondary to fat necrosis manifested as liponecrosis, oil cysts, or a lipophagic granuloma
4. Calcifications caused by any of the above-mentioned reasons

These various changes are only partially separable, and together they determine the mammographic pattern. For didactic reasons, these changes are treated separately.

Diffuse Changes of the Parenchymal Structure

(See **Fig. 19.9a–c.**)
Hyperemia with increased transudation as well as edema secondary to axillary dissection and radiotherapy cause mammographically:
- Diffusely increased parenchymal density
- Diffusely increased trabecular markings
- Thickening of the skin and areola

These acute changes can resolve slowly during the first 2 years after therapy. Chronic edema can resolve or undergo fibrotic transformation, which produces a similar mammographic pattern to that seen with edema.

The slow transformation of a chronic persistent edema into fibrosis (**Fig. 19.10a–c**) can be recognized mammographically by:
- Slight resolution of the diffusely increased parenchymal density corresponding to the replacement of fluids with connective tissue and partial resorption of the edema
- Thinner and sharper demarcation of the increased trabecular markings
- Some resolution of the initial thickening of the skin and areola
- Calcifications that can develop owing to cell necrosis

If the described resolution and transformation is reversed by a renewed increase in the diffuse changes, or if the diffuse changes remain unchanged without recognizable resolution, the following conditions have to be considered in the differential diagnosis:
- Secondary mastitis
- Venous stasis (heart failure, mediastinal or axillary space-occupying lesion)
- Carcinomatous lymphangiosis

Localized Changes of the Cutaneous and Parenchymal Structures

These may occur with:
- Scar formation following surgery
- Fat necrosis that can transform into oil cysts, calcifications, or a lipophagic granuloma secondary to radiation-compromised microcirculation and subsequent development of necrosis, (partial) resorption, or formation of granulation tissue

Scar formation is characterized by:
- Parenchymal asymmetry
- Associated architectural distortion and spiculations that can have extensions to the skin, the pectoral muscle or chest wall (see **Figs. 19.3a,b** and **19.4b**)

Fig. 19.9a–i

a–c Diffuse acute structural changes of the parenchyma. **a** Status post-segmentectomy (tylectomy): 5 days after surgery, diffusely increased density in the lateral half of the breast with air pocket (arrow) and skin thickening. **b** Three weeks after completion of radiation therapy: Thickening of the skin and areola, diffusely increased reticular markings, and delicate cicatricial radial structural transformation at the site of the excision. **c** Four years after completion of radiation therapy: Almost complete resolution, with skin thickening confined to the region of the scar and underlying radial structural transformation.

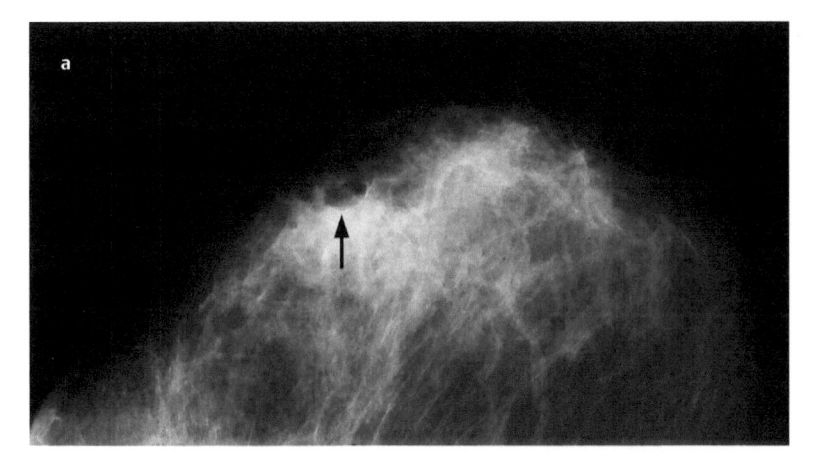

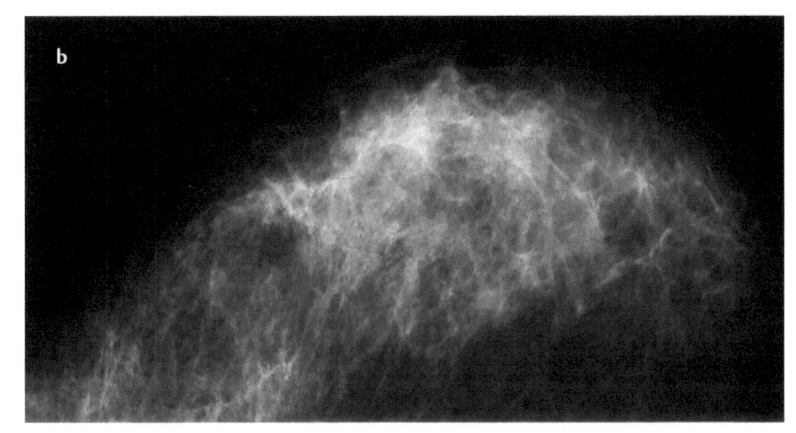

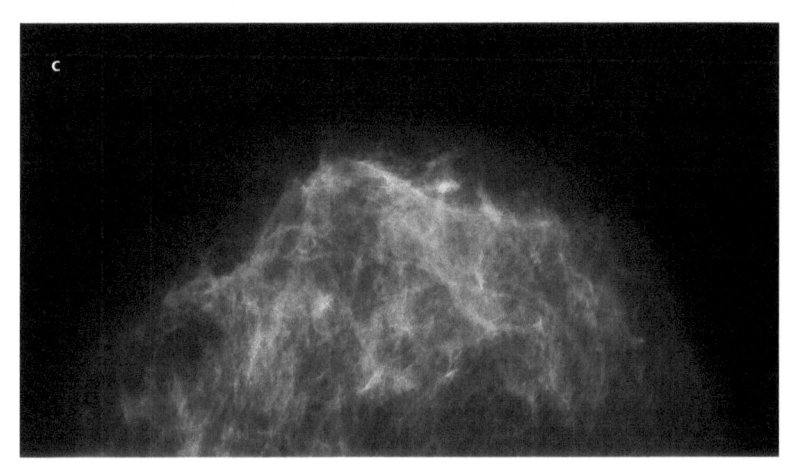

Fig. 19.9d–i ▷

19 Post-Traumatic, Post-Surgical, and Post-Therapeutic Changes

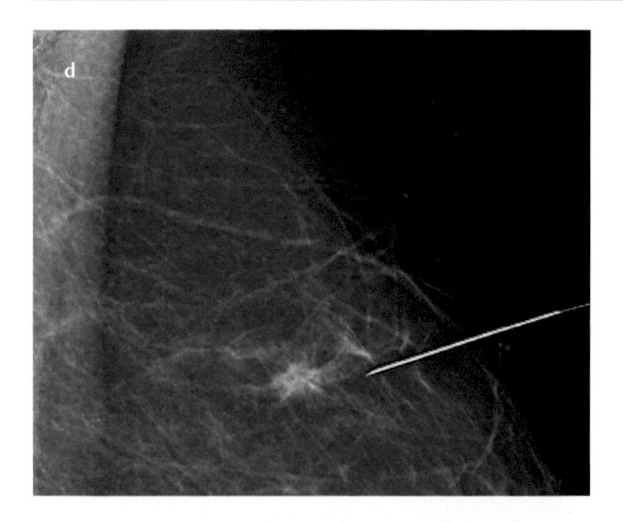

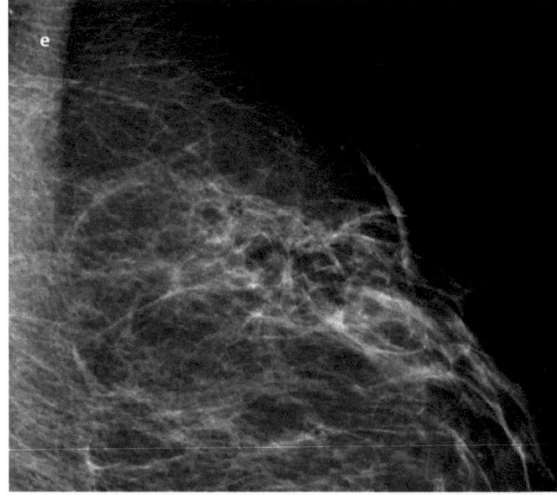

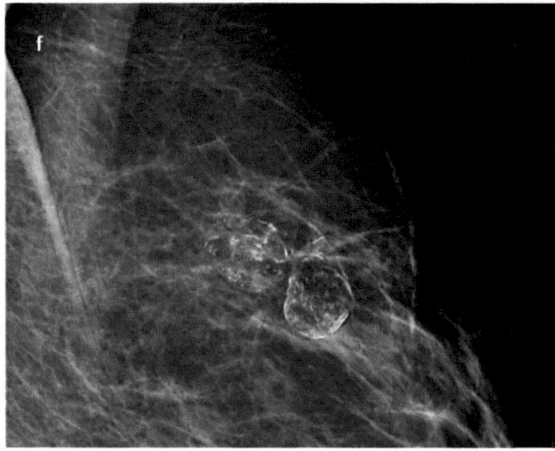

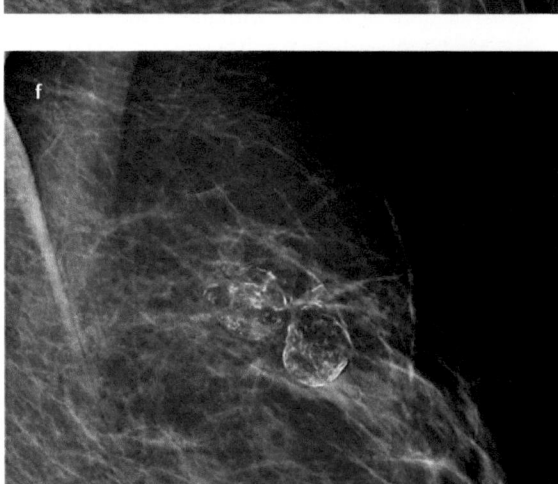

◁ continued

d–f Preoperative localization image of a small, nonpalpable invasive cancer. One year later at the first follow-up examination a group of round fat-equivalent nodules is visible at the segmentectomy region. Another year later these oil cysts calcify.

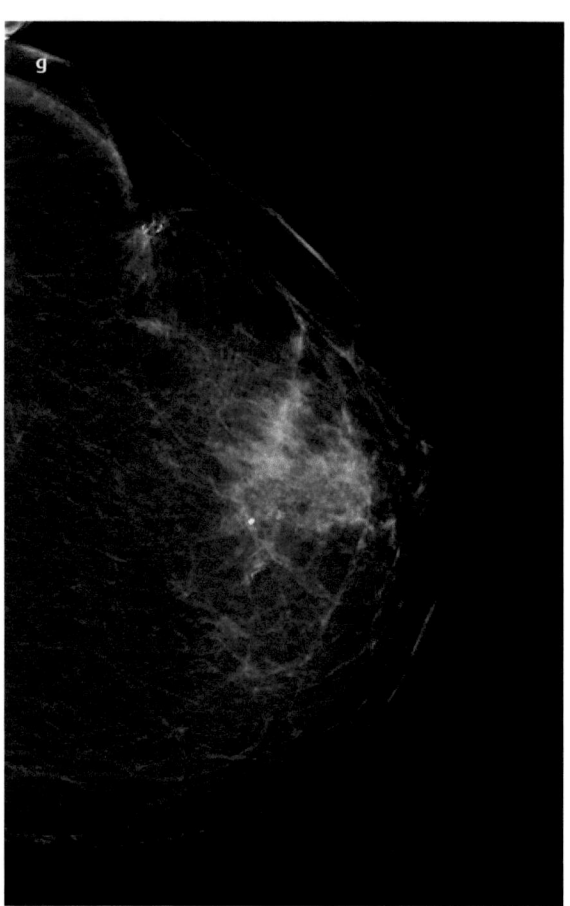

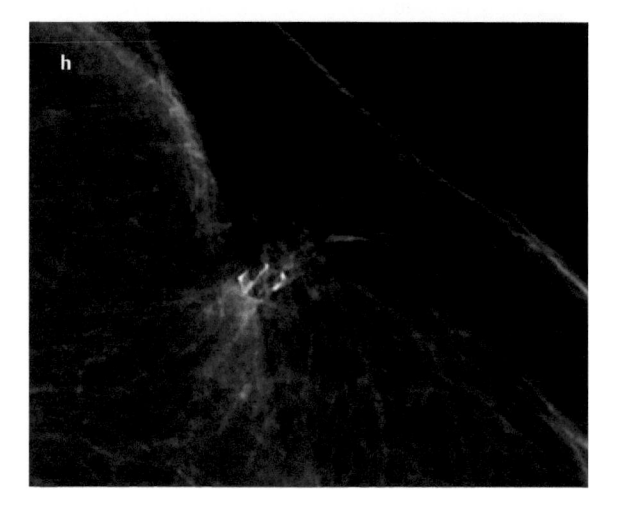

g,h 3.5 years after therapy, increased density and retraction of the scar and some skin thickening have persisted. A new dystrophic egg shell-like calcification indicates a small calcified oil cyst in the scar.

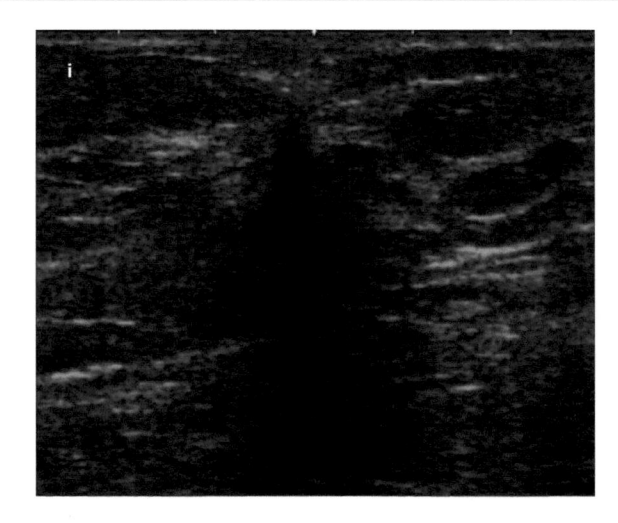

i On ultrasound a moderate skin thickening is seen, architectural distortion, small calcifications and some increased shadowing are compatible with the mammographic finding of architectural distortion and development of a typical small calcified oil cyst.

- Masses caused by delayed resorption of large hematomas or seromas (**Fig. 19.11a–d**), by dense fibrosis, or by lipophagic granulomas (**Fig. 19.12**)
- Calcifications
- Localized thickening or retraction of the skin along the scar (**Fig. 19.13**)

Evaluating the temporal course of these changes is of great importance for their correct interpretation.

In case of uncertainty concerning margins or residual microcalcifications a postoperative mammogram can be obtained before the initiation of radiation therapy. If residual suspicious microcalcifications are present, re-excision is indicated. The mammogram may be obtained shortly after surgery and can often be tolerated as early as 1–2 weeks post surgery. These studies usually show hematomas or seromas. Large hematomas may not resolve completely, resulting in a persistent mass of variable extent. Characteristically, follow-up examinations will document decrease in size and increase in scar formation with spiculation.

A parenchymal scar seen as a spiculated structure without central density can be recognized by its variable morphologic presentation on different projections, in contrast to a spiculated cancer which mostly extends in all spatial directions. The radial structure of a mature scar remains constant in configuration and density.

After the completion of radiation, a new baseline mammogram of the treated breast should be obtained about 6 months after radiation therapy. It should be followed by bilateral mammograms, which should be performed at least yearly (Khatcheressian et al. 2006, National Institute for Health and Clinical Excellence 2006).

In the United Kingdom the National Institute for Health and Clinical excellence (NICE) has critically appraised all existing literature available regarding follow-up and has made the following evidence-based recommendations:
- Annual mammography (including DCIS) until the patient enters the National Screening Programme
- If the patient is already eligible for screening: annual mammography for 5 years.
- On reaching screening age or after 5 years of annual mammography follow-up, the screening frequency should be stratified in line with the patient's risk category

Oil Cysts

Oil cysts can arise from areas of fat necrosis. They are characterized by:
- Round or oval radiolucencies of fat density (**Fig. 19.9d,e**)
- A smooth capsule
- Eggshell-like calcifications within the capsule (**Fig. 19.4d,f,g**). They are very characteristic but are not always present. During their evolution, less characteristic thin calcifications may be observed.

Oil cysts are often clinically palpated as moderately moveable, suspicious nodules or indurations, but they do not require further evaluation if they exhibit a mammographically typical appearance.

Lipophagic Granuloma

(See **Figs. 19.12** and **19.3c.**)

Lipophagic granuloma can be the manifestation of a post-therapeutic fat necrosis within scar tissue but may also develop at any other site within the irradiated breast outside the scar. It generally presents as a newly developing mass with an irregular outline and cannot generally be distinguished from a recurrence. It may also present as a round solid mass or nodule with slightly irregular contour, sometimes indistinct outline and sometimes even smooth outline (Holli et al. 1998, Harrison et al. 2000) Therefore, biopsy is usually necessary.

Calcifications

Dystrophic calcifications frequently occur in conjunction with therapy-induced cell and tissue necrosis.

Concerning the individual configuration and arrangement, the following calcifications can be classified as typically benign (therapy-induced):
- Large, elongated, and coarse as well as round, amorphous calcifications of the stroma (**Fig. 19.4a,b**)
- Typical ringlike calcifications occasionally beginning as semicircles as manifestation of a calcifying liponecrosis

19 Post-Traumatic, Post-Surgical, and Post-Therapeutic Changes

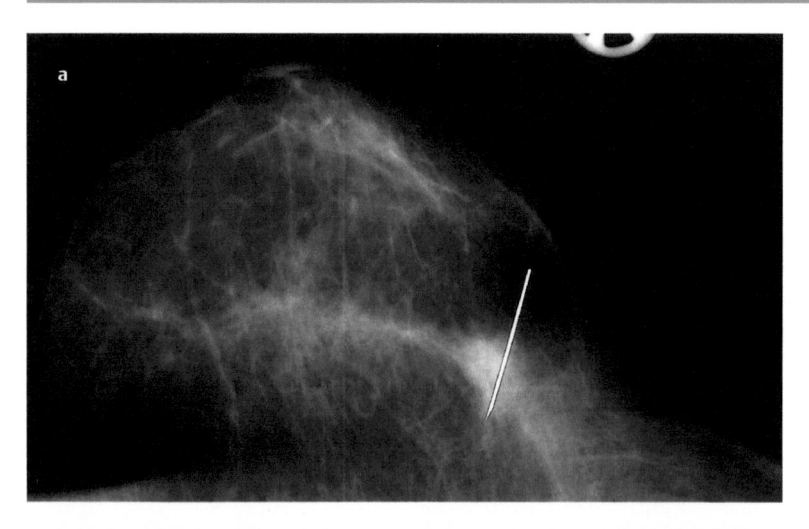

Fig. 19.10a–c Diffuse chronic structural changes of the parenchyma.

a Localization mammogram of the primary tumor (1982).
b Mammography 3 weeks after completion of radiation therapy: Swelling of the entire breast, thickening of the skin and areola, diffusely increased reticular markings.
c Six years after therapy of the primary tumor, a thickening of the skin and areola persisted. The diffusely increased reticular markings are more distinct now, compatible with fibrosis. Calcified suture material at the site of the excision (arrowheads).

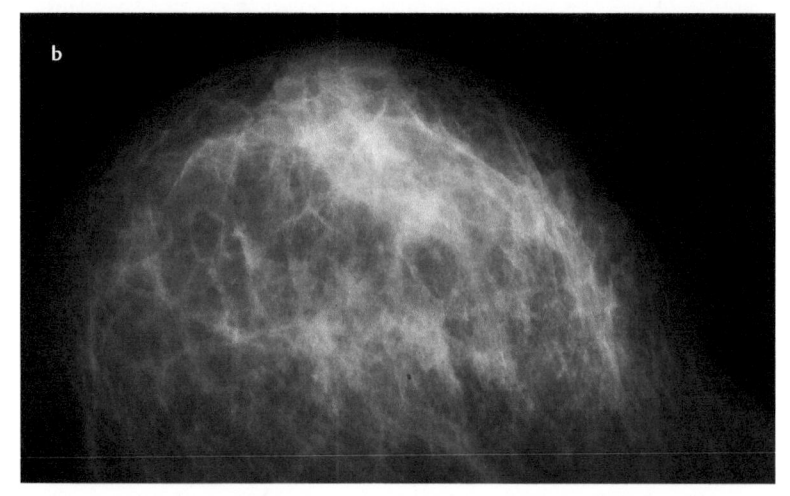

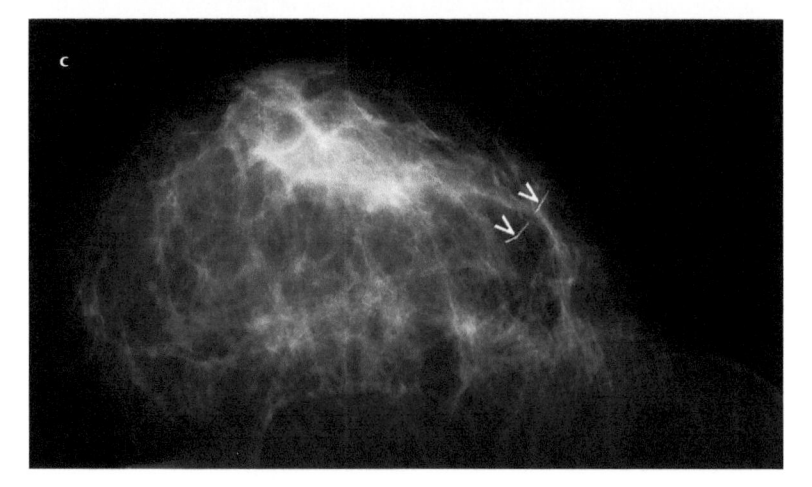

Fig. 19.11a–g Changes after breast-conserving therapy may be focal and/or diffuse. ▷

a,b Mediolateral and mediolateral oblique views of a postlumpectomy breast at 6 and 18 months after breast conservation. The rounded mass with adjacent surgical clips is a postoperative seroma. Note that it slowly involutes with time.

c,d In this patient a diffuse increased density is seen 6 months after breast-conserving therapy. Eighteen months after therapy the increased density has partly subsided. However, retraction is visible around the scar.

Changes Following Breast-Conserving Therapy with Irradiation

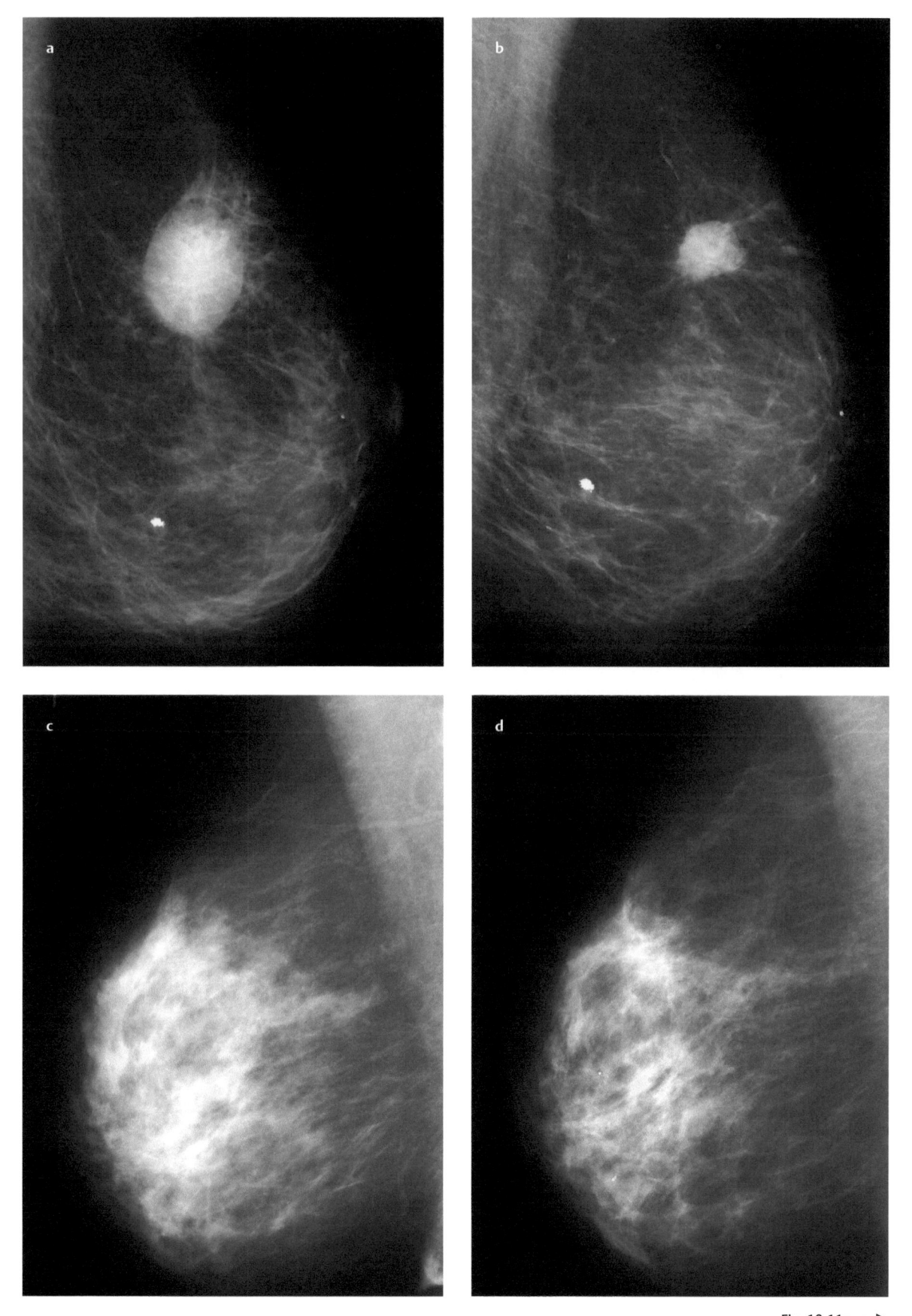

Fig. 19.11e–g ▷

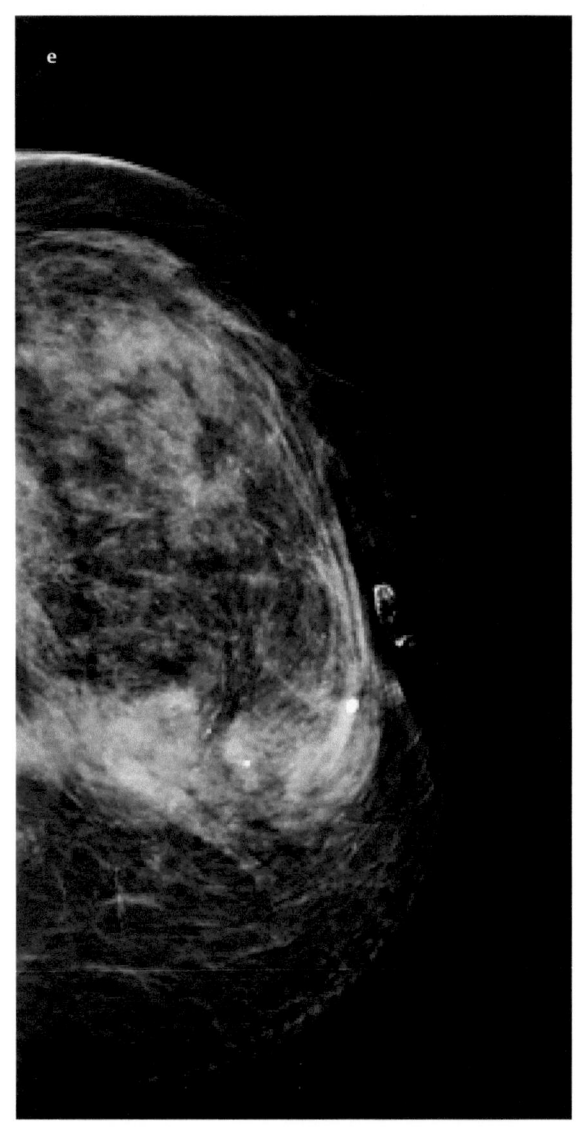

◁ continued

e–g After breast-conserving surgery this patient developed a large hematoma that never did absorb. Even years after primary treatment two masses remained, skin thickening and retraction. On ultrasound (**g**) two complex masses had developed, representing oil cysts.

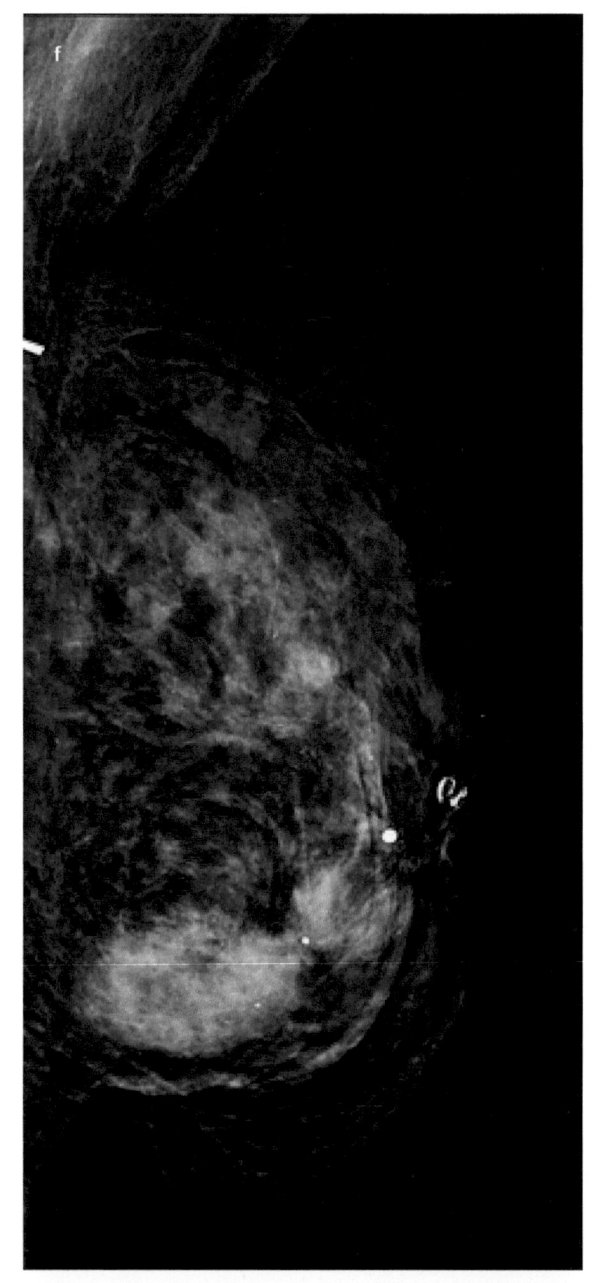

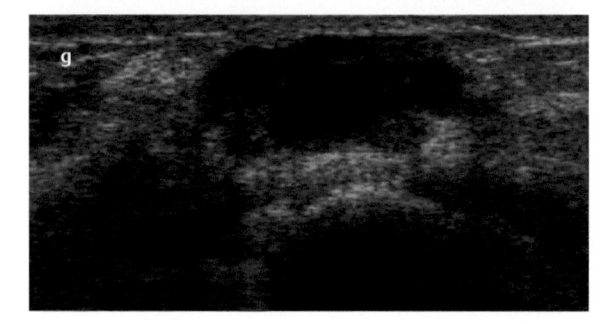

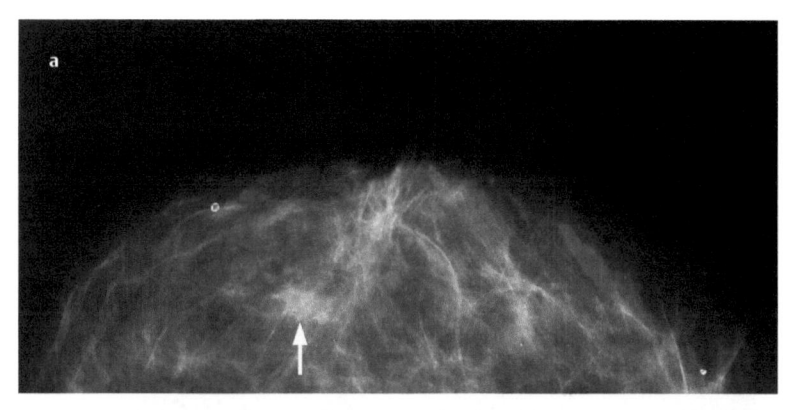

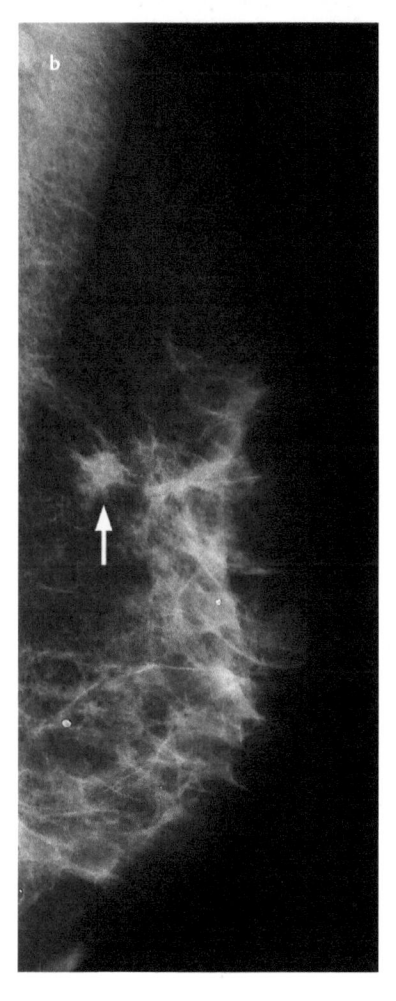

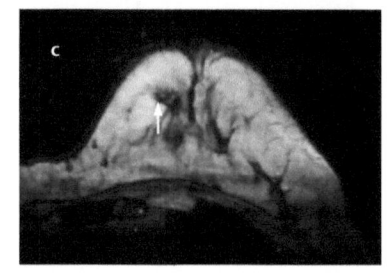

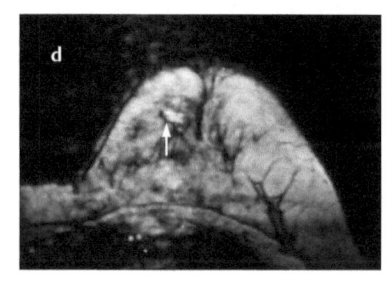

Fig. 19.12a–d Lipophagic granuloma mimicking a malignancy.

a,b This patient had a mammogram 18 months after biopsy of a suspicious finding that turned out to be a proliferative mastopathy. A previous postoperative mammogram was not obtained. This mammogram again shows a suspicious density in the region of the scar (arrow): **a** craniocaudal view; **b** mediolateral view.

c,d Because of the suspicious finding, an excisional biopsy was recommended. A supplemental contrast-enhanced magnetic resonance image was obtained as part of a trial designed for preoperative patients. **c** Representative section through the lesion before intravenous administration of contrast medium. **d** Shows the same section as in (**c**) after injection of the contrast medium Gd-DTPA. The lesion shows a rapid intense enhancement with irregular margins to be considered as suspect. *Histology*: Lipophagic granuloma. (From Heywang-Köbrunner SH, Beck R. Contrast-enhanced MRI of the breast. Berlin; Heidelberg: Springer; 1996. With kind permission of Springer Science+Business Media.)

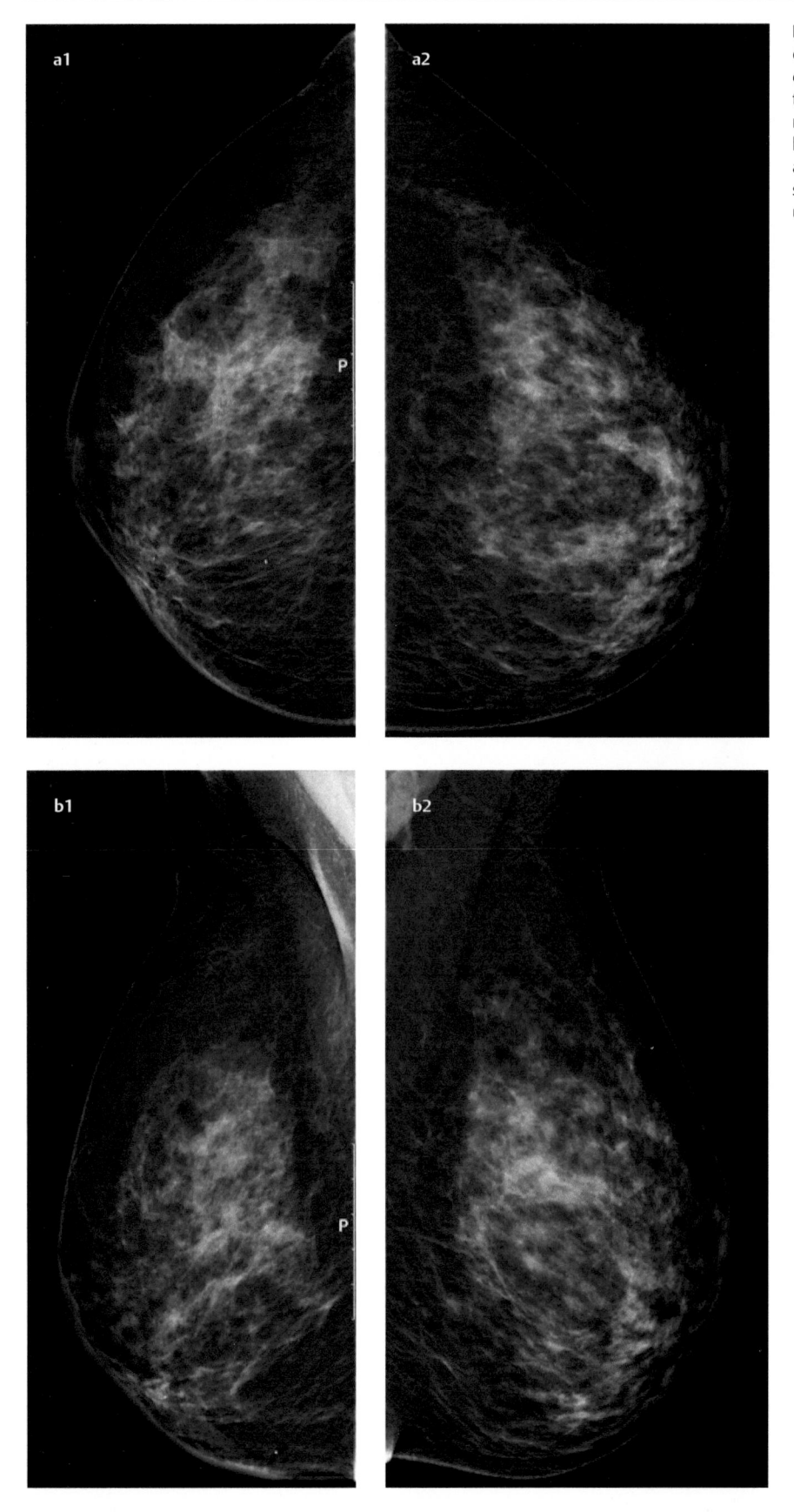

Fig. 19.13a,b Localized cutaneous and parenchymal changes after breast-conserving therapy. Skin thickening and retraction in the right inner lower quadrant and in the axillary tail, scarring of the subcutaneous tissue and the underlying breast parenchyma.

- Eggshell-like calcifications around the radiolucency of an oil cyst (**Fig. 19.4d** and **Fig. 19.9d,e**)
- Scattered dystrophic microcalcifications
- Fine, punctate calcifications at the site of tumorectomy

Calcifications evolving in the capsule of an oil cyst, a local aggregation of dystrophic calcifications, or calcifying liponecrosis can produce small pleomorphic clusters of microcalcifications. These are difficult to distinguish from malignant microcalcifications. Magnification mammography and short-term follow-up examinations may provide additional information (**Fig. 19.4g**).

Magnification mammography is necessary for an exact analysis of the contour and for finding all worrisome calcifications.

Detection of Recurrence and Differential Diagnosis

Recurrences can become mammographically visible as:
- A nodular or ill-defined mass
- Increasing size or density of the scar
- Suspicious or newly developing uncharacteristic microcalcifications
- Diffusely increased density (diffusely growing recurrence)

Focally Growing Recurrence

(See **Fig. 19.14a,b**.)

About 80–90% of intramammary recurrences develop in the vicinity of the scar, and early treatment failures tend to be at the biopsy site. The most important feature of focal recurrences and also the best criterion for distinguishing them from post-therapeutic changes is the temporal evolution:
1. Newly occurring mass or density and/or newly developing uncharacteristic or suspicious microcalcifications
2. Enlarging mass or scar
3. Increasing radiodensity
4. Increasing architectural distortion

These changes can be very discrete and can be underestimated or overlooked with variations in technique (different exposures).

A newly occurring mass and suspicious calcifications in quadrants other than the one harboring the primary tumor are mostly recognized with the same accuracy as in the untreated breast. Apart from recurrence, the differential diagnosis also includes benign changes, such as cysts or fibroadenomas. Cysts can be diagnosed sonographically. A new lipophagic granuloma occurring after therapy cannot be distinguished from recurrent disease by any imaging method and therefore usually requires biopsy.

Microcalcifications as Evidence of Recurrence

Mammography is necessary to detect microcalcifications that can be an early sign of recurrence. Since microcalcifications can develop as benign post-therapeutic changes after radiation, thorough analysis of their individual configuration and their distribution is of great importance (**Fig. 19.14c,d**).

The criteria for the analysis of microcalcifications are also applicable to recognizing recurrent disease (see Chapter 24). Calcifications associated with recurrent breast cancer have a pattern identical to those found with de novo breast cancers.

It is important to consider the time of the appearance in the differential diagnostic consideration.

If the entire tumor was removed, documented by specimen radiography, histopathologic examination, and postoperative mammogram, a recurrence within 12–18 months after irradiation would be unusual. Instead, dystrophic calcifications tend to evolve during this time span.

Diffusely Increased Density as Evidence of Recurrence

Diffusely growing recurrences are most difficult to diagnose. They can be multicentric or present as carcinomatous lymphangiosis or they can even be manifested by the growth of dispersed small-cell malignancies. They can be diagnosed as recurring, increasing, or (which is most difficult) persisting diffuse density and structural coarsening, and as areas of increasing parenchymal density, together with a clinical increased consistency and possibly with a reduction in size and retraction of the breast (**Fig. 19.14e,f**). In our experience, more than half of diffusely growing recurrent tumors were early recurrences with unusually rapid tumor growth, primarily affecting young women.

Sonography

Diffuse Structural Changes

Radiation induces varying degrees of skin thickening. In the acute stage, the edema-related echogenicity increases in the subcutaneous space and decreases in the parenchyma, leading to a loss of the normal echo pattern (**Fig. 19.15**).

Over a period of 1–2 years, skin thickening and other early changes slowly regress. Some skin thickening may persist. Increased fibrosis found in the irradiated tissue frequently causes diffusely increased echogenicity.

Focal Structural Changes

These can occur as:
- Scar formation
- Fat necroses in the form of *oil cysts* or *lipophagic granuloma*

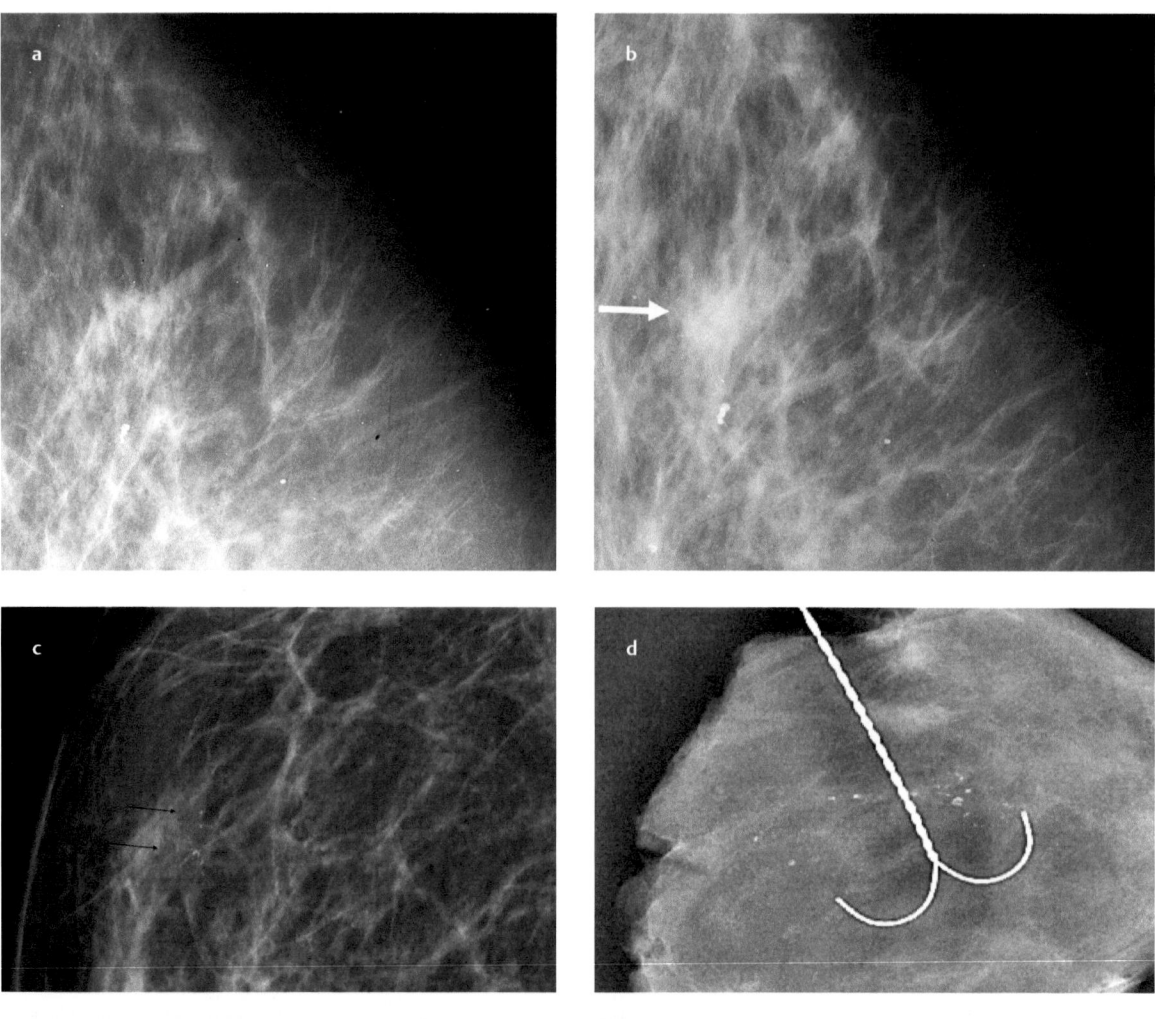

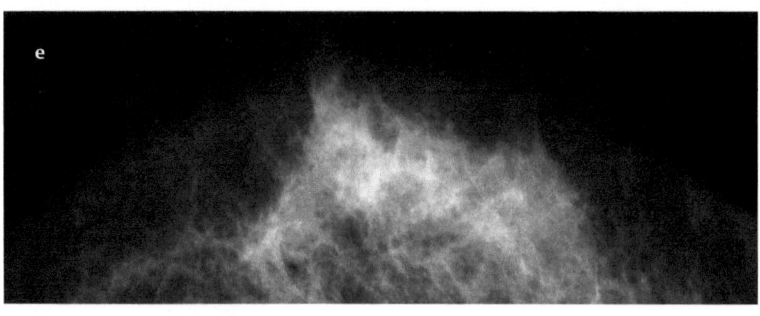

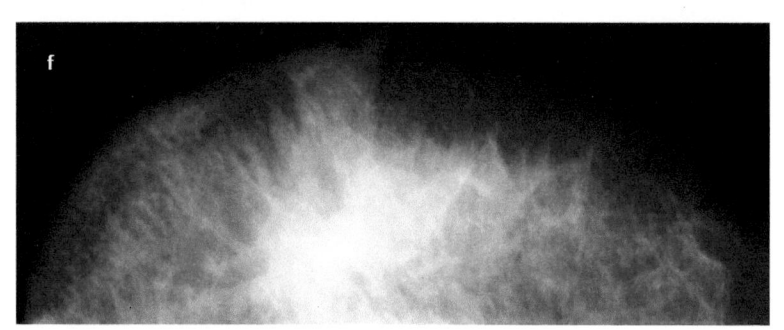

19 Post-Traumatic, Post-Surgical, and Post-Therapeutic Changes

Fig. 19.14a–i Mammographic presentations of recurrences.

a Four years after breast conservation, a few coarse calcifications are present at the surgical site due to fat necrosis.

b Three years later, a new mass (arrow) has developed at the scar: a 1-cm recurrent infiltrating ductal carcinoma.

c,d Two years after breast conservation for a ductal carcinoma in situ (DCIS) associated with microcalcifications, very few new pleomorphic linear calcifications (arrows) have developed. **d** Specimen radiography: these calcifications were due to new DCIS.

e,f Two years after breast-conserving therapy, scar-induced cutaneous thickening in the medial half of the breast, ill-defined reticular markings. Because of edematous changes and dense parenchyma, it is difficult to assess. Eleven months later (**f**): Clinically decreased size and increased consistency of the right breast. Corresponding increase in the mammographic density throughout the entire remaining parenchyma and progressing spiculation: Diffusely growing recurrence.

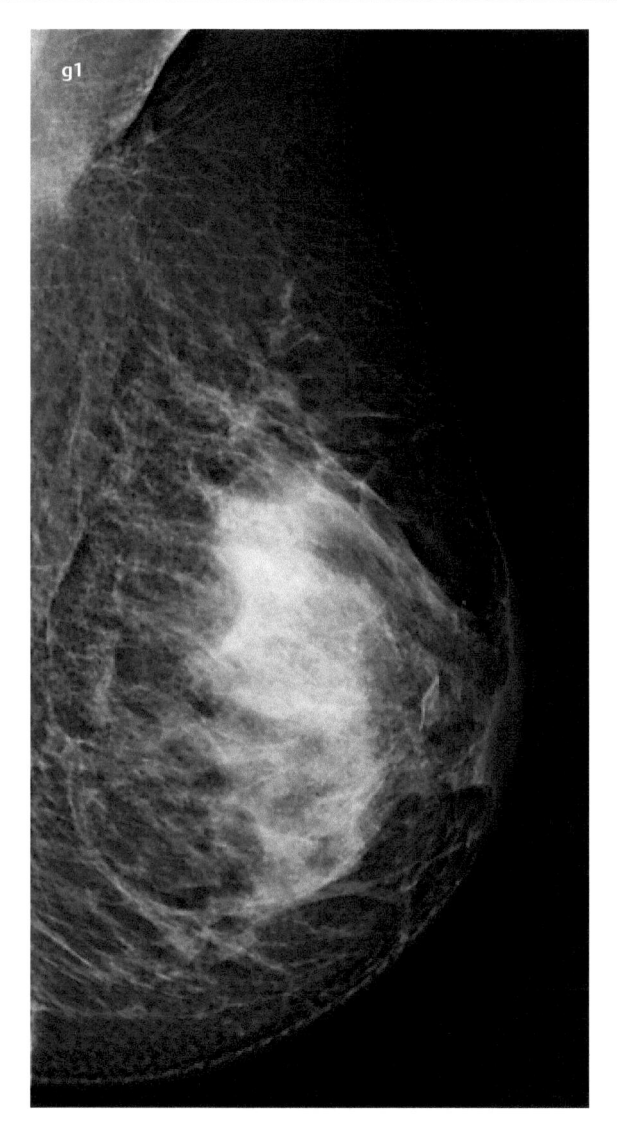

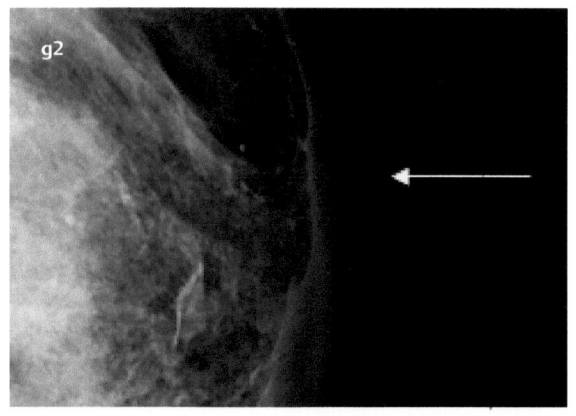

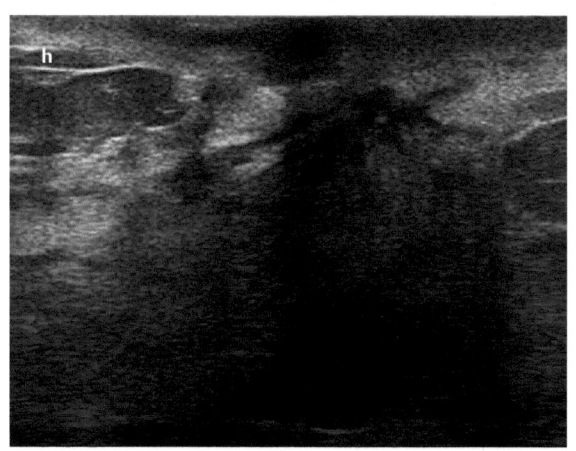

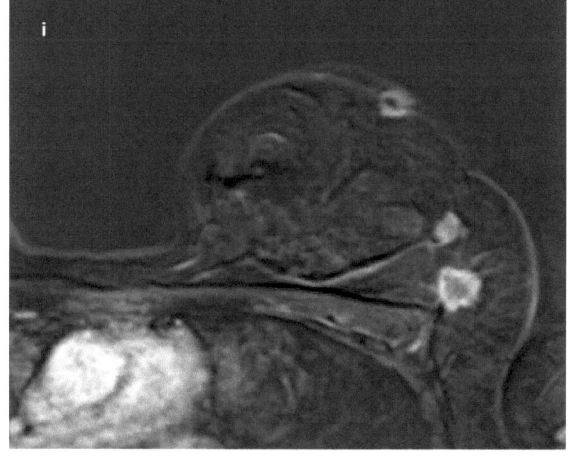

g,h This 42-year-old patient previously treated with neoadjuvant therapy (chemotherapy and trastuzumab) and breast-conserving surgery presented 2.5 years after primary treatment with a slight palpable thickening of the skin and the subcutaneous tissue in an area of 1.5–2 cm from the nipple. She had noted the thickening herself 6 months after a normal mammogram and sonogram. **g** The diagnostic mammogram (obtained at the time of the clinical finding) shows dense tissue, no visible mass, no suspicious microcalcifications. The only change compared with the previous mammogram is a skin thickening at the 2 o'clock position from the nipple in the area of the palpable abnormality, located 4 cm antero-medial to the scar. **h** On ultrasound a diffuse hypoechoic infiltration of the skin and diffusely spreading hypoechoic ductlike and nodular structures are seen in the tissue underlying the skin. *Histology*: Invasive ductal carcinoma grade 2–3.

i MRI demonstrates multifocal invasive recurrence involving the outer quadrants between 2 and 5 o'clock.

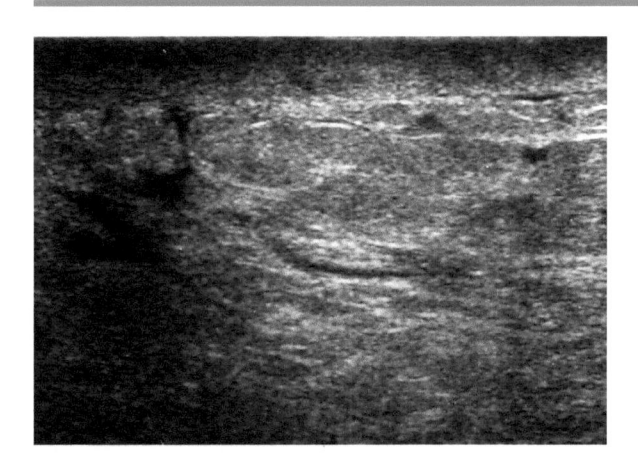

Fig. 19.15 Sonographic presentation of the breast after tumorectomy (lumpectomy) and radiation (see also **Fig. 19.6**). Extensive lymphedema 3 months after completion of radiation therapy. Increased echogenicity is seen in the subcutaneous tissue as well as in the prepectoral fat, with loss of the demarcation between the subcutaneous soft tissue and thickened dermis as well as poor separation of parenchyma from fatty tissue.

In its early stage, the scar region, similar to nonirradiated scars, often contains a seroma or hematoma; the resolution of either can be well-monitored sonographically. With increasing granulation tissue and fibrosis, small or large hypoechoic areas, and acoustic shadows—as also seen after surgery alone (see also **Fig. 19.6**)—can develop in the region of the scar and compromise the evaluation. Well-documented serial examinations may be helpful.

Oil cysts (compare p. 117) are in general correctly diagnosed only when the sonography is interpreted together with mammography.

On Doppler imaging a lipophagic granuloma is visualized as a hypoechoic lesion with or without acoustic shadowing, with or without increased perfusion, and cannot be sonographically distinguished from a primary or recurrent carcinoma.

Utility

In the follow-up of patients after breast conservation and irradiation, sonography:
- Can be helpful to distinguish the mammographically visible or palpable hematoma from a mass, if doubts exist
- Can be helpful to detect a recurrence (visible as a persistent mass that does not resolve) if the breast tissue is very dense. However, sensitivity and specificity are reduced due to post-therapeutic hypoechoic areas and shadowing.
- Is helpful in determining whether a new mass is due to a cyst

In case of doubts and impaired or inconclusive assessment by ultrasound and mammography, contrast-enhanced MRI should be considered. It is superior to sonography in the detection or exclusion of small recurrences in severely scarred breast tissue. These advantages of MRI are well proven for diagnostic problems more than 1 year after irradiation (Viehweg et al. 1998, Drew et al. 1998, Belli et al. 2006, Sardanelli et al. 2010).

Magnetic Resonance Imaging

Acute Stage

Immediately after radiation (Heywang-Köbrunner et al. 1993) as well as within the subsequent 12 months, the irradiated tissue and the scar may show enhancement. Often a moderate and diffuse, but sometimes also patchy, strong enhancement is seen. This enhancement usually decreases within the initial 12 months with considerable individual variation. Some authors (Müller et al. 1998) have reported such changes early after radiation therapy to a lesser degree, and thus also apply MRI earlier after irradiation (> 6 months). Later than 12 months after radiotherapy, the irradiated tissue can still exhibit some diffuse, usually progressive enhancement.

Cutaneous thickening and enhancement usually regress more slowly than the parenchymal enhancement.

Late Stage

More than 12 months after therapy, diffuse and progressive enhancement is seen only in individual cases. In the vast majority of cases only minimal ("absent") enhancement exists. Residual skin thickening and focal, scar-related architectural distortion can be diagnosed by absent contrast enhancement and do not interfere with the evaluation by MRI (**Fig. 19.16c,d**).

Utility

Within the first 12 months after radiotherapy, the information provided by MRI may be compromised by diffuse enhancement. Patchy and sometimes focal enhancement (probably due to ongoing granulation) may cause false positive calls.

With increasing fibrosis, the enhancement markedly decreases. From 12 months after radiotherapy, detection and exclusion of recurrent disease in irradiated tissue is considerably improved.

From approximately 12 months after radiotherapy, evaluation by MRI is generally excellent, since the fibrosed

Changes Following Breast-Conserving Therapy with Irradiation

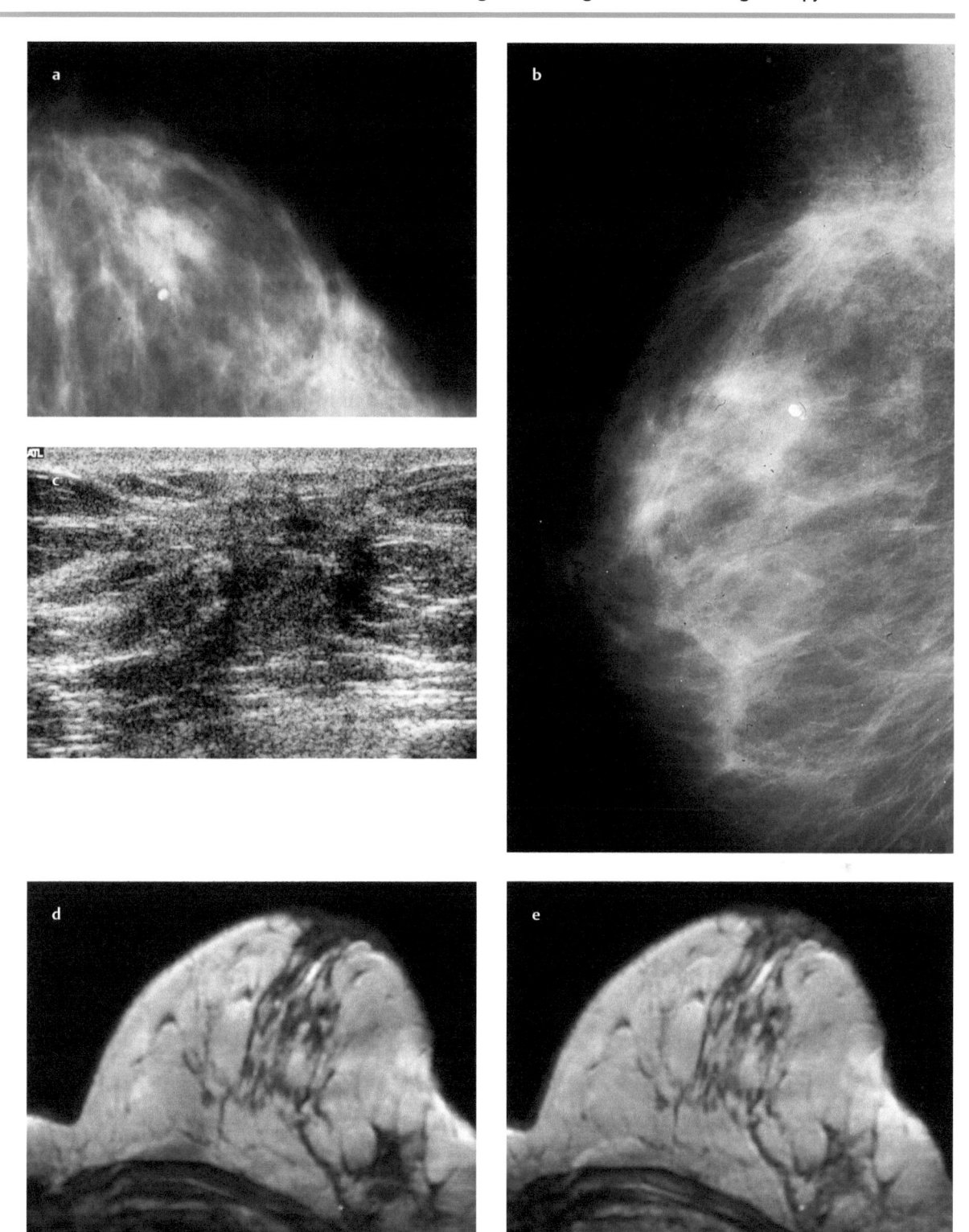

Fig. 19.16 a–e Indeterminate palpable finding in the region of the scar 14 months after breast-conserving therapy.

a,b Craniocaudal and mediolateral views (suboptimal positioning due to extensive scar formation): the central radiolucency within the scar is consistent with a scar rather than a recurrent cancer.

c On ultrasound the scar is imaged as an indeterminate hypoechoic area with some shadowing.

d Representative section through the scar region before administration of contrast medium.

e The same section after intravenous administration of Gd-DTPA shows no appreciable enhancement: no evidence of a recurrence. Conclusion confirmed by clinical–mammographic follow-up for more than 3 years.

parenchymal tissue enhances even less than normal mammary parenchyma. Supplemental MRI can detect very small recurrent tumors in dense or even irregularly structured tissue with great sensitivity (**Fig. 19.17b–d**), or exclude them with a high degree of certainty. Furthermore, MRI is generally able to visualize all the tissue including the chest wall. This is particularly advantageous in cases with severe scarring which is adhering to the chest wall. In such cases the significant parts of the scar may not be evaluated mammographically, since they cannot be adequately included on the mammogram (even with the best possible positioning).

Therefore, contrast-enhanced MRI is the ideal method to complement mammography for otherwise difficult-to-evaluate scar tissue and for solving problems more than 12 months after breast-conserving therapy. However, mammography remains the modality of choice to detect suspicious microcalcifications, should they develop.

Possibly owing to different radiation techniques and individually differing responses to radiation therapy, different observations have been reported during the first year after irradiation and the use of MRI during this period is controversial (Müller et al. 1998, Viehweg et al. 1998). We would recommend using MRI more than 12

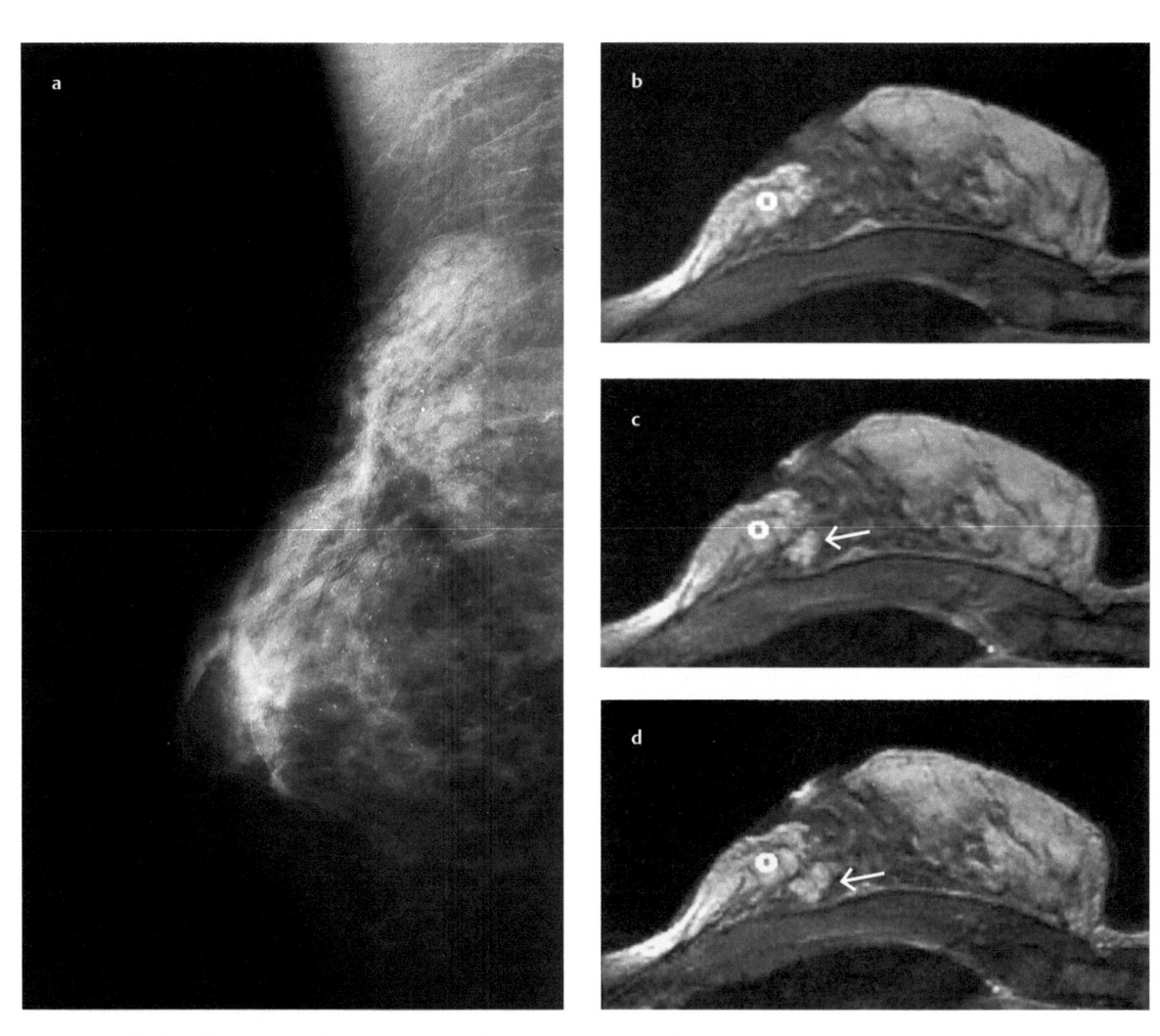

Fig. 19.17 a–d Clinically, status post breast-conserving therapy 5 years ago, unchanged palpable finding.

a The mammogram shows spiculation in the upper half of the breast at the lumpectomy site, unchanged since the previous examination, and diffuse microcalcifications known for years, unchanged (the primary tumor had no microcalcifications). Supplementary magnetic resonance imaging (MRI) was offered as part of a clinical trial.

b–d MRI: representative section through the scar before (**b**) as well as immediately after (0–5 min) (**c**), and delayed (6–11 min) (**d**) after Gd-DTPA. Suggestive focal enhancement (arrow) is apparent in the scar region. It characteristically enhances early and shows so-called washout (**d**). The focus discovered by MRI was excised after MR-guided localization. *Histology*: Recurrence of an invasive ductal carcinoma.

months after therapy, whenever possible. Only if severe diagnostic problems concerning the presence of residual tumor cannot be solved by conventional imaging should MRI be considered.

Percutaneous Biopsy

Percutaneous biopsy can be diagnostically helpful in the therapeutic decision, particularly since diagnostic excisional surgery on nonmalignant post-therapeutic changes should be avoided due to the possibility of impaired healing.

The patient should be informed that the rate of infectious complications may be increased, particularly early after irradiation. With percutaneous biopsy, however, fewer complications may be expected than with surgical biopsy.

Note:
- Accuracy can decrease in markedly fibrosed tissue due to needle deviation and insufficient or non-representative tissue.
- Histologic accuracy may be reduced owing to procuring smaller specimens in the presence of marked fibrosis or as a result of early post-therapeutic cellular changes (inflammation, necrosis).

If sampling is difficult on account of to severe scarring, a biopsy method that allows acquisition of sufficient tissue may be preferable. In the case of very small findings VABB may be preferable to core needle biopsy (Heywang-Köbrunner et al. 2009).

Thus—in experienced hands—percutaneous biopsy is able to differentiate recurrent cancer from fibrosis, fat necrosis, and granuloma with high accuracy.

> **Summary**
>
> Depending on whether a hematoma, seroma, or fat necrosis is present, acute post-traumatic and post-surgical changes can have a variable mammographic presentation. After plastic surgery the typical course of the scars should be known. Also, comparison with prior imaging is very helpful to achieve the best possible sensitivity and specificity within scarred tissue.
>
> If a malignancy (residual tumor) has to be excluded in freshly traumatized or surgical tissue, mammography should always be used. Its major contribution to the differential diagnosis concerns exclusion or demonstration of suspicious microcalcifications. However, carcinomas without microcalcifications may also be correctly diagnosed depending on the underlying post-therapeutic changes.
>
> Scar-related changes in their late stage after trauma or surgery (more than 3 months) or after radiation (more than 12 months) can cause characteristic mammographic features (architectural distortion or spiculated areas mostly without central density, coarse, or ringlike dystrophic calcifications) or sonographic phenomena (acoustic shadowing or hypoechoic areas). Because of architectural distortion following surgery and increased density following radiation, the overall evaluation can be compromised, and the differential diagnosis can pose problems. For the scarred breast following surgery as well as for the breast with radiation changes, mammography remains the primary diagnostic method, together with clinical examination.
>
> In addition to the selected use of additional projections, coned-down compression, and magnification views, an important diagnostic role is given to serial mammograms, whereby the accuracy can be improved by keeping exposure conditions constant.
>
> In the breast that is difficult to evaluate, the selected use of contrast-enhanced MRI is important. In particular, if the evaluation is impaired owing to increased density and scars, contrast-enhanced MRI permits a markedly improved and earlier detection of recurrence and a correct identification of scar-related fibrotic changes starting 1 year after radiotherapy. Furthermore, it usually allows inclusion of all the breast tissue including the chest wall, an area which, owing to scarring adhering to the chest wall, sometimes may not be possible to include on the mammogram.
>
> Percutaneous biopsy is the most important next step for differentiation of indeterminate or suspicious findings. As for other indications core needle biopsy is generally able to solve questions concerning lesions that can be visualized by ultrasound. Discrete indeterminate changes or microcalcifications may require more extended sampling. In these cases VABB may be the method of choice.

References and Recommended Reading

Barnsley GP, Grunfeld E, Coyle D, Paszat L. Surveillance mammography following the treatment of primary breast cancer with breast reconstruction: a systematic review. Plast Reconstr Surg 2007;120(5):1125–1132

Beer GM, Kompatscher P, Hergan K. Diagnosis of breast tumors after breast reduction. Aesthetic Plast Surg 1996;20(5):391–397

Belli P, Costantini M, Malaspina C, Magistrelli A, Latorre G, Bonomo L. MRI accuracy in residual disease evaluation in breast cancer patients treated with neoadjuvant chemotherapy. Clin Radiol 2006;61(11):946–953

Bock E, Bock C, Belli P, Campioni P, Manfredi R, Pastore G. Role of diagnostic imaging of the breast in patients treated with postsurgical radiotherapy or presurgical radiotherapy or chemotherapy. [Article in Italian] Radiol Med (Torino) 1998;95(1-2):38–43

Dao TH, Rahmouni A, Campana F, Laurent M, Asselain B, Fourquet A. Tumor recurrence versus fibrosis in the irradiated breast: differentiation with dynamic gadolinium-enhanced MR imaging. Radiology 1993;187(3):751–755

Denis F, Desbiez-Bourcier AV, Chapiron C, Arbion F, Body G, Brunereau L. Contrast enhanced magnetic resonance imaging underestimates residual disease following neoadjuvant docetaxel based chemotherapy for breast cancer. Eur J Surg Oncol 2004;30(10):1069–1076

Dershaw DD. Mammography in patients with breast cancer treated by breast conservation (lumpectomy with or without radiation). AJR Am J Roentgenol 1995;164(2):309–316

Drew PJ, Kerin MJ, Turnbull LW, et al. Routine screening for local recurrence following breast-conserving therapy for cancer with dynamic contrast-enhanced magnetic resonance imaging of the breast. Ann Surg Oncol 1998;5(3):265–270

Eidelman Y, Liebling RW, Buchbinder S, Strauch B, Goldstein RD. Mammography in the evaluation of masses in breasts reconstructed with TRAM flaps. Ann Plast Surg 1998;41(3):229–233

Fisher B, Anderson S, Bryant J, et al. Twenty-year follow-up of a randomized trial comparing total mastectomy, lumpectomy, and lumpectomy plus irradiation for the treatment of invasive breast cancer. N Engl J Med 2002;347(16):1233–1241

Flamm CR, Ziegler KM, Aronson N. Technology Evaluation Center assessment synopsis: use of magnetic resonance imaging to avoid a biopsy in women with suspicious primary breast lesions. J Am Coll Radiol 2005;2(6):485–487

Ghossein NA, Alpert S, Barba J, et al. Breast cancer. Importance of adequate surgical excision prior to radiotherapy in the local control of breast cancer in patients treated conservatively. Arch Surg 1992;127(4):411–415

Giess CS, Keating DM, Osborne MP, Rosenblatt R. Local tumor recurrence following breast-conservation therapy: correlation of histopathologic findings with detection method and mammographic findings. Radiology 1999;212(3):829–835

Gilles R, Guinebretière JM, Shapeero LG, et al. Assessment of breast cancer recurrence with contrast-enhanced subtraction MR imaging: preliminary results in 26 patients. Radiology 1993;188(2):473–478

Gluck BS, Dershaw DD, Liberman L, Deutch BM. Microcalcifications on postoperative mammograms as an indicator of adequacy of tumor excision. Radiology 1993;188(2):469–472

Godinez J, Gombos EC, Chikarmane SA, Griffin GK, Birdwell RL. Breast MRI in the evaluation of eligibility for accelerated partial breast irradiation. AJR Am J Roentgenol 2008;191(1):272–277

Grosse A, Schreer I, Frischbier HJ, et al. Results of breast conserving therapy for early breast cancer and the role of mammographic follow-up. Int J Radiat Oncol Biol Phys 1997;38(4):761–767

Günhan-Bilgen I, Oktay A. Mammographic features of local recurrence after conservative surgery and radiation therapy: comparison with that of the primary tumor. Acta Radiol 2007;48(4):390–397

Harrison RL, Britton P, Warren R, Bobrow L. Can we be sure about a radiological diagnosis of fat necrosis of the breast? Clin Radiol 2000;55(2):119–123

Harvey JA, Moran RE, Maurer EJ, DeAngelis GA. Sonographic features of mammary oil cysts. J Ultrasound Med 1997;16(11):719–724

Hattangadi J, Park C, Rembert J, et al. Breast stromal enhancement on MRI is associated with response to neoadjuvant chemotherapy. AJR Am J Roentgenol 2008;190(6):1630–1636

Heywang-Köbrunner SH, Beck R. Contrast-Enhanced MRI of the Breast. Heidelberg, New York: Springer; 1996

Heywang-Köbrunner SH, Schlegel A, Beck R, et al. Contrast-enhanced MRI of the breast after limited surgery and radiation therapy. J Comput Assist Tomogr 1993;17(6):891–900

Heywang-Köbrunner SH, Heinig A, Hellerhoff K, Holzhausen HJ, Nährig J. Use of ultrasound-guided percutaneous vacuum-assisted breast biopsy for selected difficult indications. Breast J 2009;15(4):348–356

Hogge JP, Zuurbier RA, de Paredes ES. Mammography of autologous myocutaneous flaps. Radiographics 1999;19(Spec No):S63–S72

Holli K, Saaristo R, Isola J, Hyöty M, Hakama M. Effect of radiotherapy on the interpretation of routine follow-up mammography after conservative breast surgery: a randomized study. Br J Cancer 1998;78(4):542–545

Houssami N, Ciatto S, Martinelli F, Bonardi R, Duffy SW. Early detection of second breast cancers improves prognosis in breast cancer survivors. Ann Oncol 2009;20(9):1505–1510

Houssami N, Macaskill P, Marinovich ML, et al. Meta-analysis of the impact of surgical margins on local recurrence in women with early-stage invasive breast cancer treated with breast-conserving therapy. Eur J Cancer 2010;46(18):3219–3232

Houssami N, Abraham LA, Miglioretti DL, et al. Accuracy and outcomes of screening mammography in women with a personal history of early-stage breast cancer. JAMA 2011;305(8):790–799

Kaufmann M, Minckwitz G, Bear HD, et al. Recommendations from an international expert panel on the use of neoadjuvant (primary) systemic treatment of operable breast cancer: new perspectives 2006. Ann Oncol 2007;18(12):1927–1934

Khatcheressian JL, Wolff AC, Smith TJ, et al; American Society of Clinical Oncology. American Society of Clinical Oncology 2006 update of the breast cancer follow-up and management guidelines in the adjuvant setting. J Clin Oncol 2006;24(31):5091–5097

Kim HJ, Im YH, Han BK, et al. Accuracy of MRI for estimating residual tumor size after neoadjuvant chemotherapy in locally advanced breast cancer: relation to response patterns on MRI. Acta Oncol 2007;46(7):996–1003

Kim SJ, Moon WK, Cho N, Chang JM. The detection of recurrent breast cancer in patients with a history of breast cancer surgery: comparison of clinical breast examination, mammography and ultrasonography. Acta Radiol 2011;52(1):15–20

Kontos M, Allen DS, Agbaje OF, Hamed H, Fentiman IS. Factors influencing loco-regional relapse in older breast cancer patients treated with tumour resection and tamoxifen. Eur J Surg Oncol 2011;37(12):1051–1058

Krämer S, Schulz-Wendtland R, Hagedorn K, Bautz W, Lang N. Magnetic resonance imaging in the diagnosis of local recurrences in breast cancer. Anticancer Res 1998;18(3C):2159–2161

Krishnamurty R, Whitman GJ, Stelling CB, Kushwaha AC. Mammographic findings after breast conservation therapy. Radiographics 1999;19(Spec No):S53–S62; quiz S262–S263

Lee CH, Dershaw DD, Kopans D, et al. Breast cancer screening with imaging: recommendations from the Society of Breast Imaging and the ACR on the use of mammography, breast MRI, breast ultrasound, and other technologies for the detection of clinically occult breast cancer. J Am Coll Radiol 2010;7(1):18–27

Leibman AJ, Styblo TM, Bostwick J III. Mammography of the postreconstruction breast. Plast Reconstr Surg 1997;99(3):698–704

Lewis-Jones HG, Whitehouse GH, Leinster SJ. The role of magnetic resonance imaging in the assessment of local recurrent breast carcinoma. Clin Radiol 1991;43(3):197–204

Lin K, Eradat J, Mehta NH, et al. Is a short-interval postradiation mammogram necessary after conservative surgery and radiation in breast cancer? Int J Radiat Oncol Biol Phys 2008;72(4):1041–1047

Mandrekas AD, Assimakopoulos GI, Mastorakos DP, Pantzalis K. Fat necrosis following breast reduction. Br J Plast Surg 1994;47(8):560–562

Montgomery DA, Krupa K, Jack WJ, et al. Changing pattern of the detection of locoregional relapse in breast cancer: the Edinburgh experience. Br J Cancer 2007;96(12):1802–1807

Müller RD, Barkhausen J, Sauerwein W, Langer R. Assessment of local recurrence after breast-conserving therapy with MRI. J Comput Assist Tomogr 1998;22(3):408–412

Mussurakis S, Buckley DL, Bowsley SJ, et al. Dynamic contrast-enhanced magnetic resonance imaging of the breast combined with pharmacokinetic analysis of gadolinium-DTPA uptake in the diagnosis of local recurrence of early stage breast carcinoma. Invest Radiol 1995;30(11):650–662

Nakamura S, Kenjo H, Nishio T, Kazama T, Doi O, Suzuki K. Efficacy of 3D-MR mammography for breast conserving surgery after neoadjuvant chemotherapy. Breast Cancer 2002;9(1):15–19

National Institute for Health and Clinical Excellence, National Collaborating Centre for Primary Care. Clinical Guideline 80. Breast cancer (early and locally advanced): diagnosis and treatment. London: National Institute for Health and Clinical Excellence (www.nice.org.uk); 2006

Orel SG, Reynolds C, Schnall MD, Solin LJ, Fraker DL, Sullivan DC. Breast carcinoma: MR imaging before re-excisional biopsy. Radiology 1997;205(2):429–436

Pinsky RW, Rebner M, Pierce LJ, et al. Recurrent cancer after breast-conserving surgery with radiation therapy for ductal carcinoma in situ: mammographic features, method of detection, and stage of recurrence. AJR Am J Roentgenol 2007;189(1):140–144

Poggi MM, Danforth DN, Sciuto LC, et al. Eighteen-year results in the treatment of early breast carcinoma with mastectomy versus breast conservation therapy: the National Cancer Institute Randomized Trial. Cancer 2003;98(4):697–702

Ruch M, Brade J, Schoeber C, et al. Long-term follow-up findings in mammography and ultrasound after intraoperative radiotherapy (IORT) for breast cancer. Breast 2009;18(5):327–334

Sardanelli F, Boetes C, Borisch B, et al. Magnetic resonance imaging of the breast: recommendations from the EUSOMA working group. Eur J Cancer 2010;46(8):1296–1316

Sidibé S, Coulibaly A, Traoré S, Touré M, Traoré I. Role of ultrasonography in the diagnosis of axillary lymph node metastases in breast cancer: a systematic review. [Article in French] Mali Med 2007;22(4):9–13

Soderstrom CE, Harms SE, Farrell RS Jr, Pruneda JM, Flamig DP. Detection with MR imaging of residual tumor in the breast soon after surgery. AJR Am J Roentgenol 1997;168(2):485–488

Soo MS, Kornguth PJ, Hertzberg BS. Fat necrosis in the breast: sonographic features. Radiology 1998;206(1):261–269

Tendulkar RD, Chellman-Jeffers M, Rybicki LA, et al. Preoperative breast magnetic resonance imaging in early breast cancer: implications for partial breast irradiation. Cancer 2009;115(8):1621–1630

Untch M, Thomssen C, Costa SD, Eds. Colloquium Senologie 2011. [Article in German] Munich: Aegileum Verlag; 2011

van Dongen JA, Voogd AC, Fentiman IS, et al. Long-term results of a randomized trial comparing breast-conserving therapy with mastectomy: European Organization for Research and Treatment of Cancer 10801 trial. J Natl Cancer Inst 2000;92(14):1143–1150

Veronesi U, Cascinelli N, Mariani L, et al. Twenty-year follow-up of a randomized study comparing breast-conserving surgery with radical mastectomy for early breast cancer. N Engl J Med 2002;347(16):1227–1232

Viehweg P, Heinig A, Lampe D, Buchmann J, Heywang-Köbrunner SH. Retrospective analysis for evaluation of the value of contrast-enhanced MRI in patients treated with breast conservative therapy. MAGMA 1998;7(3):141–152

Voogd AC, van Tienhoven G, Peterse HL, et al. Local recurrence after breast conservation therapy for early stage breast carcinoma: detection, treatment, and outcome in 266 patients. Dutch Study Group on Local Recurrence after Breast Conservation (BORST). Cancer 1999;85(2):437–446

Wöckel A, Kreienberg R. First Revision of the German S3 Guideline 'Diagnosis, Therapy, and Follow-Up of Breast Cancer'. Breast Care (Basel) 2008;3(2):82–86

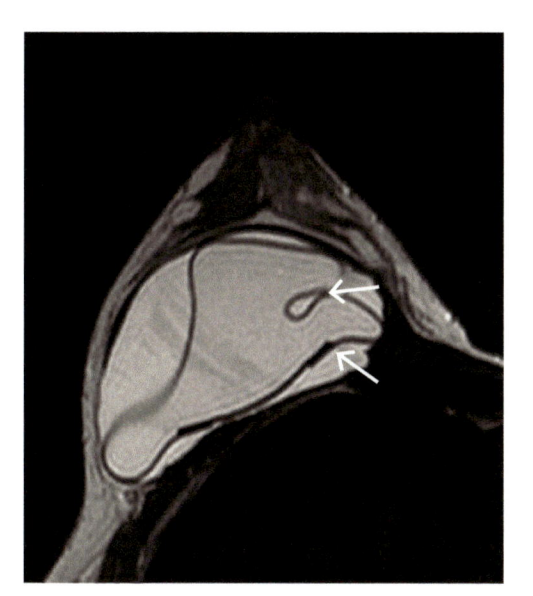

20 Radiologic Assessment of Women with Breast Implants

Types of Implants → *534*
Structure → *534*

Anatomy → *535*

Imaging → *535*
Mammography → *535*
Ultrasound → *539*
Magnetic Resonance Imaging → *540*
Histopathologic Assessment in Women with Implants → *540*

Complications of Breast Implants → *541*
Surveillance of Women with an Implant Following Oncoplastic Surgery → *544*
Screening of Asymptomatic Women who have had Breast Augmentation → *547*
Imaging Assessment of Women with Implants after Oncoplastic Surgery → *547*
Imaging Assessment of Women after Augmentation Implant → *547*
Histopathologic Assessment in Women with Implants → *547*

References and Recommended Reading → *552*

20 Radiologic Assessment of Women with Breast Implants

S. Barter, S. H. Heywang-Koebrunner

Cosmetic augmentation of the breast with implants is performed widely, and breast reconstruction using implants is increasingly offered to women who need surgery for breast cancer. Imaging of women with breast implants presents a challenge to the radiologist.

There are four main scenarios in which imaging is utilized:
1. Assessment of women presenting symptomatically with a breast lump
2. Assessment of the implant for complications and possible rupture
3. Surveillance of women with an implant following oncoplastic surgery
4. Screening of asymptomatic women who have had breast augmentation

It is important to understand the different types of implant available, their possible location, and their composition to understand normal and abnormal imaging appearances.

Types of Implants

There are many different designs and manufacturers of breast implants, but their contents fall into four basic types: Saline filled, silicone gel filled, filled with a combination of saline and silicone, and filled with an alternative (e.g., soybean oil). At least 14 different types of implants have been classified, and women should be informed about the type of implanted prostheses by the plastic surgeon and written information should be available for the radiologist, but in practice this is rarely the case.

Structure

- Implants may be single, double, or even triple lumen, and smooth or textured.
- Saline implants have a silicone shell, and have a less natural feel.
- Folds and valves are normal findings on imaging—not to be confused with leakage.
- Double lumen implants have a chamber within a chamber, usually consisting of an outer chamber of silicone and an inner chamber of saline.

Saline-Filled Breast Implants

The three types of saline-filled breast implants are as follows:
- One type is a single lumen implant that is filled during the operation with a fixed volume of saline through a valve. There are no adjustments to the saline volume after surgery.
- A second type is a single lumen implant that is filled during the operation with saline through a valve. This type of implant allows for adjustments of the saline volume after the operation.
- A third type is a single lumen implant that is prefilled by the manufacturer with a fixed volume of saline. There are no valves for filling during the operation or for adjustments of the saline volume after the operation. Saline-filled breast implants have a silicone rubber shell.

Silicone Gel-Filled Breast Implants

The three types of silicone gel-filled breast implants are as follows:
- One type is a single lumen implant that is prefilled by the manufacturer with a fixed volume of silicone gel.
- A second type is a double lumen implant with (1) an inner lumen prefilled by the manufacturer with a fixed volume of silicone gel, and (2) an outer lumen that is filled during the operation with a fixed volume of saline through a valve.
- A third type is a double lumen implant with (1) an outer lumen prefilled by the manufacturer with a fixed volume of silicone gel, and (2) an inner lumen that is filled during the operation with saline through a valve. This type of implant allows for adjustments of the saline volume after the operation.

In double lumen implants the signal intensity of the two chambers usually differs.

A silicone gel-filled breast implant has a silicone rubber shell with the same general composition as the saline-filled breast implant.

Alternative Breast Implants

An alternative breast implant typically has a silicone rubber shell with a filler made from soya bean oil rather than saline or silicone gel. The filler material may or may not be a gel.

Collagen or silicone has been injected freely into the breast in the past, and a new method of breast augmentation has recently been introduced whereby hyaluronic acid (Macrolane, Restylane) or free polyacrylamide gel is injected into the breast. Free injection of filler material produces a bizarre appearance on mammography and ultrasound scan making interpretation very difficult for the radiologist (**Fig. 20.1**).

Anatomy

Implants can be placed in one of two areas, retroglandular or subpectoral. Seventy-five percent of breast implants are retroglandular, the remaining 25% of implants are subpectoral (**Fig. 20.2**).

Imaging

(See **Fig. 20.3**.)

Mammography

In women who received implants for reconstruction after mastectomy, the layer of skin and subcutaneous tissue is mostly very thin and may therefore not allow performance of a mammogram of adequate quality. Therefore mammography is usually not performed for surveillance in patients after mastectomy.

If, however, only a partial mastectomy has been performed and significant amounts of residual tissue exist, mammographic surveillance should be considered and attempted.

In symptomatic cases mammography is indicated. If mammography is impossible due to the tissue covering the implant being too thin, special mammographic views should be attempted in addition to or instead of the usual ones. Whatever special view or angulation is chosen, the only goal is to optimally include the area of concern with as little overlap by the implant as possible. Thus special mammographic views have to be adapted to the individual anatomy. As in women without implants, mammography can demonstrate or exclude suspicious microcalcifications or other findings indicative of malig-

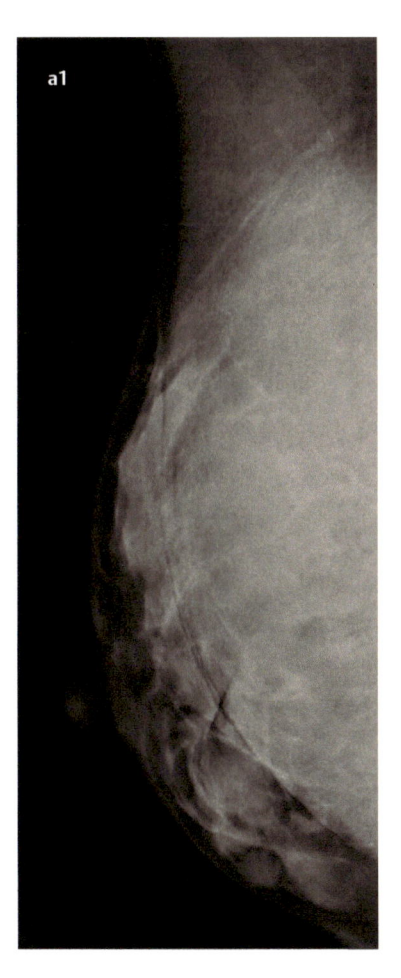

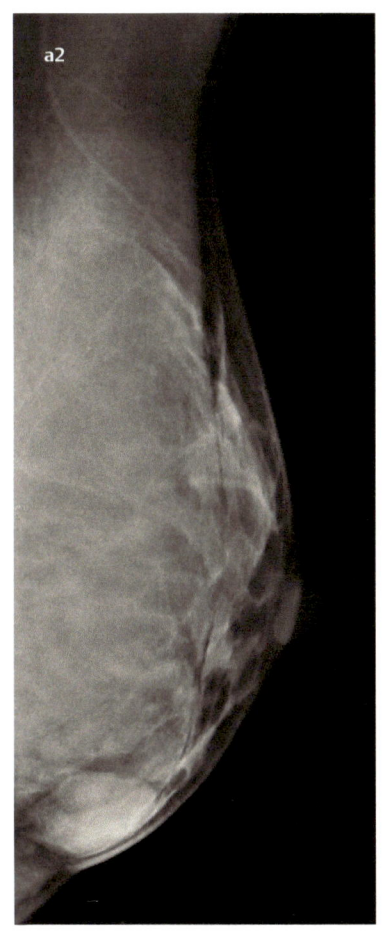

Fig. 20.1a–e

a,b Mammograms (**a**) and ultrasound (**b**) of a patient with a hyaluronic filler (Macrolane) injected into the breast.

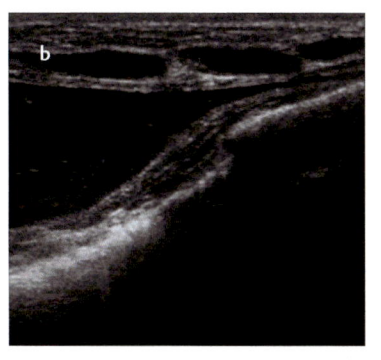

Fig. 20.1c–e ▷

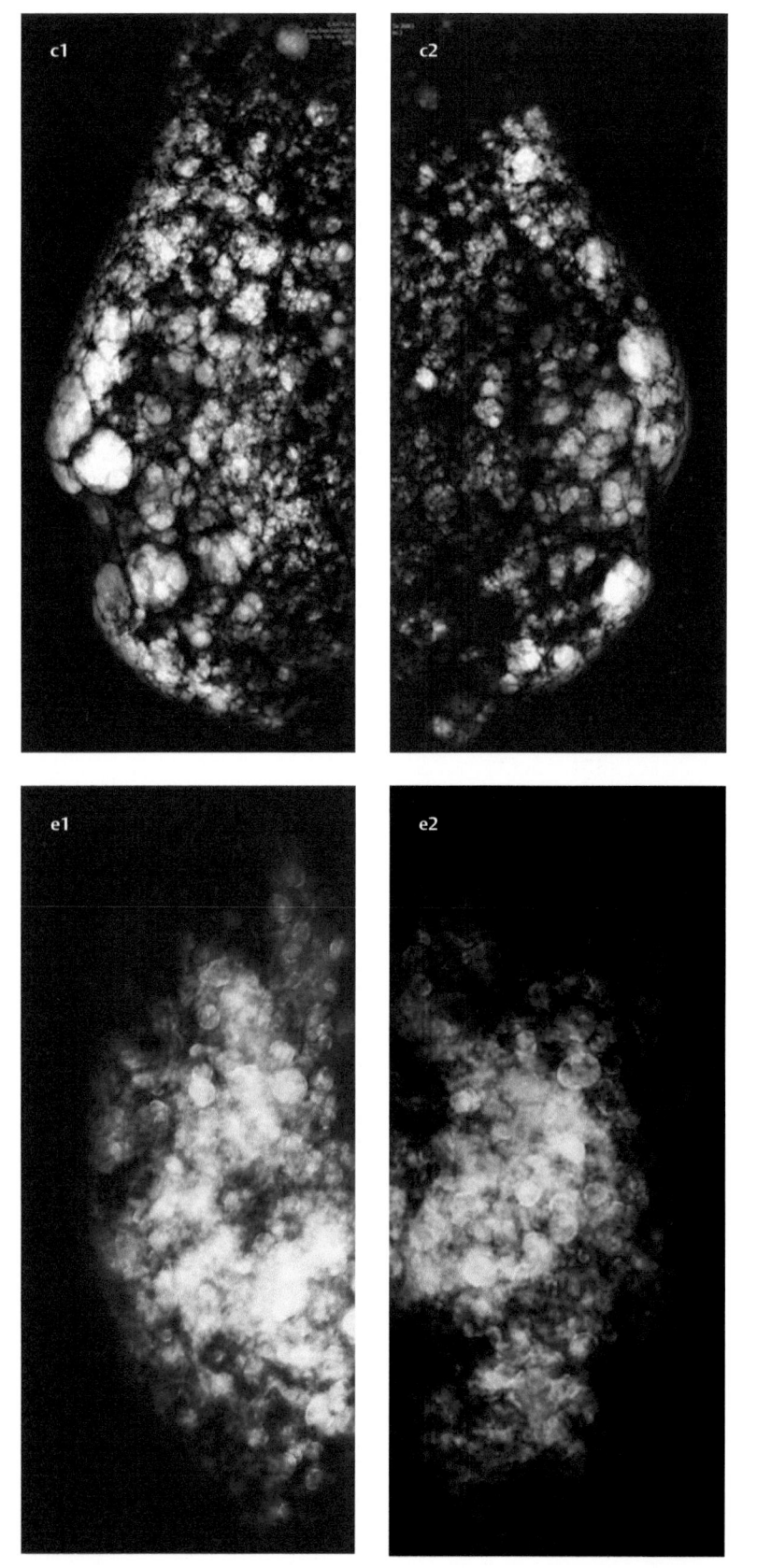

20 Radiologic Assessment of Women with Breast Implants

◁ continued

c,d Mammographic (**c1,c2**) and ultrasound (**d**) appearances of breast augmentation following injection of free collagen.

e Mammograms of a patient with free silicone breast augmentation. Interpretation following such procedures is almost impossible.

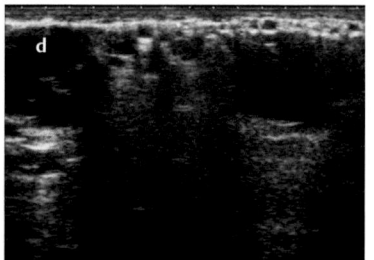

Imaging

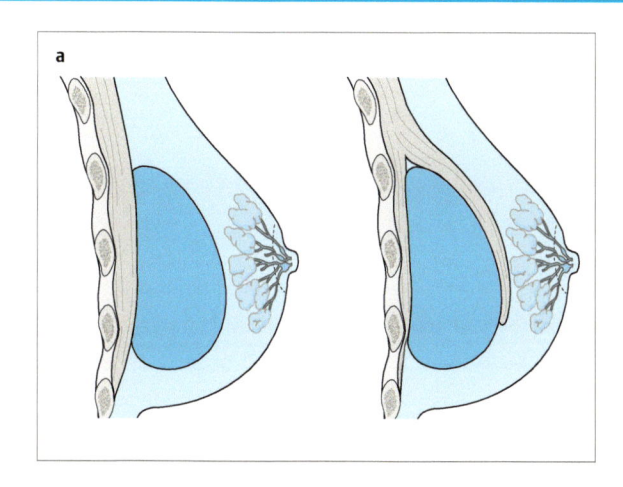

Fig. 20.2a–c

a Diagram showing subglandular and subpectoral location of implants.

b,c Mammograms (**b**: mediolateral oblique view using standard technique; **c**: craniocaudal view using Eklund technique) showing subpectoral implants. Arrows show pectoral muscle overlying implant.

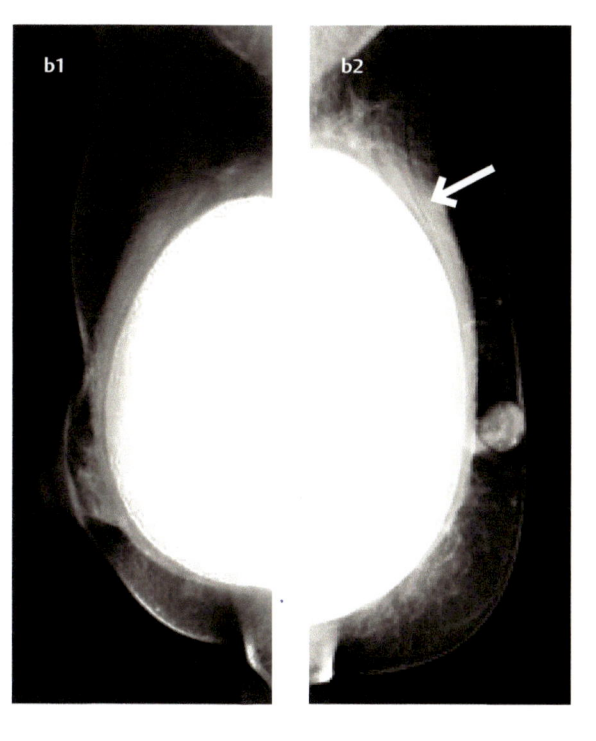

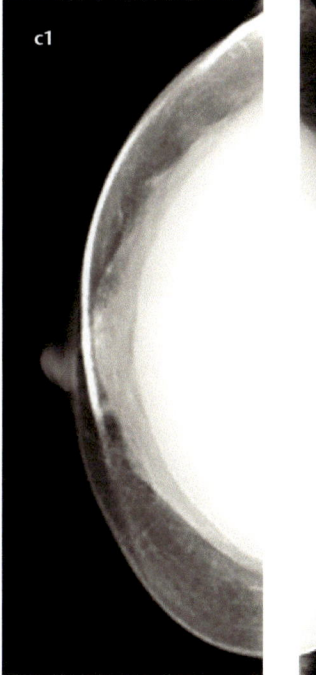

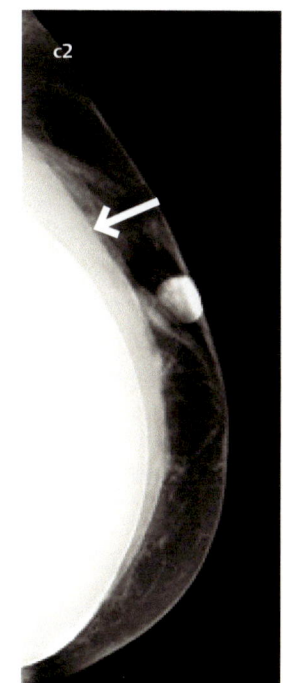

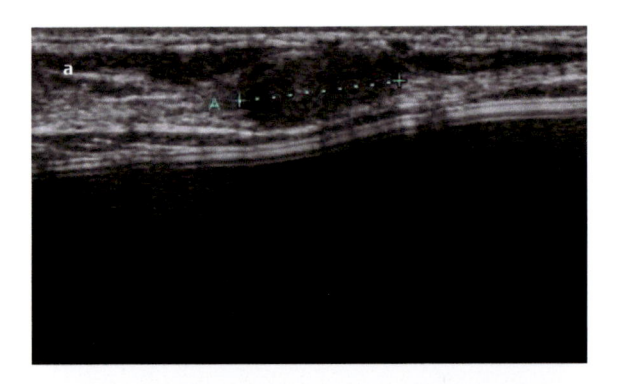

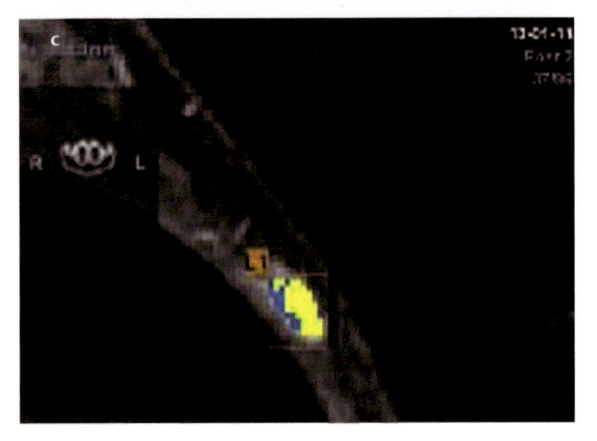

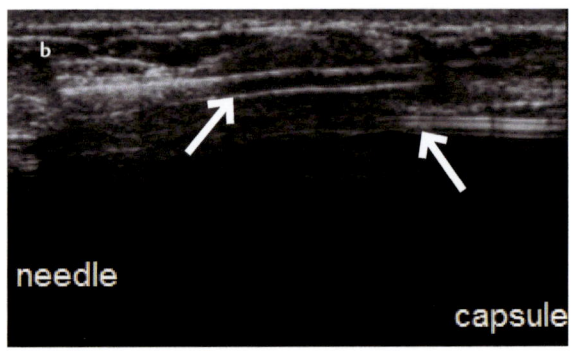

Fig. 20.3a–c Triple assessment of a 49-year-old woman with breast implants and a palpable mass in the left upper outer quadrant. Mammograms failed to show an abnormality.
a Ultrasound shows a poorly defined 8-mm mass.
b Note how the needle is directed away from the implant capsule during ultrasound-guided biopsy.
c Magnetic resonance images showing an 8-mm enhancing mass. *Histology*: invasive lobular carcinoma.

nancy. Or it may help to identify a benign change such as a typically calcified fibroadenoma or a pathognomonic oil cyst, for example.

Mammography is indicated for assessment of symptomatic women with implants *after augmentation.* Implants are not a contraindication for screening of women after augmentation mammoplasty, although the sensitivity of screening will be reduced. The X-rays used for mammographic imaging of the breasts cannot penetrate silicone or saline implants well enough to image the overlying or underlying breast tissue. Therefore, some breast tissue (~25%) will not be seen on the mammogram, as it will be covered up by the implant.

However, special techniques for augmented breasts have been developed to maximize the amount of breast tissue visualized if implants are present. The Eklund technique (see Chapter 3) should be employed wherever possible to maximize the amount of breast tissue visualized. (**Fig. 3.29**)

To visualize as much breast tissue as possible, women with implants may undergo additional views as well as the four standard images taken during diagnostic mammography. Conventional oblique and superior–inferior views may be supplemented with a lateral and Eklund technique (implant displacement view). In the Eklund technique the implant is pushed back against the chest wall and the breast is pulled forward over it. This allows better imaging of the anterior part of each breast (**Fig. 20.4**).

Implant ruptures may occur very occasionally following mammography.

Some increased risk of implant rupture has been described in women with very old implants (> 10–15 years) and in women with fixed implants that cannot be mobilized.

When association of an implant rupture with a preceding mammogram is considered, it should be remembered that the average mammogram generates less than 4 psi. The examining finger generates about 6 psi. Old implants may be leaky anyway. Leakage of silicone through the pores of an implant is called "sweating." Furthermore old implants may also be fragile.

When an association between mammography and implant rupture is suspected, a correlation of onset of symptoms (during or shortly after a mammogram) should be assured.

The patient should generally be informed that (depending on the individual anatomy) even with adequate technique up to 25% of the tissue cannot be visualized. She should also understand that nevertheless mammography remains the best method to screen for breast cancer (except for high-risk groups). She should know that there exists a small risk of rupture with mammography, which appears to be very low for intact implants.

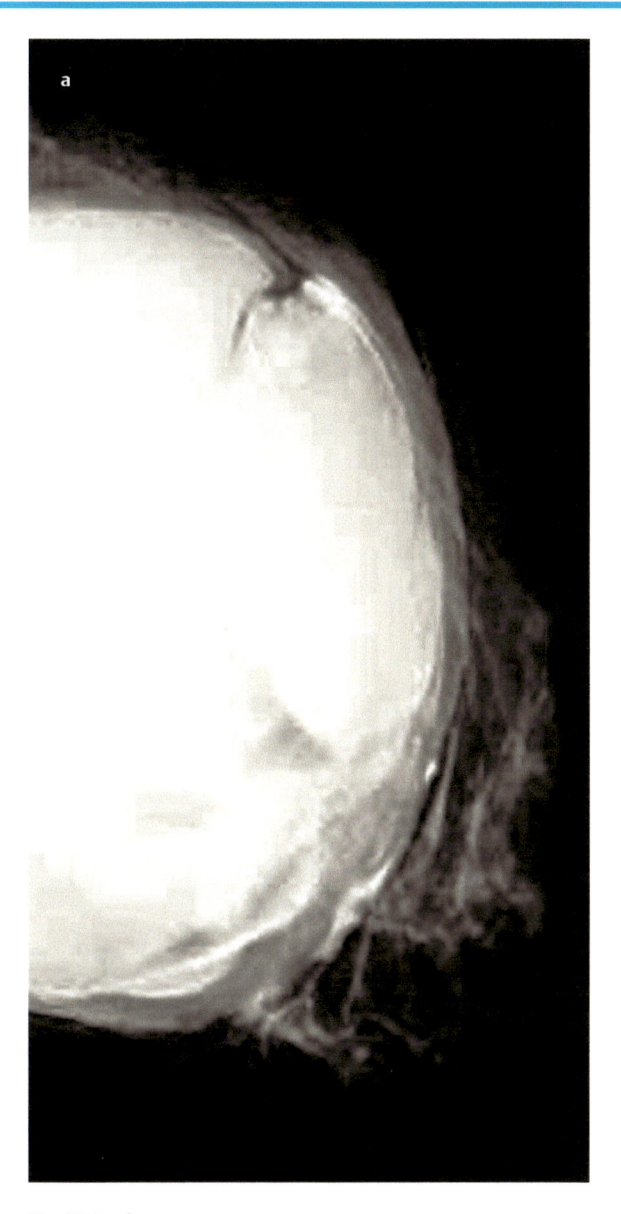

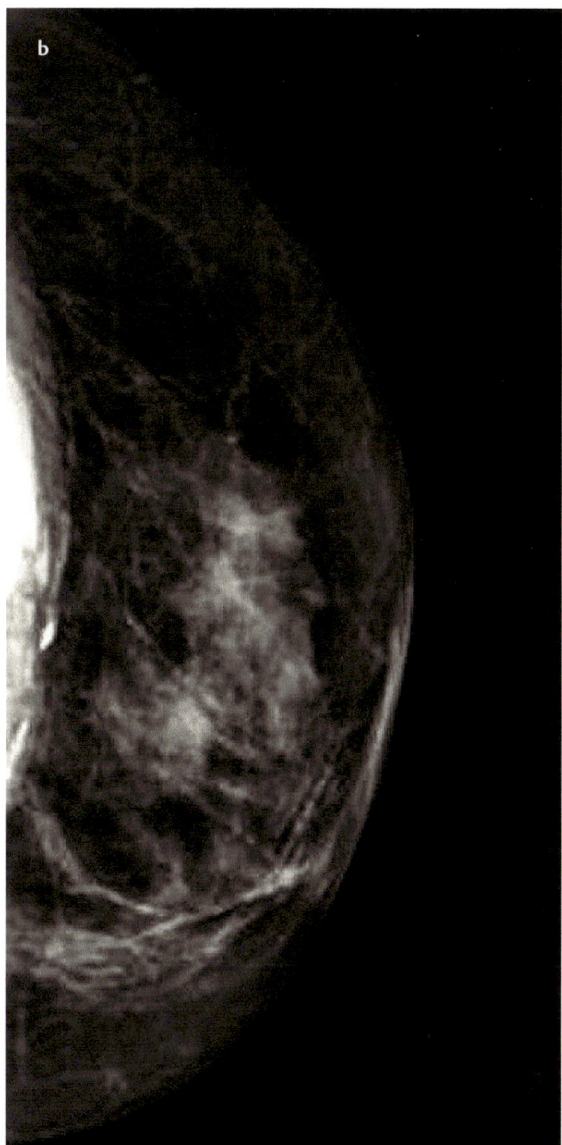

Fig. 20.4a–b

a,b Mammograms showing effect of the Eklund technique (see also **Fig. 3.29** and pp. 71–72): Without implant displacement (**a**); with implant displacement (**b**). Note calcification of implant capsule.

Ultrasound

Ultrasound is indicated in assessment of women with implants who present with a focal abnormality, and it may be considered to complement mammography in women in whom large parts of the breast tissue are obscured on the screening mammogram. So far it is not (yet) generally standard to recommend ultrasound for screening of implants.

It is indicated for early complications of implant insertion, e.g. infection, hematoma.

Ultrasound may be used for the detection of implant rupture or leakage, but is not as sensitive or specific as magnetic resonance imaging (MRI) for detection of implant rupture (Steinbach et al. 1993).

When ultrasound imaging is performed, it should be attempted to include the chest wall. However, depending on the size of the implant and owing to shadowing behind the implant it is often impossible to reliably evaluate tissue behind the implant. Scarring can mostly be identified correctly, since scarring is in most cases discrete. Also, shadowing or hypoechoic areas due to scarring often show a connection to the scar of the skin. In cases with extensive scarring (after surgical complications or in patients with focal fibrosis or granulomas) assessment may be severely impaired by shadowing and hypoechoic tissue. Overall, ultrasound is less sensitive than MRI and it cannot distinguish reliably between nodular scarring or granuloma and malignancy, which in many cases is possible by MRI. Even though Doppler ultrasound has been suggested for distinguishing between scarring and malignancy, according to our experience this distinction is unreliable.

Magnetic Resonance Imaging

For evaluation of implant integrity, MRI without contrast agent is sufficient. The usual unenhanced MRI study should be performed using thin slices and high resolution and at least two different orientations. If implant rupture is suspected or fluid is detected between the implant shell and the fibrous capsule, silicone-only and water-only or silicone-suppressed images should be used to distinguish between silicone leakage or "sweating of the implant" and other fluid collections.

Contrast-enhanced breast MRI is needed to detect or exclude malignancy. For this purpose the usual dynamic sequences with fat suppression or subtraction technique should be acquired. Unless cardiac artifacts can be adequately suppressed by spiral image acquisition or other types of artifact suppression, coronal imaging should be preferred to transverse imaging, since with transverse image acquisition the cardiac artifact usually crosses either the left breast (phase encoding anterior–posterior) or both axillas (phase encoding left–right). This can be avoided with coronal image acquisition, as here phase encoding can be chosen in the craniocaudal direction. With this technique, cardiac artifacts cross neither the axilla nor the breast. This issue is important, since the implants are usually fixed to the chest wall and thus reach further posteriorly in the prone position than breast tissue does.

For further details of this technique see Chapter 5.

The EUSOMA group has made the following evidence-based recommendations regarding breast MRI for women with implants (Sardanelli et al. 2010):
1. MRI is not recommended as a screening tool for implant rupture in asymptomatic women with breast implants. (Considering that implants or implant leakage is associated neither with an increased rate of breast cancer nor with any type of generalized disease such as autoimmune disease or reaction, there is no general indication for increased surveillance for breast cancer or for leakage due to the implant).
2. In patients with symptoms suggesting of implant rupture (pain, asymmetry, change in shape, etc.), after conventional imaging, noncontrast MRI is recommended to confirm or exclude rupture. This recommendation is based on the much higher sensitivity and specificity of MRI for implant rupture or leakage compared with mammography or ultrasound.
3. In patients with implants and signs/symptoms of parenchymal disease (e.g., breast lump), when conventional imaging is not diagnostic, noncontrast MRI and dynamic contrast-enhanced MRI are indicated to exclude implant rupture and to evaluate the breast gland parenchyma. This recommendation is based on literature showing a higher sensitivity and specificity of contrast-enhanced MRI compared with all other imaging modalities for this special indication. It may be explained by tomographic imaging and the excellent distinction of scarring and invasive malignancy by contrast-enhanced MRI (Boné et al. 1995, Heinig et al. 1997, Belli et al. 2002).
4. In symptomatic patients who have undergone breast augmentation with direct polyacrylamide gel injection, noncontrast MRI and dynamic contrast-enhanced MRI are indicated.

Therefore MRI is indicated for problem-solving in a woman who presents with a focal abnormality where triple assessment has failed to resolve the diagnosis. It is considered by many as the "gold standard" for assessment of implant rupture.

Histopathologic Assessment in Women with Implants

Ultrasound-guided biopsy is invaluable in women with implants, as it is for other indications.

When performing percutaneous breast biopsy, the needle path should be parallel to the implant. For firing the needle tip should be guided away from the implant capsule (Fig. 20.3b).

If suspicious microcalcifications only are detected in a woman with an implant, vacuum-assisted breast biopsy under stereotactic guidance may be possible if an angulation exists that allows separation of the implant from the suspicious area. In this case we recommend insertion of the needle at the side of the suspicious area that is proximal to the implant and cutting and suction toward the side distal to the implant.

If a lesion cannot be approached by percutaneous breast biopsy, MRI may be helpful for additional evaluation. Unless the probability of malignancy is very low, surgical biopsy after adequate marking may be needed.

Any lesion that can be visualized by ultrasound can usually be marked using ultrasound guidance. If this is impossible without risking injury to the implant, however, it may be useful to mark the skin that directly overlies the lesion. (In such cases the space between skin and implant is usually very thin. The surgeon should be instructed to excise all the tissue between the skin mark and the implant.) For lesions visible by mammography alone, mammographically guided marking is necessary. In patients with little tissue, manual marking may be preferable to a stereotactic approach, since the former approach can be better adapted to the individual anatomy. Marking of the skin is another option, if the lesion is situated directly between the skin and the implant. If a lesion is visualized only by MRI, marking with the usual breast biopsy coil may be difficult, since using this approach the needle path mostly will point toward the implant. In such cases either skin marking may be considered, if skin adjacent to the lesion can be approached under MR-guidance. Alternatively, marking under computed tomographic guidance may be an option (see Chapter 8).

Before any intervention patients should be informed about possible complications (see Chapters 7 and 8), which in patients with implants may also include injury to the implant.

Complications of Breast Implants

1. Hematoma and Infection

Hematoma and infection can occur in the early postoperative period and are best assessed by ultrasound with aspiration of any collection for bacterial analysis.

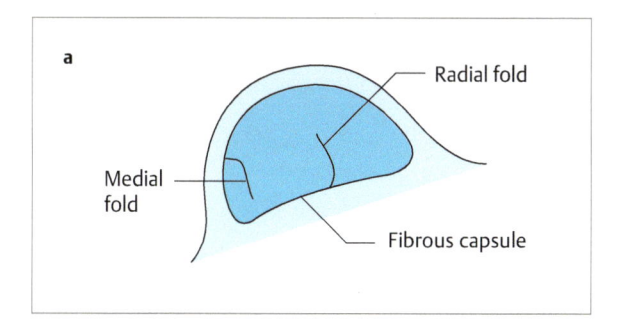

2. Capsule Contracture

Formation of a fibrous capsule is a normal process.

Within the first year after surgery the body produces a capsule of firm fibrosis that surrounds the implant. This fibrotic capsule is usually thicker than the outer capsule of the implant and is directly adjacent to it. Therefore, on imaging the outer capsule of the implant is usually not distinguishable from the thick, adjacent fibrotic capsule.

With time the capsule of the body tends to shrink. This may cause radial folds in the implant. These radial folds extend from the surface and run in a radial direction toward the center of the implant. Radial folds are a normal finding (Steinbach et al. 1993) (**Fig. 20.5**).

If fibrotic shrinkage continues, a *pathologic capsular contracture* may result. This will affect the shape of the breast and may cause increasing pain. According to Baker clinicians distinguish four degrees (Baker I: Soft breast no significant scarring; Baker II: Contracture palpable but not visible; Baker III: Visible and palpable hardening; deformed shape; Baker IV: Visible and palpable hardening, very painful). Open capsulotomy or implant removal may be indicated depending on the severity of the symptoms (see **Fig. 20.4c,d**).

Sometimes capsular contracture may be associated with increased calcification of the capsule.

On imaging a rounded implant indicates shrinkage of volume and is often the only sign of capsular fibro-

Fig. 20.5a,b Diagram and MRI showing radial folds (arrows), not to be confused with rupture.

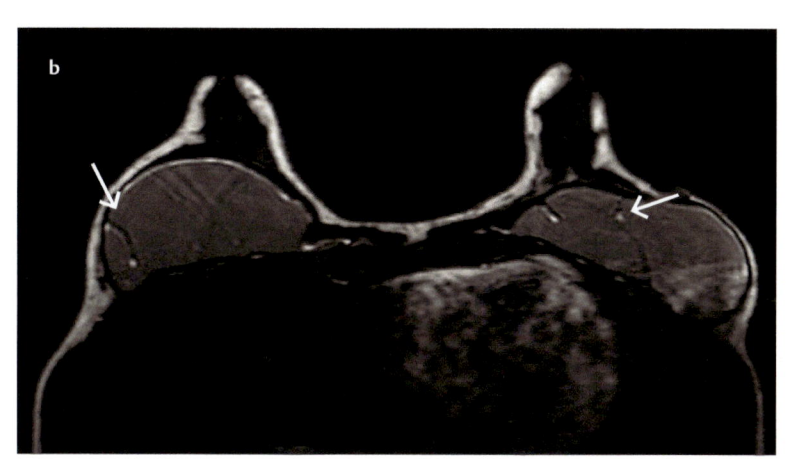

sis. (Usually the thickness of the fibrotic capsule does not change.) Sometimes the number of radial folds may increase.

3. Capsular Herniation

Focal herniation of an intact implant through the fibrous capsule may develop. This causes a lump or bulge in the contour of the implant. On mammography a focal bulge cannot be distinguished from an implant rupture (**Fig. 20.6**). The correct diagnosis is usually possible by checking with the finger under ultrasound observation. (The fluid in the implant will move when pressing the bulge. Also, examination in different planes will usually demonstrate that the herniation is part of the implant.)

4. Reactive Fluid and Implant Sweating

Due to slight local reaction to the implant and mechanical stress there may be a small amount of tissue fluid that surrounds the implant. This tissue fluid may be detectable by ultrasound or MRI. It may surround the implant or collect between the shell of the implant and the fibrous capsule that is built by the body around the implant. On ultrasound or MRI morphologically it cannot be distinguished from a small intracapsular leak of the implant (see below). Therefore, if fluid is detected in this location MRI may be indicated.

With the usual T1- and T2-weighted pulse sequences fluid usually exhibits the same signal as simple cysts. The distinction between reactive fluid and silicone is made by use of silicone-only sequences (see below). Reactive fluid should have no signal intensity (in contrast to the contents of a silicone implant).

With older implants the implant capsule may become increasingly permeable and liquid silicone may extrude through the pores of the implant shell. Unless a single hole can be identified, this is called "sweating" of the implant. Sweating of the implant occurs with increasing age of the implant and indicates that implants tend to become leaky. At surgery a definite defect in the implant cannot be found, but the explanted implant is sticky from the extruded silicone. On imaging differentiation between sweating of an implant and a small intracapsular rupture (see below) is impossible.

5. Intracapsular Rupture

Liquid silicone leaks outside the shell of the implant, usually through a small pin-size hole but is contained within the fibrotic capsule of the body. No further complications are associated with this type of rupture. However, the risk of an extracapsular rupture (with possible local complications) is increased.

Mammography is often normal with intracapsular rupture since the silicone is contained within the fibrous capsule. If imaged en face a localized leak may also present like local bulging. Mammographically a distinction between bulging and intracellular or extracapsular rupture is mostly not possible or at least uncertain (**Fig. 20.7**). In this case the bulging was caused by extracapsular silicone (see also **Fig. 20.8c**).

Ultrasound may show disorganization of the implant contents (**Fig. 20.8a**). The collapsed implant shell can give the "stepladder sign" on ultrasound whereby the collapsed shell is seen as several parallel folds (**Fig. 20.8b**). This is the equivalent of the linguini sign on MRI.

If free silicone extrudes beyond the capsule of the body into surrounding tissue, usually granulation tissue forms which surrounds tiny droplets of silicone. This appearance presents with high echogenicity and some acoustic shadowing. The echogenicity decreases with increasing distance from the transducer (the so-called "snowstorm" pattern).

The following MRI signs have been described in association with intracapsular rupture:
- "Keyhole" sign or "noose" sign and "reversed C" sign indicate that silicon is shown inside and outside the capsule of an implant. Thus the outer capsule of the implant becomes visible as a fine line which is separate from the thick capsule of the body. If discrete, these signs may be associated with sweating of the implant.

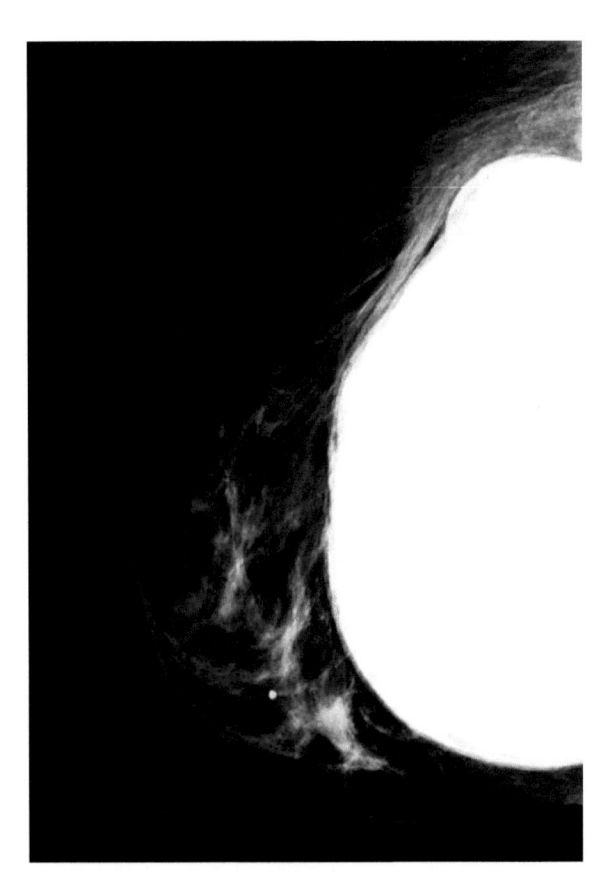

Fig. 20.6 Mammogram showing focal bulge in an implant.

Complications of Breast Implants

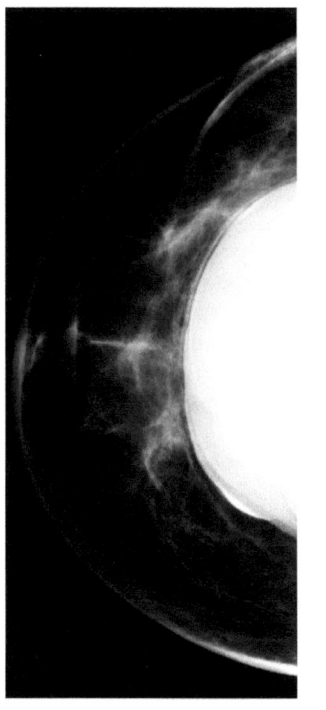

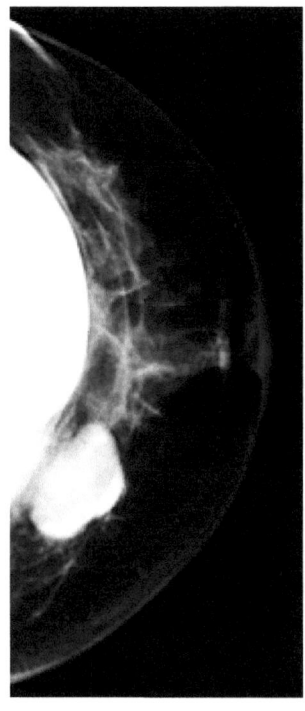

Fig. 20.7 50-year-old woman presented to a symptomatic breast clinic with a mass in the lower inner quadrant of her left breast. She had had breast implants for 14 years. Craniocaudal views showing an extracapsular rupture with silicone outside the implant on the left.

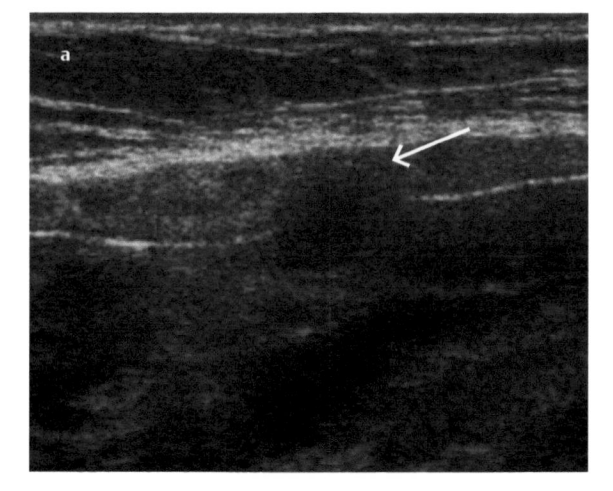

Fig. 20.8a–c

a Ultrasound of extracapsular rupture showing disorganization of implant contents and free silicone outside the implant capsule (arrow).

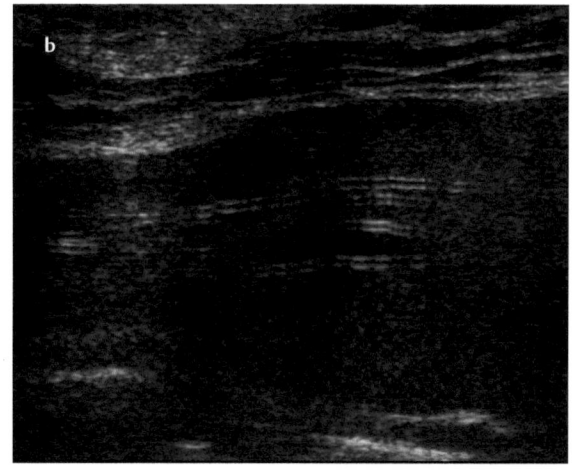

b Intracapsular implant rupture showing the stepladder sign. The collapsed implant shell is seen as a series of parallel linear echoes. The magnetic resonance imaging equivalent is called the "linguini sign".

Fig. 20.8c ▷

◁ continued

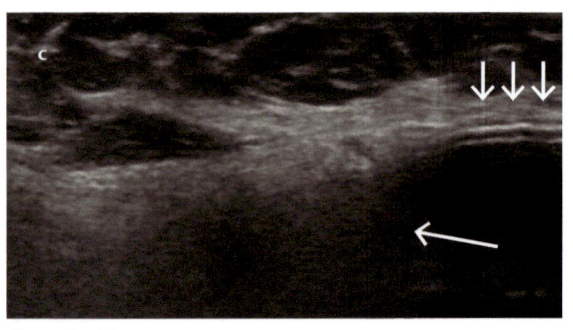

c Extracapsular silicone and silicone granuloma on ultrasound showing "snowstorm" pattern due to free silicone (large arrow). Small arrows indicate implant capsule. Same patient as **Fig. 20.7**.

Usually they indicate intracapsular rupture (**Figs. 20.9** and **20.10**).
- The "linguini sign" indicates intracapsular rupture, and occurs when there is rupture of the capsule of the implant associated with its complete collapse. The collapsed capsule is seen as a fine line swimming within the lake of silicone that is contained within the thick capsule of the body (**Fig. 20.11a,b**).
- The "salad oil" sign occurs if the inner capsule of a double lumen implant ruptures. Saline and the oily silicone mix, leading to droplets, as is seen when salad oil and vinegar are mixed. As long as the outer capsule remains intact, this has no consequence for the patient (**Fig. 20.12a,b**).

6. Extracapsular Rupture

This occurs when both the capsule of the implant and the fibrotic capsule surrounding it are ruptured. Free silicon deposits can be visualized in the surrounding breast parenchyma and sometimes in the axillary nodes. The patients usually complain of a lump, or a change in shape of the implant. Extracapsular rupture should in general lead to removal of the implant, though there is no evidence to indicate that free silicone causes breast cancer or generalized reactions.

According to official data published in the United States, implant rupture is estimated to occur in around 15% of the implants within the first 10 years (McLaughlin et al. 2007). Thus imaging to assess implant integrity may be an important diagnostic question in women with implants. However, there is no evidence on the impact of implant rupture on morbidity. Thus there is no basis to strive for early detection of implant rupture and recommend regular MR screening for this purpose (Sardanelli et al. 2010).

On mammography, free silicone is seen as a radiodense mass or masses. These may calcify, and the calcification can persist after the implant has been removed. (**Figs. 20.7** and **Fig. 20.13**, and see **Fig. 13.6e**).

On ultrasound silicone is highly echogenic, with posterior attenuation giving a "snowstorm" appearance. Nodes that contain silicone are enlarged and echogenic with a similar "snowstorm" appearance (**Figs. 20.8c** and **20.14**).

On MRI an extracapsular rupture is diagnosed if silicone is present outside the fibrous capsule surrounding the implant (**Fig. 20.15**). Extracapsular ruptures need to be distinguished from other fluid collections such as simple or complicated cysts, hematomas, or seromas. Silicone-selective pulse sequences are used to make this distinction. Whenever a silicone deposit is seen outside the implant, it should be ascertained that it is not a residual deposit from a preceding implant (see **Fig. 13.6e**).

MRI is more accurate than clinical breast examination and conventional imaging for assessing implant integrity: While radiographic mammography is expected to detect around 25–30% of implant ruptures, MRI will detect the rupture in the region of 78–89% (Herborn et al. 2002, Hölmich et al. 2005). In particular, Herborn et al. reported 87% sensitivity and 89% specificity, Holmich et al. 89% and 97%, respectively. MRI is also the most accurate technique for differentiating intracapsular from extracapsular rupture and for assessing the extent of silicone leakage into the breast and granuloma formation (Topping et al. 2003).

Surveillance of Women with an Implant Following Oncoplastic Surgery

Mammographic surveillance is not indicated in the reconstructed breast after mastectomy. A rare exception may concern patients with partial mastectomy and significant residual tissue (**Fig. 20.16**).

Distinction of scarring or postsurgical granulomas may be difficult with conventional imaging. However, typical changes with scarring should be known (**Fig. 20.17**).

Ultrasound may be considered for this special indication (**Fig. 20.18**).

For women at high genetic risk and in selected cases at high risk of recurrence (previous recurrences or multicentric disease), MRI may be considered because of its excellent sensitivity, its tomographic technique, and its very good capability for distinguishing scarring and recurrence (**Fig. 20.19**).

The EUSOMA group has made the following evidence-based recommendations regarding breast MRI for women with an implant following oncoplastic surgery (Sardanelli et al. 2010):

1. In patients with tissue expanders, MR compatibility should be evaluated.
2. In asymptomatic patients routine surveillance with dynamic contrast-enhanced MRI is not recommended for the average risk group. It is recommended for higher-risk groups that would qualify for MR screening, for example, patients carrying the *BRCA* gene.
3. In symptomatic women, when conventional imaging is negative or equivocal, noncontrast MRI and dynamic contrast-enhanced MRI are indicated.

Complications of Breast Implants

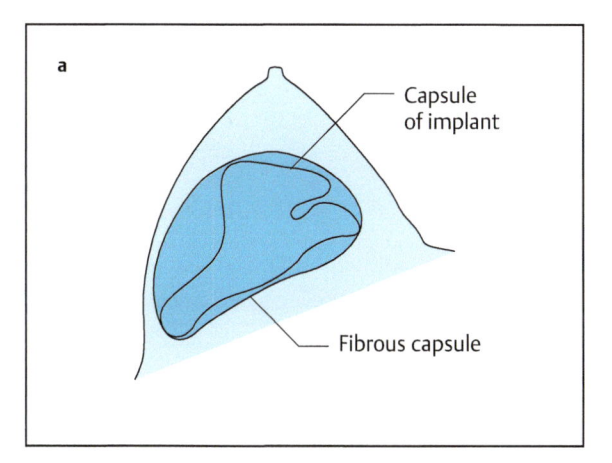

Fig. 20.9a,b Diagram (**a**) and magnetic resonance image (**b**) of a "keyhole" sign (top arrow). The implant capsule (bottom arrow) is seen as a fine line which is separate from the fibrous capsule. Intracapsular rupture.

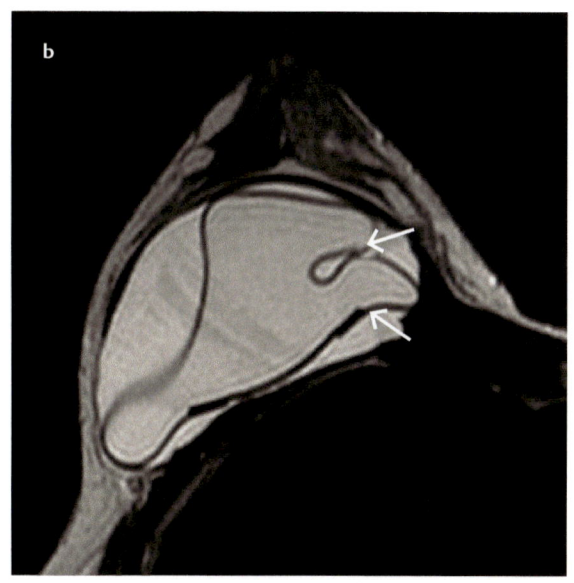

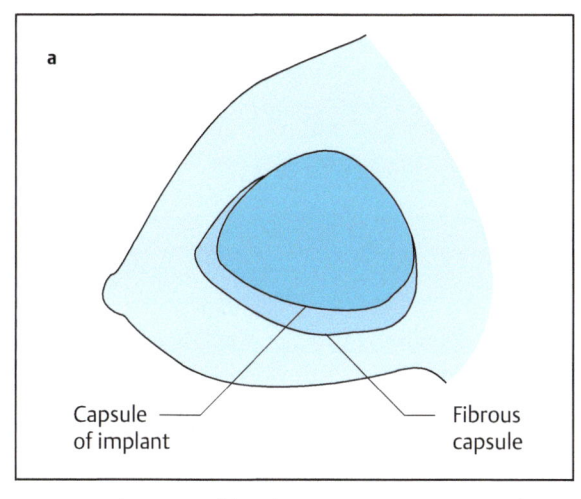

Fig. 20.10a,b Diagram (**a**) and magnetic resonance image (**b**) of "reverse C" sign. Silicone is shown inside and outside the capsule (arrow) of an implant.

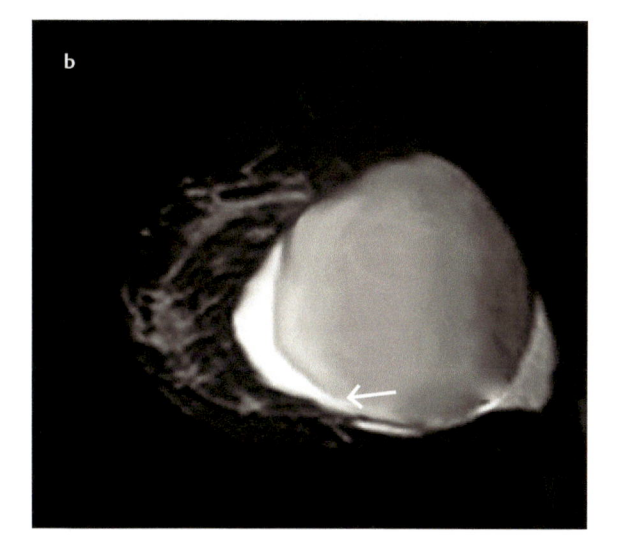

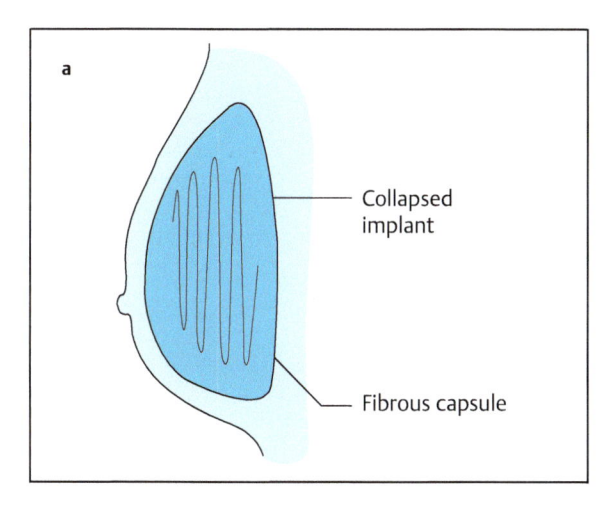

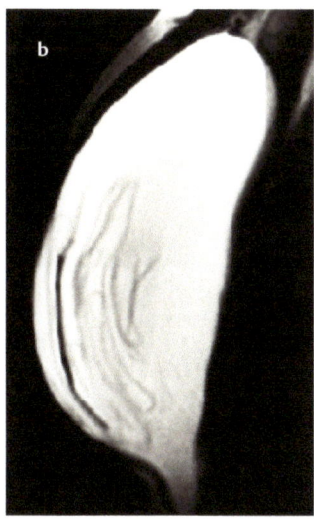

◁ **Fig. 20.11a,b** The "linguini sign". Diagram (**a**) and magnetic resonance image (**b**) of intracapsular rupture. The collapsed implant shell is seen as a series of parallel linear structures resembling linguini.

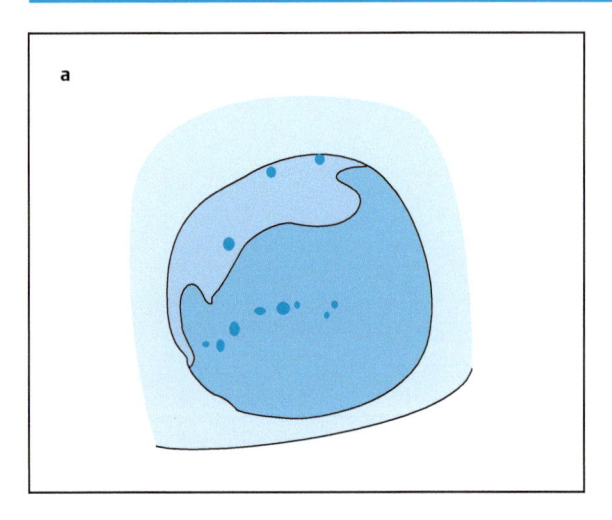

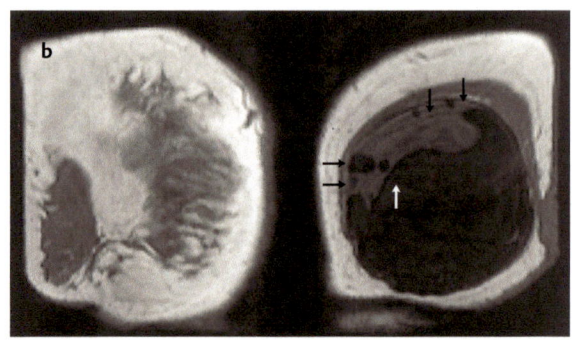

Fig. 20.12a,b Diagram (**a**) and magnetic resonance image (**b**) of the "salad oil" sign. The inner capsule of a double lumen implant has ruptured. Saline and the oily silicone have mixed, leading to droplets, as is seen when salad oil and vinegar are mixed.

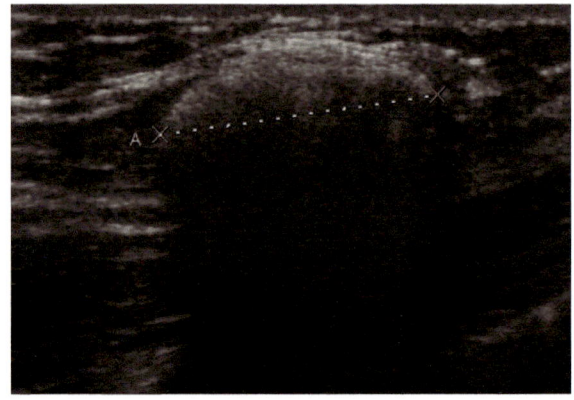

Fig. 20.14 Ultrasound image showing silicone deposits in an axillary lymph node after extracapsular rupture.

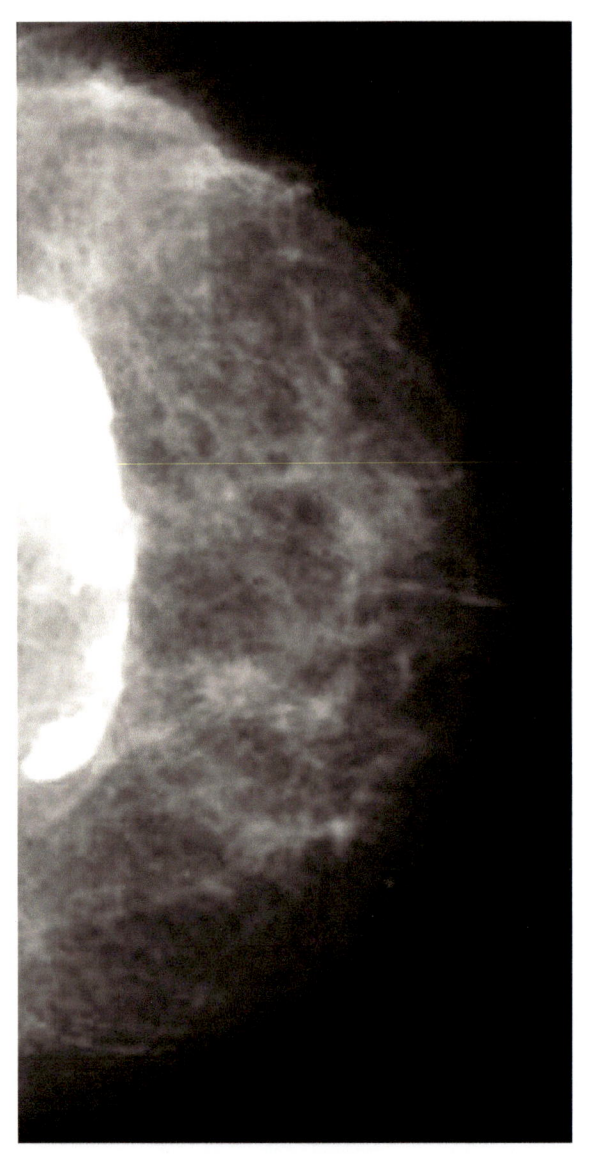

Fig. 20.13 Mammograms showing dystrophic calcification following implant removal.

Complications of Breast Implants

Imaging Assessment of Women with Implants after Oncoplastic Surgery

Any woman with implants who is symptomatic or who has a clinical abnormality in the breast should undergo imaging assessment and—in case of a BI-RADS (Breast Imaging Reporting and Data System) 4 or 5 finding—histopathologic assessment as for a woman with no implants (**Fig. 20.3**). Thus the lesion(s) in question should be imaged by ultrasound and mammography.

Whenever a focal lesion is noted, however, histopathologic assessment is indicated.

This is feasible in most cases. If breast biopsy is not possible owing to the individual anatomy or the imaging finding (lesion not visible by ultrasound), percutaneous MRI may ideally complement the diagnostic information.

Considering that no imaging method is 100% sensitive, great care is necessary when excluding malignancy. Usually short-term follow-up should be performed in cases with very low probability of malignancy, whereas surgical biopsy will be necessary if this is not possible and percutaneous biopsy cannot be performed. In cases with impaired diagnostic assessment due to severe scarring, MRI may, however, be very helpful.

Imaging Assessment of Women after Augmentation Implant

In women who have had an augmentation implant imaging assessment is identical to that of women without implants. It should always include a complete mammogram and high-resolution ultrasound. Special views may need to be adapted to the individual anatomy.

The next step for indeterminate or suspicious lesions is percutaneous breast biopsy, which is technically feasible in most cases. Only for selected exceptions may MRI be needed for supplementary information concerning lesions close to the implant or the chest wall.

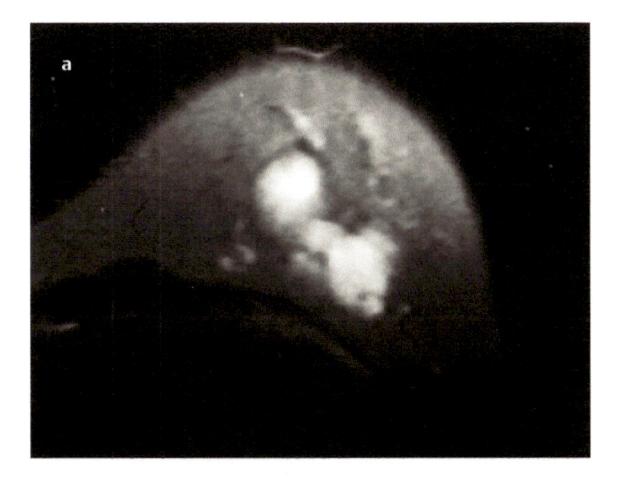

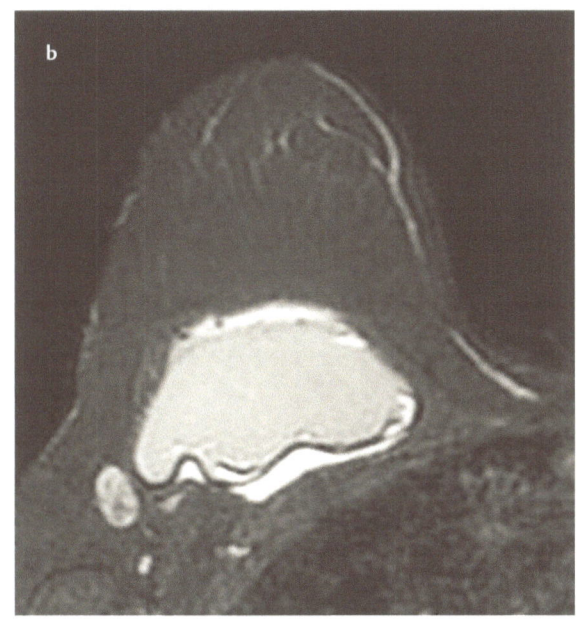

Fig. 20.15a,b Magnetic resonance image of extracapsular ruptures showing free silicone (**a**) and silicone in the axillary node (**b**).

Screening of Asymptomatic Women who have had Breast Augmentation

Screening mammography remains the best method of detecting breast cancer in asymptomatic women with implants, although the sensitivity is reduced. Digital mammography, by allowing manipulation of the image is preferred to radiographic mammography.

There is no evidence in the literature for routine breast screening with ultrasound or MRI in women with breast implants. MRI screening is indicated in such patients, if they are at high genetic risk.

Histopathologic Assessment in Women with Implants

As described above, histopathologic assessment is the next step for all patients with implants with a suspicious or indeterminate finding. Core needle biopsy is possible in most patients, while stereotactic vacuum-assisted breast biopsy may be limited to patients with sufficient tissue surrounding the implant. MRI may support a decision for or against histopathologic assessment. However, caution is necessary. If percutaneous breast biopsy is not feasible, surgery after adequate marking is unavoidable for patients with BI-RADS category 4 or 5 lesions. Depending on the anatomy imaging guidance may have to be individually adapted.

20 Radiologic Assessment of Women with Breast Implants

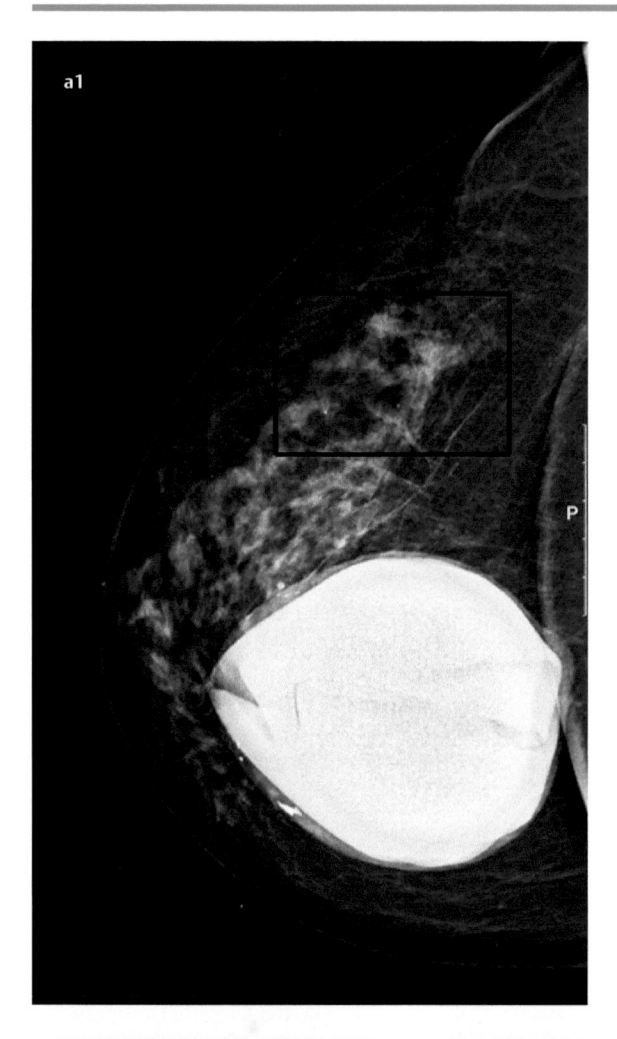

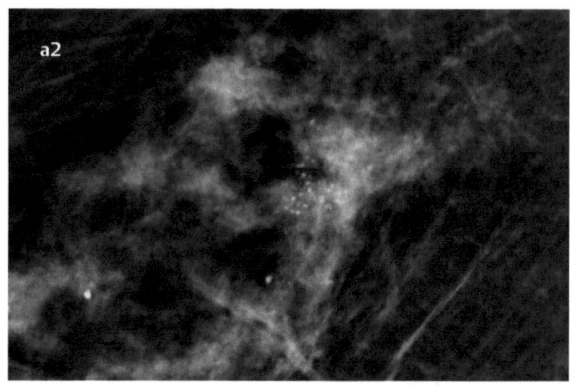

Fig. 20.16a–c

a Invasive breast cancer detected by mammographic microcalcifications in a patient who had obtained a small implant after a benign surgical excision long ago.
b Ultrasound does not show the full extent of the lesion. However, one larger focus and some further tiny foci of invasion are visualized by this high-resolution sonographic examination.
c On magnetic resonance imaging the ductal distribution of the extensive intraductal component is nicely seen. In this case the invasive foci appear to exhibit a slightly earlier and stronger enhancement than the extensive intraductal component.
Histology: Ductal invasive carcinoma pT1c.

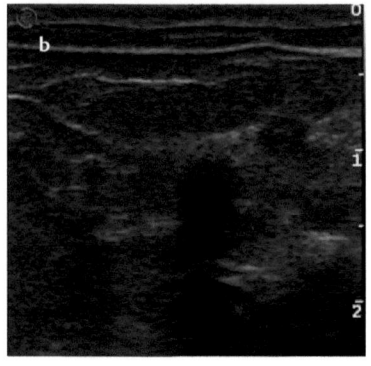

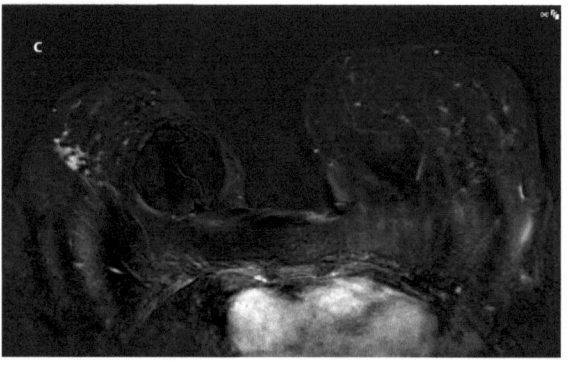

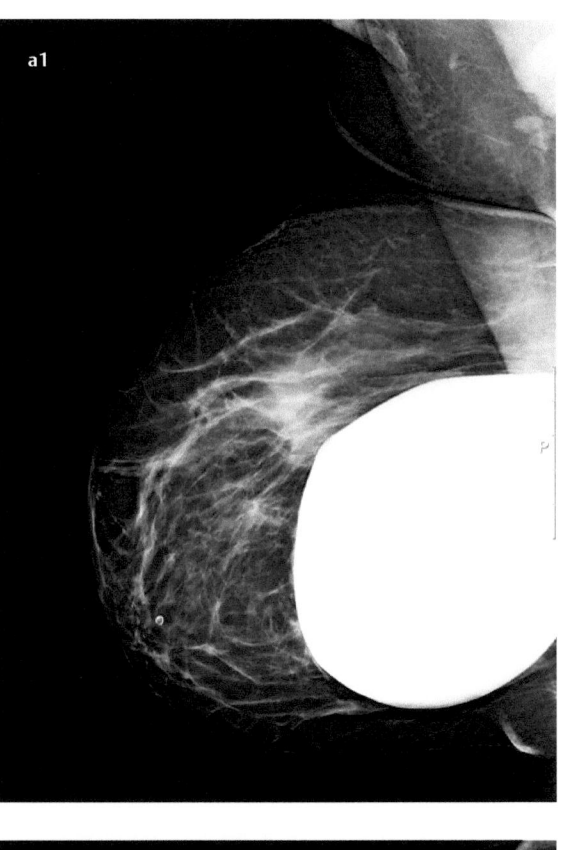

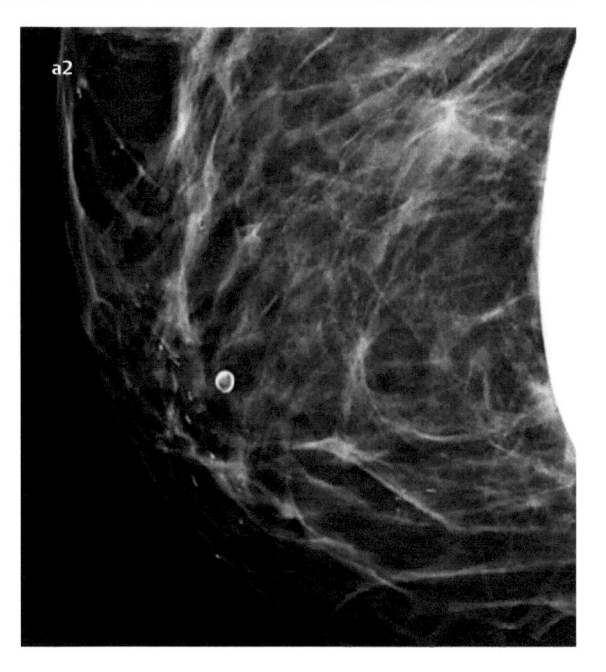

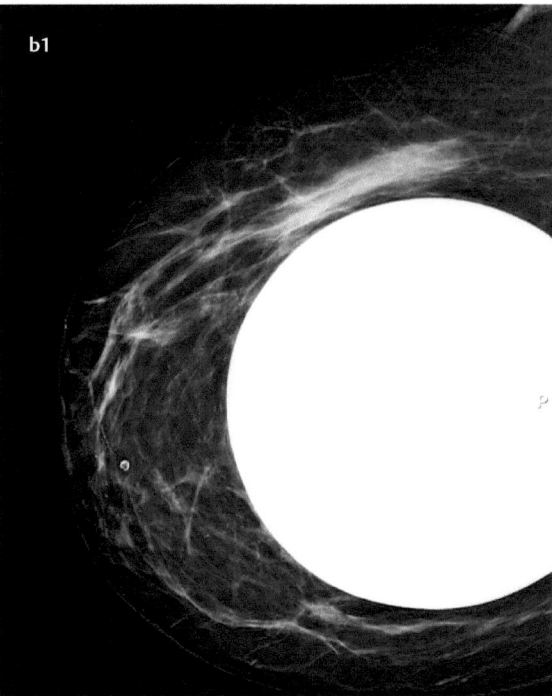

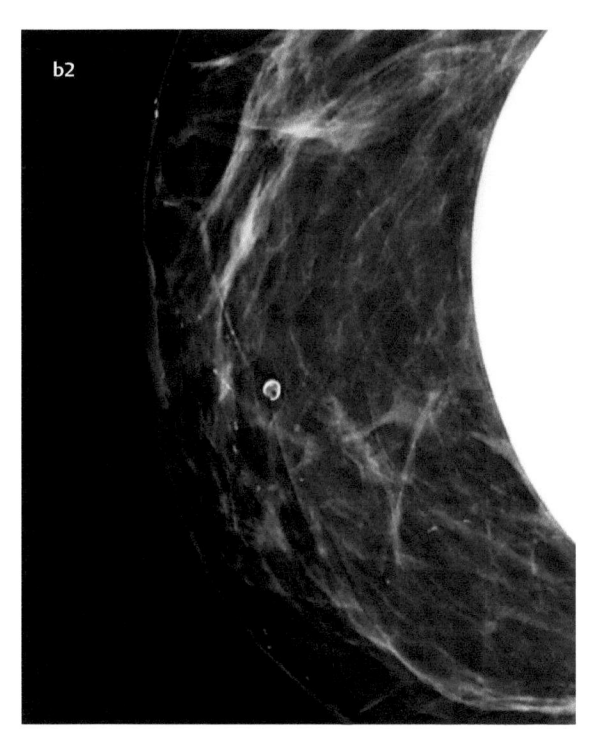

Complications of Breast Implants

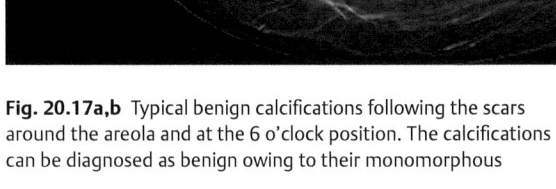

Fig. 20.17a,b Typical benign calcifications following the scars around the areola and at the 6 o'clock position. The calcifications can be diagnosed as benign owing to their monomorphous punctate shapes and their distribution following the scar. **a** Mediolateral oblique view; **b** craniocaudal view.

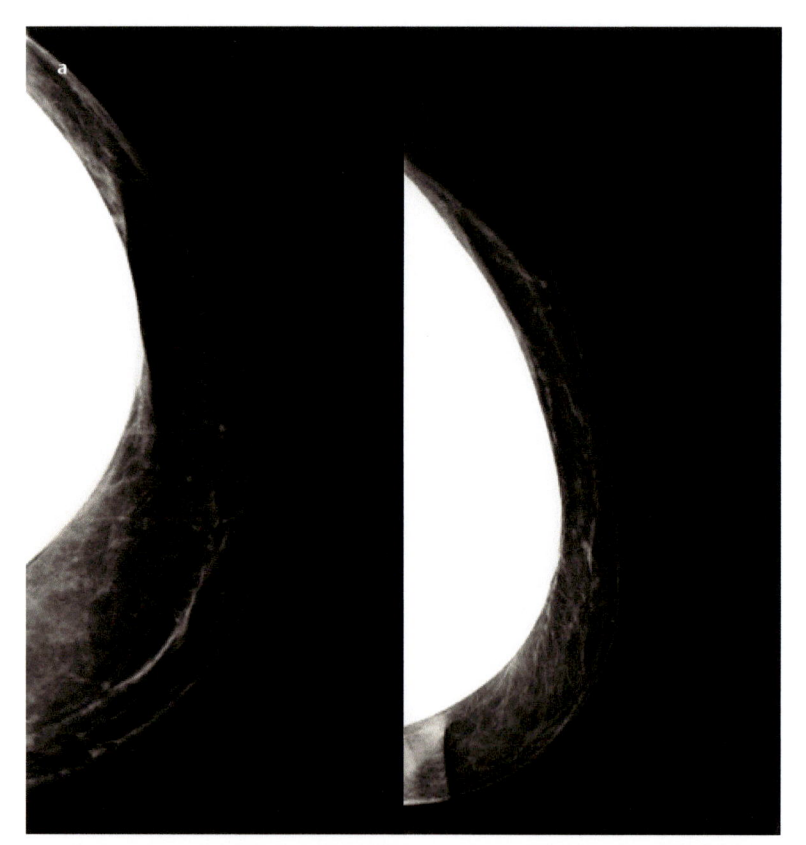

20 Radiologic Assessment of Women with Breast Implants

Fig. 20.18a–c
a Craniocaudal and mediolateral oblique views did not show an abnormality in this patient who underwent surveillance imaging after bilateral breast cancer and implant surgery 6 months before.
b Incidentally an oval lesion that retrospectively corresponded to a discrete area of palpable thickening was detected by ultrasound. The lesion exhibited very little perfusion and was therefore considered to possibly correspond to post-therapeutic fibrosis. But histopathologic assessment was recommended and performed.
c As shown the needle that penetrates the lesion is angled away from the implant. *Histology* revealed a G3 ductal invasive breast cancer.

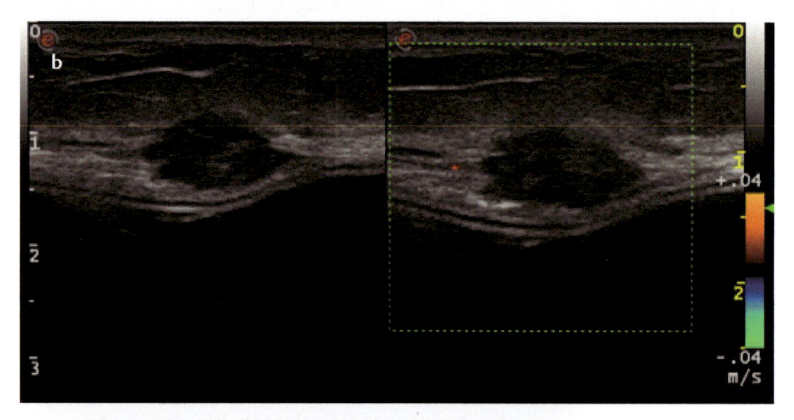

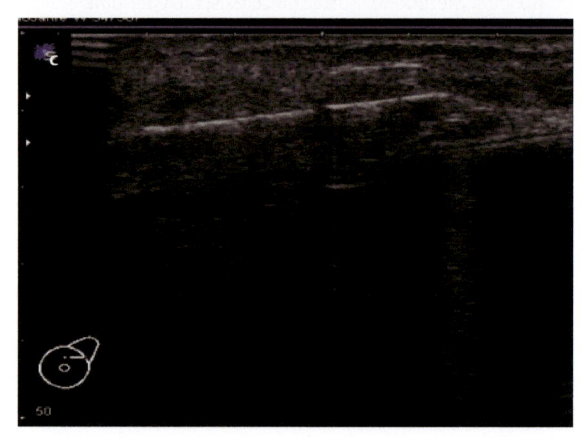

Complications of Breast Implants

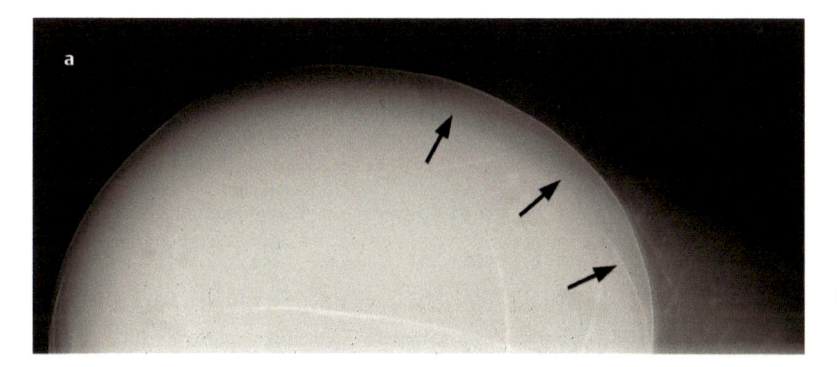

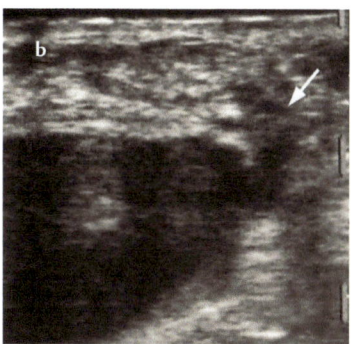

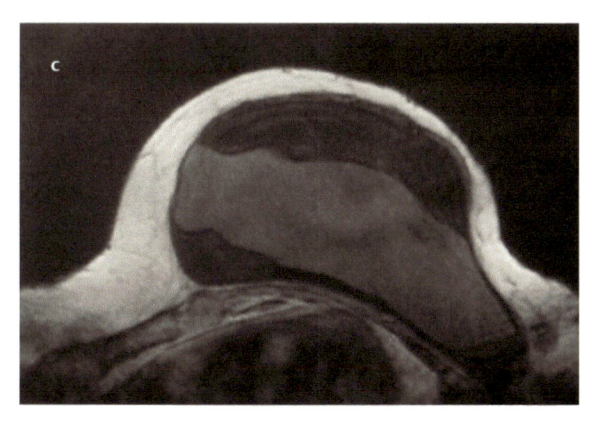

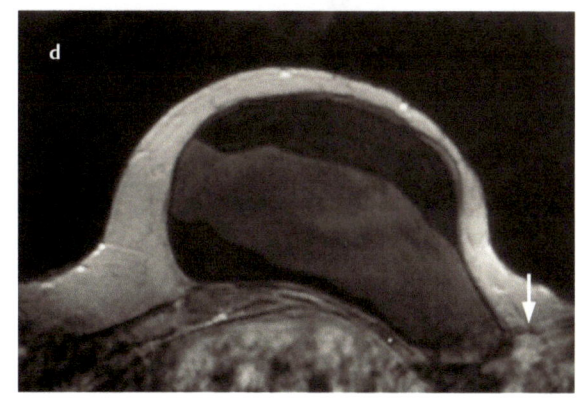

Fig. 20.19a–d Detection of the carcinoma in the presence of a silicone prosthesis.

a The mammographic evaluation is considerably compromised by the narrow mantle of tissue surrounding the prosthesis. The mobility is impaired because of scarring along the thoracic wall. There is no evidence of densities or calcifications suspicious for malignancy in several projections with the craniocaudal view shown here (the arrows point at the outline of the inner compartment of the double lumen prosthesis).

b The small carcinomatous focus at the dorsolateral aspect of the outer margin of the prosthesis was not noted clinically or sonographically. It was apparently mistaken as part of the prosthesis itself. Only retrospectively could a corresponding area be identified on the sonogram (arrow).

c,d Representative magnetic resonance imaging section before administration of contrast medium (**c**) at the level of subsequent enhancement (**d**). After application of contrast medium, highly suspicious enhancement adjacent to the prosthesis (arrow) was seen. *Histology*: Recurrence of a ductal carcinoma. (Reproduced with kind permission of Springer Science+Business Media from Heywang-Köbrunner and Beck 1996.)

Summary

Imaging of implants is challenging for the radiologist. Familiarity is needed with the types of implant, technical prerequisites, typical appearances of implant imaging in general, scarring and implant complications, possibilities and limitations of the imaging, and interventional methods.

Patients after augmentation who are not at increased genetic risk should generally undergo screening mammography, which in the event of doubt may be supplemented by ultrasound.

For patients with silicone implants after mastectomy no ideal method for surveillance exists. Depending on the clinical assessment and additional risk factors (personal or family history) ultrasound or MRI may be useful.

However, for women at low risk no recommendation for routine MRI exists.

In cases of indeterminate or suspicious findings, percutaneous breast biopsy is the next step. In the event of difficulties MRI may be useful to support a recommendation for or against histopathologic assessment versus short-term follow-up. It will, however, only rarely be needed for the assessment of women after augmentation mammoplasty.

The approach for interventions may have to be individually adapted.

References and Recommended Reading

Belli P, Romani M, Magistrelli A, Masetti R, Pastore G, Costantini M. Diagnostic imaging of breast implants: role of MRI. Rays 2002;27(4):259–277

Boné B, Aspelin P, Isberg B, Perbeck L, Veress B. Contrast-enhanced MR imaging of the breast in patients with breast implants after cancer surgery. Acta Radiol 1995;36(2):111–116

Heinig A, Heywang-Köbrunner SH, Viehweg P, Lampe D, Buchmann J, Spielmann RP. Value of contrast medium magnetic resonance tomography of the breast in breast reconstruction with implant. [Article in German] Radiologe 1997;37(9):710–717

Herborn CU, Marincek B, Erfmann D, et al. Breast augmentation and reconstructive surgery: MR imaging of implant rupture and malignancy. Eur Radiol 2002;12(9):2198–2206

Heywang-Köbrunner SH, Beck R. Contrast-enhanced MRI of the breast. Heidelberg, New York: Springer; 1996

Hölmich LR, Vejborg I, Conrad C, Sletting S, McLaughlin JK. The diagnosis of breast implant rupture: MRI findings compared with findings at explantation. Eur J Radiol 2005;53(2):213–225

McLaughlin JK, Lipworth L, Murphy DK, Walker PS. The safety of silicone gel-filled breast implants: a review of the epidemiologic evidence. Ann Plast Surg 2007;59(5):569–580

Sardanelli F, Boetes C, Borisch B, et al. Magnetic resonance imaging of the breast: recommendations from the EUSOMA working group. Eur J Cancer 2010;46(8):1296–1316

Steinbach BG, Hardt NS, Abbitt PL, Lanier L, Caffee HH. Breast implants, common complications, and concurrent breast disease. Radiographics 1993;13(1):95–118

Topping A, George C, Wilson G. Appropriateness of MRI scanning in the detection of ruptured implants used for breast reconstruction. Br J Plast Surg 2003;56(2):186–189

21 Skin Changes

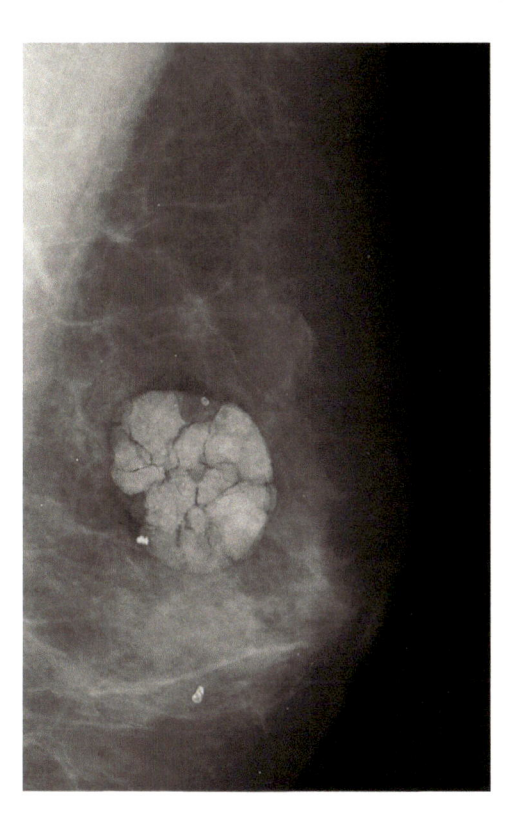

Nodular Changes of the Skin and Subcutaneous Tissue ⇢ 554
Clinical Findings ⇢ 554
Diagnostic Strategy ⇢ 554

Skin Thickening ⇢ 554
Definition ⇢ 554
Incidence ⇢ 554
Diagnostic Strategy ⇢ 555
Clinical Findings ⇢ 561

References and Recommended Reading ⇢ 562

21 Skin Changes

I. Schreer, S. H. Heywang-Koebrunner, S. Barter

Nodular Changes of the Skin and Subcutaneous Tissue

Nodular changes of the skin and subcutaneous tissue can be visualized on the mammogram and, if not seen in profile, can be mistaken for intramammary lesions. Therefore, mammographic interpretation should always include the results from inspection and palpation of the skin.

Most frequent are:
- Fibroepitheliomas (usually at the areola/mamilla)
- Moles
- Epithelial cysts (atheromas)
- Lipomas
- Keloids
- Hemangiomas, lymphangiomas, neurofibromas, histiocytomas, and leiomyomas, which are rare nodular cutaneous or subcutaneous lesions

Clinical Findings

While fibroepitheliomas most frequently account for small, sometimes pedunculated lesions at the nipple, moles and epithelial cysts can occur anywhere on the skin of the breast. Epithelial cysts (atheromas) form nodular tumors of variable size within the skin and occasionally become infected. Lipomas present as soft, subcutaneous nodules of variable size with more or less pronounced bulging of the overlying skin.

Diagnostic Strategy

All nodular changes of the skin and subcutaneous tissue are accessible to direct examination and therefore can be evaluated clinically. Since they can mimic intramammary lesions, imaging studies should always be interpreted in conjunction with the clinical findings.

Mammography

Moles and epithelial cysts can generally be assigned to a cutaneous location by their pattern of a mass surrounded by a radiolucent rim, which is caused by air between the tumor, skin, and compression device (**Fig. 21.1a,b**) and accounts for the characteristic mammographic appearance. The size and density of the focal findings are subject to wide individual variability. Moles also can contain calcific particles, potentially imitating an intramammary lesion with microcalcifications (**Fig. 21.1d,l,m**).

In general, the correct diagnosis is established by combining clinical and mammographic findings. If questions remain, a repeat view with a marker placed on the cutaneous finding is recommended for clarification.

Skin Thickening

Definition

The thickness of the skin can vary from individual to individual. Furthermore, small breasts presumably have a slightly thicker skin than larger breasts. According to Willson et al. (1982) and Pope et al. (1984), the lateral and cranial skin thickness as seen in the normal mammogram (craniocaudal projection and mediolateral projection, respectively) should not exceed 2.5 mm. Medially and caudally, the skin thickness can be up to 3 mm. However, in an individual patient skin thickness is best assessed by comparing both sides, since skin thickening is rarely bilateral and its presence is usually suspected based on clinical or other mammographic findings. Discrete pathologic skin thickening cannot always be distinguished from a normal variant. Findings suggesting a pathologic process are: localized skin thickening; asymmetry in comparison with the contralateral side; a change with time (assuming comparable mammographic technique); and an association with increased trabecular markings in the subcutaneous tissue or elsewhere in the breast.

Incidence

Skin thickening can involve the breast locally (confined to one area) or diffusely (**Fig. 21.2a–e**).

The most important causes of *localized skin thickening* include:
- Dermatologic conditions such as circumscribed scleroderma, psoriasis, etc.
- Band-like skin thickening as a manifestation of Mondor disease, which is a thrombophlebitis of a superficial vein. It presents as cordlike skin thickening along the course of the vein, associated with slight retraction if seen in the stage of scar formation.
- Skin thickening in scarring (**Fig. 21.2g–i**)
- Concomitant thickening of the skin overlying a localized process (representing localized reaction or direct infiltration), as seen, for instance, with an abscess, fat necrosis, carcinoma, metastasis, and hematologic malignancy (see also **Fig. 16.5a**)

The most important causes of diffuse skin thickening are:
- Mastitis
- Inflammatory carcinoma, diffuse metastatic spread to the breast, diffuse infiltration of the breast as seen with hematologic malignancies
- Iatrogenic edema following surgery, radiotherapy (see pp. 489, 509), later evolving into a scar, and anticoagulation therapy (as manifestation of an acute mammary necrosis)
- Lymphatic stasis caused by interruption of the lymphatics (mainly axillary), secondary to axillary nodal metastases, inflammatory processes and status post axillary dissection, or radiation
- Generalized edema due to cardiac decompensation, obstructed venous drainage, fluid overload, renal insufficiency, severe hepatic disease, or hypoalbuminemia

Diagnostic Strategy

The differential diagnosis for localized skin thickening can generally be narrowed down on the basis of the physical examination. The clinical findings must be incorporated in the interpretation of the imaging findings to establish the correct diagnosis of an imaged localized skin thickening. The nature of any underlying focal finding determines the differential diagnosis of the accompanying localized skin thickening.

Except for exclusively dermatologic conditions, diffuse skin thickening is invariably associated with edema of the connective tissue. It can be classified as follows:
- Symmetric appearance in both breasts can be evidence of generalized edema (cardiac decompensation, fluid overload, etc.), to be confirmed clinically. Important exceptions are asymmetric generalized edema following preferential lying on one side, or bilateral edema due, for example, to bilateral lymphatic stasis secondary to axillary metastases bilaterally or superior vena cava syndrome with obstructed venous drainage (**Fig. 21.2a**).

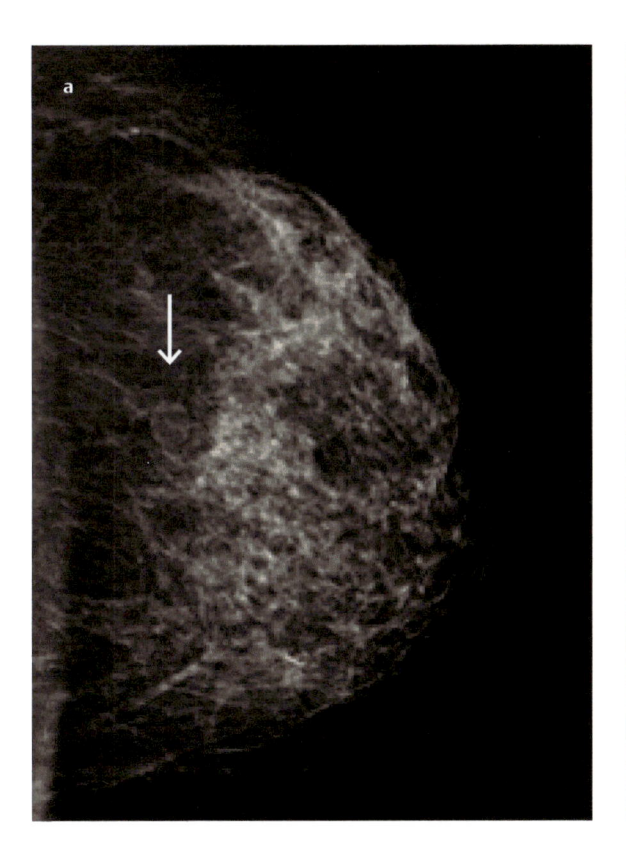

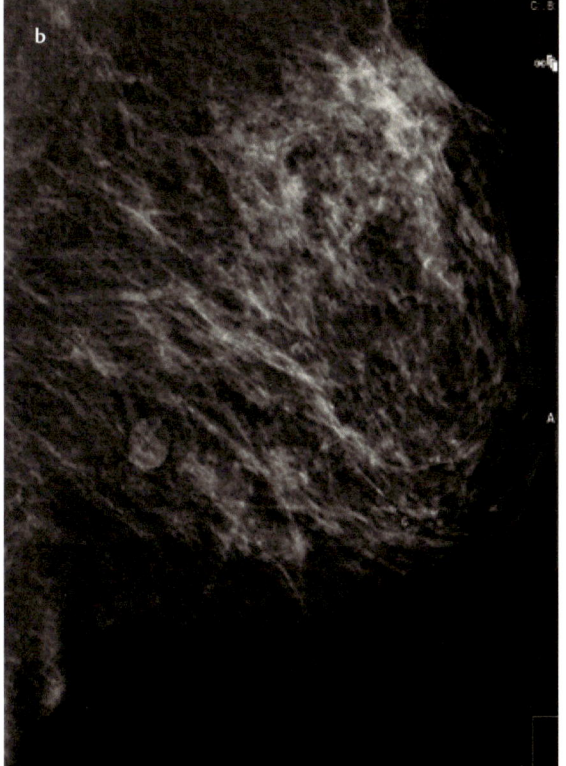

Fig. 21.1a–o
a,b Round, smoothly outlined mass measuring 10 mm in diameter, surrounded by a radiolucent halo in the 6 o'clock position: Verruca.

Fig. 21.1c–h ▷

21 Skin Changes

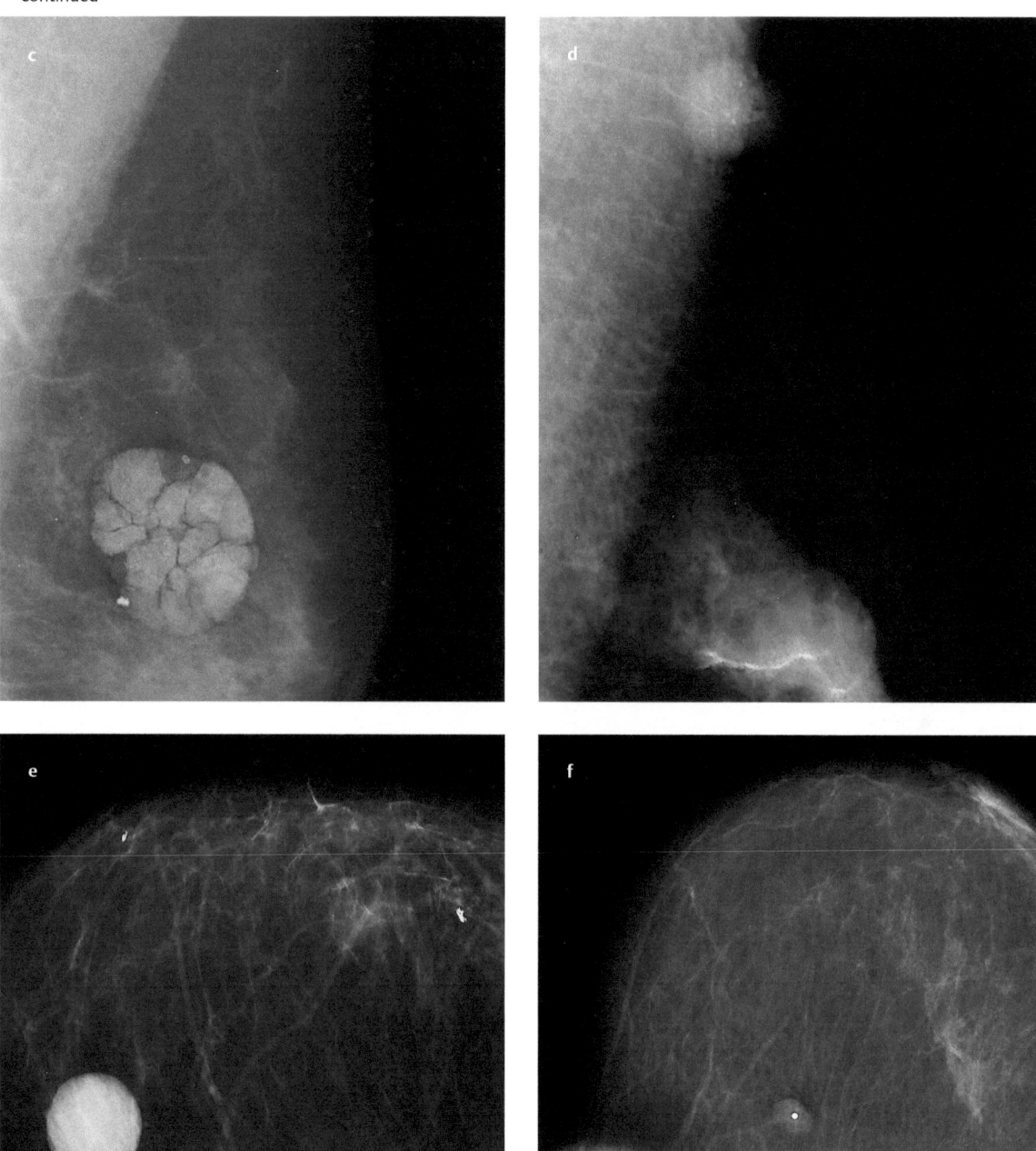

◁ continued

c   A 77-year-old woman with a large mole on her breast.
d   Smoothly outlined mass, measuring 14 mm in diameter, with central microcalcifications, in the extended axillary view, corresponding to a verruca senilis.
e   Very dense, round, smoothly outlined mass, measuring 23 mm in diameter, craniocaudal view of the medial half of the breast, corresponding to an atheroma in the inner lower quadrant.
f   To resolve diagnostic uncertainties, a lead pellet placed as marker on the skin can confirm the suspected diagnosis.

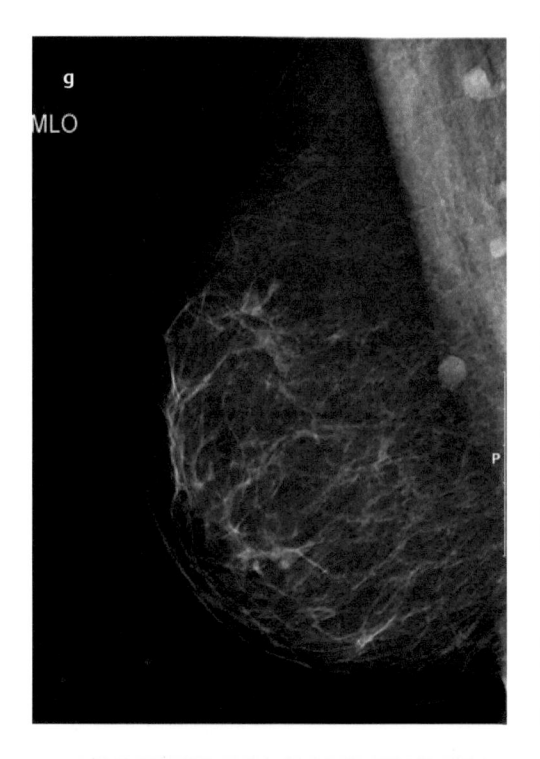

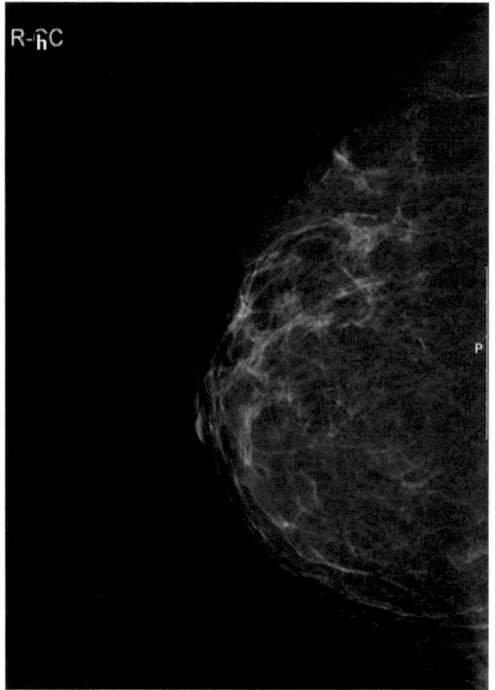

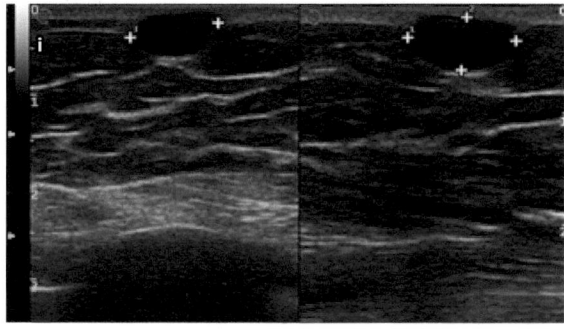

g–i There was a well-circumscribed nodule which had newly appeared on the screening mammogram, visible only on the mediolateral oblique (MLO) view (**g**), but not on the original craniocaudal view (**h**). Inspection and ultrasound demonstrated a skin lesion, which was not thought to correspond to the nodule, since it was located in the right lower quadrant (**i**).

Fig. 21.1j–o ▷

◁ continued

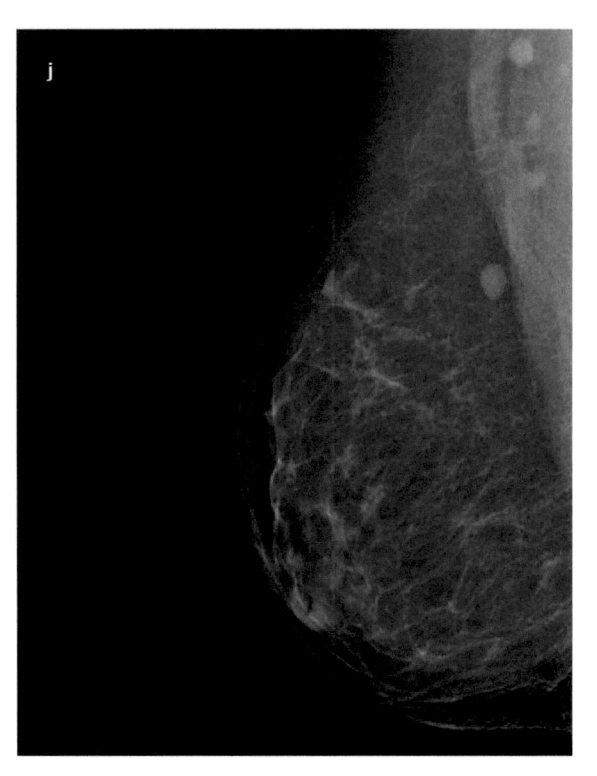

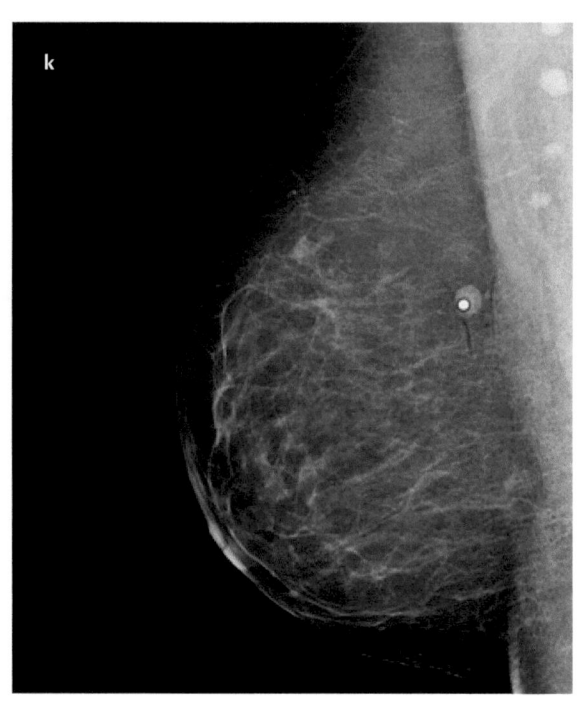

The extended craniocaudal view shows that the lesion is located laterally (**j**). The lesion still did not appear to correspond to the sonographic and clinical finding. To countercheck another MLO view was taken with a marker (**k**). It proved that the lesion, which was located in the right lower quadrant projected cranially on the MLO view and indeed corresponded to the skin lesion (**l**).
The confusing projection is explained by the oblique angle of image acquisition of the MLO view. Furthermore some variation in the position may also be explained by the different position, in which the mammogram (upright) and the sonogram (supine) is acquired. The proof that the newly occurring lesion corresponds to an intracutaneous nodule (probably a retention cyst) obviates the need for further assessment or short-term follow-up. The patient went back to screening.

l,m Skin warts containing very fine microcalcifications (arrows): craniiocaudal view (**l**); MLO view (**m**).

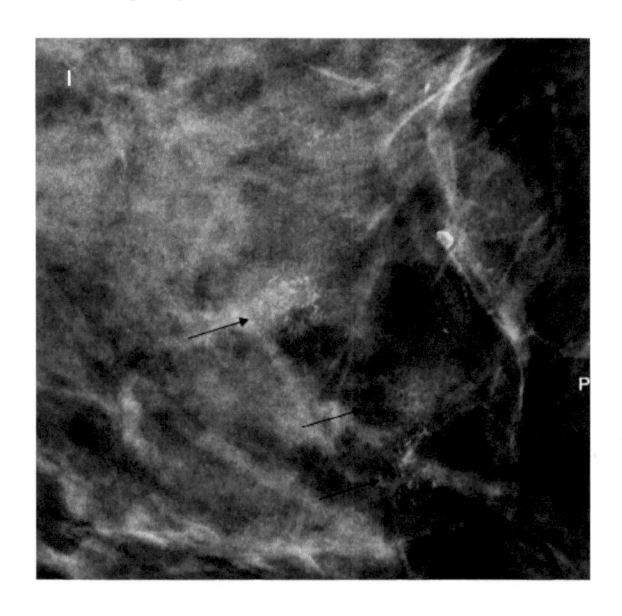

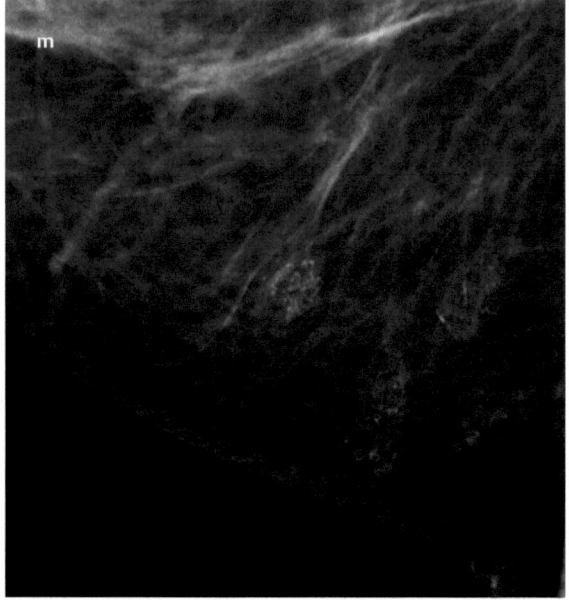

Skin Thickening

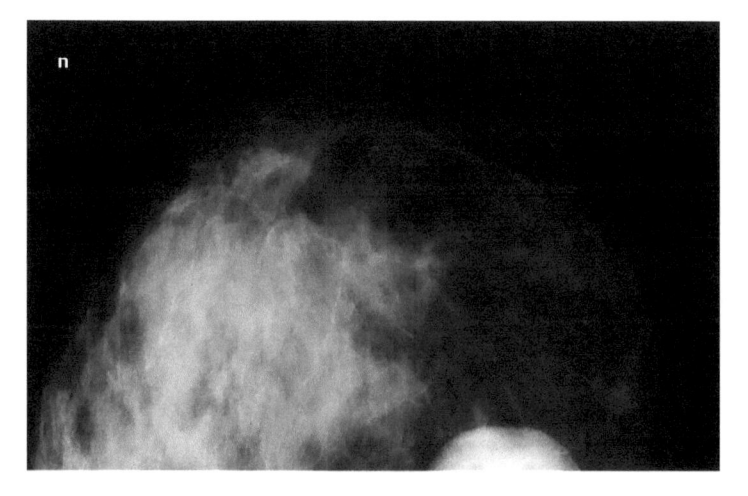

n Convex mass with two central, partially visualized radiolucencies in projection of the medial half of the breast along the thoracic wall: Partially visualized tip of the nose.
o Patient with known neurofibromatosis. The large neurofibromas are partially superimposed on the breast tissue. They are clearly identified as pendulating superficial skin lesions.

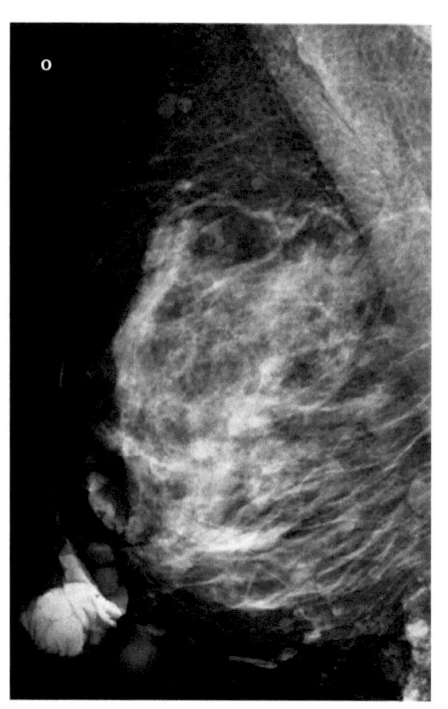

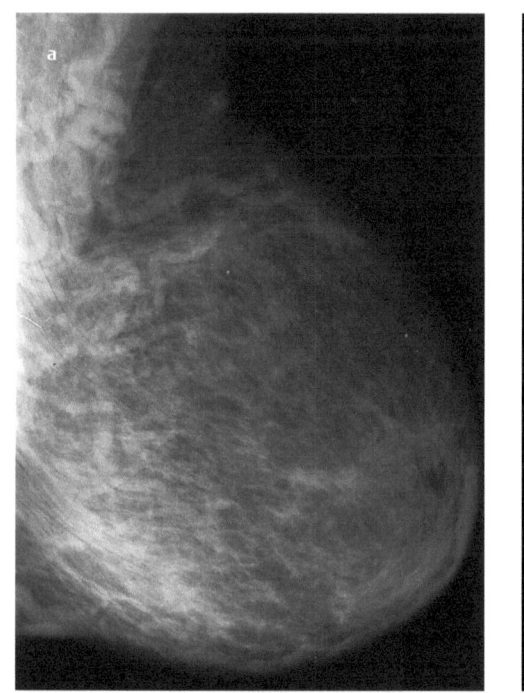

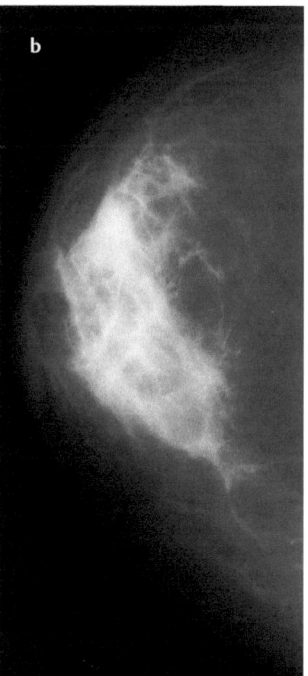

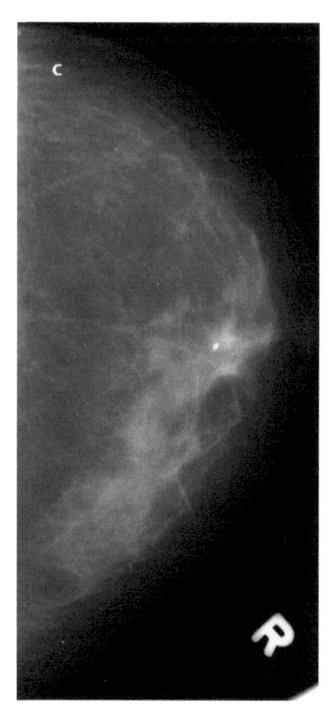

Fig. 21.2a–h
a This patient has developed superior vena cava obstruction due to central venous catheters. Skin thickening, trabecular coarsening, and multiple dilated veins serving as collaterals are shown.
b,c Skin thickening and diffuse increase in breast density are seen on the left due to bacterial mastitis, which resolved following antibiotic therapy.

Fig. 21.2d–f ▷

◁ continued

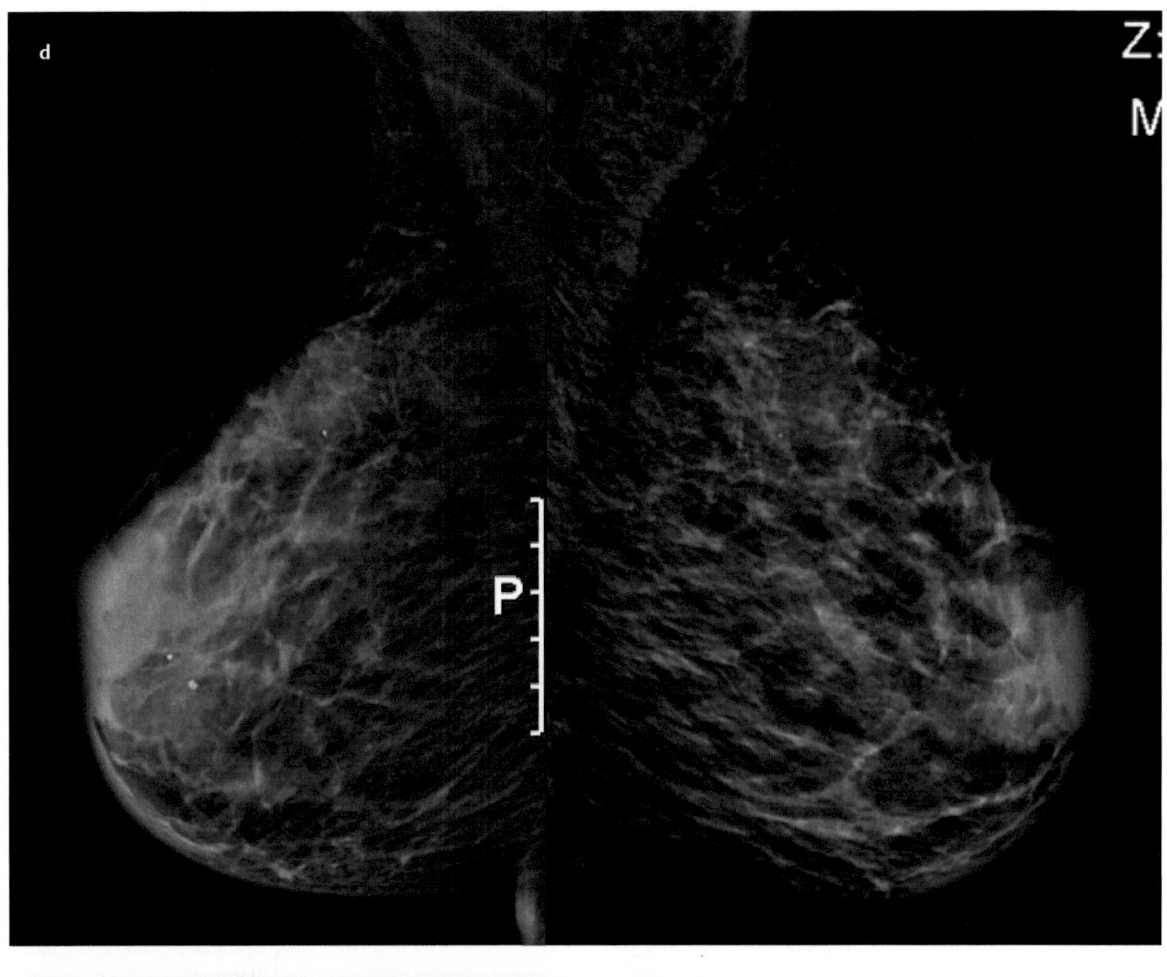

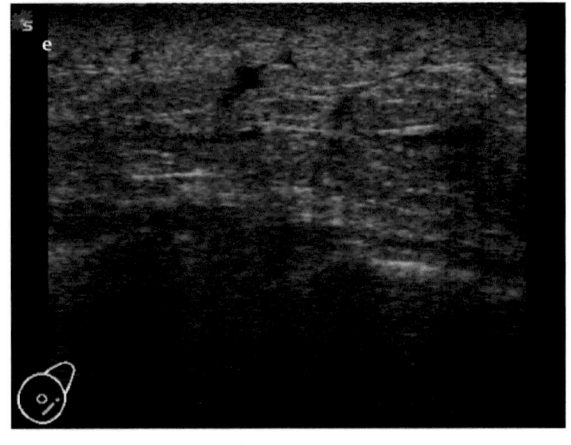

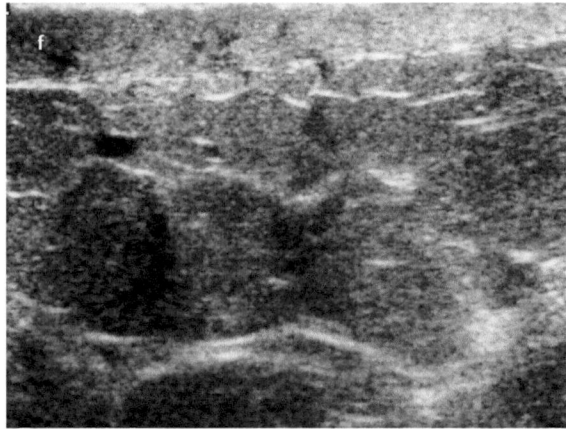

d–f Edema and skin thickening due to mediastinal obstruction. The patient, who had been invited for a first-round screening mammogram reported increased thickening and size of the left breast which had developed during the preceding 9 months. **d** The left breast is enlarged and exhibits increased interstitial and reticular densities, as well as a global skin thickening.

e On ultrasound imaging pronounced skin thickening is seen. The borders between the skin, subcutaneous tissue and glandular tissue are completely blurred and overall increased echogenicity is seen. Hypoechoic wormlike structures correspond to enlarged lymphatic vessels. Edematous changes were also seen in the axilla, but no enlarged or suspicious lymph nodes.

A more extensive history revealed that the patient suffered from metastatic bronchial carcinoma. The findings are compatible with lymphedema due to mediastinal obstruction.

f Ultrasound image at the end of radiation therapy: Diffuse skin thickening and edema.

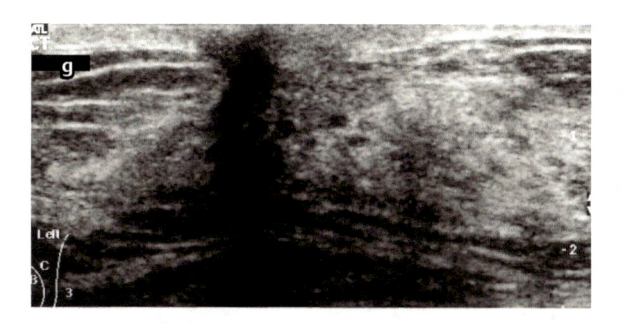

g,h Sonography of typical scar. Broad interruption and hypoechogenicity of the skin level and irregular posterior shadowing, horizontal view (**g**). Sagittal view of the same patient (**h**), where the interruption of the skin, subcutaneous fat layer, and breast tissue is visible together with retraction phenomena.

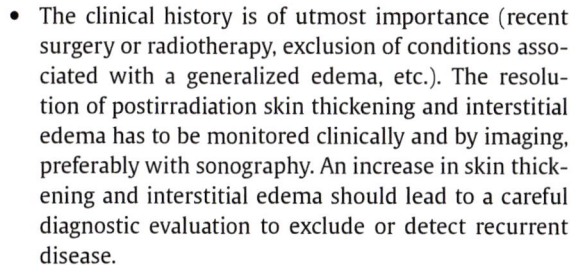

- The clinical history is of utmost importance (recent surgery or radiotherapy, exclusion of conditions associated with a generalized edema, etc.). The resolution of postirradiation skin thickening and interstitial edema has to be monitored clinically and by imaging, preferably with sonography. An increase in skin thickening and interstitial edema should lead to a careful diagnostic evaluation to exclude or detect recurrent disease.
- For the difficult differential diagnosis between inflammatory carcinoma and mastitis (see pp. 316 and 402 and **Figs. 13.1** and **15.7**), imaging has to be used, as it should be used for newly suspected venous or lymphatic stasis (sonography or contrast-enhanced computed tomography (CT) or magnetic resonance imaging (MRI) are useful for evaluating the axillary findings).
- If imaging cannot establish a definitive diagnosis (as would be the case if microcalcifications suggestive of malignancy are present), imaging can be helpful to select the most appropriate site for the excisional biopsy, with punch biopsy of the skin (see p. 402).
- If inflammatory skin thickening is suspected, a trial of anti-inflammatory therapy should be considered (to be monitored by serial imaging, using sonography).

Clinical Findings

For the differential diagnosis, a carefully obtained clinical history (underlying malignancy, related to surgery or radiotherapy) is of great importance, as are inspection (in dermatologic conditions), general physical examination (in the presence of generalized edema), and clinical evaluation of the breast (erythema, hyperthermia, peau d'orange).

To detect skin thickening, imaging is superior to the clinical examination since inflammatory carcinoma, for instance, can cause skin thickening that is visible on imaging studies weeks prior to its clinical manifestation.

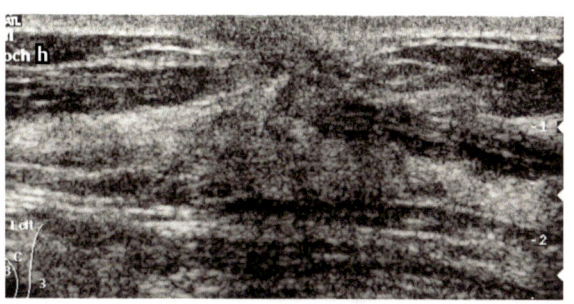

Mammography

With correct exposure, skin thickening is reliably and readily seen mammographically.

In addition to detecting or documenting skin thickening (important, for instance, for monitoring changes following radiotherapy), mammography is mainly used to detect signs of malignancy (suspicious microcalcifications or a suspicious lesion). Absence of a lesion or microcalcifications, however, does not exclude an otherwise suspected malignancy.

Sonography

Sonography (Liu et al. 2008) can also be employed to detect or document skin thickening. Detecting a hypoechoic focus in mammographically dense tissue can be relevant for the differential diagnosis.

Contrast-Enhanced MRI

MRI (Kalli et al. 2010) can also reveal skin thickening. Wormlike enhancement in and around tumorous foci found in subcutaneous lymphatic vessels can be evidence of lymphangiomatosis but is not visible in all cases. Otherwise, skin thickening and enhancement in the thickened skin are nonspecific. Contrast-enhanced MRI can make an important contribution to the differential diagnosis by detecting or excluding otherwise occult focal lesions in mammographically dense tissue (e.g., after radiotherapy). But for the differentiation between mastitis and inflammatory carcinoma, contrast-enhanced MRI is less suitable because enhancement is found in both conditions.

Biopsy Methods

Excisional biopsy including skin is the most suitable method for further evaluation of skin thickening. The histologic finding that is diagnostic for inflammatory carcinoma is the presence of tumor emboli in the dermal lymphatics. Imaging can be useful in selecting the site to be biopsied.

Summary

Skin thickening can be detected and documented with all imaging methods. For the differential diagnostic classification, clinical history, course of the skin thickening (status post radiotherapy), clinical findings (evidence of generalized edema), and inspection (dermatologic origin) are of particular importance.

While skin thickening with or without edema is generally nonspecific, imaging is used to search for signs suggestive of malignancy, such as microcalcifications or additional highly suggestive focal findings, or to identify suspicious areas for biopsy.

References and Recommended Reading

Britton CA. Mammographic abnormalities of the skin and subcutaneous tissues. Crit Rev Diagn Imaging 1994;35(1):61–83

Crowe DJ, Helvie MA, Wilson TE. Breast infection. Mammographic and sonographic findings with clinical correlation. Invest Radiol 1995;30(10):582–587

Kalli S, Freer PE, Rafferty EA. Lesions of the skin and superficial tissue at breast MR imaging. Radiographics 2010;30(7):1891–1913

Kushwaha AC, Whitman GJ, Stelling CB, Cristofanilli M, Buzdar AU. Primary inflammatory carcinoma of the breast: retrospective review of mammographic findings. AJR Am J Roentgenol 2000;174(2):535–538

Liu T, Zhou J, Osterman KS, et al. Measurements of radiation-induced skin changes in breast-cancer radiation therapy using ultrasonic imaging. Proc IEEE Eng Med Biol Soc 2008;2(2):718–722

Pluchinotta AM, De Min V, Presacco D, Reschiglian E, Tasinato R. Unilateral edema of the breast secondary to congestive heart failure. Report of 2 cases. [Article in Italian] Minerva Chir 1994;49(11):1171–1174

Pope TL Jr, Read ME, Medsker T, Buschi AJ, Brenbridge AN. Breast skin thickness: normal range and causes of thickening shown on film-screen mammography. J Can Assoc Radiol 1984;35(4):365–368

Skaane P, Bautz W, Metzger H. Circumscribed and diffuse skin thickening (peau d'orange) of the female breast. [Article in German] Rofo 1985;143(2):212–219

Willson SA, Adam EJ, Tucker AK. Patterns of breast skin thickness in normal mammograms. Clin Radiol 1982;33(6):691–693

22 The Male Breast

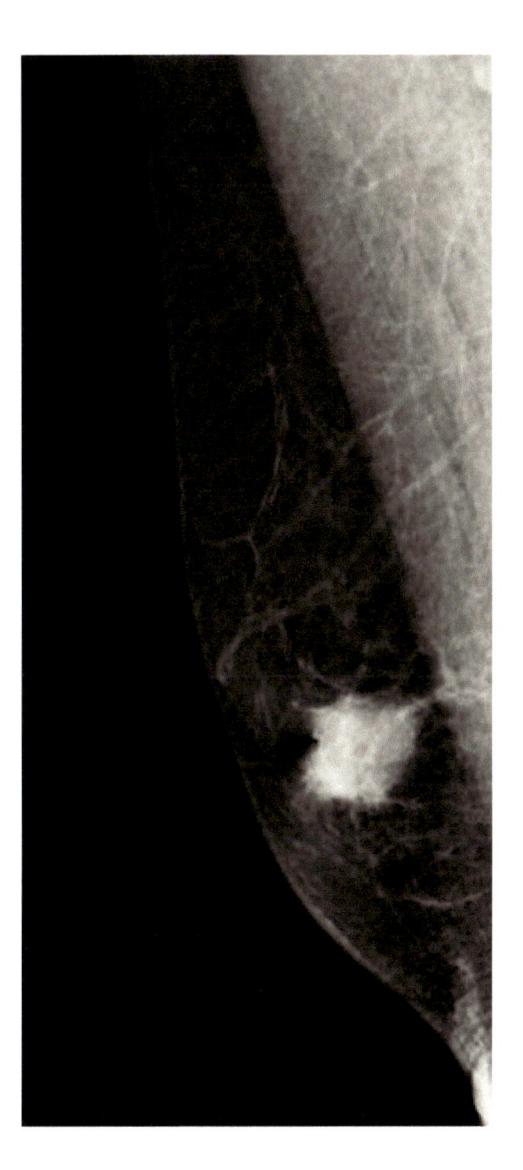

Anatomy 564
Clinical Examination 564
Mammography 564
Ultrasound 564
Magnetic Resonance Imaging 564

Gynecomastia 565
Definition 565
Histology 565
Clinical Findings 565
Diagnostic Strategy 565

Breast Cancer 567
Definition 567
Histology 567
Clinical Findings 569
Diagnostic Strategy 569

Miscellaneous 571

References and Recommended Reading 573

22 The Male Breast
S. Barter

Although still relatively uncommon, the attendance of men at symptomatic breast units is increasing. The most common presenting complaints remain those of pain and a breast lump. Despite the small numbers of men presenting, it is remains paramount that we understand the salient clinical and imaging findings to ensure we optimize patient management.

Male breast cancer constitutes about 1% of all breast cancer diagnoses. The spectrum of breast disease in men is similar to that in women, though given the absence of lobules in the male breast, breast cancer is almost exclusively ductal. Breast carcinoma and gynecomastia are the two principal diagnoses, with other pathologies significantly less common (Iuanow et al. 2011). Consequently, the main role of examination and investigation of the symptomatic male breast is to differentiate between these two processes.

Anatomy

The male breast extends from the second to the sixth anterior ribs with the sternum as the medial border and the midaxillary line as the lateral border.

When interpreting male breast symptoms, it is important to understand the anatomy. The normal male breast consists of predominantly fatty tissue with few ducts and stroma (Johnson and Murad 2009), which is distinctly different from women's breasts, where ducts, stroma, and glandular tissue predominate. This classically lies in a central retroareolar location. Given the sensitivity of the male breast to hormonal change, temporary or permanent increases in size can occur during the patient's life, such as in puberty or old age.

Clinical Examination

The standard protocol for the investigation of men presenting at the breast clinic has not been universally agreed. However, as with the female patients, it is generally accepted that it should begin with full bilateral clinical examination. The volume of palpable tissue can vary between men, ranging from no distinguishable mammary tissue, to a small area of retroareolar resistance. It has been reported that about 57% of men aged over 44 years old, have palpable breast tissue (Johnson and Murad 2009).

Mammography

The incidence of male breast cancer is too low to justify screening; therefore all mammography in male patients is diagnostic. Mammography has been shown to be a sensitive and specific method for distinguishing gynecomastia from breast carcinoma in men (Evans et al. 2001).

Dependent on the history, clinical findings, and age, mammography should be considered an essential component of the investigatory pathway. The standard views are as for female patients, with bilateral craniocaudal and mediolateral oblique projections. If there is persistent clinical concern or a discrete clinical or mammographic abnormality, then targeted ultrasound should be performed (Appelbaum et al. 1999, Evans et al. 2001, Günhan-Bilgen et al. 2002).

Normal Findings

At mammography, in many men, there is only fat-density within the breast on mammography, with no significant retroareolar soft tissue. If present, glandular tissue usually takes the form of a few strands of ductal or connective tissue extending from the nipple, or a more homogenous funnel-shaped soft tissue density in the central retroareolar region. If glandular tissue is present, it is surrounded by fatty tissue, which can vary from patient to patient (Appelbaum et al. 1999) (**Fig. 22.1**).

Ultrasound

The role of ultrasound imaging in further defining the characteristics of normal and abnormal breast tissue is well described, and it is as sensitive and specific in the male patient for evaluation of the breast, being superior to clinical examination or mammography in isolation (Günhan-Bilgen et al. 2002).

Ultrasound is the preferred technique in the male patient for guidance of biopsies since stereotaxis may be difficult due to the small breast size. Also, because of the method of detection (these are symptomatic patients), microcalcifications only or a tiny mass located in fatty tissue will rarely be the presenting mammographic finding.

It is evidentially clear from the literature that to date we still require all described modalities to maximize our diagnostic potential and accuracy in male breast disease.

Magnetic Resonance Imaging

No large studies are available on MRI in the male breast.

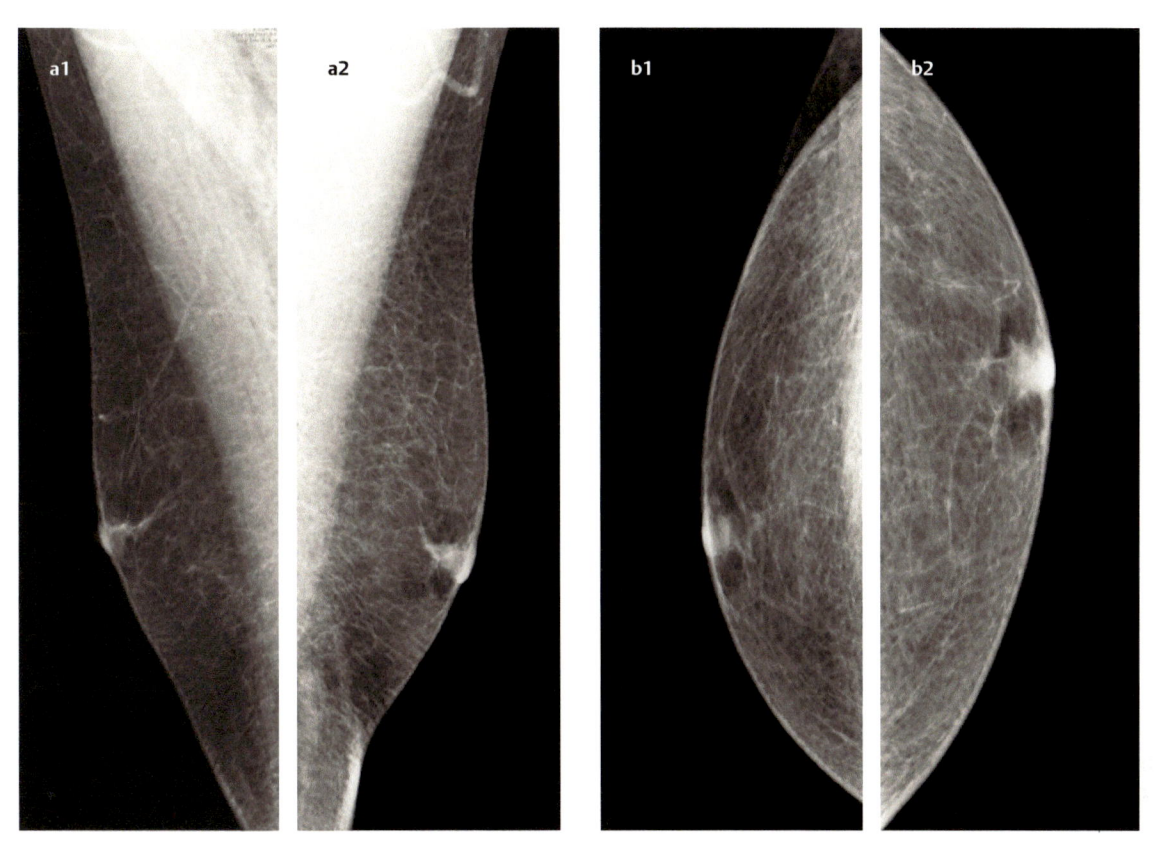

Fig. 22.1a,b Normal male mammograms. Mediolateral oblique (**a**) and craniocaudal (**b**) views.

Gynecomastia

Definition

Gynecomastia is the most common breast diagnosis in men, in which a unilateral or bilateral enlargement of the male breast occurs secondary to the influence of estrogens or substances that produce an estrogenic effect (Johnson and Murad 2009).

The etiologies are varied, ranging from idiopathic to secondary causes such as Klinefelter syndrome, endocrine and liver disorders, and drugs—both prescribed and recreational (**Table. 22.1**).

Approximately 60% of men with gynecomastia provide a medical history of a medical condition related to it or of medications known to cause it (Appelbaum et al. 1999, Johnson and Murad 2009, Iuanow et al. 2011).

Histology

Proliferation of the ductal system occurs with development and growth of alveoli, hyperplasia of the glandular epithelium, and an increase in stromal tissue.

Clinical Findings

Gynecomastia often presents as a soft mobile tender or painful mass in the subareolar region. Pseudogynecomastia is the result of deposition of fat in the subcutaneous tissue. It occurs bilaterally and is characterized by the soft consistency typical of fatty tissue. In genuine gynecomastia, the proliferative glandular tissue will be palpable unilaterally or bilaterally as a generalized or nodular localized area of increased soft, tender subareolar thickening.

Diagnostic Strategy

The most important diagnostic investigation aside from clinical examination is mammography. It has been shown to be accurate in discriminating between gynecomastia and male breast carcinoma (Evans et al. 2001).

Sonography may provide complementary information. It is indicated in young men, or to guide biopsy, but is not specific enough to identify solid findings as benign or malignant.

22 The Male Breast

Table 22.1 Causes of gynecomastia

Physiologic
Neonatal
Puberty
Senescence
Genetic
Klinefelter syndrome
Hormonal
Hypogonadism
Anabolic steroids
Exogenous estrogen
Systemic disease
Chronic liver disease
Chronic renal insufficiency
Neoplasia
Para-neoplastic syndrome
Adrenal carcinoma
Hepatocellular carcinoma
Pituitary adenoma
Drugs
Cimetidine
Diazepam
Marijuana
Omeprazole
Spironolactone
Thiazide diuretics
Tricyclic antidepressants

Mammography

Bilateral mammography should be performed unless the patient is under 35 years old in which case sonography should be performed to exclude a focal mass lesion. Three mammographic patterns of gynecomastia have been described representing various degrees and stages of ductal and stromal proliferation (Michels et al. 1977, Chantra et al. 1995, Appelbaum et al. 1999, Chen et al. 2006). These are the nodular, dendritic, and diffuse glandular patterns.

- Nodular gynecomastia corresponds to a pathologic classification of florid gynecomastia, which is thought to be the early phase, seen in patients with gynecomastia for less than 1 year. Mammography demonstrates a small nodular subareolar density which may be unilateral, but is usually bilateral, even if there are only unilateral symptoms (**Fig. 22.2**).
- Dendritic gynecomastia is thought to represent the pathologic correlation of fibrous gynecomastia which is seen in patients with long-standing symptoms. Dense fibrotic stroma is present histologically, which is seen on mammography as a subareolar soft tissue density with radiating projections, particularly into the upper outer quadrants (**Fig. 22.3**). This should not be confused with malignancy, since the mass arises directly from beneath the nipple with no associated nipple distortion or skin thickening.
- Diffuse glandular gynecomastia is commonly seen in patients receiving exogenous estrogen (e.g., for treatment of prostate cancer), and appears on mammography as a heterogeneous enlarged dense breast, similar to a female breast (**Fig. 22.4**).

Calcifications are not associated with gynecomastia (Chantra et al. 1995).

Ultrasound

In nodular gynecomastia there is a subareolar fan or disc-shaped mass which is hypoechoic surrounded by normal fatty tissue. A lobular margin can usually be perceived, but the zone of transition between the area of gynecomastia and normal fatty tissue may be poorly defined (**Fig. 22.5a**). The mass may be hypervascular on color flow sonography and therefore may be confused with a malignant process. For this reason, ultrasound-guided biopsy is required in the presence of clinical or mammographic evidence of a suspected malignancy.

Sonography in chronic dendritic gynecomastia demonstrates a subareolar hypoechoic lesion with an anechoic stellate posterior border. Fingerlike projections or "spider legs" protruding into the surrounding echogenic breast tissue may be seen (**Fig. 22.5b**). Unless familiar with this appearance, it may look suspicious for malignancy. However, a useful feature that suggests its benignity is that this mass arises directly from the undersurface of the nipple without causing any overlying skin thickening or nipple retraction. If there is any clinical doubt, however, biopsy is mandatory.

In diffuse glandular gynecomastia, both dendritic and nodular features may be seen at sonography surrounded by diffuse, hyperechoic, fibro-glandular breast tissue. This is distinguished from malignancy by the extensive disease without a discrete mass (**Fig. 22.5c**).

Therefore, because of the confusing appearances of ultrasound imaging, it is indicated only if there is clinical suspicion of malignancy, since mammography will usually be diagnostic.

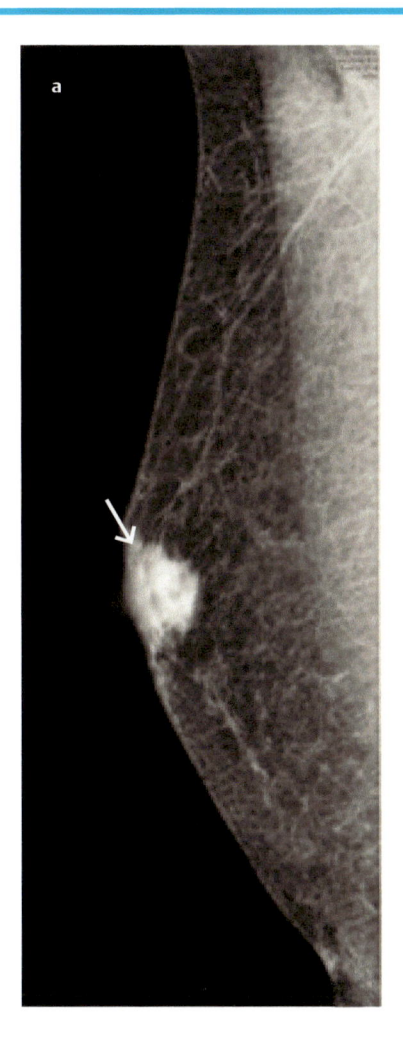

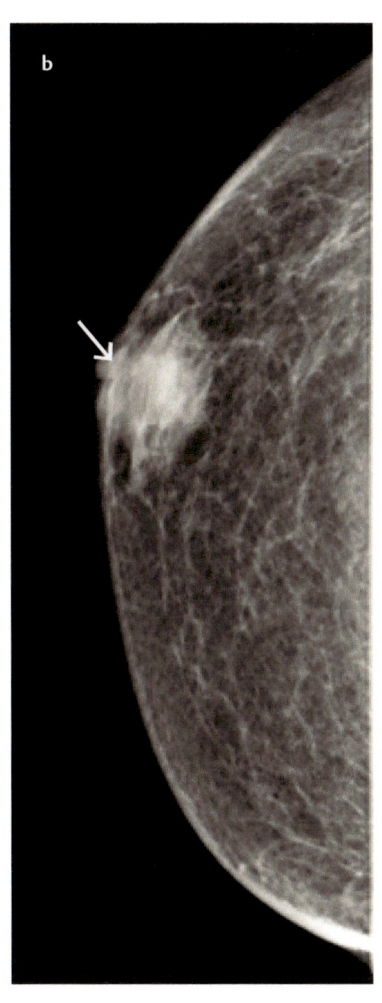

Fig. 22.2a,b Nodular gynecomastia. Right mediolateral oblique and craniocaudal views. Note small subareolar nodular density.

Breast Cancer

Definition

Breast carcinoma in men is rare, representing only 0.2% of male cancers and 1% of breast cancer (Chantra et al. 1995).

Breast awareness in men is improving but continued education of male patients is crucial to ensure that pathology presents early, because, as in women, early diagnosis is associated with an improved outcome (Chantra et al. 1995). The risk factors for breast cancer are similar to those for women, for example, genetic predisposition from *BRCA1* and *BRCA2*, increased age, exposure to ionizing radiation at a young age, and additional gender-specific factors such as cryptorchidism and Klinefelter syndrome. Klinefelter syndrome is a rare genetic condition (XXY) characterized by reduced or absent sperm production, small testes, and enlarged breasts. These patients have an elevated blood estrogen-to-androgen ratio and therefore a 3% risk and 20-fold increased incidence of breast cancer and are also more likely to have bilateral breast cancer. A family history of breast cancer in a first-degree relative increases the risk 2- to 4-fold.

Histology

Approximately 85% of primary breast cancers in men are invasive ductal carcinomas or ductal carcinoma in situ (DCIS). Men do not have lobules, even those with gynecomastia, so lobular cancer is not seen in men. All other histologic subtypes of carcinoma seen in women have also been described in men (Thomas 1993).

22 The Male Breast

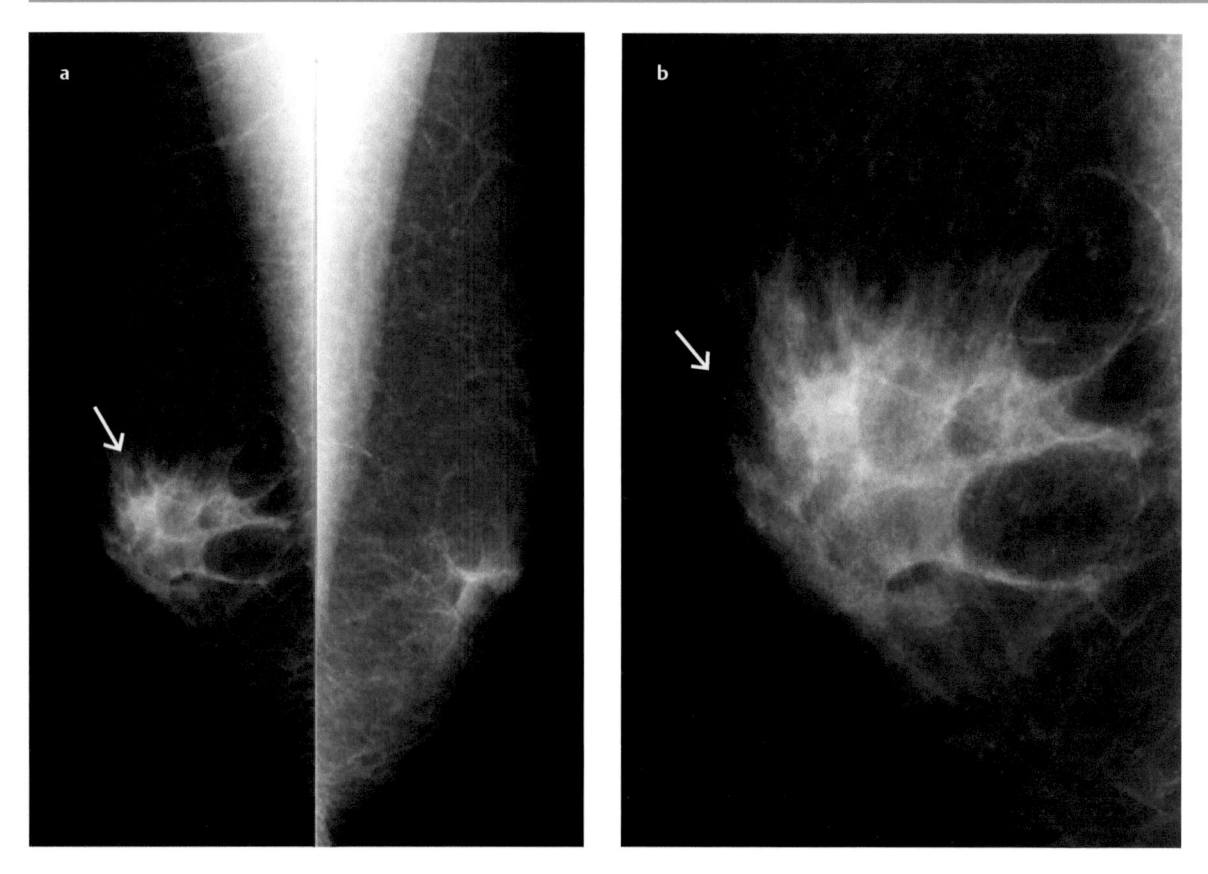

Fig. 22.3a,b Dendritic gynecomastia. Oblique views and magnification right oblique showing unilateral changes of a subareolar soft tissue density with radiating projections.

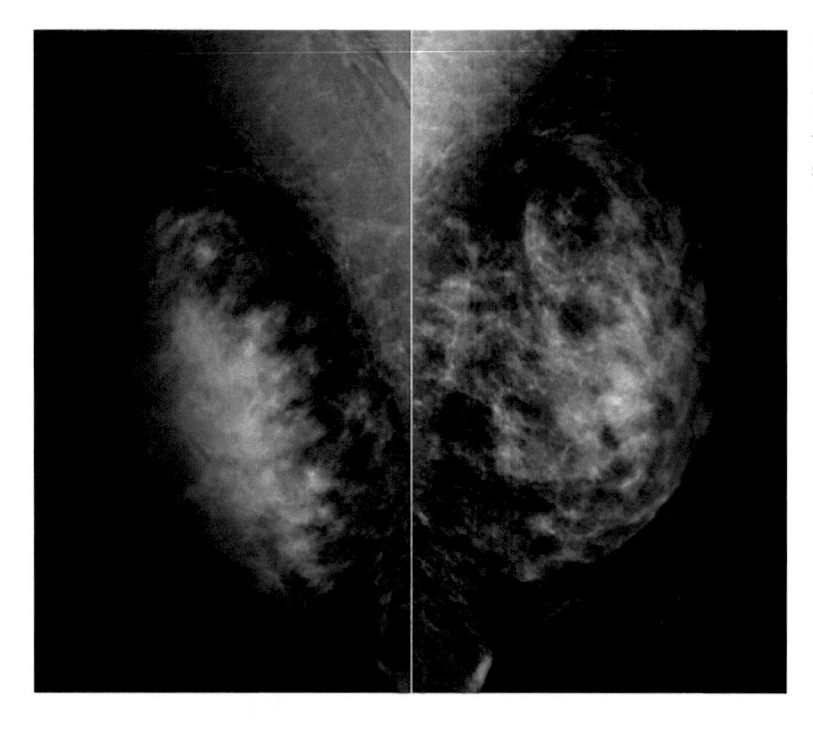

Fig. 22.4 Diffuse glandular gynecomastia. Patient is under the care of the endocrinology team for hypogonadotrophic hypogonadism and is being treated with Testogel (testosterone). Oblique views showing heterogeneous enlarged dense breast tissue, similar to a female breast.

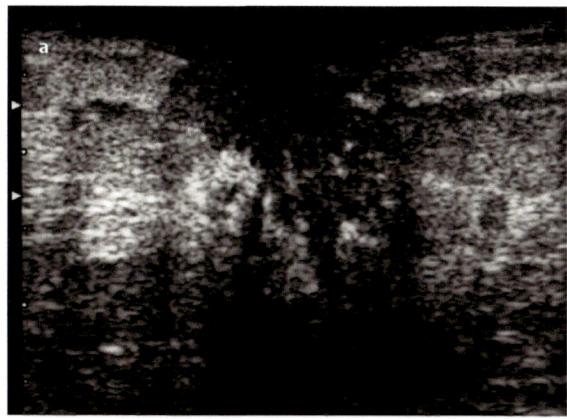

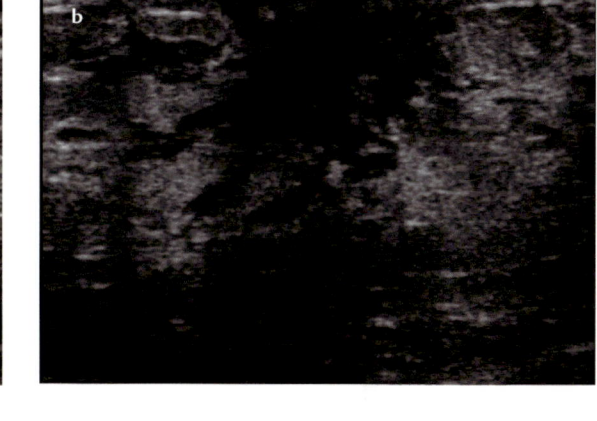

Fig. 22.5a–c Sonography of of gynecomastia.
a Nodular gynecomastia showing hypoechoic subareolar fan-shaped mass.
b Dendritic gynecomastia with an anechoic mass with a stellate border and fingerlike projections or "spider legs" protruding into the surrounding echogenic breast tissue.
c Massive gynecomastia showing diffuse benign breast changes with no focal mass.

Clinical Findings

Male breast cancer usually presents as a discrete firm mass, with or without bloody nipple discharge. Breast cancer in men is usually subareolar, and skin thickening and changes in the nipple are commonly present. The palpable mass is hard and nontender, not soft and tender as in gynecomastia. A bloody discharge from the nipple is always strongly suggestive of breast cancer in the male. Palpable axillary nodes are present in about 50% of cases at presentation (Chantra et al. 1995, Chen et al. 2006).

Diagnostic Strategy

Imaging strategies are the same as in the female patient. Bilateral mammography should always be performed since risk factors predisposing one breast to developing cancer will also affect the other breast.

Ultrasound scan of the breast and axilla is used to characterize the breast mass and evaluate axillary nodes for involvement. Ultrasound-guided biopsy is useful in men because the smaller breast size allows good penetration with high frequency transducers, affording good visualization of the needle. Stereotactic-guided biopsy is not usually feasible in the male patient because of the smaller breast size.

Mammography

Male breast cancer usually occurs in a subareolar location or just eccentric to the nipple, since male breast cancer commonly originates from central ducts. Occasionally, cancers may arise in a peripheral location. Eccentric and peripheral location is not typical for benign gynecomastia and is suspicious for carcinoma (Appelbaum et al. 1999, Günhan-Bilgen et al. 2002, Chen et al. 2006).

At mammography, these are typically high-density irregular masses. The margins are usually spiculated, lobulated, or microlobulated and may be well defined or ill defined, and may be associated with pleomorphic microcalcifications (**Fig. 22.6a–c**). They can be distinguished from benign gynecomastia because carcinoma appears as a discrete mass, commonly with secondary features. Secondary features are seen in a larger percentage of men and occur at a smaller lesion size than in women because the male breast is smaller. Nipple retraction, skin thickening, and increased trabeculation are helpful in diagnosis and carry a poor prognosis (**Fig. 22.7a**).

Microcalcification is less commonly seen in males than in females. It occurs primarily in DCIS components of tumors (Appelbaum et al. 1999, Günhan-Bilgen et al. 2002, Chen et al. 2006).

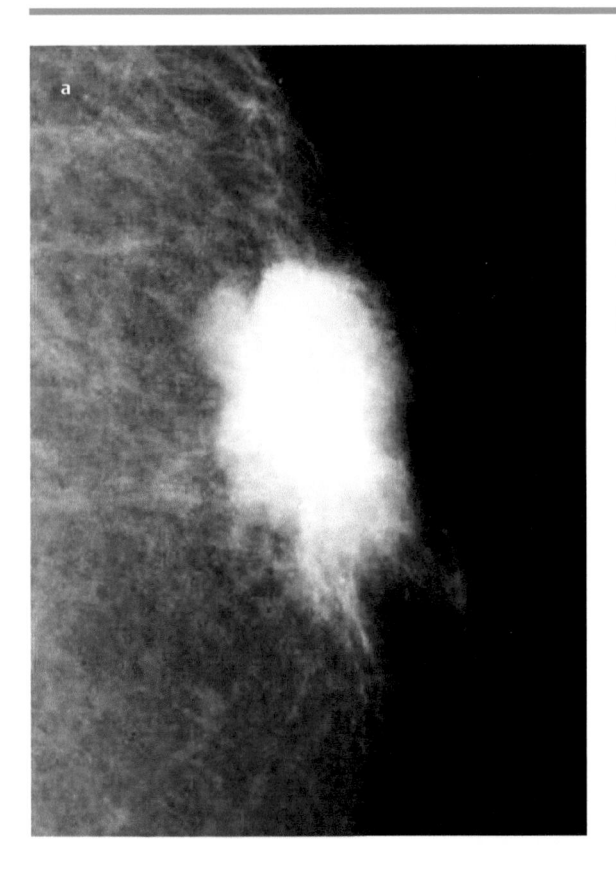

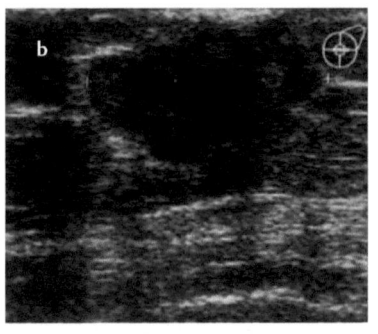

Fig. 22.6a,b Imaging of a 68-year-old male patient with a clinically suspicious mass in the left breast. The magnified section of the craniocaudal mammogram (**a**) was a subareolar dense spiculated mass. The ultrasound scan (**b**) confirms an irregular mass. Note lack of posterior acoustic effect.

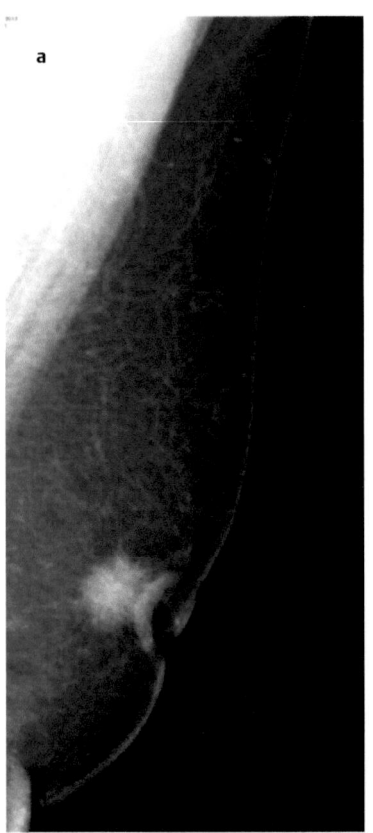

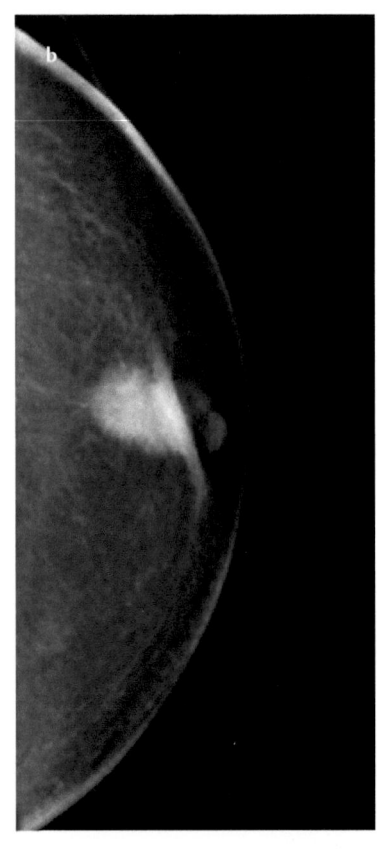

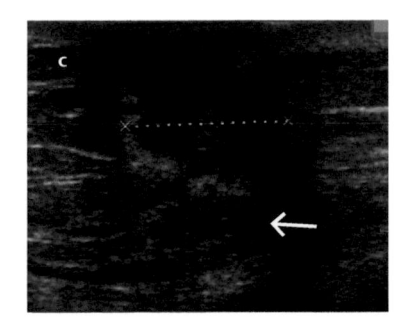

Fig. 22.7a–c Imaging of a 73-year-old man with a hard discrete nodule at the edge of the left nipple and nipple distortion.

a,b Mediolateral oblique (**a**) and craniocaudal (**b**) views show a spiculated mass and retraction of the nipple.

c The ultrasound scan shows a microlobulated mass with skin thickening (larger arrow). Note there is posterior acoustic enhancement (smaller arrow). *Histology*: 18-mm grade 3 invasive ductal carcinoma, 10 of 18 nodes positive.

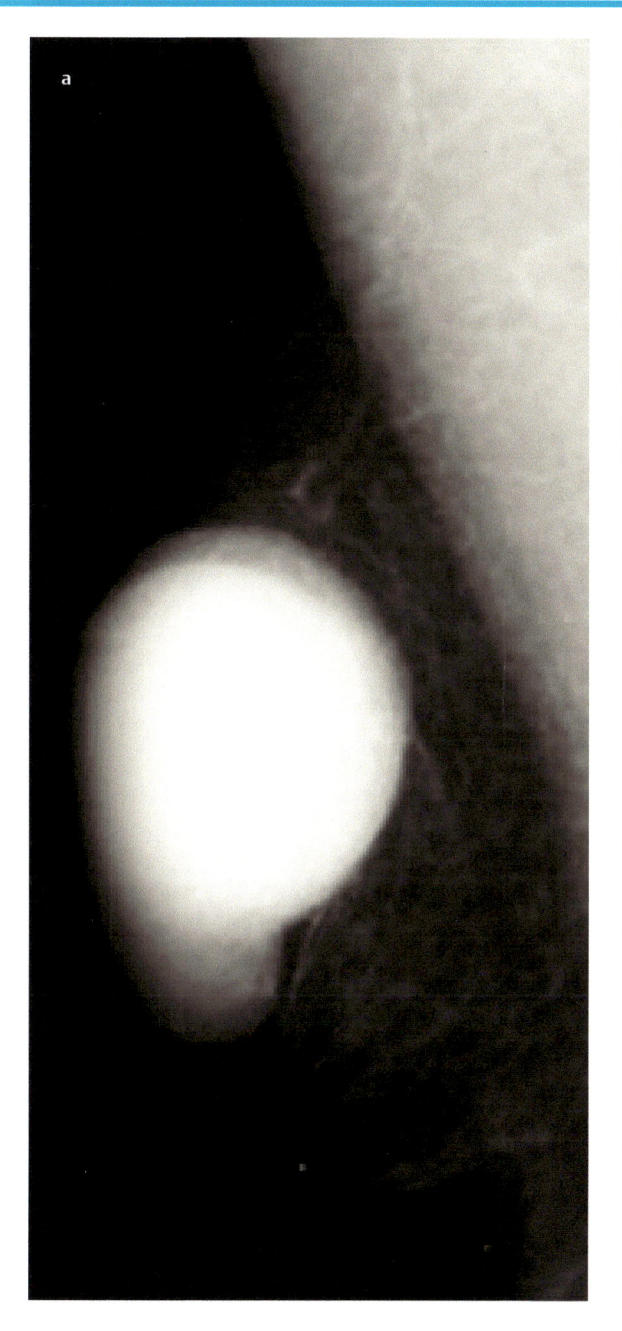

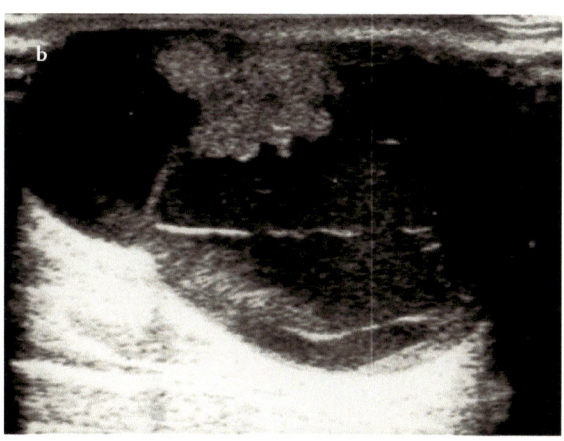

Fig. 22.8a,b Intracystic papillary carcinoma.
a Oblique view shows a large clearly circumscribed mass.
b Ultrasound scan shows complex cystic components suggestive of malignancy. Biopsy confirmed intracystic papillary carcinoma.

attenuation (**Fig. 22.6d**), and some may show acoustic enhancement (Günhan-Bilgen et al. 2002, Chen et al. 2006) (**Fig. 22.7c**). Sonography is helpful in assessing the relationship of the mass to the nipple and skin thickening, and nipple retraction can also be easily appreciated at ultrasound (**Fig. 22.7c**). Sonography is also useful for lesions located deep in the breast, which may be difficult to see at mammography.

When evaluating a suspicious breast lesion, ultrasound scanning of the axillary region should be routinely performed, as in the female patient. Enlarged axillary lymph nodes occur in 50% of male patients with breast cancer (Chen et al. 2006).

Male breast malignancy may also present as a complex mass on sonography, with the majority of histopathologic outcomes being papillary DCIS. Therefore, a circumscribed mass at mammography with cystic components at sonography in a male patient must be considered suspicious for malignancy (**Fig. 22.8**).

Men can, however, present with circumscribed masses that can be partially cystic or homogeneously hypoechoic on ultrasound (Iuanow et al. 2011) (**Fig. 22.8**).

Ultrasound

Male breast cancers have similar sonographic features to those in women. Invasive ductal carcinomas appear as nonparallel, discrete, hypoechoic masses (**Fig. 22.6d**). The margins may be angulated, microlobulated (**Fig. 22.7c**), or spiculated. Posterior acoustic features are not helpful for distinguishing benign versus malignant lesions, since in some male breast cancers there is no posterior acoustic

Miscellaneous

Other benign lesions include sebaceous cysts, hematomas, lipomas, abscesses, and fat necrosis. Sebaceous cysts are usually readily diagnosed clinically by their typical appearance, and do not require imaging. On mammography they are well defined, and on ultrasound they are seen in the subcutaneous tissues with a typical track leading to the punctum on the skin. In patients with hematomas, there is typically a history of trauma, anticoagulant use, or a clotting disorder. On mammography, hematomas are usually circumscribed and dense but may be irregular, and can be difficult to distinguish from malignancy. On

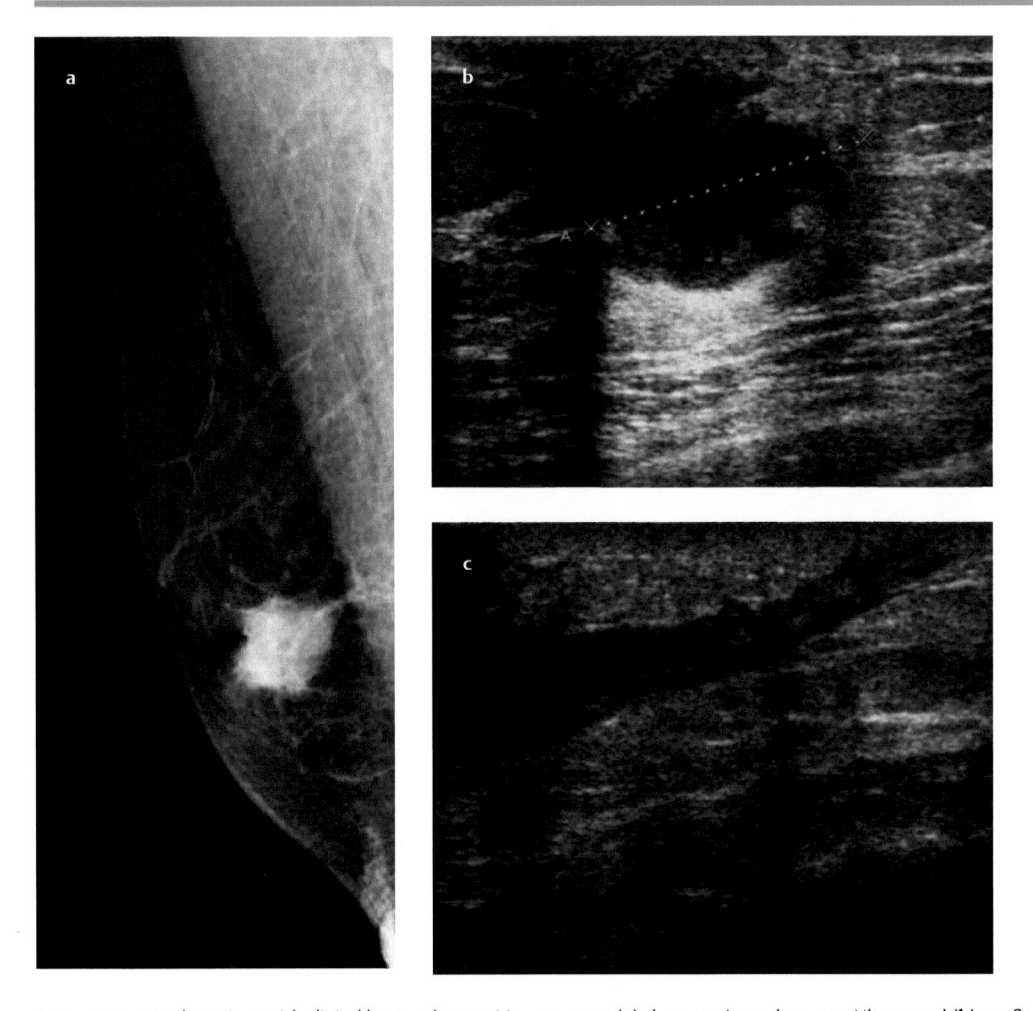

Fig. 22.9a–c Male patient with clinical breast abscess. Mammogram (**a**) shows an irregular mass. Ultrasound (**b**) confirms a complex fluid collection and demonstrates the discharging track to the skin (**c**). This resolved completely with ultrasound-guided drainage and antibiotics.

ultrasound, acute hematomas typically are hyperechoic often becoming more hypoechoic over time. Fine needle aspiration or core needle biopsy will confirm the diagnosis if there is any doubt.

Lipomas are the second most common benign lesion in the male breast, and on imaging have identical features to lipomas in the female breast. They are typically radiolucent on mammography and have a thin radiopaque capsule, which is characteristic in making the diagnosis. On ultrasound lipomas are circumscribed and most often are echogenic. Biopsy is not usually indicated if there are typical appearances.

Breast abscesses may be seen in the male, and are thought to arise within areas of ductal ectasia. On mammography an abscess, as in the female breast is seen as an irregular mass, associated with skin thickening, and can be difficult to distinguish from malignancy. Ultrasound imaging will show an irregular hypoechoic fluid collection which may contain internal echoes and debris (**Fig. 22.9**).

As in women, management is often by percutaneous drainage of abscesses, but in resistant cases, surgical excision of both the abscess and the ducts may be necessary.

Fat necrosis may occur following blunt or penetrating trauma and can present as a tender mass. Mammography may demonstrate a radiolucent circumscribed mass, sometimes with coarse and lucent-centered calcifications as in the female breast. On ultrasound, fat necrosis usually has typical features which enable the diagnosis to be made in the clinical context of trauma, avoiding biopsy.

There are other malignant neoplastic processes affecting the male breast, but with significantly lower incidence. Tumors can arise from any tissue within the breast, from the skin and subcutaneous tissue to the lymphatic and neurovascular structures. However, given the relative rarity of these pathologies, we will not cover them in depth in this book. It is of importance to include metastases when considering the presence of a breast mass in a male patient, most commonly from lymphoma, lung cancer, and melanoma. Ultrasound-guided biopsy is indicated for any mass not obviously benign.

> **Summary**
>
> Gynecomastia is usually evident by clinical examination. However, the poor sensitivity and specificity of the clinical examination determines the need to use mammography, sonography, and image-guided biopsy to confirm clinical suspicion. Gynecomastia is usually bilateral, with varying degrees of asymmetry.
>
> The imaging features of male breast cancer are as seen in females. If an underlying breast cancer is suspected, irrespective of the presence or absence of gynecomastia, image-guided biopsy of the abnormality is required.

References and Recommended Reading

Appelbaum AH, Evans GF, Levy KR, Amirkhan RH, Schumpert TD. Mammographic appearances of male breast disease. Radiographics 1999;19(3):559–568

Chantra PK, So GJ, Wollman JS, Bassett LW. Mammography of the male breast. AJR Am J Roentgenol 1995;164(4):853–858

Chen L, Chantra PK, Larsen LH, et al. Imaging characteristics of malignant lesions of the male breast. Radiographics 2006;26(4):993–1006

Evans GF, Anthony T, Turnage RH, et al. The diagnostic accuracy of mammography in the evaluation of male breast disease. Am J Surg 2001;181(2):96–100

Günhan-Bilgen I, Bozkaya H, Ustün EE, Memiş A. Male breast disease: clinical, mammographic, and ultrasonographic features. Eur J Radiol 2002;43(3):246–255

Iuanow E, Kettler M, Slanetz PJ. Spectrum of disease in the male breast. AJR Am J Roentgenol 2011;196(3):W247–W259

Johnson RE, Murad MH. Gynecomastia: pathophysiology, evaluation, and management. Mayo Clin Proc 2009;84(11):1010–1015

Michels LG, Gold RH, Arndt RD. Radiography of gynecomastia and other disorders of the male breast. Radiology 1977;122(1):117–122

Thomas DB. Breast cancer in men. Epidemiol Rev 1993;15(1):220–231

III Application of Diagnostic Imaging of the Breast

23 Screening

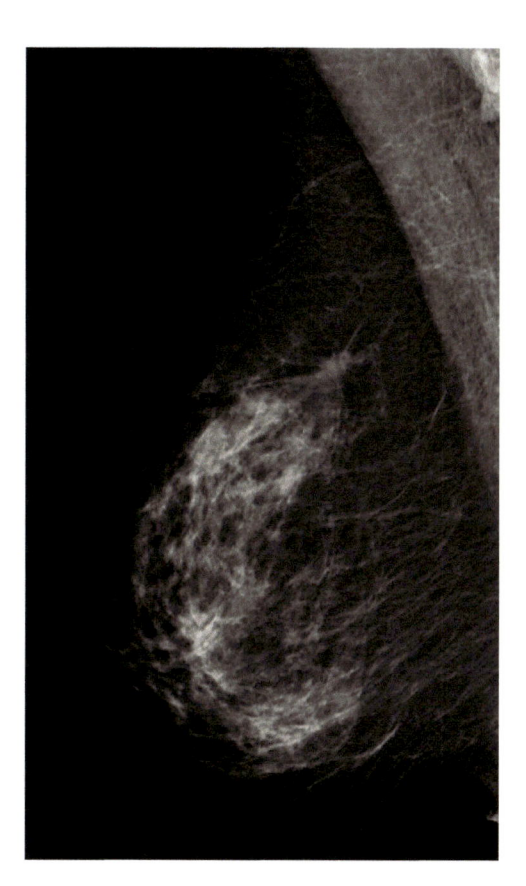

Definition → *578*
Quality Assurance → *578*

The Special Task of Screening → *578*

The Data and Discussions → *579*
Other Age Groups → *581*
Other Tests for Breast Cancer Screening → *582*
Absolute Numbers → *582*
Potential Risks and Limitations → *583*
Expected Advantages → *586*

References and Recommended Reading → *589*

23 Screening

S. H. Heywang-Koebrunner, I. Schreer, S. Barter

Definition

Screening refers to examinations performed regularly on asymptomatic women. According to European guidelines this term implies that screening is performed in a population-based screening program. In such programs all entitled women are systematically invited for mammography (mostly based on population registry data). This program is associated with strict quality assurance, exact prospective documentation, and systematic follow-up (optimally linked with the cancer registry). The goal is to ensure detection of breast cancer in the examined population at the earliest possible stage to reduce breast cancer mortality and to allow the reduction of unnecessary diagnostic steps and aggressive treatments to minimize potential side effects for the screened population.

Quality Assurance

Quality assurance of a screening program has to include the complete diagnostic chain. It should ideally also include the subsequent therapeutic chain, since only adequate therapy can warrant that a benefit from early detection can be transferred into a reduction in mortality. It is important not only to check the early available process parameters but also to eventually assess the desired outcome, which should include assessment of mortality reduction. For mortality evaluation, complete documentation of both the screening and the cancer registration including adequate statistics on causes of death are indispensable. Outcome is calculated by matching these data. Based on the delay between diagnosis of early malignancy and the expected time span between diagnosis and death, the full effect of a functioning screening program may be assessable only after up to 15 years of follow-up. The outcomes concerning mortality reduction, other advantages, and possible risks need to be continuously monitored to justify regular screening of the asymptomatic population.

The Special Task of Screening

Although breast *cancer affects 1 out of 8–10 women during her lifetime*, and even though breast cancer is the most frequent malignancy among women, the number of incident cancers per year or per screening round is very low. Between ages 50–69 *only 2–3 out of 1,000 women are affected per year*. At age 40 years this number is around 1 per 1,000 examined women. However, the addition of these yearly incident cancer cases results in more than 100 cancer cases occurring during the lifetime of 1,000 women. This number is equivalent to the statement that *1 out of 8–10 women is affected by breast cancer during her life.*

Considering the very low numbers of incident cancers per year, the difficulty of breast cancer screening becomes understandable. In a biennial screening program in women aged 50–69, for example, after the first round (during which prevalent cancers of the same and previous years may be detected) only 5–6 cancers are expected to occur among every 1,000 women screened. *The demanding diagnostic task thus is to correctly recognize the few cancers among the large number of women with normal or benign findings.* Considering the many normal variants, early detection is a difficult task. It is also completely different from the task of diagnostic breast imaging, where interpretation may be heavily influenced by the prospective or retrospective knowledge of a clinical abnormality, by the redundant information from several imaging modalities, and by the possibility of targeted evaluation.

No mammography screening program is capable of detecting all cancers that are expected to arise during the time period of the subsequent screening interval. Depending on the type of breast cancers and the type of surrounding breast tissue, some cancers are not detectable by mammography, since their mammographic features are not sufficiently different from those of the surrounding tissue. These comprise 10–15% of the breast cancers in the screened population. It is important to understand that sometimes even larger breast cancers may not be detectable by mammography. Furthermore, by their nature, in a population breast cancers will grow continuously, whereas any screening will assess the state only at given time points (mostly at 2-year intervals). Therefore with the given intervals and the limitations of mammography, to date *interval cancers—that is, cancers that are detected between the screening rounds—cannot be avoided.*

The main task of mammography screening, namely mortality reduction, is closely related to reduction of the incidence of late (life-threatening) stages of breast cancer. In mammography screening this is attempted by detecting as many cancers as early as possible. However, mammography screening is not designed or able to exclude breast cancer.

Even though it is known that screening will not be able to detect all breast cancers within the complete (2-year) interval, the sensitivity of screening mammography is calculated as the proportion of the cancers detected at screening divided by the number of all carcinomas that become apparent during the complete time period of the subsequent (2-year) interval. This is different from the calculation that is used for diagnostic imaging.

In a good biennial screening program (as defined in the European guidelines) it is possible to detect more than 1.5 times of the annually expected incident cancer cases during a screening round. Interval cancers make up less than 25% of the cancers detected during a biennial interval. To avoid delayed diagnoses in women with interval cancers, all screened women must be adequately informed that mammography is not able to detect all cancers. They should be encouraged to report any interim findings and should know who should be contacted for further assessment, if a change is noted.

For the screeners, the art is to detect as many small cancers as possible but not to simultaneously raise suspicion in the remaining 997/1,000 women who are healthy.

In quality-assured European screening programs it is possible to achieve good sensitivity while recalling around 30–40 out of 1,000 examined women per biennial follow-up round. This specificity (97%) is excellent for a diagnostic imaging modality. However, for a screening test this implies that on average during 20 years of screening (10 rounds) about 30–40% of the screened women (3–4% per round) will be recalled once. If histopathologic assessment is recommended in 1% of the screened women per round, 10% of the screened population will undergo histopathologic assessment once during the 20 years. Even though every second breast biopsy will yield a breast cancer, the added number of women undergoing at least one breast biopsy (mostly a needle biopsy) in a screened population (1 out of 10) is significant.

These numbers may explain the *importance of specificity* for any method that is considered to be used for population screening and the extraordinary *importance of quality assurance*.

The Data and Discussions

Mammography screening is one of the most intensively investigated fields of medicine. Our existing knowledge is based on randomized studies, on large case–control studies, on nonrandomized multicenter studies, and on the evaluation of several service screening programs. The vast majority of all studies showed a significant benefit and could prove a statistically significant mortality reduction.

The results of the most important *eight randomized studies*, as initially published are summarized in **Table 23.1**. As shown, the studies had different designs (single- vs. two-view mammography, with or without palpation and with screening intervals ranging from 12 to 33 months). They also concerned different age groups. The largest database exists for screening of women between ages 50 and 65.

Six of the eight randomized trials reported a significant reduction in mortality (Becker and Junkermann 2008, Nelson et al. 2009, Smith et al. 2010). One study (from Malmö) reported a nonsignificant mortality reduction of only 19%, which, however, was consistent with a significant crossover between the study and the control group. (Up to 30% of the invited women did not undergo screening, whereas 20% of the cancers in the control group were detected by screening mammography.) Another study from Canada showed no mortality reduction. For this study, however, severe deficiencies have been reported (Baines et al. 1990, Tarone 1995, Kopans 2009), namely: only volunteers were examined; there were serious problems with the randomization (assignment to the mammography group *after* clinical examination; predominant inclusion of symptomatic women and advanced stages in the study group); and an independent review of mammographic technique classified 50% of the mammograms as of poor or unacceptable image quality (Baines et al. 1990).

In 2000, Gøtzsche re-evaluated the eight randomized studies (Gøtzsche and Olsen 2000). Using formal criteria (small imbalances in the age distribution of a few months between the study and control groups), he excluded all six studies that had shown significant mortality reduction. The age differences in the six discarded studies had resulted from the fact that part of the municipalities had been randomly assigned to the study group and part to the control group. He insists on his weighting of the studies, even though cluster randomization (randomization of municipalities, not of single women) is a generally accepted method of randomization. Also, age imbalances occurred in different studies in either direction without recognizable effect. In further publications Gøtzsche assumed a bias concerning the assignment of the cause of death in some of the studies. Finally he pointed out some inconsistencies concerning reported numbers or exclusions. His criticism led to extensive re-assessment of the randomized studies by the World Health Organization, including counterchecking of the process of assigning causes of death.

In 2002 the International Agency for Research on Cancer published the following: "... many criticisms were unsubstantiated. Remaining deficiencies do not invalidate the results of the trials ..." (International Agency for Research on Cancer 2002).

Irrespective of the presented additional evidence, Gøtzsche insists on his weighted interpretation of the results of the randomized studies (Gøtzsche and Nielsen 2011). His evaluation thus mainly relies on the data from Malmö and on the strongly debated data from Canada. Based on this he assumes that the reduction in mortality comparing the group of women invited to mammography screening versus those not invited makes up only 15%.

Most other authors consider the screening effect, as assessed from the randomized studies, to be higher (Becker and Junkermann 2008, Nelson et al. 2009, Smith

Table 23.1 Results of the randomized controlled trials

Study	Start	Age (yrs)	Modality	Interval (mo)	Participation (%)	Follow-up (yrs)	Relative risk (95% confidence interval)	
							All	< 50 years
HIP	1963	40–64	2-view Mx + PE	12	67	10	0.71 (0.55–0.93)	0.77 (0.50–1.16)
Two County	1977	40–74	1-view Mx	33 (> 50)	89	29 and 15.2	K⁺ 0.69 (0.56–0.84)	0.73 (0.37–1.4)
Malmö 1 and 11	1976	45–69	2-view Mx, then 1 or 2 views	18–24	74	12	0.81 (0.62–1.07)	0.64 (0.45–0.89)
Stockholm	1981	40–64	1-view Mx	24	81	11.4	0.80 (0.53–1.22)	1.08 (0.54–2.17)
Gothenburg	1982	40–59	2-view, then 1-view	18	84	12		0.56 (0.31–0.99)
All Swedish studies		40–49		18–24		12.8 (median)		0.71 (0.57–1.89)
Edinburgh	1978	45–64	2-view Mx + PE (later 1-view Mx)	12 (PE) 24 (Mx)	61	14	0.79 (0.60–1.02)	0.75 (0.48–1.18)
Canada 1 (NBSS 1)	1980	40–49	2-view Mx + PE	12	100	10.5		1.14 (0.83–1.56)
Canada 2 (NBBS 2)	1980	50–59	2-view Mx +PE vs. PE	12	86.7	13	1.02 (0.78–1.33)	
UK Age Trial	1991	39–41	2-view Mx, then 1-view Mx	12	81	10		0.83 (0.66–1.04)

Mx, Mammography; PE, Physical examination; K+, Kopparberg; O+, Ostergotland.

et al. 2010, Duffy et al. 2012, Fitzpatrick-Lewis et al. 2012, Independent UK Panel on Breast Cancer Screening 2012). Considering that only about 70% of the invited women participated, whereas up to 30% of women from the control group may also have participated, it is estimated that, based on the data of the randomized studies, *mortality reduction among women who actually participate in biennial mammography screening will range above 30%* (International Agency for Research on Cancer 2002, Tabar et al. 2003, 2011, Brenner et al. 2009).

This estimate has been confirmed by other study types and by ongoing evaluations of national and regional screening programs (Parvinen et al. 2006, Swedish Organized Service Screening Evaluation Group 2006, Coldman et al. 2007, Gabe et al. 2007, Jonsson et al. 2007, Roder et al. 2008, Schopper and de Wolf 2009, Duffy et al. 2010, Allgood et al. 2011, Euroscreen working group 2012).

Two recent publications have again doubted the effect of screening (Kalager et al. 2010, Gøtzsche and Nielsen 2011). These studies have, however, been strongly criticized for various important reasons (lacking exclusion of cancers that occurred before onset of any screening, inadequate very short observation time of only 2.5 years). Also, both evaluations stem from countries (Denmark and Norway, respectively) where significant opportunistic screening exists outside the screening program. Neither of these evaluations calculated the effect of mammography screening among true participants nor has any attempt been made to estimate the effect of opportunistic screening.

In a publication by Duffy the effect of mammography screening was re-evaluated based on the data of the Swedish Two-County Study and of the British screening program using more than 15 years' follow-up (Duffy et al. 2010). From the data of the randomized Swedish Two-County Study, Duffy estimates that 8.8 lives were saved per 1,000 women screened, which exceeds a 40% mortality reduction for true screening participants. For the British program, in which mammography screening is offered to the women every 3 years, he calculated a mortality reduction of 5.7 lives per 1,000 women screened.

Meanwhile, the original results of the randomized studies have also been confirmed by a completely independent panel (Independent UK Panel on Breast Cancer Screening 2012).

When assessing national trends in mortality reduction as documented by the cancer registries, it is difficult to assess which factors may influence the observed mortality reduction. For the Dutch screening program, Otto was able to demonstrate that mortality reduction clearly correlated with the onset of mammography screening in different municipalities (Otto et al. 2003). Berry calculated the effect of mammography screening and of adjuvant therapy using different models (Berry et al. 2005). According to his calculations both mammography screening and adjuvant therapy contribute to the achieved mortality reduction about equally.

A recent case reference study from the Netherlands, in which mortality reduction was examined in screened versus nonscreened women, confirmed the above results and showed that mortality reduction by mammography screening had significantly increased from 28% up to 65% when comparing the effects before versus after 1992 (van Schoor et al. 2011). They attribute the increased effect to improved mammographic technology, to improved diagnostic workup of screen-detected abnormalities, and to a better linkage between screening and standardized therapy in breast centers.

In summary, to date (more than 30 years after initiation of the randomized trials) there is no reason to doubt that mammography screening accounts for a significant reduction in breast cancer mortality. It is estimated that biennial mammography screening allows a reduction in mortality among participating women of 30–35%.

Other Age Groups

To date mammography screening is generally accepted and recommended for women aged 50–69. This recommendation is strongly based on the fact that the largest database exists for this group of women.

However, only around 50% of breast cancers occur between ages 50 and 69. Approximately 20% of breast cancers occur before age 50, whereas 30% occur after age 70. Overall the breast cancer incidence at age 40 amounts to about one-third of the incidence observed at age 60. It rises continuously from ages 40 to 60 and stays high throughout life after age 60.

These facts support the question as to whether mammography screening should also be offered to women below age 50 and beyond age 70.

For women aged 40–49 consideration has to be given to the fact that owing to the lower incidence of breast cancer at this age, due to the somewhat lower sensitivity of mammography in the mostly denser breast tissue of younger women, and as a result of a higher false positive rate, the benefit–risk ratio in this age group is decreased compared with that in women aged 50–69. Existing data indicate a mortality reduction that is lower than that expected in women age 50–69: the AGE trial (which studied the value of mammography at age 40) yielded a statistically nonsignificant mortality reduction of 17% when comparing invited versus noninvited groups. Analysis of true participants, however, resulted in a statistically significant mortality reduction of 24% after a 10-year observation time (Moss et al. 2006).

A recent analysis of the Swedish screening program for young women (SCRY) yielded a mortality reduction of 29% among participants. However, these women had been screened at intervals of 1.5 years (Hellquist et al. 2011). A recent meta-analysis of all data from randomized studies in women age 40–49 reported an average mortality reduction of 17% (Magnus et al. 2011). Based on the data of a systematic review by Nelson, the US Preventive Services Task Force advised against screening before age 50 (Nelson et al. 2009), while the American College of Radiology explicitly recommended yearly mammography screening starting at age 40 and strongly supported shorter intervals (Lee et al. 2010, Hendrick and Helvie 2011). In a recent case reference study, a similar effect was proven for true participants of screening below age 50 as it was observed for women aged 50 (van Schoor et al. 2008, 2011). Even though the benefit–risk ratio (comparing mortality reduction with false positive ratio) is lower at age 40–49 than after age 50, due to the younger age the calculated years of saved lifetime may be even higher for ages 40–49.

So screening should further be considered for this age group. However, diligent consideration should be given to the optimum regimen. It may be worth specifically testing the use of additional methods for this age group or selected subgroups.

The data for women beyond age 70 confirm a high sensitivity of mammography and a low false positive rate. Moreover, the high incidence beyond age 70 also supports a decision for mammography screening. However, with increasing age (mainly > 75) the rate of overdiagnosis will increase, since an increasing number of screened women may die from other causes and thus might not benefit from early detection of an early malignancy.

Taking the above considerations into account, recommendations vary in different countries for women below age 50 and beyond age 70. Whereas Sweden and Finland offer screening to women before age 50, the screening interval has been shortened to 1.5 years. This takes into account the faster growth rates in younger women. (Other countries are following.) Shortened screening intervals and the additional use of other methods are being discussed as potential tools to make up for the diagnostic difficulties faced in this younger age group owing to their denser breast tissue.

Based on systematic data analysis, mammography screening is offered to women up to age 75 in the Netherlands and in the United States (Fracheboud et al. 2006, Nelson et al. 2009). In the United Kingdom and Australia, women are actively invited up to age 69, but are welcome to further participate beyond age 70, if they so desire. There is an initiative commencing in 2011 in the United Kingdom to extend the invited age range from age 47 to 73. The US Preventive Services Task Force (2009) recommends screening from ages 50 to 75; the American College of Radiology recommends yearly screening starting at age 40.

Other Tests for Breast Cancer Screening

So far, insufficient data exist concerning the use of other imaging modalities for breast cancer mass screening.

Several studies performed in selected asymptomatic women showed that ultrasound is capable of detecting small nonpalpable breast cancers that are mammographically occult. The reported incremental cancer detection rate ranges from 2.8 to 4.6 cancers per 1,000 women (Berg et al. 2008, Heywang-Köbrunner et al. 2008, Nothacker et al. 2009, Corsetti et al. 2011). However, patient selection in these studies varied strongly and cannot be compared with a screening population based on reported age distribution or risk factors. The data indicate that the false positive rate might increase significantly with the additional use of ultrasound, leading to approximately three times as many biopsies and an unknown number of recommendations for short-term follow-up.

The known operator dependence and lack of an effective and tested quality assurance program for screening sonography have so far prevented its use in such a setting in a national screening program.

Based on the existing data the American College of Radiology specifically states that *sonography is not a screening study for the breast*. Also, so far, no controlled breast cancer screening program has yet used or integrated ultrasound scanning.

Contrast-enhanced breast magnetic resonance imaging (MRI) is accepted as a tool for screening women at high risk. The highest sensitivity was achieved by combining mammography and MRI in these women. In this special indication (with special types of tumors, with a high proportion of very young women) on average 10% of breast cancers were detected only by mammography, while about 33% were detected only by MRI (Lord et al. 2007, Riedl et al. 2007, Warner et al. 2008).

Unfortunately, a significant number of false positive calls leading to additional assessments (biopsy) and recommendations for the short term must be expected to occur with MRI screening. Compared with mammography alone biopsy rates may triple, which in women at high risk may be acceptable considering the proven earlier detection and the problems faced with conventional imaging in this special indication (Heywang-Köbrunner et al. 2008).

Another special problem of MRI concerns the fact that lesions that are only detected by MRI require MR-guided biopsy, a technique which requires special experience and equipment and which is associated with significant additional costs.

To date there is insufficient data to assess the value of contrast-enhanced MRI in women at intermediate risk. Thus, *there is no recommendation to use MRI for screening in women at low or intermediate risk.*

Even though some studies exist which show that breast cancers may be detected in dense breast tissue by scinti-mammography or by positron emission mammography (PEM), the high radiation dose associated with both methods is a clear argument against regular use of these technologies for breast cancer screening (Hendrick 2010).

Absolute Numbers

Even though breast cancer is the most frequent malignancy in women, its yearly or biennial incidence is low. This means that a high number of normal tests need to be performed at regular intervals to make early detection possible. Without mentioning the denominator and without clear definitions of given percentages, a false perception of true proportions may occur.

To allow the reader a better understanding of the demands and limitations of mammography screening, absolute numbers are presented. The numbers presented here have been agreed upon by several experts in Germany considering the range given in the literature. They provide a careful estimate and should serve to give an improved understanding of absolute numbers and true proportions (The German National Mammography Screening Program; Perry et al. 2006).

In a biennial screening program (which is the most common type of screening program in Europe), the following numbers are expected when *screening 1,000 women for 20 years (= 10 rounds)*:

- 1,000 women between ages 50 and 69 years are screened biennially.
- 10,000 mammograms have to be performed.
- 65 cancers are expected to occur in 1,000 women during 20 years of screening (age 50–69).
- 50 cancers are expected to be detected by screening mammography.
- Fifteen cancers are expected to occur as interval cancers.
- To detect breast cancer early, 30–40 women are recalled for additional evaluation per round. This means that on average 300–400 recalls occur among 10,000 mammograms, or 300–400 of 1,000 women will be recalled once during 20 years of screening.
- On average 100 biopsies (10 per round), mostly needle biopsies, will be performed in the 1,000 women during the 20 years of screening. These will result in 50 benign diagnoses and 50 screen-detected breast cancers.
- Five overdiagnoses will be made. (This number is lower than assumed by Gøtzsche and Nielsen [2011], but higher than calculated by Duffy et al. [2010]). That is: Instead of 45 women, who would have noted a breast cancer without any screening (probably at a later stage), 50 women will be informed about their histologically proven breast cancer and undergo treatment. Without mammography screening the additional 5 would have survived without knowing about their breast cancer.

- Fifteen women would die from breast cancer without mammography screening.
- Screening will save the lives of 5 of the 15 breast cancer patients.

Recent data, which have become available for the ongoing European screening programs, indicate that the above-mentioned side effects may even be smaller, while up to 9 lives may be saved in 1,000 women who participate (biennial screening between the ages of 50 and 69) (Euroscreen Working Group 2012).

Potential Risks and Limitations

As shown by the above absolute numbers mammography screening means systematic examination of the population at regular intervals and may be associated with potential side effects. The following paragraphs give an overview of the discussed potential side effects of mammography screening. They include radiation risk, false positive call, (interval cancers) and overdiagnosis.

Radiation Risk

The radiation dose needed for a full field digital mammogram has dropped significantly during the last few decades. Today the average glandular dose amounts to less than 4 mGy per breast. The individual dose depends on further factors such as breast size, density, and breast compression. In women above age 40 the risk of inducing a breast cancer by this low amount of radiation is by a factor of 50 to 100 lower than the yearly natural risk of being affected by breast cancer (National Academy of Sciences 2006, Hendrick 2010, Yaffe and Mainprize 2011). Since mammography, however, is able to detect breast cancer early and thus can save by far more lives than it would risk, it is unreasonable to use radiation as an argument against the use of mammography for breast cancer screening in women above age 40.

However, since radiation is applied to the healthy population, diligent use of screening mammography implies strict quality assurance and monitoring.

Other Potential Risks

Some women are afraid that compression might cause breast cancer. These women can be assured that no cancer can be caused by compression in any part of the body.

False Positive Rate

Virtually no medical test is able to solely and effectively filter out only positive findings.

According to the results published for quality assured European screening programs mammography achieves an excellent specificity of approximately 97%. This means that (during subsequent rounds) about 30–40/1,000 women are recalled for an abnormality per round (Perry et al. 2006, Heywang-Köbrunner et al. 2010). In 20–30 of these women the suspicion can be eliminated by additional mammographic views or targeted ultrasound. (According to the European guidelines a recommendation for short-term follow-up should be given to less than 10/1,000 examined women.) Ten of the 1,000 women screened per round undergo histopathologic assessment, which today in most cases (9/10) can be achieved by core needle biopsy or vacuum-assisted breast biopsy. In 5 of the 10 women (per round) a breast cancer will be detected.

When adding up the numbers of recalls from the 10 rounds, indeed 400 out of 1,000 women will on average be recalled *once* during the 20 years of screening (between age 50 and 69) and 100 of 1,000 screened women will experience a needle biopsy at least once. In 50 of the 1,000 screened women, breast cancer will be verified.

Hendrick and Helvie calculated the risks per woman. Using the above data the risk of each woman with the above screening regimen equals a risk of being recalled (for imaging) of 1 recall every 50 years, one biopsy with a benign result every 150–200 years and one radiation-induced death in more than 200,000 years (calculation following the model of Hendrick and Helvie 2011). The above numbers demonstrate that, depending on the presentation, identical numbers may yield a completely different perception of risks.

From the medical aspect, the advantage clearly outweighs the disadvantages associated with recalls and with further assessments. This clear benefit is further supported by the new possibilities of minimally invasive procedures, which are only rarely associated with medically important side effects. A well-organized screening program ensures that the number of recalls and assessments is as low as possible and that the best tolerated minimally invasive methods are applied following state-of-the-art recommendations.

The psychological stress of a recall cannot be avoided. It is, however, limited to the time between informing the woman and the time of the final diagnosis. In the vast majority of cases the diagnosis is established within 2–3 weeks and women without breast cancer can definitely be assured of not having breast cancer.

Even though the limited time period of stress is experienced differently, this stress is comparable to many other situations of stress during life. Long-term negative effects caused by short-term stress that is subsequently resolved are rarely expected to occur in healthy women (Armstrong et al. 2007, Brewer et al. 2007, Salz et al. 2010).

According to our own experience the vast majority of recalled women are capable of dealing with this situation. They confirm that they prefer being recalled to taking any unnecessary risk (Heywang-Köbrunner et al. 2011). Nevertheless, the exact wording of any invitation and the way of handling anxious patients require adequate consideration and special training of personnel.

"Short-term" follow-up (mostly after 6 months), however, may require special consideration, since the long-lasting uncertainty may not be tolerated as well as short-term stress (e.g. of a needle biopsy), which then resolves (Armstrong et al. 2007, Brewer et al. 2007, Salz et al. 2010). In the individual case any recommendation for short-term follow-up should thus diligently be considered and explained to the patient. Some screening programs do not allow short-term follow-up.

Interval Cancers

Overall interval cancers do not represent a side effect of screening but a limitation of screening.

By definition interval cancers are cancers which occur in screening participants and become clinically apparent between two screening rounds. Considering that a screening round may last 22–26 months, in Germany a cancer will be registered as an interval cancer if it occurs within 24 months of the previous screening examination. In other programs both the definition and the screening interval may vary. These facts have to be considered when comparing results from different countries or programs.

Considering that cancers can grow and surface continually at any time, whereas screening assesses only the situation at given time points, interval cancers are unavoidable with any type of screening unless a method were able to prospectively detect all breast cancers which are visible at the time point of screening *and* predict all those that might become apparent during the complete subsequent screening interval (of 2 years, for example). So far no such method is known. This shows that the definition of sensitivity used for screening may differ strongly from the definition used in other fields of medicine.

Theoretically the following situations may describe the possible presentations of interval cancers (Boyer et al. 2004, Hofvind et al. 2008, Kirsh et al. 2011, Pellegrini et al. 2011):

1. A cancer newly develops during the interval starting from nothing or from some microscopic change, which is occult to all methods or tests (example: fast-growing tumor).
2. An existing breast cancer (that might be visible by other methods or might even be palpable) is mammographically occult or causes an unspecific change only, which cannot be diagnosed prospectively. During the interval (possibly even directly after mammography screening) the cancer becomes clinically apparent (example: limitation of the screening method).
3. The breast cancer is mammographically visible but it is not detected or is misinterpreted by the screeners (missed breast cancer; human error).

Since neither an exact definition of the onset of tumor growth nor a clear-cut border between an unspecific change and a discrete sign of malignancy exist, the three situations cannot always be clearly separated.

In theory, *situation 1* describes the true interval cancer. Such true interval cancers more often concern fast-growing cancers, usually cancers of a histopathologic high grade (grade 3). Grade 3 tumors make up less than 30% of the tumors in women aged 50–69 and less than 20% of the T1 tumors in these women.. Whereas the screening interval of 2 years may be sufficient for most G1 or G2 tumors, for those fast-growing cancers that start growing early after the last screen a biennial screening interval may be too long. Detection of a fast growing tumor in a biennial screening program may depend on the onset of tumor growth with respect to the time-point of the screening examination. Shorter screening intervals, as are used in some countries for screening younger women, will increase the probability of detecting more cancers with fast tumor growth at the screening examination.

Situation 2 demonstrates the limitations of mammography as a screening test. Missing larger cancers can be avoided by asking women to report any noted changes. Even though other methods have proven capable of detecting some of the mammographically occult cancers, no other imaging method has so far been accepted as a test for mass screening of women at usual risk. Reasons include as yet unsolved problems of quality assurance, expected significantly higher rates of false positive calls, and cost–benefit considerations. The required quality assurance would, for example, need to warrant reliable early detection of at least some of those cancers that cannot be detected by mammography screening.

Situation 3 is one that should be minimized in good screening programs. Tools to achieve this include blinded double reading, reader training, and continuous feedback (training on interval carcinomas and participation of readers in interdisciplinary screening conferences with histopathology–imaging correlation) and finally monitoring of the accuracy of all involved readers. As is other aspects of life, human errors may thus be reduced, but can never be eliminated.

Owing to the large spectrum of normal variants certain changes may be seen in retrospect (knowing where the palpable finding is, or where it is seen on subsequent mammography) but cannot be expected to be diagnosed prospectively (see **Fig. 16.8a**). For discrete and minimal changes prospective diagnosis could be compared to not being able to see the wood for the trees.

It must be understood that, depending on the histology of the cancer and depending on the surrounding tissue, sometimes even large cancers may be undetectable by mammography or may be suspected only based on very subtle changes. Also some large cancers may suddenly become palpable in large areas even though no clinical (or imaging) sign existed before. It is assumed that such cancers may arise from large areas of pre-existing, premalignant changes (atypical ductal hyperplasia or non-calcified ductal carcinoma in situ [DCIS]). They suddenly present as a palpable finding when the extended premalignant lesion changes into an invasive cancer. This may occur simultaneously and multifocally within the large area and is then usually associated with reactive changes such as fibrosis, edema, or rarely even inflammation, which causes the clinical signs. Fortunately, such sudden and unpredictable presentation of extended (interval) cancers only concerns a few percent of all cancers.

Considering that any retrospective diagnosis is heavily biased, the distinction between no sign, minimal sign, and missed cancer is quite difficult and should be made only by persons with significant experience with both reading of interval cancers and prospective mammography screening.

To assess the correct function of a screening program, the European guidelines for mammography screening suggest thresholds for recommended detection rates and for acceptable rates for interval cancers. Furthermore, interval cancers need to be analyzed by those responsible for the program and should be discussed with all persons involved in the screening and assessment chain. This process serves to identify potential weak links in the screening chain and allow optimization by continuous feedback.

In each screening program interval cancers should be assessed and classified as "true interval cancer" (not visible prospectively, newly appearing), as "minimal sign" (this usually means that at least some uncharacteristic change is seen in retrospect, which, however, cannot be expected to be prospectively identifiable as a sign indicating malignancy), or as a "missed cancer." Those interval cancers classified as "missed" or "minimal sign" should be presented to the screening team at regular intervals for training and optimization.

Errors may occur at any point along the diagnostic or therapeutic chain. They may include organizational deficits concerning information transfer (of reported clinical symptoms) from the patient to the screeners, from screening to assessment, or from assessment to further treatment (intra- or interdisciplinary information), or from screening to the patient (reporting the result). They may concern reading errors, errors of the consensus conference or of the assessment process, or inadequate treatment. Any error may compromise the effect of early detection. Therefore, analysis of the origin of errors and identification of any systematic error is essential to success.

Overall, screening is a difficult task. Considering the known advantages of mammography screening, the unavoidable occurrence of interval cancers may not be easy to understand and communicate. Any interval cancer means frustration and disappointment for both the patient and for the screening team.

Therefore, open and honest communication of the possibilities and limitations of mammography screening is of great importance.

To avoid delayed diagnoses in the case of interval carcinomas we recommend systematically and prospectively communicating the following message to all screened women:
- Even though mammography screening allows detection of most breast cancers early, some cancer cannot be diagnosed by mammography. Therefore, whenever a change occurs (even after a normal screening examination), the woman should be encouraged to see her doctor or present to the screening unit for further assessment.

Overdiagnosis

Overdiagnosis of breast cancer in a screening program describes the fact that in a screened population more breast cancers are detected than in a comparable unscreened population. Most of the additional cancers detected at screening would have presented later on as a clinical finding. Some of the additional cancers, however, would never have become apparent without screening. Thus, their detection does not contribute to mortality reduction. These additionally detected, histopathologically correctly designated true malignancies are called "overdiagnoses." The name originates from the fact that the "overdiagnosed" cancer would not have threatened the woman's life, since the woman will die of a different cause before the cancer had become apparent (without screening).

Since the individual life span of each woman is not known ahead, and since the natural history of each cancer can be estimated (based on tumor stage and grading) but can never be exactly predicted for the individual case, it is impossible to foresee therefore which breast cancer would or would not threaten the patient's life, had it not been detected and treated. While the possibility of overdiagnosis increases with the detection of early disease, the probability of saving a life by detection at a still curable stage increases as well. Overall, overdiagnosis is a statistically calculated number that deals with an extreme form of length–time bias.

Even though overdiagnosis is mostly mentioned as a side effect of mammography screening it must be pointed out that there is no reason to believe that overdiagnosis is less important for opportunistic screening. Owing to a lack of documented data on women undergoing opportunistic screening, a lack of data on control groups and a lack of systematic long-term follow-up (> 10 years) outside organized screening programs, it is impossible to *calculate* overdiagnosis, even though overdiagnosis does exist for any test that is sufficiently effective to detect cancer earlier than clinically.

The most extreme assumption would be that a screening program selectively detects breast cancers that would never progress or would even regress without treatment.

The latter assumption was made by Zahl et al. (2008), who (based on ecological data only) compared a screened Norwegian population from one region with a control group from a different region and from a 5-year earlier period. This publication has had a major impact on the results of a meta-analysis published by Jørgenssen and Gøtzsche in 2009, even though the results have been very critically debated by renowned epidemiologists and other experts (Ciatto 2009, Euler-Chelpin et al. 2009, Kopans 2009, Paci and Kalager 2009, Pisani et al. 2009, de Gelder et al. 2011, Puliti 2012). The criticism concerned the calculation model and doubted the comparability of the chosen study and control groups. Doubts focus on inadequate adjustment for lead time (i.e., insufficient observation time and follow-up time were used to correctly include the postponed diagnoses of the control group, and thus observe the expected compensatory drop) and insufficient comparability of the chosen study and control groups (risk, age, other factors) is assumed (Puliti 2012).

While regression of a breast cancer or extreme numbers of overdiagnoses, as assumed by Zahl, Jørgenssen and Gøtzsche (Zahl et al. 2008, Jørgensen and Gøtzsche 2009, Gøtzsche and Nielsen 2011), are unlikely, the phenomenon of overdiagnosis does and must exist. It is associated with any test that is sufficiently sensitive to detect cancers years before they might become clinically apparent and for any population for which the expected life span is limited (e.g., beyond age 60–70). For mammography screening the full effect concerning mortality reduction will be apparent after 15 years of follow-up. (This is due to the detection of some very early or premalignant stages.) Any death in a woman with screen-detected cancer that occurs for reasons other than breast cancer within these 15 years might contribute to the number of cases counted as "overdiagnoses."

The interval between screens causes some filtering toward lower-grade cancers. This filtering influences the proportion of low-/higher-grade malignancies among screen-detected cancers and thus has an effect on mortality reduction. However, it should not increase the absolute number of overdiagnoses in a population.

It should also be pointed out that the process of establishing a screening diagnosis—which after the first round is based on comparison with previous studies—filters out those lesions that develop newly or grow. There is no logical explanation why (as assumed by some opponents of screening) malignancies that are detected based on their increase in size or new growth would regress without any treatment. Furthermore, mere comparison of grading among screen-detected cancers versus clinically apparent cancers is certainly not adequate, since progression from lower to higher grades is known to occur with time and with increasing tumor size, from histopathology and epidemiological data.

Overall, calculation of overdiagnosis is difficult due to the large possibilities of bias and the partly limited information available from existing data sources. Thus, to date, published results diverge significantly ranging from 1% to 50% (de Koning et al. 2006, Zackrisson et al. 2006, Zahl et al. 2008, Puliti et al. 2009, Duffy et al. 2010). The best founded calculations report rates around 5–10% (Puliti 2012). However, owing to the uncertainty of all underlying data, the many possible assumptions and the resulting extreme variations, the existing level of evidence on this subject is extremely low.

Overall, overdiagnosis can never be avoided if a test is sufficiently sensitive to diagnose a disease before it becomes clinically apparent, since during the gained time span (which may exhibit a wide range) other events may limit the patient's life. Overdiagnosis probably concerns less than 10% of the detected breast cancers. The risk of overdiagnosis appears to be low for women before age 60. It increases after age 60 and further increases after age 70, since other risks of death increase. The possibility of overdiagnosis also increases with small and slow-growing cancers. Since some DCIS lesions (even though being a precursor of invasive disease) may not develop into invasive breast cancer during the remaining life span of a woman, DCIS must be considered an important potential source of overdiagnosis and thus requires special attention.

The major side effect of overdiagnosis is that the patient who does not benefit from the diagnosis is informed about her diagnosis and thus undergoes treatment (so-called overtreatment).

Today in most fields of medicine neither therapy nor diagnosis is possible without risking overdiagnosis or overtreatment. Being aware of the possibility of overdiagnosis, diagnosticians should not strive for detection of minimal pre-invasive disease, but rather for detection of significant disease as early as possible to reduce life-threatening late stages. Detection of prognostically favorable cancers and cancer stages implies the potential of life saving but may also be associated with overdiagnosis in patients with a limited life span. Therefore patients with early breast cancer and low-grade DCIS should also be adequately informed about their excellent survival prognosis and treatment should be adapted as well as is possible to the patient's individual risk.

Expected Advantages

Advantages of mammography screening include mortality reduction and improved therapeutic options, such as reduced rate of axillary dissections, reduced need for chemotherapy, reduction of mastectomy, and better cosmetic results. Reassurance in the case of a negative test has falsely been a neglected advantage. Furthermore, there are other positive advantages of a complete quality-assured diagnostic and therapeutic chain on the health system, which have been observed and are predicted for science and research into breast cancer.

Mortality Reduction

Mortality reduction is considered to be the main effect of mammography screening and has thus been the incentive for the introduction of mass screening.

Even though detection of early breast cancer is one component, a much better estimate for mortality reduction is achieved if the incidence of late stages (T2+, T2 or N+ stages) decreases compared with the incidence before onset of screening.

The following biases may explain why *early detection need not be equivalent to life saving.*

Certain cancers may be lethal with or without early detection. *Lead time bias* describes the fact that earlier detection in these cases falsely improves 5-year survival statistics owing to the advanced date of diagnosis. Overall mortality, however, is not affected.

Prognostically very favorable cancers, however, may be curable with or without screening. Since prognostically favorable cancers grow more slowly, their preclinical stage lasts longer than that of fast-growing malignancies. Owing to the longer time span of the preclinical stage the chance of detecting prognostically favorable cancers (using any periodical examination) is generally somewhat higher than for fast-growing cancers. This selection bias might be enhanced by choosing too long screening intervals. This type of bias is called *length–time bias*. Detection of prognostically very favorable cancers including cancers that otherwise might not have been detected (overdiagnoses) will improve the stage distribution among the detected cancers. Absolute breast cancer mortality in the population, however, will not be influenced.

Finally, various types of *selection bias* (such as preferential selection of certain socioeconomically selected parts of the population) may occur when screening participants are compared with nonparticipants.

Thus correctly assessing the effect of a screening measure requires direct assessment or estimation of mortality reduction.

Proof of mortality reduction, however, is not trivial, since the diagnostic screening test precedes the endpoint (death) by 8–15 years. All evaluations (including randomized trials) have limitations. Thus combined analysis of available data and evaluations may yield the best possible answer. Limited information available from the usual sources (screening databases, cancer registries, and death statistics) and privacy legislation complicate the necessary and important evaluations.

In spite of existing difficulties and limitations, ample data are available to date, rendering mammography screening one of the most intensively investigated fields of medicine.

Based on these data there is no reason to doubt that *quality-assured mammography screening is capable of significantly reducing breast cancer mortality.*

According to the existing range of results it may be assumed that using quality-assured biennial screening mammography performed at age 50–69 the following mortality reduction may be achieved:

- Among 1,000 women screened for 20 years about 65 cancers are expected, of which 15 are expected to be lethal. For screening participants it may be expected that 5 of the 15 deaths can be prevented.
- This implies that biennial screening saves approximately 1 life in 200 screening participants (most of whom will never be affected by breast cancer) or 1 life per 2,000 screening mammograms. However, it also implies that breast cancer mortality among true participants is reduced by at least 30%.

Some authors insist on communicating to women a so-called benefit ratio of 1 life saved per 200 or per 2,000, meaning 1 life saved among 200 screening participants or among 2,000 mammograms. We explicitly warn against communicating the former ratios without exactly defining and explaining the denominator. One typical example is the following message used by some opponents of screening: "Only one out of 2,000 women will benefit from screening." This information may be at least as misleading as the simple message of a mortality reduction of greater than 30%. (Mathematically all this information is equivalent.) The reason for misunderstanding this information is that no woman expects to learn about a ratio of benefit that is calculated *including* women who will never be affected by breast cancer. The message furthermore disregards all other positive effects of early detection and quality assurance (see below).

Communicating such rates could instead lead to the false belief that screening might save only 1 of 200 or even 2,000 affected women. This could erroneously discourage women from attending for mammography screening. Conversely, according to our own experience, women wish to learn about the benefit from screening, which may only be expected for those women who are affected by breast cancer. The correct answer for the latter question is: 3 out of 10 women affected by breast cancer will die from their disease. Among screening participants one of those three lives can be saved.

It should be added that during the 20 years of screening, only approximately 65 cancers are expected to occur in 1,000 women.

Improved Therapeutic Options

Despite significant advantages of therapy (including the possibilities of breast conservation, of limited axillary surgery, of plastic surgery, of adjuvant and neoadjuvant therapy), therapy of breast cancer is associated with significant mid-term and long-term side effects. Therapy, too, is only able to save some of the threatened lives.

For most women with invasive breast cancer or DCIS early detection allows a reduction in the aggressiveness of the treatment. A decreasing need for certain therapies with earlier detection is thus mostly associated with improved therapeutic options, less fear, and fewer side effects.

Improved treatment options include:

- *Reduced need for mastectomy.* Cancer registry data show impressively decreased rates of mastectomies among T1 stages versus late stages (T2–4). Most DCIS can be treated with breast conserving therapy. However, for extensive DCIS (which is known to be associated with a significant risk of developing into or containing invasive breast cancer) breast conserving therapy may not be an adequate option. Even though some mastectomies cannot be avoided by mammography screening—or might even be the consequence of a certain number of overdiagnoses—up-to-date results from the Dutch screening programs confirm an overall reduction of mastectomies associated with screening mammography. Similar trends are being reported from regions of the young German screening program (Health Council of the Netherlands 2002, Holland et al. 2007, Schrodi 2011).
- *Reduced chemotherapy.* Detection at an early stage offers the unique chance of decreasing the need for chemotherapy. The reduced need for chemotherapy for most small tumors (< 1 cm) is part of most treatment guidelines. With the high percentage of early cancers detected at screening, reduced need for chemotherapy is a logical consequence of the screening results. Such trends, concerning the screened age groups, have been observed parallel to the introduction of mammography screening by population registries (Vervoort et al. 2004, Schrodi 2011). A reduced need for chemotherapy is perceived as a decisive advantage of early detection by most women.
- *Reduced need for axillary dissection.* With the introduction of sentinel node biopsy, axillary dissection can be avoided today in a high percentage of women, whose lymph nodes are not involved. Decreased N+ stages have been documented in several screening programs (Health Council of the Netherlands 2002, Schrodi 2011). Trends towards reduced axillary dissections in the screening age groups parallel to the introduction of mammography screening are being observed. The side effects of axillary dissection mostly exceed the side effects of breast conservation or mastectomy, as reported and rated by most breast cancer patients. Therefore, reduction of axillary dissection is an important advantage.
- *Better cosmetic results.* Better cosmetic outcome may naturally be expected with earlier detection since removal of a small tumor can be more easily handled than removing large parts of the breast tissue (tumor including safety margin). Considering that surgery of nonpalpable lesions is somewhat more demanding than surgery of palpable lesions, it becomes obvious that quality-assured screening must be followed by quality-assured further treatment. Only if both are utilised may the potential advantage of early detection be fully realised.

Patient Reassurance

Most opponents of mammography screening deny that *a correctly reported negative finding* constitutes an important advantage of a screening program. This contradicts our experience with thousands of screened women. Even though women should know and are informed by us that a negative mammogram cannot guarantee absence of malignancy in all cases or for the complete subsequent interval, most women are grateful and relieved to receive this information. The reason is that most women know about other women who are affected by breast cancer or who even died of breast cancer. (This is unavoidable when considering that 1 out of 8–10 women is affected during her life time). Thus they are concerned. They perceive a negative test finding as a relief and consider the possibility of reassurance an important incentive and advantage of mammography screening.

Further Effect on Health System

The strict *quality assurance* associated with mammography screening and assessment and the linkage of most European programs to quality-assured therapy (performed in certified breast centers) has allowed improvement in the overall quality and transparency of breast cancer care.

Support of Scientific Progress

Finally, the *databases*, which are created for quality assurance and surveillance of screening programs, contain important information concerning imaging and histopathologic tumor features. Their linkage with treatment data and outcome data from cancer registries includes an enormous pool of information. Evaluation of such correctly linked anonymous data may provide invaluable and objective information that may help to significantly improve our understanding and knowledge and may thus contribute to further optimize diagnosis and treatment among all or selected subgroups of patients.

When assessing the effects and side effects of mammography screening, opponents tend to refer to prostate cancer screening. However, prostate cancer screening using prostate-specific antigen (PSA) testing is absolutely not comparable to mammography screening. The side effects of a false positive PSA test may be unacceptable considering that—contrary to mammography screening—it may be impossible to find the exact reason for elevated PSA levels. This indeed means long-term uncertainty. In addition prostate cancer occurs 10–15 years later in life than does breast cancer and its treatment may be associated with even more severe side effects and reduced quality of life than most treatments of early breast cancer. Combined with the shorter life expectancy of men, the potential for overdiagnoses and unacceptable increase in overtreatment is much higher than with mammography screening.

Thus, overall, the benefit–risk ratio of PSA screening is very different from that of mammography screening. Its comparison to mammography screening is not adequate or justified.

Summary

Mammography screening is one of the most intensively investigated fields of medicine.

Thoroughly investigated data consistently confirm that mammography screening is capable of significantly reducing breast cancer mortality. Even though breast cancer may affect 1 out of 8–10 women, early detection is demanding, since the yearly incidence corresponding to this ratio is below 0.5% for women without increased risk. This means that mortality reduction can be achieved only by regular (mostly biennial) mammography screening of large numbers of healthy women. A high level of quality assurance is needed to facilitate early detection of the few incident cancers per round and reliable distinction from numerous normal variants. Considering the high number of healthy women who are regularly examined by screening, potential side effects must be carefully weighed against expected advantages.

Side effects cannot be avoided. They include a low risk associated with the radiation, false positive calls (which for mammography are much lower than for most other diagnostic tests), and a debated number of overdiagnoses, which must be considered, as in most other fields of medicine.

Advantages include mortality reduction and improved therapeutic options with the need for fewer aggressive therapies.

Even though the disadvantages may affect all women while the benefit will mostly concern women affected by breast cancer, the quality of the advantages (saved lives and a reduced need for aggressive therapies) certainly outweigh the unavoidable disadvantages.

Awareness of the potential side effects and of the small overall number of cancers that can be detected per round, but whose detection is a prerequisite to saving lives or avoiding aggressive therapies, is essential. There must be understanding of both the need for excellent quality assurance and for individually adapted therapy and counseling of patients with screen-detected breast cancer.

The occurrence of interval cancers and the fact that a significant number of lethal cancers still occur in spite of screening demonstrate the need for further optimization and development of the methodology. For women at increased risk biennial mammographic screening is generally not considered sufficient.

Instead, for intermediate risk most health systems recommend yearly imaging by mammography and ultrasound. This scheme should start at age 40 or 10 years before the earliest age of cancer involvement in the family. For high-risk patients, yearly screening by MRI and mammography is recommended (see also Chapter 5, p. 154).

Further possibilities for improving the effect of screening may include shortening of the screening interval, further improvement in mammographic technique, and hopefully in future support from improved computer-aided detection programs or the complementary use of further tests for all or selected women in the population. However, the effects and potential side effects of suggested changes or other methods will require very critical testing before they may be recommended for use in large parts of the population.

References and Recommended Reading

Allgood PC, Warwick J, Warren RM, Day NE, Duffy SW. A case-control study of the impact of the East Anglian breast screening programme on breast cancer mortality. Br J Cancer 2008;98(1):206–209

Allgood PC, Duffy SW, Kearins O, et al. Explaining the difference in prognosis between screen-detected and symptomatic breast cancers. Br J Cancer 2011;104(11):1680–1685

Armstrong K, Moye E, Williams S, Berlin JA, Reynolds EE. Screening mammography in women 40 to 49 years of age: a systematic review for the American College of Physicians. Ann Intern Med 2007;146(7):516–526

Baines CJ, Miller AB, Kopans DB, et al. Canadian National Breast Screening Study: assessment of technical quality by external review. AJR Am J Roentgenol 1990;155(4):743–747, discussion 748–749

Becker N, Junkermann H. Benefit and risk of mammography screening: considerations from an epidemiological viewpoint. Dtsch Arztebl Int 2008;105(8):131–136

Berg WA, Blume JD, Cormack JB, et al; ACRIN 6666 Investigators. Combined screening with ultrasound and mammography vs mammography alone in women at elevated risk of breast cancer. JAMA 2008;299(18):2151–2163

Berry DA, Cronin KA, Plevritis SK, et al; Cancer Intervention and Surveillance Modeling Network (CISNET) Collaborators. Effect of screening and adjuvant therapy on mortality from breast cancer. N Engl J Med 2005;353(17):1784–1792

Boyer B, Hauret L, Bellaiche R, Gräf C, Bourcier B, Fichet G. Retrospectively detectable carcinomas: review of the literature. [Article in French] J Radiol 2004;85(12 Pt 2):2071–2078

Brenner H, Heywang-Köbrunner S, Becker N. Re: Public knowledge of benefits of breast and prostate cancer screening in Europe. J Natl Cancer Inst. 2010;102(5):356; Author reply 356-7.

Brewer NT, Salz T, Lillie SE. Systematic review: the long-term effects of false-positive mammograms. Ann Intern Med 2007;146(7):502–510

Ciatto S. The overdiagnosis nightmare: a time for caution. BMC Womens Health 2009;9:34

Coldman A, Phillips N, Warren L, Kan L. Breast cancer mortality after screening mammography in British Columbia women. Int J Cancer 2007;120(5):1076–1080

Corsetti V, Houssami N, Ghirardi M, et al. Evidence of the effect of adjunct ultrasound screening in women with mammography-negative dense breasts: interval breast cancers at 1 year follow-up. Eur J Cancer 2011;47(7):1021–1026

de Gelder R, Heijnsdijk EA, van Ravesteyn NT, Fracheboud J, Draisma G, de Koning HJ. Interpreting overdiagnosis estimates in population-based mammography screening. Epidemiol Rev 2011a;33(1):111–121

de Gelder R, Draisma G, Heijnsdijk EA, de Koning HJ. Population-based mammography screening below age 50: balancing radiation-induced vs prevented breast cancer deaths. Br J Cancer 2011b;104(7):1214–1220

de Koning HJ, Draisma G, Fracheboud J, de Bruijn A. Overdiagnosis and overtreatment of breast cancer: microsimulation modelling estimates based on observed screen and clinical data. Breast Cancer Res 2006;8(1):202

Duffy SW, Tabar L, Olsen AH, et al. Absolute numbers of lives saved and overdiagnosis in breast cancer screening, from a randomized trial and from the Breast Screening Programme in England. J Med Screen 2010;17(1):25–30

Duffy S, Yen MF, Chen T, et al. Long-term benefits of breast screening. Breast Cancer Manag 2012;1(1):31–38

Euler-Chelpin, et al. Overdiagnosis in publicly organised mammography screening programmes: systematic review of incidence trends. Author reply. BMJ 2009;339:b2587

Euroscreen Working Group. Summary of the evidence of breast cancer service screening outcomes in Europe and first estimate of the benefit and harm balance sheet. J Med Screen 2012;19(Suppl 1):5–13

Fitzpatrick-Lewis D, Hodgson N, Ciliska D, Peirson L, Gauld M, Liu Y. Breast cancer screening. Canadian Task Force. http://canadiantaskforce.ca/wp-content/uploads/2012/09/Systematic-review.pdf?9d7bd4 2011

Fracheboud J, Groenewoud JH, Boer R, et al. Seventy-five years is an appropriate upper age limit for population-based mammography screening. Int J Cancer 2006;118(8):2020–2025

Gabe R, Tryggvadóttir L, Sigfússon BF, Olafsdóttir GH, Sigurdsson K, Duffy SW. A case-control study to estimate the impact of the Icelandic population-based mammography screening program on breast cancer death. Acta Radiol 2007;48(9):948–955

Gøtzsche PC, Nielsen M. Screening for breast cancer with mammography. Cochrane Database Syst Rev 2011;1:CD001877

Gøtzsche PC, Olsen O. Is screening for breast cancer with mammography justifiable? Lancet 2000;355(9198):129–134

Health Council of the Netherlands. The benefit of population screening for breast cancer with mammography (Publication no. 2002/03E). The Hague: Health Council of the Netherlands; 2002

Hellquist BN, Duffy SW, Abdsaleh S, et al. Effectiveness of population-based service screening with mammography for women ages 40 to 49 years: evaluation of the Swedish Mammography Screening in Young Women (SCRY) cohort. Cancer 2011;117(4):714–722

Hendrick RE. Radiation doses and cancer risks from breast imaging studies. Radiology 2010;257(1):246–253

Hendrick RE, Helvie MA. United States Preventive Services Task Force screening mammography recommendations: science ignored. AJR Am J Roentgenol 2011;196(2):W112-6

Heywang-Köbrunner SH, Schreer I, Heindel W, Katalinic A. Imaging studies for the early detection of breast cancer. Dtsch Arztebl Int 2008;105(31-32):541–547

Heywang-Köbrunner SH, Hacker A, Sedlacek S, Hertlein M. State of mammography screening: results of the reference center Munich 2011 and review. [Article in German] In: Untch M, Thomssen C, Costa S-D (eds). Munich: Aegileum Publishers; 2011, pp. 1-15.

Heywang-Köbrunner SH, Hacker A, Sedlacek S. Advantages and disadvantages of mammography screening. Breast Care (Basel) 2011;6(3):199–207

Hofvind S, Geller B, Skaane P. Mammographic features and histopathological findings of interval breast cancers. Acta Radiol 2008;49(9):975–981

Holland R, Rijken H, Hendriks J. The Dutch population-based mammography screening: 30-year experience. Breast Care 2007;2:12–18

Independent UK Panel on Breast Cancer Screening. The benefits and harms of breast cancer screening: an independent review. The Lancet. October 30, 2012

International Agency for Research on Cancer (WHO). Press release no. 139: Mammography screening can reduce deaths from breast cancer. www.iarc.fr/en/media-centre/pr/2002/pr139.html 2002

Jørgensen KJ, Gøtzsche PC. Overdiagnosis in publicly organised mammography screening programmes: systematic review of incidence trends. BMJ 2009;339:b2587

Jonsson H, Bordás P, Wallin H, Nyström L, Lenner P. Service screening with mammography in Northern Sweden: effects on breast cancer mortality—an update. J Med Screen 2007;14(2):87–93

Kalager M, Zelen M, Langmark F, Adami HO. Effect of screening mammography on breast-cancer mortality in Norway. N Engl J Med 2010;363(13):1203–1210

Kirsh VA, Chiarelli AM, Edwards SA, et al. Tumor characteristics associated with mammographic detection of breast cancer in the Ontario breast screening program. J Natl Cancer Inst 2011;103(12):942–950

Kopans DB. Why the critics of screening mammography are wrong. Diagn Imaging (San Franc) 2009;31(12):1–5

Kopans DB, Smith RA, Duffy SW. Mammographic screening and "overdiagnosis". Radiology 2011;260(3):616–620

Lee CH, Dershaw DD, Kopans D, et al. Breast cancer screening with imaging: recommendations from the Society of Breast Imaging and the ACR on the use of mammography, breast MRI, breast ultrasound, and other technologies for the detection of clinically occult breast cancer. J Am Coll Radiol 2010;7(1):18–27

Lord SJ, Lei W, Craft P, et al. A systematic review of the effectiveness of magnetic resonance imaging (MRI) as an addition to mammography and ultrasound in screening young women at high risk of breast cancer. Eur J Cancer 2007;43(13):1905–1917

Magnus MC, Ping M, Shen MM, Bourgeois J, Magnus JH. Effectiveness of mammography screening in reducing breast cancer mortality in women aged 39-49 years: a meta-analysis. J Womens Health (Larchmt) 2011;20(6):845–852

Miller AB, To T, Baines CJ, Wall C. Canadian National Breast Screening Study-2: 13-year results of a randomized trial in women aged 50-59 years. J Natl Cancer Inst 2000;92(18):1490–1499

Moss SM, Cuckle H, Evans A, Johns L, Waller M, Bobrow L; Trial Management Group. Effect of mammographic screening from age 40 years on breast cancer mortality at 10 years' follow-up: a randomised controlled trial. Lancet 2006;368(9552):2053–2060

National Academy of Sciences. Health risks from exposure to low levels of ionizing radiation: BEIR VII—phase 2. Washington, DC: National Academies Press; 2006

Nelson HD, Tyne K, Naik A, et al. Report No. 10-05142-EF-1: Screening for Breast Cancer: Systematic evidence review update for the US Preventive Services Task Force. Rockville, MD: Agency for Healthcare Research and Quality; 2009

Nothacker M, Duda V, Hahn M, et al. Early detection of breast cancer: benefits and risks of supplemental breast ultrasound in asymptomatic women with mammographically dense breast tissue. A systematic review. BMC Cancer 2009;9:335

Otto SJ, Fracheboud J, Looman CW, et al; National Evaluation Team for Breast Cancer Screening. Initiation of population-based mammography screening in Dutch municipalities and effect on breast-cancer mortality: a systematic review. Lancet 2003;361(9367):1411–1417

Paci W-F, Kalager M. Overdiagnosis in publicly organised mammography screening programmes: systematic review of incidence trends. BMJ 2009;339:b2587 (author reply)

Parvinen I, Helenius H, Pylkkänen L, et al. Service screening mammography reduces breast cancer mortality among elderly women in Turku. J Med Screen 2006;13(1):34–40

Pellegrini M, Bernardi D, Di Michele S, et al. Analysis of proportional incidence and review of interval cancer cases observed within the mammography screening programme in Trento province, Italy. Radiol Med (Torino) 2011;116(8):1217–1225

Perry N, Broeders M, De Wolf C, et al, Eds. European Guidelines for Quality Assurance in Mammography Screening. 4th ed. Luxembourg: Office for Official Publications of the European Communities; 2006

Pisani P et al. (Rapid Responses to Jørgensen KJ, Gøtzsche PC BMJ 2009) BMJ, Aug 20 and Sept 8, 2009

Porter GJR, Evans AJ, Burrell HC, Lee AH, Ellis IO, Chakrabarti J. Interval breast cancers: prognostic features and survival by subtype and time since screening. J Med Screen 2006;13(3):115–122

Puliti D, Zappa M, Miccinesi G, Falini P, Crocetti E, Paci E. An estimate of overdiagnosis 15 years after the start of mammographic screening in Florence. Eur J Cancer 2009;45(18):3166–3171

Puliti D, Duffy SW, Miccinesi G, et al. Overdiagnosis in mammographic screening for breast cancer in Europe: a literature review. J Med Screen 2012;19(Suppl 1):42–56

Riedl CC, Ponhold L, Flöry D, et al. Magnetic resonance imaging of the breast improves detection of invasive cancer, preinvasive cancer, and premalignant lesions during surveillance of women at high risk for breast cancer. Clin Cancer Res 2007;13(20):6144–6152

Roder D, Houssami N, Farshid G, et al. Population screening and intensity of screening are associated with reduced breast cancer mortality: evidence of efficacy of mammography screening in Australia. Breast Cancer Res Treat 2008;108(3):409–416

Salz T, Richman AR, Brewer NT. Meta-analyses of the effect of false-positive mammograms on generic and specific psychosocial outcomes. Psychooncology 2010;19(10):1026–1034

Schopper D, de Wolf C. How effective are breast cancer screening programmes by mammography? Review of the current evidence. Eur J Cancer 2009;45(11):1916–1923

Schrodi S. Epidemiological changes in the population with introduction of mammography screening in Bavaria. Research Project of the German Cancer Association; 2011

Smith RA, Duffy SW, Tabar L. Screening and early detection. In: Babiera GV, Esteva FJ, Skoracki R, eds. Advanced therapy of breast disease. 3rd ed. Shelton, CT: People's Medical Publishing House; 2010

Swedish Organised Service Screening Evaluation Group. Reduction in breast cancer mortality from organized service screening with mammography: 1. Further confirmation with extended data and 2. Validation with alternative analytical methods. Cancer Epidemiol Biomarkers Prev 2006;15(1):45–51 and 52–56

Tabar L, Yen MF, Vitak B, Chen HH, Smith RA, Duffy SW. Mammography service screening and mortality in breast cancer patients: 20-year follow-up before and after introduction of screening. Lancet 2003;361(9367):1405–1410

Tabar L, Vitak B, Chen TH et al. Swedish two-county trial: impact of mammographic screening on breast cancer mortality during 3 decades. Radiology 2011;260(3):658–663

Tarone RE. The excess of patients with advanced breast cancer in young women screened with mammography in the Canadian National Breast Screening Study. Cancer 1995;75(4):997–1003

The German National Mammography Screening Program. www.mammo-programm.de [In German]

Tumor registry data, Munich: http://www.tumorregister-muenchen.de/facts/spec/spec_C50f_G.pdf

US Preventive Services Task Force. Screening for breast cancer: US Preventive Services Task Force recommendation statement. Ann Intern Med 2009;151(10):716–726, W-236

van Schoor G, Broeders MJ, Paap E, Otten JD, den Heeten GJ, Verbeek AL. A rationale for starting breast cancer screening under age 50. Ann Oncol 2008;19(6):1208–1209

van Schoor G, Moss SM, Otten JD, et al. Effective biennial mammographic screening in women aged 40-49. Eur J Cancer 2010;46(18):3137–3140

van Schoor G, Moss SM, Otten JD, et al. Increasingly strong reduction in breast cancer mortality due to screening. Br J Cancer 2011;104(6):910–914

Vervoort MM, Draisma G, Fracheboud J, van de Poll-Franse LV, de Koning HJ. Trends in the usage of adjuvant systemic therapy for breast cancer in the Netherlands and its effect on mortality. Br J Cancer 2004;91(2):242–247

Warner E, Messersmith H, Causer P, Eisen A, Shumak R, Plewes D. Systematic review: using magnetic resonance imaging to screen women at high risk for breast cancer. Ann Intern Med 2008;148(9):671–679

Yaffe MJ, Mainprize JG. Risk of radiation-induced breast cancer from mammographic screening. Radiology 2011;258(1):98–105

Zackrisson S, Andersson I, Janzon L, Manjer J, Garne JP. Rate of over-diagnosis of breast cancer 15 years after end of Malmö mammographic screening trial: follow-up study. BMJ 2006;332(7543):689–692

Zahl PH, Maehlen J, Welch HG. The natural history of invasive breast cancers detected by screening mammography. Arch Intern Med 2008;168(21):2311–2316

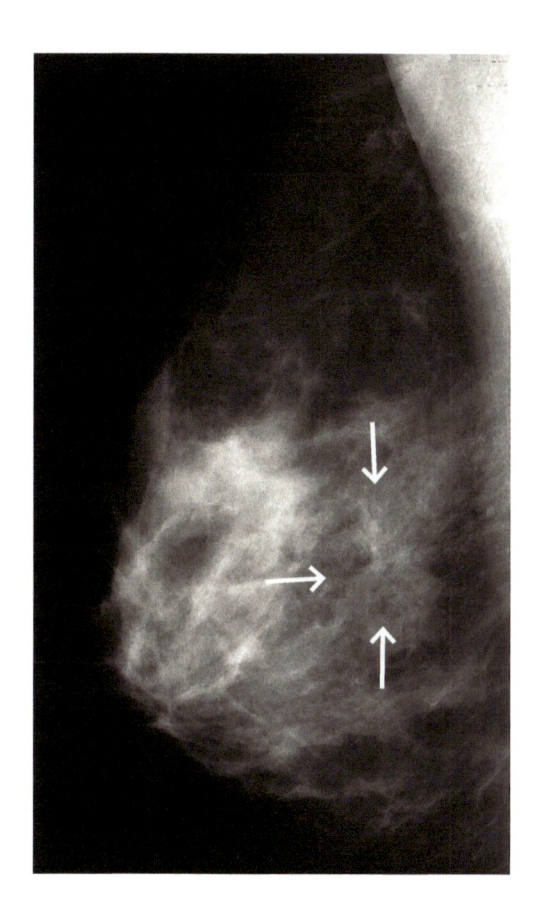

24 Additional Diagnostic Evaluation of Screening Findings and Solving of Problems in Symptomatic Patients

Pathognomonic Findings ⇢ *594*
Imaging Assessment ⇢ *595*
Histopathologic Assessment ⇢ *596*

Differential Diagnosis and Assessment ⇢ *597*
Smoothly Outlined Density ⇢ *597*
Mass Not Smoothly Outlined, Focal Asymmetry ⇢ *604*
Architectural Distortion ⇢ *615*
Asymmetry ⇢ *626*
The Mammographically Dense Breast ⇢ *632*
Other Clinical Abnormalities ⇢ *640*
Microcalcifications ⇢ *642*
Nipple Discharge ⇢ *657*
Inflammatory Changes ⇢ *661*
The Young Patient ⇢ *663*

References and Recommended Reading ⇢ *673*

24 Additional Diagnostic Evaluation of Screening Findings and Solving of Problems in Symptomatic Patients

I. Schreer, S. H. Heywang-Koebrunner, S. Barter

Abnormalities may be detected either clinically or by imaging. Only some of these abnormalities eventually prove to be malignant, whereas the others eventually prove to be benign.

A few abnormalities may not require further assessment since their presentation at imaging is pathognomonic. Such presentations should be known.

To correctly classify abnormalities that are not pathognomonic—that is, correctly diagnose breast cancers as early as possible (when changes may still be uncharacteristic) or exclude malignancy using the least invasive measures—international standards demand that any abnormality first undergoes state-of-the art *imaging assessment*. If malignancy can reliably be excluded based on such imaging assessment, no further measures are needed.

If this is not possible, *histopathologic assessment* must be considered. According to international guidelines, histopathologic assessment should whenever possible be performed using minimally invasive methods.

The goal is to avoid unnecessary diagnostic open surgery in cases that eventually prove to be benign. Due to the smaller volume of tissue removed by minimally invasive procedures (percutaneous breast biopsy) morbidity is reduced. General anesthetic and associated perioperative risks (bleeding, infection, cardiac risks, etc.) can thus be avoided or reduced. Visible scarring and diagnostic problems due to imaging changes caused by scarring are usually minimized with percutaneous breast biopsy.

In cases of malignancy percutaneous breast biopsy allows the optimal surgical and therapeutic approach. For this purpose it may be necessary to perform percutaneous breast biopsy in more than one location within the breast. It is proven that percutaneous breast biopsy allows a reduction in the number of surgical procedures needed to obtain clear margins, resulting in better cosmetic results, fewer recurrences, and overall a better outcome for the patient. Also, based on proven histology, therapeutic options can be discussed preoperatively with the informed patient.

Pathognomonic Findings

(See **Table 24.1**.)

Definition

The term pathognomonic refers to findings that, without further tests, are diagnostic of a certain histology and consequently do not require surgical confirmation.

Incidence

Pathognomonic findings are rare. There are certain entities that may have pathognomonic presentations. But even among these entities often only a proportion of the presentations are pathognomonic. For example, some fibroadenomas may be recognized by pathognomonic coarse bizarre calcifications (see **Fig. 12.2a,f,i**). Most fibroadenomas, however, fail to show the mammographically typical calcifications.

Pathognomonic presentations that allow prediction of a benign lesion do not require further workup.

Typical Findings, Probably Benign Findings, and Diagnostic Strategy

Pathognomonic findings have to be distinguished from typical findings, which are strongly suggestive of the underlying histology but cannot unequivocally prove it.

Typical findings on mammography (multiple cysts, multiple benign well-circumscribed masses, scattered microcalcifications, and so on) noted during screening can often be monitored at the usual screening intervals (depending on the patient's age or risk), if the patient is asymptomatic and—in particular—if comparison with previous imaging does not show a significant change.

For probably benign findings, comparison with previous examinations is indicated. Centrally organized screening programs, which follow the European guidelines, also suggest that if a probably benign lesion is not associated with a low risk of malignancy based on its presentation and/or comparison with previous films, the lesion should undergo imaging (and if needed) histopathologic assessment.

Table 24.1 Pathognomonic images

Histologic diagnosis	Characteristic findings
Mammography	
Lipoma	Focal, round, or oval lesion of fat density with delicate rim (capsule)
Hamartoma	Focal, smoothly outlined lesion containing areas of lipomatous and water density
Oil cyst	Focal radiolucency with surrounding rim (capsule) without/with eggshell-like calcifications
Lymph node	Focal, oval, smoothly outlined density, with—depending on the projection—central or marginal, round radiolucency
Galactocele	Focal, smoothly outlined lesion, composed of fatty components and water-equivalent structures (layering possible), history of pregnancy or lactation
Calcified fibroadenoma	Smoothly outlined, focal density with/without halo, oval, or polylobulated, if containing characteristic calcifications
Cyst containing milk of calcium	Smoothly outlined, focal, round density with calcifications that project centrally in the craniocaudal view and layer inferiorly on the mediolateral view
Verruca	Smoothly outlined mass exhibiting a cauliflower-like structure (multilobulated) and frequently very sharp borders (soft tissue–air)
Sonography	
Cyst	Anechoic, smoothly outlined thin-walled lesion with good distal acoustic enhancement and good compressibility

Short-term follow-up (BI-RADS [Breast Imaging Reporting and Data System] 3) should be recommended only in selected cases—according to the European guidelines, to less than 1% of the screened women—if the probability of malignancy is very low (< 2%) and histopathologic assessment thus does not appear justified. The patient should be well informed and understand this decision. The reason is that a well performed percutaneous breast biopsy may for most patients eventually be better tolerated than long-term uncertainty (for 6 months or longer).

Considering that some malignancies exhibit slow growth, follow-up should usually include a survey of at least 2 years. A usual scheme is follow-up at 6, 12, and 24 months. Rarely, however, lesions (probably corresponding ductal carcinoma in situ [DCIS] or B3 lesions or low-grade invasive carcinoma) may stay unchanged for a long time period and suddenly start growing. The sudden growth can be explained by transition from pre-invasive to invasive or by a shift of the grading with time. Considering these facts, follow-up should be limited to a small number of patients with probably benign lesions. Except for suspected post-therapeutic changes or calcifying fibroadenomas, the changes in which become more characteristic with time, we are quite reticent about following up microcalcifications, preferring a definitive percutaneous biopsy.

Suspicious or indeterminate findings should be confirmed histologically (usually by percutaneous biopsy) before any therapy is initiated.

Imaging Assessment

State-of-the-art imaging assessment must be completed before considering biopsy. It usually includes double-view mammography, further mammographic techniques (views in other planes, rolled views, spot compression, magnification views, galactography, etc., when indicated) and high-resolution breast ultrasound. Views of the lesion in further planes may not be necessary if, for example, ultrasound unequivocally proves a benign cyst or confirms a suspicion that requires biopsy. On the other hand, ultrasound of the breast may not be necessary if the lesion in question is located in a fatty breast and concerns a small group of microcalcifications without associated mass.

The main goal of imaging assessment is to reliably exclude malignancy in lesions or demonstrate changes that can safely be diagnosed as being normal or benign. Normal findings may include changes proven to be due to superimposition or a benign asymmetry. Other definitely benign findings may include simple cysts or typically calcified fibroadenomas, hamartomas, or oil cysts. Lesions that are considered indeterminate or suspicious after imaging assessment is completed always require further workup.

Considering the higher proportion of benign lesions and the somewhat higher sensitivity of breast tissue to radiation, it is recommended that *ultrasound is used first in symptomatic women below age 40 years*, whereas mammography should generally be performed first in women beyond age 40 (exception: suspected cyst). Unless the first method can reliably exclude malignancy the other method (mammography in the case of ultrasound and vice versa) needs to be added. Additional views are needed to complement mammography before considering biopsy in all cases, because these views may provide further clarification.

Magnetic resonance imaging (MRI) does not belong to state-of-the-art imaging assessment of abnormalities that are accessible for percutaneous breast biopsy. The reason is that the sensitivity (90–95%) and negative predictive value of MRI are inferior to state-of-the-art percutaneous breast biopsy (> 95–98%). Thus MRI assessment may be associated with an increased risk of a false negative diagnosis. Furthermore, the specificity of MRI is lower than that of percutaneous breast biopsy. Since many benign changes (such as fibroadenomas, areas of adenosis, granulomas, etc.) enhance with MRI, and exclusion of early malignancy is thus often not possible, the false positive rate of an MRI study performed to exclude malignancy would far exceed that of percutaneous breast biopsy. False positive calls from MRI may concern the leading lesion. They may, however, also occur in other areas within the same or contralateral breast. Such findings usually cannot be ignored, even though it is known that—in patients, who do not belong to a high-risk population—the probability of malignancy among MR-only detected malignant lesions is very low.

In selected cases, however, MRI may be helpful. Such cases may concern one of the following situations:
- Abnormalities visible on one mammographic view only. Here MRI may aid in the exclusion of a true lesion or localize it in the third dimension, which may thus allow targeting for percutaneous breast biopsy.
- Multiple lesions. In cases where there are multiple lesions, MRI may help determine the lesion(s) with the highest suspicion that require histopathologic assessment. It may also help exclude malignancy in the case of multiple cystic lesions, which on ultrasound appear hypoechogenic as they contain protein or blood components.
- Rarely, mammography and ultrasound may be extremely difficult to interpret due to multiple lesions or extensive scarring.
- Rare diffuse changes that cannot be targeted (e.g., increasing nipple retraction without further abnormality on conventional imaging or unusual regional changes without an exact target). Here, MRI may exclude an underlying lesion or may help to target the area of greatest concern.

According to the authors' experiences such lesions will make up less than 2–3% of all assessment cases in a screening population.

If more than one lesion is identified, *a concept should be made* as to which workup might be needed for each lesion and how further workup should begin. Usually histopathologic assessment should commence with the lesion of highest suspicion. The exact location of each important lesion should be unequivocally documented (clock-position, distance to the nipple) before histopathologic assessment starts.

Ultrasound of the axilla should be performed, whenever a lesion requiring histopathologic assessment is identified. It is usually recommended that axillary ultrasound scanning be performed before percutaneous breast biopsy, since after percutaneous breast biopsy reactive changes might cause sonographic appearances imitating lymph node involvement. A recent study by Britton, however, has shown that this is usually not the case (Britton et al. 2009).

Histopathologic Assessment

As mentioned above, histopathologic assessment is required whenever malignancy cannot be excluded or is suspected based on completed imaging assessment. Whenever possible, percutaneous biopsy should be performed using minimally invasive techniques. The reasons include a better outcome for patients with a preoperative histopathologic diagnosis of malignancy, avoidance of unnecessary surgery on benign lesions, and the possibility of discussing precise therapeutic options with the informed patient preoperatively. If, however, individual factors (severe other diseases, uncooperative patient, contraindications to local anesthetic) do not allow percutaneous breast biopsy or indicate that the patient might not benefit (e.g., due to limited life expectancy in the case of other severe diseases), an individual decision may be needed. European guidelines (Perry et al. 2006), for example, demand that at least 70% of histopathologic assessments be performed using minimally invasive methods, optimally > 90%.

Unless a very highly experienced cytology facility is available, core needle biopsy (CNB) is the method of choice for percutaneous breast biopsy of masses and architectural distortions that can be visualized by ultrasound (or rarely larger masses which are visualized by mammography only and can be targeted stereotactically). Vacuum-assisted breast biopsy (VABB) is the method of choice for the assessment of microcalcifications without associated mass and for MR-guided percutaneous breast biopsy. Based on the known limitations of stereotactically guided CNB, according to our experience, VABB should also be considered for small masses or architectural distortions visualized by mammography only. The reasons for this approach are fewer problems resulting from tissue shift due to needle insertion, local anesthetic, or bleeding, and better assessment of representative removal of tissue due to visualization of lesion reduction or a well-centered cavity.

Surgical biopsy should be considered for cases in

which percutaneous breast biopsy is impossible (see above), for suspicious palpable abnormalities without correlating imaging findings (since targeting and counter-check by imaging is not possible), and for diffuse changes (for which a truly representative area cannot be defined).

Finally, the patient has to be adequately informed and has to agree with the intervention.

Differential Diagnosis and Assessment

Smoothly Outlined Density

(See **Fig. 24.1**.)

Diagnostic Question

A smooth outline of a density generally supports the diagnosis of a benign lesion.

Smoothly outlined localized findings seen on screening mammography most frequently represent cysts or fibroadenomas, but 2–7% of all breast carcinomas can be expected to present as a nodule with a partially well-circumscribed margin and 2% with a well-defined outline.

Owing to displacement of surrounding fat by their growth, medullary, papillary, or mucinous carcinomas can give the impression of a capsule and even might have a halo sign (see **Fig. 16.3r,s**). The most frequent malignancy presenting as a well-circumscribed mass is a ductal carcinoma (mostly grade 3). Some DCISs and, rarely, lobular carcinoma may also present as a well-circumscribed mass. Furthermore, intracystic carcinomas, metastases, involved lymph nodes, lymphomas, or sarcomas can present as smoothly outlined focal lesions.

Diagnostic Strategy

In most screening programs the patient is not seen by a medical doctor. In such screening programs a significant number of assessment studies can be avoided if the technologist diligently describes the location of significant skin lesions, marks scars, and documents important history data (such as proven histology or proven absence of change of known masses).

Unless the technologist has indicated a skin lesion or a known benign lesion at the exact location of the mammographic abnormality, or unless mammography clearly indicates the presence of a benign skin lesion, image analysis is the next step to decide for or against recalling the patient.

1. After excluding an obvious skin lesion, the analysis should check for typical benign features, mainly the presence of fatty components or calcifications pathognomonic of a calcifying cyst or fibroadenoma. If based on fatty components and the typical imaging features, a lipoma, a hamartoma, a galactocele, an oil cyst, or a lymph node can be diagnosed and no further assessment is indicated.
2. If previous films exist these should be obtained if possible. In order not to miss change in a slowly growing lesion, it is always advisable to compare the current with the earlier films as well, and not only with the most recent ones. If a well-circumscribed lesion is stable for more than 2–3 years, malignancy is improbable (rare exceptions of malignancies that are unchanged for years and then start growing exist, but will mainly concern a transforming well-circumscribed DCIS or papillary lesion).

   For lesions with less than 2 years follow-up, an individual decision has to be made based on the available follow-up period, lesion morphology, and the patient's risk. Well-circumscribed malignancies (usually ductal invasive carcinoma grade 3) are more frequent in women at high risk; therefore well-circumscribed solid lesions detected in women at high risk should usually undergo histopathologic assessment.

   In patients at low risk, low density supports the diagnosis of a benign lesion (a cyst that due to its compressibility is flat and should exhibit low density on both mammographic views; old fibroadenomas may exhibit low density caused by fatty involution). Also the presence of multiple lesions supports the diagnosis of benign changes.

   Depending on the imaging presentation of a well-circumscribed mass and its density and the patient's risk, further assessment or usual screening may be adequate in the individual case and is considered acceptable for asymptomatic women in international screening programs. As mentioned before, short-term follow-up should be considered only after complete imaging evaluation and after the patient has been adequately informed.

   Any well-circumscribed lesion that increases in size should undergo further assessment. Unless imaging assessment can prove that it is benign (e.g., a simple cyst, an extramammary benign skin lesion, or a benign lymph node), histopathologic assessment must be considered.
3. Even if at first glance (based on the two screening views) a lesion may appear to be intramammary, one of the first questions of the imaging assessment should address this question once more, since intracutaneous or other extramammary lesions may appear to project into the parenchyma based on two views.

   Intracutaneous lesions can mostly be diagnosed by inspection, palpation, or ultrasound.

   In case this is not clear or if correlation (of multiple changes) is uncertain, views with skin markers or

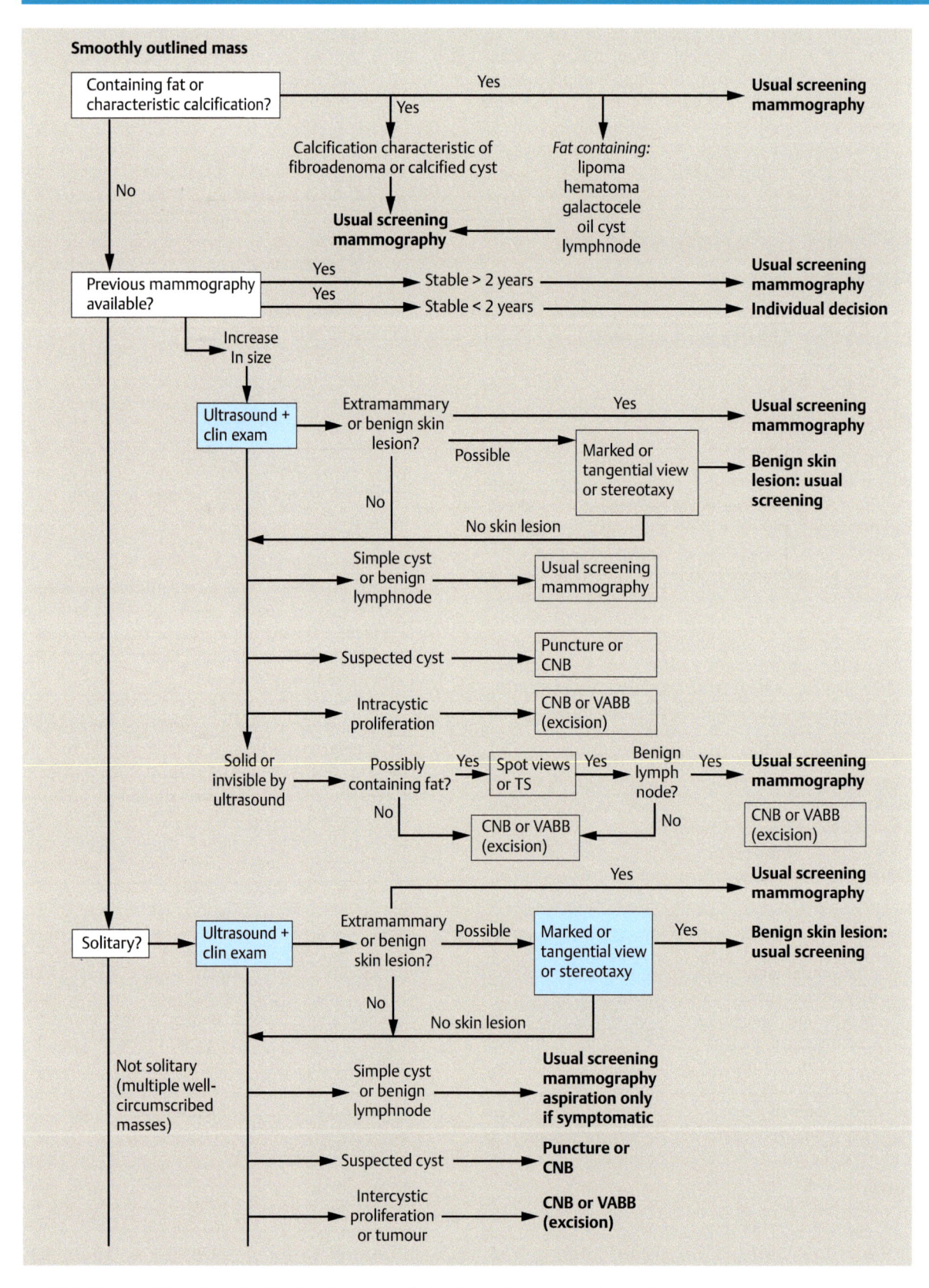

Fig. 24.1 The smoothly outlined focal finding: flow chart outlining diagnostic workup and evaluation.

Differential Diagnosis and Assessment

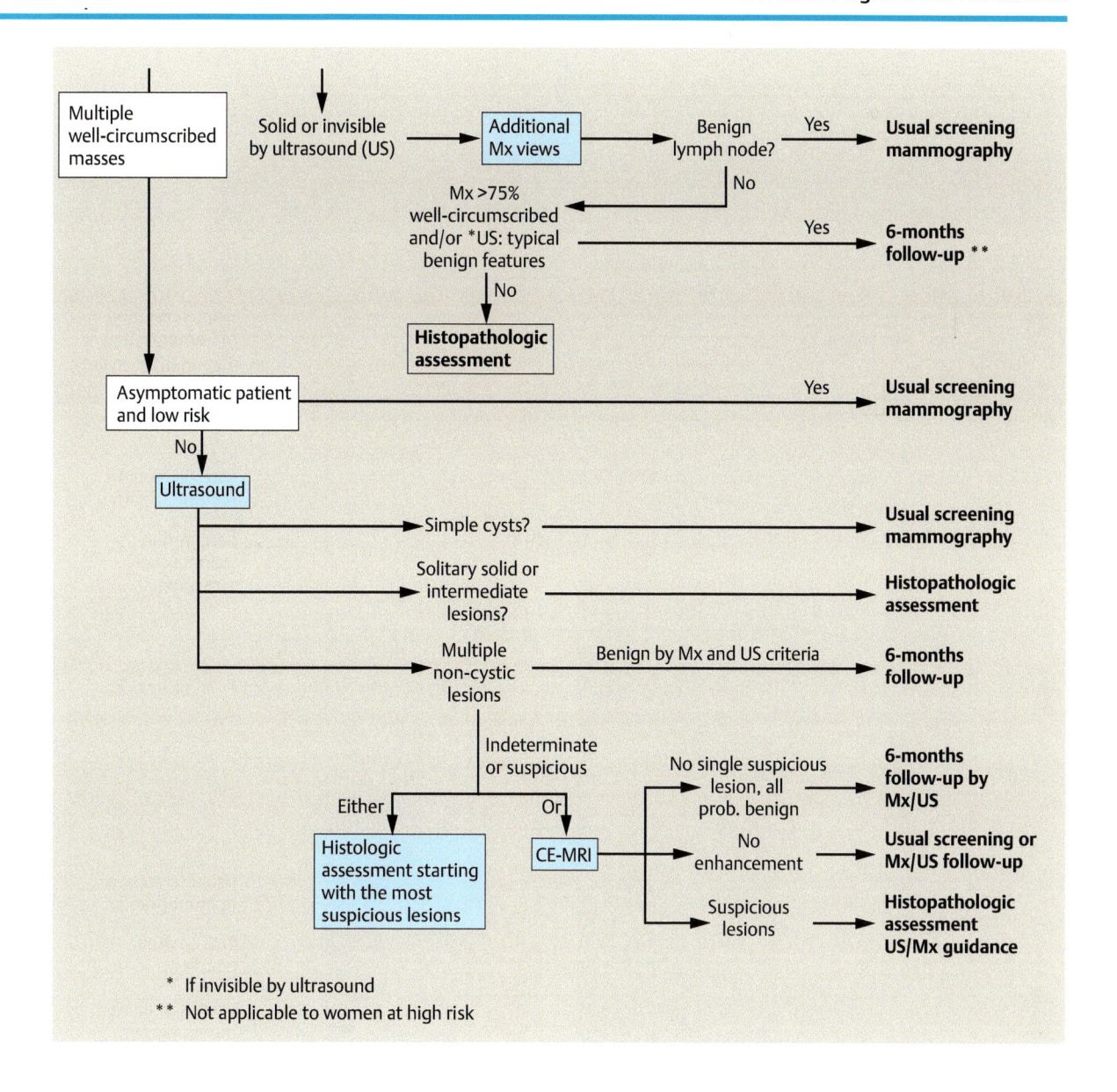

```
Multiple                Solid or invisible      Additional          Benign           Yes     Usual screening
well-circumscribed  →   by ultrasound (US)  →   Mx views       →    lymph node?   →          mammography
masses                                                               │
                                              Mx >75%                │ No
                                              well-circumscribed  ←──┘              Yes     6-months
                                              and/or *US: typical                 →         follow-up **
                                              benign features
                                              │ No
                                              ▼
                                              Histopathologic
                                              assessment

Asymptomatic patient                                                                Yes     Usual screening
and low risk                                                                      →         mammography
│
│ No
▼
Ultrasound
│
├─→ Simple cysts?                                                                           Usual screening
│                                                                                 →         mammography
│
├─→ Solitary solid or                                                                       Histopathologic
│   intermediate lesions?                                                         →         assessment
│
└─→ Multiple                Benign by Mx and US criteria                                    6-months
    non-cystic           ────────────────────────────────→                                  follow-up
    lesions
         │
         │ Indeterminate
         │ or suspicious
         │
    Either │  Or
    ┌──────┴──────┐        ┌──────────────→ No single suspicious       6-months
    │             │        │                lesion, all          →     follow-up by
    ▼             ▼        │                prob. benign               Mx/US
Histologic      CE-MRI ────┤
assessment                 │                No                         Usual screening or
starting with              ├──────────────→ enhancement         →     Mx/US follow-up
the most                   │
suspicious lesions         │                Suspicious                 Histopathologic
                           └──────────────→ lesions             →     assessment
                                                                       US/Mx guidance
```

* If invisible by ultrasound
** Not applicable to women at high risk

a tangential view (acquired after marking the skin) may answer the question (**Fig. 24.2**).

As for skin changes, see Chapter 21. Most well-circumscribed skin changes are benign and breast cancer can be ruled out. If there is any doubt, a dermatologist may be consulted.

Extramammary structures may include an incidentally visualized contralateral nipple (**Fig. 24.3**) or even the tip of the nose (see **Fig. 21.1q**) that may project into the breast. They may be recognized as typical artifacts by image analysis seen as a semicircular density shown on one view only.

4. Among intraparenchymal lesions, ultrasound imaging is usually able to correctly identify simple cysts and benign lymph nodes. Care should be taken not to confuse a hypoechoic malignancy with a benign simple cyst (absent to very low echogenicity, smooth wall, adequate posterior enhancement, adequate elasticity and mobility). Benign lymph nodes are identified by the high echogenicity of the hilum, the smooth and thin hypoechoic cortex, and the vessels that enter the hilum. Patients in whom a well-circumscribed mass can be identified as a simple cyst or benign (intramammary) lymph node can go back to usual screening.

Lesions that correspond to probable cysts, which may be echogenic due to their proteinaceous contents, may be punctured. If a solid or complex cystic lesion is suspected, percutaneous histopathologic assessment using CNB (or in the case of a suspected papillary lesion or very small lesions, VABB) will answer the question. If a small lesion is (mostly)

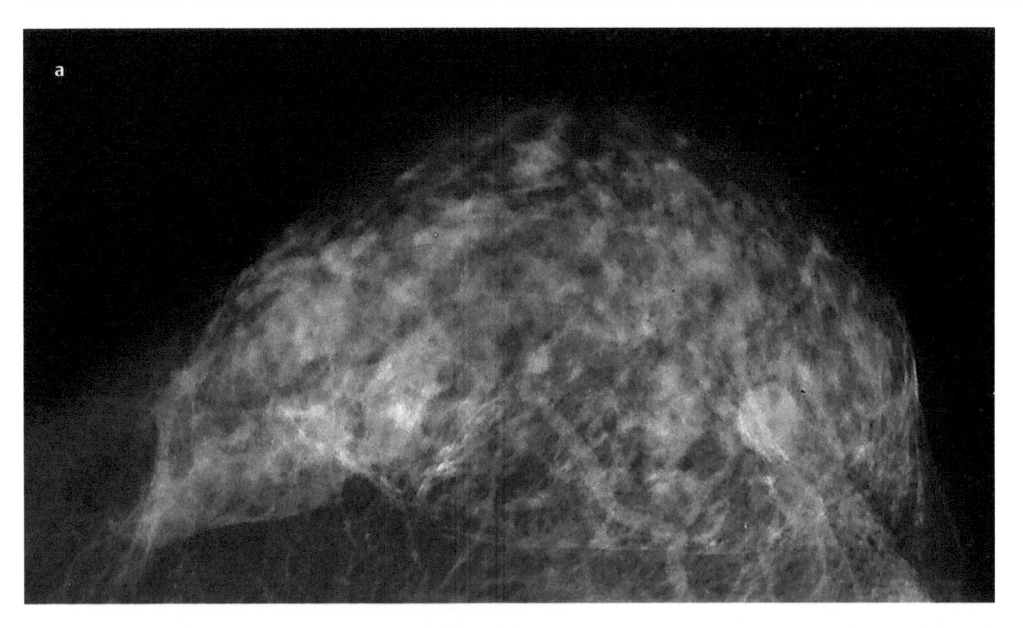

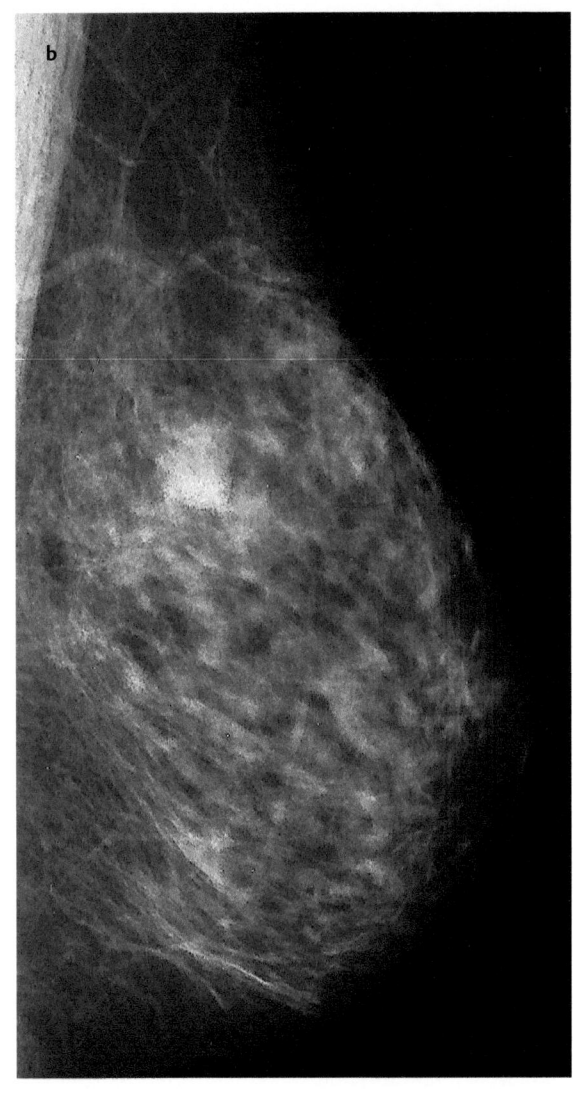

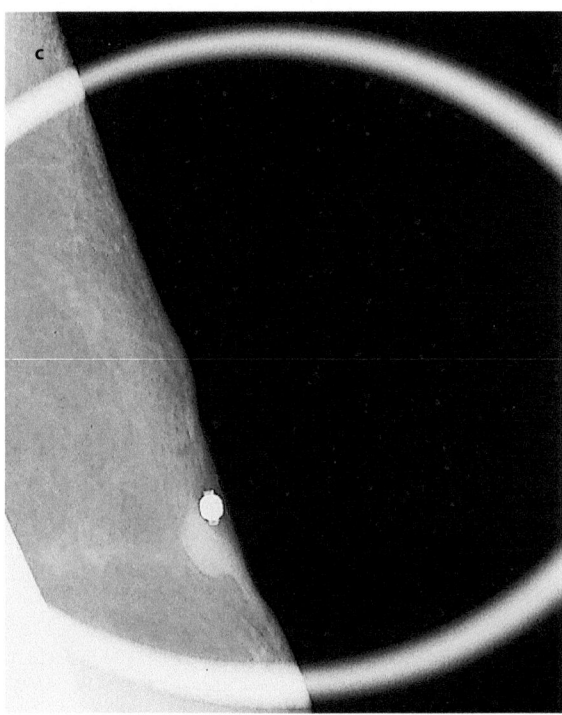

24 Additional Diagnostic Evaluation of Screening Findings and Solving of Problems in Symptomatic Patients

Fig. 24.2a–e

a–c The craniocaudal view (**a**) shows a 10-mm round lesion projecting on the medial half of the breast, which can be localized in the upper half of the breast on the mediolateral view (**b**). A tangential compression spot view after marking of the palpable atheroma (**c**) shows superimposition of marker and lesion (underexposed view to visualize the skin).

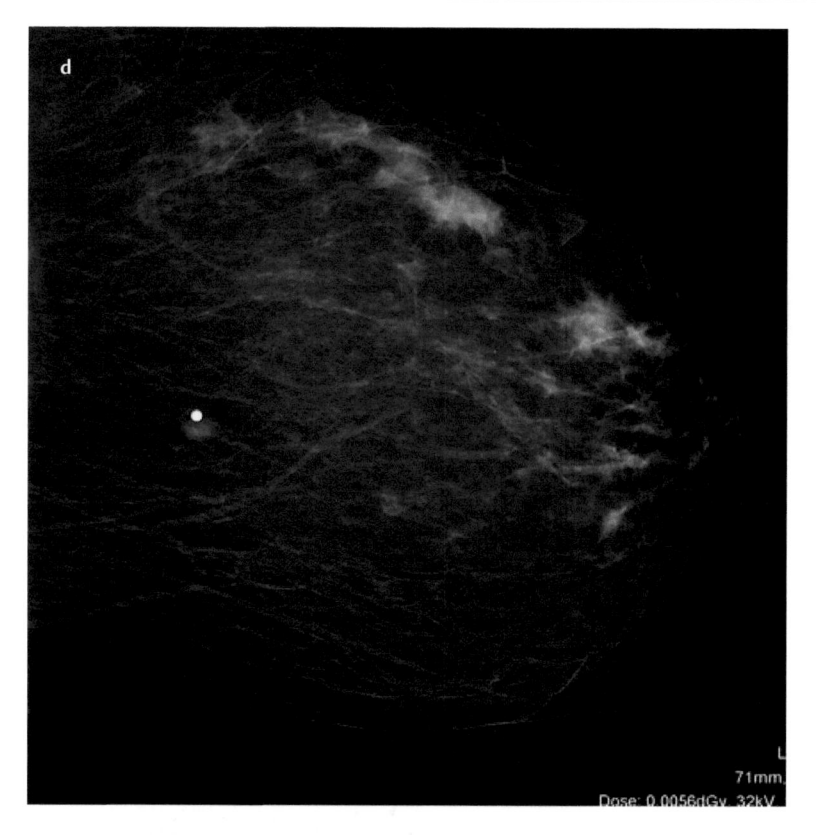

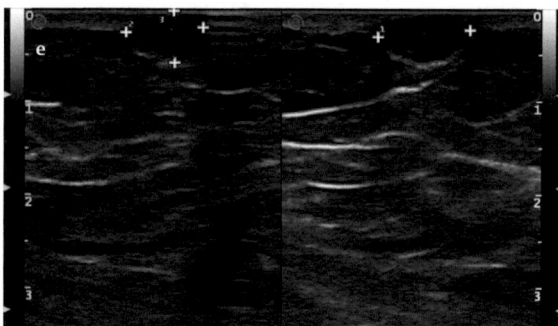

d,e Another case of a screen-detected well-circumscribed nodule that projected into the breast. Since the lesion had newly developed, the patient was recalled. Based on the clinical examination the possibility of a skin lesion was discussed. **d** To prove this etiology in this very large and mobile breast another craniocaudal view was taken with a skin marker placed in the area of the suspected skin lesion. **e** An additional ultrasound image showed the intracutaneous location, which information made further studies unnecessary. *Diagnosis*: Definitely benign skin lesion compatible with a retention cyst.

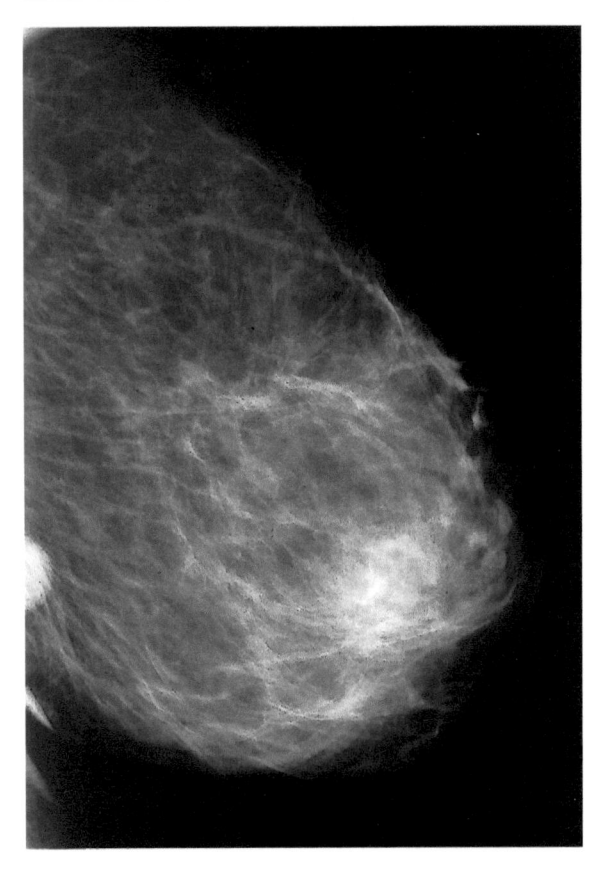

24 Additional Diagnostic Evaluation of Screening Findings and Solving of Problems in Symptomatic Patients

Fig. 24.3 Incidental visualization of the contralateral nipple, seen as convex density close to the chest wall (mediolateral view).

removed by percutaneous breast biopsy, clip marking should be considered after sampling the lesion.

For solid masses showing typical benign sonographic features (see Chapter 4) short-term follow-up or even usual screening may be adequate. The risk of malignancy is usually very low (< 2%) in asymptomatic women at low risk. These features are not reliable, however, for women at high risk (familial breast cancer) due to the higher incidence of well-circumscribed malignancies in such patients. In symptomatic patients with a newly detected lesion and in all patients with newly developing or increasing masses, percutaneous breast biopsy should be considered.

5. Lesions that cannot be identified by ultrasound are most probably solid.
6. The remaining intramammary solid lesions and lesions not identified by ultrasound should undergo complete mammographic imaging evaluation to visualize or exclude presence of a lucent hilum, to assess the borders of the lesion without superimposition. Mostly this can be achieved by additional views (spot views, views at different angles, rolled views). When assessing lesion borders, the lesion should be imaged as close to the image receiver as possible (e.g., medial lesions should be imaged using a lateromedial projection, lateral lesions on a mediolateral projection) to minimize geometric unsharpness. Tomosynthesis may be quite helpful in identifying a central fatty hilum in a lymph node, in determining the exact location of a lesion visible

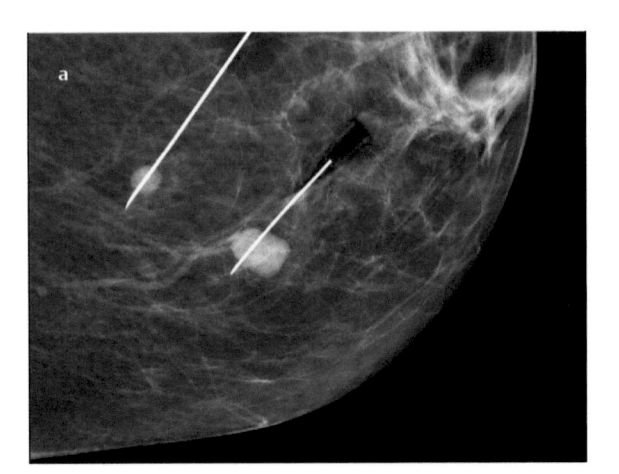

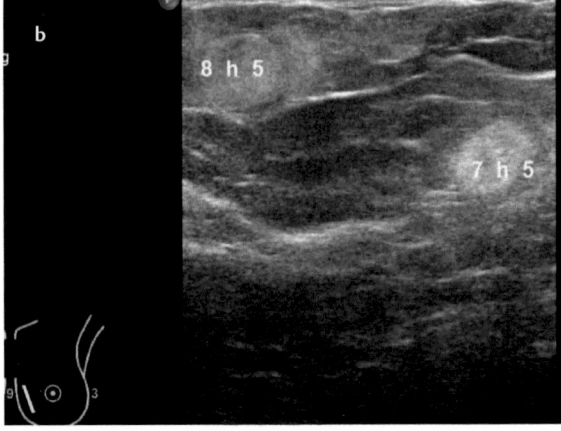

Fig. 24.4a,b Well-circumscribed nodules detected on a diagnostic mammogram, which was performed due to a palpable finding which corresponded to one of the nodules.

a Craniocaudal mammogram showing several well-circumscribed masses which had newly developed compared with a preceding screening mammogram 1.5 years ago.

b Sonographically the masses appeared well-circumscribed and hyperechoic. Ultrasound-guided core needle biopsy followed by a search for the primary tumor proved metastases of an undifferentiated carcinoma of unknown origin.

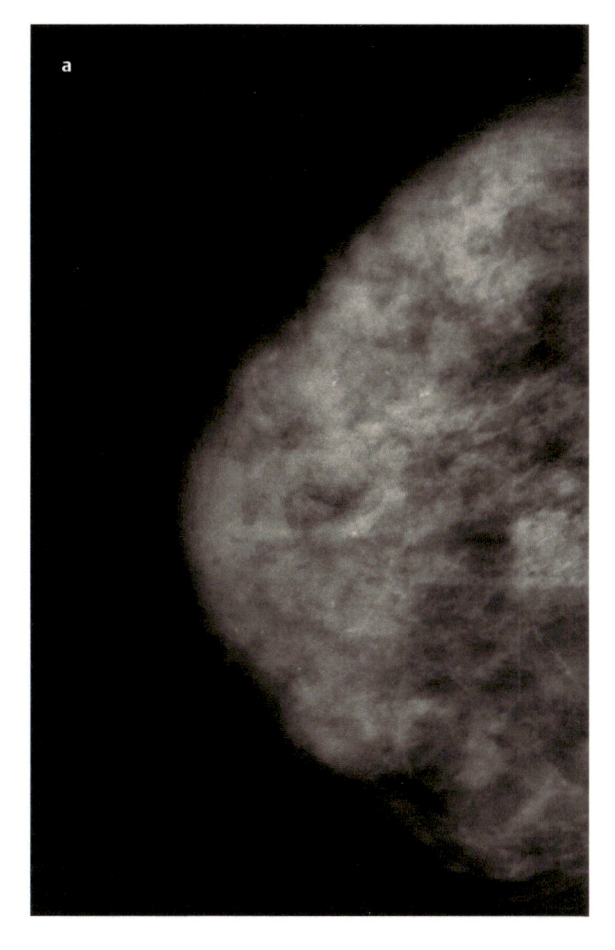

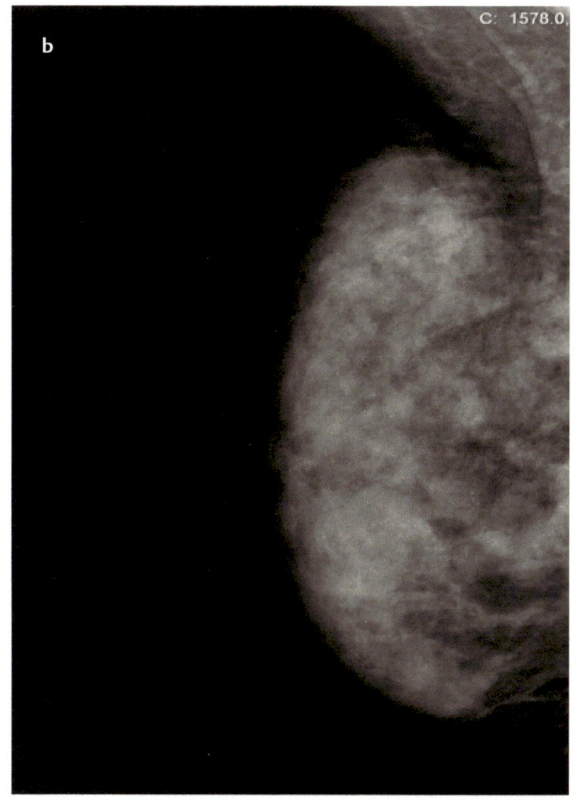

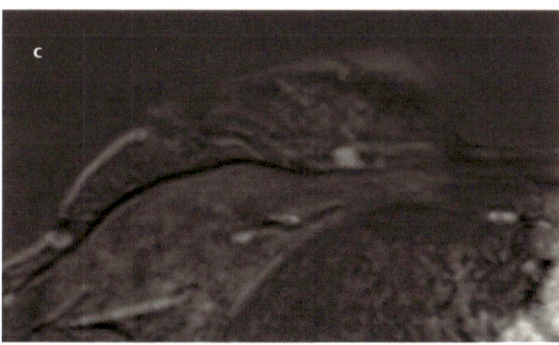

Differential Diagnosis and Assessment

Fig. 24.5a–d Magnetic resonance imaging (MRI)-detected well-circumscribed small mass in a very nodular dense breast. Based on an abnormality of the contralateral (left) breast, this patient was recalled for further assessment. Since the abnormality on the left side could not unequivocally be solved by conventional imaging, an MRI study was performed, which solved the problem on the left side, but a small, well-circumscribed mass was detected on the right side.

- **a,b** Craniocaudal (**a**) and mediolateral oblique (**b**) mammograms of the right breast. Very nodular dense breast tissue is shown. Even though assessment is impaired in such breasts, there was no indication for a recall based on the screening mammogram in a patient without any clinical suspicion and without risk. (Multiple nodules usually indicate benignity.)
- **c** By chance on MRI (performed for the left side) a small 4-mm nodule with progressive enhancement was detected without correlation on ultrasound. The patient refused immediate further workup and chose follow-up assessment after another 4–6 months.
- **d** Five months later the lesion was visible by ultrasound (US) and corresponded to an oval (no more) well-described nodule of 6 mm. *Histology* after US-guided core needle biopsy yielded a ductal invasive breast cancer G1.

24 Additional Diagnostic Evaluation of Screening Findings and Solving of Problems in Symptomatic Patients

on one view only, and in assessing lesions without superimposition in breasts with a density of ACR2–3. The exact role of tomosynthesis in assessing lesion borders is under investigation.

7. Solid lesions which (if visible by ultrasound) exhibit the typical benign sonographic features and which (if mammographically visible) exhibit smooth contours (of which > 75% can be assessed without superimposition) are associated with a high probability of benignity (> 98%). In these women a 6-month follow-up (or even routine screening) may be adequate. (For symptomatic patients and for women at high risk percutaneous breast biopsy is preferable to short-term follow-up).

8. Lesions which, based on complete mammographic–sonographic evaluation, are not typically benign or associated with a very high probability of benignity (> 98%) should undergo histopathologic assessment using percutaneous breast biopsy. MRI is usually not part of the imaging evaluation of solid masses (**Fig. 24.4**).

9. Multiplicity (of well-circumscribed lesions) usually supports a diagnosis of benignity (multiple cysts, fibroadenomas, or papillomas). Indeterminate or suspicious lesions, however, require further assessment (**Fig. 24.5**). Rarely, multiple well-circumscribed lesions may correspond to intramammary metastases. This diagnosis should be considered in the case of multiple nodules of high density and in patients with multiple nodules of similar size (or classes of similar size). The diagnosis is, however, often not helpful for the patient's management, since these patients usually cannot be cured.

In rare cases with multiple lesions with benign to indeterminate imaging features, contrast-enhanced MRI may be helpful. It is able to exclude malignancy in cases with multiple hypoechoic cysts and it may help to identify lesions that require histopathologic assessment.

10. The method of choice for histopathologic assessment of solid masses visible by ultrasound (US) is US-guided CNB. For suspected papillary lesions, VABB may be considered. If the lesion can be completely removed by VABB and proves to be a benign papillary lesion (which in the case of US-guided CNB—owing to the smaller sampled tissue volume—would usually be classified as a B3 lesion), surgical excision may be avoided. Small well-circumscribed masses not visualized by ultrasound are ideally assessed using stereotactically guided VABB, since lesion removal can prove benignity. Rare larger lesions which are not visible by ultrasound can be assessed using stereotactic CNB. According to our experience the reliability of stereotactic VABB exceeds that of stereotactic CNB for masses as well, and allows the exclusion of malignancy even in cases with unspecific histopathologic findings. With the new interventional methods surgical biopsy is very rarely needed for histopathologic assessment of well-circumscribed masses.

Mass Not Smoothly Outlined, Focal Asymmetry

(See **Figs. 24.6, 24.7, 24.8, 24.9, 24.10, 24.11, 24.12, 24.13.**)

Definition

A mass is a space-occupying lesion visible in two planes. A focal asymmetry is a focal lesion visible in one plane. It may correspond to superimposition, a focal parenchymal asymmetry, or a true mass.

Diagnostic Question

The spectrum of masses and focal asymmetries not smoothly demarcated includes parenchymal lobules, benign tumors (cyst, fibroadenoma, phyllodes tumor, papilloma, nodular adenosis), localized post-traumatic and post-therapeutic changes (hematoma, fat necrosis, scar), and malignancies.

Diagnostic Strategy

1. Before deciding on the necessity for a recall or further assessment, previous mammograms should be obtained for comparison of size and radiodensity.
   - A finding that is stable over more than 2–3 years favors a benign process. For shorter observation periods, individual decisions based on the imaging presentation and individual risk factors are recommended. Based on all available information in the individual case, usual screening or further assessment may be adequate. After imaging assessment, possible options may range from usual screening to short-term follow-up to histopathologic assessment (see below).
   - Lesions that are clearly suspicious usually require further histopathologic workup. In the case of long-term follow-up (for many years) of a lesion that shows no change, or if the imaging finding can be unequivocally be explained (e.g., by scarring), the patient can be returned to usual screening.
   - Any increase in size mandates further evaluation.
2. Clinical history and physical examination determine whether the findings are post-traumatic or post-therapeutic. In the presence of scarring, the following approach is recommended:
   - As long as clinical and mammographic findings concur, follow-up examinations are adequate.
   - If serial examinations reveal an increase in size, progressing radial configuration (combined with

Differential Diagnosis and Assessment

Ill-defined mass or focal asymmetry

```
Comparison with previous mammography
├── Stable or decrease in size and density for more than 3 years → Usual screening mammography
├── Stable or decrease in size and density for less than 3 years → Depending on observation period, follow-up in 6–12 months
├── Decrease in size with retraction or increasing density → HA
└── Increase in size or new findings → Recent history: post-surgical or post-traumatic?
        ├── Yes → Uncertain? Residual tumor? Compromised evaluation → Contrast-enhanced MRI
        │         ├── Suspicious → Histological assessment
        │         └── Negative → Usual screening mammography
        └── No → Scar based on history and mammographic findings → Usual screening mammography

Not available → History + clin. exam: post-surgical or post-traumatic?
        ├── Yes → Suspicious → Histological assessment
        └── No → Proliferation during hormone replacement therapy possible?
                    → Ultrasound
                        ├── Simple cysts? → Usual screening mammography
                        ├── Suspicious or indeterminate sonographic findings → HA ultrasound-guided
                        └── No finding or probably benign → Real mass or super-imposition
                                → Additional views and/or tomosynthesis
                                    ├── Suspicious or indeterminate mass → HA
                                    ├── Super-imposition → Usual screening mammography or follow-up
                                    └── Indeterminate and visible on one view only
                                        Either: 6-month follow-up*
                                        Or: HA stereotactic
                                        Or: MRI
                                            ├── No enhancement → Follow-up or screening mammography
                                            └── Suspicious enhancement → HA
```

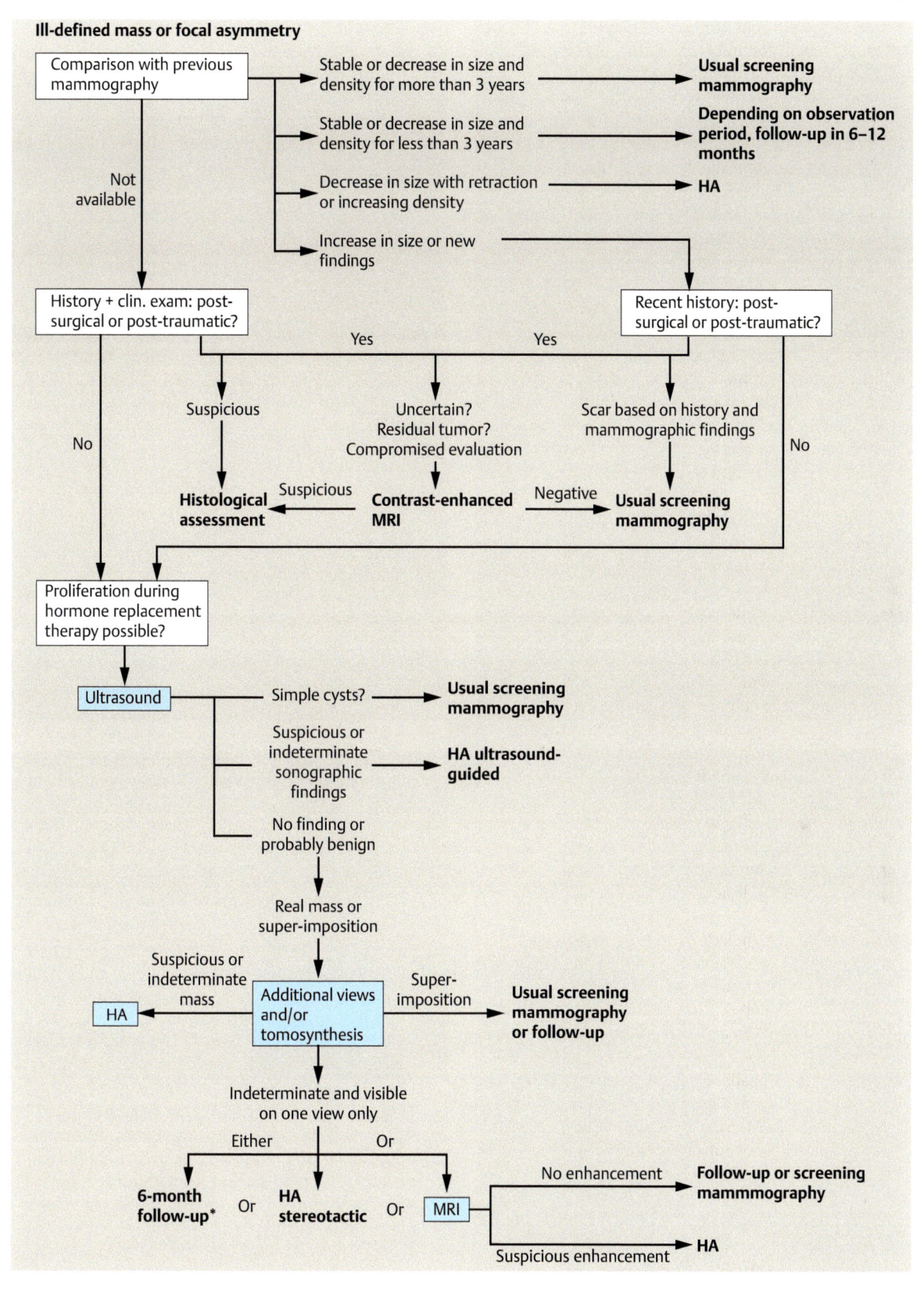

Fig. 24.6 Assessment of ill-defined mass and focal asymmetry. HA, histopathologic assessment (usually CNB or VABB, rarely excision required). *Suspected superimposition or hormonal influence.

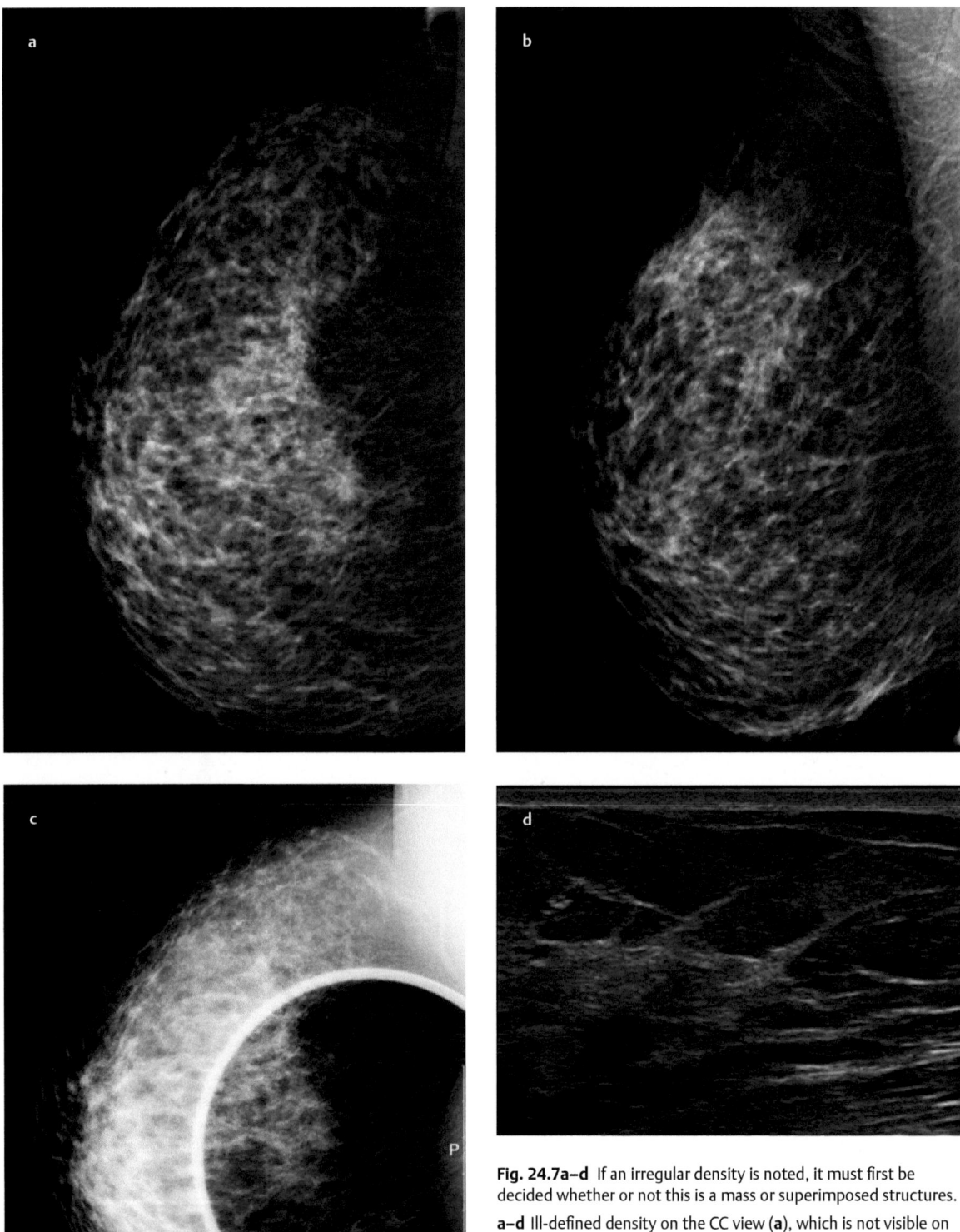

Fig. 24.7a–d If an irregular density is noted, it must first be decided whether or not this is a mass or superimposed structures.

a–d Ill-defined density on the CC view (**a**), which is not visible on the MLO view (**b**). The density could not be reproduced on CC spot compression (**c**), but on ultrasound an ill-defined mass was detected (**d**), which after core needle biopsy turned out to correspond to an invasive ductal carcinoma.

Differential Diagnosis and Assessment

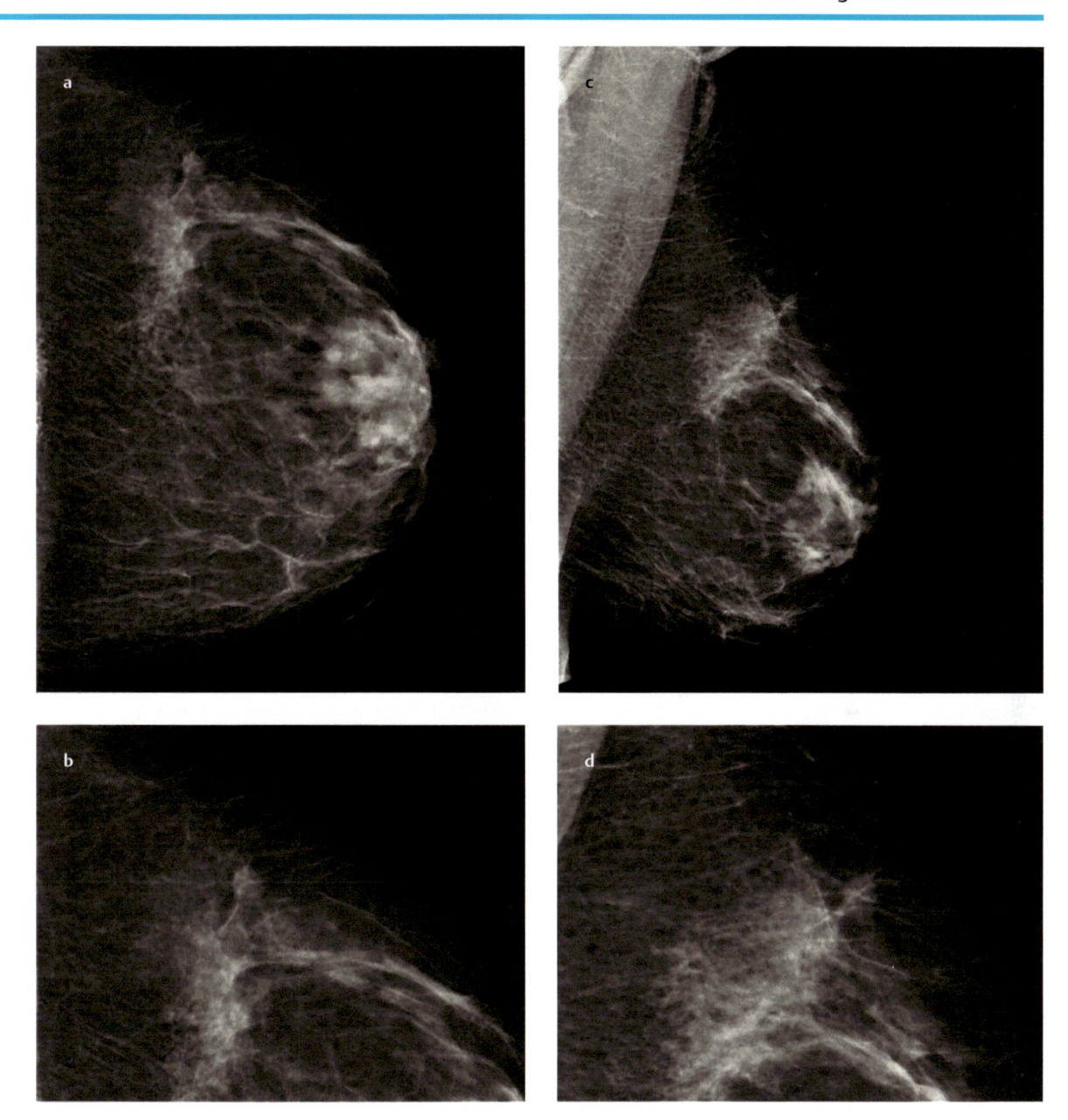

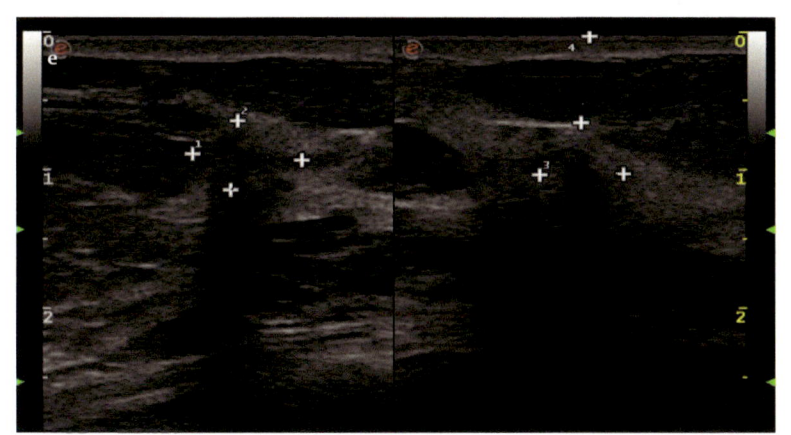

Fig. 24.8a–e

a Screening mammography showing a round transparent nodule posteriorly and laterally on the craniocaudal view.
b The magnified craniocaudal view shows that—even though the nodule is round—the posterior border may exhibit slight unsharpness.
c,d On the mediolateral oblique view (c), again the nodule is fairly transparent, however its caudal border is blurred and there is a suggestion of retraction (d).
e The lesion was detected on ultrasound when searching the area, knowing its location from the mammogram. *Histology*: Invasive ductal carcinoma.

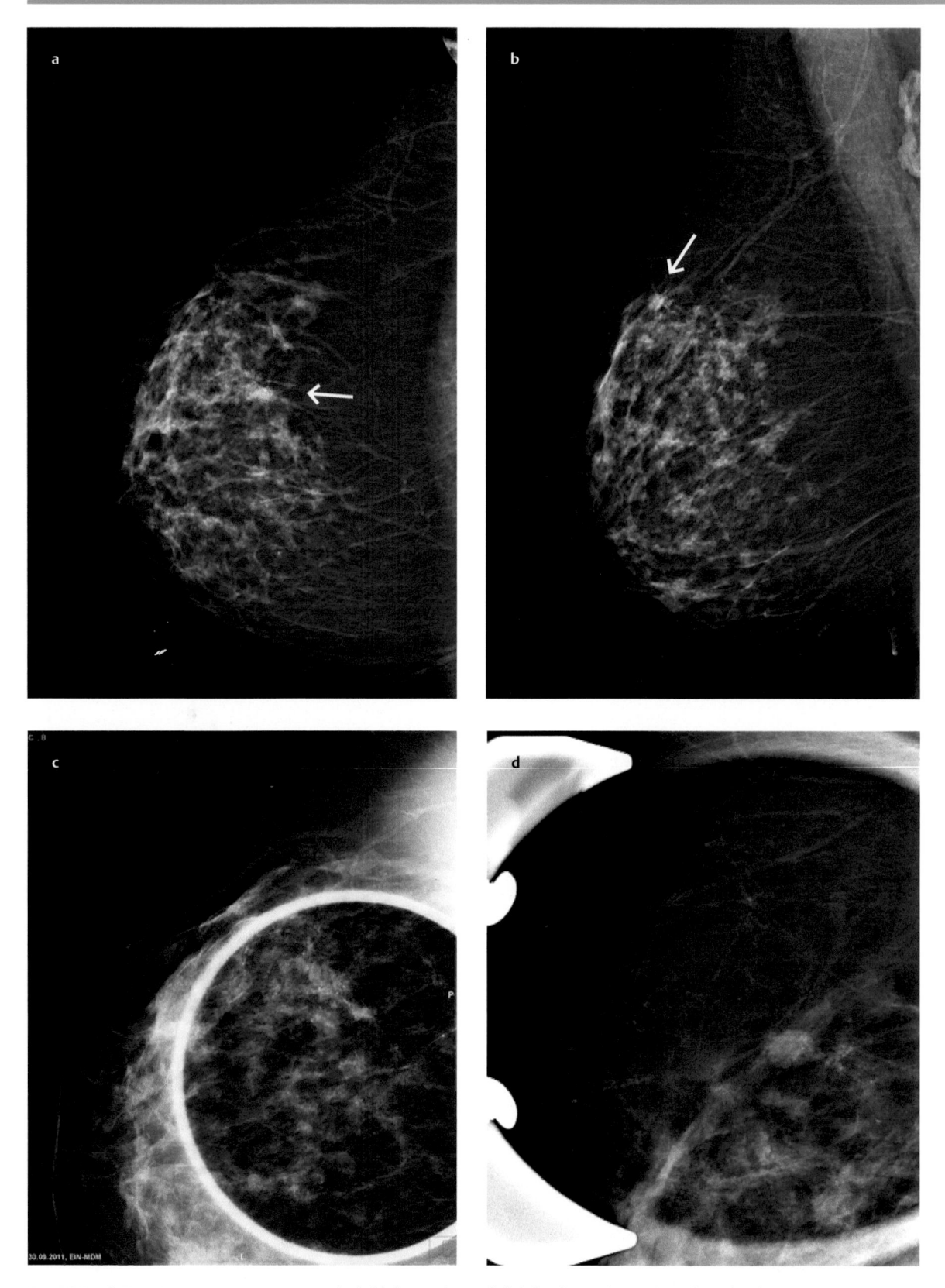

Fig. 24.9a–d Two-view screening mammography (**a,b**) detected a small ill-defined mass (arrows), confirmed with spot compression (**c**) and magnification (**d**). Ultrasound-guided core needle biopsy yielded a 5-mm nodular adenosis.

Differential Diagnosis and Assessment

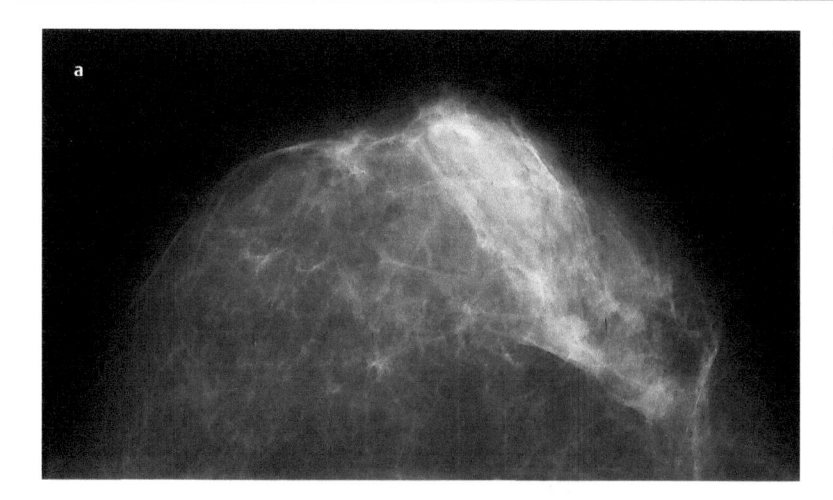

Fig. 24.10a–d Multiple round lesions. This patient had supraclavicular nodal metastases and was being investigated to find the primary tumor.

a,b Mammographically (craniocaudal view), several indeterminate masses are seen in the outer quadrants.

c,d A representative magnetic resonance imaging section shows two nodules before (**c**) and after (**d**) intravenous administration of Gd-DTPA. Neither nodule shows any appreciable enhancement. These findings are compatible with old fibroadenomas. An excisional biopsy was deferred. Follow-up mammography revealed the lesions to be stable. Further tumor search discovered a gastric carcinoma.

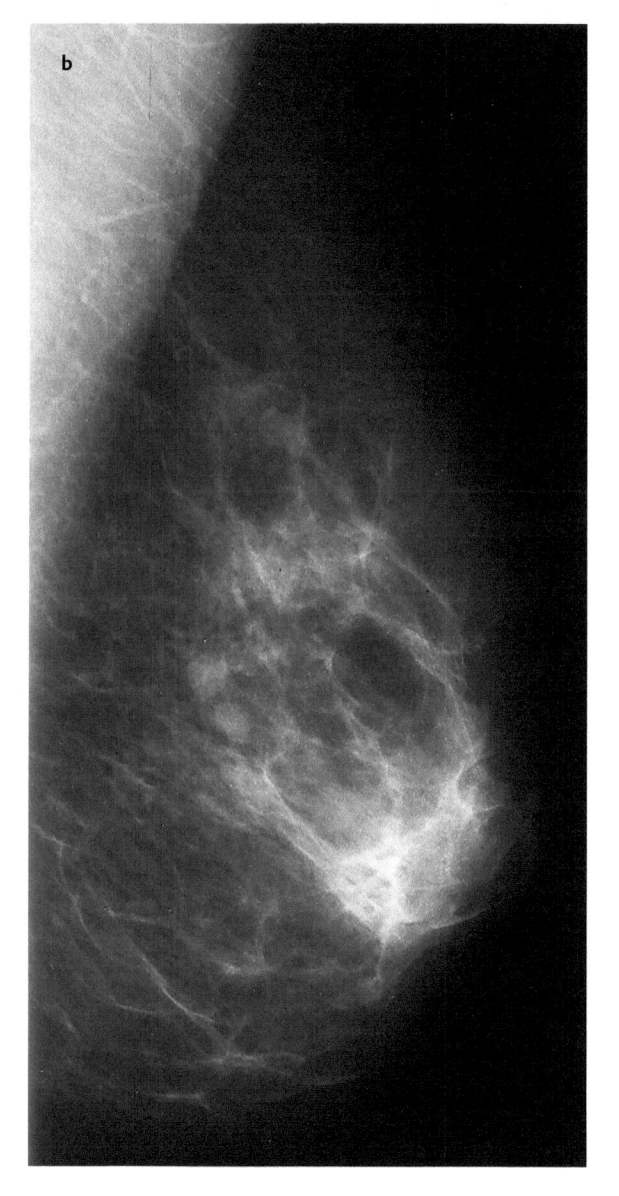

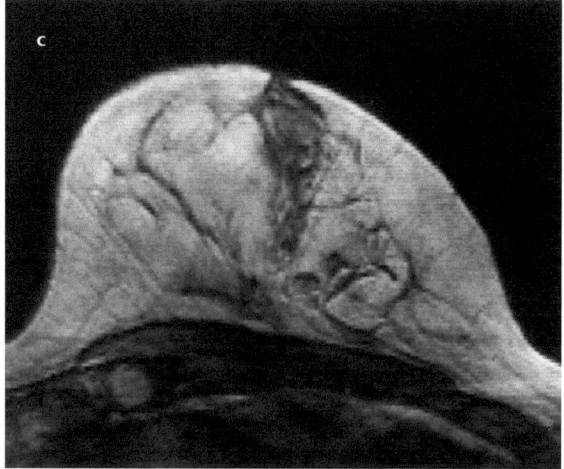

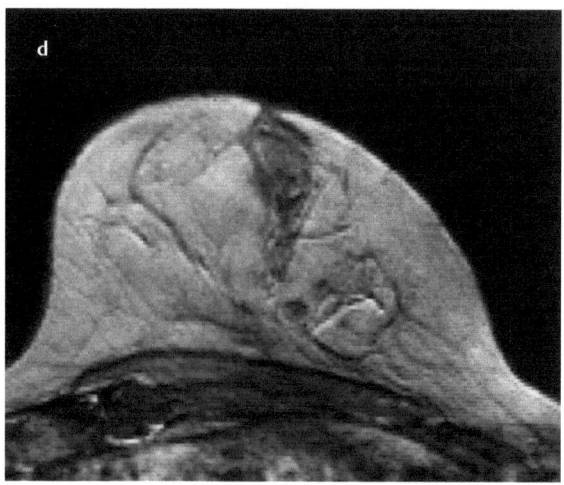

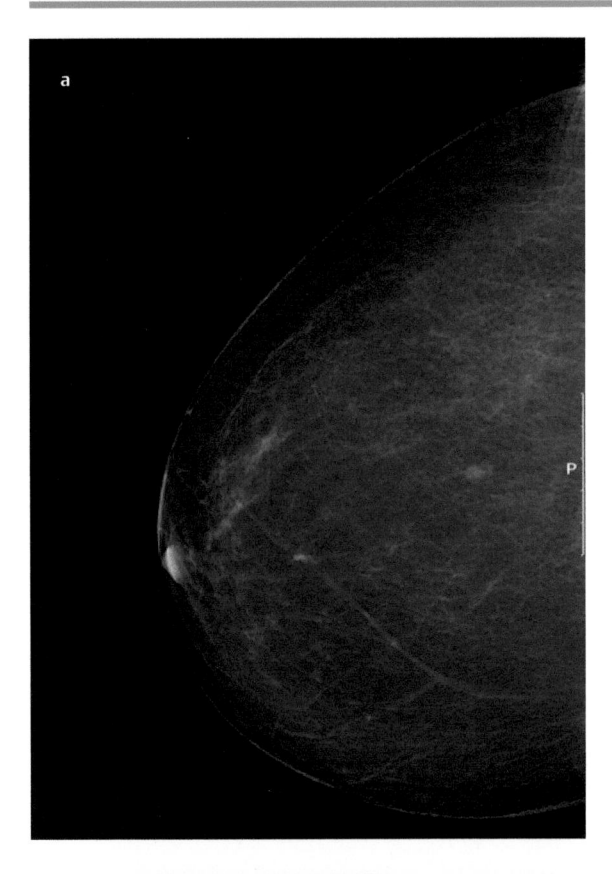

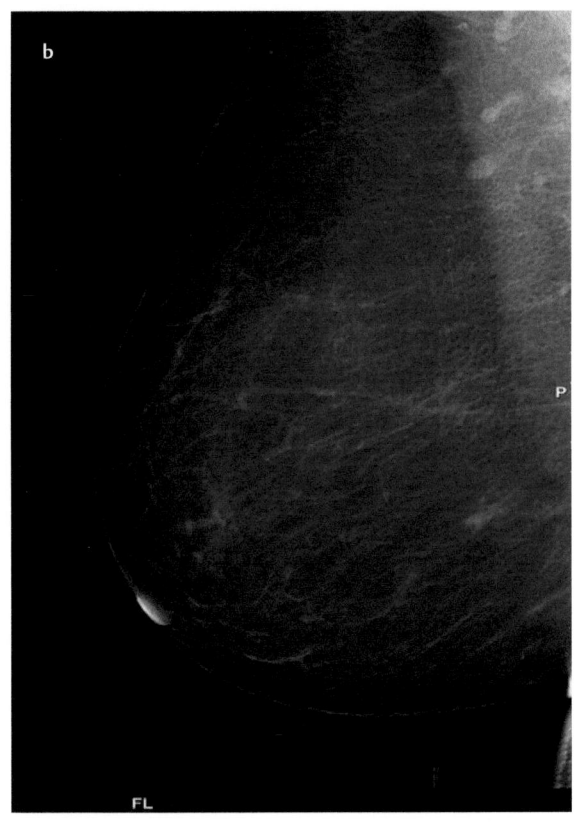

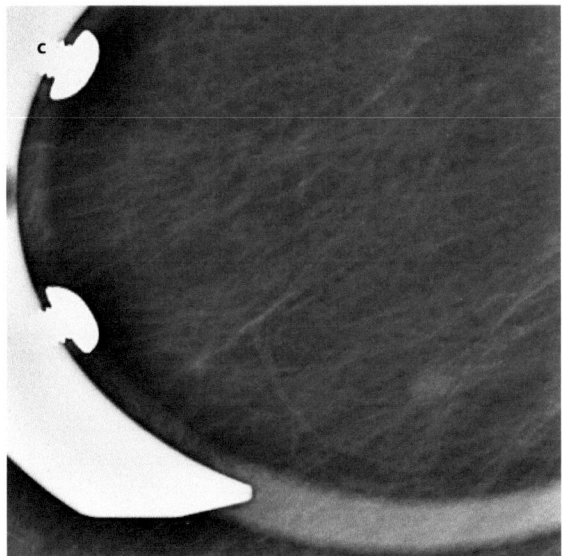

24 Additional Diagnostic Evaluation of Screening Findings and Solving of Problems in Symptomatic Patients

Fig. 24.11a–c New density.

a A faint nodular density had newly developed compared with the previous mammogram (craniocaudal view).
b On the mediolateral oblique (MLO) view it is very uncharacteristic and even less prominent. However, it did not appear sharp.
c The MLO spot compression shows a small nodule which is very transparent and might falsely suggest defined margins. Since the density was new, we decided to suggest stereotactic vacuum-assisted breast biopsy to the patient. The very small nodule could not be detected on retrospective ultrasound, as might be suspected anyway within this large fatty breast. *Histology* revealed a 5-mm ductal invasive breast cancer G2.

Differential Diagnosis and Assessment

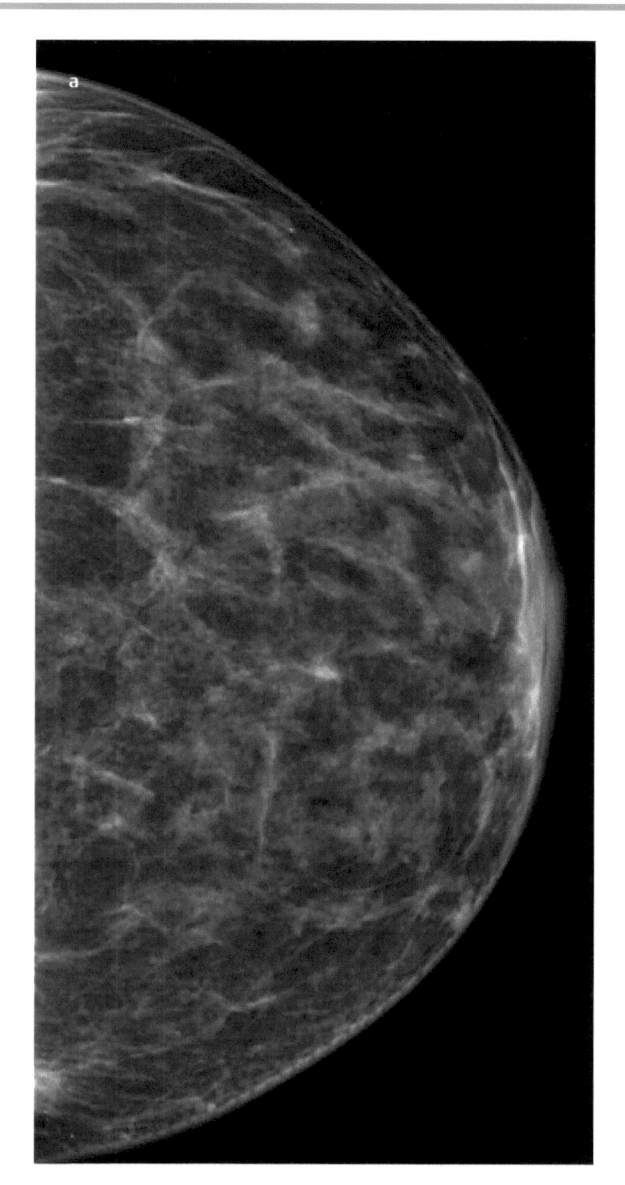

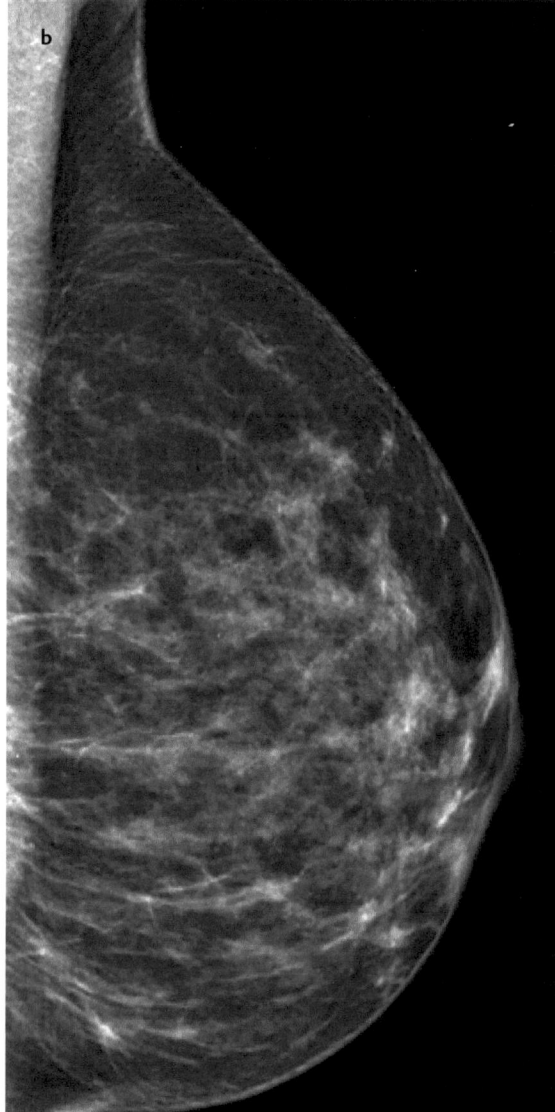

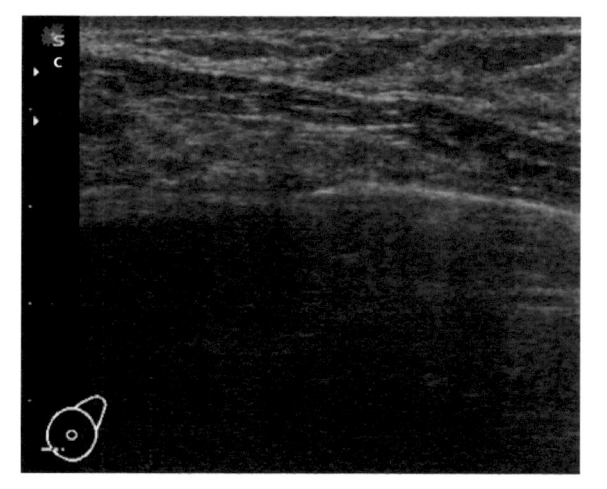

Fig. 24.12a–c

a,b Focal density shown medially and posteriorly on a craniocaudal screening mammogram (**a**). Neither the mediolateral oblique view (on which a medial lesion close to the chest wall might escape) nor the lateromedial view shown here (**b**)—which is the best view to demonstrate pathology that is located medially and far posteriorly—shows a mass.

c The targeted search by ultrasound yields normal soft and moveable breast tissue anterior to the chest wall throughout both inner quadrants.

All imaging findings indicate that the density on the initial craniocaudal view corresponds to an isolated bundle of muscle, imaged en face on this view. This isolated bundle of muscle is called the sternal muscle.

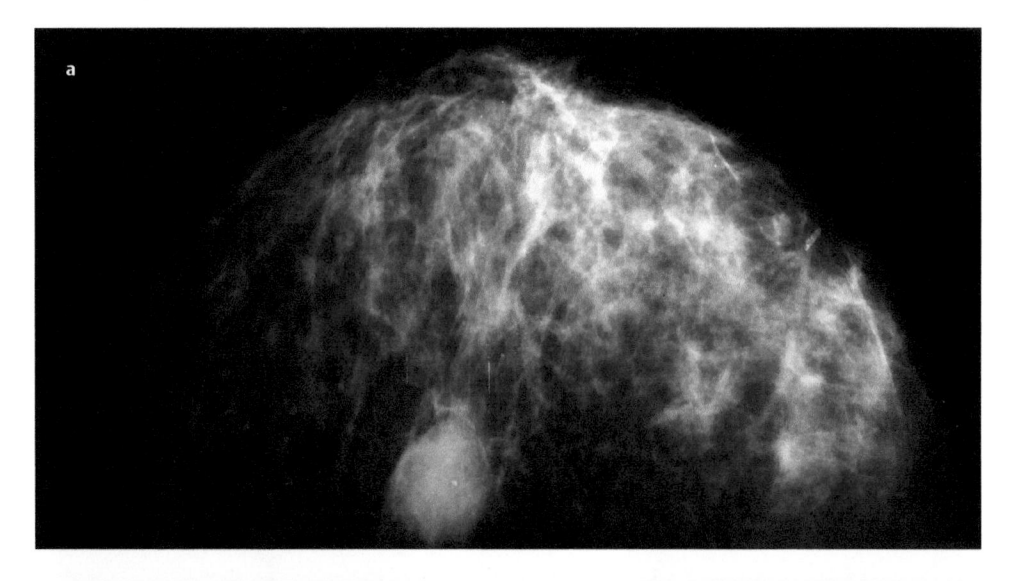

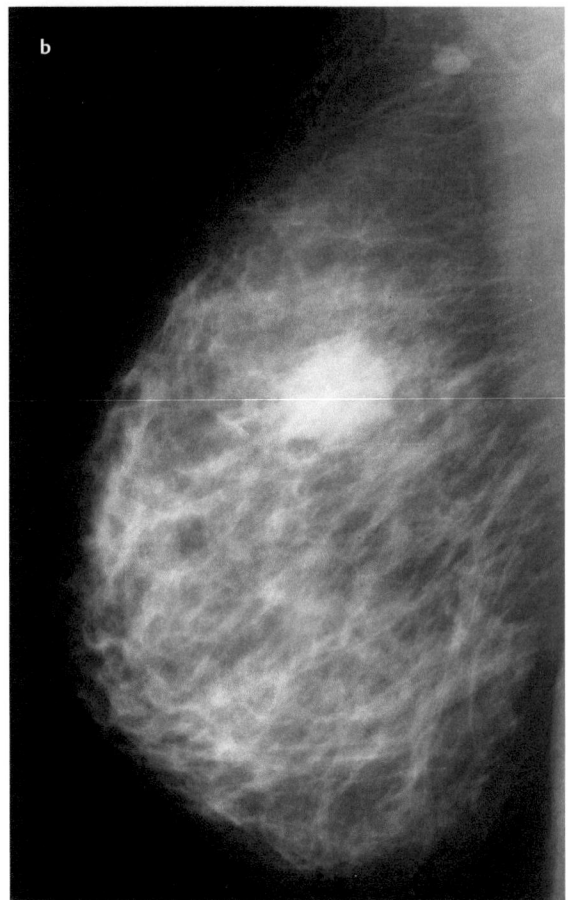

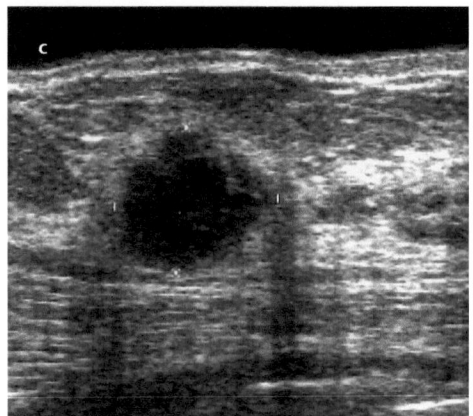

24 Additional Diagnostic Evaluation of Screening Findings and Solving of Problems in Symptomatic Patients

Fig. 24.13a–h This 61-year-old patient presented with a palpable lump of approximately 3 cm. Based on the patient's age, and on the lesion's partly smooth borders, which were to some degree superimposed by breast tissue, the lesion had to be considered suspicious (BI-RADS 4).

a,b Craniocaudal and mediolateral oblique outside mammograms.
c Ultrasound was performed to guide percutaneous core needle biopsy. No additional focus was noted.

Differential Diagnosis and Assessment

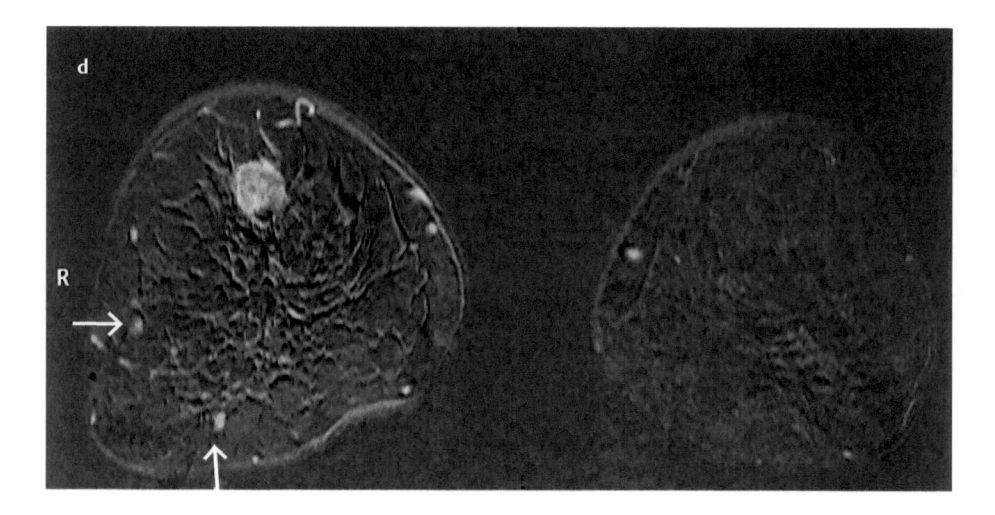

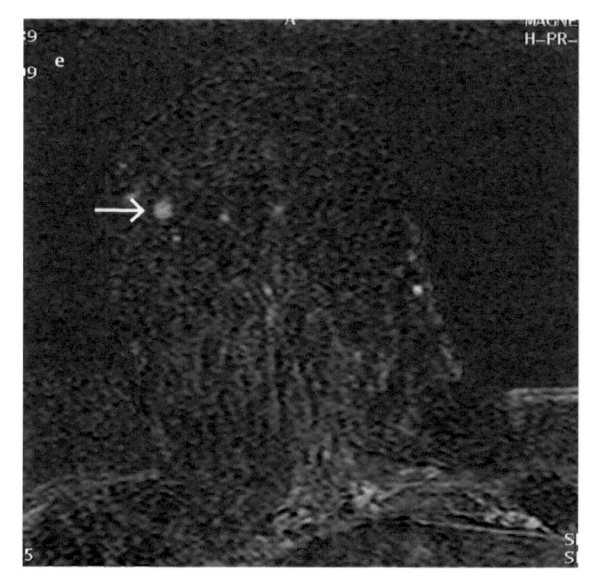

d Contrast-enhanced magnetic resonance imaging (MRI) was performed to check for multicentricitiy. A coronal MR subtraction image is shown, which demonstrates the tumor in the 12 o'clock position and two small additional foci in the 9 and 6 o'clock positions. (Further enhancing foci were noted in other areas as well.)

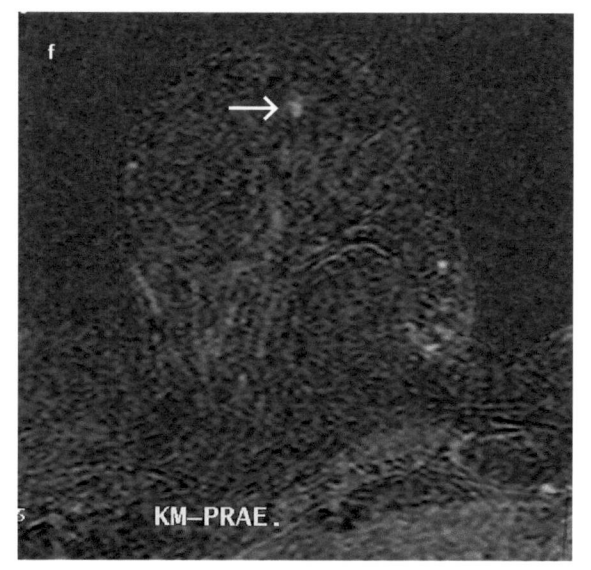

e,f Small enhancing foci may be caused by malignancy or benign changes. Therefore, histologic proof is necessary before further therapeutic decisions are made.
In this case, two representative foci were marked under MR guidance. First the breast was positioned in the biopsy coil using moderate compression and imaging performed to find lesion 1 (**e**) and lesion 2 (**f**) (arrows). Both lesions are shown on transverse subtraction images (postcontrast minus precontrast).

Fig. 24.13 g–h ▷

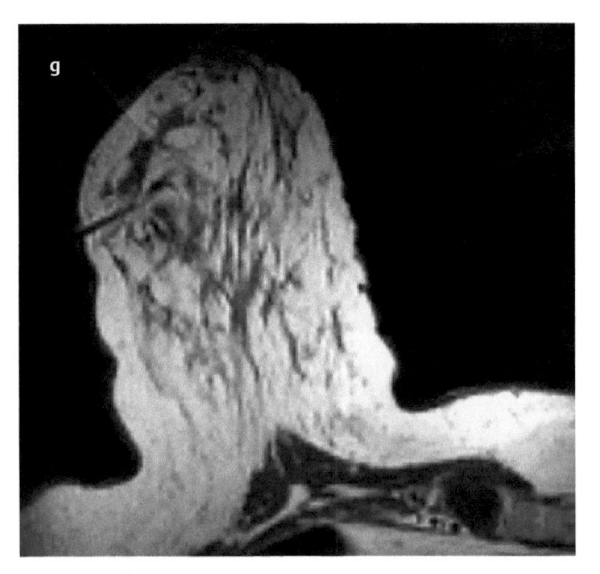

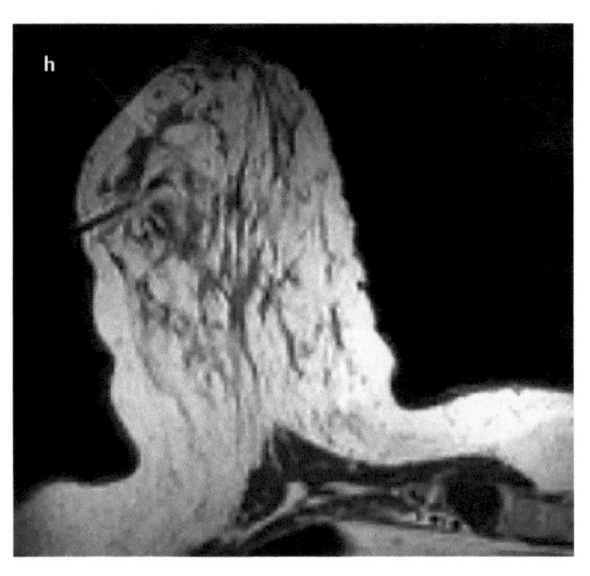

g,h The needle was then positioned and another MR sequence obtained showing the wire in place in lesion 1 (**g**) and in lesion 2 (**h**) *Histology* of the main tumor showed invasive ductal carcinoma. The additional foci proved to be ductal carcinoma in situ. The patient decided against breast conservation and was treated by mastectomy and breast reconstruction.
The value of detecting very small additional foci is presently under discussion (see Chapter 5).

increased density, development of a new mass or nodule in the scar, or suspicious microcalcifications, biopsy is indicated.
- In the case of questionable findings or impaired mammographic evaluation or both, MRI can be very helpful, since it is able to detect tumors, even within severe scarring, and since it can differentiate between a tumor and fibrosis quite reliably.
3. Next, it must be decided whether the finding represents a true lesion or is caused by superimposition.
    - A true mass must be unambiguously assigned a spatial dimension in both projections.
    - If seen in one projection only, its focal nature can be confirmed or excluded by one or several additional mammographic views and/or by ultrasound. Additional mammographic views may include spot views, rolled views, or further projections.

Considering that a significant number of mammographically detected small breast cancers (often breast cancers surrounded by fatty breast tissue or DCIS) may not be visible sonographically (even in retrospect), ultrasound alone should not be used to exclude malignancy in the presence of a suspicious mammographic focal finding. Thus additional mammographic evaluation is strongly recommended for indeterminate focal findings.

Considering that a significant number of early breast cancers may be visible on one mammographic view only, malignancy should not be excluded based on additional views only. Due to a better compressibility of early lobular carcinomas, such malignancies may falsely disappear on spot views. Therefore, we recommend always using both additional mammographic views (including rolled views and different projections) *and* high-resolution ultrasound for excluding malignancy in the case of indeterminate focal findings.

Tomosynthesis may be quite helpful for distinguishing true lesions from superimposition, for assessing focal lesions without superimposition, and for determining the exact location of findings visible on one view only. The highest benefit may probably be expected in breasts with a density of ACR2–3. The exact role of tomosynthesis is still under investigation.

In rare cases with difficult distinction between superimposition and a true finding or in the case of suspicious findings visible on one view only that cannot be localized in three dimensions, MRI may be very helpful.

Any lesion that is not well circumscribed and cannot be diagnosed as unequivocally benign (e.g., superimposition, scarring, for which usual screening may be recommended) should undergo histopathologic assessment if it can be targeted. For rare lesions that probably correspond to superimposition, short-term follow-up or additional MRI may be adequate.

Indeterminate or suspicious focal lesions visible by ultrasound should be biopsied under sonographic guidance, usually US-guided CNB. According to our experience, small focal lesions visible by mammography only, can ideally be assessed using stereotactic VABB. Larger lesions, which rarely cannot be detected by retrospective ultrasound imaging, can be assessed using stereotactic CNB.

For lesions that can be visualized or targeted by MRI alone, MR-guided VABB is required.

Architectural Distortion

(See **Fig. 24.14**.)

Diagnostic Questions

Architectural distortion may be the only early sign of a carcinoma. Carcinomas most frequently presenting as an architectural distortion include lobular breast carcinomas, tubular carcinoma, and sometimes ductal invasive carcinomas or DCIS. Absence of a central density (so-called "black star") increases the probability of a benign entity. However, it is not a reliable sign of benignity. Scarring usually presents with architectural distortion and characteristically is imaged very variably using different projections. Thus for changes compatible with scarring evaluation of any change with time is most important. In women without clinical findings and without a history compatible with scarring, neoplastic changes must be distinguished from superimposition. Differentiation from radial scar (synonyms: sclerosing radial lesion, infiltrating epitheliosis), which represents a special manifestation of fibrocystic and proliferative changes, is mostly impossible by imaging. A histopathologic diagnosis of a radial scar based on CNB corresponds to a B3 lesion. A diagnosis based on CNB only usually requires excision, since radial scars may coexist with DCIS, tubular carcinoma, or invasive carcinoma that may be located peripherally. For small radial scars without atypias which are diagnosed and completely excised by VABB follow-up may be adequate if agreed in a multidisciplinary conference. For larger radial scars which are only sampled by VABB, we usually recommend excision.

Diagnostic Strategy

(See **Figs. 24.15 and 24.16**.)
1. First, a scar should be excluded by clinical history and physical examination. Even small incisions for abscess drainage can induce intraparenchymal scars.
   - If clinical and mammographic findings do not completely agree with this diagnosis, previous examinations, including preoperative mammograms, should, if possible, be obtained for comparison. Knowing the original location of an excised finding is helpful. Periareolar scars are usually not helpful in localizing the site of prior breast surgery.
   - If previous mammograms are not available, if the region of interest is not included, or if the radial structure does not unequivocally coincide with the scar, further imaging assessment is usually indicated.
   - Imaging evaluation should start with additional mammographic views and ultrasound. Since early lobular carcinomas may be easily compressible and can falsely disappear on spot compression views, we recommend always checking with both high-resolution ultrasound and with various views including a rolled view or a view in a different projection.
   - In the event of remaining doubt short-term follow-up or MRI may be helpful.
   - MRI may be very helpful for assessing changes that due to severe scarring may be uncertain (or impossible) to target under sonographic or stereotactic guidance.
   - An evolving or progressing new focal density, newly developing suspicious microcalcifications, or combined increased retraction and density of the scar are indications for histopathologic assessment. In addition to a carcinoma, post-traumatic fat necrosis may manifest as an ill-defined mass or as an architectural distortion with or without central density. Granulation tissue in fat necrosis is usually impossible to distinguish from malignancy using any imaging modality.
2. Architectural distortions that cannot be explained by scarring need to be distinguished from superimposition. Additional views including rolled views and views in different projections plus ultrasound scanning should be used. Spot views may be helpful, but architectural distortions that resolve on spot views must be analyzed very carefully. Stretched and straight lines visualized on mammography (in the absence of scarring) have to be considered suspicious.
   - Architectural distortions seen in one projection only are more likely to represent a superimposition or a benign change (small radial scar). Since some early malignancies may be visible only on one view, a careful search in other planes and by ultrasound is always indicated to exclude or support a suspicion.
   - When comparing with prior films it must be considered that some malignancies presenting as architectural distortion (tubular carcinoma, carcinoma in situ, or early lobular carcinoma) may be stable for a long time. Therefore, older films (of sufficient quality) are mostly more helpful than more recent films for comparison.
   - Tomosynthesis is proving another valuable tool for distinguishing architectural distortion from neoplastic changes.
   - In the event of remaining doubts or problems targeting an architectural distortion, contrast-enhanced MRI may help by tomographic identification of the area of distortion or by displaying its enhancement behavior. But it should be kept in mind that even faintly enhancing spiculated structures should be excised, since radial scars can harbor carcinomas in situ that might not show strong enhancement.

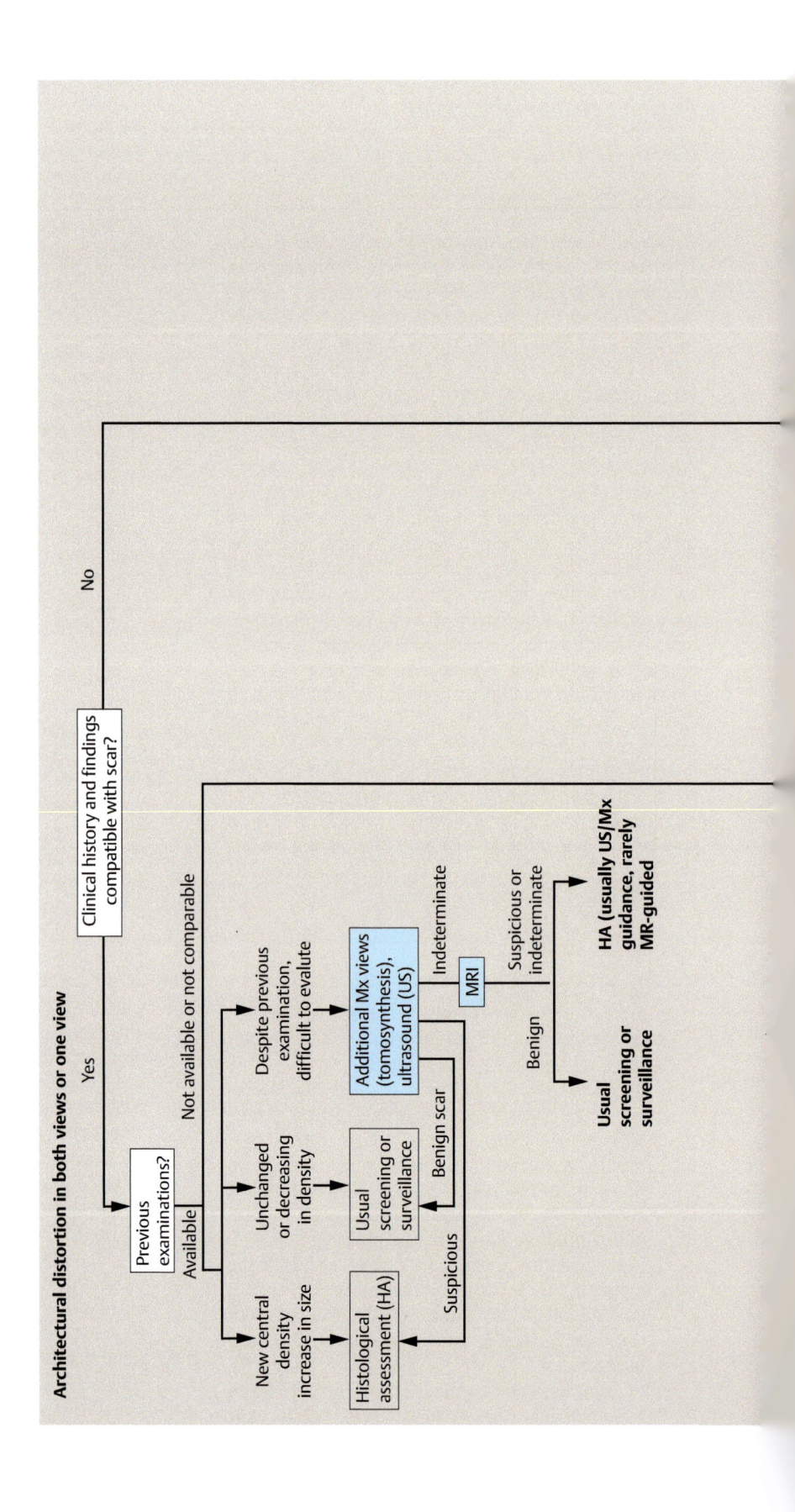

24 Additional Diagnostic Evaluation of Screening Findings and Solving of Problems in Symptomatic Patients

Architectural distortion in both views or one view

- Clinical history and findings compatible with scar?
  - Yes → Previous examinations?
    - Available
      - Unchanged or decreasing in density → Usual screening or surveillance
      - New central density increase in size → Histological assessment (HA)
    - Not available or not comparable
      - Despite previous examination, difficult to evaluate → Additional Mx views (tomosynthesis), ultrasound (US)
        - Benign scar → Usual screening or surveillance
        - Suspicious → Histological assessment (HA)
        - Indeterminate → MRI
          - Benign → Usual screening or surveillance
          - Suspicious or indeterminate → HA (usually US/Mx guidance, rarely MR-guided)
  - No → (Additional Mx views (tomosynthesis), ultrasound (US))

Differential Diagnosis and Assessment

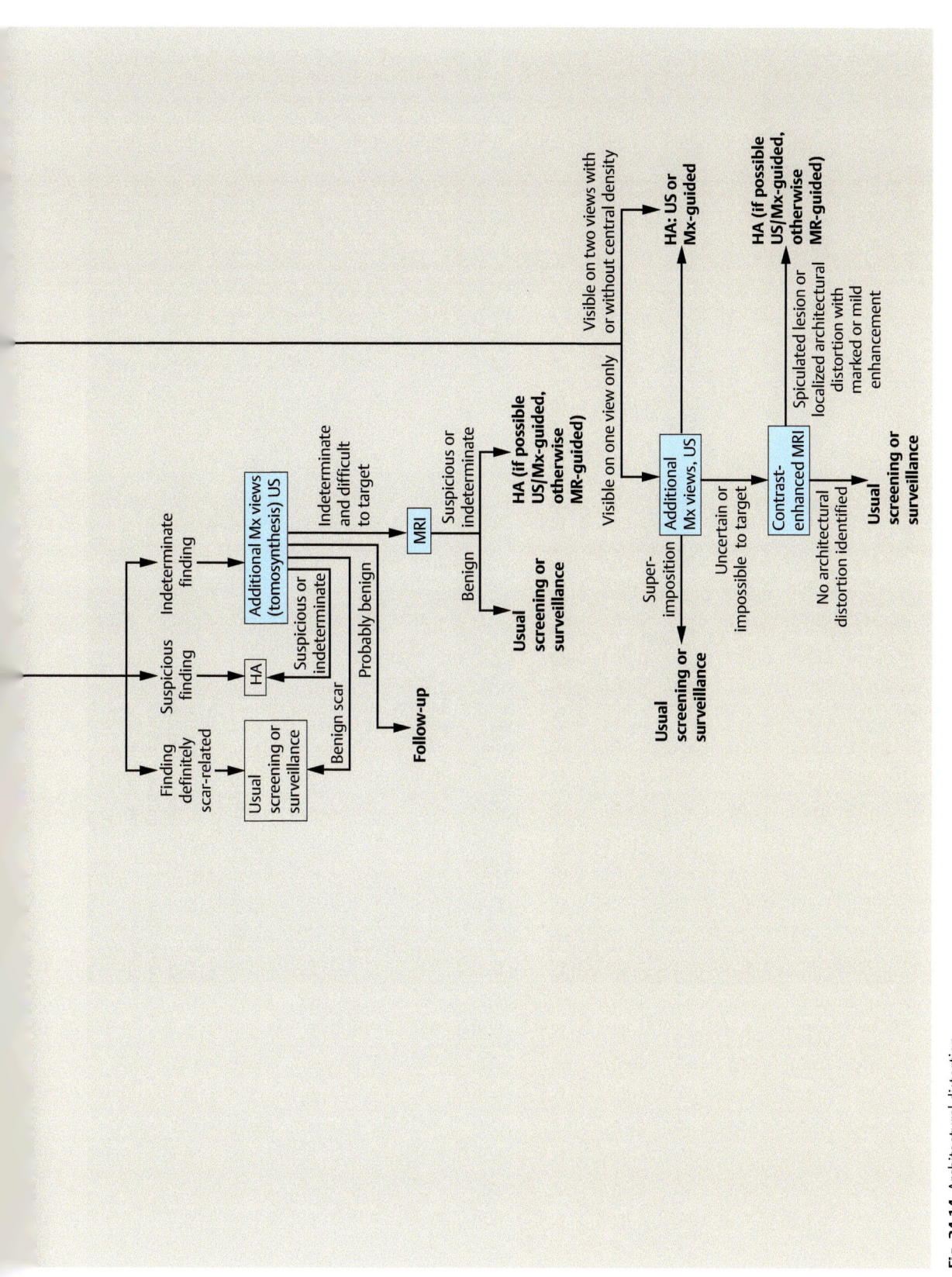

Fig. 24.14 Architectural distortion.

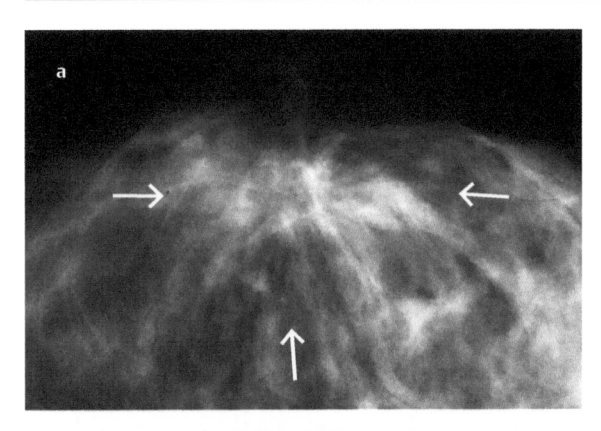

24 Additional Diagnostic Evaluation of Screening Findings and Solving of Problems in Symptomatic Patients

Fig. 24.15a–g Differential diagnosis of architectural distortion.
- **a** Patient A: Delicate architectural distortion in the retroareolar area, with interposed fat lobules centrally: Periareolar scarring.
- **b** Patient B: A delicate architectural distortion was suspected in this asymptomatic patient on the mediolateral oblique (MLO) view of the screening mammogram only (arrow).
- **c** The architectural distortion seen on the MLO view was not seen on the craniocaudal (CC) view and could thus neither be confirmed nor precisely localized.

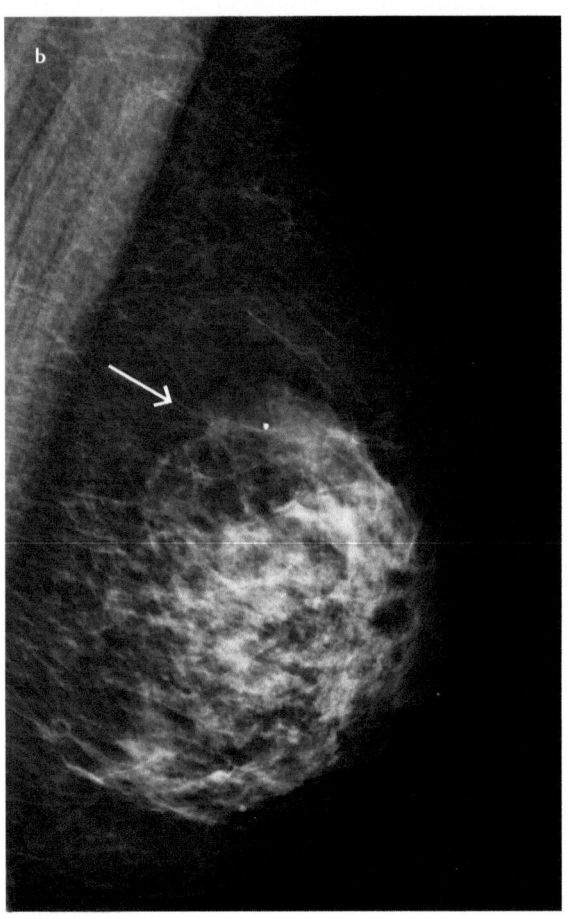

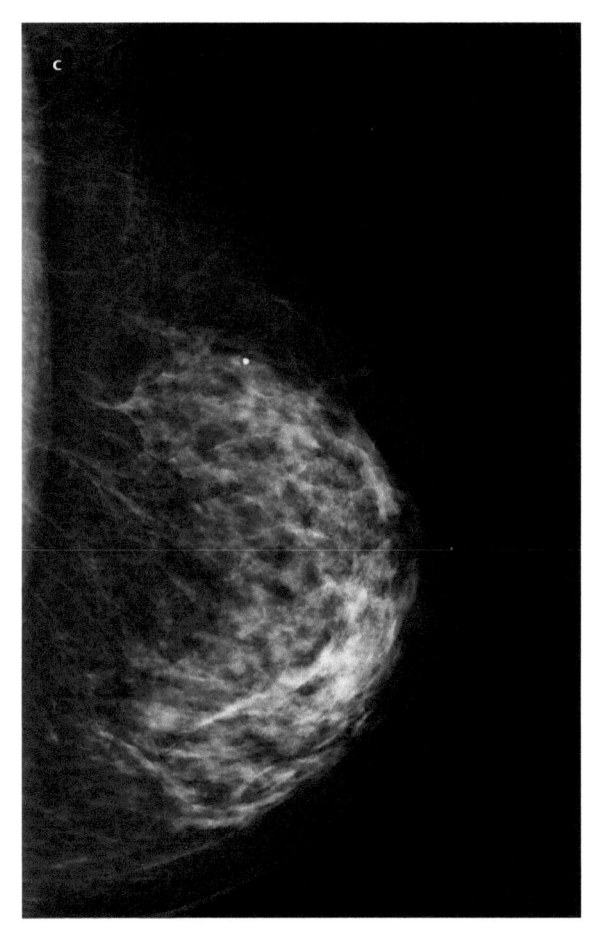

Differential Diagnosis and Assessment

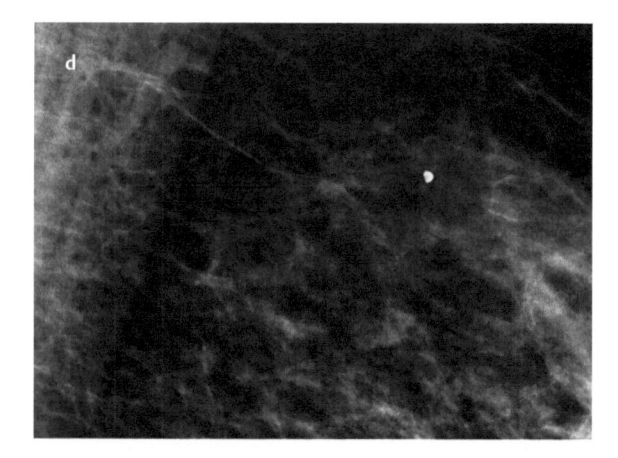

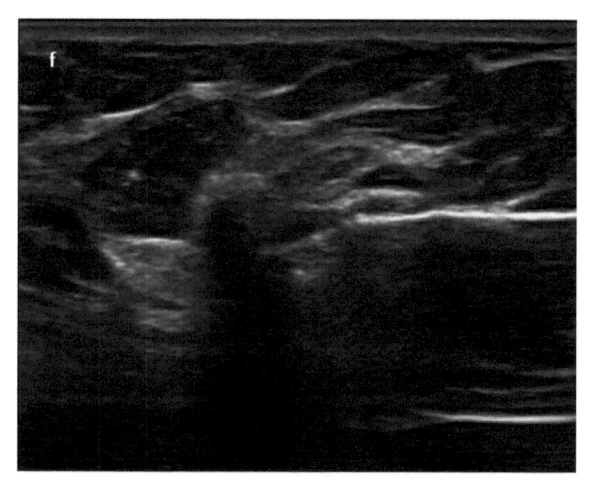

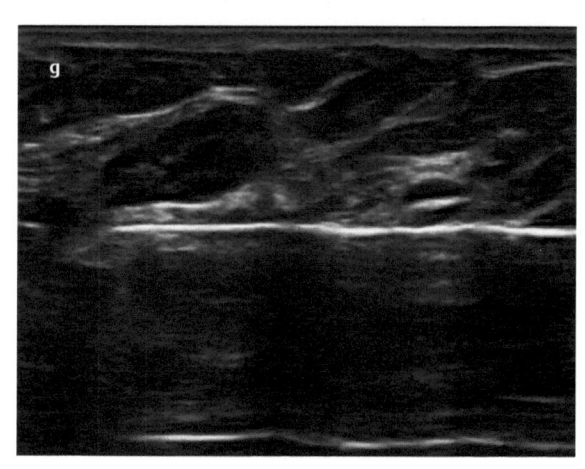

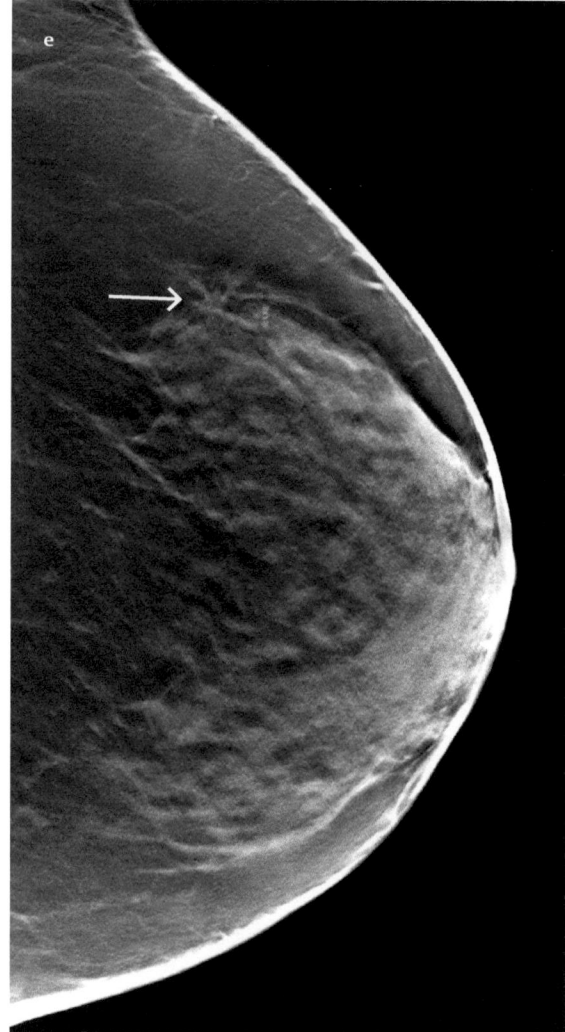

- **d** On the MLO spot view some converging lines could be seen. But, owing to the absence of straight lines, retraction could not be proven and superimposition was difficult to exclude.
- **e** On this section of a tomosynthesis slice both the lesion and its dense center of only 3-4 mm are clearly displayed.
- **f** As stereotactic visualization appeared very difficult, an intensive search was made by ultrasound and, knowing its exact location from the tomosynthesis, the lesion could be located. The image demonstrates the pre-shot image before core needle biopsy (CNB).
- **g** Post-shot image of ultrasound-guided CNB. *Histology*: Invasive ductal carcinoma, grade 1.

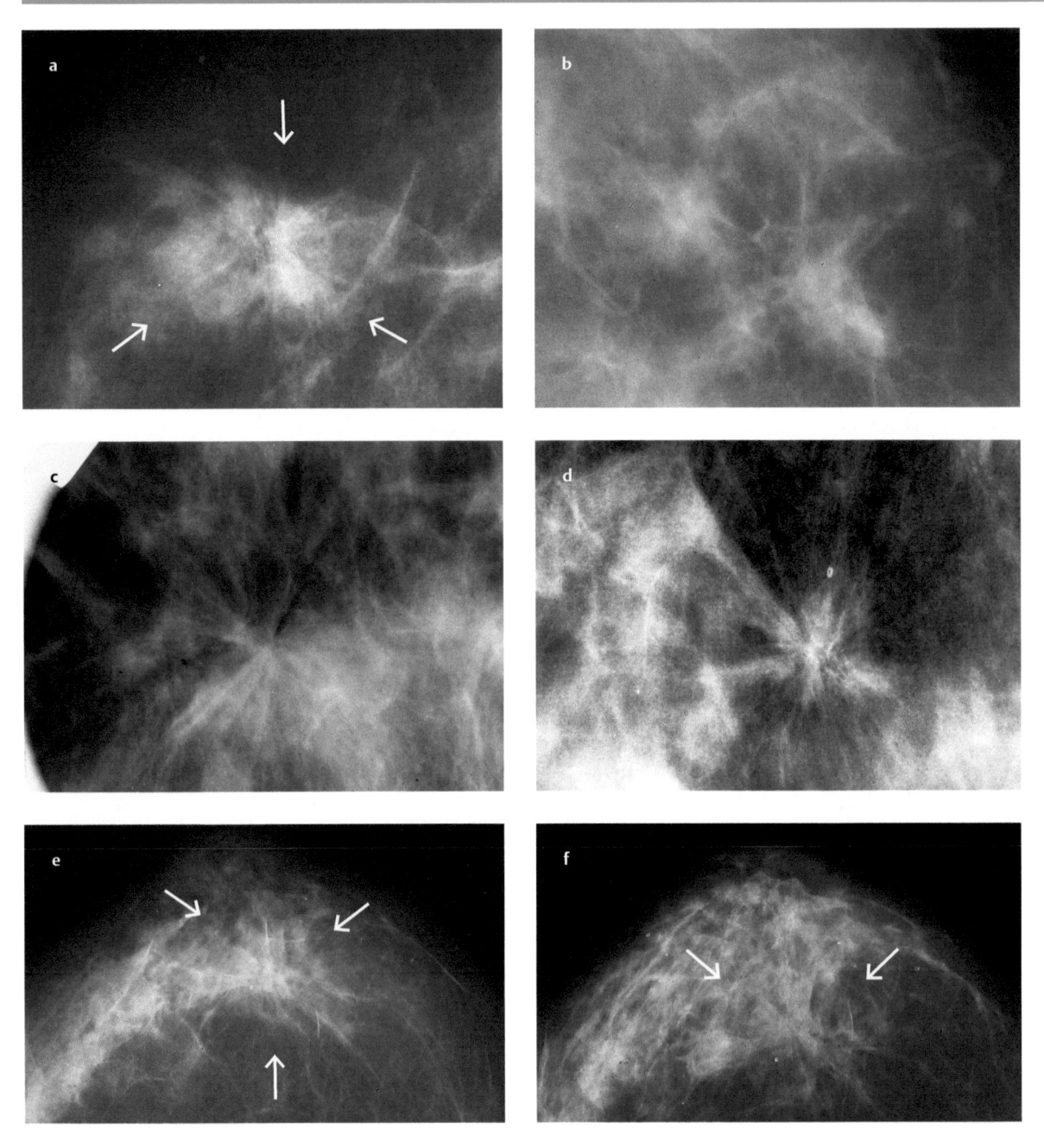

Fig. 24.16a–w Differential diagnosis of architectural distortion.

a Patient A: Architectural distortion without central focal density. *Histology*: Sclerosing adenosis.

b Patient B: Relatively thick extensions radiate from an irregularly outlined mass. *Histology*: Regressively altered fibroadenoma.

c Patient C: This spiculated mass without central density has the characteristic pattern of a radial scar. Biopsy confirmed this diagnosis.

d Patient D: This spiculated mass has a similar pattern to (**c**). However, greater central density and thicker spicules suggest the true diagnosis of infiltrating ductal carcinoma. Definitive differentiation of malignancy from radial scar is not possible based on imaging findings. Biopsy needs to be done to make the final diagnosis.

e Patient E: Clinically, no palpable abnormality was found. Mammographically, there is marked architectural distortion.

f The same patient as (**e**), mammography 6 years later. The radial extensions are longer. *Histology*: Radial scar.

Differential Diagnosis and Assessment

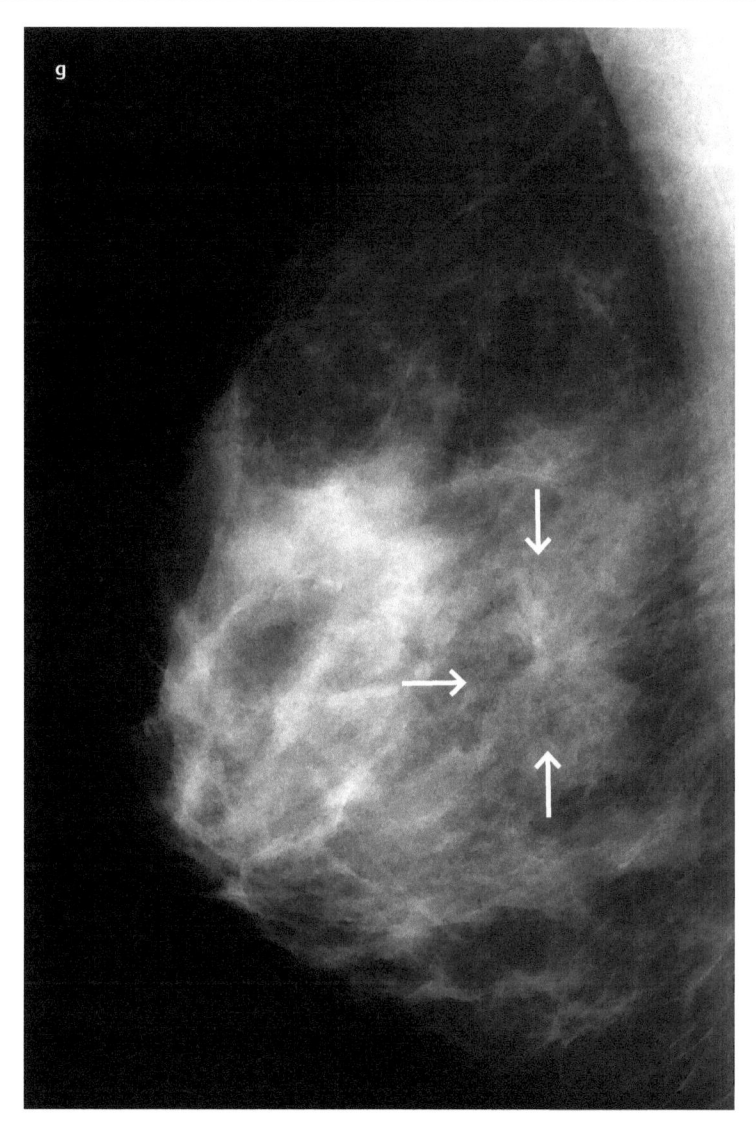

g–i Patient F: Discrete architectural distortion in the upper half of the breast close to the chest wall with very few round calcifications (**g**). On specimen radiography the architectural distortion as well as the microcalcifications are clearly visible (**h**). Sonography shows a hypoechoic irregularly outlined area, measuring 9 mm in diameter, with acoustic shadowing (**i**) *Histology*: Atypical ductal epithelial hyperplasia with ductal carcinoma in situ measuring 7 mm diameter.

Fig. 24.16j–w ▷

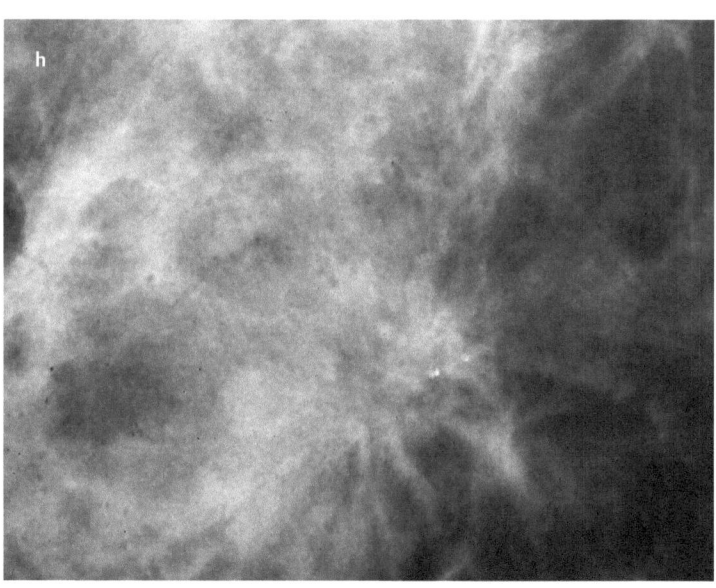

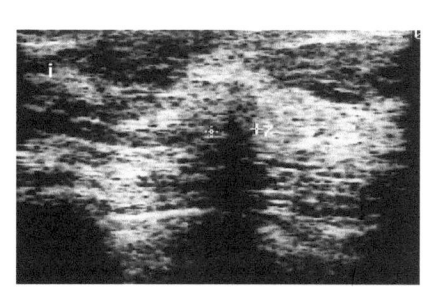

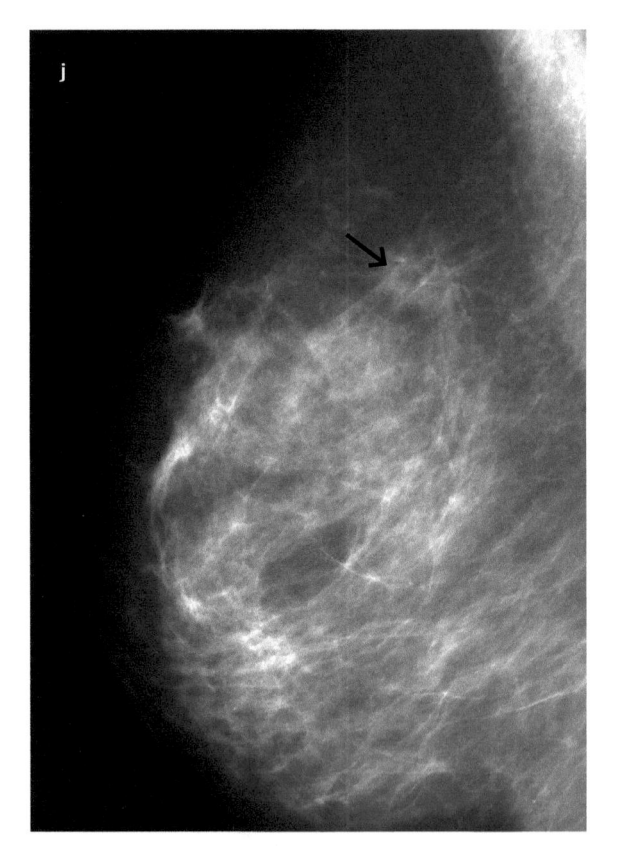

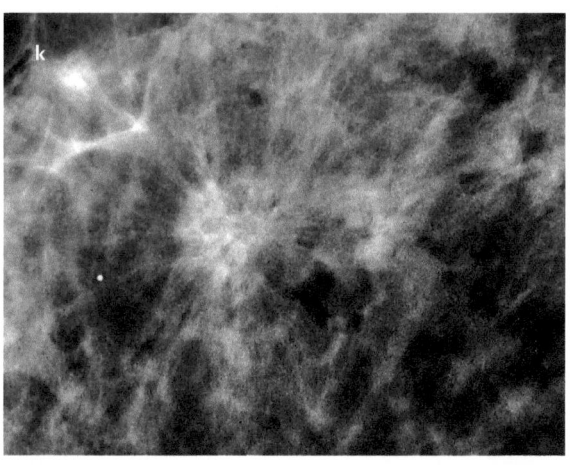

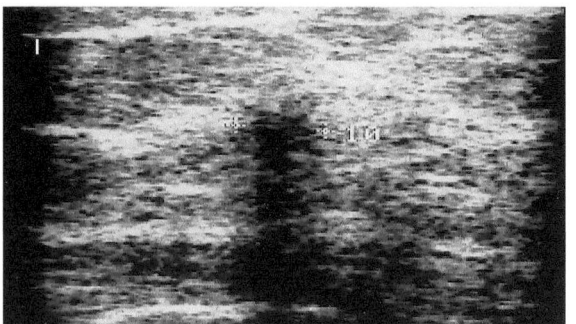

◁ continued

j–l Patient G: Architectural distortion with spicules and a definite central lucency (**j**). Even though a central lucency is more often associated with benign radial scars than with malignancy, histopathologic workup remains necessary. Specimen radiography (**k**); sonographically, a 10-mm hypoechoic irregularly outlined focus with acoustic shadowing corresponds to the mammographic finding (**l**). *Histology*: Infiltrating lobular carcinoma measuring 13 mm in diameter.

Differential Diagnosis and Assessment

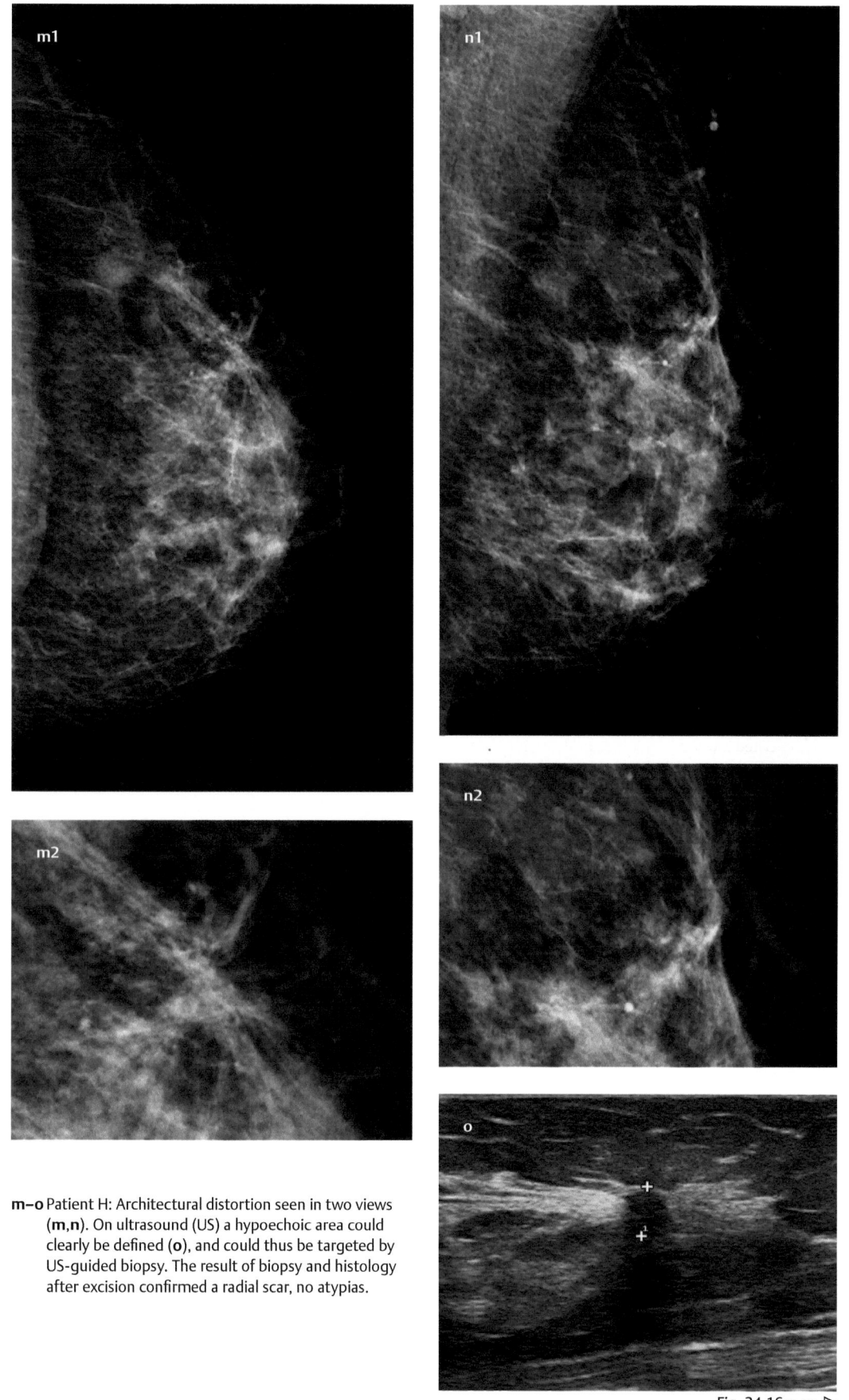

m–o Patient H: Architectural distortion seen in two views (**m,n**). On ultrasound (US) a hypoechoic area could clearly be defined (**o**), and could thus be targeted by US-guided biopsy. The result of biopsy and histology after excision confirmed a radial scar, no atypias.

Fig. 24.16 p–w ▷

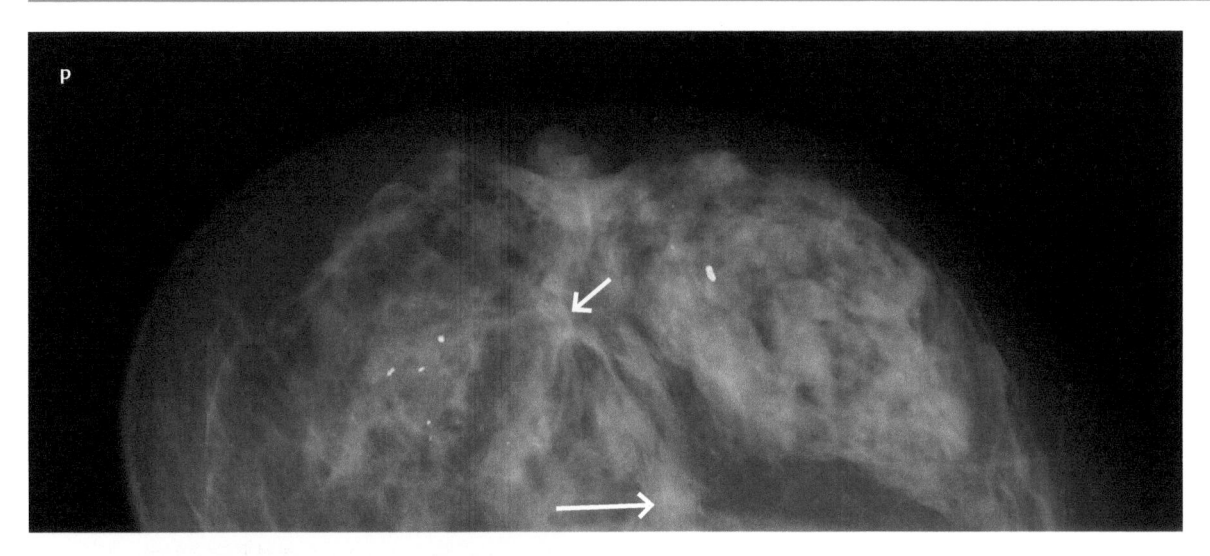

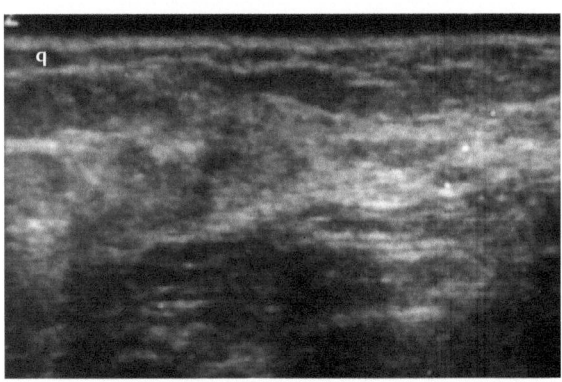

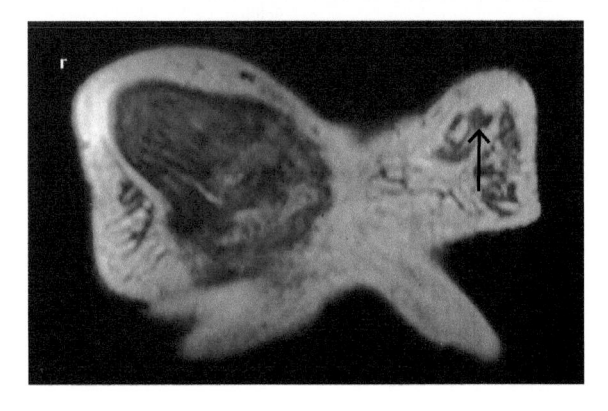

p–s Patient I: In addition to extensive scarring (short arrow), a suspicious nodular density is noted very close to the chest wall (long arrow) (**p**). Despite numerous attempts, this finding could not be reproduced in any other view because of compromised positioning due to the scarring. This region was not included on previous mammograms. Magnetic resonance imaging (MRI) was recommended for further localization of the finding after it could not be delineated sonographically because of the scarring and resultant limited evaluation (sonographic visualization of scar tissue, no focal findings) (**q**). Prepectoral coronal slice of MRI before (**r**) and after (**s**) administration of contrast medium. While the pectoral muscle is predominantly seen on the right, a highly suspicious enhancement is seen on the left in the prepectoral parenchyma (arrow). The finding was successfully excised after MR-guided localization. *Histology*: Ductal carcinoma, 1 cm.

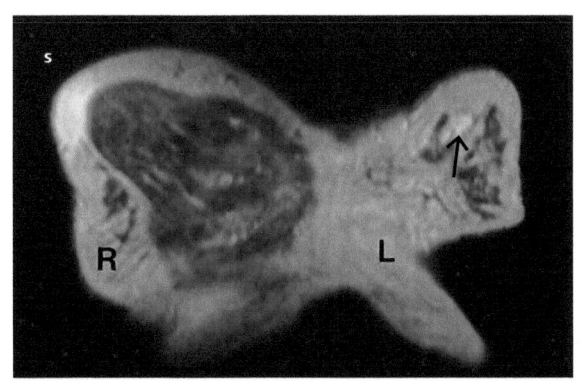

Differential Diagnosis and Assessment

◁ continued

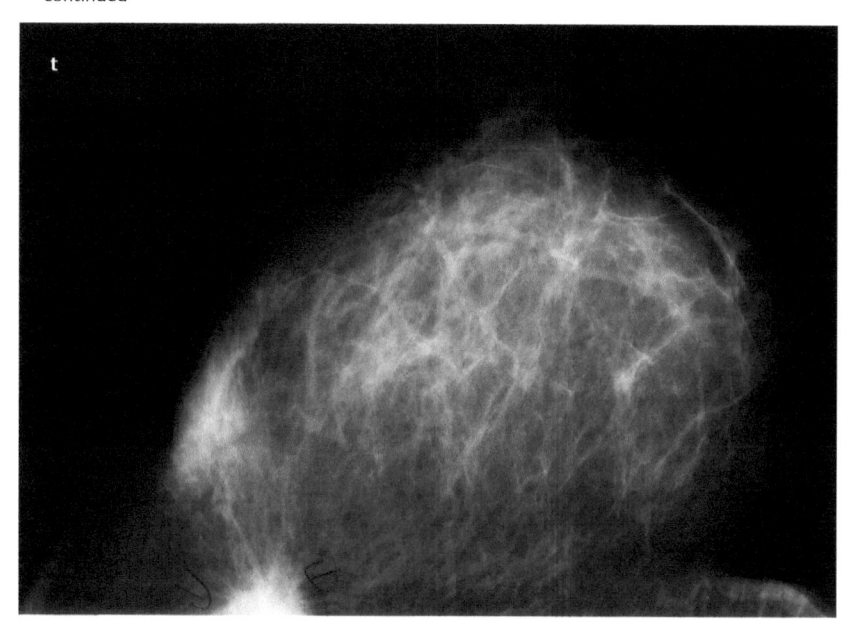

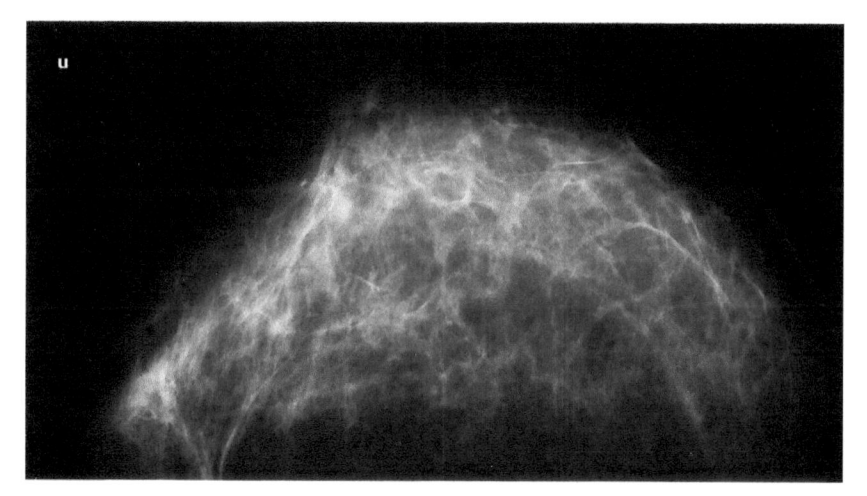

t–w Patient J: Use of contrast-enhanced MRI in a patient with a worrisome finding after breast-conserving therapy. This patient had been referred 1 year after tumorectomy and radiotherapy because of a spiculated focal finding in two projections. (The primary carcinoma did not contain any microcalcifications). Current mammography delineates a spiculated density consistent with a scar, but recurrence could not be excluded (**t**). The preceding mammogram was not helpful in this patient, because the area in question had not been included (**u**). Contrast-enhanced MRI, corresponding section before Gd-DTPA (**v**). A spiculated lesion is visualized with high signal in the center before administration of contrast medium. This high signal intensity can be attributed to resolving products of hemoglobinolysis. The same section as in (**v**) after intravenous administration of Gd-DTPA is shown (**w**). There is no appreciable increase in signal intensity, excluding a malignancy with a high degree of certainty. The finding corresponds to scarring with increased signal intensity due to centrally deposited products of hemoglobinolysis.

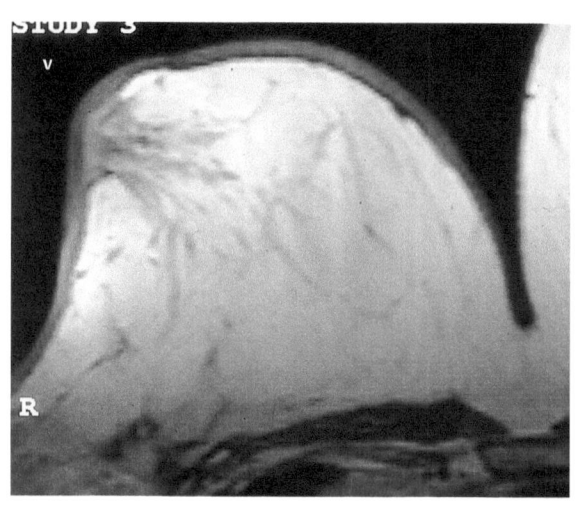

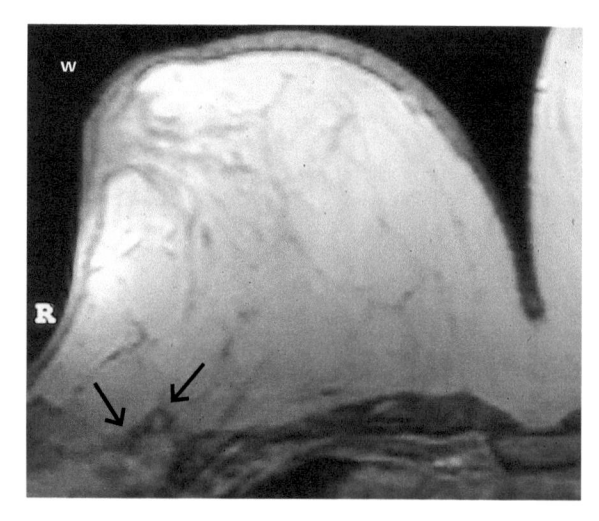

Asymmetry

(See **Fig. 24.17**.)

While asymmetry can be a subtle sign of malignancy, occasionally the only sign, most global asymmetries are due to normal parenchymal asymmetry with or without underlying benign changes (**Fig. 24.18**).

Diagnostic Strategy

If asymmetry is present, it should be closely scrutinized: previous mammograms, if available, are quite helpful. To correctly assess differences in density (right breast vs. left breast, present compared with prior mammograms, a critical check of technical comparability is necessary (compression, exposure, and film contrast).

Special attention is necessary for any area that increases in size and density, that increases in density and decreases in size (check for retractive signs?) or that persists while other areas of the breast decrease in density. Any of the latter signs may be a hint of underlying malignancy.

On mammography interposed fat supports a benign diagnosis but does not always exclude malignancy.

Correlation with the findings of the physical examination and mammography is important, since diffusely growing invasive carcinomas are often palpable. It should

---

Global mammographic asymmetry (asymptomatic patient)

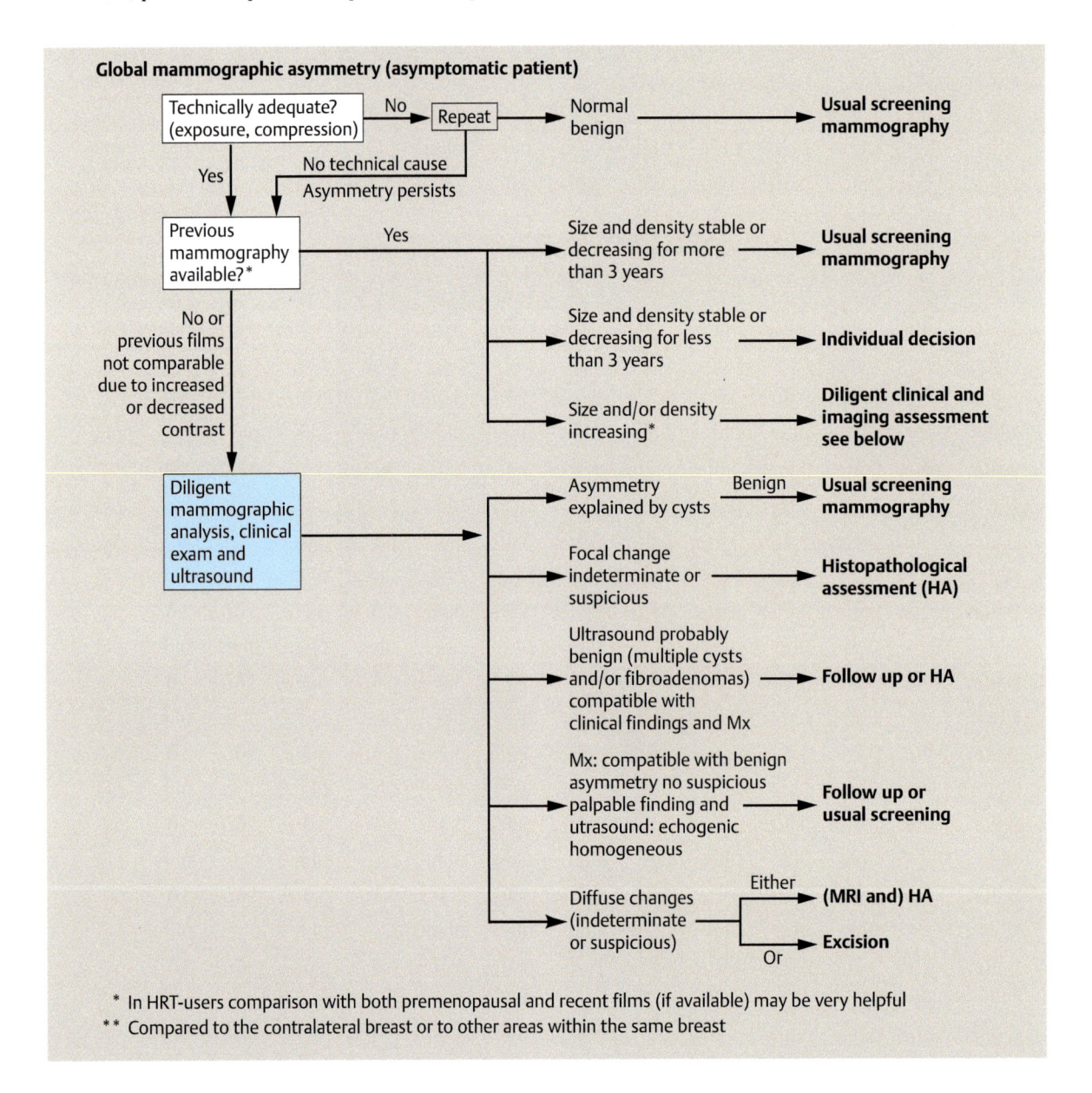

- Technically adequate? (exposure, compression)
  - No → Repeat → Normal benign → Usual screening mammography
  - Yes / No technical cause, Asymmetry persists
- Previous mammography available?*
  - Yes →
    - Size and density stable or decreasing for more than 3 years → Usual screening mammography
    - Size and density stable or decreasing for less than 3 years → Individual decision
    - Size and/or density increasing** → Diligent clinical and imaging assessment see below
  - No or previous films not comparable due to increased or decreased contrast →
- Diligent mammographic analysis, clinical exam and ultrasound →
  - Asymmetry explained by cysts → Benign → Usual screening mammography
  - Focal change indeterminate or suspicious → Histopathological assessment (HA)
  - Ultrasound probably benign (multiple cysts and/or fibroadenomas) compatible with clinical findings and Mx → Follow up or HA
  - Mx: compatible with benign asymmetry no suspicious palpable finding and utrasound: echogenic homogeneous → Follow up or usual screening
  - Diffuse changes (indeterminate or suspicious) → Either → (MRI and) HA / Or → Excision

* In HRT-users comparison with both premenopausal and recent films (if available) may be very helpful
** Compared to the contralateral breast or to other areas within the same breast

Fig. 24.17 Global asymmetry.

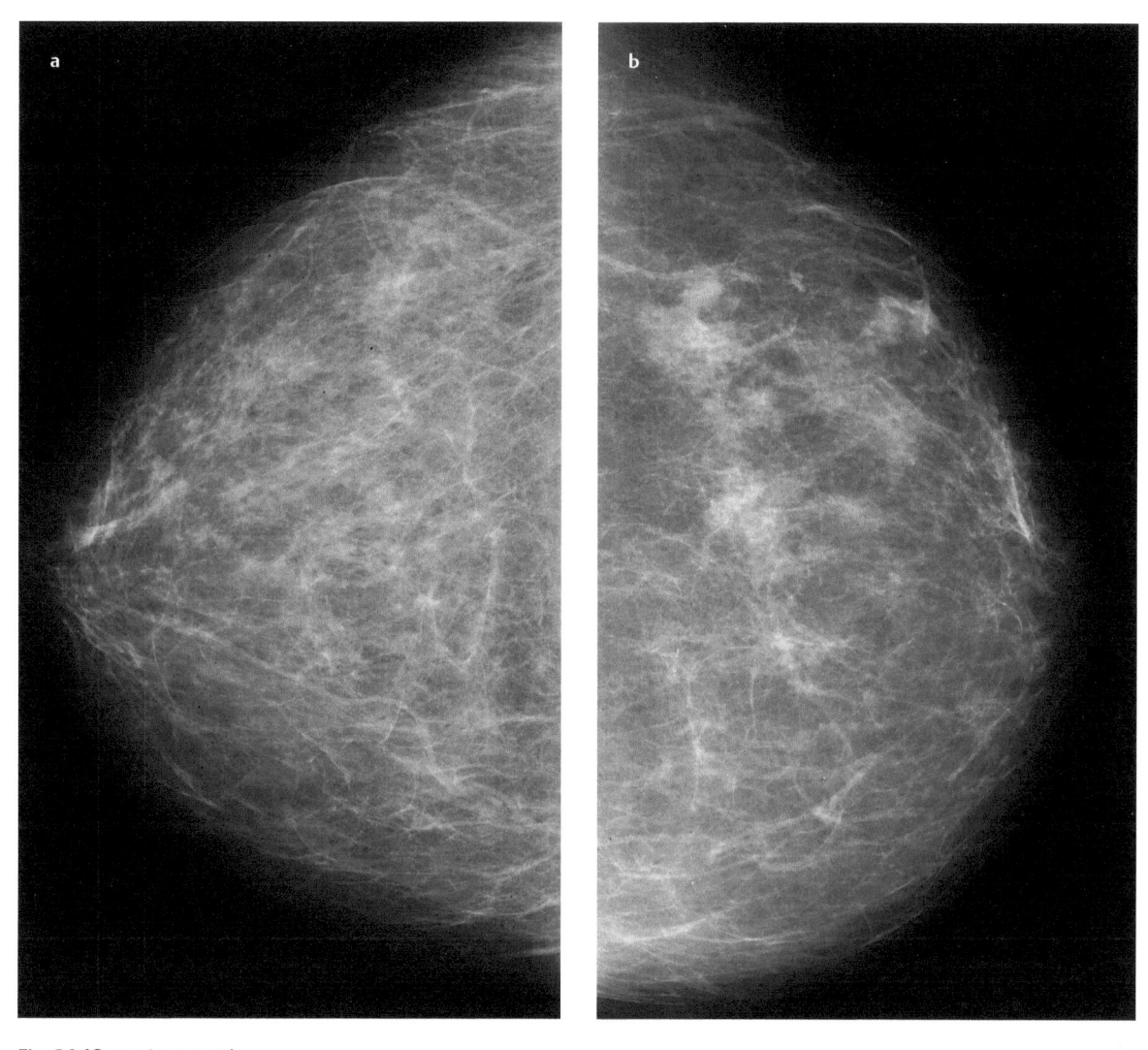

Fig. 24.18a–o Asymmetries.

a,b Routine mammography in craniocaudal view of the right breast (**a**) and left breast (**b**) reveals a definite asymmetry mediocentrally on the left. The presence of regularly distributed fat lobules and the absence of a sonographic and clinically palpable finding supports the diagnosis of a benign asymmetry with a high degree of certainty.

Fig. 24.18c–o ▷

◁ continued

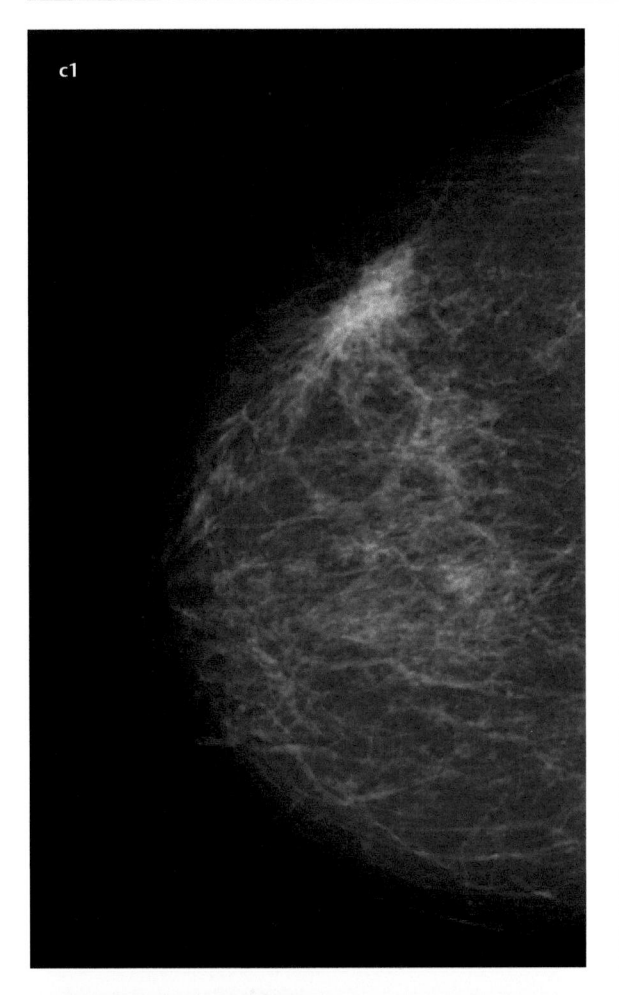

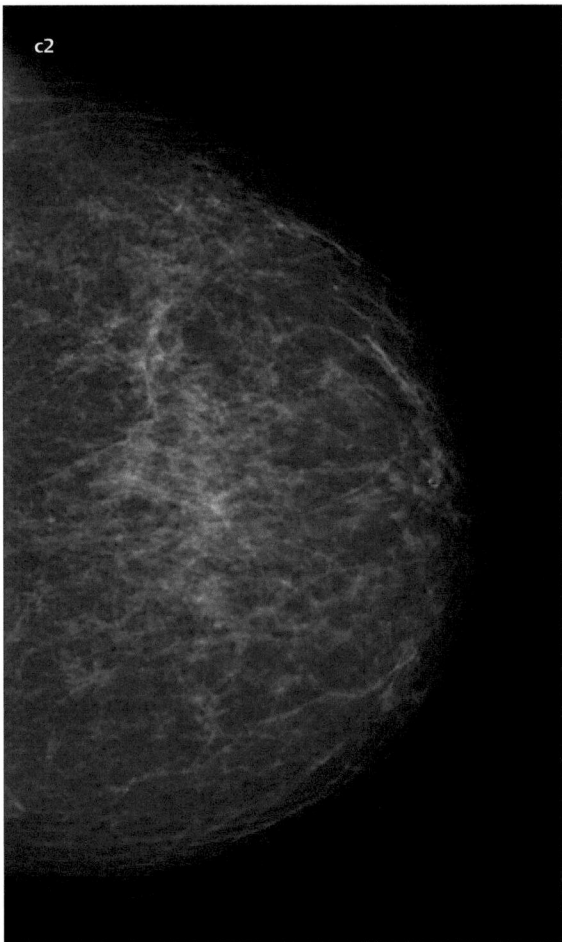

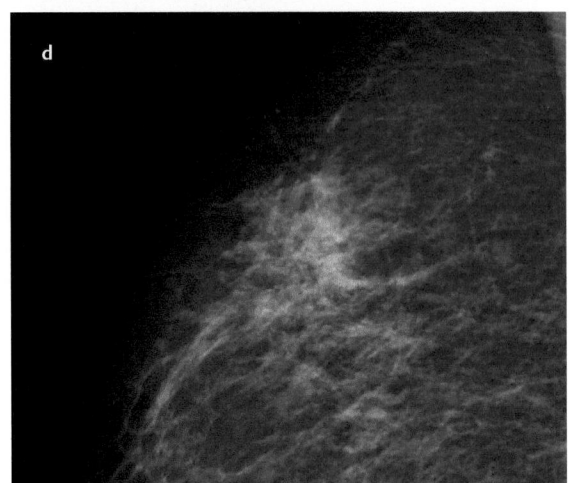

c,d Ductal carcinoma in situ (DCIS) presenting as an asymmetry, which is more striking on the craniocaudal views (**c**). On the mediolateral oblique view (magnified section) (**d**) the asymmetry contains fat lobules, but does not resolve completely.
Sonographically no abnormality was seen. Stereotactically guided vacuum-assisted breast biopsy yielded an intermediate grade DCIS.

Differential Diagnosis and Assessment

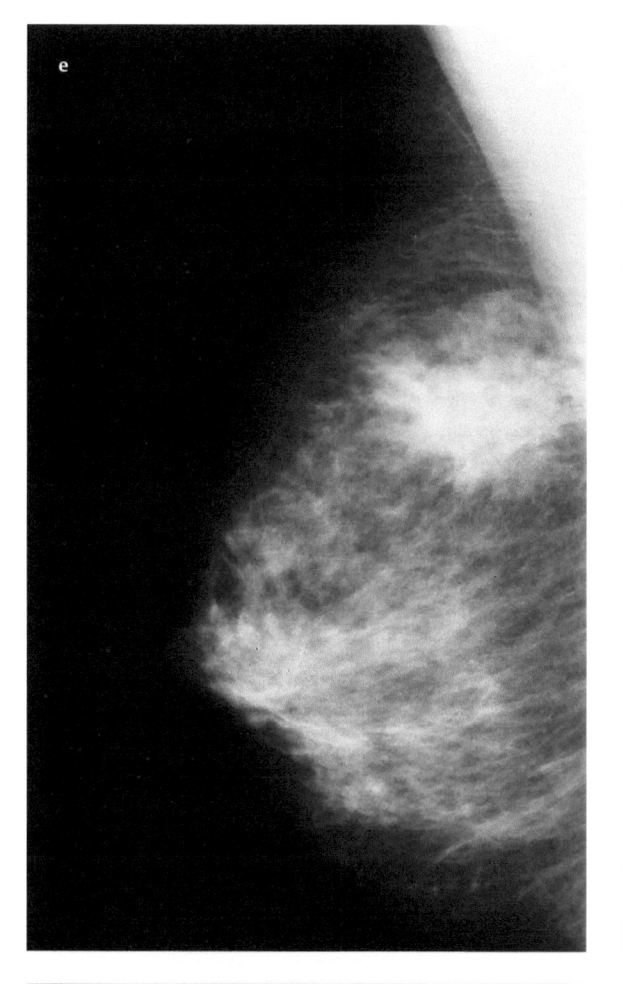

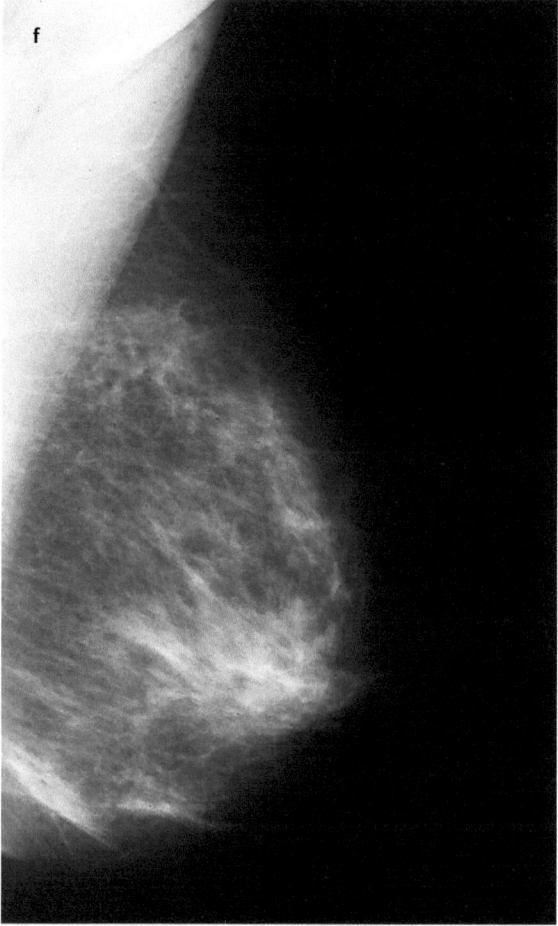

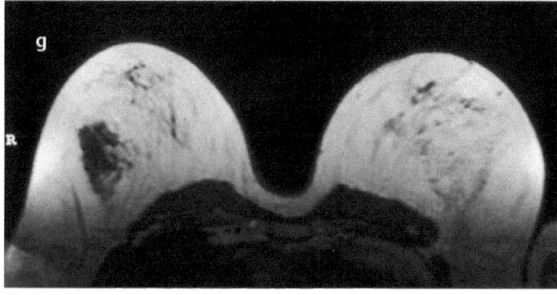

e–h This 57-year-old patient shows a pronounced mammographic asymmetry. The fat islands within the asymmetry as well as the palpable fibrocystic finding support the diagnosis of a benign asymmetry. **e,f** Mammography shows a pronounced asymmetry on the right (**e**) in comparison with the left. **g** Representative section through the asymmetric area before intravenous administration of Gd-DTPA. **h** The same section as in (**g**) after intravenous injection of Gd-DTPA shows no appreciable enhancement, supporting the diagnosis of a benign asymmetry. The diagnosis was proven by follow-up.

Fig. 24.18i–o ▷

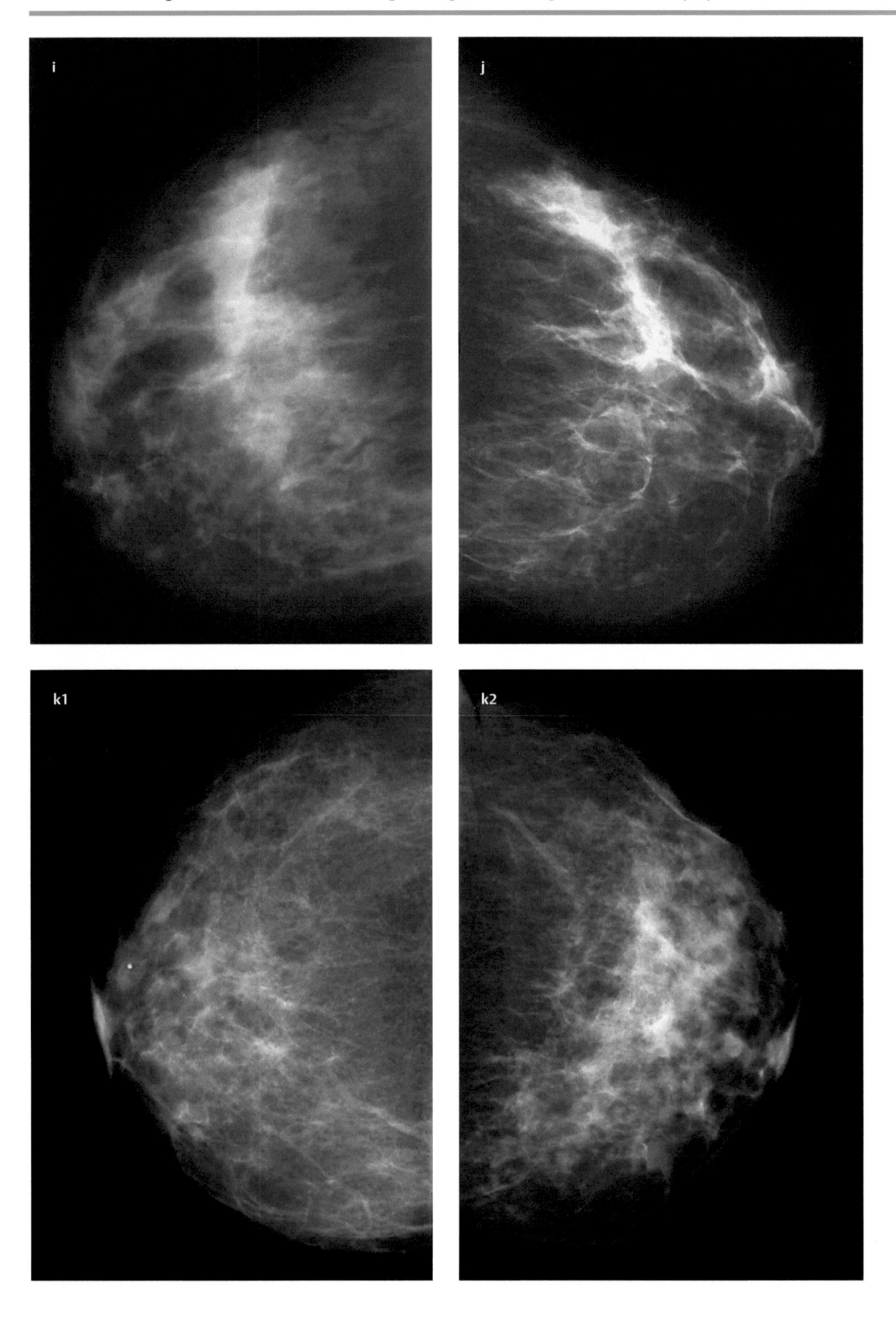

24 Additional Diagnostic Evaluation of Screening Findings and Solving of Problems in Symptomatic Patients

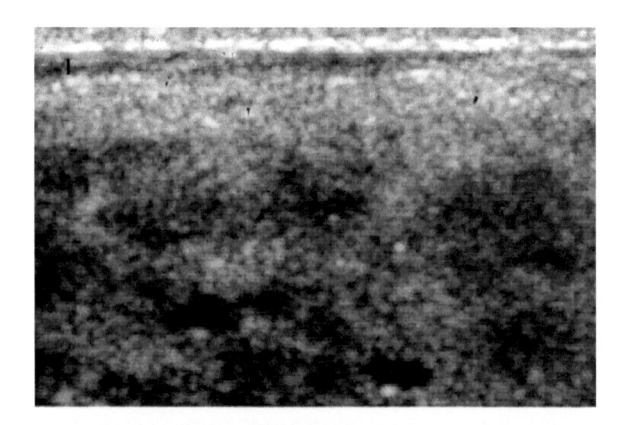

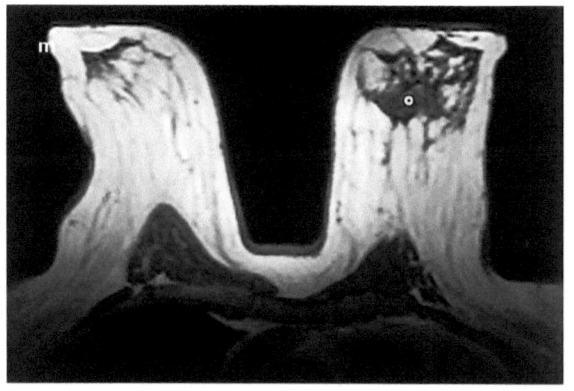

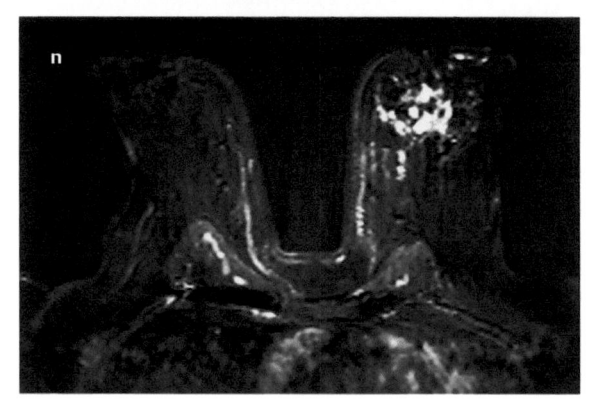

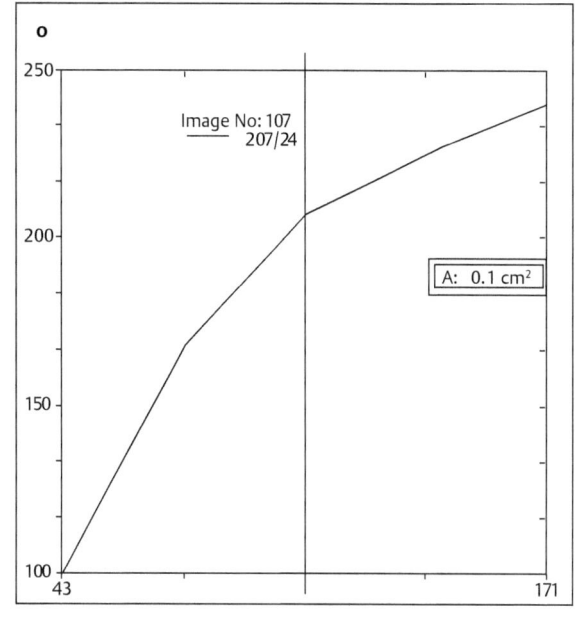

i, j The craniocaudal mammograms of a patient with a striking asymmetry are shown. The breast tissue on the right is denser and less distinct. *History*: Unilateral breast-feeding for 2 years.

k–l Patient with a striking mammographic and a mildly palpable asymmetry. Craniocaudal views show a striking mammographic asymmetry and no microcalcifications (**k**). Ultrasound showed dilated ducts, but was considered inconclusive (**l**).

m–o To determine the best area for percutaneous biopsy, an MRI was performed. A representative image before (**m**) intravenous application of Gd-DTPA is shown, as well as the subtraction image of the same slice (**n**) (= postcontrast minus precontrast).
Strong enhancement is seen which, however, exhibits a progressive enhancement curve (**o**). Even though enhancement is diffuse and delayed and therefore unspecific, malignancy may be suspected, particularly in view of the striking asymmetry of enhancement. *Histology* revealed a DCIS with micro-invasion. The latter may explain the unusually discrete clinical findings.

be remembered that diffusely growing carcinomas, such as lobular carcinomas or less common diffusely growing ductal invasive carcinomas, usually do not present as palpable focal lesions but as generalized rubbery, increased consistency or as a focal palpable ridge of tissue. Known asymmetry without a palpable abnormality supports a benign diagnosis. However, diffusely growing noncalcified DCIS may be a less common malignant cause of a developing or persisting asymmetry without significant palpable findings. Owing to the subtle clinical, mammographic, and sonographic changes it is probably not possible to reliably diagnose all noncalcified DCIS. And it may be unavoidable that sometimes even extended DCIS may be missed by state-of-the-art assessment using conventional imaging.

Sonography may be very valuable, as it may demonstrate benign cysts that can explain a mammographic asymmetry (justifying usual further screening). If ultrasound scanning reveals echogenic soft and mobile tissue, malignancy is improbable. Benign focal changes (that explain the asymmetry) can be biopsied under sonographic guidance or may be followed. Suspicious focal findings require histopathologic assessment, usually US-guided CNB.

Diffuse changes may occur in cases with diffuse malignancy or pronounced benign changes or in patients with chronic inflammatory changes (diffuse chronic or subacute specific or unspecific mastitis, see Chapter 13). Their distinction from malignancy may be quite difficult both clinically, by imaging, *and by histopathology*. Therefore, if percutaneous sampling of diffuse changes is attempted, special attention must be paid to adequate sampling (acquisition of multiple cores, adequate fanning of US-guided biopsy, representative VABB of the most suspicious area). Benign results require interdisciplinary discussion. Sometimes immunostaining may be helpful. Pre-interventional MRI may be helpful for choosing the area of the highest suspicion or (in combination with percutaneous breast biopsy) excluding malignancy in possibly benign findings. Excision of the suspicious asymmetric tissue will usually yield the most reliable diagnosis and may—in view of the difficult differential diagnosis and percutaneous histopathologic assessment—be worth considering, depending on the degree of suspicion after complete imaging evaluation.

Postmenopausal hormone replacement therapy (HRT) can produce a pronounced proliferation of the parenchyma, with formation of cysts, lumps, or renewed growth of fibroadenomas. This can accentuate known pre-existing asymmetries or lead to the formation of new solid masses or cysts. In many cases with mammographic asymmetry caused by HRT, the mammographic presentation will resemble the mammographic presentation before menopause. Therefore comparison with premenopausal films may be helpful.

If MRI is considered, HRT containing progesterone should be discontinued at 4–6 weeks before the scheduled MRI examination. MRI is able to correctly diagnose approximately 90% of diffusely growing invasive carcinomas and probably a significant proportion of the diffusely growing, noncalcified, high-grade DCIS. Owing to the possibility of false positive calls the role of MRI in the assessment of asymmetries is disputed. If malignancy is to be excluded in indeterminate asymmetric findings we recommend combining MRI and percutaneous breast biopsy.

The Mammographically Dense Breast

Dense tissue is encountered in a high percentage of patients under the age of 40 years (> 50%) and with decreasing frequency in patients over the age of 50 (30–50%) (see **Table 10.1**). Also, the proportion of women with dense tissue increases with the number HRT users. Furthermore, increased use of HRT is associated with significantly higher rates of false positive calls (mostly caused by newly developing or growing cysts or fibroadenomas) (see Chapter 10).

Diagnostic Questions

The problem of the mammographically dense breast is inherent in the inverse relationship between mammographic sensitivity in detecting carcinomas without microcalcifications and increasing radiographic density.

Dense Breast in Asymptomatic Patients without Increased Risk

Diagnostic Strategy and Goals

Screening the mammographically dense breast is worthwhile. Even in the very dense breast, microcalcifications can be reliably detected as important evidence of a carcinoma. Noncalcified carcinomas can become visible if they have induced retraction or parenchymal bulging, or if they are of increased density relative to the surrounding tissue, or located at the periphery of the cone of dense breast tissue.

Because of the more difficult detection of noncalcified carcinomas within mammographically dense tissue, mammography achieves a lower sensitivity, which may be as low as 50% in very dense breasts. In some screening programs, which include women below age 50, this disadvantage may partly be compensated by shorter screening intervals (1–1.5 years instead of bi-annual screening which is often used in women above age 50).

However, the sensitivity of digital mammography exceeds that of conventional mammography. Further improvements are expected from tomosynthesis, and its role in women with dense breasts is presently being investigated.

Owing to both the limited sensitivity of mammography in the dense breast and the higher incidence of breast cancer in dense and very dense breasts, the use of an additional screening method beyond mammography may be desirable and is currently being discussed.

Unfortunately, so far neither sonography nor contrast-enhanced MRI have proven suitable or been approved to replace or routinely complement mammography. Even though some interesting results have been presented by a few very experienced sonographers in preselected groups of patients, there exists no validation yet that would justify the general use of sonography for screening asymptomatic women at low risk. Sonography is time-consuming. A significant number of false positive results have to be expected. Due to its high operator dependence and problems of quality assurance, an acceptable relation of benefit (reproducible added detection) to risks and costs (false positives and added assessments) is not considered proven.

Contrast-enhanced MRI is not useful in this patient group either. Apart from the high costs, an unacceptably large number of false positive findings may be expected in asymptomatic patients at low risk. Also high-quality histopathologic assessment is not widely available or affordable for such high numbers of patients.

Even though the problem of the limited sensitivity of mammography in dense breasts is not yet solved, to date neither sonographic nor MRI screening of asymptomatic women appears justified. There is no international recommendation that supports sonographic or MRI screening (alone or as an adjunct to mammography) in asymptomatic women at low risk (see Chapter 23).

Dense Breast in Asymptomatic Patients with High or Intermediate Risk

Diagnostic Strategy and Goals

If the risk of developing a breast carcinoma is definitely increased because of a positive family history in close relatives or because of a history in a previous breast, an individually tailored surveillance strategy may be appropriate.

In the United States high risk is defined as a life-time risk greater than 20% of being affected by breast cancer; in Europe high risk is usually defined as a life-time risk greater than 30%.

In women at *high risk* for familial breast cancer intensified surveillance with yearly mammography (starting at age 30) and yearly MRI (age 25–55) is internationally recommended.

This recommendation is valid for all types of breast tissue. Beyond age 55, MRI may no longer be necessary due to the lower incidence of familial breast cancer beyond age 55 and due to decreasing breast density with age. According to international results the role of added ultrasound is questionable. (The additional use of ultrasound in these women is only recommended in Germany.)

Constellations with a more than 10% probability of being at high familial risk are summarized in **Table 1.2**. It is recommended that these patients undergo genetic counseling and in cases of high risk, intensified surveillance. Furthermore the above-mentioned scheme is also recommended for women who had been exposed to mantle field irradiation before age 30.

Even though this has not been separately investigated, similar surveillance schemes may be valuable for women at high risk due to combined personal and family history of breast cancer, who present with dense breast tissue.

There is no unique recommendation for women at *intermediate risk* (life-time risk of breast cancer ranging between 15% and 30%).

Usually, yearly mammography, starting at the age of 40 or 5 years before the age at which the youngest family member was affected, is recommended. Ultrasound may be used as a supplementary investigation in the case of diagnostic problems.

In patients at intermediate or low risk and with difficult-to-assess breast tissue the supplementary method of choice is sonography.

MRI has proven to be the most sensitive imaging modality—a fact which has been impressively proven for staging of preoperative patients (**Figs. 24.19 and 24.20**). In spite of this fact, for the average patient an improved outcome (fewer re-excisions or fewer recurrences) has not been proven so far (Sardanelli et al. 2010). Possibly, this might be due to the parallel effects of radiation therapy and adjuvant therapy, which may be able to eliminate many of the small, only MR-detected foci.

Other indications where (in dense breast tissue) MRI may be helpful include:
- Search for primary tumor in patients with dense breast tissue (a well-proven indication, see Chapter 5)
- Diagnostic problems that cannot be adequately solved by conventional imaging and percutaneous breast biopsy (see Chapter 5)

Palpable Findings in the Dense Breast

Diagnostic Problem

Numerous breast cancers are still detected as palpable findings. Some of these breast cancers occur in age groups that do not undergo screening (women below age 40 or 50, or beyond age 70–75). Other palpable breast cancers are detected in women who do not participate in screening. Interval cancers are mostly detected clinically and correspond to fast-growing cancers—for which the chosen screening interval may be too short—and to cancers which are mammographically occult and these missed at screening.

Even though clinical examination has by far the lowest sensitivity, no imaging method is capable of demonstrating all breast cancers and—in particular—so far no imaging method is capable of recognizing all cancers that are expected to occur within the subsequent one or two years (which are the usual screening intervals). While the vast majority of palpable breast cancers are visible by mammography or sonographically, or both, rarely palpable breast cancer is not shown by either method or may even be misdiagnosed by MRI. However, a small number of such cases exists (example: rare non-enhancing diffuse lobular breast cancer). Therefore diligent consideration and weighing of the suspicion is necessary for all cases with clinical abnormalities.

Clinical examination is the simplest method available. Its sensitivity for detecting early malignancy is limited. But a significant number of breast cancers is presently detected clinically and will continue to be so. Unfortunately, clinical changes (unless large) are also associated with a moderate specificity ranging around 20%.

To avoid unnecessary biopsy of clinical findings it is standard practice to diligently assess any clinical findings

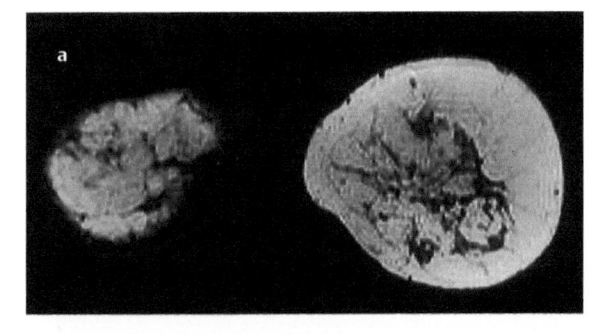

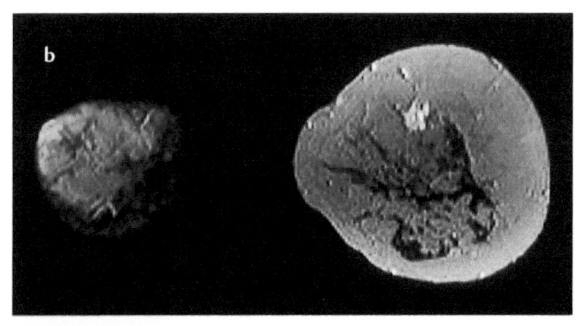

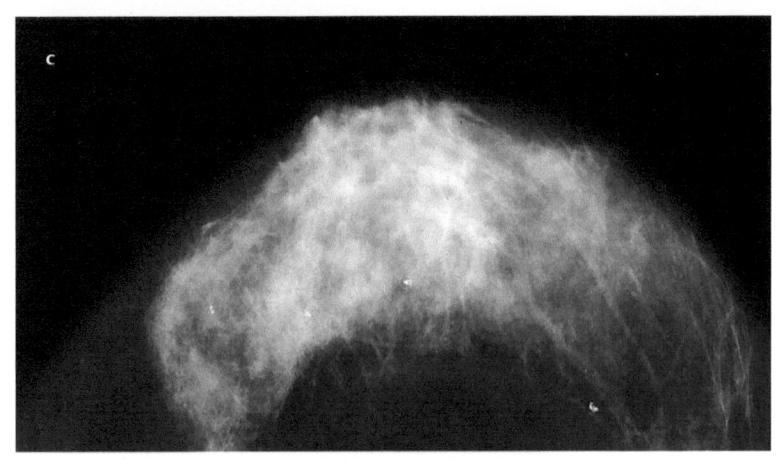

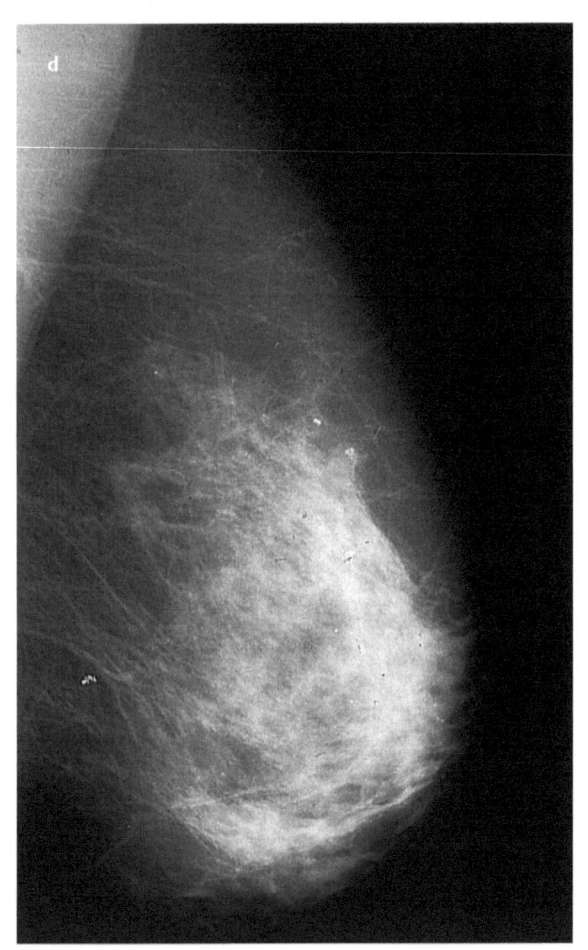

24 Additional Diagnostic Evaluation of Screening Findings and Solving of Problems in Symptomatic Patients

Fig. 24.19a–d Advantages of contrast-enhanced magnetic resonance imaging (MRI) for following the dense breast (increased risk). This patient is status after right breast carcinoma and underwent bilateral mammography. Because of an indeterminate finding in the irradiated right breast, contrast-enhanced MRI was performed, incidentally visualizing a suspicious finding in the left breast.

a Contrast-enhanced MRI before intravenous application of Gd-DTPA. This is the same slice as shown in (**b**). The section of the irradiated right breast is only partially imaged on this slice because of post-therapeutic volume loss and retraction toward the chest wall.
b After intravenous injection of contrast medium, an early irregularly outlined and thus suspicious enhancement is seen at the 12 o'clock position in the left breast.
c Craniocaudal mammography, left breast. *Histology*: 1-cm ductal carcinoma.
d Mediolateral view, left breast. Outside mammography, which was obtained without clinical suspicion, reveals no evidence of malignancy and would not have prompted any further investigation. Retrospectively reviewed, sonography revealed no focal finding. *Histology*: Ductal carcinoma.

Differential Diagnosis and Assessment

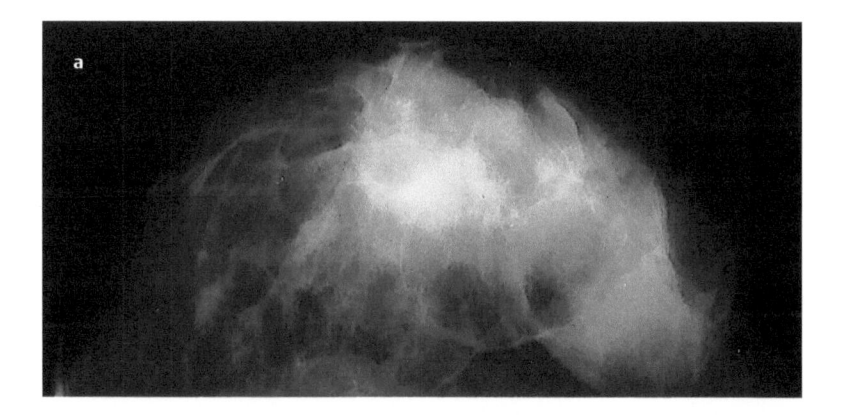

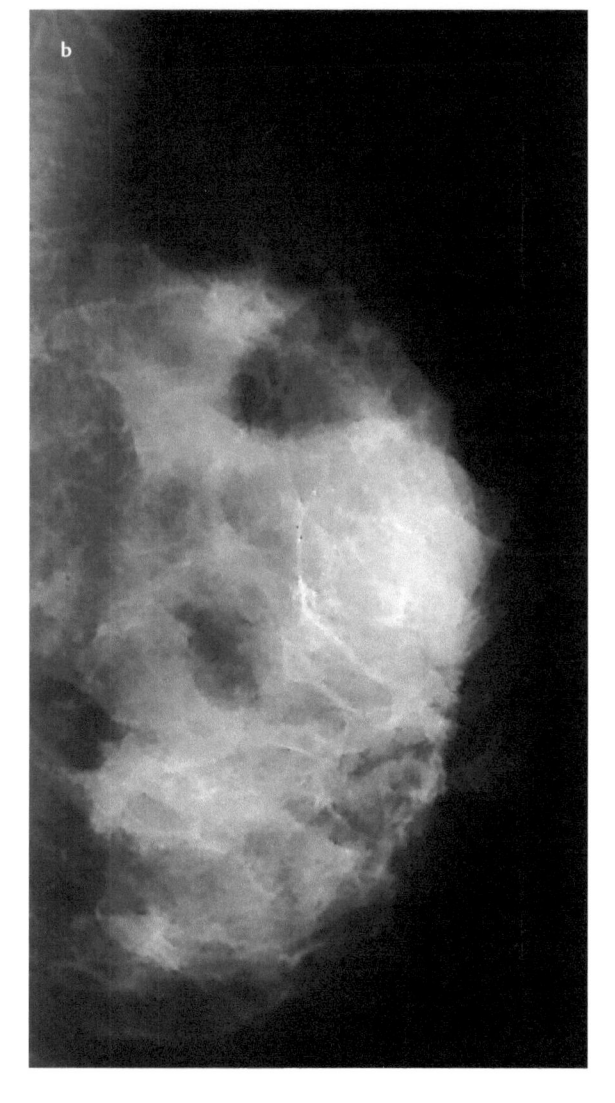

Fig. 24.20a–d Assessing the extent of and detecting additional foci in the mammographically dense breast. Patient with a suspicious palpable finding behind the nipple following excisional biopsy of a benign lesion 3 years ago. Although the area is sonographically hypoechoic and thus considered suspect, magnetic resonance imaging (MRI) was performed because of impaired evaluation of the surgically altered retroareolar region.

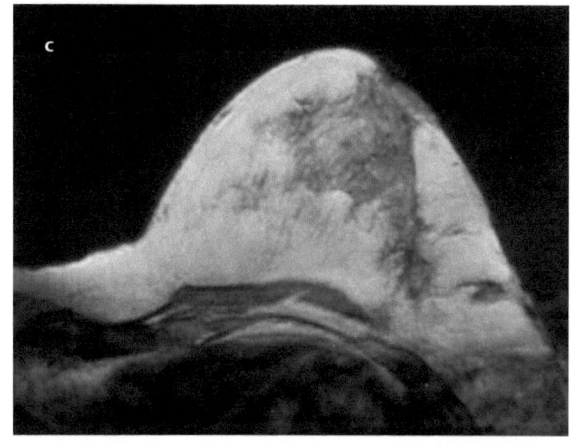

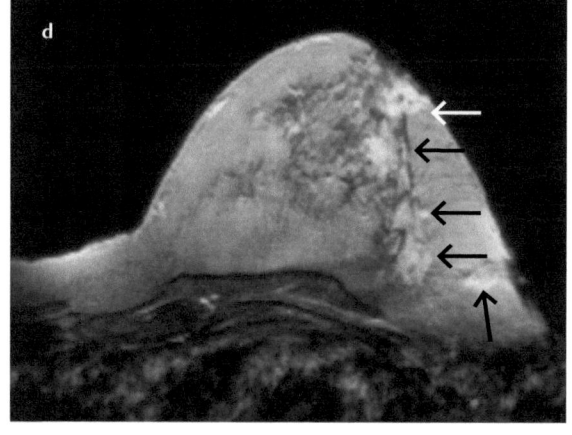

a,b Mammographic craniocaudal (**a**) and mediolateral oblique (**b**) views show very dense tissue with retraction due to scarring.
c MRI section at the level of the palpable finding in the region of the scar before administration of Gd-DTPA.
d The same level after Gd-DTPA shows highly suspicious enhancement in the palpable finding. Also visualized are several additional foci of suspicious enhancement, suspected neither clinically nor by any other method. *Histology*: Multifocal papillary carcinoma.

by imaging and—if needed—histopathologic assessment before further decisions are made.

Imaging evaluation of any palpable abnormality is recommended for several reasons:
- If malignancy can be excluded with high reliability, unnecessary interventions or surgery can be avoided.
- In case of a suspicious finding image-guided percutaneous breast biopsy has a higher accuracy than blind biopsy of palpable findings.
- Irrespective of the final diagnosis of the lesion in question, imaging evaluation is needed to exclude other important findings while pursuing the leading lesion, which itself might even turn out to be benign.

Diagnostic Strategy

Owing to the lower sensitivity of mammography in dense breast tissue and young patients, due to the higher prevalence of benign changes and the low prevalence of malignancy in younger women and because of the increased sensitivity of juvenile tissue to radiation, *it is recommended that the assessment of clinical findings begins with ultrasound in women below age 40. For women beyond age 40 state-of-the-art assessment usually starts with mammography* (Albert et al. 2009).

Mammography

Many palpable lesions may be characterized by *mammography*:
- Most breast cancers are seen as a mass, density, asymmetry, or architectural distortion with or without microcalcifications, or as an area of microcalcifications. Even in mammographically dense breasts, carcinomas are quite reliably diagnosed if they contain microcalcifications. Some may also be visible as an obvious mass, by an area of increased density, parenchymal asymmetry, or architectural distortion, or bulging of the parenchyma. Others may be diagnosed correctly by combining the mammographic and clinical information.
- Opaque skin markers may be placed over palpable lesions so they can be localized on the mammogram. Even unspecific mammographic abnormalities that might correspond to the clinical finding as well as any significant finding in other areas of the same or contralateral breast should undergo further state-of-the-art evaluation.
- If a palpable finding corresponds to a mammographic abnormality (rarely the case) that exhibits the pathognomonic features of a lipoma, calcified fibroadenoma, lymph node, galactocele, or oil cyst, mammography allows exclusion of a malignancy.
- While the sensitivity of mammography in fatty areas of the breast (provided exact correlation is warranted) approaches almost 100% and thus may also allow exclusion of malignancy, the sensitivity of mammography for detecting a carcinoma without microcalcifications decreases with increasing radiodensity of the tissue, and the sensitivity of mammography alone may be as low as 50% in breasts with ACR4 density.

> Except for the rare benign findings that are pathognomonic mammography cannot exclude malignancy in the presence of a questionable or definite palpable abnormality within breast tissue that is not equivalent to fat. In most cases ultrasound is able to ideally complement mammography within dense breast tissue or dense areas of breast tissue.

Sonography

Even though it is less reliable concerning the detection of *nonpalpable lesions*, ultrasound is able to visualize a high percentage (usually > 90%) of palpable lesions.
- Definitive demonstration of cysts can avoid unnecessary biopsy.
- Hypoechoic (and rare hyperechoic) focal lesions can be biopsied percutaneously under sonographic guidance. By documenting the correct position of the needle to the lesion sonographically, accuracy can be considerably improved in comparison with conventional puncture of palpable lesions without image guidance. Otherwise, small and deep-lying palpable lesions can be missed, as they may escape the advancing needle.
- Very easily moveable, smoothly outlined lesions with a pseudocapsule, homogeneous echo texture, and good distal enhancement are very suggestive of a fibroadenoma. In young patients without high risk and in patients with compatible (probably benign) clinical findings, short-term follow-up may be justified. However, in the event of any increase in size, of clinically indeterminate or suspicious findings, or in patients at increased risk, percutaneous breast biopsy may be preferable.

Thus, for all other hypoechoic findings that are not definitely benign based on clinical, mammographic or sonographic findings, biopsy should be considered (**Fig. 24.21**; see also **Fig. 16.13b**). As recommended in the European guidelines biopsy should be performed percutaneously whenever possible to avoid unnecessary surgery.

Percutaneous Biopsy

To warrant exact correlation, all palpable findings which are visible by ultrasound should be biopsied under sonographic guidance.

In the case of clinically probably benign findings (elastic and moveable tissue), absence of mammographically suspicious findings and sonographically homogeneous hyperechoic tissue, the probability of malignancy is very low and follow-up can mostly be justified. In cases of clinically suspicious findings, however, biopsy should be considered even in hyperechoic tissue without a definite lesion.

Differential Diagnosis and Assessment

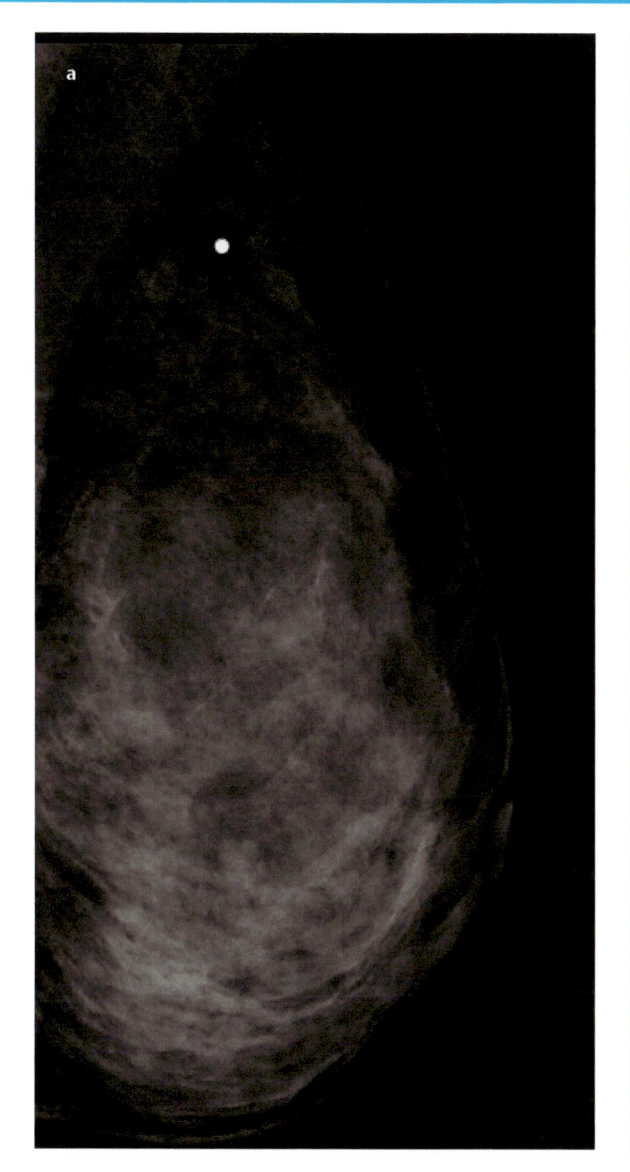

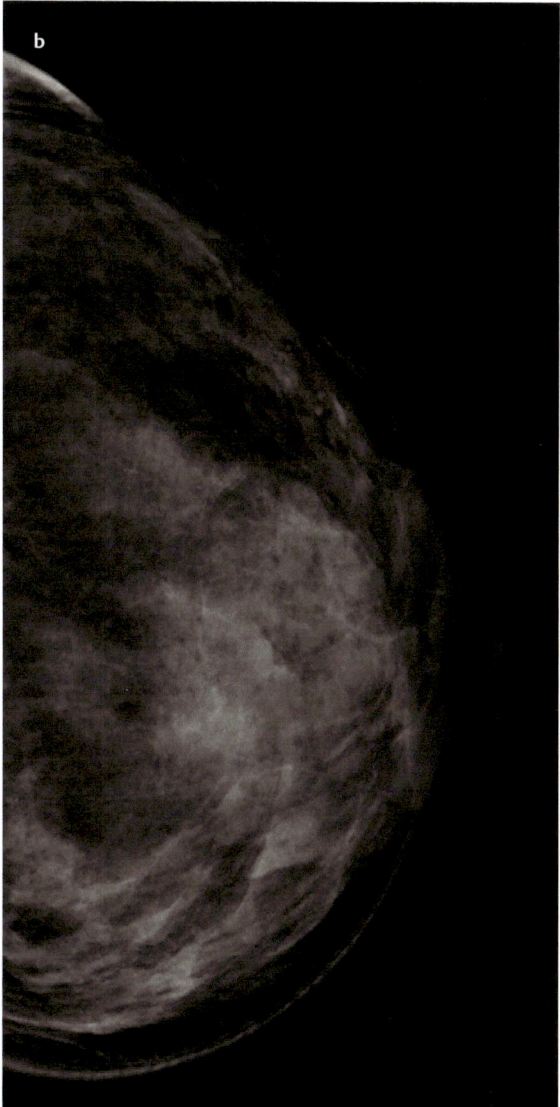

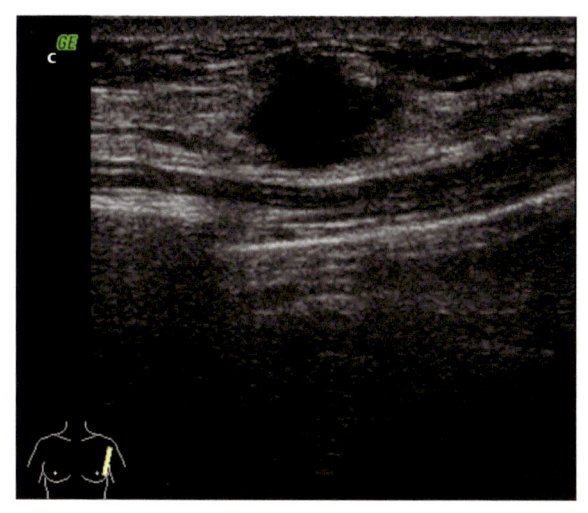

Fig. 24.21a–i Palpable findings in the dense breast.

a–c This 44-year-old patient noted a 1-cm palpable, hard but mobile mass in the axillary tail of her left breast. **a** The skin marker was placed to check that the lesion was included on the mammogram. As shown, the area of the palpable finding is included on the mediolateral oblique view. However, no mass could be delineated within the dense tissue (ACR3–4). No suspicious microcalcifications were noted. **b** The palpable finding is probably not included on the craniocaudal view (or is obscured by dense surrounding tissue). **c** On ultrasound (US) a hypoechoic ill-defined mass is seen. US-guided core needle biopsy (CNB) revealed a ductal invasive breast cancer G2.

Fig. 24.21 d–i ▷

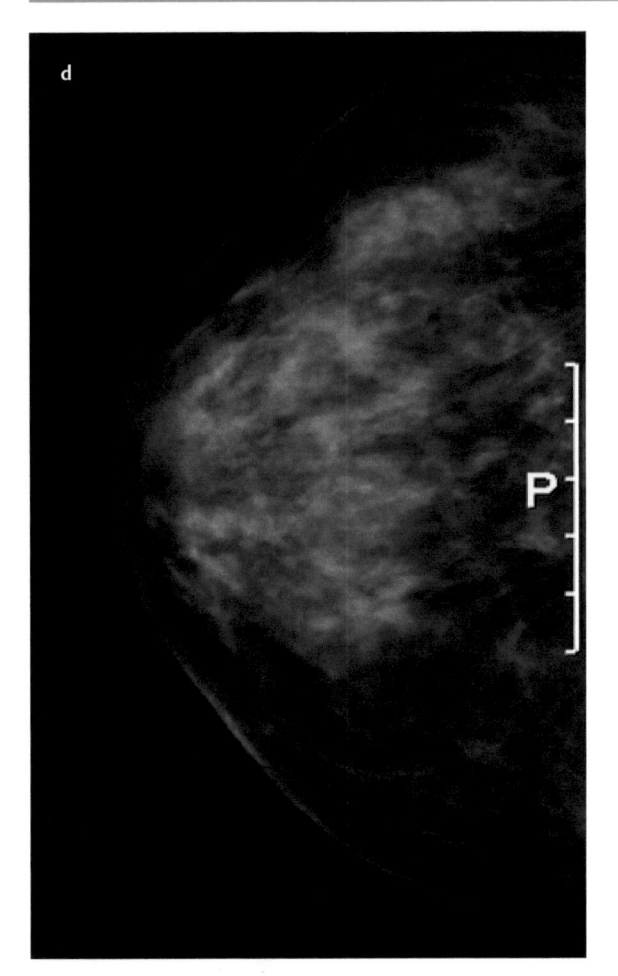

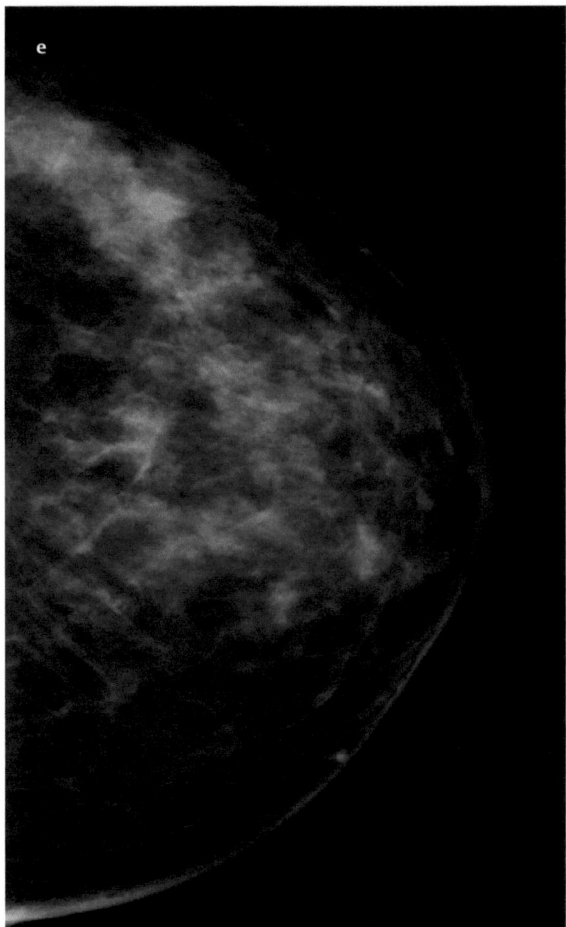

◁ continued

d–i This 47-year-old patient presented with a diffuse palpable thickening of her left upper outer quadrant but no distinct mass. Craniocaudal (**d,e**) and mediolateral oblique (**f,g**) views showed dense breast tissue (ACR3). Mammography confirmed some asymmetry. However, no microcalcifications, no mass, and no architectural distortion were seen.

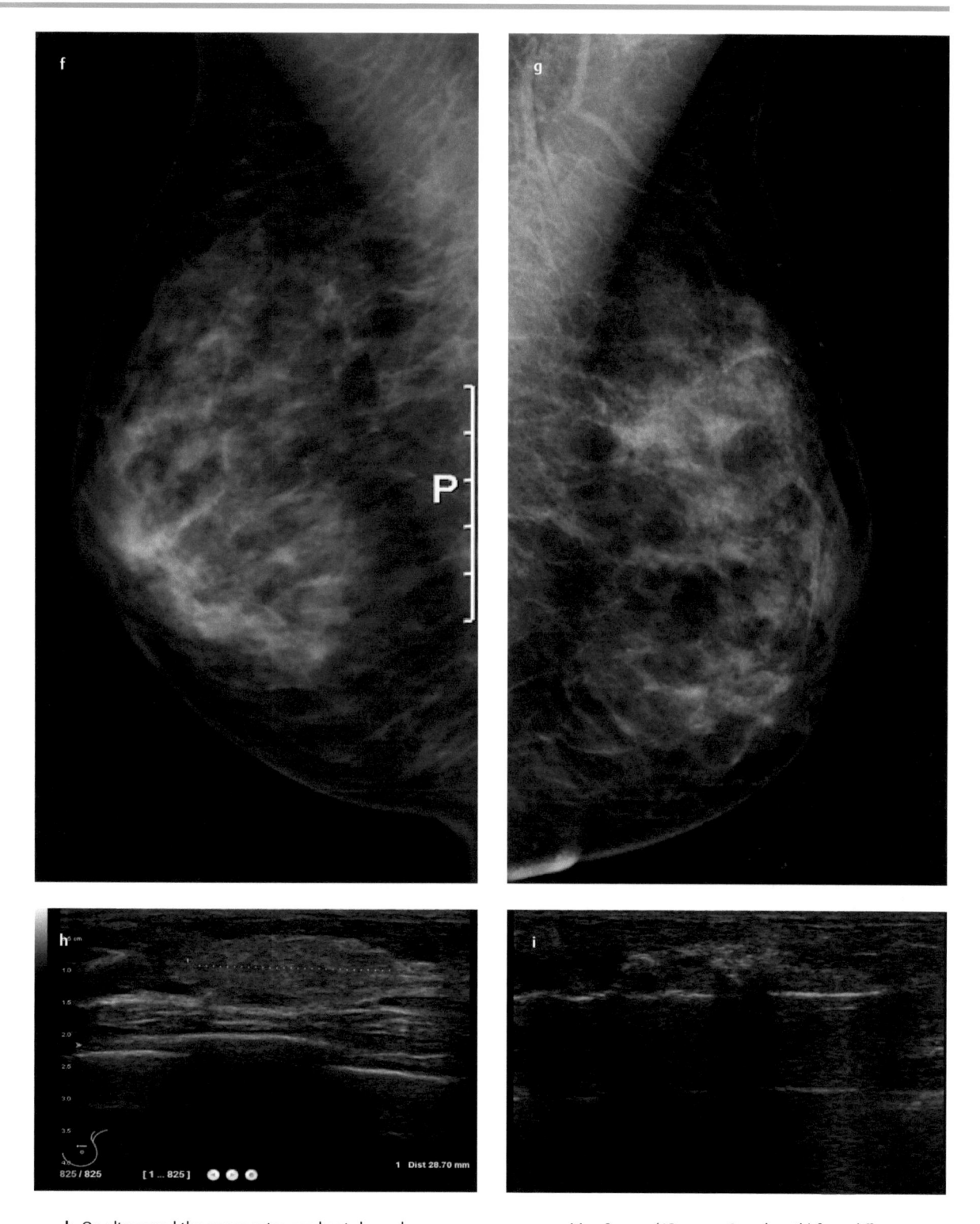

h On ultrasound the upper outer quadrant showed homogeneous echogenicity and decreased elasticity compared with the contralateral side. (In most cases such imaging findings are indicative of benign asymmetry.) **i** In this case percutaneous breast biopsy was performed based on the palpable asymmetry and because the patient had reported a change with time. Since the palpable finding corresponded to a diffuse thickening, US-guided CNB was performed by acquiring 8 cores (12 gauge, 2 cm length) from different areas (fanning). *Histology* revealed a lobular carcinoma.

This presentation is a rare presentation of a diffusely growing carcinoma. The case emphasizes the difficulties observed with diffusely growing malignancy and the importance of diligent assessment of any clinical finding in areas with nonfatty mammographic density and of findings which appear to change.

As mentioned before, the vast majority of palpable findings can and should be biopsied under sonographic guidance (usually US-guided CNB). If a palpable lesion is not visible by ultrasound, a guidance method should be chosen that demonstrates the lesion and can thus reliably countercheck sampling from the correct area.

Lesions visible by mammography should only therefore undergo stereotactically guided biopsy. If, rarely, a suspicious lesion (e.g., if detected incidentally by MRI when evaluating a clinical abnormality) is visible by MRI only, MR guidance will be necessary.

In patients with diffuse palpable abnormalities caution and critical analysis of representative biopsy is necessary in all cases for which percutaneous breast biopsy is considered or performed. While excision of the lesion will usually yield a reliable answer, it must be kept in mind that some of the entities, which may cause diffuse changes (diffusely growing lobular breast cancer or non-calcified DCIS), may exhibit a discontiguous growth pattern with only small nests of cells contained within the large palpable areas. Even if the area is sampled correctly, the cellular changes decisive for the correct histopathologic diagnosis may be missed using percutaneous breast biopsy. Therefore in critical cases additional evaluation by MRI, short-term follow-up or excision may need to be discussed. All cases with uncertain correlation of clinical findings, imaging and histopathology or discrepant findings should be discussed in a multidisciplinary conference. For further clarification additional imaging (MRI), short-term follow-up or preferably re-biopsy or excision should be considered as options.

For indeterminate or suspicious palpable findings with no imaging correlation we usually recommend considering excision instead of percutaneous breast biopsy, since monitoring of sampling from the correct area is not possible.

Contrast-Enhanced MRI

Although the combination of mammography and contrast-enhanced MRI is highly sensitive and detects even small carcinomas, the latter should not be considered the primary method to supplement mammography in the evaluation of a palpable finding. Apart from the costs, the reasons are the considerably higher false positive rate of contrast-enhanced MRI in comparison with percutaneous biopsy and the relatively high proportion of patients (~25%) with diffuse enhancement that may preclude a definitive diagnosis.

The use of contrast-enhanced MRI is appropriate in patients with:
- Extensive scars and unclear palpable findings (status, post surgery, implants, or radiation)
- Multiple questionable findings, in particular when the results of other modalities are contradictory—the pattern of enhancement can serve to find or select suspicious areas for a targeted percutaneous biopsy

Other Clinical Abnormalities

Pain

Pain, especially when it varies with the menstrual cycle, is a frequent manifestation of fibrocystic alteration. It is usually bilateral and more severe in the upper outer quadrants. If a thorough mammographic and clinical evaluation is negative, the patient should be informed of the probable hormonal cause and be reassured. In general, this pain is not a manifestation of a malignancy.

If the patient complains of localized pain, experienced as "crawling ants or a "creeping sensation and it appears essentially unrelated to the menstrual cycle, it should be taken seriously and deserves further evaluation, just like a palpable abnormality.

Search for Primary Tumor

In the woman with an axillary nodal metastasis and no palpable lesion in the breast to suggest a primary mammary carcinoma, clinical imaging in the usual order is indicated.

If mammography fails to identify the primary lesion in the breast, supplemental methods, such as sonography and, if negative, contrast-enhanced MRI can be helpful (see also Chapter 5, p. 168 and **Fig. 16.16**).

If contrast-enhanced MRI is negative or inconclusive because of diffuse enhancement, breast imaging has reached its limitation, or the primary tumor is not in the breast. (We are aware of only two published single cases, for which the question could then be answered by positron emission tomography. In one of these cases the quality of MRI was severely impaired.) In the majority of these rare cases, the primary tumor is indeed found in other organs and, consequently, searching for a primary tumor in other organs is appropriate in the presence of an axillary nodal metastasis. This also applies to adenocarcinomatous or even hormone receptor-positive metastases. (Depending on the method used for hormone receptor analysis, carcinomas of other origin, rarely even lymphomas, can be hormone receptor positive).

Nipple Retraction

Nipple retraction has to be evaluated carefully. Since unilateral nipple retraction may be caused by an underlying carcinoma, supplemental mammographic views (retroareolar spot views in two planes), sonography, and, if needed, contrast-enhanced MRI, should be employed. (**Fig. 24.22**; see also **Fig. 16.5a**).

The differential diagnosis of retroareolar malignancy mainly includes chronic inflammatory changes (or scarring), rarely a radial scar (or scarring papillary lesion), DCIS, or invasive carcinoma.

Differential Diagnosis and Assessment

Nipple retraction

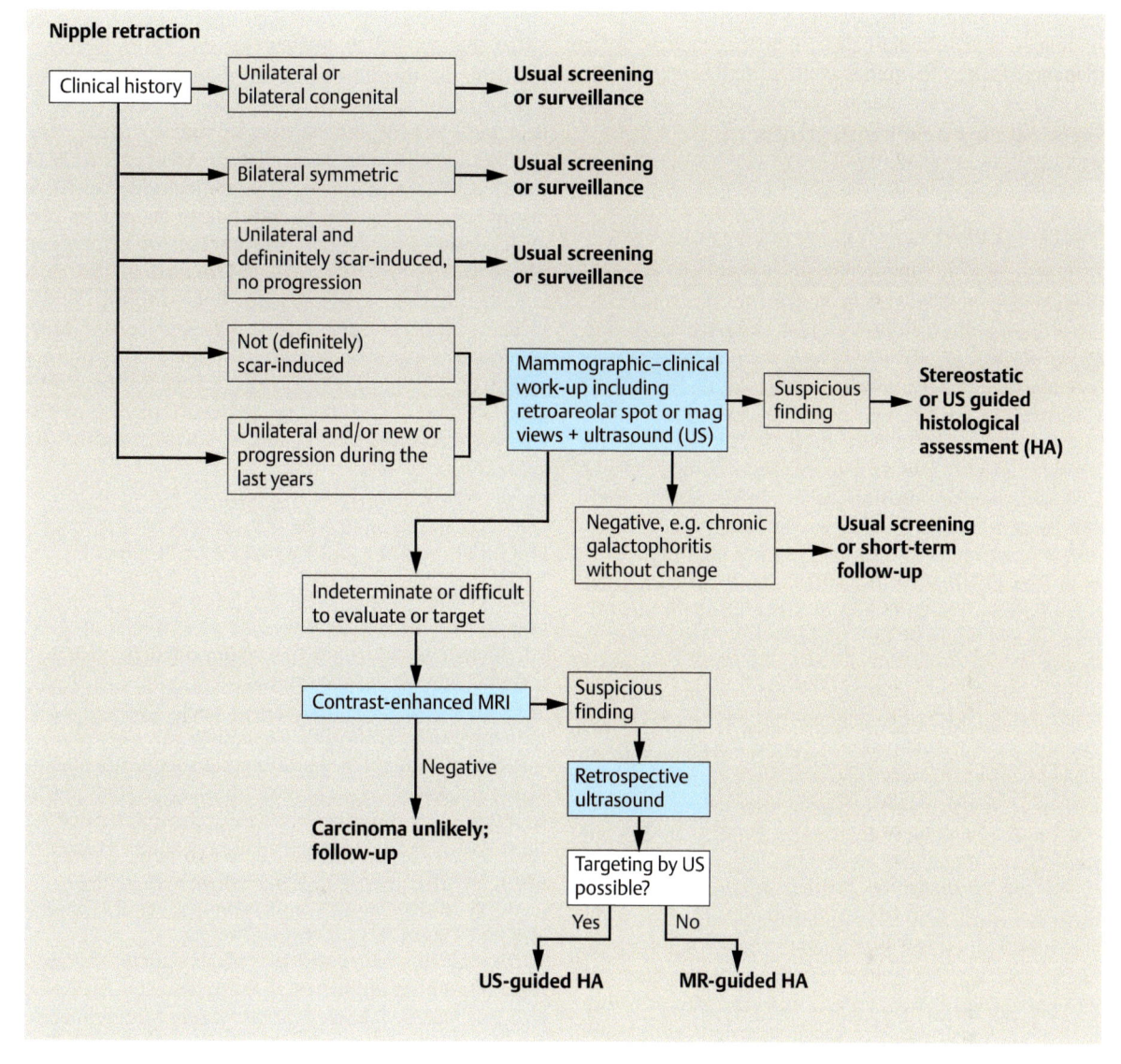

```
Clinical history
├─► Unilateral or bilateral congenital ──► Usual screening or surveillance
├─► Bilateral symmetric ──► Usual screening or surveillance
├─► Unilateral and definitively scar-induced, no progression ──► Usual screening or surveillance
├─► Not (definitely) scar-induced ─┐
└─► Unilateral and/or new or progression during the last years ─┤
                                   ▼
                    Mammographic–clinical work-up including retroareolar spot or mag views + ultrasound (US)
                          │
                          ├─► Suspicious finding ──► Stereostatic or US guided histological assessment (HA)
                          ├─► Negative, e.g. chronic galactophoritis without change ──► Usual screening or short-term follow-up
                          └─► Indeterminate or difficult to evaluate or target
                                   ▼
                            Contrast-enhanced MRI
                             │          │
                      Negative          Suspicious finding
                         │                  ▼
                         ▼            Retrospective ultrasound
               Carcinoma unlikely;         │
                 follow-up          Targeting by US possible?
                                     Yes ──► US-guided HA
                                     No ──► MR-guided HA
```

Fig. 24.22 Nipple retraction.

Microcalcifications

(See **Fig. 24.23**.)

Possibilities and Limitations of Diagnostic Methods

Mammography

Mammography is the only diagnostic method that can reliably detect calcifications suggestive of malignancy. Detecting calcifications is of great importance because about 30–40% of carcinomas harbor microcalcifications and because these carcinomas, because of the microcalcifications, are often discovered at a very early stage, frequently at a pre-invasive stage (DCIS). The problem, however, is that a considerable number of benign changes also contain microcalcifications. The indiscriminate excision of all microcalcifications would yield a carcinoma in only 1 of every 10–20 excisions. Such a high number of diagnostic biopsies can be justified neither medically nor economically. Therefore, the presence of microcalcifications should not invariably lead to a recommendation to biopsy.

In spite of the importance of detecting early breast cancer (preferably breast cancer in the pre-invasive stage) the question of overdiagnosis and unnecessary therapy associated with the detection of DCIS (or even B3 lesions) and the assessment of microcalcifications should be considered. Only a proportion of cases of DCIS (25–50%) (if untreated) are assumed to develop into invasive breast cancer, and in the individual case it will never be possible to predict which DCIS will turn into invasive breast cancer and which cancer will eventually threaten the patient's life. By and large, however, it must be acknowledged that low-grade DCIS and B3 lesions may be associated with invasive breast cancer in a much lower percentage and after much longer time spans (on average > 10 years) than DCIS grade 2–3. At the same time some invasive breast cancers may develop a new and grow fast and may thus represent a more important unpredictable threat. While DCIS grade 3 may become invasive in more than 50% of the cases within on average 5 years, around 80% of patients with DCIS grade 1 and B3 lesions may undergo therapy (with the associated side effects and psychological stress) with uncertain benefit to the patient.

In view of these problems aggressive detection of small (and very small) foci of low-grade DCIS or minor B3 lesions may not be associated with any significant benefit to the patient, while follow-up may detect significant changes, indicating the early development of invasive disease.

While detection of DCIS grade 3, early invasive cancer, and extended areas of DCIS (with the risk of extended invasion) remain of great importance, one should be aware that even DCIS grade 3 can only partly be recognized by the development of microcalcifications (some DCIS grade 3 are occult by imaging, others might be detectable by MRI—if it were performed).

Thus it will never be possible to detect all DCIS or invasive disease. In view of potential side effects an overly aggressive policy of detection of low-grade DCIS or B3 lesions should not be the goal of responsible diagnostics.

One should be aware that the finer and less characteristic the microcalcifications and the smaller the group, the lower the probability of malignancy or significant malignancy (grade 2–3 or invasive). Thus finding a sensible diagnostic threshold is an important task of the radiologist involved in screening, which in the future may gain even more importance.

Technical Requirements for Mammographic Detection and Differential Diagnosis of Microcalcifications

Correct exposure (a problem mainly associated with screen film–mammography) is particularly important since underexposure can render microcalcifications undetectable within dense tissue.

Compared with screen–film mammography digital mammography is further increasing the detection of microcalcifications. In dense breasts sometimes significant microcalcifications become visible by the new digital technique only. However, the rate of fine microcalcifications also increases and the specificity appears to drop—a fact which may also carry disadvantages (see above).

Adequate compression is mandatory since it improves sharpness and contrast (see pp. 52–54).

Magnification mammography yields a better morphologic evaluation and often the detection of additional fine calcifications. Thus, it improves the differentiation between calcifications judged to be benign or suspicious for malignancy, increases the identification of carcinomas, and helps to reduce the number of unnecessary biopsies. Moreover, determining the exact extent of the carcinoma may be decisively improved by magnification mammography.

Sonography

Because of its limited detection of DCIS owing to its inability to image microcalcifications, sonography does not provide any relevant diagnostic information to the differential diagnosis of microcalcifications.

Individual cases of microcalcifications with sonographic visualization of thickened ducts or of the larger microcalcifications are known, but this does not justify the conclusion that sonography can reliably diagnose microinvasive or carcinomas in situ.

Magnetic Resonance Imaging

MRI does not appear to be suitable for the differential diagnosis of small areas of microcalcifications.

The reason is that most proliferative changes associated with microcalcifications enhance with a pattern similar to that of carcinomas in situ with microcalcifications, and are therefore indistinguishable. Furthermore, it can be assumed that only 80–85% of carcinomas in situ show enhancement (which can be uncharacteristic, i.e., delayed or diffuse). However, if large areas of asymmetric uncharacteristic microcalcifications exist within dense breast tissue, MRI may be helpful, as focal, segmental, dendritic, or asymetric fast enhancement may correctly indicate the presence of malignancy.

Percutaneous Biopsy

Probably due to the discontiguous growth of DCIS, the accuracy of CNB is lower for the assessment of microcalcifications than that for masses. Therefore, if core needle biopsy is used for assessment of microcalcifications, diligent correlation between imaging and histopathology is critical. A negative core biopsy or fine needle biopsy cannot exclude malignancy or replace surgical biopsy. Based on its proven higher sensitivity and its usually good tolerance and limited side effects, VABB is generally considered the method of choice for the histopathologic assessment of microcalcifications. Open biopsy after wire localization is recommended in indeterminate cases, if vacuum biopsy is not available or appropriate (depending on the lesion type or location, or on patient factors).

- Mammography is the method of choice for the detection and differential diagnosis of microcalcifications.
- Meticulous analysis of mammographically visualized microcalcifications is the prerequisite for accurate detection of up to 50% of early breast cancers and avoiding high numbers of unnecessary biopsies or inadequate overdiagnosis.

Analysis of Microcalcifications

The goal of analyzing calcifications is to categorize them as:
- Definitely benign, versus
- Indeterminate or suspicious of malignancy

Principal Considerations

Systematic investigations have shown that typically malignant microcalcifications arise almost exclusively in invasive and noninvasive ductal carcinomas, while lobular carcinomas calcify only very rarely and fail to develop a mammographically typical calcification pattern.

Since DCIS grows along the ductal system it is understandable that segmental or ductal distribution is one of the most important potential indicators of malignancy. This also explains the high positive predictive value of so-called "casting-type" microcalcifications. These microcalcifications typically occur in comedo-type DCIS (grade 2 or 3) or comedo-type invasive ductal carcinoma. They correspond to casts (consisting of abundant necrotic malignant cells which are produced by the DCIS in small lactiferous ducts), which calcify. Casting-type microcalcifications are often fragmented and may assume V or Y shapes.

Another typical shape of suspicious microcalcifications corresponding to central ductal necrosis in DCIS grade 2–3 and comedo-type invasive ductal carcinoma concerns coarse granular and so-called pleomorphic microcalcifications. These microcalcifications are very variable in size, shape, and density and have been described as resembling crushed stone. The individual calcification within a group can be extremely irregular, sometimes even bizarre in shape and ranges from fine to 2 mm in size.

In contrast, the probability of malignancy decreases with rounded groups (lobular pattern), diffuse spread, and very fine microcalcifications. For these shapes and distribution patterns a significant overlap with benign changes exists.

However, experience has shown that developing or increasing microcalcifications (even if fine) and ductal or segmental distribution (even of uncharacteristic microcalcifications) is associated with a higher rate of malignancy and therefore should be assessed more aggressively.

Finally, there are certain morphologies and distribution patterns which may clearly indicate a certain (mostly benign) entity (so-called special types) and some patterns supporting the diagnosis of benign disease in the absence of other suspicious findings ("teacup" calcifications, symmetric distribution, etc.).

Overall, calcifications are analyzed as to:
- Their location (malignant calcifications are implicitly intramammary),
- Their individual shapes, and
- Their distribution pattern

Fig. 24.23 shows our algorithm for assessing microcalcifications. Following this algorithm we first "check" for "special" types (of characteristically benign calcifications); next we check for signs which might indicate the presence of malignancy and thus require histopathologic assessment; finally the remaining calcifications are checked concerning features supporting a benign diagnosis.

24 Additional Diagnostic Evaluation of Screening Findings and Solving of Problems in Symptomatic Patients

A. Check for "special types" (typical benign calcifications)

1. Localization
- Unequivocal intracutaneous (extramammary) → Benign usual screening
- Possibly intracutaneous (some ringlike calcifications, round grouping, possible location in scar) → Uncertain → Tangential view or marked views or stereotaxy or tomosynthesis → Intracutaneous → Benign usual screening
- Intraparenchymal: No / Yes

2. Individual shape: coarse smooth elongated ("needles") — Yes → Such calcifications (being intra and periductal) follow the ductal system (and may even have a central lucency); coarse v or y shapes are acceptable → Benign secretory disease usual screening

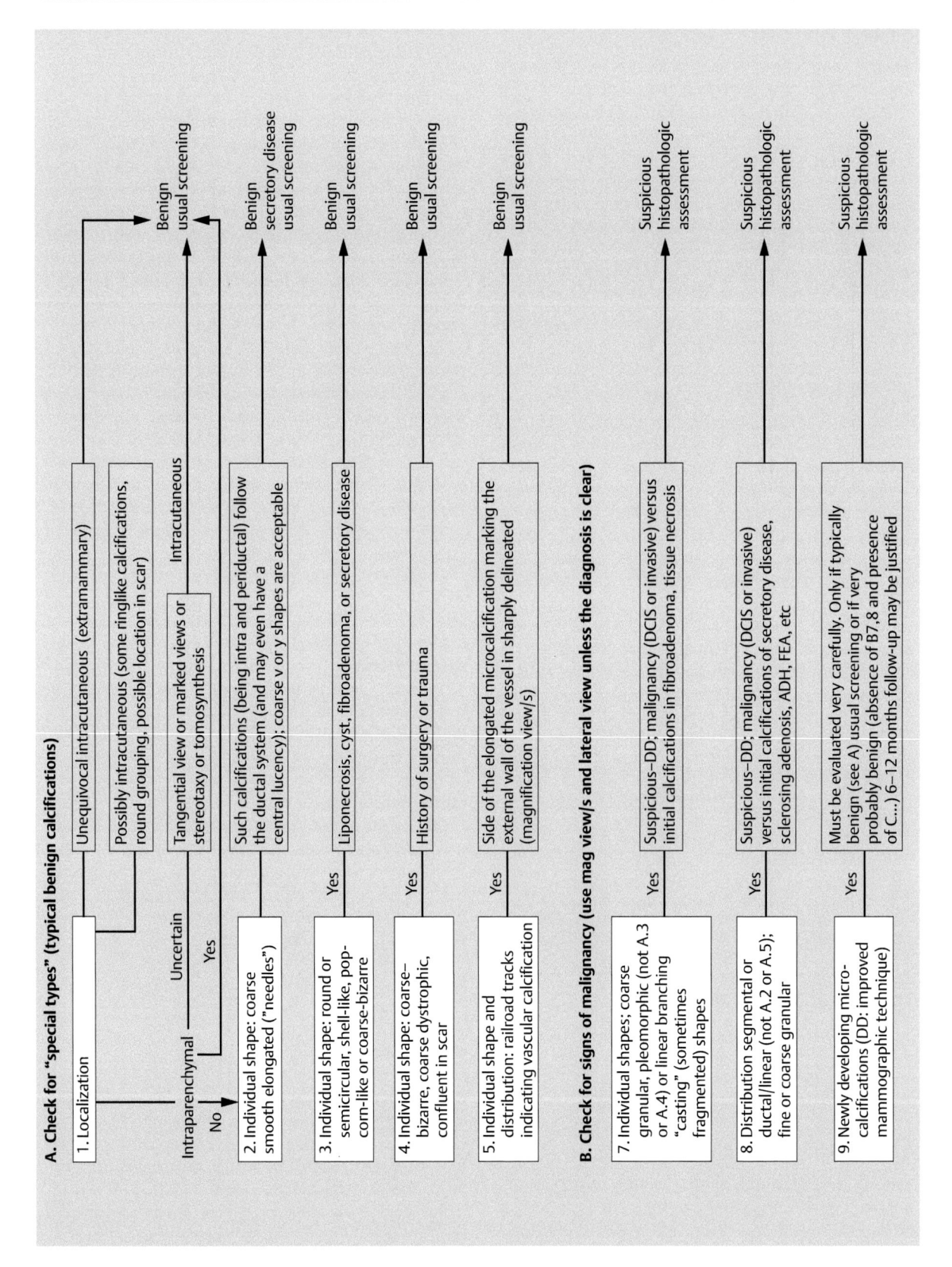

3. Individual shape: round or semicircular, shell-like, popcorn-like or coarse-bizarre — Yes → Liponecrosis, cyst, fibroadenoma, or secretory disease → Benign usual screening

4. Individual shape: coarse-bizarre, coarse dystrophic, confluent in scar — Yes → History of surgery or trauma → Benign usual screening

5. Individual shape and distribution: railroad tracks indicating vascular calcification — Yes → Side of the elongated microcalcification marking the external wall of the vessel in sharply delineated (magnification view/s) → Benign usual screening

B. Check for signs of malignancy (use mag view/s and lateral view unless the diagnosis is clear)

7. Individual shapes; coarse granular, pleomorphic (not A.3 or A.4) or linear branching "casting" (sometimes fragmented) shapes — Yes → Suspicious–DD; malignancy (DCIS or invasive) versus initial calcifications in fibroadenoma, tissue necrosis → Suspicious histopathologic assessment

8. Distribution segmental or ductal/linear (not A.2 or A.5); fine or coarse granular — Yes → Suspicious–DD; malignancy (DCIS or invasive) versus initial calcifications of secretory disease, sclerosing adenosis, ADH, FEA, etc → Suspicious histopathologic assessment

9. Newly developing microcalcifications (DD: improved mammographic technique) — Yes → Must be evaluated very carefully. Only if typically benign (see A) usual screening or if very probably benign (absence of B7,8 and presence of C...) 6–12 months follow-up may be justified → Suspicious histopathologic assessment

Fig. 24.23 Microcalcifications.

Differential Diagnosis and Assessment

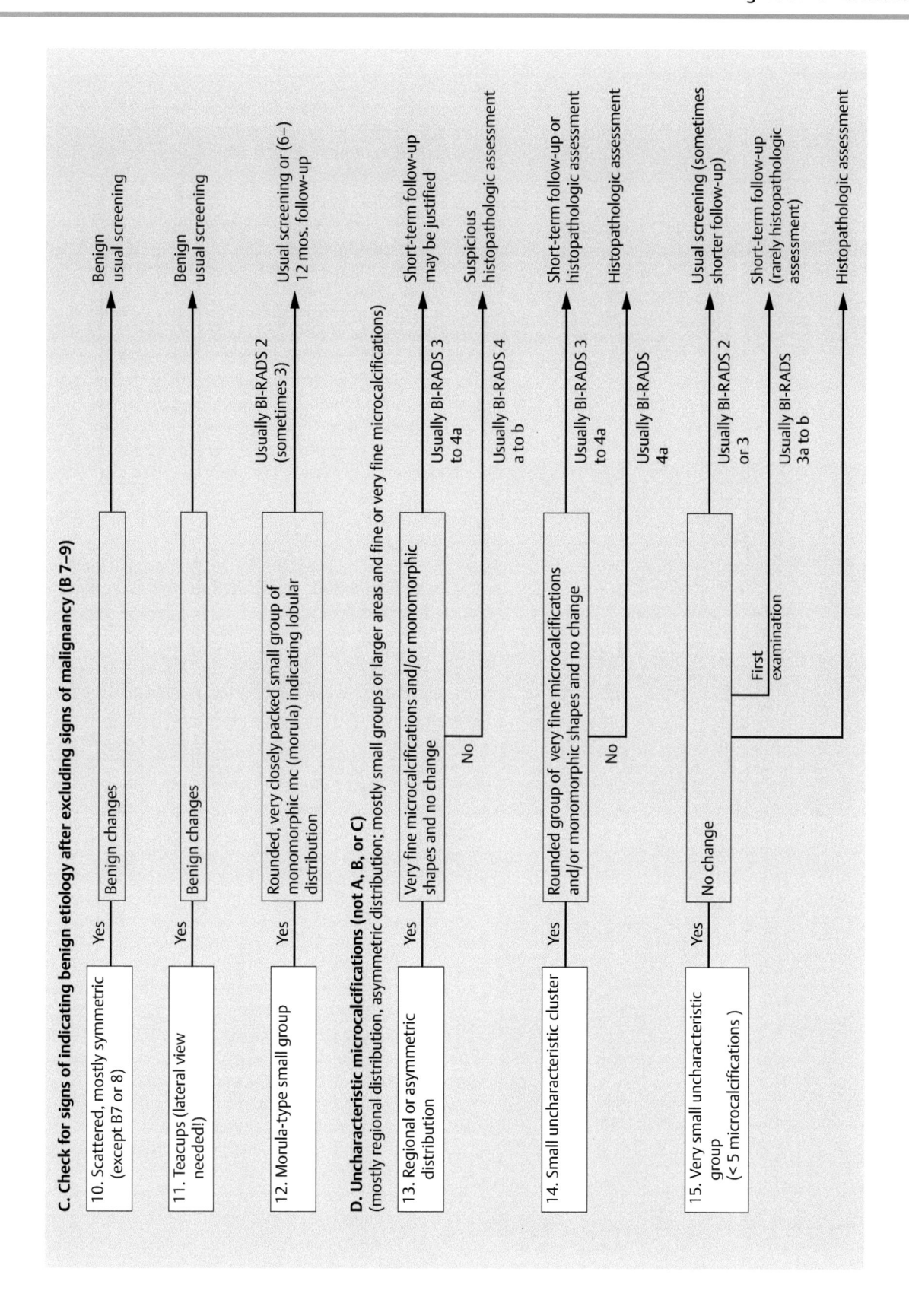

C. Check for signs of indicating benign etiology after excluding signs of malignancy (B 7–9)

Item	Yes →	Recommendation
10. Scattered, mostly symmetric (except B7 or 8)	Benign changes	Benign usual screening
11. Teacups (lateral view needed!)	Benign changes	Benign usual screening
12. Morula-type small group	Rounded, very closely packed small group of monomorphic mc (morula) indicating lobular distribution	Usually BI-RADS 2 (sometimes 3) → Usual screening or (6–) 12 mos. follow-up

D. Uncharacteristic microcalcifications (not A, B, or C)
(mostly regional distribution, asymmetric distribution; mostly small groups or larger areas and fine or very fine microcalcifications)

Item	Yes →	Sub-criterion	Recommendation
13. Regional or asymmetric distribution	Very fine microcalcifications and/or monomorphic shapes and no change	—	Usually BI-RADS 3 to 4a → Short-term follow-up may be justified
		No →	Usually BI-RADS 4 a to b → Suspicious histopathologic assessment
14. Small uncharacteristic cluster	Rounded group of very fine microcalcifications and/or monomorphic shapes and no change	—	Usually BI-RADS 3 to 4a → Short-term follow-up or histopathologic assessment
		No →	Usually BI-RADS 4a → Histopathologic assessment
15. Very small uncharacteristic group (< 5 microcalcifications)	No change	—	Usually BI-RADS 2 or 3 → Usual screening (sometimes shorter follow-up)
		First examination	Usually BI-RADS 3a to b → Short-term follow-up (rarely histopathologic assessment)
			Histopathologic assessment

645

Extramammary Location and Special Types Indicating Benign Calcifications

Artifacts

Artifacts mimicking microcalcifications may be caused by defects or dust on the image receiver or film; they may be caused by film development or by powder or ointment on the skin. The last (**Fig. 24.24**) usually produce characteristic, punctate, or streaky calcific densities arranged along dermal lines. Recognizing such structures is generally not problematic. The same applies to artifacts on the intensifying screen caused by fingerprints, dust, and defects of the screen (**Fig. 24.25**). Furthermore, dotlike or linear artifacts can be imprinted on the film by the rolls in the automatic processor.

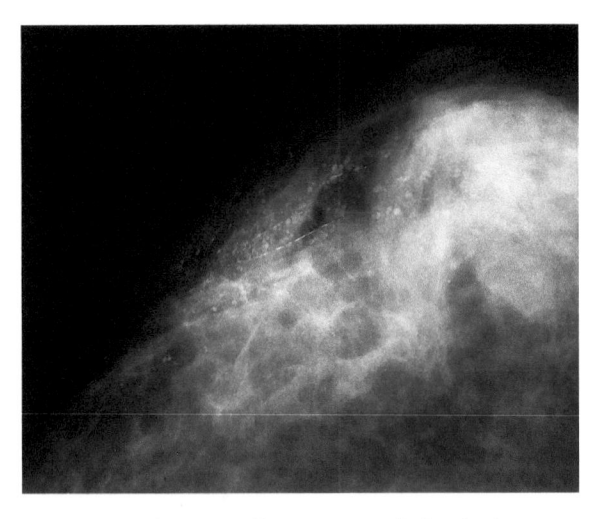

Fig. 24.24 Artifacts caused by ointment applied to the skin.

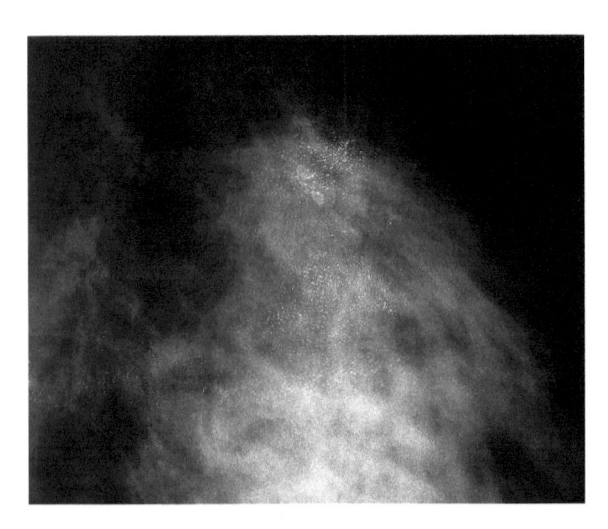

Fig. 24.25 Artifact of the intensifying screen: Fingerprint.

Extramammary Benign Calcifications

Calcifications located outside the breast parenchyma—that is, intracutaneous calcifications—are usually benign (unless, rarely, such calcifications are associated with a suspicious skin abnormality which, however, would be obvious at inspection).

Most dermal calcifications are in the sebaceous glands of the skin. They are round, usually ringlike, sometimes dumb-bell–like, and correspond to the size of skin pores (**Fig. 24.26**). They are often found in the dermis of the inner half of the breast.

In general, dermal calcifications can be easily diagnosed on the basis of their location and configuration. If they appear in groups, the diagnosis might be questioned, in particular when their round and ringlike contours are not clearly discernible. If a cutaneous origin (which could prove their benignity) is suspected, either views with skin markers or a tangential view may be obtained for clarification (**Fig. 24.26b,c**) (p. 640). Unless recognized by the usual imaging assessment and the above measures, dermal location may also be proven by a stereotactic calculation.

Special Types Indicating Benign Intramammary Calcifications

(See **Figs. 24.27, 24.28, 24.29, 24.30, 24.31, 24.32, 24.33**.) *Coarse, needlelike calcifications* are typical of chronic secretory disease (so-called plasma cell mastitis). Like ductal calcifications, they follow the ductal system. Histologically, they are intraductal and periductal. Despite a ductal or segmental, V-shaped and Y-shaped arrangement, they can be clearly identified as benign as long as they are large, coarse, and smooth. A central radiolucency within the needles or a combination with round, coarse calcifications with or without radiolucency is considered definitive proof. Caution is advised when evaluating needlelike, fine and fragmented calcifications since in these cases the differentiation between a primary ductal carcinoma and "plasma cell mastitis" can be difficult (**Figs. 24.34 and 24.35**).

Other elongated (mostly curved) calcifications may occur in scars and correspond to suture calcifications. They can be unequivocally diagnosed as benign if their curves clearly indicated the shape of sutures. Calcified worms (filiariasis) may also be a rare cause of coarse elongated calcifications. Even though these calcifications may be quite typical, they are extremely rare.

Large (> 1 mm), rounded calcifications with or without central radiolucency can develop in scars or fat necroses (subcutaneous without trauma, usually bilateral with calcifying liponecrosis), "plasma cell mastitis," and calcified fibroadenomas or papillomas (whereby the soft tissue density may or may not be visible). They are invariably benign.

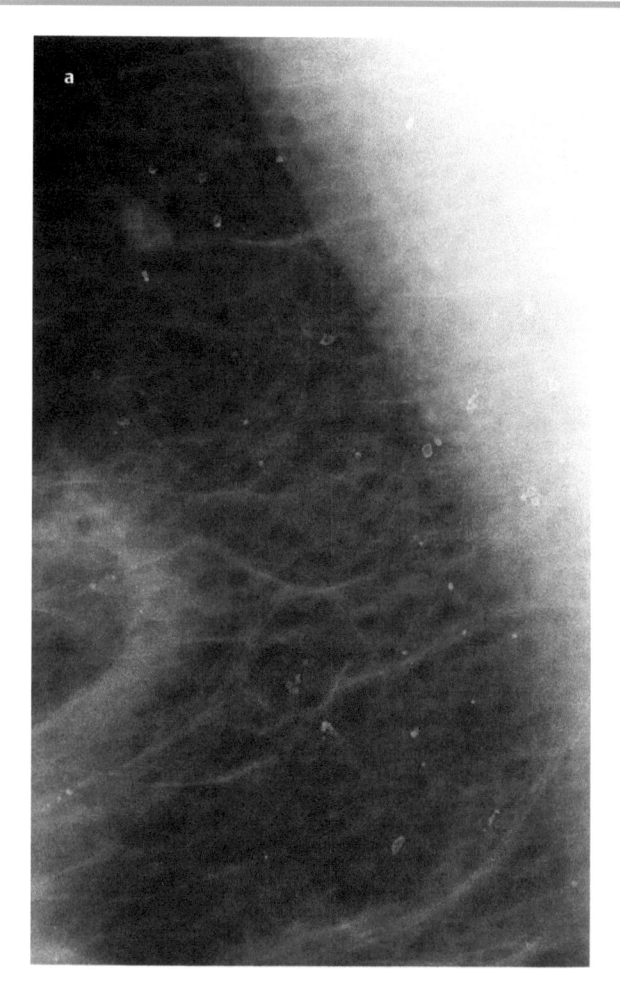

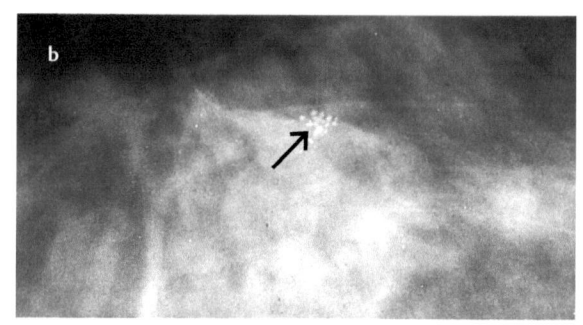

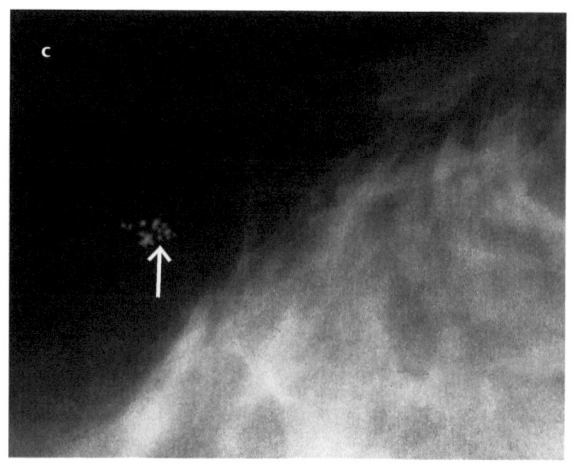

Differential Diagnosis and Assessment

Fig. 24.26a–c
a Punctate and ringlike calcifications projecting diffusely throughout the entire breast. Several of the calcifications can clearly be assigned to skin pores. The finding corresponds to calcifications in the sebaceous glands.
b The craniocaudal view shows several round calcifications close together in the retroareolar region (arrow).
c These calcifications are projected over the subcutaneous region (arrow) in the tangential view.

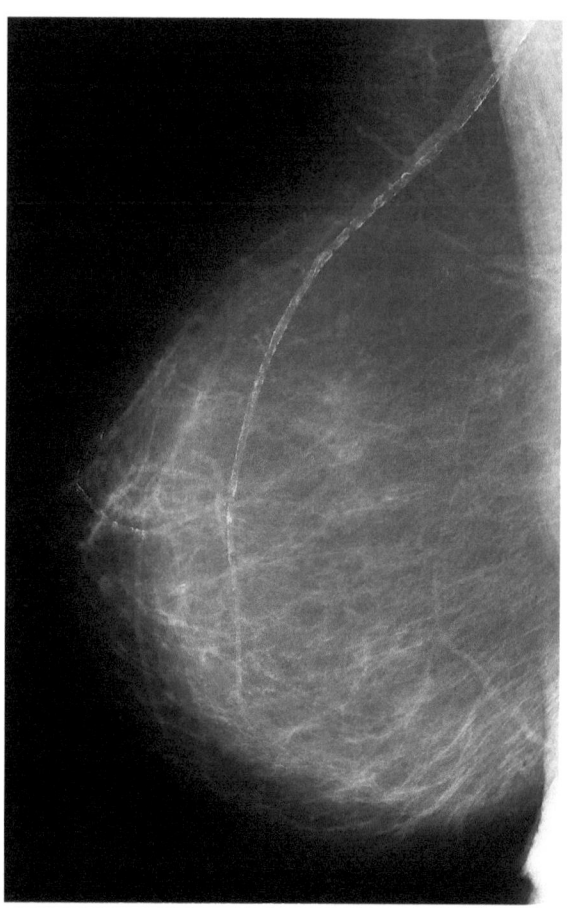

Fig. 24.27 Linear and round calcifications directly following a narrow, vascular structure: Arteriosclerosis.

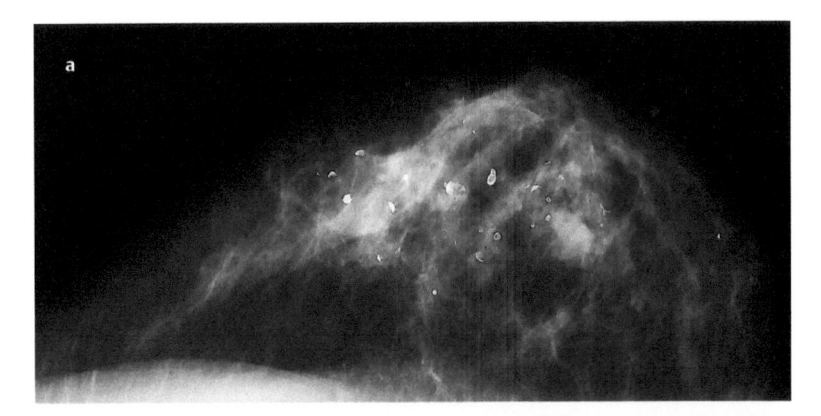

Fig. 24.28a–c

a Multiple elongated, curved, crescentic, and ringlike calcifications following recurrent mastitis with abscess incision and drainage.
b Almost symmetrically arranged "idiopathic" calcifying liponecrosis without known preceding trauma.
c Large calcified fat necrosis following breast augmentation with transplanted autogenous adipose tissue (mediolateral views).

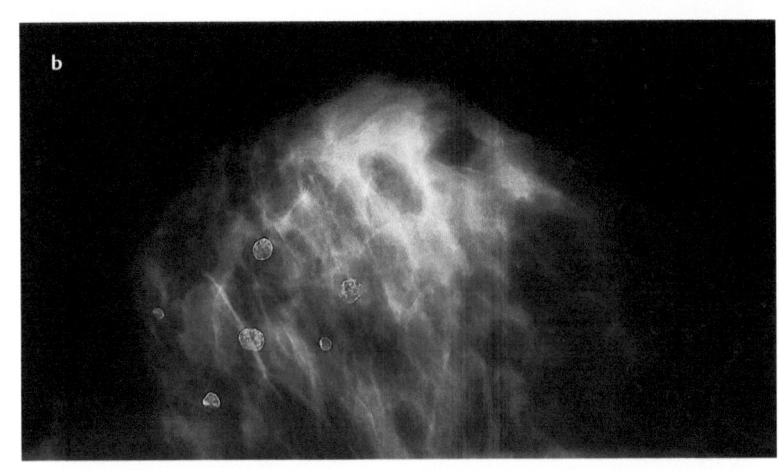

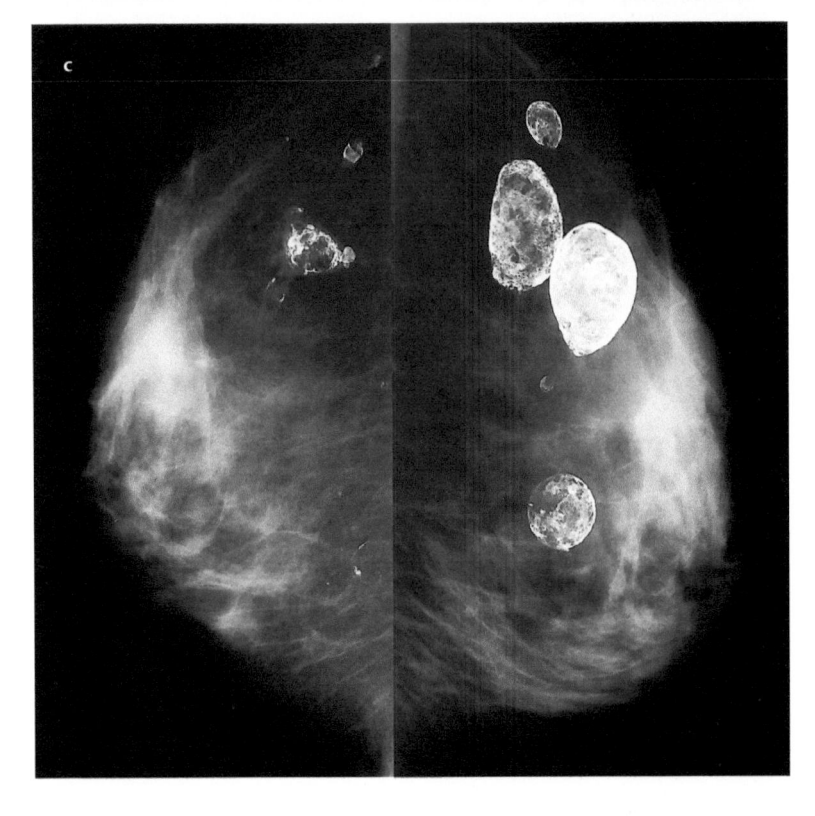

Differential Diagnosis and Assessment

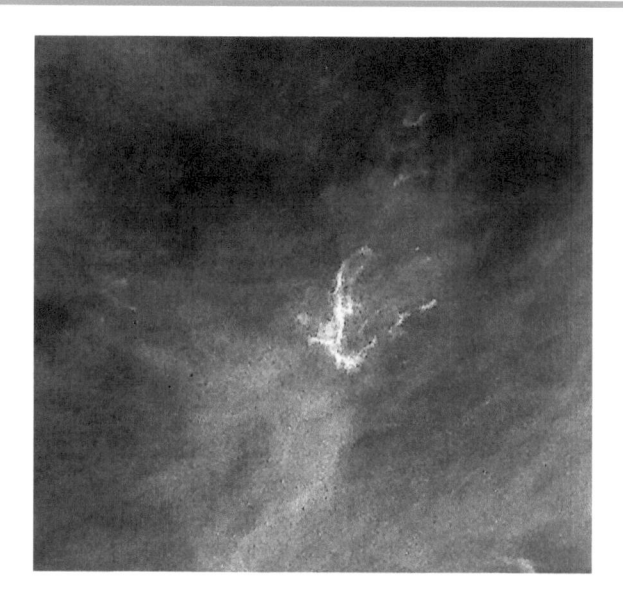

Fig. 24.29 Elongated, in part linear, dystrophic calcifications within scar-induced architectural distortion.

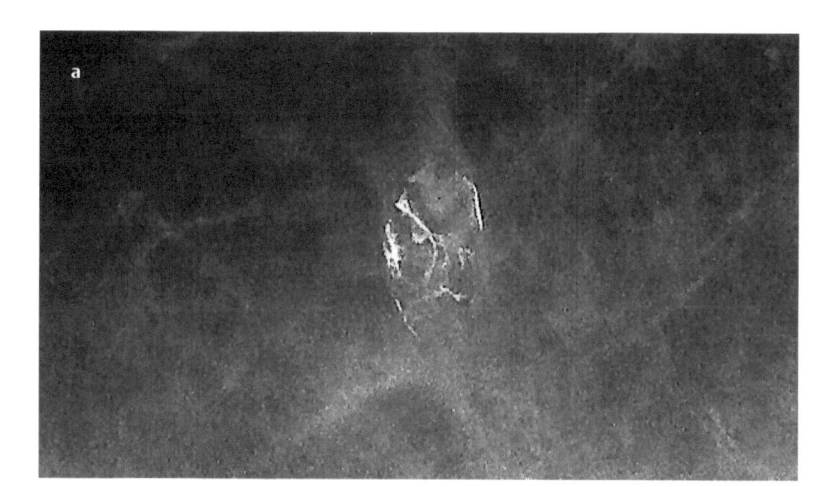

Fig. 24.30a,b
a Fine eggshell-like calcifications projected over an oval radiolucency: Calcifying oil cyst.
b Subtle shell-like (in part, punctate) calcifications around droplike deposits of wax, injected for augmentation.

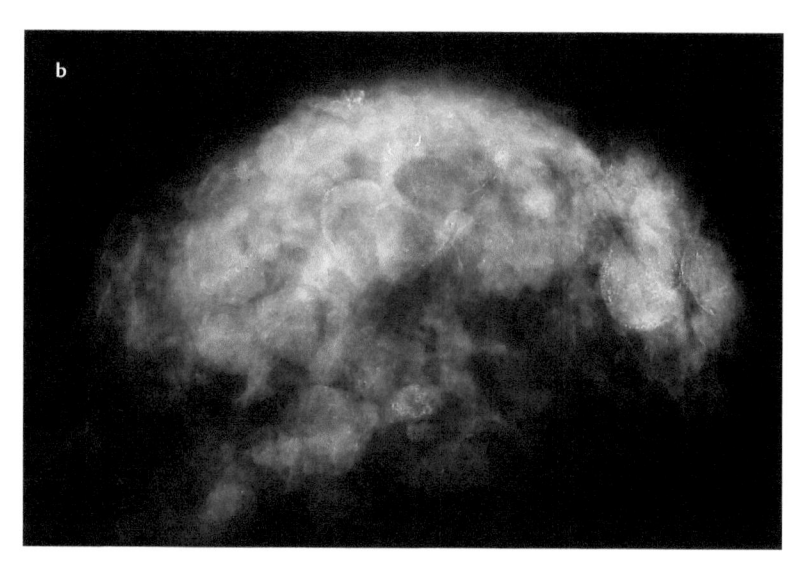

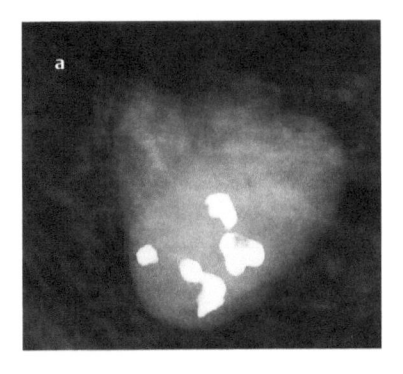

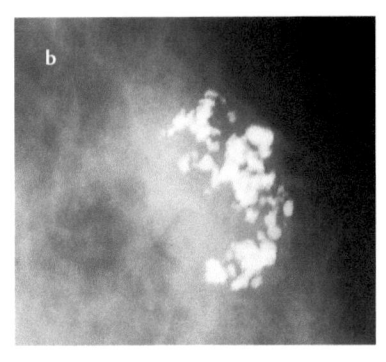

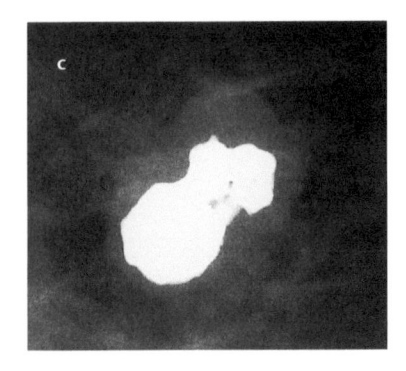

24 Additional Diagnostic Evaluation of Screening Findings and Solving of Problems in Symptomatic Patients

Fig. 24.31a–c
a Several coarse, irregularly outlined calcifications within a lobulated lesion: Typical fibroadenoma.
b Barely discernible oval density with typical coarse bizarre fibroadenomatous calcifications.
c Macrocalcifications of an almost completely calcified fibroadenoma.

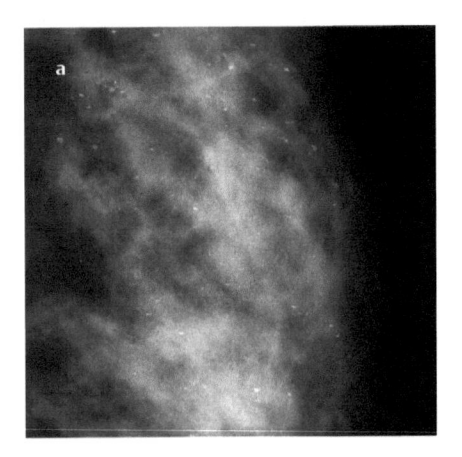

Fig. 24.32a,b
a In part round, in part linear and multiple crescentic, "teacup" calcifications due to sedimentation of calcific particles within milk of calcium cysts, seen only in the mediolateral view.
b Unilateral, relatively monomorphic, fine microcalcifications without typical distribution. *Histology*: Simple fibrocystic changes without proliferations containing psammomatous calcifications.

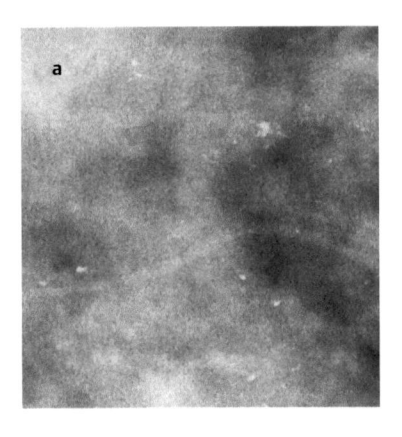

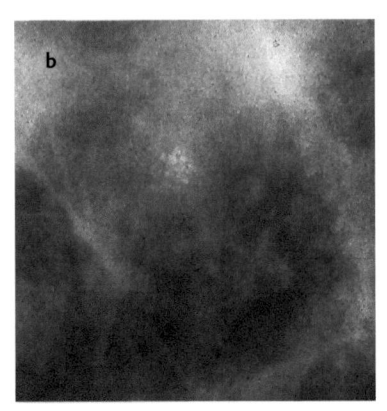

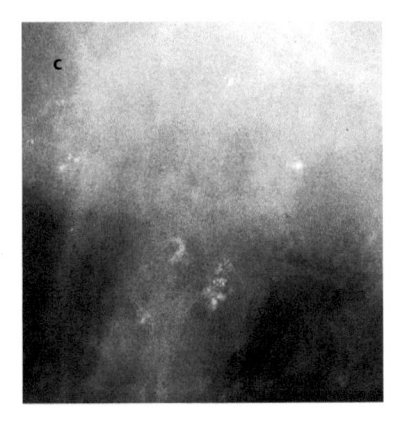

Fig. 24.33a–c
a Punctate scattered calcifications in blunt duct adenosis.
b Several punctate, clustered calcifications in a round group (morula-like): Small cystic adenosis.
c Typical image of multiple, morula-like calcifications with intralobular distribution in sclerosing adenosis.

Semicircular or shell-like calcifications around radiolucent lesions can develop in oil cysts, scars, and fat necrosis, as part of a foreign body reaction around droplets of silicone or wax injected for augmentation, in calcifying liponecrosis, and in "plasma cell mastitis." They too are always benign.

Fibroadenomas or papillomas may calcify starting from the periphery (whereby the soft tissue density may or may not be visible). Some may completely calcify and are then invariably benign. Other fibroadenomas or papillomas may present with the combined calcifications confined to an oval or round area, a smoothly outlined soft tissue density, and evolving peripheral calcification. Such presentations are also characteristic of benign fibroadenomas or papillomas. (In cases with only subtle peripheral calcifications, follow-up examinations at 6-, 12- and 24-month intervals may prove progression to coarse calcifications that are typical of benign fibroadenomas or papillomas. However, in the case of additional suspicious findings—e.g., indistinctly outlined surrounding density—further evaluation of individual cases is indicated.)

In cysts. Calcifications in the wall can develop in oil cysts or milk of calcium cysts but can also indicate a complex cyst. If an oil cyst (radiographically visualized central radiolucency) or a simple milk of calcium cyst ("teacups" on mediolateral mammogram or, in the case of large cysts, sonographically moveable sedimentations) has been documented, further diagnostic steps are unnecessary.

As a foreign body reaction around deposits of silicone or wax that have been injected for augmentation. These shell-like calcifications are definitely benign. The usually increased density due to fibrosis, silicone, and calcifications, however, compromises the overall evaluation of the breast tissue (**Fig. 24.30b**).

Coarse, popcornlike, or bizarre calcifications larger than 2 mm can be found in fibroadenomas and papillomas. The larger these calcifications, the more characteristic they are. Such characteristic popcorn-like or bizarre calcifications support the diagnosis of a fibroadenoma or papilloma with a high degree of certainty.

It is, however, important to keep in mind that bizarre calcifications smaller than 2 mm can resemble pleomorphic granular calcifications found in carcinomas.

Consequently, bizarre calcifications can only establish the diagnosis of a fibroadenoma if they are large enough and show an arrangement uncharacteristic of malignancy.

If, however, smaller calcifications suggestive of malignancy are found next to these calcifications or if coarse calcifications are surrounded by an irregularly outlined density, the differential diagnosis must consider necrotic calcifications in a carcinoma or a calcified fibroadenoma surrounded by a carcinoma.

In scars, *coarse needles, linear curved suture calcifications or bizarre large dystrophic calcifications* are characteristically seen along the scars. Again, caution should be observed when evaluating delicate calcifications and possible ductal distribution, since a new or residual carcinoma within or adjacent to the scar has to be excluded.

Parallel microcalcifications are characteristic of *vascular calcifications*. They do not follow (in two projections) the course of ductal structures. Even if these calcifications appear amorphous or fragmented, the correct diagnosis can usually be established as long as the parallel lines resemble railroad tracks. The outer contour of the lines is smooth and sharply delineated, but the lines need not be completely calcified. The vascular nature is further supported when the vessels are delineated as tubular soft tissue densities within the surrounding adipose tissue.

Typical Morphologies and Distribution Suggestive of Malignancy

The following individual shapes are typical of carcinomas.

Casting Microcalcifications

(See **Fig. 24.34.**)

These microcalcifications, which can branch and assume V or Y shapes, correspond to calcified casts which are often associated with comedo-type DCIS or a comedo-type invasive ductal carcinoma. These calcifications are to be differentiated from the needlelike or branching calcifications of the so-called plasma cell mastitis that are generally larger and may have smooth parallel walls. Less frequently, microcalcifications in benign fibrocystic changes may assume elongated shapes (**Figs. 24.35 and 24.36**), for example secretory calcifications or calcifications associated with sclerosing adenosis. Because the branching and casting microcalcifications are frequently a sign of carcinoma, the suspicion of malignancy should be raised whenever such calcifications are observed following the ductal system or within a cluster of microcalcifications.

Pleomorphic and Larger Granular Calcifications

These microcalcifications are very variable in size, shape, and density and have been described as resembling crushed stone. The individual calcification within a group can be extremely irregular, sometimes even bizarre in shape (**Figs. 24.37 and 24.38**) and range in size from fine to 2 mm. Usually each calcification is different from the others. (Usually the larger calcifications correspond to necrotic casts within the dilated ducts of comedo-type malignancy.)

These calcifications have to be differentiated from the bizarre calcifications in fibroadenomas, which usually (but not always) are larger and coarser, frequently exhibit a different distribution pattern, and often are associated with a large, coarse dystrophic calcification. If such calcifications are contained in a completely well-circumscribed soft tissue mass, this can be diagnostically

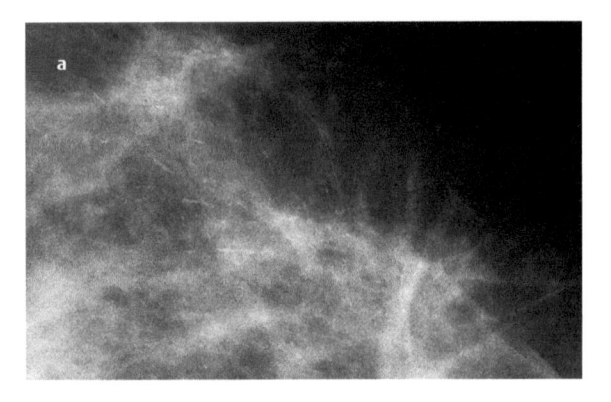

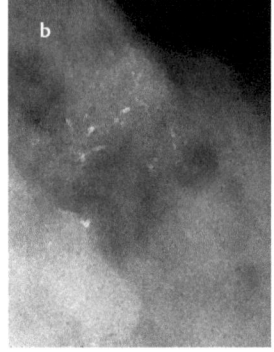

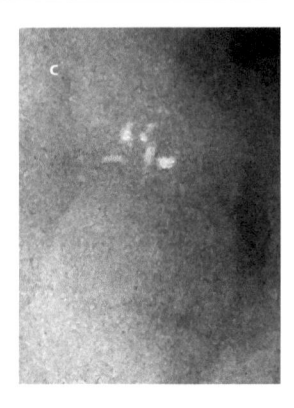

24 Additional Diagnostic Evaluation of Screening Findings and Solving of Problems in Symptomatic Patients

Fig. 24.34a–c

a Multiple needlelike and fine microcalcifications in a ductal distribution (magnification view). *Histology*: Ductal carcinoma in situ (DCIS), comedo-type.

b Group of microcalcifications including several elongated or V-shaped calcifications: Highly suspicious. *Histology*: DCIS, comedo-type with microinvasion.

c Group of elongated and very polymorphic, suspicious microcalcifications. *Histology*: DCIS, comedo-type.

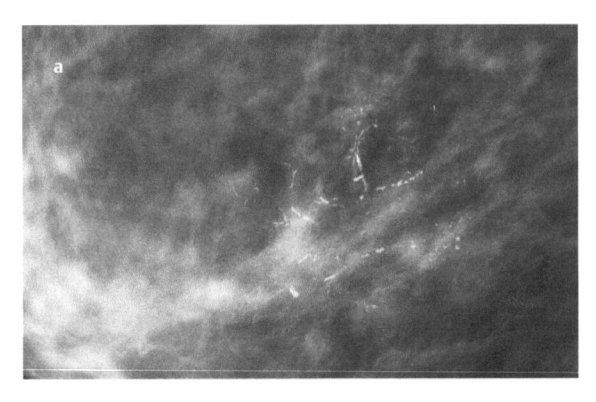

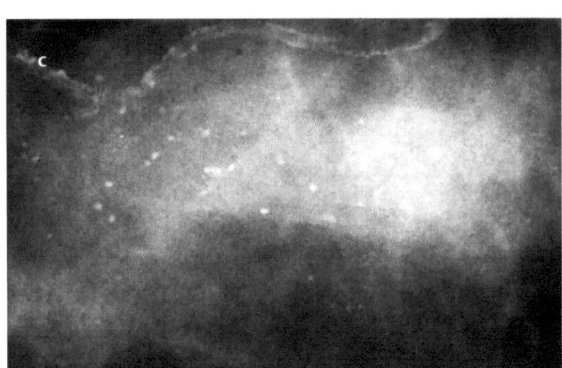

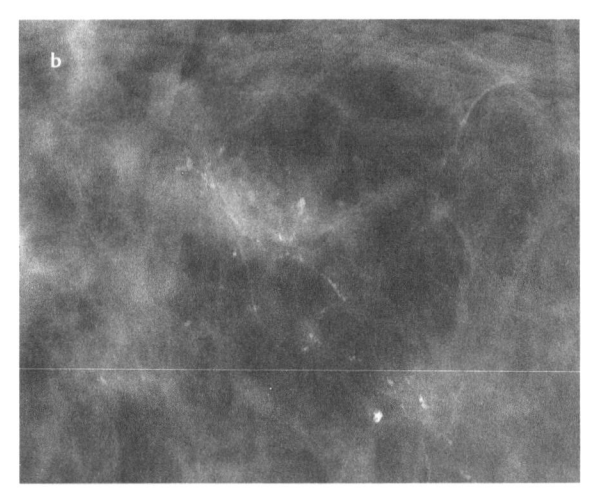

Fig. 24.35a–c Pleomorphic, linear calcifications must be considered strongly suggestive of malignancy, while smooth, linear calcifications can be a manifestation of a benign condition.

a Relatively coarse, elongated, partially V-shaped or Y-shaped casting calcifications that grow along the ducts. In addition to these coarse calcifications, fine and tiny microcalcifications suggest the correct diagnosis: Ductal carcinoma in situ.

b Calcifications with similar morphology and distribution as in (**a**). *Histology*: So-called "plasma cell mastitis," no malignancy.

c Diffusely distributed microcalcifications with slight polymorphism including individual elongated forms. *Histology*: Fibrocystic disease including secretory-type calcifications.

Differential Diagnosis and Assessment

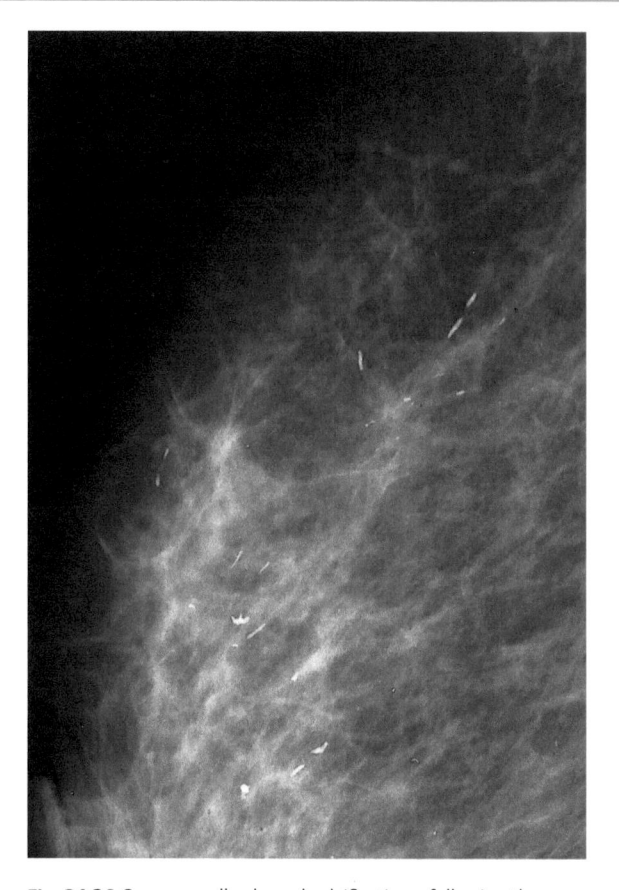

Fig. 24.36 Coarse needle-shaped calcifications, following the ducts and oriented toward the nipple: "Plasma cell mastitis."

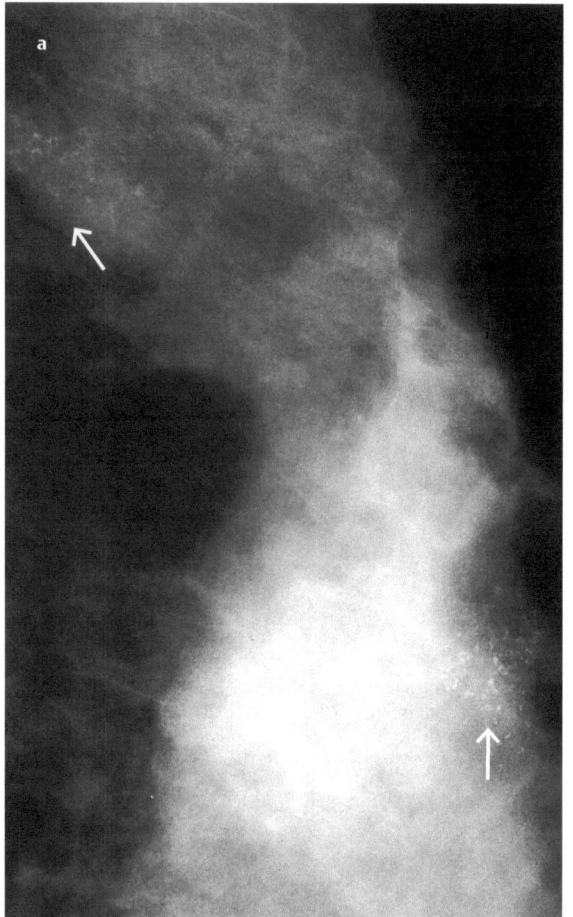

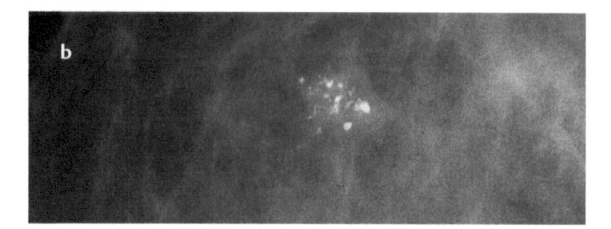

Fig. 24.37a,b Pleomorphic microcalcifications suggestive of malignancy can be both very fine and very coarse (> 1 mm).

a The mediolateral view shows two groups of very fine pleomorphic microcalcifications, 4 cm apart, in the lateral aspect of the breast: Multicentric ductal carcinoma in situ (DCIS).

b Delineation of a small group of considerably coarser pleomorphic calcifications, so-called granular mircrocalcifications. Despite the accompanying soft tissue density, these calcifications should not be mistaken for bizarre calcifications of a fibroadenoma. Furthermore, the somewhat irregular contour of the accompanying soft tissue density should be noted. *Histology*: DCIS.

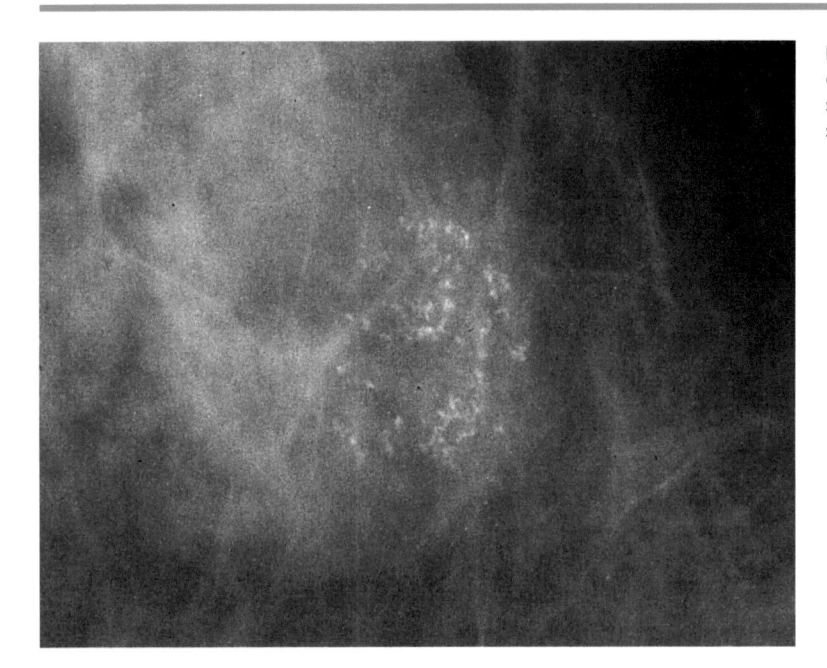

Fig. 24.38 Large group of polymorphic and casting microcalcifications that are highly suspicious. *Histology*: Ductal carcinoma in situ.

helpful by indicating a fibroadenoma. However, any less characteristic group of pleomorphic microcalcifications requires further assessment. In addition to fibroadenomas, the larger granular calcifications may less frequently be observed in benign changes or initial fat necrosis.

Fine Granular Calcifications

(See **Fig. 24.39**.)

Fine granular calcifications do not belong to calcifications typical of malignancy. They can be a manifestation of a carcinoma. However, the positive predictive value (PPV) mostly ranges around 10–15%. Malignancy is more probable with linear shapes or pleomorphism. Most fine granular microcalcifications are smaller than 50 μm—that is, very delicate—and are visible by summation on mammography if they are clustered in small groups. Fine granular calcifications occur in micropapillary and cribriform subtypes of the noncomedo DCIS and in the corresponding invasive carcinomas. These very fine granular calcifications precipitate in the secretion-filled interspaces between the papillary or cribriform cellular proliferations.

Since fine granular calcifications are also frequently associated with benign changes, these calcifications have to be considered uncharacteristic.

They should, however, raise concern about malignancy if they exhibit a segmental or ductal distribution (see below), have increased in number, or are new. For small groups of fine granular calcifications, the decision to perform a biopsy should be made less aggressively, as these are more likely due to benign proliferative changes and—if malignant—may just be associated with low-grade DCIS.

Typical Distribution Pattern of Malignant Calcifications

Ductal Arrangement of Calcifications

(See **Figs. 24.34a, 24.35a, 24.39a**.)

Any ductal arrangement is considered strongly suggestive of an intraductal origin of the calcifications and requires biopsy because of the high suspicion of malignancy. Biopsy should be considered for any type and size of microcalcifications presenting with such distributions (except unequivocal secretory disease, see above).

Segmental Distribution of the Calcifications

The suspicion of malignancy increases with the conspicuity of the segmental arrangement (**Figs. 24.34a** and **24.40**). So-called "club" or "butterfly" forms of segmental arrangement may result from subsegments visualized in differing projections.

Newly Developing Microcalcifications

Experience (gained mainly from analysis of interval cancers) has shown that newly developing microcalcifications are associated with a higher probability of malignancy and therefore require special attention. Newly developing microcalcifications may not yet present with typical suspicious shapes or distribution.

Since both benign and malignant calcifications may develop, it may not possible to assess all newly developing microcalcifcations. However, the threshold for biopsy should be lowered for newly developing microcalcifications. For less suspicious newly developing microcalcifications, short-term follow-up may be considered.

Differential Diagnosis and Assessment

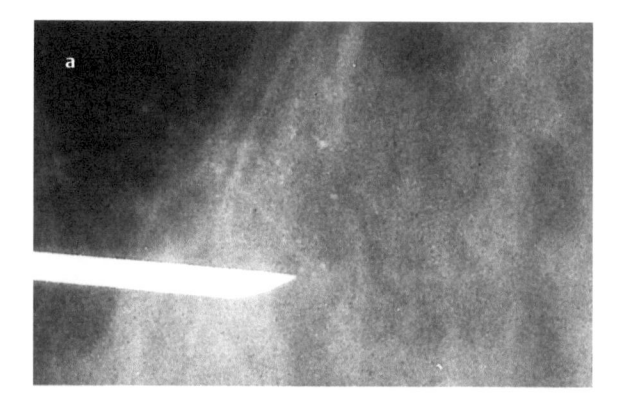

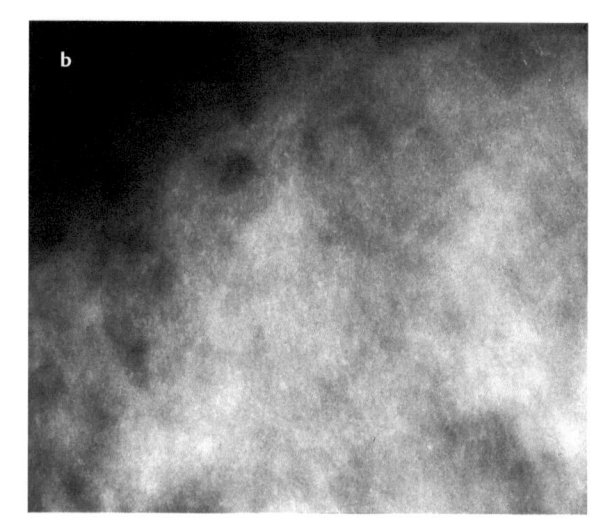

Fig. 24.39a,b

a Fine-granular calcifications. The triangular arrangement is suggestive of malignancy. *Histology*: Small invasive ductal carcinoma.

b Very fine calcifications diffusely distributed throughout the entire breast, new since the previous examination and therefore suggestive evidence of a possible carcinoma. No palpable abnormality or difference compared with the contralateral side: *Histology*: Ductal carcinoma diffusely spread throughout the breast.

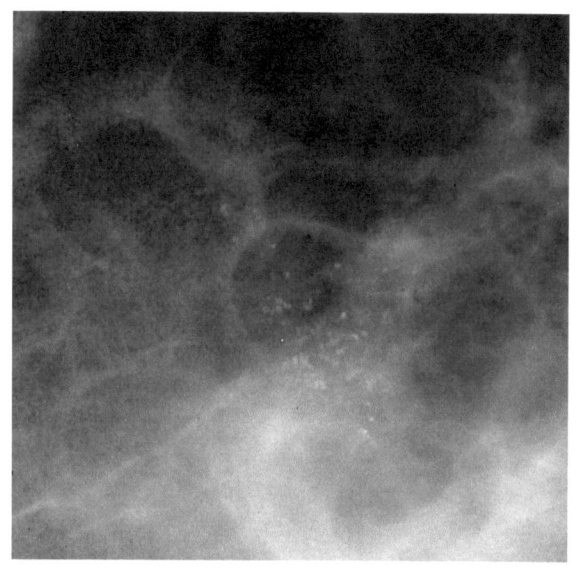

Fig. 24.40 Typical triangular group, with its apex pointing toward the nipple (not imaged, right lower corner). *Histology*: Ductal carcinoma in situ, comedo-type.

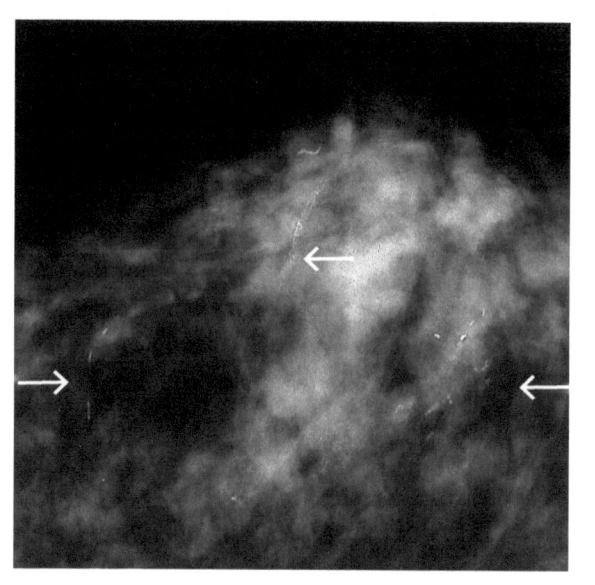

Fig. 24.41 Left arrow: Calcifications as part of a plasma cell mastitis. Middle arrow: Vascular calcifications. Right, Open arrow: segmentally arranged, pleomorphic calcifications of ductal carcinoma in situ.

Lack of Symmetry

Malignant calcifications rarely appear in symmetric locations in the right and left breasts. Therefore, the suspicion of malignancy is strengthened if calcifications are found at one location in one breast only. However, asymmetric distribution is not a typical sign of malignancy.

Signs Indicating Benign Calcifications after Excluding (the above) Signs of Malignancy

A prerequisite for assuming microcalcifications to be caused by benign changes is absence of signs that may indicate malignancy.

Under this condition the following findings support calcifications associated with benign changes.

Symmetric and Scattered Distribution

Both symmetry and scattered distribution (evenly distributed throughout the parenchyma; see also **Fig. 24.33**) support the diagnosis of benignity.

Diffusely distributed, mostly symmetric calcifications are typically associated with certain types of fibrocystic changes, mainly sclerosing adenosis. The symmetric appearance of malignant microcalcifications is extremely rare.

The calcifications in benign changes are frequently punctate, stippled, or round.

If amorphous calcifications show a symmetric distribution, a predominantly monomorphic appearance and, in particular, the teacup phenomenon, the diagnosis of fibrocystic changes is supported.

Teacup Phenomenon

(See **Fig. 24.32**.)

The teacup phenomenon is caused by sedimentation in microcysts (cysts containing milk of calcium) (see also pp. 265–268), as seen with benign fibrocystic changes. Since the teacup phenomenon may be detectable only on the 90° lateral view, obtaining a 90° lateral view—if possible, with magnification—is mandatory for the assessment of indeterminate microcalcifications.

In the craniocaudal view, these calcifications frequently appear amorphous, and accurate diagnosis cannot be made on this view. The teacup phenomenon is usually seen in a small part of the microcalcifications associated with benign disease only. The diagnosis of a benign process can be made with a high degree of certainty if neither calcifications suggestive of malignancy nor suspicious masses (as evidence of a carcinoma that coexists with the described benign changes) are observed amid these calcifications (**Fig. 24.41**).

Morula-Type Small Group

In microcystic or blunt duct adenosis (**Fig. 24.33b,c**) small calcifications that are round, punctate, or stippled and have a uniform monomorphous shape may be arranged in a small rounded group with a rosette-like arrangement ("morula"). This arrangement is indicative of a lobular distribution (and thus a benign change). The diagnosis of benignity is further supported by the multiplicity and symmetry of such small groups and by relatively uniform morphology.

Uncharacteristic Microcalcifications

Microcalcifications, which neither exhibit any of the above signs suspicious of malignancy nor definite signs indicating a benign change, mostly are classified as indeterminate (BI-RADS 4a) or probably benign (BI-RADS 3).

Most uncharacteristic microcalcifications are fine granular or amorphous and thus may in a small percentage (mostly 5–15%) be an indicator of (mostly low-grade) malignancy. The majority will, however, be associated with benign changes.

Based on the existing gray zone it will not always be possible to find the right decision.

To find the best possible individual decision, each area or group must be diligently analyzed (including high-quality mammography, lateral and magnification views; previous images should be available). Analysis should consider:

- The individual risk of the patient (family history, individual history)
- Patient age
- Exact distribution pattern of microcalcifications
- Morphology of microcalcifications
- Any associated changes
- Change with time (whenever possible previous films should be obtained!)
- Histology from previous biopsies (if available) should be considered (Is it representative? Can it explain an underlying disease that may also be compatible with the present changes?)

Overall, the more symmetrical the appearance and the finer and more widely spread the microcalcifications, the higher the probability of benign changes. In cases with significant asymmetry, pleomorphism, increase in number or size of the microcalcifications, or possible ductal or segmental arrangement, histopathologic assessment needs to be considered. Excision of the complete area in question will in general provide a reliable answer, but in cases with a high probability of a benign change this may be an aggressive measure leading to significant scarring.

Thus even for larger areas of (asymmetric) microcalcifications, percutaneous biopsy of the most suspicious area might be considered (which may be associated with some loss of sensitivity). Selection of the most representative area may be crucial. In very difficult cases, pre-interventional MRI may be helpful to exclude the presence of an invasive malignancy or enhancing higher-grade DCIS, or to select the area of the highest suspicion.

Any significant change—increase in number or size of microcalcifications, development of a soft tissue density (sometimes associated with a decrease in microcalcifications, even in cases of malignancy!), any sign of retraction—requires histopathologic assessment. Failure to observe any appreciable changes for less than 1–2 years, unfortunately, raises the likelihood of a benign diagnosis only slightly. Since DCIS may stay unchanged for a long time but may suddenly start to progress to invasive disease, caution is necessary and only long-term absence of a change (> 5–10 years) may significantly support a benign diagnosis.

Follow-up examinations may be useful when the compilation of all findings suggest a benign lesion with a high degree of certainty. Some benign changes (particularly calcifications in scarring or fibroadenomas) tend to become more characteristic with time.

Clustered calcifications should be carefully evaluated. To determine whether microcalcifications are clustered, the cluster must be visualized in two projections. Only an evaluation in two projections can separate a true cluster from a coincidental superimposition of calcifications that are at different locations but seen next to each other in one view. Such "pseudogroups" are not indicative of malignancy.

Considering the lower probability of significant malignancy in cases with very fine microcalcifications or little pleomorphism, follow-up may be justified for small probably benign groups of microcalcifications. In cases that exhibit any significant change or significant pleomorphism, histopathologic assessment should be considered. When informing the patient, it should be remembered that percutaneous breast biopsy may be better tolerated than long-term follow-up and uncertainty.

For very small groups of uncharacteristic microcalcifications (mostly fewer than five calcifications) follow-up is mostly considered adequate.

Appendix: Differential Diagnostic Significance of a Soft Density Surrounding Microcalcifications

(See **Figs. 24.42, 24.43, 24.44, 24.45, 24.46.**)

A surrounding or accompanying soft tissue density is often not helpful. Presence or absence of a soft tissue density can by no means substitute for a meticulous analysis of the microcalcifications.

A surrounding soft tissue density is contributory if:
- It is identifiable as a vessel (best if seen in two projections) with beginning mural calcifications.
- It is round and entirely smooth in outline: This can support the diagnosis of a fibroadenoma. However, in the case of suspicious microcalcifications, DCIS within a fibroadenoma must be considered.
- It is ill defined or spiculated and consequently unequivocally suspect.
- It is of fat density and consequently has a pattern diagnostic of a benign entity, for example, an oil cyst.

Less contributory is:
- Finding uncharacteristic densities around microcalcifications, since they may be caused by infiltration, reactive changes, uncharacteristic benign changes, or superimposition.
- Finding nodular densities around microcalcifications. They can suggest an early calcifying fibroadenoma or papilloma. But this is not conclusive because invasive carcinomas or carcinomas in situ can be nodular and calcify.

Finally, the presence or absence of a soft tissue density around microcalcifications permits no reliable differentiation between invasive carcinoma and carcinoma in situ. On the one hand, a soft tissue density accompanying an invasive carcinoma can be overlooked amid surrounding dense parenchyma. On the other hand, a reactive fibrosis can produce a soft tissue density around a pure carcinoma in situ.

Nipple Discharge

(See **Fig. 24.47.**)

Definition

A pathologic discharge refers to a spontaneous, usually unilateral, nonmilky secretion from one or a few lactiferous ducts. Spontaneous means that it should not be provoked by the patient compressing the breast. (If patients express the breast regularly, this causes production of prolactin and discharge; in the case of chronic discharge possibly acute or chronic inflammatory changes may be provoked.)

Diagnostic Problems

The first diagnostic challenge is to distinguish discharge requiring further assessment of the breast from other types of discharge.
- Causes of discharge include increased level of prolactin (usually caused by a prolactinoma). The latter diagnosis is established by blood tests and by MRI of the brain. It requires targeted treatment of the hyperprolactinemia.

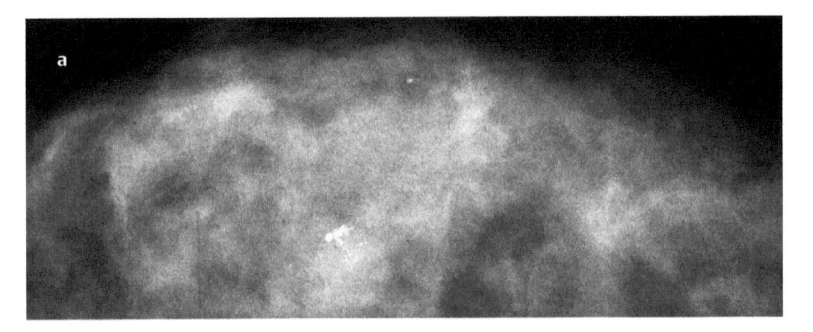

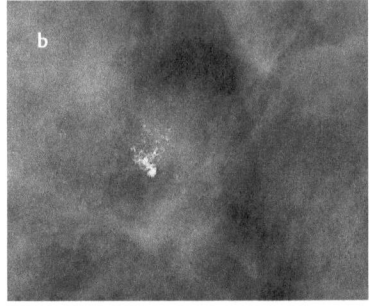

24 Additional Diagnostic Evaluation of Screening Findings and Solving of Problems in Symptomatic Patients

Fig. 24.42a,b

a Very fine calcifications as well as a coarse calcification with a bizarre outline are seen within a barely discernible round density measuring 7 mm located within dense parenchyma.

b Magnification mammography. *Diagnosis*: Fibroadenoma, confirmed by increasing coarseness of the calcifications on follow-up.

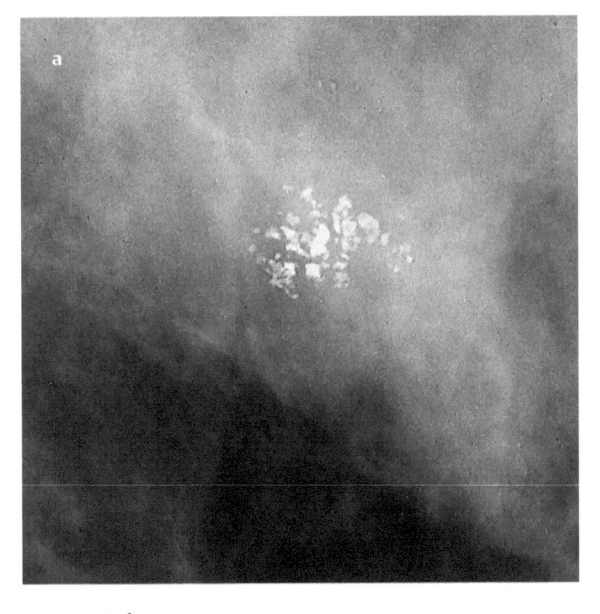

Fig. 24.43a,b

a Pleomorphic bizarre calcifications in a subtle oval area. *Histology*: Fibroadenoma.

b Granular and irregular linear calcifications forming an oval group with a pointed extension. Note the calcifications outside the soft-tissue density. *Histology*: Ductal carcinoma in situ.

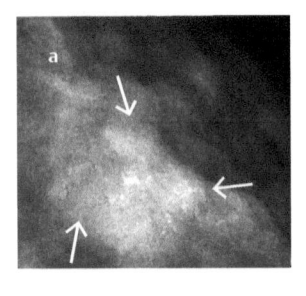

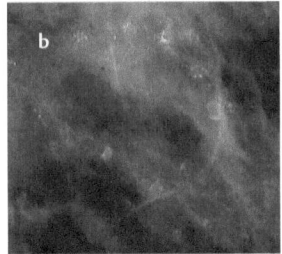

Fig. 24.44a–c Specimen radiography.

a Round lesion (arrows) measuring 8 mm, with multiple, somewhat pleomorphic calcifications that are closely aggregated: papilloma.
b Multiple tiny round groups, almost forming a circle, of punctate calcifications: papillomatosis.
c Multiple groups of microcalcifications are delineated within an indistinctly outlined soft-tissue density, with two groups unmistakably punctate. In addition, there are many granular, pleomorphic calcifications: papillary carcinoma.

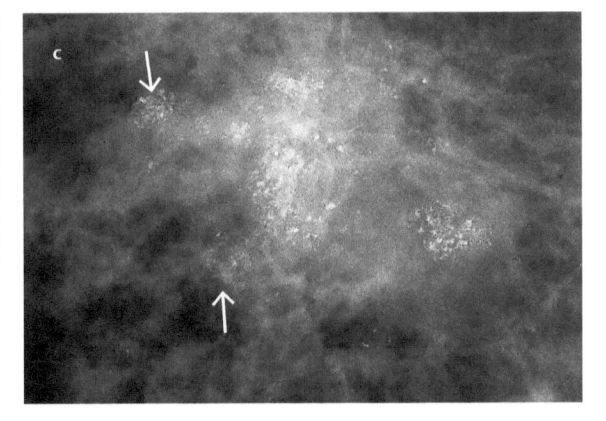

Differential Diagnosis and Assessment

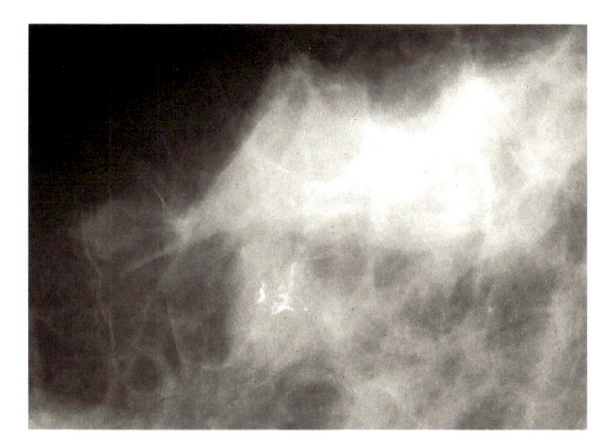

Fig. 24.45 Oval, partially sharply outlined lesion measuring 11 mm, with relatively large, pleomorphic, bizarre calcifications centrally. Despite the relatively coarse structure, not a fibroadenoma but an intraductal carcinoma.

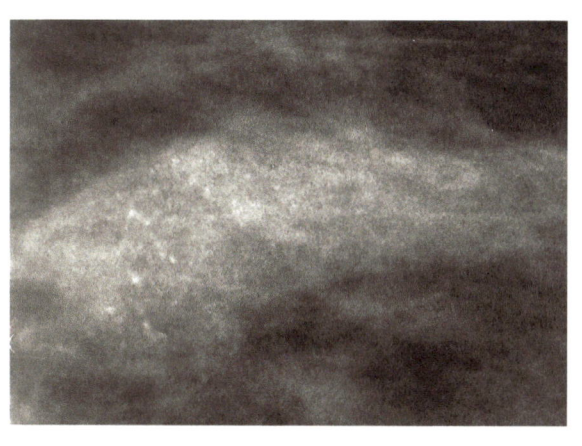

Fig. 24.46 Multiple fine-granular microcalcifications. Biopsy was recommended because of suggested segmental distribution (magnification ×3): DCIS.

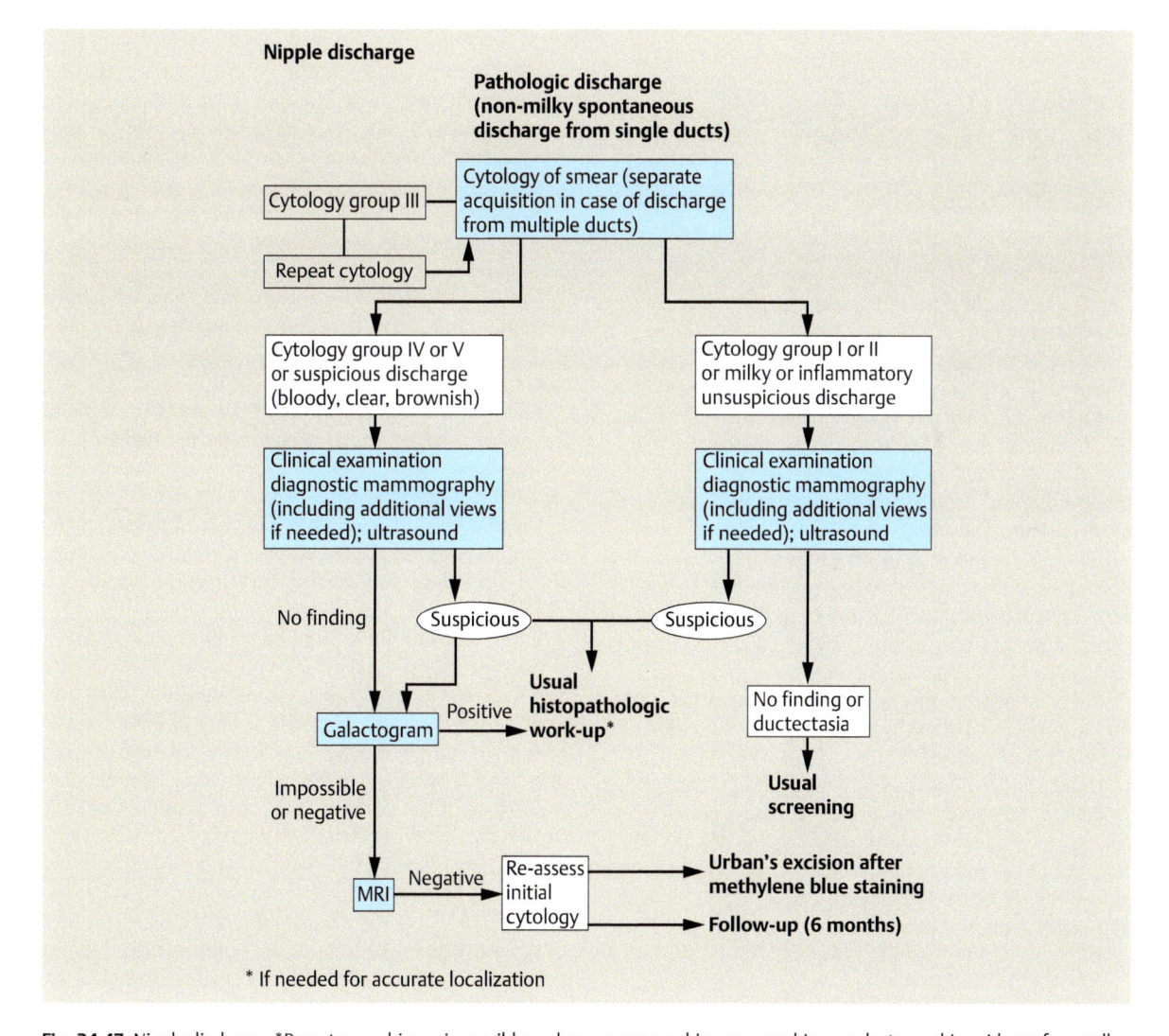

Fig. 24.47 Nipple discharge. *Percutanous biopsy is possible under mammographic, sonographic, or galactographic guidance for small areas or suspected lesions. For the other cases, excisional biopsy needs to be considered.

- Discharge that occurs only with strong pressure, or that occurs only when provoked by the patient, also does not require further assessment of the breast.
- If chronic discharge occurs and the patient expresses her breast regularly, further diagnostic assessment is often necessary. However, simultaneously the patient must be instructed to stop expressing her breast.
- Discharge can be caused by benign changes and chronic inflammation (secretory disease), by one or multiple papillomas, by a rare lactating fibroadenoma, or by DCIS or invasive carcinoma.
- Whenever a type of discharge is diagnosed or suspected that requires further assessment of the breast, the next problem concerns localizing the lesion in question and differentiating benignity from malignancy.
- Whenever excision is indicated the exact extent of the lesion in question needs to be assessed.
- The extent may range from a few millimeters in size (e.g., a small papilloma) to one or more segments (in the case of uncertain findings or a DCIS or invasive carcinoma that causes the discharge). Some DCIS or even invasive cancers may cause pathologic discharge as the only or leading symptom.

Diagnostic Strategy

Deciding For or Against Assessment of the Breast

Decide whether the discharge is spontaneous or occurs only when provoked.

As a rule, any spontaneous discharge calls for a cytologic smear. Only a positive cytologic smear (papillary cells, suspicious cells, blood) is diagnostically useful. A reliable distinction between papilloma and (papillary) carcinoma is not cytologically possible. Since the sensitivity of a cytologic smear is very low, *a negative cytologic smear can never exclude malignancy.*

Bilateral discharge is generally a manifestation of a hormonal dysfunction and consequently not an indication for galactography. Only the case of a hemorrhagic or cytologically suspicious discharge warrants further evaluation of the breast(s) in question.

A discharge from several ducts more often has a hormonal cause, and checking the status of the endocrine system is recommended.

Unilateral spontaneous discharge must be further evaluated whenever one or several lactiferous ducts secrete spontaneously and the discharge is neither milky nor definitely inflammatory (based on cytology and inspection). Further assessment is also necessary if the cytologic smear is suspicious.

Searching for the Origin of Secretion

(See also Chapter 14.)

The assessment starts with *clinical examination, ultrasound, and mammography.*

Clinically in some cases a trigger point may indicate the location of a papilloma or lactating fibroadenoma. This area should then be checked very thoroughly. Any suspicious finding on mammography or ultrasound requires the usual assessment as indicated for the type of lesion (e.g., mass or microcalcifications). Any focal lesion should be assessed histologically (usually by percutaneous breast biopsy) using the guidance method that allows the easiest and best tolerated approach. On ultrasound, radial scanning may demonstrate dilated ducts which may help define the area in question. If a localized area with dilated ducts can be defined, percutaneous breast biopsy may be considered. In order not to miss a diffusely growing malignancy, however, ample sampling should be performed. Alternatively US-guided VABB may be considered. A critical interdisciplinary countercheck of representative biopsy is necessary for any nonmalignant result.

In the case of unspecific or widely distributed findings (diffusely dilated ducts) or of absent findings we recommend performing *galactography or MRI.* The value of galactography is generally accepted; the value of MRI is being investigated. MRI is necessary if galactography is not possible.

For *galactographically* documented duct ectasia or a normal ductal system, follow-up imaging at the age-specific intervals is adequate (unless there are cytologically suspicious findings).

Any galactographic filling defect with or without irregularities of the ductal wall or any truncated duct is a manifestation of an intraductal process and requires histopathologic assessment.

Histopathologic assessment can be performed directly after galactography, for example, by stereotactic targeting of the filling defect or the ductal system in question and VABB.

In the case of diffuse findings, surgical excision might be considered. Surgical excision, however, also requires adequate marking of the area in question. Thus wire marking might require another galactogram. Stereotactic marking is quite possible, if the lesion had been marked by a clip following the initial galactography (see **Fig. 8.7**) since the clip can serve to guide preoperative marking. Finally, the secreting ductal system may be marked and followed intraoperatively by the surgeon after using methylene blue or it might be analyzed using galactoscopy. It should, however, be noted that the success rate of galactoscopy is lower than that of galactography, that it allows the acquisition of only very small amounts of tis-

Differential Diagnosis and Assessment

sue, and that it mostly only allows access to the proximal 4 cm of the ductal system.

MRI may be able to demonstrate an enhancing mass, duct or segment, which—unless detectable by retrospective ultrasound—may also be targeted under MR guidance. Presently the false positive rate of MRI for this indication is not exactly known.

Assessing the Extent of a Lesion Associated with Nipple Discharge

The extent of a focal lesion can often be assessed quite correctly by imaging. It must be remembered that some DCIS may be mammographically occult and that mammographically the area of microcalcifications may (more frequently) underestimate and (sometimes) overestimate the extent of a DCIS. MRI more frequently overestimates the extent of a DCIS, but may also underestimate its extent. Not all cases of DCIS enhance on MRI. In the case of diffuse or patchy enhancement (due to benign changes) MRI may not allow any reliable estimate. Also a galactographic stop may indicate only the proximal end of the area of involvement, whereas the ductal system distal to the stop cannot be assessed at all. Therefore in the case of nonmass lesions excision of the complete ductal system that may be involved should usually be attempted. In the case of DCIS, excision should include a sufficient safety margin.

Inflammatory Changes

(See **Figs. 24.48** and **24.49**; see also **Fig. 16.7**.)

Definition

If localized erythema or diffuse changes with erythema or hyperthermia, or both, are noticed clinically, the differential diagnosis must center around the differentiation between malignancy (carcinoma with inflammatory component, inflammatory carcinoma, and, rarely, hematologic malignancy or metastases) and inflammation (mastitis, abscess).

Diagnostic Problems

Above all, the differentiation between subacute or chronic inflammatory processes can be difficult.

Diagnostic Strategy

The *clinical history* usually supports an inflammatory origin in context with a pregnancy, with lactation, or with prior or recurrent inflammations. In the presence of nipple discharge, the microbiologic and cytologic examination of the discharge can be helpful.

Mammography is of special importance here. It is true that malignancy and inflammation generally cannot be distinguished in a focal mass or diffuse density without

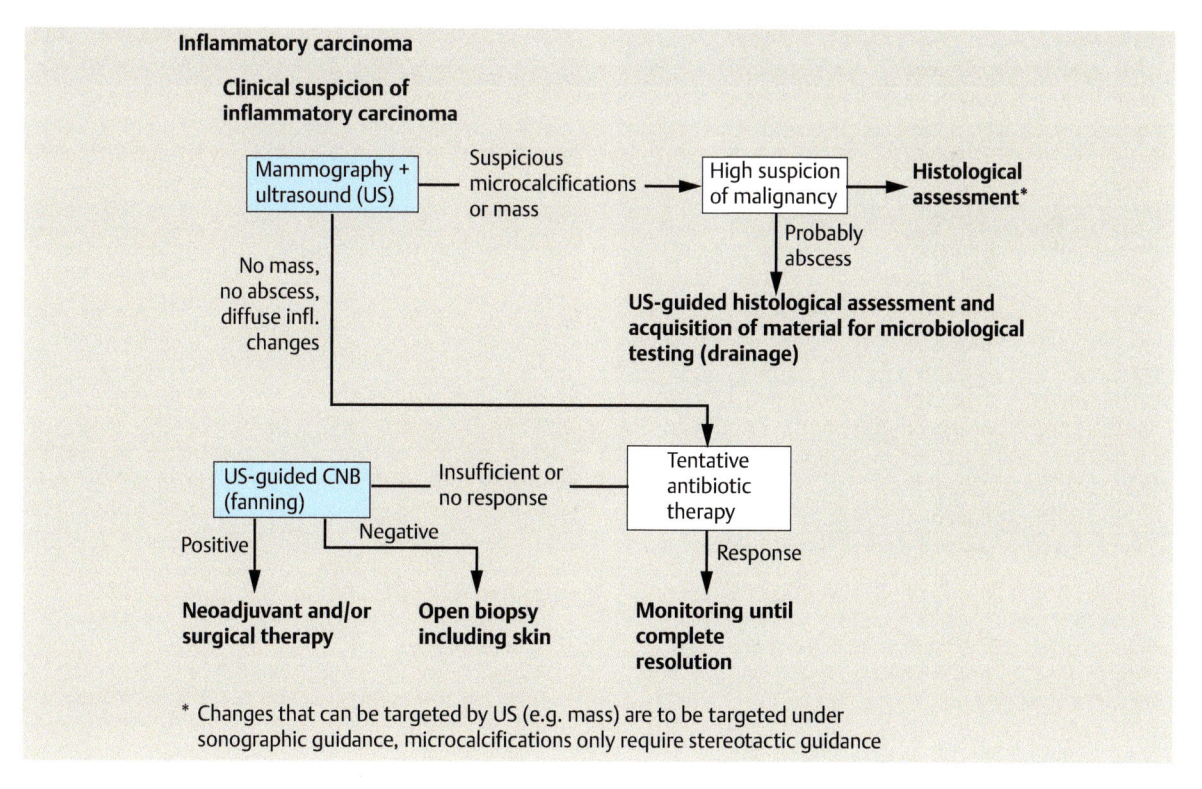

* Changes that can be targeted by US (e.g. mass) are to be targeted under sonographic guidance, microcalcifications only require stereotactic guidance

Fig. 24.48 Inflammatory changes.

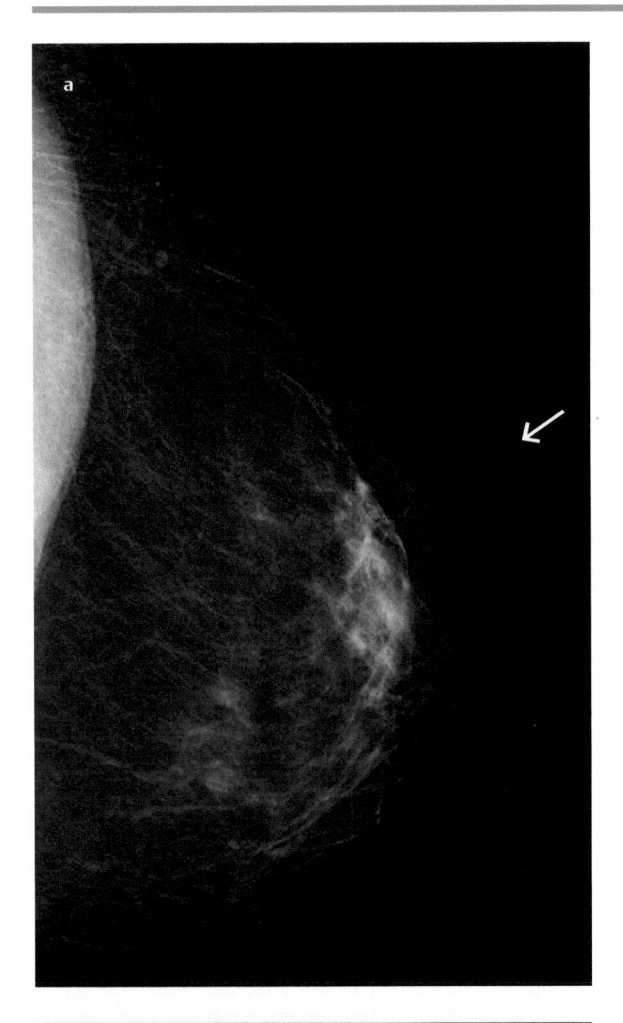

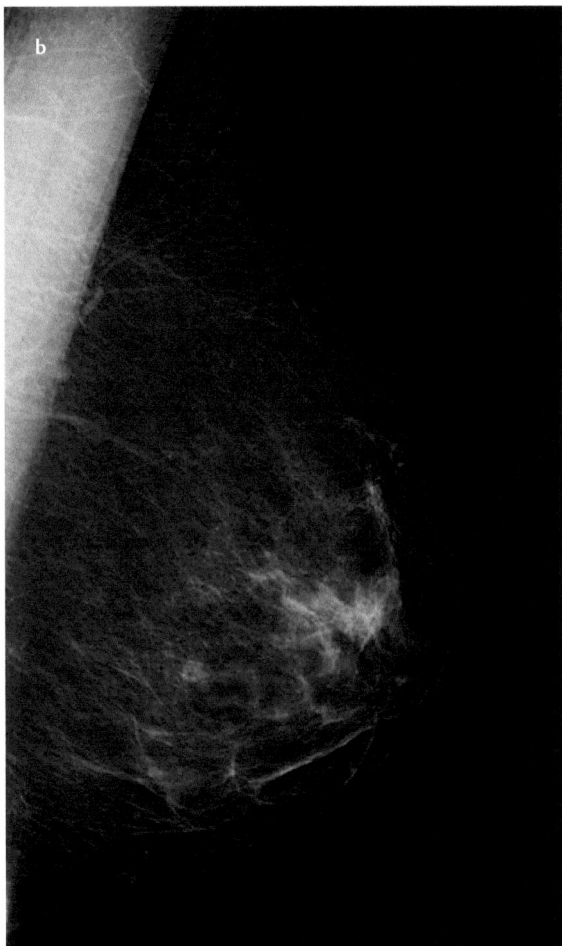

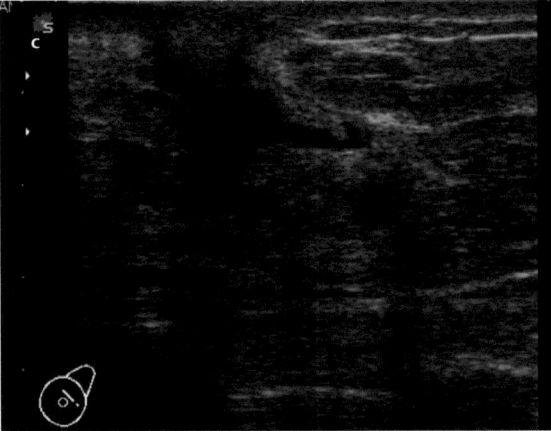

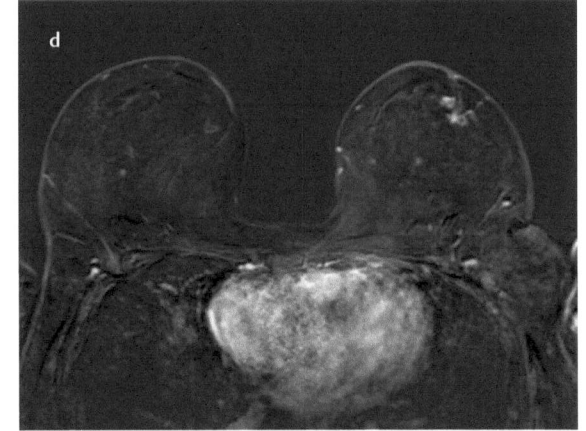

24 Additional Diagnostic Evaluation of Screening Findings and Solving of Problems in Symptomatic Patients

Fig. 24.49a–d This 68-year-old patient presented for a screening mammogram. When examining the patient a faint reddening of the skin in an area of about 2 cm was noted, 4–5 cm from the nipple in the 2 o'clock position. No palpable finding, no skin retraction, no peau d'orange.

a,b The screening mammogram does not show a significant change. The tissue in the area of question (arrow) is moderately dense (ACR2–3).

c On ultrasound a diffusely hypoechoic area was noted underneath the skin extending to the skin, which showed slight thickening.

d Magnetic resonance imaging was performed to assess the extent of this uncharacteristic change. *Histology* revealed a diffusely growing ductal invasive carcinoma (G2–3), growing in nests of cells.

microcalcifications, but if suspicious microcalcifications can be identified, a malignancy is very probable.

Sonographically demonstrated hypoechoic or anechoic spaces with fluctuation would indicate an inflammatory process. An abscess, which is characterized by a relatively smooth inner wall, has to be distinguished from a carcinoma with central necrosis, which usually exhibits nodular thickening and an irregular inner surface.

Mammographically or sonographically suspicious or indeterminate findings should be assessed histologically primarily using percutaneous breast biopsy. Whenever an inflammatory process is considered in the differential diagnosis some material should be gained for microbiological testing of aerobic or anaerobic bacteria.

Without conclusive evidence provided by mammography or sonography and in cases with significant inflammation, tentative *anti-inflammatory therapy* (using a usual antibiotic combination for mastitis) for 1–2 weeks is considered as the next diagnostic step. The resolution of the finding has to be monitored until inflammation resolves completely. The necessary short-term follow-up can be performed sonographically/clinically.

It should be mentioned that some inflammatory processes fail to elicit any clinical inflammatory signs, as found in so-called cold abscesses caused by tuberculosis or fungus and in some granulomatous conditions, as well as in chronic inflammations that may occur in association with fibrocystic changes. Their diagnosis is generally only established histologically after biopsy of a lesion that was discovered as a palpable finding or mammographic density.

Any suspicious or indeterminate change that persists after 1–2 weeks of antibiotic therapy requires histopathogical and microbiologic assessment as described above.

Percutaneous breast biopsy is the desirable method since inflammatory carcinoma is usually managed with neoadjuvant chemotherapy and does not require primary surgery. However, it must be remembered that some diffuse malignancies (some diffuse lobular carcinomas and some diffusely growing inflammatory carcinomas) may be very difficult to diagnose by percutaneous breast biopsy owing to dispersed growth of single cells or nests of cells, which may be missed due to sampling error. Therefore sampling of diffuse changes always requires acquisition of significant amounts of tissue (fanning with acquisition of multiple thick cores or VABB of a sufficiently large area), critical interdisciplinary correlation of imaging and histopathology, and analysis of agreement.

Any discordant finding requires excisional biopsy which should also include some of the overlying skin.

The Young Patient

Special Considerations and Problems

Diagnosis of breast cancer can be more difficult in younger patients (below age 35–40 years) than in those who are older.

There are several reasons for this:
- The incidence of breast cancer in this age group is very low. Less than 7.5% of all breast cancers occur before age 40 and 0.6% in women who are less than 30 (Winchester 1996, Ries et al. 2008).
- In patients who are affected before age 30, hereditary breast cancer should be considered.
- There is a high incidence of benign breast disease (lumpiness, fibroadenomas).
- Mammography is less sensitive in some of these patients.
- There is an increased, yet still small, radiation risk in those at a young age compared with older age groups. Whether the otherwise very low risk of radiation-induced breast cancer may be increased for certain hereditary types of breast cancer (due to specific gene changes) has been discussed (Den Otter et al. 1996, Bebb et al. 1997, Sharan et al. 1997). Being the only method suitable for screening and the only method that can reliably detect DCIS, mammography remains indispensable in these patients.

These factors have led to an increased rate of delayed diagnoses of carcinoma among younger patients compared with older patients. Furthermore, the positive biopsy rates (the number of carcinomas per recommended biopsies) are much lower in younger patients (Kerlikowske et al. 1993, Gillett et al. 1997, Gajdos et al. 2000, Kushwaha et al. 2000, Ries et al. 2008).

Few women in this age group undergo mammographic screening. This is usually limited to women with first-degree relatives with premenopausal breast cancer, a history of treatment for Hodgkin disease, a prior breast biopsy revealing a high-risk lesion, or a previous history of breast cancer. A recent study has evaluated screening mammography performance in the United States for women of less than 40 years of age (Yankaskas et al. 2010).

Data from 6 mammography registries was pooled resulting in data from over 100,000 women. Young women have very low breast cancer rates, but after mammography they experience high recall rates, high rates of additional imaging, and low cancer detection rates. No cancers were found in women younger than 25 years and there was poor performance for the large group of women aged 35–39 years. In a theoretical population of 10,000 women aged 35–39 years, 1,266 women who are screened will receive further workup, with 16 cancers detected and 1,250 women receiving a false positive result.

In younger women, most cancers present as clinically evident masses, which need to be distinguished from the numerous benign masses and lumps detected in the young patient. These should be viewed with suspicion and the workup of these lesions individually tailored to each patient. The screening for the detection of lesions in these women is performed as in older women. A sensitivity to the real or perceived risk of radiation-induced cancer should be part of the treatment of these younger women. Even in pregnant women, however, suspicious lesions should be appropriately worked up.

Breast Changes in the Younger Patient and Their Histology

The appearance of the normal breast beginning from childhood to adult age has been reviewed in Chapter 9. Based on age-related physiologic changes, the breast of the younger patient on palpation is denser and lumpier than that of older patients (> 50 years). This higher consistency or lumpiness in itself does not imply disease. It does, however, impair clinical and, if performed, mammographic evaluation. Large individual variations exist; sometimes the breast of even very young patients (in their twenties) can contain ample amounts of fat.

The following benign entities are typically found in young patients (Blaker et al. 2010):

Fibrocystic, hyperplastic, and proliferative changes can occur. When proliferative changes with atypia are detected, this entity is associated with an increased risk of malignancy (see Chapter 10), as it is in older women.

Fibroadenomas. Even though fibroadenomas have a wide age distribution, the greatest incidence is in women between the ages of 25 and 35, and the fibroadenoma is the most frequent breast mass in children. Both pericanalicular and intracanalicular types are seen. In young patients, they largely consist of ample myxoid stroma with a high water content and are vascular. Some are cellular and adenomatous. Fibrosed fibroadenomas do not usually occur in young women. Multiple fibroadenomas are frequently encountered.

The *juvenile fibroadenoma or giant fibroadenoma* is a special type of fibroadenoma that occurs almost exclusively in young patients (maximum incidence around menarche). It is a well-circumscribed tumor, typically with rapid growth. Histologically, it consists of proliferating stroma and often epithelial hyperplasia. It is completely benign and not associated with an increased risk of malignancy.

The *phyllodes tumor* is much rarer in the young patient than the juvenile fibroadenoma. It can, however, be encountered, albeit rarely, in the young patient as well as a rapidly growing, well-circumscribed mass.

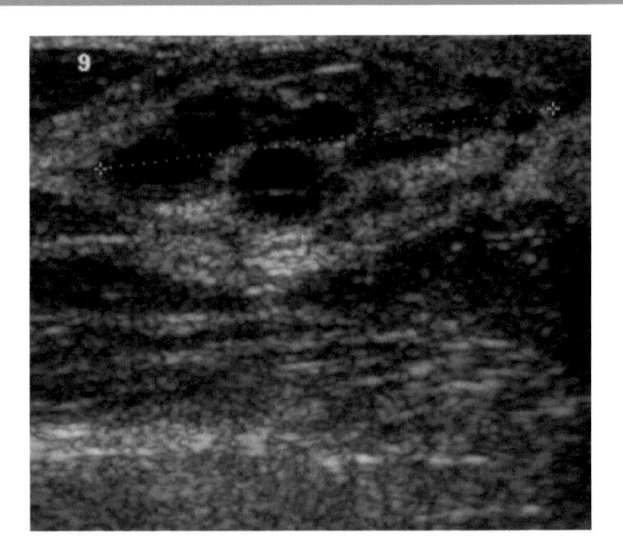

Fig. 24.50 A 15-year old patient with a family history of breast cancer presented with a palpable mass in the upper outer quadrant. The sonogram displays a hypoechoic mass including small cystic spaces. *Histology*: Juvenile papillomatosis.

Papillomas can occur in young patients.

Juvenile papillomatosis is an infrequent finding, which is typically diagnosed in adolescents and young women (**Fig. 24.50**). Histologically, the lesion, which generally becomes apparent as a palpable mass or nipple discharge, is characterized by ductal papillomatosis, papillary apocrine hyperplasia, multiple (micro)cysts, often cellular atypia, and sometimes even necrosis. About 30–40% of the cases are associated with a family history of breast carcinoma. Local recurrence and bilaterality have been reported. Whether the individual risk of breast carcinoma is increased is debatable. An association between juvenile papillomatosis and juvenile secretory carcinoma has been reported (Bazzocchi et al. 1986, Ferguson et al. 1987, Rosen and Kimmel 1990, Nonomura et al. 1995).

Overall *malignancy* is less frequent in younger patients than in patients above 40 years of age. Various types of malignancy, including breast carcinomas, hematologic malignancy, and sarcomas, have been encountered.

During pregnancy the following benign and malignant entities can also be encountered (Sabate et al. 2007):

Benign

- The fibroadenoma is the most frequent benign mass occurring during pregnancy. It is followed by papillomas, fibrocystic disease, galactocele, abscess, puerperal mastitis, and—rarely—breast infarct or phyllodes tumor (see Chapters 11–13).
- Many fibroadenomas increase in size during pregnancy, becoming apparent and necessitating further workup. Sometimes infarction may occur.

- Breast infarct, which can affect any part of the breast tissue as well as sometimes a fibroadenoma, is histologically characterized by a mass consisting of or containing coagulation necrosis. The exact etiology of breast infarcts during pregnancy is not known.

Malignant

- About 1–2% of breast cancers are considered concurrent with pregnancy or lactation. These include cancers that are detected during or within 1 year of pregnancy. Unfortunately, diagnosis of these cancers is often too late, probably because of the difficult distinction between neoplastic growth versus physiologic changes during pregnancy and lactation (Gorins et al. 1996, Ayyappan et al. 2010). Besides breast cancer, an association with pregnancy has been described for some rare lesions such as benign and malignant phyllodes tumor, Burkitt lymphoma, and angiosarcoma.

Risk of Breast Cancer

Breast cancer is an unusual disease in young women. Even though malignancies have been described in the teenage group and women in their early twenties, a relevant increase of risk starts after about 25 years of age. At age 25, the incidence of breast cancer is approximately 1/10,000. Breast tumors in young women usually show more aggressive features including larger tumor size, a higher incidence of poorly differentiated tumors, positive lymph nodes, high proliferation rates, higher expression of epidermal growth factor receptor 2 (HER2), higher expression of basal-like histologic subtype, and absence of endocrine receptors. Because of these factors, breast cancer in young patients is often associated with a poor prognosis (Pollán 2010).

If a younger woman (< 30 years) has breast cancer, she has a significant risk of being a *BRCA* gene carrier. Genetic counseling may be indicated to offer optimum future monitoring to her and, if desired, her relatives (Tse and Tan 2010).

After age 30 the risk of breast cancer in young women rises rapidly to approximately 1/1,000 at age 40. Although malignant lesions are rare in these younger women, they do occur, and an attempt should be made to avoid unnecessary delay in diagnosis. In patients with genetic risk factors and in those with a family history of premenopausal breast cancer, the risk of breast cancer increases significantly even before 35–40 years of age.

The following paragraphs will summarize special issues in the diagnostic workup of young patients. Based on these considerations, recommendations for a diagnostic strategy will be made.

Clinical Findings

The great majority of young patients with breast problems present with a lump, lumpiness, localized pain, and occasionally with pathologic nipple discharge or other rare findings. Some young patients are referred because of an individual or strong family history of breast cancer or because of known genetic risk factors.

Benign causes of a palpable abnormality in the young patient include normal breast tissue, fibroadenoma, fibrocystic changes, papilloma, cyst, and, infrequently, juvenile papillomatosis. During pregnancy or lactation, benign causes include a galactocele, an abscess, puerperal mastitis, or a breast infarct.

Juvenile papillomatosis can present on palpation as an indeterminate mass or can be palpable like a fibroadenoma. Breast infarct becomes apparent as an indeterminate or suspicious mass of rubbery consistency. Unfortunately, in situ and invasive carcinoma, as well as other rare malignancies, have to be included in the differential diagnosis.

The differential diagnosis of very large masses should include the juvenile fibroadenoma, virginal hypertrophy, and rare phyllodes tumor, lymphoma (e.g., Burkitt lymphoma during pregnancy), and sarcoma (periductal fibrosarcoma or angiosarcoma during pregnancy).

The causes of pathologic discharge are similar in younger women to those in the older age group and include papillomas, papillomatosis, duct ectasia, or fibrocystic changes, a lactating fibroadenoma (rarely), or, in less than 10% of the cases, a carcinoma.

As in the older patients, the sensitivity of the clinical examination for the detection of carcinoma varies with the lesion size and decreases strongly with smaller tumor size. As reported by Reintgen 1993 on a large series of over 500 breast carcinomas, only about 50% of the carcinomas in the size range of 11–15 mm are palpable, and even experienced clinicians do not detect the majority of breast cancers until they are greater than 15 mm.

Overall, clinical evaluation of the younger patient is more difficult because of the increased firmness and nodularity of the breast tissue. Because of the even greater pronounced nodularity and firmness of the breast tissue, evaluation frequently is significantly impaired during pregnancy and lactation.

Furthermore, the high prevalence of benign disease impairs assessment. During pregnancy and lactation, detection and diagnosis of malignancy and its differentiation from the physiologic hypertrophic changes become even more difficult, as documented by the commonly encountered delays in diagnosis.

Mammography

Mammographic evaluation in the young patient is often impaired by dense glandular tissue that can obscure both benign and malignant masses. Therefore, the value of mammography is limited. However, because of the variability of parenchymal patterns, about 30% of the patients have sufficient amounts of interposed fat to be readily assessed mammographically. Because of its unique capability to image microcalcifications (which may be the only sign of malignancy in ~30% of the carcinomas), mammography can be useful (see **Figs. 24.51, 24.52, 24.53, 24.54, 24.55**) below 35 years of age. It should therefore be utilized whenever indicated (see below).

When not obscured by dense tissue, benign lesions display large variations, as described in the respective chapters. Juvenile papillomatosis, an infrequent lesion seen predominantly in the young patient, usually cannot be distinguished from dense glandular tissue on mammography (**Fig. 24.51b,c**). This appearance, together with the usually encountered palpable abnormality, does not allow exclusion of malignancy. Breast infarct, a rare finding associated with pregnancy or lactation, can be obscured by dense tissue or present as an ill-defined mass or asymmetry mammographically. It usually cannot be distinguished from malignancy. For lesions with typical benign features (fat-containing lymph node, hamartoma, etc.), no further assessment is needed. For those with a high probability of benignity (> 98%), follow-up is justified. In the other cases, which unfortunately constitute the large majority in young patients, biopsy remains necessary. However, the vast majority of these cases can be solved by percutaneous breast biopsy, mostly core needle biopsy.

As to detection and diagnosis of malignancy, many authors have reported a decreased sensitivity of mammography and a lower PPV for patients under 35 years of age.

The increased number of reported false positive calls is explained by the high prevalence of benign lesions (nodular breast tissue or fibroadenomas), where malignancy cannot be excluded because of their uncharacteristic appearance or overall high density (see **Fig. 24.52b,c**).

Mammographic false negative interpretations have mainly been attributed to two facts:
- Owing to the higher amount of glandular or dense breast tissue, carcinomas without microcalcifications may be obscured (**Fig. 24.53**).
- A relatively high percentage of carcinomas (15–20%) in young patients has been reported as having been misinterpreted as benign masses (like fibroadenomas) (see **Fig. 16.13c,d**) (Dawson et al. 1998, Foxcroft et al. 2004).

In spite of these problems, mammography is able to detect nonpalpable carcinomas even in young patients (see **Fig. 24.54**) (Ayyappan et al. 2010, Otto et al. 2012):
- In those younger patients (approximately 30%) who have fatty or mixed dense/fatty breast patterns, accuracy is comparable to that achieved in older patients.
- Detection of carcinomas presenting with suggestive microcalcifications is excellent in any breast type.

During pregnancy and lactation (Ayyappan et al. 2010, Taylor et al. 2011), mammographic evaluation, which is only indicated in symptomatic patients, is even more difficult than in the nonpregnant young patient. This is caused by further increase in density due to glandular proliferation, increased water content, and hyperemia. Even though numerous lesions can be obscured mammographically and benign lesions can only rarely be unequivocally diagnosed by mammography, mammography should be performed for all indeterminate or suspicious lesions; mostly because of its capability to image microcalcifications, a definite diagnosis of malignancy will be possible in at least some cases (**Fig. 24.55**). In these cases, mammography can accelerate the diagnosis of carcinoma instead of unnecessarily waiting for completion of pregnancy. In addition, in the case of suspected malignancy, further foci may be detected, which can be important for adequate treatment planning.

When mammography is applied in the young patient, it must be remembered that the potential risk of radiation is higher for younger patients than for older patients. Consideration of this potential increased risk of breast cancer is important when mammography is applied in asymptomatic patients. It is not important in those symptomatic patients whose symptoms cannot be explained by clinical or sonographic findings. Because of the low energy of the mammographically used X-rays, virtually no radiation will reach the fetus, particularly when the abdomen is shielded. Therefore, pregnancy is not a contraindication to mammography. To decrease mammographic density and thus improve mammographic evaluation during lactation, mammograms should be taken directly after breast-feeding.

Based on the above considerations and the experiences reported in the literature, the following recommendations are given for the *use of mammography*:
- *Routine mammographic screening is not advocated in the asymptomatic normal risk patient younger than 40 years* (Yankaskas et al. 2010).
- In women with a first-degree relative with premenopausal breast cancer and in women with positive genetic testing, with a history of Hodgkin disease, a prior breast cancer, and mediastinal irradiation, or with a high-risk lesion for breast biopsy, routine screening before age 40 is indicated. In women with a first-degree relative with breast cancer, screening should begin at an age 5 years younger than the cancer was diagnosed in that relative but not earlier than 25 years of age. In women treated for Hodgkin disease, screening should commence no later than 8 years after the completion of treatment (Dershaw et al. 1992).

Differential Diagnosis and Assessment

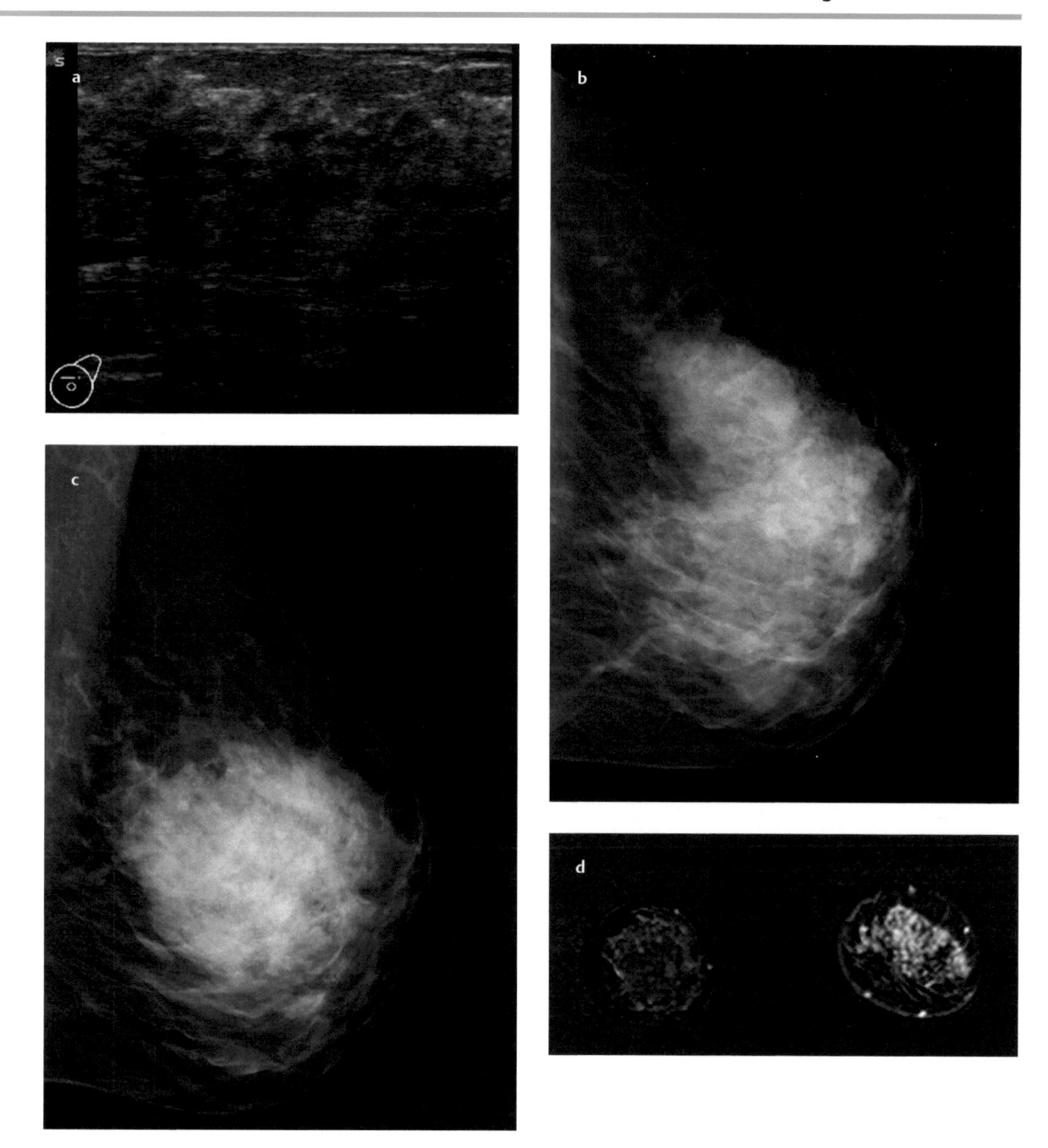

Fig. 24.51a–d A 39-year-old patient with very lumpy breasts presented with brownish nipple discharge on the left for 2 years. (Examination in an external breast center 1 year earlier for the same symptoms had resulted in a diagnosis of benign changes.)

- **a** The ultrasound scan shows echogenic tissue with hypoechoic ductal structures, homogeneously distributed throughout the left breast. No focal abnormality. Overall this is quite an uncharacteristic finding, which could indeed be compatible with benign changes.
- **b,c** Mammography (**b**, craniocaudal view; **c**, mediolateral oblique view) shows dense lumpy breast tissue, no mass, no microcalcifications and no significant asymmetry (compared with the contralateral side, not shown).
- **d** Magnetic resonance imaging was performed instead of galactography, since the nipple discharge came from multiple ducts. The subtraction series showed extended enhancement throughout the left breast. Based on these findings ultrasound-guided percutaneous breast biopsy was performed from multiple areas (fanning) and yielded an extensive noncalcified ductal carcinoma in situ (DCIS) grade 3. *Final histology*: Extended high-grade noncalcified DCIS of the left breast with microinvasion (pT1a, N0).

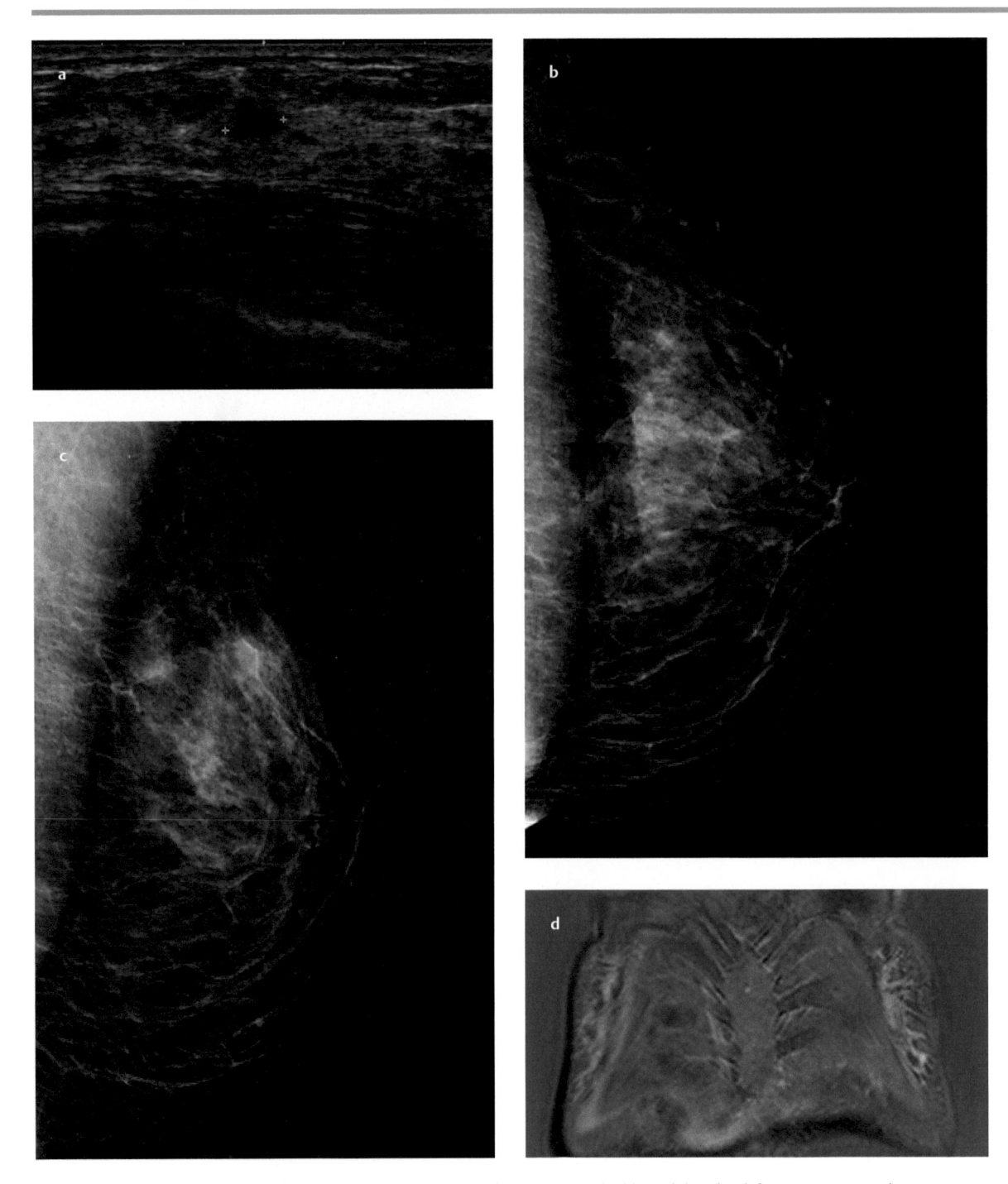

Fig. 24.52a–d This 31-year-old patient presented with a small uncharacteristic palpable nodule in her left upper outer quadrant (moderate family history of breast cancer).

- **a** Ultrasound revealed an ill-circumscribed hypoechoic area of 5–7 mm in diameter.
- **b,c** Mammographically the small lesion is obscured by dense tissue (ACR3). No microcalcifications. The nodularity seen in the upper quadrant on the mediolateral oblique view (**b**) resolves on the craniocaudal view (**c**) and is uncharacteristic.
- **d** Since percutaneous breast biopsy had revealed an invasive ductal carcinoma (G2), magnetic resonance imaging was performed to exclude multicentricity. Owing to diffuse, patchy, bilateral enhancement, assessment was impaired and the lesion was not visible. Four years after breast conservation (wide excision of a unifocal cancer) there is no sign of further lesions. (Subtraction image of the representative slice is shown.) The proven carcinoma exhibits an uncharacteristic morphology and enhancement curve (plateau-type). No further suspicious lesion was noted. *Histology*: Invasive ductal carcinoma G2.

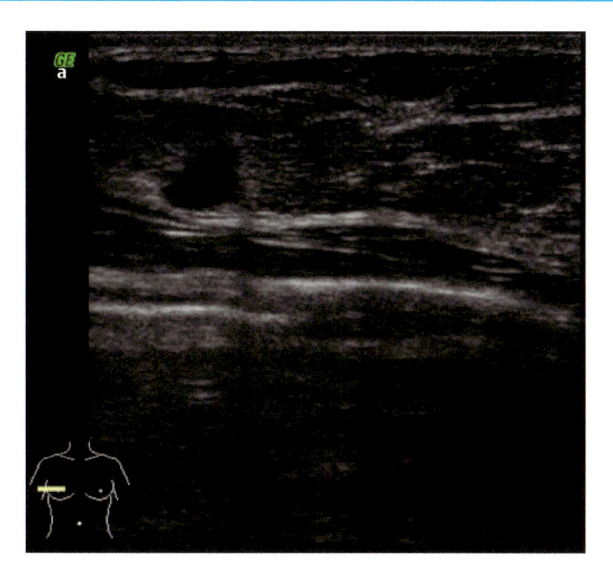

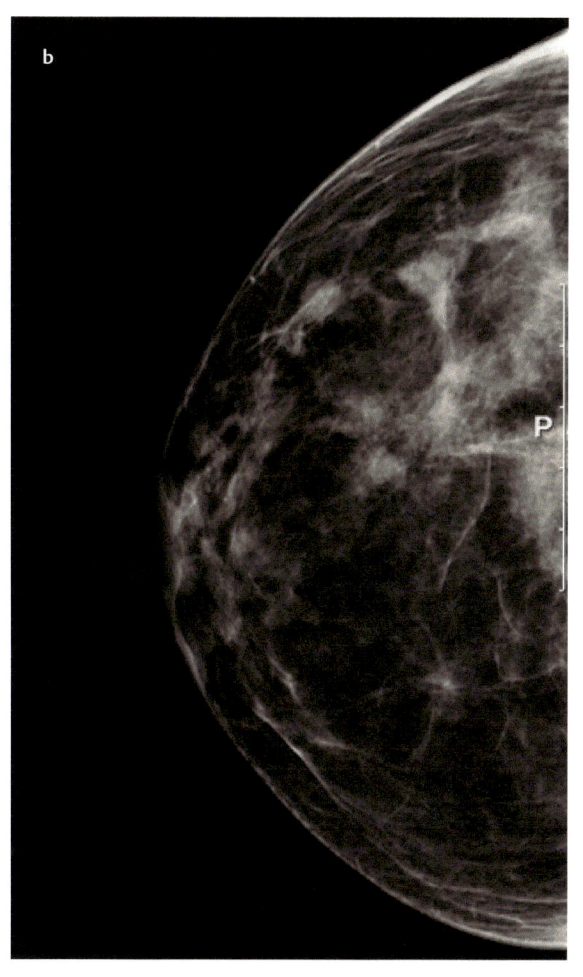

Differential Diagnosis and Assessment

Fig. 24.53a,b Breast cancer in young patients.

A 35-year-old patient with a strong family history of breast cancer presented with a palpable mobile nodule of about 8 mm in her right upper outer quadrant.
a Even though the mass was mobile, ultrasound revealed an ill-defined roundish mass with a slightly hyperechoic rim. Based on the ultrasound findings, biopsy was indicated.
b On mammography (craniocaudal view) the nodule corresponded to an uncharacteristic nodular density within overall nodular asymmetrically distributed breast tissue (ACR2).
Percutaneous breast biopsy revealed a 7-mm invasive ductal carcinoma G3, ER/PR negative, Her2neu 3+. An additional magnetic resonance image showed no further foci. Subsequent testing proved a *BRCA1* mutation.

- Considering the high prevalence of benign problems (e.g., cysts) that can at least partly be solved by ultrasound scanning, *in symptomatic patients mammography should be used after sonography.*
- In all symptomatic patients whose finding cannot unequivocally be explained as a sonographically typical benign lesion (cyst, galactocele, freely moveable typical benign solid mass as defined on pp. 120–123, mammography is strongly recommended, since in some cases mammography may prove the only method able to correctly detect and diagnose a malignancy by visualization of suspicious microcalcifications, architectural distortion, or sometimes even a suspicious mass (e.g., within larger breasts or fatty tissue).
- The previous recommendation also applies to symptomatic patients during pregnancy. Pregnancy is no contraindication to mammography. Shielding should be used in these patients, and the patients should be adequately informed and reassured.
- In the case of *absent mammographic findings in dense tissue or potentially benign mammographic findings*, a negative mammogram should not dissuade the clinician from *further workup* of suspicious or indeterminate clinical findings.

Sonography

In view of the difficulties surrounding mammographic detection and diagnosis of breast cancer in the young patient, sonography has been proposed as the method of choice. Indeed, the use of sonography is recommended as the first method for the workup of symptomatic patients below the age of 35 years. The reasons are as follows:
- As sonography is not associated with any radiation, it is completely harmless for the patient.
- In the case of a simple cyst, a definitive diagnosis is possible by sonography, and no further workup is necessary.
- In patients with mammographically dense tissue, a hypoechoic suspicious mass detected in an area of an indeterminate palpable finding supports the diagnosis of malignancy and immediate further workup (**Figs. 24.52a** and **24.53a**)

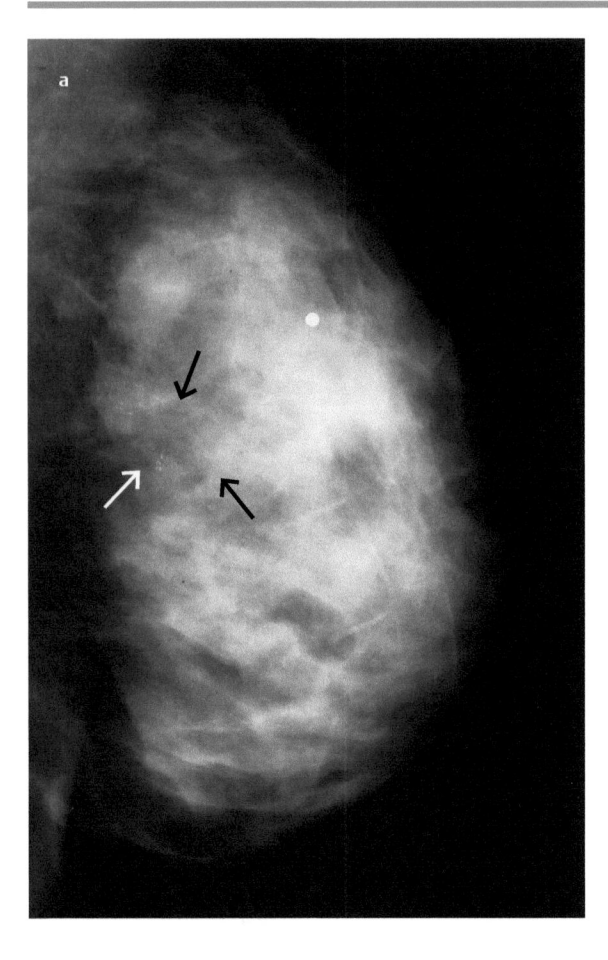

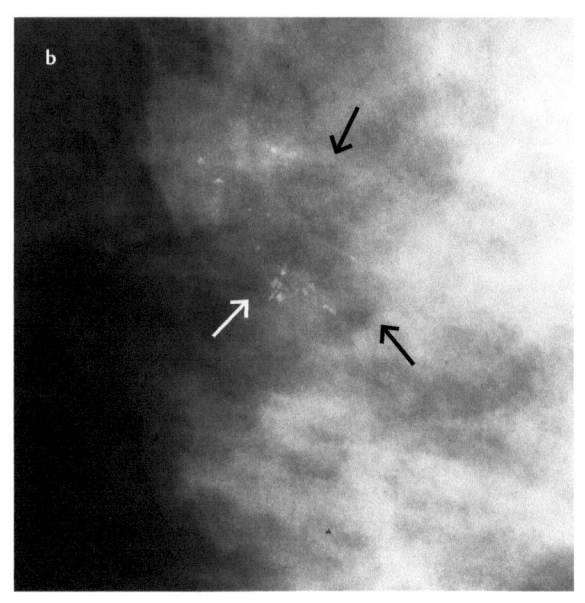

Fig. 24.54a,b Breast cancer in young patients.
A 22-year-old patient who presented with bone metastases. Search for primary tumor revealed mammographically suggestive microcalcifications, which are excellently seen in spite of the dense tissue: oblique view (**a**); magnification of the area of microcalcifications (**b**).

- In the pregnant or lactating patient, a galactocele can be suspected if a hypoechoic lesion shows fluctuation of the echoes with palpation or if septations are seen (**Fig. 11.4**). The diagnosis can easily be established by aspiration of milk.

As with mammography, many of the benign and malignant lesions unfortunately exhibit a wide range of sonographic findings and considerably overlap in their sonographic appearance (**Fig. 16.13; Figs. 24.51a and 24.52a**).

Juvenile papillomatosis can present as a hypoechoic mass, which can be more or less well circumscribed or can resemble a fibroadenoma. With high-resolution sonography, numerous, mostly small cysts and dilated ducts may be visible within the lesion (so-called typical Swiss cheese appearance) that can be a hint to this diagnosis (**Fig. 24.50**). Since cystic spaces can also be encountered with fibrocystic changes and in phyllodes tumors, this appearance cannot be considered pathognomonic, and further workup remains necessary. Breast infarct presumably will present as an indeterminate hypoechoic, hyperechoic, or complex mass of mixed echogenicity with or without attenuation and therefore cannot be distinguished from malignancy.

Overall, the sonographic appearance cannot be considered sufficiently characteristic for the majority of solid lesions to warrant a final diagnosis. Workup must be continued:
- If the above-mentioned criteria of a simple cyst or typical fibroadenoma are not fulfilled
- If there are no sonographic findings

As with older women, the general limitations of sonography concerning the detection of small and preinvasive carcinomas also apply to younger patients (see Chapter 4). Sonographic differentiation between benign and malignant masses is usually not reliable (see **Fig. 16.13**).

Percutaneous Biopsy

Percutaneous biopsy appears a most valuable adjunct, particularly in young patients with indeterminate changes. Its increased use may help to both avoid a large number of diagnostic excisional biopsies and decrease the cases with a delayed diagnosis.

Owing to the widely varying sensitivity of fine needle aspiration, CNB or VABB (in case of microcalcifications or other small lesions visible by mammography only) may be the more appropriate procedure at most facilities.

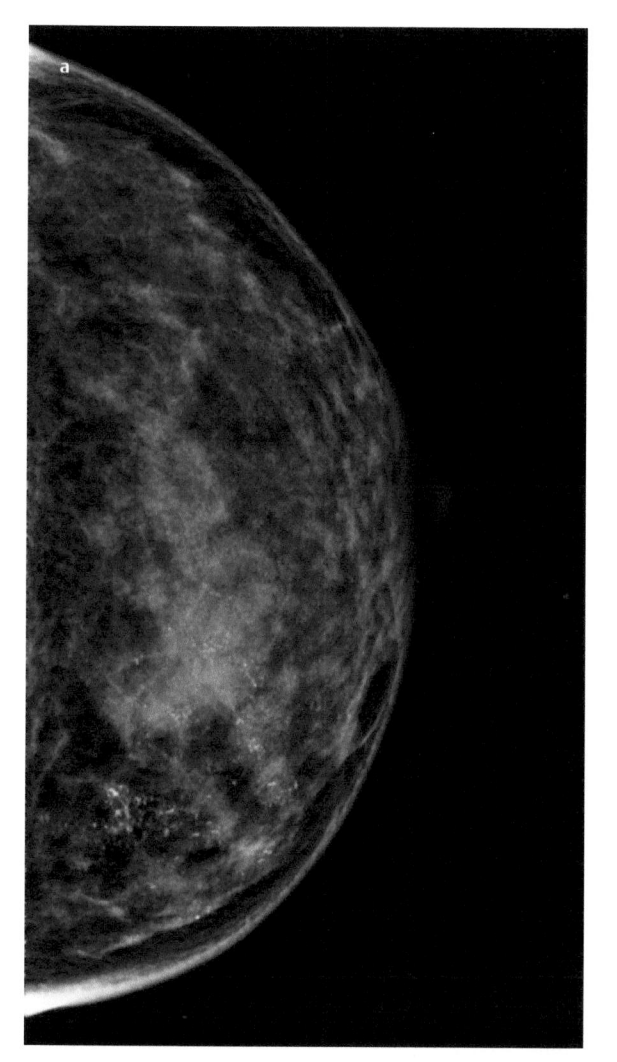

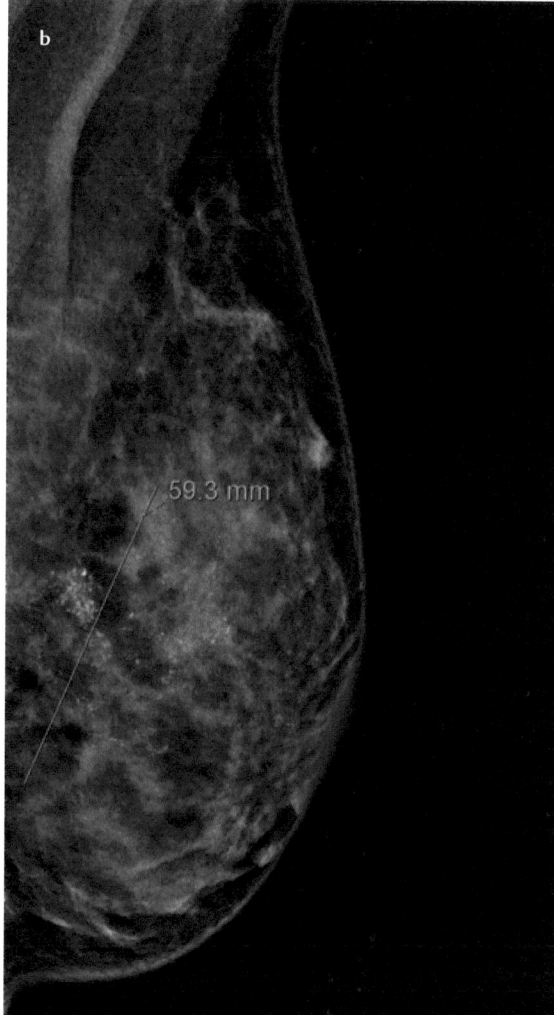

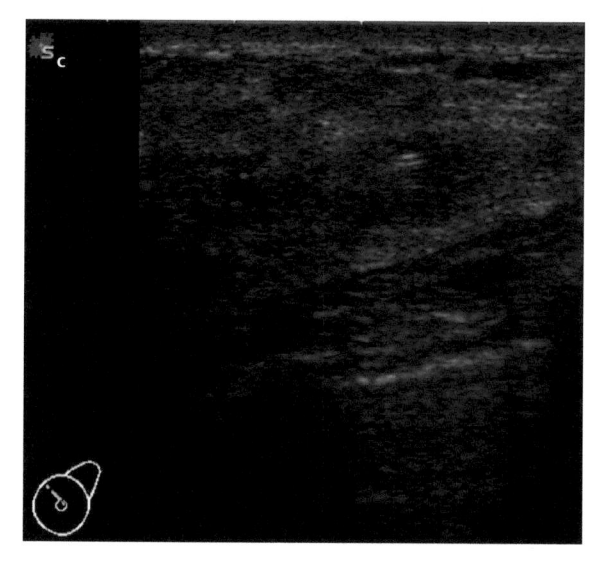

Fig. 24.55a–c This 34-year-old patient presented for a checkup without any clinical findings. Her sister had been affected by an inflammatory breast cancer 2 years before at age 35.

Owing to the positive family history mammography, ultrasound, and magnetic resonance imaging were recommended to her. Mammography revealed extended areas of suspicious microcalcifications (**a,b**). Since there was no ultrasound finding (**c**), histopathologic assessment was performed using stereotactic vacuum-assisted breast biopsy, which yielded an extended ductal carcinoma in situ (DCIS) grade 3.

Based on the family history and the extended microcalcifications, the patient underwent skin-sparing mastectomy, which revealed extended DCIS grade 3 and two unexpected foci of invasive breast cancer of 13 mm and 5 mm in diameter. The patient opted against genetic testing.

This case demonstrates both the value of mammography in women at high risk and the limitations of all imaging modalities compared to final histology.

Sufficient material must be obtained, and the results of percutaneous biopsy must be counterchecked with the clinical and imaging findings.

In the event of indeterminate results, insufficient material, or results that are not concordant with imaging findings, repeat biopsy must be undertaken.

During pregnancy or lactation, an increased tendency to bleed exists due to physiologic hyperemia. This can usually be taken care of by firm compression, even during the procedure. The authors are not aware of any reports concerning an increased risk of infection or milk fistulas, as reported for surgical biopsy. However, it may be best taken care of by cessation of breast-feeding before biopsy (Harris et al. 1991). The radiologist should be aware of the possibility of fistula formation if biopsy of a galactocele is attempted.

Magnetic Resonance Imaging

Contrast-enhanced MRI is not indicated as a screening method for young patients with dense or lumpy breast tissue. The reasons are as follows:
- MRI has a high sensitivity for detection of occult benign changes (e.g., fibroadenomas, areas of adenosis) in at least 15% of patients.
- Areas of transient enhancement due to hormonal influences, which may be another cause of false positive calls, may be more frequent in this age group.
- At the same time, the prevalance of malignancy is by far lower than that of benign disease.

Therefore, contrast-enhanced MRI might necessitate an unacceptably high number of workups for benign changes in young patients without high genetic risk, while detecting very few, if any, malignancies.

Finally, MRI is generally not necessary for evaluation of palpable, mammographically or sonographically visible masses, since percutaneous biopsy—owing to its lower false positive rate —is much more cost-effective.

Contrast-enhanced MRI for early detection of malignancy is, however, indicated for screening of young women at high-risk, who (after diligent counseling) opt for imaging surveillance. (For definition of this very limited group, see Chapters 1 and 5; imaging of women at high risk, see Chapter 5). Considering that both mammography and MRI may offer complementary information while neither method alone has 100% sensitivity, alternating screening using MRI and mammography every 6 months may be the most effective alternative (Lowry et al. 2012).

Diagnostic Strategy

Based on the different situations concerning the prevalence of breast cancer and the capabilities of each method, and based on different estimations of potential radiation hazards in this age group, the following diagnostic strategy should be adopted:
- Screening is not recommended for asymptomatic patients without significantly increased risk.
- The definition of a high-risk situation should be made by specialists (geneticists) based on genetic testing and algorithms based on family history and individual risk factors. Before imaging surveillance is offered the patient should be informed about possibilities, limitations and potential side effects of imaging surveillance as compared to primary prevention (mastectomy, ovarectomy; see Chapters 1 and 5).
- In high-risk patients, screening mammography is presently recommended at yearly intervals starting from age 30. Yearly MRI is recommended (starting from age 25–30 (depending on the national program) up to about age 55. The additional use of ultrasound (every 6 months) is recommended only in the German program (based on expert opinion).
- For the evaluation of palpable masses in patients under 40 years of age, sonography should be used first. If a benign diagnosis can be made with a high degree of accuracy, no further workup is necessary, and follow-up is sufficient.
- In all other cases, a mammogram should follow. A single-view mammogram for detection of microcalcifications may be sufficient. Additional views should be obtained as needed.
- Pregnancy or lactation is no contraindication to mammography. During lactation, mammography should be performed immediately after breast-feeding because the breast density is lower than before breast-feeding. Based on its capability to visualize suspicious microcalcifications, mammography, even in very dense breasts, can help to avoid a delay in diagnosis or may be able to detect additional foci. It should therefore be used whenever indicated.
- In all cases with negative or benign-appearing findings with imaging, the diagnosis must be critically correlated with the clinical findings. In view of the limited sensitivity of all modalities in young patients, percutaneous biopsy should be generously used in case of any doubt.
- As usual, percutaneous biopsy has to be performed diligently and its results critically checked to determine whether the diagnosis is appropriate for the imaging and clinical findings.

References and Recommended Reading

Albert US, Altland H, Duda V, et al. 2008 update of the guideline: early detection of breast cancer in Germany. J Cancer Res Clin Oncol 2009;135(3):339–354

Alleva DQ, Smetherman DH, Farr GH Jr, Cederbom GJ. Radial scar of the breast: radiologic-pathologic correlation in 22 cases. Radiographics 1999;19(Spec No):S27–S35, discussion S36–S37

Ayyappan AP, Kulkarni S, Crystal P. Pregnancy-associated breast cancer: spectrum of imaging appearances. Br J Radiol 2010;83(990):529–534

Ballesio L, Maggi C, Savelli S, et al. Role of breast magnetic resonance imaging (MRI) in patients with unilateral nipple discharge: preliminary study. Radiol Med (Torino) 2008;113(2):249–264

Bazzocchi F, Santini D, Martinelli G, et al. Juvenile papillomatosis (epitheliosis) of the breast. A clinical and pathologic study of 13 cases. Am J Clin Pathol 1986;86(6):745–748

Bebb G, Glickman B, Gelmon K, Gatti R. "AT risk" for breast cancer. Lancet 1997;349(9068):1784–1785

Berg WA, Blume JD, Cormack JB, et al; ACRIN 6666 Investigators. Combined screening with ultrasound and mammography vs mammography alone in women at elevated risk of breast cancer. JAMA 2008;299(18):2151–2163

Berg WA, Gutierrez L, NessAiver MS, et al. Diagnostic accuracy of mammography, clinical examination, US, and MR imaging in preoperative assessment of breast cancer. Radiology 2004;233(3):830–849

Bernard JR Jr, Vallow LA, DePeri ER, et al. In newly diagnosed breast cancer, screening MRI of the contralateral breast detects mammographically occult cancer, even in elderly women: the Mayo Clinic in Florida experience. Breast J 2010;16(2):118–126

Bird RE, Wallace TW, Yankaskas BC. Analysis of cancers missed at screening mammography. Radiology 1992;184(3):613–617

Blaker KM, Sahoo S, Schweichler MR, Chagpar AB. Malignant phylloides tumor in pregnancy. Am Surg 2010;76(3):302–305

Bluemke DA, Gatsonis CA, Chen MH, et al. Magnetic resonance imaging of the breast prior to biopsy. JAMA 2004;292(22):2735–2742

Boetes C, Strijk SP, Holland R, Barentsz JO, Van Der Sluis RF, Ruijs JH. False-negative MR imaging of malignant breast tumors. Eur Radiol 1997;7(8):1231–1234

Bouté V, Goyat I, Denoux Y, Lacroix J, Marie B, Michels JJ. Are the criteria of Tabar and Dean still relevant to radial scar? Eur J Radiol 2006;60(2):243–249

Brenner RJ, Fajardo L, Fisher PR, et al. Percutaneous core biopsy of the breast: effect of operator experience and number of samples on diagnostic accuracy. AJR Am J Roentgenol 1996;166(2):341–346

Britton PD, Provenzano E, Barter S, et al. Ultrasound guided percutaneous axillary lymph node core biopsy: how often is the sentinel lymph node being biopsied? Breast 2009;18(1):13–16

Ciatto S, Rosselli del Turco M, Catarzi S, Morrone D, Bonardi R. The diagnostic role of breast echography. [Article in Italian] Radiol Med (Torino) 1994;88(3):221–224

Dawson AE, Mulford DK, Taylor AS, Logan-Young W. Breast carcinoma detection in women age 35 years and younger: mammography and diagnosis by fine-needle aspiration cytology. Cancer 1998;84(3):163–168

DeMartini W, Lehman C, Partridge S. Breast MRI for cancer detection and characterization: a review of evidence-based clinical applications. Acad Radiol 2008;15(4):408–416

Den Otter W, Merchant TE, Beijerinck D, Koten JW. Breast cancer induction due to mammographic screening in hereditarily affected women. Anticancer Res 1996;16(5B):3173–3175

Dennis MA, Parker SH, Klaus AJ, Stavros AT, Kaske TI, Clark SB. Breast biopsy avoidance: the value of normal mammograms and normal sonograms in the setting of a palpable lump. Radiology 2001;219(1):186–191

Dershaw DD, Yahalom J, Petrek JA. Breast carcinoma in women previously treated for Hodgkin disease: mammographic evaluation. Radiology 1992;184(2):421–423

Eby PR, Demartini WB, Peacock S, Rosen EL, Lauro B, Lehman CD. Cancer yield of probably benign breast MR examinations. J Magn Reson Imaging 2007;26(4):950–955

Egyed Z, Péntek Z, Járay B, et al. Radial scar-significant diagnostic challenge. Pathol Oncol Res 2008;14(2):123–129

Facius M, Renz DM, Neubauer H, et al. Characteristics of ductal carcinoma in situ in magnetic resonance imaging. Clin Imaging 2007;31(6):394–400

Ferguson TB Jr, McCarty KS Jr, Filston HC. Juvenile secretory carcinoma and juvenile papillomatosis: diagnosis and treatment. J Pediatr Surg 1987;22(7):637–639

Foxcroft LM, Evans EB, Porter AJ. The diagnosis of breast cancer in women younger than 40. Breast 2004;13(4):297–306

Gajdos C, Tartter PI, Bleiweiss IJ, Bodian C, Brower ST. Stage 0 to stage III breast cancer in young women. J Am Coll Surg 2000;190(5):523–529

Gillett D, Kennedy C, Carmalt H. Breast cancer in young women. Aust N Z J Surg 1997;67(11):761–764

Gorins A, Lenhardt F, Espie M. Breast cancer during pregnancy. Epidemiology—diagnosis—prognosis. [Article in French] Contracept Fertil Sex 1996;24(2):153–156

Graf O, Helbich TH, Fuchsjaeger MH, et al. Follow-up of palpable circumscribed noncalcified solid breast masses at mammography and US: can biopsy be averted? Radiology 2004;233(3):850–856

Grunwald S, Heyer H, Kühl A, et al. Radial scar/complex sclerosing lesion of the breast—value of ultrasound. Ultraschall Med 2007;28(2):206–211

Gutierrez RL, DeMartini WB, Eby PR, Kurland BF, Peacock S, Lehman CD. BI-RADS lesion characteristics predict likelihood of malignancy in breast MRI for masses but not for nonmasslike enhancement. AJR Am J Roentgenol 2009;193(4):994–1000

Harris JR, Hellman S, Henderson C, Kinne DW. Breast Diseases. 2nd ed. Philadelphia: JB Lippincott; 1991

Harvey JA, Fajardo LL, Innis CA. Previous mammograms in patients with impalpable breast carcinoma: retrospective vs blinded interpretation. 1993 ARRS President's Award. AJR Am J Roentgenol 1993;161(6):1167–1172

Heywang-Köbrunner SH, Bick U, Bradley WG Jr, et al. International investigation of breast MRI: results of a multicentre study (11 sites) concerning diagnostic parameters for contrast-enhanced MRI based on 519 histopathologically correlated lesions. Eur Radiol 2001;11(4):531–546

Heywang-Köbrunner SH, Schreer I, Heindel W, Katalinic A. Imaging studies for the early detection of breast cancer. Dtsch Arztebl Int 2008;105(31–32):541–547

Heywang-Köbrunner SH, Viehweg P, Heinig A, Küchler C. Contrast-enhanced MRI of the breast: accuracy, value, controversies, solutions. Eur J Radiol 1997;24(2):94–108

Hong AS, Rosen EL, Soo MS, Baker JA. BI-RADS for sonography: positive and negative predictive values of sonographic features. AJR Am J Roentgenol 2005;184(4):1260–1265

Hrung JM, Sonnad SS, Schwartz JS, Langlotz CP. Accuracy of MR imaging in the work-up of suspicious breast lesions: a diagnostic meta-analysis. Acad Radiol 1999;6(7):387–397

Hwang ES, Kinkel K, Esserman LJ, Lu Y, Weidner N, Hylton NM. Magnetic resonance imaging in patients diagnosed with ductal carcinoma-in-situ: value in the diagnosis of residual disease, occult invasion, and multicentricity. Ann Surg Oncol 2003;10(4):381–388

Institute for Clinical Systems Improvement. Health Care Guideline: Diagnosis of Breast Disease 2012 www.icsi.org

Jackson VP, Dines KA, Bassett LW, Gold RH, Reynolds HE. Diagnostic importance of the radiographic density of noncalcified breast masses: analysis of 91 lesions. AJR Am J Roentgenol 1991;157(1):25–28

Kerlikowske K, Grady D, Barclay J, Sickles EA, Eaton A, Ernster V. Positive predictive value of screening mammography by age and family history of breast cancer. JAMA 1993;270(20):2444–2450

Kneeshaw PJ, Turnbull LW, Smith A, Drew PJ. Dynamic contrast enhanced magnetic resonance imaging aids the surgical management of invasive lobular breast cancer. Eur J Surg Oncol. 2003;29(1):32–37

Kushwaha AC, Whitman GJ, Stelling CB, Cristofanilli M, Buzdar AU. Primary inflammatory carcinoma of the breast: retrospective review of mammographic findings. AJR Am J Roentgenol 2000;174(2):535–538

Lee CH, Dershaw DD, Kopans D, et al. Breast cancer screening with imaging: recommendations from the Society of Breast Imaging and the ACR on the use of mammography, breast MRI, breast ultrasound, and other technologies for the detection of clinically occult breast cancer. J Am Coll Radiol 2010;7(1):18–27

Lee E, Wylie E, Metcalf C. Ultrasound imaging features of radial scars of the breast. Australas Radiol 2007;51(3):240–245

Liberman L, Mason G, Morris EA, Dershaw DD. Does size matter? Positive predictive value of MRI-detected breast lesions as a function of lesion size. AJR Am J Roentgenol 2006;186(2):426–430

Liberman L, Morris EA, Benton CL, Abramson AF, Dershaw DD. Probably benign lesions at breast magnetic resonance imaging: preliminary experience in high-risk women. Cancer 2003;98(2):377–388

Linda A, Zuiani C, Furlan A, et al. Radial scars without atypia diagnosed at imaging-guided needle biopsy: how often is associated malignancy found at subsequent surgical excision, and do mammography and sonography predict which lesions are malignant? AJR Am J Roentgenol 2010;194(4):1146–1151

Lord SJ, Lei W, Craft P, et al. A systematic review of the effectiveness of magnetic resonance imaging (MRI) as an addition to mammography and ultrasound in screening young women at high risk of breast cancer. Eur J Cancer 2007;43(13):1905–1917

Lowry KP, Lee JM, Kong CY, et al. Annual screening strategies in BRCA1 and BRCA2 gene mutation carriers: a comparative effectiveness analysis. Cancer 2012;118(8):2021–2030

Mainiero MB, Goldkamp A, Lazarus E, et al. Characterization of breast masses with sonography: can biopsy of some solid masses be deferred? J Ultrasound Med 2005;24(2):161–167

Meissnitzer M, Dershaw DD, Lee CH, Morris EA. Targeted ultrasound of the breast in women with abnormal MRI findings for whom biopsy has been recommended. AJR Am J Roentgenol 2009;193(4):1025–1029

Mendelson EB. Problem-solving ultrasound. Radiol Clin North Am 2004;42(5):909–918, vii

Menell JH, Morris EA, Dershaw DD, Abramson AF, Brogi E, Liberman L. Determination of the presence and extent of pure ductal carcinoma in situ by mammography and magnetic resonance imaging. Breast J 2005;11(6):382–390

Morrogh M, Morris EA, Liberman L, Van Zee K, Cody HS III, King TA. MRI identifies otherwise occult disease in select patients with Paget disease of the nipple. J Am Coll Surg 2008;206(2):316–321

Moy L, Noz ME, Maguire GQ Jr, et al. Role of fusion of prone FDG-PET and magnetic resonance imaging of the breasts in the evaluation of breast cancer. Breast J 2010;16(4):369–376

Nakahara H, Namba K, Watanabe R, et al. A comparison of MR imaging, galactography and ultrasonography in patients with nipple discharge. Breast Cancer 2003;10(4):320–329

National Breast Cancer Centre. Magnetic resonance imaging for the early detection of breast cancer in women at high risk: a systematic review of the evidence. Camperdown, NSW: NBCC; 2006

National Institute for Health and Clinical Excellence. Clinical Guideline 41. Familial Breast Cancer: the classification and care of women at risk of familial breast cancer in primary, secondary and tertiary care. London: National Institute for Health and Clinical Excellence; 2006

NCCN Clinical Practice Guidelines in Oncology. Breast Cancer Screening and Diagnosis Guidelines V.I 2008 www.nccn.org

Nonomura A, Kimura A, Mizukami Y, et al. Secretory carcinoma of the breast associated with juvenile papillomatosis in a 12-year-old girl. A case report. Acta Cytol 1995;39(3):569–576

Nothacker M, Duda V, Hahn M, et al. Early detection of breast cancer: benefits and risks of supplemental breast ultrasound in asymptomatic women with mammographically dense breast tissue. A systematic review. BMC Cancer 2009;9:335–344

Otto SJ, Fracheboud J, Verbeek AL, et al; National Evaluation Team for Breast Cancer Screening. Mammography screening and risk of breast cancer death: a population-based case-control study. Cancer Epidemiol Biomarkers Prev 2012;21(1):66–73

Pediconi F, Occhiato R, Venditti F, et al. Radial scars of the breast: contrast-enhanced magnetic resonance mammography appearance. Breast J 2005;11(1):23–28

Perfetto F, Fiorentino F, Urbano F, Silecchia R. Adjunctive diagnostic value of MRI in the breast radial scar. Radiol Med (Torino) 2009;114(5):757–770

Perry N, Broeders M, de Wolf C, Toernberg S, Holland R, von Karsa L, eds. European Guidelines for Quality Assurance in Breast Screening an Diagnosis. Luxembourg: Office for Official Publications of the European Communities; 2006: 221–56

Peters NH, Borel Rinkes IH, Zuithoff NP, Mali WP, Moons KG, Peeters PH. Meta-analysis of MR imaging in the diagnosis of breast lesions. Radiology 2008;246(1):116–124

Pollán M. Epidemiology of breast cancer in young women. Breast Cancer Res Treat 2010;123(Suppl 1):3–6

Raza S, Goldkamp AL, Chikarmane SA, Birdwell RL. US of breast masses categorized as BI-RADS 3, 4, and 5: pictorial review of factors influencing clinical management. Radiographics 2010;30(5):1199–1213

Reintgen D, Berman C, Cox C, et al. The anatomy of missed breast cancers. Surg Oncol 1993;2(1):65–75

Ries LAG, Melbert D, Krapcho M, et al, Eds. SEER Cancer Statistics Review, 1975–2005. Bethesda, MD: National Cancer Institute; 2008

Roelofs AA, Karssemeijer N, Wedekind N, et al. Importance of comparison of current and prior mammograms in breast cancer screening. Radiology 2007;242(1):70–77

Rosen EL, Smith-Foley SA, DeMartini WB, Eby PR, Peacock S, Lehman CD. BI-RADS MRI enhancement characteristics of ductal carcinoma in situ. Breast J 2007;13(6):545–550

Rosen PP, Kimmel M. Juvenile papillomatosis of the breast. A follow-up study of 41 patients having biopsies before 1979. Am J Clin Pathol 1990;93(5):599–603

Rosenberg RD, Hunt WC, Williamson MR, et al. Effects of age, breast density, ethnicity, and estrogen replacement therapy on screening mammographic sensitivity and cancer stage at diagnosis: review of 183,134 screening mammograms in Albuquerque, New Mexico. Radiology 1998;209(2):511–518

Saarenmaa I, Salminen T, Geiger U, et al. The visibility of cancer on earlier mammograms in a population-based screening programme. Eur J Cancer 1999;35(7):1118–1122

Sabate JM, Clotet M, Torrubia S, et al. Radiologic evaluation of breast disorders related to pregnancy and lactation. Radiographics 2007;27(Suppl 1):S101–S124

Sardanelli F, Boetes C, Borisch B, et al. Magnetic resonance imaging of the breast: recommendations from the EUSOMA working group. Eur J Cancer 2010;46(8):1296–1316

Saslow D, Boetes C, Burke W, et al; American Cancer Society Breast Cancer Advisory Group. American Cancer Society guidelines for breast screening with MRI as an adjunct to mammography. CA Cancer J Clin 2007;57(2):75–89

Schelfout K, Van Goethem M, Kersschot E, et al. Preoperative breast MRI in patients with invasive lobular breast cancer. Eur Radiol 2004;14(7):1209–1216

Schmutzler R, Schlegelberger B, Meindl A, et al. Spezielle Strategie – familiäre Belastung. In: Schulz KD, Albert U (Hrsg). Stufe 3 Leitlinie. Brustkrebsfrüherkennung in Deutschland. 1. Aktualisierung 2008. Munich: W. Zuckschwerdt Verlag; 2008: 237

Schnall MD, Blume J, Bluemke DA, et al. Diagnostic architectural and dynamic features at breast MR imaging: multicenter study. Radiology 2006;238(1):42–53

Schouten van der Velden AP, Boetes C, Bult P, Wobbes T. The value of magnetic resonance imaging in diagnosis and size assessment of in situ and small invasive breast carcinoma. Am J Surg 2006;192(2):172–178

Schwartz GF, Hughes KS, Lynch HT, et al; Consensus Conference Committee. Proceedings of the international consensus conference on breast cancer risk, genetics, & risk management, April, 2007. Breast J 2009;15(1):4–16

Sharan SK, Morimatsu M, Albrecht U, et al. Embryonic lethality and radiation hypersensitivity mediated by Rad51 in mice lacking Brca2. Nature 1997;386(6627):804–810

Shin HJ, Kim HH, Kim SM, et al. Papillary lesions of the breast diagnosed at percutaneous sonographically guided biopsy: comparison of sonographic features and biopsy methods. AJR Am J Roentgenol 2008;190(3):630–636

Shiraishi A, Kurosaki Y, Maehara T, Suzuki M, Kurosumi M. Extension of ductal carcinoma in situ: histopathological association with MR imaging and mammography. Magn Reson Med Sci 2003;2(4):159–163

Sickles EA. Nonpalpable, circumscribed, noncalcified solid breast masses: likelihood of malignancy based on lesion size and age of patient. Radiology 1994;192(2):439–442

Skaane P, Engedal K. Analysis of sonographic features in the differentiation of fibroadenoma and invasive ductal carcinoma. AJR Am J Roentgenol 1998;170(1):109–114

Skaane P, Sauer T. Ultrasonography of malignant breast neoplasms. Analysis of carcinomas missed as tumor. Acta Radiol 1999;40(4):376–382

Skaane P. The additional value of US to mammography in the diagnosis of breast cancer. A prospective study. Acta Radiol 1999;40(5):486–490

Skandarajah AR, Field L, Yuen Larn Mou A, et al. Benign papilloma on core biopsy requires surgical excision. Ann Surg Oncol 2008;15(8):2272–2277

Soo MS, Rosen EL, Baker JA, Vo TT, Boyd BA. Negative predictive value of sonography with mammography in patients with palpable breast lesions. AJR Am J Roentgenol 2001;177(5):1167–1170

Stavros AT, Thickman D, Rapp CL, Dennis MA, Parker SH, Sisney GA. Solid breast nodules: use of sonography to distinguish between benign and malignant lesions. Radiology 1995;196(1):123–134

Stavros AT. Breast Ultrasound. Philadelphia: Lippincott Williams and Wilkins; 2003

Sumkin JH, Holbert BL, Herrmann JS, et al. Optimal reference mammography: a comparison of mammograms obtained 1 and 2 years before the present examination. AJR Am J Roentgenol 2003;180(2):343–346

Swayampakula AK, Dillis C, Abraham J. Role of MRI in screening, diagnosis and management of breast cancer. Expert Rev Anticancer Ther 2008;8(5):811–817

Tabár L, Fagerberg G, Day NE, Duffy SW, Kitchin RM. Breast cancer treatment and natural history: new insights from results of screening. Lancet 1992;339(8790):412–414

Taylor D, Lazberger J, Ives A, Wylie E, Saunders C. Reducing delay in the diagnosis of pregnancy-associated breast cancer: how imaging can help us. J Med Imaging Radiat Oncol 2011;55(1):33–42

Thurfjell MG, Vitak B, Azavedo E, Svane G, Thurfjell E. Effect on sensitivity and specificity of mammography screening with or without comparison of old mammograms. Acta Radiol 2000;41(1):52–56

Trecate G, Tess JD, Vergnaghi D, et al. Lobular breast cancer: how useful is breast magnetic resonance imaging? Tumori 2001;87(4):232–238

Tse GM, Tan PH. Diagnosing breast lesions by fine needle aspiration cytology or core biopsy: which is better? Breast Cancer Res Treat 2010;123(1):1–8

Uematsu T, Yuen S, Kasami M, Uchida Y. Dynamic contrast-enhanced MR imaging in screening detected microcalcification lesions of the breast: is there any value? Breast Cancer Res Treat 2007;103(3):269–281

van Gils CH, Otten JD, Verbeek AL, Hendriks JH, Holland R. Effect of mammographic breast density on breast cancer screening performance: a study in Nijmegen, the Netherlands. J Epidemiol Community Health 1998;52(4):267–271

Van Goethem M, Schelfout K, Kersschot E, et al. Comparison of MRI features of different grades of DCIS and invasive carcinoma of the breast. JBR-BTR 2005;88(5):225–232

Varela C, Karssemeijer N, Hendriks JH, Holland R. Use of prior mammograms in the classification of benign and malignant masses. Eur J Radiol 2005;56(2):248–255

Wagner TD, Wharton K, Donohue K, et al. Pure tubular breast carcinoma: a 34 year study of outcomes. Breast J 2008;14(5):512–513

Warner E, Messersmith H, Causer P, Eisen A, Shumak R, Plewes D. Systematic review: using magnetic resonance imaging to screen women at high risk for breast cancer. Ann Intern Med 2008;148(9):671–679

Weinstein SP, Hanna LG, Gatsonis C, Schnall MD, Rosen MA, Lehman CD. Frequency of malignancy seen in probably benign lesions at contrast-enhanced breast MR imaging: findings from ACRIN 6667. Radiology 2010;255(3):731–737

Winchester DP. Breast cancer in young women. Surg Clin North Am 1996;76(2):279–287

Wojcinski S, Farrokh A, Weber S, et al. Multicenter study of ultrasound real-time tissue elastography in 779 cases for the assessment of breast lesions: improved diagnostic performance by combining the BI-RADS®-US classification system with sonoelastography. Ultraschall Med 2010;31(5):484–491

Yankaskas BC, Haneuse S, Kapp JM, Kerlikowske K, Geller B, Buist DS; Breast Cancer Surveillance Consortium. Performance of first mammography examination in women younger than 40 years. J Natl Cancer Inst 2010;102(10):692–701

Index

Note: Illustrations are comprehensively referred to in the text. Therefore, significant material in illustrations has usually been given a page reference only in the absence of its concomitant mention in the text referring to that figure. Page references to figures are in italic and those to tables are in bold.

A

abnormalities (general aspects)
  assessment of 19
  description of 79
  seen on one view only, MRI with 169
abscesses 321–326
  males 572
accessory breast tissue 244
accuracy
  biopsy 187–189, **189**
  mammography 22
    DCIS 379
    fibroadenoma 297–298
  MRI 128–129
    augmented breast and implant complications 162
    cysts 282
    DCIS 384–385
    fibroadenoma 304
    in preoperative local staging 156–158, 396
    in problem-solving after conserving therapy 159
    in problem-solving after reconstruction 162
  sonography
    carcinoma 440–441
    cysts 281
    DCIS 381
    fibroadenoma 299–304
acoustic shadows *see* shadowing
ACR *see* American College of Radiology
add-on units in stereotactic biopsy 203
adenofibrolipoma 290
adenofibroma 292–306
adenoma 292, 293
  nipple 349
adenomyoepithelioma 480
adenosis 257
  cystic *650*
  nodular *263*, *608*
  sclerosing 266, 268, *620*, *650*
adolescent breast 235
age 241–242
  changes with 241–242

mammographic density and cancer risk related to 258
screening mammography 50, 581, 663, 666
screening MRI 154
allergy and hypersensitivity
  contrast media 86
  local anesthetic 192
American College of Radiology (ACR)
  on mammography
    benign disorders 258
    BI-RADS *see* BI-RADS
    density/parenchymal pattern (ACR1–4) **8**, 9, 79, 241, 258, 259
    equipment/hardware 74, 75
    label abbreviations for breast positioning 62
  on MRI 134–135, 148
amorphous selenium 34–35
amorphous silicon 35–36
amyloidosis 310
anatomy
  breast *see* normal breast
  lymph nodes 459
angiolipoma 308
angiomas 308–309
angiomatosis 308
angiosarcoma 308, 480, 481, *482*, 484
anisomastia 242
anticoagulants and biopsy 192, 192–193
antiestrogen therapy 403
anxiety in biopsy 192
apparent diffusion coefficient 132, 181–182
architectural distortion 615–625
  biopsy performed due to 212
  differential diagnosis 431–432, 615–625
  mammography 82, 431–432
    carcinoma *406*, 407, 439
    radial scar 261
  scar *649*
    radial 261
  sonography 113, **121**
    carcinoma 433

areola
  area behind/under *see* subareolar/retroareolar region
  in Paget disease 404
artifacts
  mammography
    mimicking calcifications 646
    responsibility for evaluation of 77
  MRI, cardiac 144–145
aspirated cyst *see* cysts
assessment of imaging 186
  clinical abnormalities 19
  pathognomonic findings and 595–596
  state-of-the-art 595–596
asymmetry *see* symmetry
asymptomatic women
  with breast cancer, lower axilla examination 104
  with dense breast tissue 632–633
    with intermediate or high risk 633
  MRI 269–272, 632–633, **633**
  global mammographic asymmetry in 626
  intramammary lymph nodes 311
  screening *see* screening
attenuation
  mammography/X-rays 75
    carcinoma 405–407
  sonography, carcinoma 433–439
atypia (cellular) 188
  benign proliferative lesions 272
  flat epithelial (columnar cell hyperplasia with atypia) 338, 341–345
atypical intraductal ductal epithelial proliferations 338, 340–346, 366, *621*
atypical lobular hyperplasia (ALH) 345–346
augmented breasts *see* implanted/augmented breasts
autogenous tissue transfer 509
autoimmune granulomatous disorders 327, 327–328, 328, 329, 331, 334

677

Index

automated whole breast ultrasound 181
automatic exposure control systems 30–33, 47, 75
  manual adjustment 47, 75
  performance assessment 77
  quality of 75
axial resolution in sonography 102
axilla
  ectopic glandular tissue 19, 244
  MRI of benign lesions 143
  sonography 99–100, 186, 596
    in biopsy guidance 197
    examination 103–104
    normal findings 113
    suspicious findings 124
axillary lymph nodes *see* lymph nodes
axillary view 60

B

B3 lesions (of BI-RADS) *see* uncertain malignant potential
bar pattern 74
basal-type carcinoma 401, 402
benign disorders/lesions (non-neoplastic or in general) 255–274
  biopsy 272
  calcifications with *see* calcifications
  classification 260
  clinical examination/findings 258, 272, 273
  definition 256
  diagnostic strategy and objectives 260–261
  European guidelines for classification of lesions 211
  histopathology 256–258, 272
  incidence 256
  lymphadenopathy due to 329, 469
  males 571–572
  mammography 261–266, 272
    BI-RADS categorization 83
    density and risk 258–260, 261–265, 272
  MRI 268–272, 272
    BI-RADS categorization 151
  pathogenesis 256
  pathognomonic finding of 594–595
  sonography 266–268, 272
    BI-RADS categorization 123
  lesions with high/very high probability of benignity 118–120
  males 571–572
  in younger patients 665
  in pregnancy 664–665
benign tumors 289–293
  phyllodes tumor as 476, 479
  rare 306–309
biopsy, ductoscopic, nipple discharge and papillary lesions 350
biopsy, percutaneous (for histopathology) 185–214, 596
  abscesses 326
  accuracy 187–189, 189
  B3 lesions (of uncertain malignant potential) 340
    atypical intraductal epithelial proliferations 340–341
    fibroepithelial lesions 360, 479
    lobular neoplasia and proliferations 346, 368–370
    papillary lesions 354
    radial scar 190, 346, 348
  benign non-neoplastic disorders 272
  benign tumors/tumor-like lesions
    fibroadenoma 298
    focal fibrosis 310
    hamartoma 290, 304
    intramammary lymph nodes 312
    rare types 306
  calcifications 643
    sonographic guidance 189
  care following 193
  complications 192
  contraindications 192
  DCIS 385
  fistulas 326
  granulomatous lesions 334
  guidance *see* guidance
  HRT and 248
  indications 191–192
  inflammatory change 663
  in local preoperative staging 157
  lymph nodes 471
    sentinel 398, 458
  malignancy/semi-malignancy
    carcinoma *see* carcinoma
    hematologic tumors 486
    metastases (in breast) 489
    phyllodes tumor 360, 479
    sarcoma 484
  MRI not recommended over 151–152
  of palpable lesions in dense breast 636–640
  patient information 5, 192
  patient information/preparation 192
  possibilities/limitations 189–192
  techniques 193–212
  trauma (incl. surgery)-related changes 507
    conserving therapy + irradiation 529
    reduction mammoplasty 507
  types/methods 187
    choice 189–192
    see also specific types
  vacuum-assisted *see* vacuum-assisted biopsy
  younger patient 670–672, 672
  see also specimen
biopsy, surgical/excisional/non-percutaneous 191, 597
  B3 lesions (of uncertain malignant potential)
    atypical ductal hyperplasia 341
    flat epithelial atypia 343
    lobular neoplasia and proliferations 346
  fibroadenoma 298
  mastitis 319
  skin thickening 561
"biopsy" coils 216
BI-RADS (Breast Imaging Reporting and Data System)
  B3 *see* uncertain malignant potential
  mammography 79, 83–85, 186
    density 80
    mass 80
  MRI 144, **147**, 151
  phyllodes tumor and 476
  sonography 127
bizarre calcifications 651, *658*, *659*
bleeding/hemorrhage 504
  in preoperative localization 217
  see also hyperemia
blood vessel (vascular) calcifications 651
blurring *see* sharpness or blurring
body mass index as risk factor 10
borderline lesions 210
  atypical ductal hyperplasia as 340
  phyllodes tumor as 356, 476
  see also uncertain malignant potential
BRCA1 and *BRAC2* (cancers linked to) 392, 403

Index

special diagnostic problems 430
breast coils (MRI) 129, 130, 131
breast-feeding, unilateral asymmetry related to 629
breast-feeding 11
Breast Imaging Reporting and Data System *see* BI-RADS

C

calcifications and microcalcifications 642–657
  analysis 643–657, 651
    algorithm *644–645*
    benign causes 256, 265–266, *644, 645*, 646–651, 656
      fibroadenoma 293–298, 299
      granulomatous lesions 328
      typical benign calcifications *644*
  differential diagnosis 642–657
  ductal carcinoma in situ 370, 372–373, 372–379, 381, 501, 643, 651, *652, 653,* 654, *655, 658, 659*
    regression on turning into invasive malignancy 420
  in views
    90° lateral view 58
    tangential view, subcutaneous calcifications 60
  lymph node 469–471
    with metastases 466, 471
  malignancy/cancer/carcinoma 399, *406,* 420, 501, *655, 658, 659, 670*
    differentiation from benign changes 431
    diffusely growing 420
    focally growing 416–417
    hereditary 430
    males 569
    recurrences (after conserving therapy + radiation) 523
    signs suggesting malignancy *644, 645,* 651–656
  mammography 642
    sonographic guidance of biopsy following 189
  MRI 272, 643
  newly developing 654
  reporting and documentation 82–83
    of decreases 79
  sharpness 41
  sonography of 641
    BI-RADS and 123
    in biopsy guidance of mammographically detected 189
  specimen radiography 73, 206
  stereotactic biopsy 206
  teacup 58, 265, *650,* 651, 656
  trauma (incl. surgery)-related changes 495–504
    conserving surgery with irradiation 517–523
    reduction mammoplasty 507
  uncharacteristic *643,* 656–657
Canadian randomized controlled trials of screening **580**
cancer
  breast
    carcinoma *see* carcinoma
    other than primary carcinoma 475–491
  childhood 9
  ovarian *see* ovarian cancer
capsule, fibrous (with implants)
  contracture 541–542
  herniation 542
  rupture of 544
  rupture within 542–544
carbon solution as preoperative localization marker 226
carcinoma, invasive (often referred to in text as "malignancy" or "cancer") 391–455, 475–491
  benign disorders and risk of 250
  in BI-RADS (= B5) 211
  biopsy (percutaneous) for 191, 395, 445, 448–450, 450
    males 569
  calcifications *see* calcifications
  clinical examination 403
  clinical manifestations 402
  definition 392–393
  diagnosis/detection 98–99, 394–400, 432, 441, 448–450
    differential *see subheading below*
    problems posted 392–393
    spectrum and 393–394
    strategy and goals 394–400
  differential diagnosis 431–432, 440–441
    scars 495
  epidemiology 392
  etiology 392
  extent/degree of extension 397
    MRI correlations with 444–445
  widespread, signs suggesting 417
  frequent types 400–401
  grading 393
  hereditary *see* hereditary/familial cancer
  histopathology 400–403, 448
    males 567
    mammographic presentation influenced by 428–430
    sonographic image presentation correlating with 440
  inflammatory change 432, *662*
  interval *see* interval cancer
  males 567–571, 572
  mammography 393, 394–395, 405–432, 450
  MRI, screening *see* screening MRI
    BI-RADS categorization 83–85
    in differential diagnosis 431–432
    extent of tumor 397
    follow-up or prior studies 420–428
    histopathology influencing 428–430
    implanted breast *538, 548, 550, 551*
    males 569, 569–571
    neoadjuvant chemotherapy monitoring 399
    sensitivity and specificity 431
    younger patient *666, 668, 669*
  MRI *135, 136, 137, 138, 139,* 441–448, 450
    absence of enhancement excluding malignancy with high probability 144
    BI-RADS categorization 151
    contrast-enhanced 393
    density 405–407
    diagnostic role 441
    extent of tumor 397
    indications 445–446
    for local staging (preoperative) 156–158, 396
    neoadjuvant chemotherapy monitoring 166, 399–400, 448
    post-reconstructive surgery 159–160
    variations and pitfalls 445
  palpation problems 19
  precursors *see* precursors; uncertain malignant potential
  in pregnancy and lactation 665

679

Index

prognosis 402–403
  prognostically very favorable cancers 587
rare types 401–402
recurrence *see* recurrence
risk factors *see* risk factors
sonography 268, 393, 394–395, 432–441, 450
  advantages and limitations 438
  BI-RADS categorization 123
  diagnostic role or value 98–99, 432
  extent of tumor 397
  features with highest positive predictive value 118
  image presentation 433–440
  indications 432
  lower axilla examination in asymptomatic women with breast cancer 104
  males 569, 571
  mammography complementing 430
  neoadjuvant chemotherapy monitoring 399
  younger patient 669, 670
staging *see* staging
symptoms hinting of 11
therapy
  changes caused by 11, 493–531
  chemotherapy *see* chemotherapy
  conservation *see* conservation
  screening and its favorable impact on 588
unknown primary *see* primary tumor, unknown
younger patient 663–668
  clinical findings 665–672
  diagnostic difficulties 663
  presentation 664
  risk 665
see also borderline lesions; metastases *and specific types of carcinoma*
carcinoma in situ (and intraepithelial neoplasia) 365–388
  carcinomas (rare types) vs 401–402
  definition/terminology/biological concept 366
  ductal *see* ductal carcinoma in situ
  histology *see* histopathology
  lobular 338, 345–346, 366–370, 386

MRI *see* magnetic resonance imaging
cardiac artifacts in MRI 144–145
casting microcalcifications 373–375, 651
  DCIS 373–375, *654*
characteristic curve (film) 30
charge-coupled devices 38
chemotherapy
  neoadjuvant *see* chemotherapy
  screening reducing need for 588
chest wall injury in preoperative localization 217
childhood
  cancer 9
  radiation treatment 9
chondroma 306
Churg–Strauss syndrome 328
circumscribed skin changes 17
cleavage view 60
clinical examination and findings *see* examination and findings
clip marking
  biopsy
    core needle 194–195
    stereotactic 206
    vacuum-assisted 195–197
  preoperative localization 227
  residual tumor after neoadjuvant chemotherapy 399
clustered calcifications 657
coaxial system in biopsy
  in core needle biopsy 194
  in MR-guided biopsy 207–210
collagen injections for augmentation 535
collimation assessment 77
colloid lesions *see* mucinous lesions
color Doppler 181
columnar cell hyperplasia with atypia 338, 341–345
comedo-type DCIS 375, 384, *418*, 643
  calcifications *652*, *655*
communication with patient *see* information
complex cystic lesions 118
complex sclerosing lesion *see* radial scar
compound imaging (sonography) 102
compressibility/elasticity, assessment *see* elastography
compression (mammography) 29, 45, 52–54
  blurring avoidance 40

calcifications and adequacy of 642
contrast improved by 45, 53
craniocaudal view 55
  exaggerated medial 60
implanted breasts 71
mediolateral oblique view 54
scattering reduced by 29, 45
semiannual tests 78
of specimen 73
spot 60, 62–64, 70
compression (sonography)
  assessment of compressibility *see* elastography
  slight 103
compression plate 217–218
computed radiography 36–37
computed tomography
  lymph nodes, combined with PET 473
  preoperative localization guided by 222
computer-aided diagnosis/detection 40
  in digital tomosynthesis 179
conservation (therapy/surgery) 512–529
  calcifications 499, 512, 513, 514, 517–523, 528
  ductal carcinoma in situ 372
  recurrence risk 371
  HRT after 248
  with irradiation 512–529
  without irradiation 512
  neoadjuvant chemotherapy and 162, 163
  problem solving after 158–159
contraceptive pills *see* oral contraceptives
contralateral breast
  comparisons with 251, 420
  malignancy in 396, 398
  metastases from 487, 489
contrast (mammographic image) 26–29, 41–49
  determining factors 44–49
  compression 45, 53
  developing time extension causing increase in 49
  high but not excessive 43, 48
  low 43
  in magnification mammography, decreased 70
  screen–film systems and 30
contrast (sonographic image), resolution 102

contrast-enhanced digital
    mammography 180
contrast-enhanced MRI (incl.
    dynamic contrast-enhanced
    MRI) 128–175
  benign disorders 268–269, 273
    not recommended 269–272
  carcinoma 393, 400, *443*
  conserving surgery with
    irradiation 514, 526, 528
  dense breasts
    asymptomatic women 269–
      272, 632–633
    palpable lesions 640
  implanted breast 540
  lymph nodes 471–472
  patient information 5
  patient selection and
    indications 151–169
  phyllodes tumor 479
  reduction mammoplasty 507
  scheduling and performing 4,
    132–134
  screening *see* screening
    mammography
  skin thickening 561
  technique 128
  younger patients 672
  see also enhancement
contrast media
  as preoperative localization
    marker 222–226
  lactiferous duct imaging 85, 87
    hypersensitivity/allergy 86
    non-ionic 86
Cooper ligaments
  anatomy 234
  mammography 236
    carcinoma, thickening 420
  sonography 237
core needle biopsy (CNB) 187,
    187–188, 190–191, 194–195, 596
  accuracy 187–188
  carcinoma 448
  DCIS 385
  European guidelines for
    classification of lesions 211
  MR-guided 189–190
  non-specific findings 212
  papillary lesions 354
  patient preparation 193
  radial scar 190, 346, 348
  stereotactic *206*
  technique 194–195
  US-guided 190, *199–200*,
    201–202

cosmetic outcome and impact of
    screening 588
couches, stereotactic biopsy 203
Cowden syndrome 292
craniocaudal view 56
  calcifications (benign causes) 265
  exaggerated lateral 58
  exaggerated medial 60
  lesion location determined in 83
  spot compression *67*, *68*, *69*
cribriform DCIS 370, 375, 654
cutaneous ... *see* skin
cyst(s) (and cystic areas/
    lesions) 257, 258, 275–287
  aspirated 193, 281–282
    pneumocystography 92–93,
      282
  calcified 651
    oil cysts *649*, 651
  clinical examination and
    findings 276
  definition 276
  dermoid 306
  diagnosis 276–284
    differential 276, 281, 599–602
    objectives in 276
    strategies 278–284
  epithelial 306, 554
  with fibroepithelial lesions 356
  histology 276
  mammography 261, 278, 282,
    286
    of aspirated cyst 92–93, 282
    galactocele 284, **595**
    oil cyst 284–286
  medical history 276
  milk of calcium in 265, **595**
  MRI 282–284
    oil cyst 286
  oil *see* oil cysts
  palpation 258
  papillary carcinoma/cancer
    within *see* papillary carcinoma
  papilloma within 281, *351*, *352*,
    440
  sebaceous, males 571
  simple vs complicated 114–118,
    276
  sonography *see* sonography
cystosarcoma *see* phyllodes tumor
cytology (incl. from fine needle
    aspiration) 190, 193
  atypia *see* atypia
  carcinoma 448
    nipple discharge 405
  classification 211

cyst 281–282
  nipple discharge 660
    carcinoma 405
    papillary lesions 349–350

D

darkroom
  cleanliness 78
  fog 78
databases for screening
    programs 588
death (mortality) reduction by
    screening 50, 578, 581, 587
demarcation *see* margins
dendritic gynecomastia 566
density, mammographic
  ACR types *8*, *9*, 79, 241, 258, *259*
  age-related changes 241
  benign lesions 258–260,
    261–265, 272
  carcinoma 405–407
  contrast related to 41
  dense breasts 632–640
    asymptomatic women with *see*
      asymptomatic women
    differential diagnosis 632–640
    palpable findings 632–640
  description 79, 80–82
  differential diagnosis of increases
    in 431
  ductal carcinoma in situ 370
  film 51
  as risk factor *8*, *9*, 258–260, 260,
    272
  smoothly outlined density,
    differential diagnosis 597–604
  soft density surrounding
    microcalcifications, differential
    diagnosis 657
dermal calcifications 646
  see also skin
dermoid cyst 306
desmoid, extra-abdominal 310, 479
development time for film 49
deviation of nipple 11, 17
diabetic mastopathy 310, 327, 328,
    329, 331, 334
diagnosis
  abscesses 321–325
  additional diagnostic evaluation
    of screening findings 594–675
  B3 lesions (of uncertain malignant
    potential) 338–339

fibroepithelial lesions 356–360, 466–469
lobular neoplasia 368–370
papillary lesions and nipple discharge 350–354
benign non-neoplastic disorders (in general) 260–261
benign tumors/tumor-like lesions
fibroadenoma 293–305
hamartoma 290
intramammary lymph nodes 312
lipoma 306
computer-aided *see* computer-aided diagnosis
cysts *see* cysts
differential *see* differential diagnosis
ductal carcinoma in situ 372–385
early, positioning for mammography and its importance in 56–57
final 83–85
fistulas 321–325
granulomatous conditions 328–334
gynecomastia 565–566
lymph node involvement 398–399, 459
malignancy/semi-malignancy
carcinoma *see* carcinoma
hematologic tumors 485–486
males 569–571
metastases (in breast) 487
overdiagnosis in screening 482, 585–586
phyllodes tumor 356–360, 466–469
sarcoma 480–484
mastitis 317
skin
nodular changes 554
thickening 555
trauma (incl. surgery)-related changes 494–507
conserving surgery with irradiation 513–529
conserving surgery without irradiation 512
reconstructive surgery 509
reduction mammoplasty 507
DICOM (Digital Imaging and Communications in Medicine) 40
Grayscale Standard Display Function 39
dietary (nutritional) risk factors 8, 10

differential diagnosis 597–671
architectural distortion 431–432, 615–625
benign disorders on MRI 269–272
calcifications 642–657
carcinoma *see* carcinoma
cysts 276, 281, 599–602
ill-defined/not smoothly outlined mass 604–615
lipoma 306
mammographically dense breast 632–640
nipple retraction 640
pain 640
skin thickening 555, 561
smoothly outlined density 597–604
trauma (incl. surgery)-related changes 495
conserving therapy without irradiation 512
reduction mammoplasty 507
younger patients with very large masses 665
diffuse architectural distortion, differential diagnosis 431–432
diffuse changes
asymmetry and 632
benign 272, 273
biopsy of 212
conserving surgery with irradiation
mammography 514
sonography 523
differential diagnosis 431
diffuse enhancement (on MRI) 269
carcinoma 400, 441–444
milky 237, 269
nonmass 149–150
diffuse fibrosis 258
diffuse glandular gynecomastia 566
diffuse growth pattern
hematologic tumors 486
invasive carcinoma, mammography 422, 423, 424
calcification 655
histology influencing mammographic presentation 430
recurrences (after conserving therapy + radiation) 523
signs **405**, 420
metastases in breast 487, 489
diffuse skin changes (incl. thickening) 555
carcinoma 404
differential diagnosis 432

diffusion-weighted MRI 132, 181–182
neoadjuvant chemotherapy monitoring 166, 400
Digital Imaging and Communications in Medicine, *see also* DICOM
digital mammography 33–39
calcifications 642
contrast 43
contrast-enhanced 180
dose and optimization of 52
image quality factors
exposure 75
resolution 74
sharpness 41
structural noise 49
tomosynthesis combined with *see* tomosynthesis
discharge, nipple 657–661
bilateral bloodless 86
galactography 86, 660
MRI compared with 169
observing 11
pathologic 86, 657–661
benign 258
cancer 404–405, 430
DCIS 379
definition 657
diagnostic problems 657–660
diagnostic strategy 660–661
papillary lesions 349–350
younger patients 665
display monitors 38
distribution patterns
benign disorders in mammography
atypical 261
typical 261, 265
calcifications 643
suggesting malignancy 651–656
documentation/recording/reporting
location of lesion 186, 227
mammography
findings 78–85
of quality control 77
sonography 105–124
US-guided biopsy 203
Doppler imaging
color 181
lipophagic granuloma 526
power 107–109
dose 50–52
compression enabling reduction in 53

noise with low-dose screen–film
systems 48, 49
optimization/minimization 51
responsibility for assessing 77
drainage of abscess,
percutaneous 326
drugs *see* medications
dual energy mammography 180
duct (lactiferous/mammary)
anatomy 234
calcification arrangement
around 654
with DCIS *140*, 383
enhancement 148, 148–150
filling defects or cutoff 660
carcinoma 430
galactography 87, 430
kinked, galactography 87
mammography 236
mass in, near to nipple,
galactography 87
MRI 91
single dilated, as rare sign of
malignancy 416
sonography 91
subareolar, importance of
determining extent of
invasion 397
see also extensive intraductal
component; terminal ducts
ductal carcinoma (of no specific
type) 400–401, 428
mammography 428, 501
architectural distortion *618*,
619, *620*
asymmetry *606*, *607*, *628*, 631
diffusely growing *see* diffuse
growth pattern
focally growing *408*, *411*, *412*,
414, *416*, *417*, *418*, *419*, *606*,
607, *610*
follow-up *425*, *426*, *427*
histology influencing 428
implanted breast *548*, *550*, *551*
inflammatory change *661*
males *570*
younger patient *667*, *668*, *669*
MRI 136, 137, 138, 442, 449, 614,
624, 634
sonography 435, 437, *440*, 637
biopsy guidance *200*
correlation with histology 440
males *571*
ductal carcinoma in situ
(DCIS) 370–385, 386, 586
calcifications *see* calcifications

carcinoma vs 401–402
clinical findings and history 372
comedo-type 375, 384, *418*, 643
definition 370
diagnostic methods 372–385
ductal enhancement with *140*,
383
histopathology 370–371
importance and natural
history 371–372
incidence 370
mammography 370, 371,
372–381, *427*
MRI 135, *140*, *141*, 370, 381–385,
604
for local preoperative size
assessment 156
non-comedo-type 375, 384
papillary *see* papillary carcinoma
in situ
sonography 381
biopsy guidance *202*
spot compression 67
therapeutic decisions 372
younger patient 671
ductal ectasia, galactography 87
ductal epithelial proliferations,
atypical 338, 340–346, 366, *621*
ductal hyperplasia, atypical
(ADH) 340–341, 366, 370, 371
ductal papilloma 349, 351–352, 354
ductography *see* galactography
ductoscopy, nipple discharge and
papillary lesions 350
dye marking for preoperative
localization 222
dynamic contrast-enhanced MRI *see*
contrast-enhanced MRI
dystrophic calcifications 651
fibroadenomas 293
granulomas 328
trauma (incl. surgery)-
related 495, 513, 517, 523

E

echoes and echogenicity 105, **122**,
237, 266–267
carcinoma 433
echogenic halo **121**
see also hyperechoic areas;
hypoechoic areas; reverberation
echoes
ectasia, ductal, galactography 87
ectopic glandular tissue, axillary 19,
244

edema, generalized and
iatrogenic 555
edematous fibroadenomas 304
edge shadows
thickened 439
thin 116
Edinburgh randomized controlled
trial of screening **580**
Eklund technique 71, *537*, 538, *539*,
539
elastography (assessment of
elasticity/compressibility)
MR 182
sonographic 106–107, **122**, 123,
181
carcinoma 439
emerging technologies 177–184
enhancement (in MRI) 143–151
carcinoma 399–400, 441–444
DCIS *140*, 383
diffuse *see* diffuse enhancement
see also contrast-enhanced MRI
epithelial atypia, flat (FEA) 338,
341–345
epithelial cysts 306, 554
epithelial proliferations
atypical ductal 338, 340–346, 366
benign 256
equipment (hardware)
mammography 26–39
image quality and 74–76
overview 26
sonography 100–103
European guidelines (in quality
assurance)
biopsy/histopathology/
cytopathology 211
screening mammography 84–85
European Society of Mastology
(EUSOMA) and implanted breast
on MRI 540
on surveillance following
oncoplastic surgery 544
exaggerated lateral craniocaudal
view 58
exaggerated medial craniocaudal
view 60
examination and findings, clinical/
physical 16–20
abscesses 321
assessment of abnormalities 19
B3 lesions (of uncertain malignant
potential)
fibroepithelial lesions 356, 476
lobular neoplasia and
proliferations 346

Index

papillary lesions 349–350
benign non-neoplastic disorders (in general) 258, 272, 273
benign tumors/tumor-like lesions
   fibroadenoma 293
   hamartoma 290
   intramammary lymph nodes 311
   lipoma 306
cysts 276
DCIS 372
dense breast and palpable findings 633
documentation and reporting 78
fistulas 321
granulomatous conditions 327
males 564
   cancer 569
   gynecomastia 565
malignancy/semi-malignancy
   carcinoma 403
   hematologic tumors 484–485
   males 569
   metastases (in breast) 487
   phyllodes tumor 356, 476
   sarcoma 480
normal breast
   adolescent 235
   age-related changes 241
   mature/adult 235–236
   pregnancy and lactation 246
   variants 242, 244
skin
   nodular changes 554
   thickening 561
trauma (incl. surgery)-related changes 494
   conserving therapy with irradiation 513
   conserving therapy without irradiation 512
younger patients 665
excision *see* biopsy, surgical/excisional; surgery
exposure (image receptor to radiation) 75
   automatic *see* automatic exposure control systems
   dose-related optimization of technique of 51
   image quality and 75
   time
      increases (= exposure creep) in digital mammography 52
      with low-sensitivity films 48
      reducing blurring 40
exposure (person to radiation) *see* radiation
extensive intraductal component (EIC) 444

F

false negative calls and interval cancer 23
false positive calls in screening mammography 23, 583–584
familial cancer *see* hereditary/familial cancer
family history-taking 9
fat (dietary), as risk factor 10
fat (fatty tissue)
   hypoechoic 112, 237, 241
   suppression (in MRI) 130
fat lobules (fat-containing lobules) 106, 237
   carcinoma vs 432, 433, 439, 441
   hamartoma 290
   lipoma 306
fat necrosis 494, 495, 504, 505, 514, 517, 523
   calcified, after breast augmentation 648
   male 572
fibroadenoma 292–306, 664
   calcified **595**, *650*, *651*, *657*, *658*
   hypercellular 293, 304, 440
   mammography 293–298, 305, *482*, **595**, *620*
   MRI *142*, *143*, 304
   sonography 299–304, 305, 433
   younger patients 663
      juvenile/giant fibroadenoma 292, 293, 664
   in pregnancy 663
fibrocystic change ("mastopathia") 236, 256, *267*, 276
   calcifications *650*, *651*, *652*, 656
   younger patient 664
fibroepithelial lesions of uncertain malignant potential 338, 356–360
fibroepithelial mixed tumors 292–306
fibroma, calcified 503
fibromatosis 310, 379
fibrosarcoma 480, 481
fibrosis (benign mammary) 258, 310–312
   in conserving surgery with irradiation 513, 514
diabetic (diabetic mastopathy) 310, 327, 328, 329, 331, 334
   in fibroadenoma 299
fibrous capsule (with implants) *see* capsule
fibrous histiocytoma 480, *481*
fiducial markers, MR-guided biopsy 207, 222
field limitation (X-ray) 75
filariasis 327
film
   density 51
   fixture retention 78
   labeling 62
   processing 33, 49
      dose and 52
      quality 76
      quality control responsibility 78
   screen combinations with 30
      blurring relating to 41
      compared with digital mammography 34
      contact optimization 78
      dose and 52
      magnification mammography 64
      quality 76
   selection 48
filter/target combination *see* target/filter combination
fine needle aspiration (FNA) 187, 190, 193
   accuracy 187
   patient preparation 193
   see also cytology
fistulas 321–326
fixture retention in film 78
flaps 509
flat epithelial atypia (FEA) 338, 341–345
focal area enhancement
   carcinoma 441–444
   DCIS 383
   nonmass 149
focal changes *see* localized changes
focal fibrosis 258, 310
focal growth (localized) pattern
   asymmetric mass 605–616
   invasive carcinoma 407–420
      additional foci 397–398; *see also* multicentricity; multifocality
      direct signs **405**, 407–417
      indirect/secondary signs **405**, 417–420

MRI 445
    recurrences (after conserving therapy + radiation) 523
  metastases in breast 487, 489
focal spot
  performance evaluation 77
  size 25–26, 40–41
focusing in sonography 102, 105
fog, darkroom 78
follow-up
  B3 lesions (of uncertain malignant potential) 339, 340
    atypical ductal hyperplasia 341
    flat epithelial atypia 343–344
  calcifications 657
  carcinoma, intervals 428
  time 79
foreign body reactions/granulomas 327, 328, 651
  calcifications 651
fungal infections 327, 331, 334

G

gadolinium (for enhanced MRI) 130–131
  lymph nodes 471–472
galactoceles 284–286, 669
galactography (ductography) 85–92
  carcinoma 430
  filling defects 87, 430, 660
  nipple discharge 169
  papillary lesions 350, 354
  preoperative localization guided by 222
galactorrhea 86
galactoscopy, nipple discharge 660–661
gamma imaging 182
gene(s), breast cancer-related 392
  testing for 404
  see also hereditary/familial cancer
generator (X-ray) 74
genetic counseling 9, 404
  and testing 404
geometry (in mammography) 25–26
  blurring relating to 40, **41**, 64
  scanned slit linear detectors 38
giant (juvenile) fibroadenoma 292, 293, 664
glandular tissue
  in axilla, ectopic 19, 244
  in mammography 235, 236
    age-related changes 241

compression and 53, 54
implanted breasts 71
photocell positioning under tissue 33, 47
visualization of small areas of pathology buried in tissue 53
MRI 237
  age-related changes 242
  benign disorders 268
normal breast
  adolescent 235
  adult 235–237
palpation 17
sonography 235, 236
  in HRT 248
gold deposits in rheumatoid arthritis 329, 471
Gothenburg randomized controlled trial of screening **580**
grading, carcinoma 393
granular calcifications *658*
  fine 654, *659*
  large 651–654
granular cell tumor 309
granulomas (and granulomatous conditions) 327–334
  foreign body *see* foreign body reactions
  lipophagic 494, 495, 507, 517, *521*, 523, 526
  MRI *143*, 331–334
Grayscale Standard Display Function (of DICOM) 39
grid (mammographic) 29, 46, 75
  dose and 52
  removal (gridless mammography) 29, 46
  for magnification mammography 69
growth patterns
  atypical intraductal ductal epithelial proliferations 340–341
  DCIS 371
  invasive carcinoma 400, **405**
    histology influencing mammographic presentation 428
  see also specific growth patterns
guidance by imaging
  for biopsy 193–212
    choice of modality 189–191
    of palpable lesions in dense breast 640
  implanted breast 540–541

male breast cancer 569
  for preoperative localization 217–222
  see also specific imaging or biopsy method
gynecomastia 565–566

H

half-value layer measurement 77
hamartoma 290, **595**
  histology 290
hardware *see* equipment
Health Insurance Plan (HIP) randomized controlled trial of screening **580**
heart causing artifacts in MRI 144–145
heel effect 28–29
hemangioendothelioma 479
hemangioma 308, 309
hemangiopericytoma 479, 480
hematologic and lymphoproliferative malignancies 466, 484–486
hematomas 494, 495, 504, 505, 517, 526
  with implantation 541
  males 571–572
hemorrhage *see* bleeding
HER2 positivity 402, 403
hereditary/familial cancer
  breast 392, 403–404, 430
    and dense breasts without symptoms, diagnostic strategy and goals 633
    MRI screening **154**
    risk assessment *8*, 9
    special diagnostic problems 430
    younger patient, mammography *669*
  ovarian 9, 154, 392, 403–404
  see also genes; genetic counseling
high-risk lesions, underestimated, lower rate with vacuum-assisted biopsy 188
high-risk women 403–404
  with dense breasts and no symptoms, diagnostic strategy and goals 633
  genetic factors *see* hereditary/familial cancer
  screening 394
    MRI 152–156, 396, 448

Index

younger 672
HIP randomized controlled trial of screening **580**
histiocytoma, fibrous 480, *481*
histology (normal breast)
  adolescents 235
  adult 235
  age-related changes 241
  pregnancy and lactation 246
histopathology (of specimen) 186, 210–212, 594, 596–597
  B3 lesions (of uncertain malignant potential) 340
    atypical ductal hyperplasia 340
    fibroepithelial lesions incl. phyllodes tumors 356
    flat epithelial atypia 341–345
    lobular proliferations/neoplasia 345, 368
    papillary lesions 349, 354
    radial scar 346
  benign non-neoplastic disorders 256–258, 272
  benign tumors/tumor-like lesions
    hamartoma 290
    intramammary lymph nodes 311
    pseudoangiomatous stromal hyperplasia 309
  biopsy for *see* biopsy
  carcinoma in situ 400
    ductal 370–371
  correlation with imaging 64, 210–212
  cysts 276
  granulomatous conditions 327
  gynecomastia 565
  implanted breast 540–541, 547–551
  interpretation 210–212
  in local preoperative staging 157
  males
    cancer 567
    gynecomastia 565
  malignant/semi-malignant lesions
    carcinoma *see* carcinoma
    hematologic tumors 484
    males 567
    metastases (in breast) 487
    phyllodes tumor 476
    sarcoma 480
  measures preceding 186
  in nipple discharge 660
  pathognomonic findings 593–597
  trauma (incl. surgery)-related changes 494
  younger patient 664–665

history-taking (incl. medical history) 5–11
  carcinoma 403
  cysts 276
  DCIS 372
  dynamic contrast-enhanced MRI and 132–134
  fibroadenoma 293
  inflammatory change 661–663
  skin thickening 561
hormonal causes of gynecomastia 566
hormonal influences on dynamic contrast-enhanced MRI 132, 145
hormonal risk factors
  endogenous 9
  exogenous *8*, 9–10, 11
hormone replacement therapy (HRT) 10, 11, 248
  asymmetry relating to 632
  mammography and 428
    screening 260
  MRI and 132, 248, 269
hypercellular carcinoma 440
hypercellular fibroadenomas 293, 304, 440
hyperechoic areas 112, 113, 237, 241
  axilla 113
  benign disorders 266, 268
  carcinoma 432, 433, *436*, *437*, *438*
  silicone granulomas 331
hyperemia 514
  in pregnancy or lactation 672
  radiation-induced 513
hyperplasia
  atypical ductal (ADH) 340–341, 366, 370, 371
  atypical lobular 345–346
  columnar cell, with atypia 338, 341–345
  pseudoangiomatous stromal 309
  younger patient 664
hypersensitivity *see* allergy and hypersensitivity
hypoechoic areas/tissue 237, 266–267, 281
  benign disorders (in general) 266–268
  carcinoma 98–99, 432, 433, *435*, *436*
    differentiation from other lesions 441
    histology and 440
  cysts 281
  fatty tissue 112, 237, 241

in mammographically dense breasts with palpable lesions 636
mastitis 319
younger patient 669

I

image (dynamic contrast-enhanced MRI) interpretation criteria 128–129
image (mammographic)
  contrast *see* contrast
  phantom, testing with 78
  presentation and processing 38–39
  quality
    hardware factors influencing 74
    responsibility for assessing 77
  receptors 29–38
    distance from source to (SID) 25–26
  repeat
    analysis 78
    avoiding too many 52
  sharpness *see* sharpness
  viewing *see* viewbox
image (sonographic)
  labeling 109
  quality 101
  near field 102
immunohistochemistry, core needle biopsy specimen 187–188
implanted/augmented breasts 535–552
  anatomical placement 535
  automatic exposure control systems with 47
  calcified fat necrosis *648*
  complications 541–544
    rupture 538, 539, 540, 542–544, 544
  histopathology 540–541, 547–551
  mammography *see* mammography
  MRI with 162, 540
    capsular complications 542, 542–544
    for evaluation of complications (incl. failure) 134, 162
    after reconstructive surgery 159–160
  positioning and views 71–72, 535, 538

Index

silicone from *see* silicone granulomas/deposits
sonography 539–540
   capsular complications 542, 544
   for guidance 540–541
   types of implants 534–535
in-phase condition (in MRI) 130
in situ carcinoma *see* carcinoma in situ
infarction of breast in pregnancy 665
infections (as cause)
   abscesses 321
   granulomas 327
   with implantation 541
   mastitis 316
inflammation, signs of (inflammatory change) 432, 661–663
inflammatory carcinoma 402
   mammography 420, *424*
      histology influencing mammographic presentation 430
   skin thickening 561
   sonographic presentation correlating with histology 440
inflammatory conditions 315–335
information, patient 4–5
   biopsy 5, 192
   mammography 4, 53
injury *see* trauma
inspection/observation 16–17
   cancer 404
   nipple 11, 17
   reporting and documentation 78
intensifying screens 29–30
   artifacts mimicking calcifications 646
   cleanliness 78
   film and *see* film
interval cancer/carcinoma 22–23, *84*, 479, 578, 582, 584–585
   breast density and risk of being detected as *259*
   self-examination for 16
interval for screening MRI 154
interventions, patient information 5
intracanalicular fibroadenoma 293, *297*, 664
intraductal lesions *see* ductal ...
intraepithelial neoplasia *see* carcinoma in situ
intralobular lesions *see* lobular ...
intramammary lymph nodes 310–312

invasive carcinoma *see* carcinoma
inversion of nipple 11, 17, 244
involution 257
   adenosis and 257
   mammography 241
   sonography 241

J

juvenile (giant) fibroadenoma 292, 293, 664
juvenile papillomatosis 664, 665, 666, 670

K

"keyhole" sign 542, *545*
kilovoltage
   accuracy and reproducibility responsibilities 77
   peak 28, 44–45
      magnification mammography 64

L

labeling
   mammographic film 62
   sonographic image 109
lactation 246
   breast cancer concurrent in 665
   hyperemia associated with 672
   mammography 246, 666, 672
   sonography 246, 669
laser in computed radiography 37
lateral craniocaudal view, exaggerated 58
lateral resolution in sonography 102–103
lateral view, 90° 58
law and carcinoma detection 395
lawnmower pattern of sonographic examination 105
lead time bias in screening mammography 587
legal issues, carcinoma detection 395
leiomyoma 306
leiomyosarcoma 480, *482*
length–time time bias in screening mammography 587
leukemia 466, 484
linear enhancement, nonmass 148
"linguini" sign 544

lipoma 306, *308*, **595**
   males 572
lipomatous metaplasia 306
lipophagic granuloma 494, 495, 507, 517, *521*, 523, 526
liposarcoma 480, 481
lobular carcinoma
   calcification, rarity 643
   mammography *423*
      architectural distortion *622*
      histology influencing 428
      implanted breast *538*
      spot compression *68*
   MRI 396, *444*
   sonography *437*, *439*, *639*
      histology correlating with 440
lobular carcinoma in situ; LCIS (and lobular intraepithelial neoplasia; LN) 338, 345–346, 366–367, 386
lobular hyperplasia, atypical 345–346
lobular pattern of calcifications 265
lobular units, terminal duct 234, 256, 276
lobulated mass, mammography *406*, 407, 431
lobules
   anatomy 234
   fat-containing *see* fat lobules
local anesthesia
   biopsy 192, 198
   galactography 86
   preoperative localization 217
   side-effects (incl. allergy) 192, 217
local staging *see* staging
localization 186, 215–229
   documentation 186
   image guidance in *see* guidance
   preoperative 215–229, 397–398
      of additional foci of carcinoma 397–398
      definition 216
      indication 216
      materials 222–227
      methods and technique 217–222
      MRI for 222, *442*, 444–445, *445*
      problems and solutions 227–228
      purpose 216
      side effects 216–217
localized changes (focal changes)
   conserving surgery with irradiation
      mammography 514, 514–517
      sonography 523–526

Index

skin
  with carcinoma 404
  thickening 554, 555
localized growth pattern *see* focal growth pattern
location (of lesion)
  describing 83
  extramammary, calcific densities 646
low-energy radiation 25, 26, 27, 44, 51, 53
Luminal A and Luminal B 402, 403
luminescence, photo-stimulable 36
lumpy breasts 258
  MRI and 672
  younger patients, mammography 667
lupus erythematosus 329
lymph node(s) (axillary) 398–399, 457–474
  anatomy 459
  biopsy *see* biopsy, percutaneous
  diagnostic value of imaging 398–399, 459
  dissection (surgery) 458
    screening reducing need for 588
  enlargement (adenopathy) 464–469
    benign causes 329, 469
    metastatic *see* lymph node metastases
  mammography 398
    metastatic nodes 464–466
    normal nodes 459–460, **595**
  MRI 471–472
    benign lesions *143*
  normal findings, sonography 113
  palpation 17, 19
  sonography 99–100, 103–104, 398
    normal/benign nodes 113, 460–463, 599
    suspicious findings 124
lymph node(s) (other than axilla)
  internal mammary *see* mammary lymph nodes, internal
  intramammary 310–312
  standard examination not necessary 103–104
lymph node metastases 464–466
  axillary 152, 448, 464–466
    calcifications 466, 471
    sonography 109
  intramammary 311
  MRI in search for primary tumor 152, 448, *609*, 640

lymphangioma 308, 309
lymphangiosarcomas 480
lymphatic stasis 489, 555, 561
lymphoproliferative malignancies (incl. lymphoma) 466, 484–486

M

macrocysts 257
macromastia 242–244
magnetic resonance elastography 182
magnetic resonance imaging (MRI) 128–175, 181–182, 237–240, 596
  abscesses 326
  accuracy *see* accuracy
  angiomas 309
  architectural distortion 615
  B3 lesions (of uncertain malignant potential)
    atypical intraductal epithelial proliferations 341
    fibroepithelial lesions incl. phyllodes tumors 359–360, 479
    lobular neoplasia and proliferations 345, 368
    papillary lesions 350, 354
    radial scar 348
  benign non-neoplastic disorders *see* benign disorders
  biopsy guided by 189, 207–210
    core needle 189–190
    for local preoperative staging 157
    vacuum-assisted 188–189, 191, 207, 210
  calcifications 272, 643
  carcinoma in situ
    ductal *see* ductal carcinoma in situ
    poorly differentiated, next to invasive carcinoma 445
  contrast-enhanced *see* contrast-enhanced MRI
  cysts *see* cysts
  dense breasts
    asymptomatic women 269–272, 632–633
    palpable lesions 640
  diagnostic criteria 134–151
  diagnostic problem solving 169
  diffusion-weighted *see* diffusion-weighted MRI
  duct 91

  fibroepithelial mixed tumors 304
  fibroadenoma *142*, *143*, 304
  fistulas 326
  focal fibrosis 310
  granulomas *143*, 331–334
  HRT and 132, 248, 269
  implants *see* implanted breasts
  lymph nodes *see* lymph nodes
  males 564
  malignancy/semi-malignancy
    carcinoma *see* carcinoma
    fibromatosis 479
    hematologic tumors 486
    metastases (in breast) 489
    phyllodes tumor 359–360, 479
    sarcoma 481
    search for unknown primary 152, 448, *609*, 640
  mastitis 319
  normal breast 237–240
    age-related changes 242
    HRT effects 248
    inverted nipple 244
    pregnancy and lactation 246
  patient information 5
  patient selection and indications 129, 151–169
  preoperative (for localization) 222, 397–398, *442*, 444–445, 445
  purpose/possibilities/limitations 128–129
  scarring 169, 505, 509, 526, 528
  scheduling 4, 132–134
  screening *see* screening MRI
  symmetry and *see* symmetry
  technique 128, 129–132
  trauma (incl. surgery)-related changes 505–507
    conserving surgery with irradiation 514, 526–529
    reconstructive surgery 509
    reduction mammoplasty 507
    younger patients 672
magnetic resonance spectroscopy (proton spectroscopy) 132, 182
neoadjuvant chemotherapy monitoring 166, 399–400, 448
magnification mammography 29, 41, 46–47, 48, 64–70, 74
  advantages 69–70
  calcifications 642
  DCIS *375*, *376*, 379
  definition 64
  disadvantages 70
  fibroadenoma *658*

Index

fundamental
 considerations 64–69
 image quality in 74
 indications 70
 scatter reduced in 29, 46–47
magnifying lens 33, 86
males 563–573
 anatomy 564
 cancer/malignancy 567–571, 572
 enlargement
  (gynecomastia) 565–566
 miscellaneous
  conditions 571–572
malignancy *see* cancer
Malmö randomized controlled trial
 of screening **580**
mammary gland
 anatomy 234
 hypoechoicity 266, 268
 supernumerary 244
mammary lymph nodes, internal
 anatomy 459
 involvement (metastases) 458
 sentinel nodes in 458
mammography 21–95, 179–181
 abscesses 321, 325, 326
  male 572
 accuracy *see* accuracy
 adenoma 293
 B3 lesions (of uncertain malignant
  potential) 340
  atypical intraductal epithelial
   proliferations 341, *621*
  fibroepithelial lesions 356–359,
   477
  flat epithelial atypia 343
  lobular neoplasia and
   proliferations 345, 368
  papillary lesions 350, 350–351
  radial scar *see* radial scar
 benign non-neoplastic disorders
  see benign disorders
 benign tumors/tumor-like lesions
  angiomas 308, 309
  fibroadenoma 293–298, 305,
   482, **595**, *620*
  focal fibrosis 310
  hamartoma 290, **595**
  lipoma 306, **595**
  pseudoangiomatous stromal
   hyperplasia 309
 calcifications *see* calcifications
 cysts *see* cysts
 density *see* density
 digital *see* digital mammography
 dual energy/spectral 180

ductal carcinoma in situ 370, 371,
 372–381, *427*
equipment overview *26*
fistulas 321, 325, 326
galactoceles 284, **595**
image *see* image
implanted breasts 535–538
 of complications 542, 544,
  544–547
 positioning and views 71–72,
  535, 538
indications/purpose 22
inflammatory change 432,
 661–663
lymph nodes *see* lymph nodes
magnification *see* magnification
 mammography
males 564
 benign lesions 571–572
 cancer 569, 569–571
 gynecomastia 565, 566
 normal findings 564
malignancy/semi-malignancy
 adenomyoepithelioma 480
 carcinoma *see* carcinoma
 fibromatosis 479
 hematologic tumors 485–486
 males 569, 569–571
 metastases (in breast) 487–489
 phyllodes tumor 356–359, 477
 sarcoma 480
mastitis 317–319
normal breast 236, 564
 adolescent 235
 age-related changes on 241
 HRT effects 248
 pregnancy and lactation 246,
  672
 variants 242, 244
of palpable lesions in dense
 breast 636
patient information 4, 53
positioning and views 54–60, 217
 additional 57–60
 implanted breasts 71–72, 535,
  538
 importance of optimized
  positioning 56–57
 labeling abbreviations 62
 in standard
  mammography 54–57
positron emission 182–183
preoperative localization by 216,
 217–221
questionnaire 5
reporting and
 documentation 80–85

scheduling 4
screening *see* screening
 mammography
sensitivity *see* sensitivity
skin
 nodular changes 554
 thickening 561
sonographic biopsy guidance of
 microcalcifications detected
 by 189
specific requirements and
 solutions 40–52
specificity *see* specificity
symmetry and *see* symmetry
symptoms and 50–51
technique 25–40
trauma (incl. surgery)-related
 changes 495–504
 conserving surgery with
  irradiation 513, 514–523
 reconstructive surgery 509
 reduction mammoplasty 507
unit assembly evaluation 77
younger patients 665–669
 pregnancy and lactation 246,
  666
see also scintimammography
Mammography Quality Assurance
 Act/MQSA (US) 76
mammoplasty
 augmentation *see* implanted/
  augmented breasts
 reduction 507–509
manual adjustment with automatic
 exposure control systems 47, 75
manual localization,
 mammographically
 guided 220–221
margins/demarcation
 mammography, description 80
 sonography
  carcinoma 433
  description **121**
masses (solid)
 cystic *see* cysts
 DCIS presenting rarely as 379,
  380
 ill-defined/not smoothly outlined,
  differential diagnosis 604–615
 interpretation/description 80
 smoothly outlined, differential
  diagnosis 597–604
 sonography 118–123, 599–602
  BI-RADS 123
  differentiation 98
 tumor-like 289–313

689

Index

younger patient 665
see also benign tumors; cancer
mastectomy
   reconstruction after *see*
      reconstructive/oncoplastic
      surgery
   screening reducing need for 588
   subcutaneous, mammography
      after 71, 72
mastitis 316–320, 663
   chronic/"plasma cell" 87, 256,
      316, 317, 319, 404, 504, 646,
      651, *652, 653*, 655
   skin thickening *560*, 562
mastodynia 258
"mastopathia" *see* fibrocystic change
medial craniocaudal view,
   exaggerated 60
mediastinal obstruction *560*
medical conditions contraindicating
   biopsy 192
medical history *see* history-taking
medical physicists' responsibilities
   (for quality) 77
medications/drugs
   biopsy and awareness of 192–193
   biopsy contraindicated with 192
   gynecomastia caused by 566
medicolegal issues, carcinoma
   detection 395
mediolateral 90° view, calcifications
   (benign causes) 265
mediolateral oblique view 54–56
   lesion location determined in 83
   spot compression *66*
medullary carcinoma 401
   histology correlating with
      sonographic presentation 440
   histology influencing
      mammographic
      presentation 428
men *see* males
menstrual cycle
   clinical examination and 236
   mammography and 54, 236, 260
   MRI and 240, 269
      dynamic
         contrast-enhanced 132
metaplasia, lipomatous 306
metastases
   in breast 487–489
   in lymph nodes *see* lymph node
      metastases
   of unknown origin *see* primary
      tumor, unknown
microbiology, granulomatous
   disease 327

microcalcifications *see* calcifications
microcysts 257
   milk of calcium in 265, **595**
microglandular adenosis 257
micropapillary DCIS 370, 371, 375,
   654
milk
   of calcium in microcysts 265, **595**
   retention 246
milky diffuse enhancement 237,
   269
minimal sign interval cancer 23
mixed tumors,
   fibroepithelial 292–306
mobility, ultrasound testing of 106,
   122, 123
   carcinoma 439
   see also motion
modulation transfer function 41
moles 554
molybdenum target and filter 27,
   44, 75
morphology *see* shape
mortality reduction by
   screening 50, 578, 581, 587
morula-type calcifications 83, 265,
   656
motion (patient)
   in mammography, blurring due
      to 40, **41**
   in MRI, incorrect subtraction due
      to 144
mucinous (colloid) lesions 360
   carcinoma 401
      histology correlating
         with sonographic
         presentation 440
      histology influencing
         mammographic
         presentation 428
      mammography *414*
mucocele-like lesions 338, 360
multicentricity
   cancer 397
      definition 397
      MRI 156, 158, 395, 396,
         396–397
   ductal carcinoma in situ *653*
multifocality (cancer) 396
   MRI 156, 158, 395, *635*
multiple lesions 604
   indeterminate, MRI 169
myoblastoma 309
myocutaneous flaps 509
myoepithelial proliferations
   (benign) 256

myofibroblastoma 306, *308*
myxoid fibroadenoma *295*

N

National Breast Screening Study
   (Canada) screening **580**
near field, sonographic image
   quality in 102
needle biopsy *see* biopsy
needlelike calcifications 646, 651,
   652, 653
negative calls in screening
   mammography 588
   false 23
neoadjuvant chemotherapy 216,
   399–400, 512
   monitoring 399–400
      MRI 162–166, 399–400, 448
neoplasms *see* benign tumors;
   cancer; tumor
Netherlands screening study 581
neu (HER2) positivity 402, 403
neurofibroma 306, *559*
new technologies 177–184
   90° lateral view 58
   90° mediolateral view,
      calcifications (benign
      causes) 265
nipples
   discharge *see* discharge
   ductal mass near,
      galactography 87
   examination/observation 11,
      17
   cancer 404
   invasion by carcinoma 417
      importance of determining 397
   inverted 11, 17, 244
   MRI 237
   Paget disease 402, 404, 430
   papillary adenoma 349
   retraction 404, 417, 420, 640
      galactography 87
      MRI 169
   sonography 237
   supernumerary 244
nodularity/nodular pattern 17, 258,
   260, 261, *262, 263*, 267
   adenosis *263, 608*
   adolescents 235
   carcinoma 400, 405, *406, 412,
      437, 439*, 440
   DCIS 401, *610*
   gynecomastia 566

hematologic tumors 485
mass (in general) 406
metastases in breast 487, *488*
pseudoangiomatous stromal hyperplasia 309
skin 554
noise 49–50
with low-dose screen–film systems 48, 49
non-comedo-type DCIS 375, 384
non-Hodgkin lymphoma 484, *485*, *486*
nonmass enhancement 148–150
normal breast 234–253
adolescent 235
adult 235–240
age-related changes 241–242
anatomy 234, 256
males 564
variant 242–244
HRT and *see* hormone replacement therapy
males 564
pregnancy and lactation 246
nuclear medicine 182–183
nutritional risk factors *8*, 10

O

obesity as risk factor 10
oblique view
with customized settings 60
mediolateral *see* mediolateral oblique view
observation *see* inspection
occult interval cancer 23
oil cysts 284–286, 310, 494, 495, 504, 507, 517, 523, 526, **595**
calcifying *649*, 651
oil-filled implants 535–536
oncoplastic surgery *see* reconstructive/oncoplastic surgery
oral contraceptives (contraceptive pill)
MRI and 132
as risk factor 10
orientation
excised specimens 228
in sonography **121**
carcinoma 433
osteoma 306
ovarian cancer
familial/hereditary 9, 154, 392, 403–404

lymph node metastases *467*
overdiagnosis in screening 482, 585–586

P

p53 (TP53) carriers, MRI screening 154
PACS (Picture Archiving and Communications System) 39, 131
pads and near field image quality in sonography 102
Paget disease of nipple 402, 404, 430
pain 640
biopsy-related 192
causes 640
palpation 16, 17–19
evaluation and findings 17–19
benign disorders 258
cancer 404, 441
dense breast 633–640
reporting and documentation 78
younger patient 672
problems 19
thickening on *410*, 432, *447*
papillary adenoma of nipple 349
papillary carcinoma (papillary cancer)
calcifications *658*
histology influencing mammographic presentation 428–430
intracystic *120*, *277*, *282*, 407, 440
males 571
MRI *143*, 407, *443*, 471, *636*
multifocal *636*
nipple discharge 661
sonography 107–109
papillary carcinoma in situ 401
ductal 428–430
spot compression 67
papillary lesions (in general) 278, 282, 306, 339, 348–355
papilloma 306, 348–355
calcifying 652
intracystic 281, *351*, *352*, *440*
nipple discharge 661
power Doppler 107–109
younger patient 665
papillomatosis
calcifications *659*
juvenile 664, 665, 666, 670

paraffin blocks of specimen, radiography 73
parasitic infestations 327, 329, 331, 334
parenchymal mammography 236
ACR1–4 categorization of density **8**, 9, 79, 241, 258, 259
conserving surgery with irradiation 514–517
focally growing invasive carcinoma 417
reporting and documentation of pattern 79
pathognomonic findings 593–597
patient
informing *see* information
motion *see* motion
outcome, MRI for preoperative local staging 158
selection
mammography 22
MRI 129, 151–171
selection bias in screening mammography 587
peak kilovoltage *see* kilovoltage
penetration (of radiation) 28–29
percutaneous biopsy *see* biopsy
percutaneous drainage of abscess 326
perforated compression plate 217–218
pericanalicular fibroadenoma 293, *297*, 664
personal history 5–9
phantom images
mammography 78
MRI 131
photocell 33, 47
positioning 33, 47, 48, 75
craniocaudal view 56
photo-stimulable luminescence 36
phyllodes tumor (cystosarcoma) 338, 356–360, 476–479
younger patient 664
physical examination *see* examination
Picture Archiving and Communications Systems (PACSs) 39, 131
"plasma cell" (chronic) mastitis 87, 256, 316, 317, 319, 404, 504, 646, 651, *651*, *653*, 655
plasminogen activator inhibitor-1 (PAI-1) 402

Index

pleomorphism
  calcifications 651–654, *655*, *658*, *659*
  LCIS 345–346, 366–370
pneumocystography 92, 282
polymastia 244
popcornlike calcifications 651
positive calls in screening mammography, false 23, 583–584
positron emission tomography (PET)
  breast 182–183
  lymph nodes 472–473
posterior enhancement of soundbeam 116
power Doppler imaging 107–109
precursors of malignancy (premalignant lesions) 366
  B3 lesions as 338, 340, 345
  DCIS as 366, *367*, 372, 385, 586
pregnancy 246
  history-taking 11
  hyperemia in 672
  lesions encountered in 664–665
  mammography 246, 666, 672
  sonography 246, 669
premalignancy *see* precursors of malignancy
preoperative/preprocedural period
  biopsy 192
  localization in *see* localization
  MRI in 444–445
  local staging 156–158, 396
    localization 222, 397–398, *442*, 444–445, 445
    neoadjuvant chemotherapy monitoring 162–166, 399–400, 448
  primary tumor, unknown *602*, 609
    search for 640, 670
    MRI in 152, 448, *609*, 640
problem-solving using mammography 22, 24–25
proliferative lesions
  benign atypical 272
  younger patients 664
  see also epithelial proliferations
prone table, stereotactic biopsy 203
prostate cancer screening and mammographic screening, comparisons 588
proton spectroscopy *see* magnetic resonance spectroscopy
pseudoangiomatous stromal hyperplasia 309
pseudocapsule
  of hamartoma 290

sonography of 120
pseudoenhancement (MRI) 144
pulse sequences
  MRI
    enhanced MRI 130
    unenhanced MRI 131
  sonography 130
punctate calcifications, scattered 265

Q

quality 75–78
  image *see* image
  radiation *see* radiation
  in views, criteria for
    craniocaudal view 56
    mediolateral oblique view 56
quality assurance in
  mammography 76–77, 578
  European guidelines *see* European guidelines
quality control
  mammography 76
    documentation 77
    film processing 78
  sonography, equipment 103
quantum noise 49
questionnaire, mammography 5

R

radial scar (complex sclerosing lesion) 257, 261, 346–348
  architectural distortion *620*, *621*, *623*
  biopsy 190, 346, 348
  mammography 348, *620*, *621*
    spot compression 67
  sonography 348, *623*
radiation
  dose *see* dose
  image receptor film exposure *see* exposure
  low-energy 25, 26, 27, 44, 51, 53
  patient exposure (and its risks) 50
    in childhood 9
    in nuclear medicine 182, 183
    patient fear 4
    protection 75
    in screening mammography 583
  quality 51, 85
    determining contrast 44

image quality and 75
  optimum 51
scattering *see* scattering
spectrum 26–29
radiation therapy (radiotherapy/irradiation)
  changes related to 11
  conserving therapy with 512–529
  DCIS 372
radio-guided occult lesion localization (ROLL) 226
radioisotopes
  dual, in preoperative localization 226
  in scintigraphy 182
radiologic technologists' responsibilities (for quality) 77, 78–79
radiotherapy *see* radiation therapy
reactive changes
  in breast cancer 420
    lymph node 469
  with implants 542
RECIST (Response Evaluation Criteria In Solid Tumors) 163
reconstructive/oncoplastic surgery (after mastectomy) 509–511
  with implants 547
    surveillance following 544–547
  problem-solving after, MRI 159–160
recording *see* documentation
recurrence
  following conservation surgery
    detection and differential diagnosis 523
    ductal carcinoma in situ, risk 371
  implanted breast *551*
reduction mammoplasty 507–509
regional enhancement (nonmass) 149
  DCIS 383
reporting *see* documentation
resolution
  mammography 74
    good compression improving 52
  sonography 101–102
Response Evaluation Criteria In Solid Tumors (RECIST) 163
retraction 431–432
  nipples *see* nipples
  parenchymal, focally growing invasive carcinoma 417
  skin
    in cancer 404

in conserving surgery with irradiation 517
retroareolar region *see* subareolar/retroareolar region
reverberation echoes 102
 cysts 102, 114, *279*, 281
"reversed C" sign 542
rheumatoid arthritis, gold deposits 329, 471
ringlike enhancement, carcinoma 443
risk assessment
 B3 lesions (of uncertain malignant potential) 339–340
 radiation dose in mammography 50–51
risk factors for cancer
 assessment 5–11, 259
 DCIS 371–372
 mammographic density as *8*, 9, 259–260, 260
 radiation *see* radiation
 younger patients 665
 see also high-risk women
rolled views 60
rosette (morula)-type calcifications 83, 265, 656
round carcinoma 400, 407, 428
rounded calcifications, large 546

S

"salad oil" sign 544
saline-filled implants 534
sarcoidosis 327, 328, 329, 334
sarcomas 480–484
 angiosarcoma 308, 480, 481, *482*, 484
scanned slit linear detectors 38
scanning laser in computed radiography 37
scars 604–614
 architectural distortion *see* architectural distortion
 calcifications 646, 651
 differential diagnosis 604–614, 615
 granulomas in 328, 331, 334
 implanted breast 539–540
 post-surgical (or other trauma) 494, 495, 505, 507, 513, 514, 517, 526
  MRI with 169, 505, 509, 526, 528
 radial *see* radial scar

scattering
 calcifications 656
 radiation 29
  reduction 29, 45–47, 53
  reduction, in magnification mammography 69
 sonography echoes 105
scheduling 4
scintillator (digital detector) 35–36
scintimammography 182
scirrhous carcinoma 242, 404, *408*, *444*, 479
scleroderma 328, 329
sclerosed fibroadenomas 205, *302*, 304
sclerosing adenosis 266, 268, *620*, *650*
scout film, stereotactic biopsy 204
screen *see* intensifying screens
screening (in general) 578–591
 data and discussions 579–581
 definition 578
 diagnostic evaluation in addition to findings on 593–674
 mortality reduction by 50, 578, 581, 587
 quality assurance 578
 special task 578–579
screening mammography and surveillance 22–23, 24, 50–51, 394, 428, 578–591
 absolute numbers 582–583
 advantages 586–589
 age and 50, 581, 663, 666, 672
 benign change in 260–261
 biennial vs annual 50
 dense breasts without increased risk 632
 false positive rate 583–584
 with implants 547
  following oncoplastic surgery 544–547
 interval cancer between *see* interval cancer
 overdiagnosis 482, 585–586
 patient information 4
 quality assurance 84–85
 risks 583
 screening sonography and 99
 sensitivity 22
screening MRI (incl. contrast) 441, 582
 high-risk women 152–156, 396, 448
 not recommended 151, 155–156, 441, 554, 672
  for implant rupture 540

screening sonography 99, 582
sebaceous cysts, males 571
secretory site of nipple discharge, search for 660–661
segmental distribution of calcifications 654
segmental enhancement (nonmass) 149
 DCIS 383
selection bias in screening mammography 587
selenium, amorphous 34–35
self-examination (BSE) 16
semicircular calcifications 651
sensitivity
 carcinoma detection 393
 mammography 22–23, 24–25
  carcinoma 431
  film development time extension causing increase in 49
  low-sensitivity screen/film systems 48
 MRI 156
sentinel node biopsy 39, 458
seromas 494, 495, 504, 505, 513, 517, 526
shadowing/acoustic shadows (in sonography)
 benign disorders 268
 carcinoma 433, 439
 cysts 281
 problems relating to 113
 thickened edge shadows 439
 thin edge shadows 116
shape/morphology (and its description and interpretation)
 of calcifications 643
 mammographic 79, 80–82
 MRI 128–129
  indeterminate, retrospective ultrasound recommended 148
 sonographic **121**
  carcinoma 433
  suggesting malignancy 651–656
sharpness (mammography) or blurring 25–26, 40–41
 screen–film systems and 30
shear wave elastography 107, 181
shell-like calcifications 651
silicon, amorphous 35–36
silicone granulomas/deposits 327, 328, 331, 334, 542, 544, 651
 calcifications 651
 lymph nodes 471

Index

silicone implants 534
 augmentation using *see* implanted/augmented breasts
silicone injections for augmentation 535
site *see* localization; location
size
 of breast 16
  automatic exposure control systems with small breasts 47
  reporting and documentation of increases in 79
 of carcinoma 397
  increase in mammogram 420
 of DCIS, MRI preoperative determination 156
skin 553–562
 calcifications 646
 in conserving surgery with irradiation, mammography of localized changes in 514–517
 examination/observation for changes 16–17
 carcinoma 404
 infiltration by carcinoma, sonography 404
 sonography 237
 thickening 554–562
  diffuse *see* diffuse skin changes
slice thickness in sonography 103
slot mammography 47
small breasts, automatic exposure control systems 47
smoothly outlined density, differential diagnosis 597–604
"snowstorm" pattern 331, 542, 544
soft density surrounding microcalcifications, differential diagnosis 657
soft tissue sarcomas 480, 481, *482*
solid lesions *see* masses
sonography (ultrasonography) 97–125, 180–181, 197–203
 abscesses 321, 325, 325–326
  male 572
 accuracy *see* accuracy
 axilla *see* axilla; lymph nodes
 B3 lesions (of uncertain malignant potential)
  fibroepithelial lesions incl. phyllodes tumors 359
  lobular neoplasia and proliferations 345, 368
  papillary lesions 350, 351–352
  radial scar 348, *623*

benign non-neoplastic disorders *see* benign disorders
benign tumors/tumor-like lesions
 angiomas 309
 fibroadenoma 299–304, 305, 433
 focal fibrosis 310
 hamartoma 290
 pseudoangiomatous stromal hyperplasia 309
biopsy guided by 100, 188, 190, 197–203
 carcinoma (females) 432
 carcinoma (males) 569
 complications 192
 core needle biopsy 190, *199–200*, *201–202*
 cyst aspiration 93
 ducts 91
 of mammographically detected microcalcifications 189
calcifications *see* calcifications
cysts 98, 266, 268, 278, 278–282, 286, **595**, 599–602
 diagnostic value 98, 278, 278–282
 differentiation from other solid lesions 98
 galactocele 284
 guidance for aspiration 93
 oil cyst 286
 pneumocystography following (with suspicious or inconclusive cysts) 92
 power Doppler 107
 reverberation echoes 102, 114, *279*, 281
dense breasts 632
documentation 105–124
duct 91
ductal carcinoma in situ *see* ductal carcinoma in situ
equipment requirements 105–111
examination technique 103
fistulas 321, 325, 325–326
granulomatous lesions 331
implanted breast *see* implanted/augmented breast
inflammatory change 663
lesions (in general) 113–124
 characteristics **121**
 retrospective ultrasound with indeterminate morphology on MRI 148
lymph nodes *see* lymph nodes

males 564
 benign lesions 571–572
 cancer 569, 571
 gynecomastia 565, 566
 malignancy/semi-malignancy
  adenomyoepithelioma 480
  carcinoma *see* carcinoma
  fibromatosis 479
  hematologic tumors 486
  males 569, 571
  metastases (in breast) 489
  phyllodes tumor 359, 479
  sarcoma 480–481
  younger patients 669, 670
mastitis 319
normal breast 112–113, 237
 adolescent 235
 age-related changes in 241–242
 HRT effects 248
 pregnancy and lactation 246
 variants 244
of palpable lesions in dense breast 636
patient information 4
preoperative localization guided by 221–222
purpose/possibilities/limitations 98–100
screening 99, 582
second look (after MRI) 156, 189, 207, 222
skin thickening 561
smoothly outlined density 599–602, 604
symmetry and *see* symmetry
technological developments 180–181
trauma (incl. surgery)-related changes 504–505
 conserving therapy + irradiation 523–526
 reconstructive surgery 509
younger women *see* younger women
source to image-receptor distance (SID) 25–26
soya bean oil-filled implants 534–535
spatial frequency filtering 39
spatial resolution in sonography 102–103
specificity
 carcinoma detection 393–394, 431
 mammography 23–24
 carcinoma 431

694

MRI 156
specimen
 handling 210
 histopathology *see* histopathology
 imaging/radiography 72–74
  DCIS 374, *375, 376, 378,* 379
  invasive carcinoma 397
  microcalcifications 73, 206
 see also biopsy
spectral mammography 180
specular echoes 105
spicules and spiculated masses 495
 axillary (metastatic)
  adenopathy 466
 DCIS 373, 379, 383
 invasive carcinoma 401, *406,* 407, *408, 419,* 428, 431
 trauma (incl. surgery)-related 495
spindle cell lesions classified as B3 lesions 360
spindle cell tumor, benign (myofibroblastoma) 306, *308*
spot compression 60, 62–64, 70
staging of cancer
 (locoregional) 395–396
 lymph nodes 459
 preoperative MRI for 156–158, 396
steatocystoma multiplex is 310
stereotactic biopsy 203–207
 complications 192
 contraindications 192
 male breast cancer 569
 palpable lesions in dense breast 640
 vacuum-assisted 191
stereotactic localization, mammographic 218–220
sternal muscle, isolated bundle *611*
Stockholm County randomized controlled trial of screening **580**
strain elastography 107
stromal hyperplasia, pseudoangiomatous 309
structure
 diffuse changes *see* diffuse changes
 localized changes *see* localized changes
 in mammography
  benign disorders, changes 261–265
  differential diagnosis with indistinctness in 431
  noise relating to 49
 in sonography, of carcinoma, internal 440

subareolar/retroareolar region (incl. ducts)
 abscess 316
 in gynecomastia 565, 566
 malignancy *618,* 640
  importance of determining involvement 397
subcutaneous mastectomy, mammography after 71, 72
subscapular artery (lateral) in lymph node sonography 461
subtraction images in MRI, patient motion affecting 144
superimposition (true lesions distinguished from)
 architectural distortion 615
 focal lesions 614
superior vena cava obstruction *559*
supernumerary mammary glands 244
surgery (incl. excision) 493–531
 B3 lesions (of uncertain malignant potential)
  fibroepithelial lesions incl. phyllodes tumors 360
  flat epithelial atypia 343
  lobular neoplasia and proliferations 346
  papillary lesions 354
  radial scar 348
 changes related to trauma of 11, 493–531
 chemotherapy before *see* neoadjuvant chemotherapy
 conserving *see* conservation
 DCIS 372
 lymph node *see* lymph nodes
 nipple discharge 660
 oncoplastic *see* reconstructive/ oncoplastic surgery
 scarring (severe) after, MRI with 169
 screening and its impact on 588
 see also preoperative/ preprocedural period *and specific procedures*
surgical biopsy *see* biopsy, surgical/ excisional
surveillance *see* screening mammography and surveillance
suture material, calcified 504
"sweating" of implants 542
Swedish screening programs 581
 randomized controlled trials **580**
symmetry or asymmetry 626–632
 calcifications 655

 focally asymmetric mass 604–615
 global 625
 mammography 604–614, 626–631
  carcinoma 407–416, 420, 431
  description 82
  MRI 632
  accessory tissue 244
 nipple 17
 size 16
 skin thickening and 555
 sonography 631–632
  accessory tissue 244
symptom(s)
 hinting of malignancy 11
 mammography and 50–51
symptomatic women
 with implants
  mammography 535–538
  MRI 540
 problem-solving in 593–674

T

tangential view 60
target/filter combination 27, 44, 44–45
 quality of radiation and 51
teacup phenomenon 58, 265, *650, 651,* 656
technetium-99m scan 182
technological developments 177–184
temporal resolution in MRI 130
 see also time-gain compensation
terminal ducts 234
 lobular units 234, 256, 276
thickened edge shadows 439
thickness (of breast)
 in mammography
  dose and 51
  increases (thickening), differential diagnosis 431, 432
 palpable thickening *410,* 432, *447*
thin edge shadows 116
thoracic artery (lateral) in lymph node sonography 461
thoracic wall (chest wall) injury in preoperative localization 217
thoraco-acromial artery in lymph node sonography 461
three-dimensional imaging
 digital mammography *see* tomosynthesis

MRI 130, 131
ultrasound 181
threshold, individual examiner's 22
thyroid hormone administration 11
time-gain compensation 104–105
see also temporal resolution
tissue transfer, autogenous 509
tomosynthesis mammography 178–179, 602–604, 614, 615
architectural distortion 615
ill-defined or focal asymmetric mass 614
smoothly outlined density 602–604
TP53 carriers, MRI screening 154
transducer (sonography) 100, 101, 102, 103, 104, 105
trastuzumab 402
trauma (injury)-related changes 493–531
surgical 11, 493–531, 493–531
triangulation via stereotaxis 203
tuberculosis 327, 331
tubular carcinoma 401
histology influencing mammographic presentation 428
tumor, gynecomastia due to 566
see also benign tumors; cancer; primary tumor, unknown
tumor-like masses 289–313
Two County randomized controlled trial of screening **580**

U

ultrasmall super-paramagnetic iron oxide (USPIO) 472
ultrasonography *see* sonography
uncertain malignant potential, lesions of (B3) 211, 337–364
definition and classification 338
diagnosis *see* diagnosis
imaging 339
prevalence 339–340
risk 339–340
specific types of lesion 340–360
therapeutic recommendations 338–339
see also borderline lesions
unknown primary tumor *see* primary tumor
urokinase plasminogen activator (UPA1) 402
USPIO contrast medium (ultrasmall super-paramagnetic iron oxide) 472

V

vacuum-assisted biopsy (VABB) 187, 188–189, 191, 195–197, 596
accuracy 188–189
carcinoma 448
cysts 278
duct 91–92
ductal carcinoma in situ 385
ultrasound-guided 91
European guidelines for classification of lesions 211
flat epithelial atypia 343
intramammary lymph nodes 312
MR-guided 188–189, 191, 207, 210
patient preparation 193
radial scar 348
stereotactic *205*, 206
technique 195–197
US-guided 191, *202*
ducts 91
variant anatomy 242–244
vascular calcifications 651
vascularity, ultrasound assessment **122**
BI-RADS and 123
vena cava obstruction, superior *559*
verruca (wart) *555*, *558*, **595**
viewbox and viewing conditions 33
responsibilities for 78
visual checklist 78
visual inspection *see* inspection

W

warts (verrucae) *555*, *558*, **595**
wax reactions/granulomas 327, 328, 331, 334, *649*, 651
Wegener granulomatosis 327, 328, 329, *330*
windowing in digital imaging 39
wire localization 217, 226–227
CT-guided *224*
MR-guided *223*
stereotactic-guided 217
work sheet, physician's *18–20*

X

X-ray beam quality assessment 77
X-ray field limitation 75
X-ray generator 74
X-ray tube 25–29
power 74

Y

younger women 663–668
changes in, and their histology 664, 672
screening mammography 50, 581, 663, 666, 672
sonography 99, 669–670
pregnancy and lactation 246, 669
special considerations and problems 663–664
see also adolescent breast; childhood